GRIFFITH'S
INSTRUCTIONS
for
PATIENTS

7th
Edition

Stephen W. Moore, M.D.
Tucson, Arizona
With the assistance of Jo A. Griffith

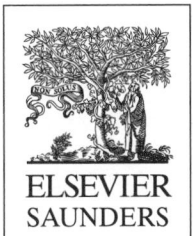

ELSEVIER
SAUNDERS

ELSEVIER
SAUNDERS

The Curtis Center
170 S Independence Mall W 300 E
Philadelphia, Pennsylvania 19106

NOTICE

Acquisitions Editor: Thomas H. Moore
Project Manager: Joan Nikelsky
Editorial Assistant: Janine Kusza
Design Coordinator: Gene Harris

Printed in the United States of America

Last digit is the print number: 9 8 7 6 5 4 3 2 1

H. Winter Griffith, M.D. (1926–1993)

Dr. H. Winter Griffith knew medicine from two perspectives—as an experienced clinician and as a patient. For twenty-five years Winter battled severe cardiovascular disease. As a patient, he received the finest medicine had to offer, including, at age 64, a heart transplant. He understood that the benefits of medical science were fully realized only when the patient was a partner with the physician in the management of illness. With this perspective, Winter devoted most of the past two decades doing what he could to improve patient education. His efforts include twenty-seven books, some for students and practitioners and some for patients themselves.

As the copier became widely available in physicians' offices, he saw the potential of clearly written, authoritative, and individualized information becoming easily available for each patient. *Instructions for Patients*, his first major effort directed to his colleagues as patient educators, was the result.

Winter passed away at age 67. His efforts continue to be perpetuated with the help of others concerned with patient education, including his publisher, Elsevier. I am sure Winter would be proud of this, the seventh edition of *Instructions for Patients*.

Daniel Levinson, M.D.
Tucson, Arizona

Preface to the Seventh Edition

As a practicing family physician, I place a tremendous amount of importance on my patients' understanding of their particular ailments. I cannot stress enough how important it is to the healing process for patients to fully comprehend all aspects of their condition. Continuing with Dr. Griffith's work, this, the seventh edition, revises and updates the topics from the sixth edition and includes 43 new topics. The majority of the written material is now at grade 8 reading level or below. You will find a wealth of appended materials, including information from various self-examinations, to diets, to simple labeled anatomical figures meant to facilitate discussions with patients about their conditions.

With these patient instruction sheets and useful appendices available in your office, you have an opportunity to provide preplanned, printed materials to patients and their families at a time when they are most motivated to learn—when there is a problem and they have come to you for help. These handouts provide quick, inexpensive, and effective supplements to personal contact. If patients perceive the materials distributed to them as an extension of the physician, the instruction sheets become a powerful teaching tool. They help to reinforce oral instructions and refresh the patient's memory with written material they can take home.

In keeping with and building upon Dr. Griffith's original intentions, we are now proud to offer physicians and their staff and patients the use of an extraordinary CD-ROM, included with the book, that contains the complete contents of the printed book (less prefatory materials and index) in both Latin American Spanish and English languages, plus a Latin American Audio Pronunciation Guide.

I know that both you and your patients will find this useful and beneficial.

Stephen W. Moore, M.D.

Contents

Diets

Appendix

Illustrations

Index

ABRUPTIO PLACENTAE

 ## BASIC INFORMATION

DESCRIPTION
The placenta (also called the after-birth) separates from the uterine wall. The placenta carries all nutrients and oxygen to the fetus. A separation can cause complications for the mother and the fetus. With a small separation, there may be no or few symptoms. Larger separations usually cause symptoms.

FREQUENT SIGNS AND SYMPTOMS
• Bleeding may be external (vaginal bleeding) or it may be concealed (bleeding remains in the uterus).
• Mild pain or discomfort, or there may be severe pain in the lower abdomen or back.
• Decreased fetal movement.
• Hard, tender abdomen.
• Uterine contractions.

CAUSES
The cause is unknown. Certain risk factors do exist.

RISK INCREASES WITH
• High blood pressure (hypertension).
• Smoking.
• Women over age 35 or younger than 20.
• Women who have had more than 4 or 5 pregnancies.
• A previous pregnancy with placental separation.
• Pregnancy with more than one fetus.
• Excess amniotic fluid (polyhydramnios).
• Chronic disorder (such as diabetes) or renal infection.
• Injury from motor vehicle accident, falls, or abuse.
• Short umbilical cord.
• Abnormal uterus or tumor.
• Premature rupture of the membranes (water breaks before delivery).
• Use of alcohol or drugs of abuse (such as cocaine).

PREVENTIVE MEASURES
• There is no sure way to prevent the problem.
• Avoid risk factors such as smoking, alcohol, or cocaine use. Get treatment for high blood pressure.

EXPECTED OUTCOME
When the separation is less severe and with immediate medical care, the outlook for mother and fetus is good.

POSSIBLE COMPLICATIONS
• Premature delivery of the child. This may lead to other complications for the newborn.
• Intrauterine growth restriction (IUGR) of the fetus.
• Shock or life-threatening bleeding in the mother.
• Blood clotting problems for the mother (disseminated intravascular coagulopathy or DIC).
• Risk of abruptio placentae in a future pregnancy.
• Uncontrolled bleeding after delivery may lead to an emergency hysterectomy.
• Death of child and/or mother.

 ## DIAGNOSIS & TREATMENT

GENERAL MEASURES
• Your obstetric provider will do a physical exam and ask questions about your symptoms. Medical tests will include blood studies and blood clotting tests. An ultrasound may be done.
• Treatment depends on the severity of the separation, the condition of the fetus, and the duration of the pregnancy. Hospital care is usually needed (except for mild cases) so the mother can be observed for any complications. If the placenta separation is slight, you may be able to return home for bed rest and close observation.
• In the hospital, fluids may be given through a vein (IV). A blood transfusion may be needed.
• Labor may be induced, if the pregnancy is at term or if there are signs of fetal distress.
• Surgery to deliver the unborn child by cesarean section, or vaginal delivery (sometimes).

MEDICATION
A drug to induce labor may be used if immediate delivery is required.

ACTIVITY
Whether you are in the hospital or have been able to return home, follow all medical instructions about any activity limits.

DIET
• A liquid-only diet may be prescribed until it is decided if surgery will be needed.
• If you are resting at home, continue with regular diet.

 ## NOTIFY OUR OFFICE IF

• You have bleeding (anything more than slight spotting) during pregnancy. This is an emergency!
• You have any other new symptoms.

Special notes:

_____

_____

_____

More notes on the back of this page ☐

ACNE
(Acne Vulgaris)

 BASIC INFORMATION

DESCRIPTION

A common skin condition. It usually affects the skin on the face, chest, and back. Acne has affected almost all people at some point during their lives. In teenagers, it is more common in males than in females. In adults, it is more common in women than men. It can last a few months, or years or for an entire lifetime.

FREQUENT SIGNS AND SYMPTOMS

• Mild acne usually causes blackheads (black spots the size of a pinhead) or whiteheads (white spots similar to blackheads).
• Pimples (also called zits). These are skin pores that have become pus-filled (clogged and infected).
• Severe acne produces many pimples.
• Redness and inflammation around pimples.
• Cysts (larger, firm swellings in the skin).

CAUSES

Glands in the skin make an oily substance called sebum. Sebum usually empties onto the skin surface through a pore (small opening) and causes no problems. With acne, the sebum becomes plugged up in the pore. Why this occurs is unclear. Sex-hormone changes during the teen years play a role. Contrary to commonly accepted myth, acne is not caused by dirt or foods.

RISK INCREASES WITH

• Teenagers and young adults.
• Endocrine disorders.
• Use of some drugs, such as cortisone.
• Family history of acne.

PREVENTIVE MEASURES

• Acne cannot be prevented at present. Certain factors can cause a flare up. Avoid them where possible.
• A flare up of acne can be caused by some make-up and lotions, certain foods, sunlight, friction (tight clothes, bicycle helmets), and hormone changes in females before their periods.

EXPECTED OUTCOMES

• Most cases respond well to treatment. It may take several months. Acne tends to disappear after teen years.
• Despite treatment, acne will sometimes flare up.

POSSIBLE COMPLICATIONS

• Poor self-image, depression and emotional stress.
• Facial scars or pitting of the skin.

 DIAGNOSIS & TREATMENT

GENERAL MEASURES

• Wash face with a mild soap once or twice a day and after exercising. Clean skin gently; don't scrub. An antibacterial soap may help. Rinse soap off completely.

• Shampoo hair daily, especially if it is oily. Don't let hair hang in the face. Use dandruff-preventing shampoo if needed.
• Avoid oil-based cosmetics. Use thinner, lotion-style, water-based products.
• Don't squeeze, scratch, pick, or rub the skin. Acne heals better without damage to the skin. Removal of comedones (blackheads) may be done by your health care provider.
• Use nonprescription acne products on your skin.
• See your health care provider if home treatments are not helping or acne is more severe. A skin exam will be done and treatment options will be discussed.
• Treatment will depend on the severity of the acne, any infection or inflammation, and if you are a female who may become pregnant. Treatment may include drugs (both for topical use or taken by mouth).
• Cosmetic surgery (dermabrasion) may be recommended to remove scars after acne heals.
• Removal or drainage of a cyst may be needed.

MEDICATIONS

• Use nonprescription creams or lotions products to treat the acne. These may contain benzyl peroxide, sulfur, salicylic acid or resorcinol.
• Antibiotics may be prescribed for bacteria infection.
• For more severe cases, topical or oral retinoids (a form of vitamin A), hormone drugs, or stronger acne drugs may be prescribed. Some drugs may increase your sensitivity to sunlight and increase the risk of sunburn.
• Caution: If you are pregnant or planning a pregnancy, tell your health care provider before using acne drugs.

ACTIVITY

No limits.

DIET

Foods don't cause acne, but some foods may make it worse. To find any food problems, stop eating foods that you think may make the acne worse. Then reintroduce them one at a time. If acne flares up 2 to 3 days after a food is eaten, leave that food out of your diet.

 NOTIFY OUR OFFICE IF

• You or a family member has acne and self-care is not helping.
• Acne recurs despite treatment.

Special notes:

_____

_____

_____

More notes on the back of this page ☐

2

ACNE ROSACEA
(Adult Acne)

 ## BASIC INFORMATION

DESCRIPTION

Chronic inflammation of skin of the nose, cheeks, forehead, and chin. Rarely, the neck, chest, ears, or scalp may be affected. Extensive nose involvement, mostly in men, is called rhinophyma. Acne rosacea tends to start between ages 30 and 50. It is more common in women, but more severe in men.

FREQUENT SIGNS AND SYMPTOMS

· Symptoms vary from person to person and sometimes in the same person. They may be mild or more severe.
· Flushing or blushing.
· Persistent redness.
· Unsightly red, thickened skin on the nose and cheeks. Small blood vessels are visible on the skin surface.
· Papules (small raised bumps) and pustules (small, white blisters with pus) on the affected skin.
· Burning, stinging, itching, swelling, dryness, or tightness of affected skin.
· Eyes may be red, burning, watery or irritated.

CAUSES

Unknown.

RISK INCREASES WITH

· Fair skinned people.
· Family history of acne rosacea.

PREVENTIVE MEASURES

Cannot be prevented. Flare-ups may be triggered by hot liquids, spicy foods, alcohol, emotional stress, some skin care products, sun exposure, hot and cold weather, heavy exercise, and hot baths.

EXPECTED OUTCOMES

There is no cure. Symptoms can be controlled with treatment and self-care. Acne rosacea is a disease of remissions and frequent flare-ups.

POSSIBLE COMPLICATIONS

· Emotional problems (such as lack of self confidence and low self-esteem).
· Eye complications.2005
· Scarring may occur, but it is rare.

 ## DIAGNOSIS & TREATMENT

GENERAL MEASURES

· Your health care provider can diagnose the condition by an exam of the affected skin area. Medical tests are usually not needed.
· Treatment will depend on each individual's needs and severity of the symptoms. Treatment may include drugs and skin treatments.
· Learn what factors cause flare-ups for you and avoid them. Keep a day-to-day diary of your activities and flare-ups to identify your trigger factors.
· Wash your face with a mild soap once or twice a day and after exercising. Clean skin gently; don't scrub. An antibacterial soap may help. Rinse soap off completely.
· Don't squeeze, scratch, pick, or rub the skin.
· Reduce stress in your life if possible. Counseling may help if the condition is adding to your stress.
· Surgery (such as laser therapy) may be recommended for visible blood vessels, to reduce redness, or to remove excess tissue from the nose.
· To learn more: National Rosacea Society, 800 S. Northwest Hwy., Suite 200, Barrington, IL 60010; (888) no-blush; website: www.rosacea.org.

MEDICATIONS

· Antibiotics (for the skin or taken by mouth) may be prescribed.
· Topical or oral retinoids (a form of vitamin A) or other drugs may be prescribed depending on the symptoms. Caution: If you are pregnant or planning a pregnancy, tell your health care provider before using acne drugs.
· Don't use nonprescription cortisone creams or lotions without medical advice. They may cause the condition to worsen.

ACTIVITY

Limit time spent in sunny, windy, very hot, or cold weather. Use a sunscreen (SPF 15 or higher).

DIET

Avoid food or drink triggers. Drink plenty of water.

 ## NOTIFY OUR OFFICE IF

You or a family member has symptoms of acne rosacea.

Special notes:

_____

_____

_____

More notes on the back of this page ☐

ADDISON'S DISEASE
(Adrenal Insufficiency)

 BASIC INFORMATION

DESCRIPTION

A rare disease that leads to failure of the adrenal glands. The adrenal glands produce hormones (cortisol and aldosterone) that affect almost every body organ and tissue. These hormones help the body respond to stress, maintain blood pressure, help heart and blood vessel function, and are involved in metabolism. Addison's can occur in all age groups. It affects men and women equally.

FREQUENT SIGNS AND SYMPTOMS

· Symptoms may develop slowly over months or years. Symptoms are caused by low levels of hormones produced by the adrenal glands.
· Weakness and fatigue.
· Nausea, vomiting, stomach pain, diarrhea, and appetite and weight loss.
· Low blood pressure causing faintness and dizziness.
· Brownish skin (looks suntanned) with white patches.
· Darkening of freckles, scars, and nipples.
· Hair loss.
· Feeling cold all the time.
· Behavior or mood changes, including aggression or depression.

CAUSES

· The cause is usually unknown, but is believed to be an autoimmune disorder.
· It also may be a result of tuberculosis, cancer, pituitary disease, or AIDS.
· Use of oral cortisone drugs for other conditions. When cortisone is stopped, normal adrenal function sometimes does not return.

RISK INCREASES WITH

· Other autoimmune diseases.
· Disorders mentioned in causes.

PREVENTIVE MEASURES

No specific preventive measures.

EXPECTED OUTCOMES

The disease can be controlled with hormone-replacement. A normal lifestyle can be expected.

POSSIBLE COMPLICATIONS

· Adrenal crisis caused by injury or illness. Symptoms may include pain, weakness, low blood pressure, high or low temperature, fainting.
· Increased risk of infections.

 DIAGNOSIS & TREATMENT

GENERAL MEASURES

· Your health care provider will do a physical exam and ask questions about your symptoms. Medical tests may include blood and urine studies, tests to measure adrenal function, and CT or MRI.
· Treatment involves replacing the hormones the adrenal glands are not making.
· This is a life-long condition. Learn how to care for yourself. Strict attention to drug schedules is vital.
· Learn about adrenal crisis and its relationship to body stress (infection, surgery or injury).
· Advise any doctor or dentist who treats you that you have Addison's disease.
· If you live or travel where medical care is not readily available, you may be given instructions on giving yourself cortisone injections in case of emergency.
· Wear a medical alert type bracelet or tag to indicate you have Addison's disease and the name of the drug and dosage that you take.
· Stay up-to-date on vaccines, such as those for influenza and pneumonia.
· Hospital care may be needed for an adrenal crisis.
· To learn more: National Adrenal Diseases Foundation, 505 Northern Blvd, Great Neck, NY 11021, (516) 487-4992 (not toll free); website: www.medhelp.org/nadf.

MEDICATIONS

Drugs to replace the hormones cortisol and aldosterone will be prescribed as needed. Never change or stop taking your drugs without medical advice.

ACTIVITY

No limits.

DIET

Special diet may be prescribed (e.g., one to maintain proper balance of sodium and potassium).

 NOTIFY OUR OFFICE IF

· You or a family member has symptoms of Addison's disease.
· After diagnosis, infection, injury, or dehydration develops. Drugs may need a dosage change.
· Swollen ankles, weight gain, or new symptoms occur.

Special notes:

_____

_____

_____

More notes on the back of this page ☐

4

ADJUSTMENT DISORDERS

 ## BASIC INFORMATION

DESCRIPTION
A person's response to a stressful life event (sometimes called a stressor) is out of proportion to what would be a normal reaction. The person is unable to adjust and this causes problems in both social and work (or school) situations or other functions of daily living.

FREQUENT SIGNS AND SYMPTOMS
- Symptoms or behavior changes occur within three months of onset of the stressor. They usually last no more than six months after the end of the stressor.
- Symptoms vary from person to person. They are often more severe in teens and the elderly.
- Changes in sleeping and eating patterns.
- Withdrawal (avoids social activities and friends).
- Fearful about the future.
- Low self-esteem and feeling emotionally numb.
- Feeling tense, anxious and depressed.
- Feelings of fear, rage, guilt or shame.
- Denial of the stressful event (acting as if it never occurred).

CAUSES
A disruption in the normal process of adapting to a stressful event. Everyone reacts differently to an event. It depends on its importance and the intensity of the event. It depends on the person's personality, temperament, age, and well-being.

RISK INCREASES WITH
- The degree of undesired change a stressor causes.
- Whether the stressor was sudden or expected.
- The importance of the stressor in the person's life.
- Lack of support systems (e.g., family, friends, religious, cultural, and social ties).
- How well a person responds to stressful life events.

PREVENTIVE MEASURES
No specific preventive measures known.

EXPECTED OUTCOME
It usually clears up on its own by the person adapting to the changed situation, or the stressor ends. Treatment can help in other cases. These disorders are common and are often only temporary.

POSSIBLE COMPLICATIONS
- Difficulty maintaining relationships or jobs.
- Lingering problems in teenagers.
- Self-treatment using alcohol or drugs to overcome undesired symptoms and feelings.
- Chronic anxiety and depression.

 ## DIAGNOSIS & TREATMENT

GENERAL MEASURES
- Your health care provider will do a physical exam and ask questions about your symptoms and the changes that are going on in your life. It is important to identify the stressor that has led to the symptoms. It can be anything that is important to you. The stressor may be only one event or a string of events. It may seem minor to some, but is important to you.
- Treatment may include self-care, counseling, and in some cases, drug therapy. This depends on severity of symptoms and impact on your lifestyle.
- Learn to cope with stress. Keeping a journal about your stressors and feelings, talking to a friend, or joining a support group may help. Take good care of your physical health (diet, exercise, and sleep).
- Counseling or psychotherapy may be recommended. Several therapy methods are effective and are often needed for a brief period. Family therapy (including marital counseling) may be recommended for some.

MEDICATION
Since adjustment disorders are usually of short duration, drugs are normally not needed. A drug may be prescribed short term for insomnia or for other specific symptoms, depending on their severity.

ACTIVITY
No limits. A routine physical exercise program is recommended. Physical activity helps reduce anxiety and stress.

DIET
Eat a well-balanced diet to maintain good health.

 ## NOTIFY OUR OFFICE IF

- You or a family member has symptoms of an adjustment disorder.
- Symptoms continue to worsen after treatment begins.

Special notes:

_____

_____

_____

More notes on the back of this page ☐

ALCOHOLISM

 BASIC INFORMATION

DESCRIPTION

A chronic, progressive disease that involves dependence on, or an addiction to, alcohol. It involves:
- Craving. A strong need or urge to drink.
- Loss of control. Not being able to stop drinking once drinking has begun.
- Physical dependence. Withdrawal symptoms, such as upset stomach, sweating, shakiness, and anxiety after stopping drinking.
- Tolerance. The need to drink greater amounts of alcohol to get "high."

FREQUENT SIGNS AND SYMPTOMS
- Need for alcohol at the start of the day.
- Use of alcohol to relieve stress or forget problems.
- Insomnia and nightmares.
- Vision, hearing, perception and alertness problems.
- Monday-morning hangovers and loss of work days.
- Makes promises to limit or stop drinking, but fails.
- Lies about drinking. Sneaks drinks at work or school.
- Anger and guilt when asked about drinking.
- Blackouts, personality and mood changes, confusion, memory loss, depression, anxiety, and fatigue.
- Tremors, violent shakes, hallucinations, or convulsions when there is no alcohol in the body.
- Poor nutrition and poor hygiene. Bad breath.
- Lack of sexual interest and loss of potency.
- Money, work, or family problems.

CAUSES
Not fully understood. It appears to be a combination of genetic, environmental, and personality factors.

RISK INCREASES WITH
- Family history of alcoholism.
- Personal history of other substance abuse.
- Genetic factors. May affect the way people's bodies process and respond to alcohol.
- Personality factors, such as needing a lot of praise and reassurance, feeling inadequate or unsure, low frustration level, being impulsive or aggressive.
- Cultural factors. Some ethnic groups have high alcoholism rates for either social or biological reasons.
- Factors such as alcohol being available, affordable, and socially acceptable.
- Personal history of emotional or psychiatric disorders.

PREVENTIVE MEASURES
Avoid or limit alcohol. Women have no more than one drink a day and men, no more than two drinks a day.

EXPECTED OUTCOMES
Treatment has varying success rates. Some people are able to quit on their own. Relapse is somewhat common, but many people have a full recovery.

POSSIBLE COMPLICATIONS
- Damage to the brain, liver, heart, and other organs.
- Fetal alcohol syndrome (children of alcoholic mothers).
- Without treatment, alcoholism can be fatal.
- Suicide or fatal motor vehicle accidents.

 DIAGNOSIS & TREATMENT

GENERAL MEASURES
- Your health care provider will do a physical exam and ask about your symptoms. You may be asked verbal questions or to fill out a written form about your alcohol use. These can help identify problem drinking. Medical tests may include blood and urine studies.
- Treatment depends on the severity of the alcohol problem, other illnesses (physical, emotional, or mental), and how motivated you are to change. Treatment usually involves withdrawal of alcohol and detoxification, and long-term support to help you remain sober.
- Specific treatment steps include counseling (may be all that is needed), drugs (in some cases), inpatient care at a hospital or treatment center, or referral to a health care provider who treats addiction problems.
- You may benefit from self-help groups such as Alcoholics Anonymous or another support group.

MEDICATIONS
- Your health care provider may prescribe:
  - Drugs that reduce the craving for alcohol.
  - Drugs that cause unpleasant physical symptoms when alcohol is consumed.
  - Drugs that reduce the pleasure of alcohol.
  - Drugs for withdrawal symptoms, as needed.

ACTIVITY
Exercise daily. It helps in maintaining your physical and mental well-being.

DIET
Eat a normal, well-balanced diet. Vitamin supplements may be recommended.

 NOTIFY OUR OFFICE IF

- You or a family member has symptoms of alcoholism. It is an illness that can be treated.
- You have a relapse after recovery.

Special notes:

_____

_____

_____

More notes on the back of this page ☐

6

ALOPECIA AREATA

 BASIC INFORMATION

DESCRIPTION

Sudden hair loss in circular patches on the scalp. The hair loss does not occur with other visible evidence of scalp disease. It can involve hair on the scalp, eyebrows, eyelashes, genital area, or sometimes underarms. Alopecia can occur at any age, from birth to older adults. Many cases start before age 20.

FREQUENT SIGNS AND SYMPTOMS

• Sudden hair loss in sharply defined circular patches. In rare cases, body hair loss may be total (alopecia universalis).
• Pain and itching may occur in some cases.
• Nails may be affected, such as pitting, in more severe cases.

CAUSES

Unknown. It is thought to be one of a group of autoimmune disorders. In these disorders, the immune system by mistake attacks the body itself. Heredity and emotional stress or psychiatric disorders may play a role.

RISK INCREASES WITH

• Family history of alopecia areata.
• Stressful life event preceding the hair loss may be a factor.
• Certain medical disorders may occur along with alopecia, but do not appear to be a cause or a risk factor.

PREVENTIVE MEASURES

Cannot be prevented at present.

EXPECTED OUTCOMES

The outcome varies depending on the amount of hair loss. There is no permanent cure and the disorder may come and go. Most people have only a few areas of alopecia and regrowth occurs in about a year.

POSSIBLE COMPLICATIONS

• Loss of all hair.
• Slow or incomplete regrowth.
• Treatment may not be effective in extensive hair loss.
• Disorder frequently recurs.

 DIAGNOSIS & TREATMENT

GENERAL MEASURES

• Your health care provider will do a physical exam of the affected scalp area. Medical tests are usually not needed unless some underlying disorder is suspected.

• In a simple, self-limited case where the alopecia is not noticeable, no treatment may be needed. In other cases, drugs may be used for treatment depending on amount of hair loss and age of patient. No one treatment helps everyone with the disorder.
• A change in hair-style may cover the affected area.
• Consider wearing a hairpiece or wig until the hair grows in again.
• For loss of eyebrow hair, dermatography may help. Small dots of colored pigment are injected into eyebrow area.
• Continue to bathe and shampoo as usual. The disorder is not contagious. Don't tug on normal hair close to areas of hair loss.
• Seek counseling if coping with the hair loss is causing emotional problems. Support groups are also available.
• To learn more: National Alopecia Areata Foundation, P.O. Box 150760, San Rafael, CA 94915; (415) 472-3780 (not toll free); website: www.naaf.org.

MEDICATIONS

• Topical steroids or topical anthralin may be prescribed. Follow instructions carefully.
• Topical minoxidil (a drug used for hair growth) may help. Its effectiveness is highly variable.
• In some cases, you may have injections of steroids into affected areas.
• Oral cortisone drugs may be recommended.
• Topical immunotherapy may be recommended. This involves producing a skin reaction to help hair growth.
• Photochemotherapy with PUVA may be recommended. It combines the use of a drug that sensitizes the skin along with a controlled dose of ultraviolet light.

ACTIVITY

No limits.

DIET

No special diet.

 NOTIFY OUR OFFICE IF

• You or a family member has symptoms of alopecia areata.
• The following occurs during treatment:
  - Hair loss increases or hair loss doesn't improve.
  - Areas show signs of infection (redness, swelling, tenderness, warmth) after injection treatment.

Special notes:

_____

_____

_____

More notes on the back of this page ☐

ALTITUDE ILLNESS
(Mountain Sickness)

 BASIC INFORMATION

DESCRIPTION
Altitude illness results from travel to higher than normal altitudes. It can affect anyone, no matter what their age or how healthy they are. Types include:
- Acute mountain sickness (AMS); the most common.
- High-altitude pulmonary edema (HAPE) and high-altitude cerebral edema (HACE). These are less common.

FREQUENT SIGNS AND SYMPTOMS
- Mild symptoms may begin when you climb or travel to around 7,000 to 8,000 feet.
    - Headache, feeling lightheaded and weak.
    - Nausea or vomiting.
    - Sleeping problems.
- As you go higher, more severe symptoms may occur.
    - Cough and trouble with breathing.
    - Unsteady walk.
    - Confusion; hallucinations (seeing things that aren't there).
    - Coma (person can not be aroused).

CAUSES
There is less oxygen in the air at higher altitudes. Symptoms start to develop when the body tries to adjust to having less oxygen than it normally has. People who live at high altitudes have adapted to these lower oxygen levels and do not get sick.

RISK INCREASES WITH
- Some people are more susceptible. It is unclear why certain people get sick while others do not. At 14,000 feet, most people will have at least mild symptoms.
- People with severe heart or lung disease or people with sickle-cell anemia.
- Going too high too quickly.

PREVENTIVE MEASURES
- Educate yourself before your trip. Find out how high the altitude will be. Know the symptoms of altitude illness. Find out if medical help will be handy.
- Ask your health care provider for advice about high altitude travel for children, for pregnant women, and for people with chronic health problems. The travel may be considered safe, but find out for sure.
- While on the trip, slowly adjust to the change in altitude. Rest for a day or two at each 1,000 to 2,000 feet. Take it easy, don't overdo, drink fluids, but not alcohol.

EXPECTED OUTCOMES
Most cases are mild and do not need medical treatment. Recovery takes only one to a few days.

POSSIBLE COMPLICATIONS
Serious outcomes, including death, are rare. They are only likely to occur if the person is unable to go down to a lower level, or is not able to get medical help.

 DIAGNOSIS & TREATMENT

GENERAL MEASURES
- If mild symptoms occur, rest for a day or two at that altitude. You may want to go back down (to descend) to a lower altitude. Do not travel higher (to ascend) until the symptoms resolve or get much better.
- If symptoms do not improve or they get worse, seek medical help. Your health care provider will ask about your symptoms, may do a physical exam, and have medical tests performed to check on your heart, lungs, and other body systems.
- Treatment steps will depend on your symptoms. You may be advised to go to a lower altitude. This is the most important and only sure treatment step.
- Symptoms should improve in a few days if you rest, drink plenty of fluids, don't drink alcohol, and avoid heavy exercise.
- For more severe symptoms, you will need to go to a lower altitude immediately. You may need pure oxygen breathed in through a mask for a period of time. A hospital stay may be necessary until you recover.

MEDICATIONS
- Ask your health care provider's advice before you travel about drugs that can help prevent or treat symptoms. Drugs do have side effects, so be cautious.
- For mild symptoms, such as headache, you may use pain relievers, such as ibuprofen or naproxen.
- In severe cases, drugs will be given to treat complications and help speed recovery.

ACTIVITY
Resume daily activities gradually upon returning to your normal altitude.

DIET
If you become ill, increase fluid intake, avoid alcohol, and eat small meals.

 NOTIFY OUR OFFICE IF

You or a family member has altitude illness symptoms, or wants to discuss symptoms that occurred on a trip.

Special notes:

_____

_____

_____

More notes on the back of this page ☐

ALZHEIMER'S DISEASE
(Presenile Dementia)

BASIC INFORMATION

DESCRIPTION
Alzheimer's disease (AD) is a brain disorder that involves gradual mental deterioration. The more gradual form, with slow development of symptoms, begins around ages 65 to 70. A rapidly progressive form begins in adults around ages 36 to 45.

FREQUENT SIGNS AND SYMPTOMS
Early stages:
- Forgetful of recent events.
- Increasing difficulty doing mental tasks, such as usual work, balancing a checkbook, or maintaining a household.
- Personality changes, including poor impulse control and poor judgment.

Later stages:
- Difficulty doing simple tasks, such as choosing clothing, solving problems.
- Failure to recognize familiar persons.
- Lack of interest in personal hygiene or appearance.
- Difficulty feeding self.
- Belligerence and denial that anything is wrong.
- Loss of usual sexual inhibitions.
- Wandering away.
- Anxiety and insomnia.

Advanced stages:
- Complete loss of memory, speech, and muscle function. This includes bladder and bowel control.

CAUSES
Damage to or loss of brain cells for unknown reasons.

RISK INCREASES WITH
- Family history of Alzheimer's disease.
- Other genetic factors.
- Aging.
- Research shows that factors related to blood circulation may be involved (such as those causing heart disease or stroke).

PREVENTIVE MEASURES
No specific preventive measures.

EXPECTED OUTCOMES
There is no cure. Treatment helps slow the progress and helps relieve the symptoms. Patients may progress from onset of symptoms to end-stage disease in 8 to 10 years. This varies from person to person. Those with end-stage disease often need the care provided in an assisted living facility that handles Alzheimer's patients.

POSSIBLE COMPLICATIONS
- Infections. They are a major cause of death in Alzheimer's patients.
- Final stages of the disease will lead to death.

DIAGNOSIS & TREATMENT

GENERAL MEASURES
- Your health care provider will do a physical exam and ask questions about the symptoms. There is no specific test to diagnose Alzheimer's. Medical tests may include cognitive tests (answering questions). Blood, urine, and spinal fluid studies, heart studies, CT, MRI, PET scans, or others help rule out other disorders. Certain genetic tests help to identify inherited forms of Alzheimer's.
- A diagnosis of Alzheimer's is overwhelming, both for the patient and the family. Educate yourselves as much as possible about what to expect and how to plan for it. With early diagnosis, the patient can take part in making decisions for the future.
- Treatment will depend on the stage of the disease. Different drugs are available that can help slow the progress of the disease.
- Drugs to treat the behavior symptoms can help make a patient more comfortable and make their care easier.
- Caring for a family member with Alzheimer's is a difficult task. Caregivers need to take care of themselves. Joining a support group for caregivers may be helpful.
- To learn more: Alzheimer's Association, 225 N. Michigan Ave., Flr. 17, Chicago. Il 60601; (800) 272-3900; website: www.alz.org.

MEDICATIONS
- Drugs that slow the progress of the disease for a limited time are usually prescribed.
- Drugs as needed to help control behavior symptoms (insomnia, agitation, wandering, depression, anxiety, and others) will be prescribed.

ACTIVITY
With time, all patient activity will require supervision.

DIET
Regular diet. Feeding help will eventually be needed.

NOTIFY OUR OFFICE IF

- You or a family member has symptoms of Alzheimer's disease.
- Caregivers have any questions or concerns about the patient, the symptoms or the treatment.

Special notes:

_____

_____

_____

More notes on the back of this page ☐

AMEBIASIS
(Amebic Dysentery; Entamebiasis)

 BASIC INFORMATION

DESCRIPTION
A parasitic infection of the intestines (bowels). Amebiasis is found worldwide, but occurs most often in developing countries. In the United States, the disease is fairly rare in the general population. It can affect all ages. Amebic dysentery is a rare, more severe form.

FREQUENT SIGNS AND SYMPTOMS
• Only about 1 in 10 persons with the infection will have symptoms. Symptoms occur when the parasites (amoebas) invade the walls of the intestine.
• Diarrhea with bad-smelling stools. Constipation may alternate with diarrhea.
• Gas and stomach bloating, cramps, and tenderness.
• Amebic dysentery may cause bloody stools, stomach pain, chills, and fever.

CAUSES
A parasite, *Entamoeba histolytica*. The infection starts when someone swallows amoeba cysts (they can't be seen) that contaminate food or water. The cysts travel to the intestines and can live there without causing symptoms. Then, for unknown reasons, the amoebas invade the intestine wall. When this happens, symptoms occur. Symptoms usually begin one to four weeks after exposure, but can take a few days or a year.

RISK INCREASES WITH
• Immigrants from developing countries.
• Travel to a foreign country. In developing countries, the drinking water may be contaminated. In addition, some places use human feces for fertilizer.
• Male homosexuals.
• Living in institutions where there are poor sanitary conditions.

PREVENTIVE MEASURES
• No specific preventive steps. No vaccine is available.
• Wash hands often to prevent spread of any germs.
• Travelers to countries where there is a risk of infection need to take proper precautions regarding food and drink.
• Avoid sexual practices that increase risk of infection.

EXPECTED OUTCOMES
In most cases, amebiasis is curable in three weeks with treatment.

POSSIBLE COMPLICATIONS
The amoebas can travel through the blood stream to other parts of the body and cause infection in different organs. This can lead to an amebic liver abscess (pus-filled area) or brain abscess.

 DIAGNOSIS & TREATMENT

GENERAL MEASURES
• Your health care provider will do a physical exam and ask about your symptoms and recent travels. Medical tests may include blood and stool studies. If liver involvement is a concern, other tests may be done.
• Treatment is with drugs. A stool sample may be rechecked after treatment is complete to be sure the infection is cleared up.
• Amebiasis is contagious. Be extra careful about personal cleanliness. Bathe frequently. Wash hands with warm water and soap after each bowel movement and before handling food.
• In severe cases of dysentery, hospital care may be needed. Fluid replacement may be necessary to manage dehydration due to diarrhea.

MEDICATIONS
Antibiotic drugs to treat amebiasis are usually prescribed. These are most often taken by mouth, but in some cases may be injected.

ACTIVITY
Get extra rest until diarrhea and other symptoms improve.

DIET
No special diet. Be sure to drink plenty of fluids to help prevent dehydration.

 NOTIFY OUR OFFICE IF

• You or a family member has symptoms of amebiasis.
• The following occur during treatment:
  - Abdominal cramps continue longer than 24 hours.
  - Diarrhea or blood in stool increases.
  - Vomiting begins.
  - Pain begins over liver or jaundice (yellow skin or eyes) occurs.
  - A skin rash appears.

Special notes:

_____

_____

_____

_____

More notes on the back of this page ☐

AMENORRHEA, PRIMARY

 BASIC INFORMATION

DESCRIPTION
Complete absence of menstruation in a young woman who is at least 16 years old, or at age 14 with a lack of normal growth or absence of secondary sexual development. It is a rare disorder, as over 95% of girls have their first menstrual period by age 15. Most girls begin menstruating by age 14, average age is 12 years, 8 months.

FREQUENT SIGNS AND SYMPTOMS
Lack of menstrual periods after puberty.

CAUSES
A failure of certain complex body functions that normally result in menstruation. There are a number of disorders or health problems that can lead to the failure.

RISK INCREASES WITH
- Delayed puberty.
- Congenital abnormalities, such as the absence or abnormal formation of female organs (vagina, uterus, and ovaries).
- Intact hymen (membrane covering the vaginal opening) has no opening to allow passage of menstrual flow.
- Disorders (tumors, infections or other problems) of the endocrine system, including the pituitary, hypothalamus, thyroid, parathyroid, adrenal, and ovarian glands.
- Chromosome disorders.
- Chronic illness.
- Polycystic ovarian syndrome (Stein-Leventhal syndrome).
- Rarely, prior gynecological surgery.
- Severe nutritional or physical stressor such as anorexia or competitive sports.
- Use of drugs, including oral contraceptives, anticancer drugs, barbiturates, narcotics, cortisone drugs, chlordiazepoxide, and reserpine.
- Family tendency to start menstruation late.
- Excessive dieting or weight loss.
- Extreme obesity.

PREVENTIVE MEASURES
No specific preventive measures. Avoid risk factors where possible.

EXPECTED OUTCOMES
- The absence of menstruation is not a health risk in itself, but the cause should be found.
- Amenorrhea is often curable with hormone treatment or treatment of the underlying cause. Treatment may be delayed to age 18, unless the cause can be identified and treated safely.
- Causes that sometimes cannot be corrected include chromosome disorders and abnormalities of the reproductive system.

POSSIBLE COMPLICATIONS
- Emotional stress about sexual development.
- May lead to infertility.
- Other complications may occur, depending on the underlying cause.

 DIAGNOSIS & TREATMENT

GENERAL MEASURES
- Your health care provider will do a physical exam and a pelvic exam. Medical tests may include urine and blood studies, hormone levels, liver, thyroid, and adrenal function studies. Other tests may be done to diagnose an underlying disorder.
- Treatment may involve hormone replacement therapy. Treatment for amenorrhea not related to hormone deficiency depends on the cause.
- Counseling may help if amenorrhea is related to stress, results from eating disorder, or for emotional concerns about sexual development.
- Surgery to correct abnormalities of the reproductive system or for cysts may rarely be needed.

MEDICATIONS
- Hormones may be prescribed if there is a hormone imbalance. They may correct the problem.
- Birth control pills may be prescribed for polycystic ovary syndrome.
- Bromocriptine may be prescribed for pituitary tumor.

ACTIVITY
Exercise regularly, but not to excess. Reduce exercise or athletic activities if they are too strenuous.

DIET
If overweight or underweight, a change in diet to correct the problem may bring on a period.

 NOTIFY OUR OFFICE IF

- You are 16 years old and have never had a period.
- Periods don't begin within 6 months, despite treatment.

Special notes:

_____

_____

_____

More notes on the back of this page ☐

AMENORRHEA, SECONDARY

 BASIC INFORMATION

DESCRIPTION
Absence of menstruation in a woman who has previously menstruated.

FREQUENT SIGNS AND SYMPTOMS
· No menstrual periods for at least 3 to 6 months.
· Other symptoms may include infertility, acne, excess hair growth (hirsutism) or hair loss, obesity, galactorrhea (breasts produce milk when not breast-feeding), headaches, and vaginal dryness.

CAUSES
A stopping of certain complex body functions that normally result in menstruation. There are a number of conditions or health problems that can lead to the failure. Pregnancy is one of the most common causes.

RISK INCREASES WITH
· Breast-feeding an infant.
· Discontinuing use of birth-control pills.
· Menopause (if a woman is over 35 and not pregnant).
· Emotional stress or psychological disorder.
· Surgical removal of the ovaries or uterus, or complications as a result of gynecological surgery.
· Disorder of the endocrine system, including the pituitary, hypothalamus, thyroid, parathyroid, adrenal, and ovarian glands.
· Hormone imbalance.
· Chronic illness, such as diabetes or tuberculosis.
· Obesity or eating disorders (anorexia or bulimia).
· Strenuous program of physical exercise, such as long-distance running, gymnastics or ballet.

PREVENTIVE MEASURES
To help avoid amenorrhea, maintain a healthy lifestyle.

EXPECTED OUTCOMES
· Amenorrhea is not a threat to health. Whether it can be corrected varies with the underlying cause.
· If from pregnancy or breast-feeding, menstruation will resume when these conditions cease.
· If from discontinuing use of oral contraceptives, periods should begin in 2 months to 2 years.
· If from menopause, periods will become less frequent or may never resume. Hysterectomy also ends menstruation permanently.
· If from endocrine disorders, hormone replacement usually causes periods to resume.
· If from eating disorders, successful treatment of that disorder will help menstruation to resume.
· If from diabetes or tuberculosis, menstruation may never resume.
· If from strenuous exercise, periods usually resume when exercise is decreased.

POSSIBLE COMPLICATIONS
· None likely, if there is no serious underlying cause.
· May experience estrogen deficiency symptoms, such as hot flashes and vaginal dryness.
· May affect fertility.

 DIAGNOSIS & TREATMENT

GENERAL MEASURES
· Your health care provider will do a physical exam and a pelvic exam. Medical tests may include a pregnancy test, blood studies of hormone levels and a Pap smear. Surgical diagnostic procedures such as laparoscopy or hysteroscopy may be recommended. These procedures use a special instrument to see inside the body's organs.
· Treatment may include lifestyle changes, drugs, treatment of underlying disorder (if one is diagnosed), and surgery (sometimes).
· Dilatation and curettage, often referred to as D & C (dilation of the cervix and a scraping out of the uterus with a curette), may be performed.
· Counseling may help if amenorrhea is related to stress or other emotional problems.
· Keep a record of menstrual cycles to aid in early detection of recurrent amenorrhea.
· To learn more, perform a web search. A good site to start with is www.4women.gov.

MEDICATIONS
· Progesterone and/or estrogen may be prescribed. If bleeding occurs after progesterone is withdrawn, the reproduction system is functional.
· Drugs to treat an underlying disorder may be prescribed.

ACTIVITY
Exercise regularly, but not to excess. Reduce exercise or athletic activities if they are too strenuous.

DIET
If overweight or underweight, a change in diet to correct the problem may be recommended.

 NOTIFY OUR OFFICE IF

· You or a family member has amenorrhea.
· Periods don't resume within 6 months.

Special notes:

_____

_____

_____

More notes on the back of this page ☐

AMYOTROPHIC LATERAL SCLEROSIS
(ALS; Lou Gehrig's Disease)

 BASIC INFORMATION

DESCRIPTION
A progressive breakdown of the cells of the spinal cord. This results in gradual loss of muscle function. It involves the central nervous system and the muscle system, especially in the hands, forearms, legs, head and neck. It usually affects people aged 40 to 60 years, and occurs more often in men than women.

FREQUENT SIGNS AND SYMPTOMS
· Muscle twitching and weakness. It begins in the hands and spreads to the arms and legs. The weakness then begins to affect muscles that control breathing and swallowing.
· Muscle cramps.
· Stiffening and spasticity of muscle groups.
· Weight loss.
· Slurring of speech.
· Mental function is rarely affected.
· Sudden involuntary bursts of laughter or crying.

CAUSES
Unknown. Research suggests that there may be more than one cause.

RISK INCREASES WITH
· Age over 40.
· Family history of ALS.
· Smoking.

PREVENTIVE MEASURES
Cannot be prevented at present.

EXPECTED OUTCOMES
· This condition is currently considered incurable. It is usually fatal in 2 to 5 years, but 20% of patients survive 5 years and 10% survive 10 years.
· Medical research into causes and treatment continues. There is hope for more effective treatment.

POSSIBLE COMPLICATIONS
· The disorder affects the patient's personal relationships, career, income, muscle coordination, sexuality, and energy.
· Progressive inability to walk and to do things involved with daily living, such as being able to feed oneself.
· Wheelchair use is needed.
· Pressure sores or skin infections due to being bedridden or in a wheelchair.
· Pneumonia due to swallowing difficulty and choking.
· The disorder is eventually fatal due to respiratory muscle weakness.

 DIAGNOSIS & TREATMENT

GENERAL MEASURES
· Your health care provider will do a physical exam and ask questions about your symptoms. No one test diagnoses ALS. Medical tests will include nerve studies (electromyography and nerve conduction velocity). Tests may include blood and urine studies, x-rays and others.
· There is no specific treatment. Supportive care is provided to relieve symptoms and for complications.
· Aids for helping with daily living are available. These can help maintain some function and quality of life.
· Counseling may be helpful in finding ways for both the patient and the family to cope with the diagnosis.
· Surgery for tracheostomy is usually required once breathing difficulties develop.
· In later stages of the disease, the patient will require complete nursing care.
· Patient and family may benefit from hospice care.
· To learn more: ALS Association, 27001 Agoura Rd., Suite 150, Calabasas Hills, CA 91301; (800) 782-4747; website: www.alsa.org.

MEDICATIONS
· Riluzole may be prescribed. It can help delay the progress of ALS for a few months.
· Antibiotics will be prescribed if infection develops.
· Baclofen or tizanidine may help reduce spasticity.
· Antidepressant may help to decrease excess saliva.

ACTIVITY
· Stay as active as possible. Weakness will gradually limit movement. A physical therapy program can help to maintain independence as long as possible.
· Obtain equipment that will aid in mobility, such as a walker or wheelchair.

DIET
· Soft, easy-to-swallow foods may be needed if swallowing is a problem.
· May require tube feedings eventually.

 NOTIFY OUR OFFICE IF

· You or a family member has symptoms of ALS (amyotrophic lateral sclerosis).
· After diagnosis, symptoms occur that cause concern.

Special notes:

_____

_____

_____

More notes on the back of this page ☐

ANAL FISSURE

 ## BASIC INFORMATION

DESCRIPTION
A laceration, tear, or crack in the lining of the anus. It affects all age groups, including infants.

FREQUENT SIGNS AND SYMPTOMS
· Sharp pain with passage of a hard or bulky stool. The pain may last up to an hour, and returns with the next bowel movement.
· Pain when sitting on a hard surface.
· Streaks of blood on the toilet paper, underwear, or diaper.
· Itching around the rectum.
· Refusal to have a bowel movement (in children).

CAUSES
The exact cause is unknown. Symptoms usually occur after the stretching of the anus from a large, hard stool.

RISK INCREASES WITH
· Constipation or prolonged diarrhea.
· Multiple pregnancies.
· Crohn's disease.
· Medical disorders of the body's immune system.

PREVENTIVE MEASURES
· Avoid constipation by:
  - Drinking at least 8 glasses of water daily.
  - Eating a diet high in fiber.
  - Using stool softeners, if needed.
· Don't strain when having a bowel movement.
· Avoid anal intercourse.

EXPECTED OUTCOMES
Most fissures heal on their own. Others can be corrected with surgery. Most infants and young children recover after the stool is softened.

POSSIBLE COMPLICATIONS
Fissure may become chronic and fail to heal.

 ## DIAGNOSIS & TREATMENT

GENERAL MEASURES
· Your health care provider will do a physical exam of the anus and rectum to confirm the diagnosis. Other medical tests are usually not needed.
· Gently clean the anus with soap and water after each bowel movement.
· To relieve muscle spasms and pain around the anus, apply a warm towel to the area.
· Sitz baths also relieve pain. Use 8 inches of warm water in the bathtub, 2 or 3 times a day for 10 to 20 minutes.
· Minor surgery may be needed to remove the fissure if conservative treatment is not successful.

MEDICATIONS
· For minor pain, use nonprescription drugs, such as acetaminophen or topical anesthetics.
· Zinc oxide ointment or petroleum jelly applied to the anal opening may help prevent any burning sensation.
· Bulk stool softeners will help to avoid the pain occurring with hard bowel movements.
· Lidocaine ointment may be recommended.
· Botox injections may be prescribed to help relax the sphincter muscles

ACTIVITY
No limits. Physical activity reduces the likelihood of constipation.

DIET
Eat a high-fiber diet and drink extra fluids to prevent constipation.

 ## NOTIFY OUR OFFICE IF

· You or your child has symptoms of an anal fissure.
· Pain continues despite treatment.

Special notes:

_____

_____

_____

More notes on the back of this page ☐

ANAL FISTULA

 ## BASIC INFORMATION

DESCRIPTION

A very small tube or tract that leads from the anal canal (the last part of the rectum) to the skin near the anal opening. Watery pus drains through this opening and causes irritation to the skin.

FREQUENT SIGNS AND SYMPTOMS

· Discharge from the anus.
· Can feel a firm and tender lump.
· Pain during or after bowel movement.
· Skin color change of the skin surrounding fistula.

CAUSES

· Infection from a tear in the anal canal lining.
· May be due to an injury, rectal infection (including chlamydia), cancer, and radiation therapy.
· Tissue damage because of an abscess (a pocket of pus).

RISK INCREASES WITH

· Puncture wound in anal canal lining (e.g., from eating an eggshell or fishbone) or injury from an enema tip.
· Injection treatment for internal hemorrhoids.
· Inflammatory bowel disease.
· Acute appendicitis or diverticulitis.

PREVENTIVE MEASURES

No specific preventive steps.

EXPECTED OUTCOMES

Some fistulas heal on their own. In others, surgical repair may be necessary and the results are usually excellent.

POSSIBLE COMPLICATIONS

· Constipation.
· Fistula may recur.

 ## DIAGNOSIS & TREATMENT

GENERAL MEASURES

· Your health care provider will do a physical exam of the anal area to confirm the diagnosis.
· Sitz baths help relieve discomfort. Sit in a tub of warm water (not hot) for 10 to 15 minutes several times a day. Dry the area carefully and completely after bathing.
· If it does not heal on its own, minor surgery can correct the fistula. It is usually done with local anesthetic on an outpatient basis. Follow your health care provider's instructions for after surgery care.

MEDICATIONS

· Stool softeners may be prescribed to prevent constipation.
· Antibiotics may be prescribed if infection is present.

ACTIVITY

Resume work and normal activity as soon as possible.

DIET

Regular diet.

 ## NOTIFY OUR OFFICE IF

· You or a family member has any symptoms of an anal fistula.
· Symptoms recur after treatment.

Special notes:

_____

_____

_____

More notes on the back of this page ☐

ANAPHYLAXIS
(Allergic Shock)

 BASIC INFORMATION

DESCRIPTION
A life-threatening allergic response to drugs or any other allergy-causing substance. Reactions that happen the fastest are often the worst.

FREQUENT SIGNS AND SYMPTOMS
Any of the following can happen within seconds or a few minutes after being exposed to something that you are very allergic to:
· Tingling or numbness around the mouth.
· Sneezing, coughing, or wheezing.
· Swelling around the face or hands.
· Feeling anxious.
· Weak, rapid pulse.
· Stomach cramps, vomiting, and diarrhea.
· Itching all over. Hives often appear.
· Watery eyes.
· Chest feels tight; trouble breathing.
· Swelling or itching in the mouth or throat.
· Pounding heartbeat.
· Faintness; loss of consciousness.
Not all symptoms occur. Seek help for any of them.

CAUSES
· Sometimes the body overreacts when it tries to rid itself of the material it is allergic to. This can be life-threatening. Things that most often cause reactions:
· Drugs of all types, especially penicillin. Shots are a bigger risk than eyedrops or drugs taken by mouth.
· Stings or bites from insects, such as bees, wasps, hornets, biting ants and some spiders.
· Vaccines.
· Pollen.
· Injected chemicals used in some types of x-ray studies.
· Foods, especially eggs, beans, seafood, and fruit.

RISK INCREASES WITH
· A previous mild allergy to things listed above.
· A history of rashes, hay fever, or asthma.

PREVENTIVE MEASURES
If you have an allergic history:
· Tell your health care provider before you accept any new drugs. Before you are given a shot, ask what it is.
· Keep a special kit, such as Ana-Kit or EpiPen, with you at all times. Be sure your family knows how to use the kit if you need it.
· If you are allergic to insect stings, wear clothing that covers all of your body when you are outside.
· Wear a medical alert bracelet or necklace warning that you have allergies.
· Always remain in a medical office 15 minutes after receiving any shot. Report any symptoms right away.
· Ask your health care provider about allergy therapy that can make you less allergic.

EXPECTED OUTCOMES
Full recovery (if treated quickly).

POSSIBLE COMPLICATIONS
If not treated quickly, anaphylaxis can cause shock, cardiac arrest, and/or death.

 DIAGNOSIS & TREATMENT

GENERAL MEASURES
· If you see signs of anaphylaxis in someone and they stop breathing:
- Call 911 (emergency) for an ambulance or medical help. If the victim is a child, perform lifesaving measures for 1 minute before calling for emergency help.
- Begin mouth-to-mouth breathing right away.
- If their heart is not beating, give CPR (cardiopulmonary resuscitation).
- Don't stop CPR until help arrives.
· Be aware that a reaction may happen when taking any medicine. Be ready to respond quickly if symptoms develop. If you have had a severe allergic reaction in the past, always carry your anaphylaxis kit.
· Long-term treatment may involve steps to make your body less sensitive to things to which you are allergic.

MEDICATIONS
· Epinephrine shots are the only immediate treatment for this condition.
· Other drugs may be given after the epinephrine that will help prevent the return of symptoms.

ACTIVITY
Return to your normal activities as soon as symptoms are better. Make sure you are not alone for 24 hours, in case symptoms come back.

DIET
Avoid foods to which you are allergic.

 NOTIFY OUR OFFICE IF

· You or a family member has symptoms of anaphylaxis. This is an emergency! Get help immediately!
· New, unexplained symptoms develop. Drugs used in treatment may produce side effects.

Special notes:

_____

_____

_____

More notes on the back of this page ☐

16

ANEMIA DURING PREGNANCY

 ## BASIC INFORMATION

DESCRIPTION

A low level of red cells and hemoglobin in the blood during pregnancy. Hemoglobin is the protein inside red blood cells that carries oxygen to body tissues. Common anemias in pregnancy include iron-deficiency anemia and folic-acid deficiency. Other anemias are glucose-6-phosphate dehydrogenase (G6PD) deficiency, thalassemia, and sickle-cell anemia.

FREQUENT SIGNS AND SYMPTOMS

- Usually no symptoms are apparent.
- Shortness of breath.
- Fatigue, weakness, or fainting.
- Pale skin, gums, eyes, and nailbeds.
- Palpitations (awareness of the heartbeat).
- Inflamed, sore tongue.
- Nausea.
- Headache.
- Jaundice (yellow skin or eyes).
- Cravings for ice, paint, or dirt (pica).

CAUSES

- Poor diet with not enough iron.
- Folic-acid deficiency.
- Loss of blood from bleeding hemorrhoids or internal bleeding.
- Even if iron and folic-acid intake are sufficient, a pregnant woman may become anemic.

RISK INCREASES WITH

- Poor nutrition, including not enough vitamins.
- Excess alcohol use, leading to poor nutrition.
- History of any disorder that reduces absorption of nutrients.
- Pregnancy with multiple babies (e.g., twins).
- Use of drugs for seizures.
- Genetic risk for some anemias.

PREVENTIVE MEASURES

- Eat foods rich in iron, such as liver, beef, dried beans, whole-grain breads and cereals, eggs, or dried fruit.
- Eat foods high in folic acid, such as wheat germ, beans, peanut butter, oatmeal, mushrooms, collards, broccoli, beef liver, and asparagus.
- Eating foods high in vitamin C, such as citrus fruits and fresh, raw vegetables.
- Take prenatal vitamin and mineral supplements, if they are prescribed.
- Get tested for certain anemias if you are at risk. Your obstetric provider will discuss the details.

EXPECTED OUTCOME

Usually curable with iron and folic-acid supplements, or other treatment if needed.

POSSIBLE COMPLICATIONS

- Premature labor, intrauterine growth restriction (IUGR), low birth weight. Folic-acid deficiency may cause birth defects (neural tube defects).
- Blood loss during labor may require blood transfusion.
- Higher risk for mother of infection after childbirth.

 ## DIAGNOSIS & TREATMENT

GENERAL MEASURES

- Your obstetric provider will do blood studies during your pregnancy. These can help diagnose anemia.
- Supplements are needed for most anemias.
- If the tongue is red and sore, rinse with warm salt water 3 or 4 times a day. Mix one-half teaspoon salt in one cup of warm water.
- Brush teeth with a soft toothbrush.

MEDICATION

- Iron, folic acid, and other supplements may be prescribed. Take iron supplements 1 hour before eating or between meals. Iron will turn bowel movements black, and often causes constipation. Iron sometimes may be taken with meals if it has caused an upset stomach.
- If you are taking a calcium supplement in addition to an iron supplement, take them at different times of day, as calcium will interfere with iron absorption.

ACTIVITY

Rest often until the anemia improves.

DIET

Eat a healthy pregnancy diet and take prescribed supplements.

 ## NOTIFY OUR OFFICE IF

- You or a family member has symptoms of anemia during pregnancy.
- You have diarrhea, nausea, abdominal pain, or constipation during pregnancy.
- You experience unexplained bleeding during pregnancy.

Special notes: _____

_____

_____

More notes on the back of this page ☐

ANEMIA, FOLIC-ACID DEFICIENCY

 BASIC INFORMATION

DESCRIPTION

Anemia that is caused by a deficiency of folic acid. It is often occurs along with iron-deficiency anemia.

FREQUENT SIGNS AND SYMPTOMS

- Fatigue and weakness.
- Red, sore tongue.
- Mouth ulcers.
- Pale skin, gums, eyes, and nailbeds.
- Shortness of breath.
- Irritability.
- Nausea, vomiting and diarrhea (rare).
- Numbness and tingling of fingers and toes.

CAUSES

- Complication of pregnancy. A woman's body needs eight times more folic acid than usual with pregnancy.
- Not enough intake or absorption of foods with a high folic-acid content. These include meat, poultry, fish, cheese, milk, eggs, green vegetables, and yeast.
- Excess alcohol use.
- Over-cooking foods, which destroys folic acid.
- Deficiency of vitamin B-12 or vitamin C.

RISK INCREASES WITH

- Adults over 60.
- Pregnancy.
- Recent surgery.
- Illness such as tropical sprue, psoriasis, acne rosacea, eczema, or dermatitis herpetiformis.
- Fad diets or general poor nutrition.
- Chronic illness.
- Surgical removal of a portion of the stomach.
- Smoking, which decreases vitamin C absorption. Vitamin C is needed for folic-acid absorption.
- Use of some drugs, such as anticonvulsants, oral contraceptives, methotrexate, triamterene, or sulfasalazine.

PREVENTIVE MEASURES

- Don't drink alcohol.
- Have regular medical checkups during pregnancy. Take prenatal vitamin supplements, if they are prescribed.
- Eat well. Include fresh vegetables, meat, and other animal proteins. Avoid fad diets. Don't over-cook food.
- Don't smoke. Smoking increases vitamin requirements.

EXPECTED OUTCOME

Usually curable in three weeks with an adequate folic-acid intake.

POSSIBLE COMPLICATIONS

- Infertility.
- Increased risk of infections.
- Congestive heart failure (severe cases only).
- Can increase the risk of conceiving a child with a neural tube defect.

 DIAGNOSIS & TREATMENT

GENERAL MEASURES

- Your health care provider may do a physical exam. Medical tests may include blood studies, a Schilling test to measure vitamin B-12 levels and a trial of taking vitamin B-12.
- Treatment consists of folic acid supplements and treating any underlying causes.
- If you smoke, find a way to quit.
- If you take oral contraceptives, consider using another form of contraception.

MEDICATION

- Folic-acid supplements will be prescribed.
- Iron supplements to take orally will be prescribed.

ACTIVITY

Anemia does cause fatigue. Schedule regular rest periods until you are able to resume normal activity.

DIET

No special diet. Eat foods daily that are high in folic acid. The liver can store folic acid for a limited time only. Foods include asparagus spears, beef liver, broccoli spears, collards (cooked), mushrooms, oatmeal, peanut butter, red beans, and wheat germ.

 NOTIFY OUR OFFICE IF

- You or a family member has symptoms of anemia.
- Symptoms don't improve in two weeks, despite treatment.
- Symptoms of infection (fever, chills, and muscle aches) occur during treatment.

Special notes:

_____

_____

_____

More notes on the back of this page ☐

ANEMIA, HEMOLYTIC

BASIC INFORMATION

DESCRIPTION

An anemia that is due to red blood cells being destroyed faster than the bone marrow can produce them. In the intrinsic type, the destruction is due to a defect in the red blood cells themselves. In the extrinsic type, healthy red blood cells are produced, but are destroyed in the spleen. Hemolytic anemia can affect all ages.

FREQUENT SIGNS AND SYMPTOMS

- Sometimes there are no symptoms. The anemia may be diagnosed on a routine health exam.
- Fatigue and weakness.
- Pale skin, eyes, and fingernails.
- Shortness of breath.
- Irregular heartbeat.
- Jaundice (yellow skin and eyes, dark urine).

CAUSES

Bone marrow cannot produce red blood cells fast enough to make up for those being destroyed. This is a process known as hemolysis. More than 200 causes for hemolysis exist. Some are due to inherited disorders and some are acquired disorders. Sometimes, the cause is unknown.

RISK INCREASES WITH

- Inherited disorders. These include hereditary spherocytosis, glucose-6-phosphate dehydrogenase (G6PD) deficiency, sickle cell anemia, or thalassemia.
- Infections such as hepatitis, cytomegalovirus, Epstein-Barr virus, typhoid fever, streptococcus, or *Escherichia coli (E. coli)*.
- Leukemia or lymphoma.
- Use of certain drugs, such as penicillin, antimalarials, sulfa, or acetaminophen.
- Various tumors.
- Family history of hemolytic anemia.

PREVENTIVE MEASURES

- Don't take any drugs that have previously caused hemolytic anemia.
- Seek genetic counseling before having children if you have a family history of hemolytic anemia (inherited forms).

EXPECTED OUTCOMES

- If hemolytic anemia is acquired, it can usually be cured when the cause, such as a drug, is stopped.
- If it is due to an underlying disorder, the outcome depends on the course of the primary disease.
- If hemolytic anemia is inherited, it is currently considered incurable. However, symptoms can be relieved or controlled.

POSSIBLE COMPLICATIONS

- Varies depending on the cause of the anemia.
- It may cause existing heart or lung disease to worsen.

DIAGNOSIS & TREATMENT

GENERAL MEASURES

- Your health care provider will do a physical exam and ask questions about your symptoms. Medical tests include blood and urine studies. Other tests may be done to help diagnose an underlying cause for anemia.
- Treatment depends on the specific hemolytic problem. Treatment may include drugs, blood transfusions, stopping drugs, or surgery.
- Blood transfusion therapy may be needed.
- Surgical removal of the spleen may be recommended.

MEDICATIONS

- Drugs will be prescribed depending on the specific cause of anemia. These may include corticosteroids, immune globulin, folic acid, iron therapy, and others.
- Drugs that are causing the anemia will be stopped.

ACTIVITY

No limits, except those caused by the symptoms.

DIET

No special diet. Fava beans should be avoided in certain patients (you will be advised).

NOTIFY OUR OFFICE IF

- You or a family member has symptoms of hemolytic anemia.
- Fever, cough, sore throat, swollen joints, muscle aches, or bloody urine occur during treatment.

Signs of infection in any part of the body (redness, pain, swelling, fever).
- New, unexplained symptoms develop. Drugs used in treatment may produce side effects.

Special notes:

_____

_____

_____

More notes on the back of this page ☐

ANEMIA, IRON-DEFICIENCY

 ## BASIC INFORMATION

DESCRIPTION
An anemia caused by inadequate amounts of iron, which is required to meet the body's needs. Iron is present in all cells and has several vital functions. The anemia can affect any age. It is more common in women of childbearing age.

FREQUENT SIGNS AND SYMPTOMS
- There may be no symptoms. It may be diagnosed on a routine health exam.
- Fatigue and weakness.
- Pale skin, eyes, and fingernails.
- General feeling of discomfort.
- Being more sensitive to cold.
- Shortness of breath.
- Dizziness.
- Restless leg syndrome (odd sensations in the legs).

CAUSES
Iron is involved with red blood cell production. When iron stores are low, fewer red blood cells are produced and this leads to anemia

RISK INCREASES WITH
- Rapid growth spurts in children and young teens.
- Heavy menstrual bleeding.
- Pregnancy.
- Not getting enough iron in the diet.
- Internal bleeding, such as from ulcers or colon polyps.
- Problems of the body in utilizing or absorbing iron.
- Kidney disease.
- Folic acid or vitamin B-12 deficiency.

PREVENTIVE MEASURES
- Adequate iron intake with a well-balanced diet.
- Correct problems causing excess blood loss.

EXPECTED OUTCOMES
Usually curable with treatment. It may take 2 months for the iron levels to return to normal. Some outcomes will also depend on the underlying cause.

POSSIBLE COMPLICATIONS
- Complications are rare in mild anemia.
- If the anemia is more severe, heart complications can occur. Children may have developmental problems.

 ## DIAGNOSIS & TREATMENT

GENERAL MEASURES
- Your health care provider will do a physical exam and ask questions about your symptoms and diet. Medical tests may include blood, urine, and stool studies. Other tests may be done to diagnose disorders that could be the cause of the anemia.
- Iron deficiency can be treated with iron supplements. Other treatment will depend on the underlying cause. The cause needs to be treated so the iron deficiency does not recur.
- Internal bleeding problems may require surgery.

MEDICATIONS
- Oral iron supplements (always follow your health care provider's instructions):
  - Take iron on an empty stomach (at least 1/2 hour before meals) for best absorption. If it upsets your stomach, take it with a small amount of food (except milk).
  - If you take other drugs, wait at least 2 hours after taking iron before taking them. Antacids and tetracyclines especially interfere with iron absorption.
  - Iron supplements may cause black bowel movements, diarrhea, or constipation.
  - Too much iron is dangerous. A bottle of iron tablets can poison a child. Keep iron supplements out of the reach of children.
- In some cases, the iron may be given by injection.

ACTIVITY
No limits. You may need to reduce activities until symptoms of fatigue are gone.

DIET
- Adults should limit milk to 1 pint a day. It interferes with iron absorption.
- Eat iron-rich foods, including meat, fish, poultry, beans, raisins, egg yolks, and leafy green vegetables.
- Increase dietary fiber to prevent constipation.

 ## NOTIFY OUR OFFICE IF

- You or a family member has symptoms of anemia.
- Nausea, vomiting, fever, stomach pain, severe diarrhea, or constipation occur during treatment.

Special notes:

_____

_____

_____

More notes on the back of this page ☐

ANEMIA, PERNICIOUS
(Vitamin B-12 Deficiency)

BASIC INFORMATION

DESCRIPTION
An anemia that results from the failure of the digestive tract to absorb vitamin B-12. Vitamin B-12 (also called cobalamin) is needed for making red blood cells and keeping the nervous system functioning. This type of anemia usually affects adults of both sexes, between ages 40 and 70.

FREQUENT SIGNS AND SYMPTOMS
- Symptoms develop slowly. It may take time to notice.
- Weakness, especially in the arms and legs.
- Sore tongue.
- Nausea, appetite loss, and weight loss.
- Numbness or tingling in the hands and feet.
- Difficulty maintaining proper balance.
- Pale lips, tongue, and gums.
- Yellow eyes and skin.
- Bleeding gums.
- Shortness of breath.
- Depression, confusion, poor memory, and dementia.
- Headache.
- Ringing in the ears (tinnitus).

CAUSES
- Pernicious anemia is due to a lack of intrinsic factor. This is a substance made by cells in the stomach that makes it possible to absorb vitamin B-12. The reason for the lack of intrinsic factor is unknown. It may be an autoimmune reaction, a genetic factor, or both.
- Other vitamin B-12 deficiency-caused anemia may be due to a variety of factors.

RISK INCREASES WITH
- Stomach surgery, stomach cancer, or gastritis.
- Diabetes and autoimmune disorders.
- Myxedema, Graves' disease, other thyroid disorders.
- Genetic factors, such as in people of Northern European ancestry. It is rare in blacks and Asians.
- Family history of pernicious anemia.
- Age over 40.
- Strict vegetarian diet or infants breast-fed by a mother on a strict vegetarian diet.
- Lack of stomach acid in older adults.
- Parasitic infections and intestinal diseases.
- Drugs such as H2 blockers, proton pump inhibitors, colchicine, neomycin, and aminosalicylic acid.
- Alcoholism.

PREVENTIVE MEASURES
Pernicious anemia cannot be prevented. In other anemias, avoiding risk factors, where possible, may help.

EXPECTED OUTCOMES
- For pernicious anemia, lifelong vitamin B-12 therapy will help symptoms and prevent complications.

- For vitamin B-12 deficiency-caused anemia, vitamin B-12 therapy or diet changes can prevent deficiency.

POSSIBLE COMPLICATIONS
- Congestive heart failure.
- Nerve damage that cannot be reversed.
- Gastric cancer.

DIAGNOSIS & TREATMENT

GENERAL MEASURES
- Your health care provider will do a physical exam and ask questions about your symptoms and your diet. Medical tests include blood tests for vitamin B-12 levels, to check for antibodies to the intrinsic factor, and to measure the body's ability to absorb vitamin B-12.
- Treatment usually involves vitamin B-12 replacement. Lifetime treatment is needed for pernicious anemia. Some symptoms should start to clear up in a few days after treatment begins, while others may take several months.
- Any underlying disorder (such as thyroid problems) will be treated also.
- Stop drinking if alcoholism led to the vitamin B-12 deficiency.

MEDICATIONS
- Vitamin B-12 replacement will be prescribed. Some patients are given injections (they can be self-administered). For other patients (or in addition to injections), the vitamin may be taken by mouth or as a nasal gel.
- Iron supplements may be prescribed.
- Avoid taking high amounts of folic acid. It can mask the signs of vitamin B-12 deficiency.

ACTIVITY
Activity may be limited until symptoms improve.

DIET
- Eat a well-balanced diet.
- People on strict vegetarian diets can change the diet or take vitamin B-12 supplements for life.

NOTIFY OUR OFFICE IF

- You or a family member has symptoms of pernicious anemia.
- Symptoms don't start to improve with treatment.

Special notes:

_____

_____

_____

More notes on the back of this page ☐

ANEURYSM

BASIC INFORMATION

DESCRIPTION
A ballooning or bulge in the wall of a blood vessel (almost always an artery). It can affect the arteries in the chest, abdomen, brain, legs, or heart wall. Aneurysms have thin, weak walls and have a tendency to rupture (burst) and cause hemorrhage (bleeding). They occur most often in adults over age 55.

FREQUENT SIGNS AND SYMPTOMS
- Usually, there are no symptoms unless the aneurysm ruptures. Symptoms that occur depend on the artery affected.
- Thoracic (chest) aneurysm produces pain in the chest, neck, back, and abdomen. The pain may be sudden and sharp.
- Cerebral aneurysm in a brain artery produces headache (often throbbing), weakness, paralysis or numbness, pain behind the eye, vision change, partial blindness, and eye pupils of different sizes.
- Abdominal aneurysm produces back pain (sometimes severe), abdomen, and groin pain.
- Peripheral aneurysm in a leg artery causes poor circulation in the leg, with weakness and paleness or swelling, and bluish color.
- Ventricular aneurysm in the wall of the heart causes irregular heartbeat, shortness of breath, and chest pain.

CAUSES
Arterial walls become weak due to defect, disease, or injury. This may be due to an acquired condition or it may be congenital (present at birth).

RISK INCREASES WITH
- Adults over 55.
- Family history of aneurysms.
- Atherosclerosis (hardening of the arteries).
- High blood pressure.
- Congenital weak artery.
- Polycystic disease or connective tissue disorders.
- Complications of blood infections.
- Fibromuscular dysplasia.
- Injury (trauma).
- Cigarette smoking.

PREVENTIVE MEASURES
No specific way to prevent aneurysms. Seek treatment for any risk factors where possible.

EXPECTED OUTCOMES
- Diagnosed, unruptured aneurysms may or may not be treated. You may be followed up with regular medical exams to watch for complications.
- Outcome of a ruptured aneurysm varies. Some persons are treated and recover with little or no damage. Others die before, during, or after treatment.

POSSIBLE COMPLICATIONS
- Stroke.
- Rupture of the aneurysm.

DIAGNOSIS & TREATMENT

GENERAL MEASURES
- Emergency treatment is needed for persons with symptoms of a ruptured aneurysm. Once the aneurysm is diagnosed, surgery may be performed. This is done to stop any bleeding and to prevent the aneurysm from recurring. Treatments called endovascular procedures can be done to plug or clog the blood vessel.
- Unruptured aneurysms may be diagnosed when a person has no symptoms. Sometimes they are found when medical tests are done for other reasons. The decision to treat or not treat these aneurysms with surgery is difficult. Both options carry risks. Your health care provider will discuss the risks and benefits of each with you. The size of the aneurysm, its location, the patient's symptoms, age, health status, and preferences must all be considered.
- Sometimes, the aneurysm can be removed and replaced with a graft (artificial blood vessel), or wrapped with a protective sleeve to prevent rupturing.
- To learn more: Search the Internet or visit a library.

MEDICATIONS
- After surgery, anticoagulants to prevent blood clots and pain relievers are usually prescribed.
- Antibiotics to prevent infection may be prescribed.

ACTIVITY
If surgery is done, you will be advised of any limits.

DIET
No special diet.

NOTIFY OUR OFFICE IF

- You or a family member has symptoms of a ruptured aneurysm. This is an emergency! Call for help; rest in bed until help arrives.
- You or a family member has minor pain or aching in the chest, abdomen, or legs. Fever or weight loss occurs for no apparent reason.

Special notes:

_____

_____

_____

More notes on the back of this page ☐

ANGINA PECTORIS

 BASIC INFORMATION

DESCRIPTION
Chest pain or discomfort due to a decrease in the blood (and oxygen) supply to the heart muscle (myocardium). Angina may be stable (symptoms are predictable), or unstable (symptoms are unexpected and usually occur while at rest). Angina affects adults of both sexes.

FREQUENT SIGNS AND SYMPTOMS
• Tightness, squeezing, pressure, fullness, ache, or pain in the center of the chest.
• Chest pain similar to indigestion.
• Discomfort or pain may also occur in the neck, jaw, shoulder, arm, or back.
• Symptoms may occur with exercise, strong emotions, heavy meals, or with temperature extremes. Some persons have angina while resting.

CAUSES
Angina occurs when the heart needs more blood and oxygen and it is unable to get what it requires. This is called ischemia. Most often it is due to coronary heart disease. With heart disease, one or more of the arteries that supply blood to the heart is narrowed or blocked. Angina also occurs if the blood does not carry enough oxygen, such as in severe anemia or carbon monoxide poisoning.

RISK INCREASES WITH
• Coronary or valvular heart disease.
• Hypertrophic cardiomyopathy (enlarged heart).
• Anemia.

PREVENTIVE MEASURES
Prevention involves preventing the coronary heart disease that leads to angina. Don't smoke. Get treatment for chronic disorders such as diabetes, high blood pressure, and obesity. Reduce high cholesterol with diet or drugs.

EXPECTED OUTCOMES
Minor angina can be relieved with rest and use of nitroglycerin and other drugs. Other treatment may be needed to correct underlying diseases.

POSSIBLE COMPLICATIONS
Heart attack, unstable angina, and/or death.

 DIAGNOSIS & TREATMENT

GENERAL MEASURES
• Your health care provider will do a physical exam and ask questions about your symptoms. A number of medical tests will be done to assess heart function and to diagnose any underlying disorder.
• Treatment usually involves drug therapy to relieve angina symptoms, slow the progress of heart disease, and prevent complications.

• If drugs cannot control the angina, there are other treatment options. They include balloon angioplasty to open blocked coronary arteries, stenting (a tiny metal tube or coil is placed in the artery to keep it open), or surgery to bypass severely blocked coronary arteries.
• Don't smoke. Find a way to quit that works for you.
• Avoid angina triggers, if possible, that increase the heart's workload, such as anger, temperature extremes, high altitude (except in commercial airline flights), or sudden bursts of activity.
• To learn more: American Heart Association, local branch listed in telephone directory, or call (800) 242-8721; website: www.americanheart.org.

MEDICATIONS
• Nitroglycerin relieves acute symptoms of angina or it can be used before activities. It does not affect symptoms of other disorders. It can work within seconds to relieve pain. Always keep it with you for immediate use.
• Drugs to prevent blood clots will be given after procedures such as balloon angioplasty or stenting.
• Other drugs for coronary disease, such as aspirin, beta-blockers, cholesterol-lowering drugs, ACE inhibitors, or calcium channel blockers may be prescribed. If they are, it is important to follow the prescribed drug regimen.

ACTIVITY
• Learn to adjust activities to lessen angina attacks.
• Don't use angina as an excuse not to exercise. A regular moderate exercise routine (determined by your health care provider) can help to control symptoms.

DIET
• Low-fat, low-cholesterol diet is often recommended.
• Weight loss diet if overweight.

 NOTIFY OUR OFFICE IF

• You or a family member has symptoms of angina pectoris.
• Angina pain lasts longer than 10 to 15 minutes, despite rest and treatment with nitroglycerin.
• You wake from sleep with chest pain that does not go away with 1 nitroglycerin tablet. If these attacks continue, report them, even if nitroglycerin relieves them.

Special notes:

_____

_____

_____

More notes on the back of this page ☐

ANIMAL BITES

 ## BASIC INFORMATION

DESCRIPTION
Bite wounds to humans from dogs, cats, or other animals (including humans).

FREQUENT SIGNS AND SYMPTOMS
· Bite wounds can be tears, punctures, scratches, ripping, or crushing injuries.
· Dog bites usually involve the hands, face, or the legs and feet.
· Cat bites usually involve the hands, followed by legs, feet, face, and trunk.

CAUSES
· Most bite wounds are from a domestic pet known to the victim. Large dogs are the most common source.
· Human bites are often the result of one person striking another in the mouth with a clenched fist.

RISK INCREASES WITH
Exposure to domestic pets or wild animals.

PREVENTIVE MEASURES
· Education on how to avoid animal bites, for children as well as adults.
· Avoid stray animals.

EXPECTED OUTCOMES
· Wounds should steadily improve and close over within 7 to 10 days.
· Dog bites rarely become infected. Cat bites and human bites frequently become infected.

POSSIBLE COMPLICATIONS
Infection, extensive soft tissue injuries with scarring, hemorrhage, rabies, and sometimes death.

 ## DIAGNOSIS & TREATMENT

GENERAL MEASURES
· Elevate the injured extremity to prevent swelling.
· If the wound is bleeding, apply pressure to the area with clean towel or cloth until bleeding stops. Clean wound with soap and water, then dry the area and cover it with sterile gauze or clean cloth.
· Do not apply antiseptic or other medicine.
· Call your health care provider, or take the patient to an emergency department if the wound is severe, it won't stop bleeding, or the bite was from a wild animal or one behaving strangely.
· Contact the local health department and consult with them about the prevalence of rabies in the species of animal involved.
· If possible the animal that caused the bite should checked for rabies. Call an animal control office for instructions.

MEDICATIONS
· Preventive antibiotic treatment may be prescribed.
· Antitetanus injection may have to be given.
· Sometimes, an antirabies vaccine or serum may have to be given.

ACTIVITY
No limits, except those caused by the injury.

DIET
No special diet.

 ## NOTIFY OUR OFFICE IF

· You or a family member suffers from an animal bite.
· The bite does not begin to heal within 2 to 3 days.
· New or unexplained symptoms develop. Drugs used in treatment may produce side effects.

Special notes:

_____

_____

_____

More notes on the back of this page ☐

ANORECTAL ABSCESS

 BASIC INFORMATION

DESCRIPTION
An abscess (collection of pus due to infection) that develops in the area around the anus and rectum. They may occur on the edge of the anal opening or deep in the rectum. They are more common in men, and are also common in people with digestion problems.

FREQUENT SIGNS AND SYMPTOMS
- Swelling around the rectum.
- Redness around the rectum.
- Dull or throbbing pain around the rectum.
- Difficulty or pain with bowel movement.
- Unable to sit comfortably.
- Fever.
- Bleeding or discharge if abscess ruptures.

CAUSES
Bacterial infection. It may occur in the glands inside the rectum that produce mucus. Bacteria in the stool can also infect a scratch or cut in the skin or in the rectum.

RISK INCREASES WITH
- Food such as egg shell or fish bone or swallowed object such as a paperclip. They can cut the skin as they pass in a stool.
- Constipation.
- Hemorrhoids, or an injection to treat them.
- Use of enemas. Enema tips can damage skin.
- Foreign objects in the rectum.
- Anal sex.
- Diseases of the bowel.
- Weak immune system due to illness or drugs.

PREVENTIVE MEASURES
Cannot always be prevented. Avoid risk factors where possible.

EXPECTED OUTCOMES
With treatment, complete healing in 6 months if no complications.

POSSIBLE COMPLICATIONS
- An extra opening (fistula) may develop between the anus and the outside of the body.
- Abscess may return if the cause is not corrected.
- Incontinence of stool (unable to control bowel movements).

 DIAGNOSIS & TREATMENT

GENERAL MEASURES
- Your health care provider can diagnose the abscess with a physical exam of the affected area. Medical tests are usually not needed, but may include an x-ray or internal exam of the rectum with a special instrument.
- Treatment most often involves outpatient surgery to open and drain the abscess. For an abscess deeper in the rectum, the patient may need hospital care.
- Follow your health care provider's instructions for changing bandages and other care after surgery. Keep that area of the body clean.
- Sitz baths every 2 to 4 hours after surgery. Sit in a bathtub with 6 to 8 inches of warm water for 20 minutes.
- Use warm compress as needed for pain.
- Have a bowel movement when you need to, even though you may anticipate pain.

MEDICATIONS
Drugs may be prescribed for pain, infection, and to help prevent constipation.

ACTIVITY
Move legs often as you recover from surgery. Return to normal activities as soon as possible after surgery.

DIET
An increase in fiber in the diet may help lower the risk of constipation. Drink plenty of fluids.

 NOTIFY OUR OFFICE IF

- You or a family member has symptoms of anorectal abscess.
- New or unexplained symptoms develop after surgery.

Special notes:

_____

_____

_____

More notes on the back of this page ☐

ANOREXIA NERVOSA

 BASIC INFORMATION

DESCRIPTION
Anorexia is a type of eating disorder. A person refuses to eat enough to maintain a normal weight for height and age. It develops over time and can occur in both sexes. It most often affects young females ages 12 to 25.

FREQUENT SIGNS AND SYMPTOMS
- Weight loss of at least 15% of ideal body weight.
- Continues to diet when not overweight. May restrict food intake or binge on food and then purge.
- Person feels fat even when extremely thin.
- Intense fear of becoming fat.
- Obsessed with food, but denies being hungry.
- Excess exercising.
- Stopping of menstrual periods or never starting.
- Uses diuretics, laxatives, emetics and amphetamines.
- Depressed, moody, irritable, withdrawn, ritual or odd behaviors, and insomnia.
- Hair loss, dry skin, feeling cold, brittle nails, low blood pressure, and poor blood circulation.

CAUSES
Unknown. There are many theories. It involves using food and weight to deal with emotional problems, such as issues of self-worth and control for the patient.

RISK INCREASES WITH
- Young females.
- Starting a normal weight-loss diet. The person refuses to stop dieting after a reasonable weight loss.
- Some personality traits such as perfectionism, obsessiveness, or low self-esteem.
- Family history of eating disorders.
- Family influence (overprotective or placing too much value on physical appearance).
- Society, cultural and peer pressure to be thin.
- Emotional stress.
- Athletes, ballet dancers, cheerleaders, or models.

PREVENTIVE MEASURES
No specific preventive measures. Early treatment may help keep it from progressing.

EXPECTED OUTCOMES
- Treatable if the patient recognizes the problem, wants help, and is compliant with treatment.
- Therapy may continue over several years. Relapses are common, especially when stressful situations occur.
- About 40% make a good recovery in 5 years, 40% have symptoms, but function fairly well, and 20% have severe, ongoing symptoms.

POSSIBLE COMPLICATIONS
Electrolyte imbalance, irregular heartbeat, esophagitis, gastritis, lack of menstrual periods, nerve disorders, anemia and weakness, infertility, osteoporosis, or suicide.

 DIAGNOSIS & TREATMENT

GENERAL MEASURE
- Your health care provider can usually diagnose anorexia with a physical exam and by asking questions about your symptoms, eating habits and weight concerns. There is no one test to diagnose anorexia. Medical tests may be done to check for possible underlying disorder, physical problems, or complications.
- Denial of the severity or even the existence of a problem is common in patients. Most patients resist treatment and behavioral change at first. Some want a quick and easy solution that is not feasible.
- The goal of treatment is for the patient to establish healthy eating patterns to regain normal weight.
- Treatment may include counseling for the patient and the family, nutrition counseling, and drug therapy if needed. Hospital care may be required if the weight is extremely low or there are life-threatening symptoms.
- A dental exam is usually recommended.
- Counseling focuses on the misconceptions that patients have of themselves (physically, mentally, emotionally). Support groups may help some patients.
- To learn more: Anorexia Nervosa and Related Eating Disorders, PO Box 5102, Eugene, OR 97405; (503) 344-1144 (not toll free); website: www.anred.org.

MEDICATIONS
- There is no one drug used to treat anorexia. Drugs may be prescribed for specific symptoms such as depression, anxiety, or agitation.
- Vitamin and mineral supplements may be prescribed.

ACTIVITY
May be limits at first until weight is gained. Then exercise for enjoyment and fitness and not to lose weight.

DIET
A dietitian will help you plan healthy meals that are not rigid, but provide food choices. Calories will be slowly increased over time to reach your individual needs.

 NOTIFY OUR OFFICE IF

- You or a family member has symptoms of anorexia.
- Weight loss continues, despite treatment.

Special notes:

_____

_____

_____

More notes on the back of this page ☐

ANXIETY DISORDER, GENERALIZED

 BASIC INFORMATION

DESCRIPTION

An illness that involves constant worry even though nothing is wrong. A person feels tense most of the time and always expects the worst to happen. They may worry about health, money, family, work, or an unknown or unspecified threat. The symptoms may be severe and interfere with daily living. Attempts to avoid the anxiety lead to more anxiety. Anxiety usually comes on slowly and can start in childhood, adolescence, or as an adult. It is more common in women.

FREQUENT SIGNS AND SYMPTOMS

- Feeling that something undesirable or harmful is about to happen.
- Constant worry about things (big and small).
- Aches and pains for unknown reasons.
- Feeling tired.
- Unable to relax.
- Muscle tension, headaches, backache.
- Trouble falling or staying asleep.
- Dry mouth, swallowing difficulty, or hoarseness.
- Twitching or trembling.
- Unable to focus or concentrate.
- Feeling irritable or grouchy.
- Nausea, diarrhea, weight loss.
- Sweating or hot flashes.
- Easily startled.

CAUSES

It is most likely a combination of hereditary factors, environmental factors (such as childhood experiences), and chemical disturbances in the brain.

RISK INCREASES WITH

- Women.
- Stressful events or crisis in one's life.
- Family history of anxiety disorders.
- Other emotional or mental illness (depression, panic disorder, phobias, or dysthymia).
- Alcohol or substance abuse.
- Lack of social connections.
- Certain personality factors (being shy or a worrier).
- Living in poverty, in a minority group, or immigrants.

PREVENTIVE MEASURES

There are no specific preventive measures.

EXPECTED OUTCOMES

Anxiety can be controlled with treatment. Overcoming anxiety often results in a richer, more satisfying life.

POSSIBLE COMPLICATIONS

- Impaired social and work functioning.
- Depression, panic disorder, or social phobia.
- Dependence on drugs or alcohol.

 DIAGNOSIS & TREATMENT

GENERAL MEASURES

- Your health care provider will do a physical exam and ask questions about your symptoms. A mental health test may be done. There is no specific test to diagnose anxiety. Medical tests may be done to rule out other medical disorders.
- Treatment may involve psychotherapy (treatment of emotional and mental problems), self-care, and drugs.
- Cognitive-behavior therapy (CBT) is often recommended. Cognitive therapy teaches how to change thoughts, behaviors, or attitudes. Behavior therapy teaches ways to reduce anxiety with deep breathing and muscle relaxation.
- Self-care steps may include:
    - Talking to a friend or family member about your feelings. This sometimes defuses your anxiety.
    - Keep a journal about your anxious thoughts or emotions. Consider the causes and possible solutions.
    - Join a self-help group.
    - Learn relaxation techniques. For some people, meditation is effective.
    - Reduce stress in your life where possible.
- To learn more: National Institute of Mental Health; 6001 Executive Blvd, Bethesda, MD 20892-9663; (800) 647-2642; website: www.nimh.nih.gov.

MEDICATIONS

- Antianxiety drugs may be prescribed.
- Antidepressants may be prescribed.

ACTIVITY

Stay active. Physical exertion helps reduce anxiety.

DIET

No special diet. Avoid caffeine and alcohol.

 NOTIFY OUR OFFICE IF

- You or a family member has symptoms of anxiety.
- Symptoms recur after treatment.

Special notes:

_____

_____

_____

More notes on the back of this page ☐

APPENDICITIS

BASIC INFORMATION

DESCRIPTION
Inflammation of the appendix. The appendix is a small tubelike pouch that is part of the large intestine. The appendix has no known function, but it can become diseased. Symptoms vary widely. It can affect all ages and both sexes.

FREQUENT SIGNS AND SYMPTOMS
- Pain that frequently begins close to the navel and moves toward the right lower abdomen. Pain becomes persistent. It worsens with moving, breathing deeply, coughing, sneezing, walking, or being touched.
- Nausea and sometimes vomiting.
- Constipation and inability to pass gas.
- Diarrhea (occasionally).
- Low fever (begins after other symptoms).
- Abdominal swelling (late stages).

CAUSES
The exact cause is unknown. The appendix may be blocked with feces from the intestinal tract which leads to infection. When infected, the appendix becomes swollen, inflamed and filled with pus.

RISK INCREASES WITH
- Viral or bacterial infection of the gastrointestinal tract.
- Family history of appendicitis.
- Cystic fibrosis.
- Diet that is low in fiber.

PREVENTIVE MEASURES
No specific preventive measures.

EXPECTED OUTCOMES
Curable with surgery. People can live a normal life without their appendix.

POSSIBLE COMPLICATIONS
- Rupture of the appendix, abscess (pus-filled area), and peritonitis. This is more common in older persons.
- Wound infection or other surgery complications.
- Bowel obstruction.

DIAGNOSIS & TREATMENT

GENERAL MEASURES
- Don't take any laxatives, enemas, or drugs for pain prior to diagnosis. Laxatives may lead to rupture, and pain or fever reducers make diagnosis more difficult.
- Your health care provider will do a physical exam and ask questions about your symptoms. Medical tests may include blood and urine studies, x-ray, CT, ultrasound, or other tests may be done to confirm the diagnosis.

- Treatment involves surgery to remove the appendix (appendectomy). Because appendicitis can be hard to diagnose, surgery may be delayed until symptoms and signs progress enough to confirm the diagnosis.
- Surgery may be done with a laparoscope (a tube-like instrument with a light on the end). Small incisions (3 to 4) are made in the abdomen. The appendix is removed using instruments inserted into the incisions.
- Open surgery may be done. This involves one larger incision in the abdomen to remove the appendix. This type of surgery is done if the appendix has ruptured (burst).
- If an abscess has formed, surgery may be delayed until the abscess is drained and has time to heal.

MEDICATIONS
- Antibiotics for infection and drugs for pain are usually prescribed after surgery.
- Stool softeners to prevent constipation may be recommended.

ACTIVITY
- Rest in a bed or chair until surgery.
- Resume normal activities gradually after surgery.

DIET
- Don't eat or drink anything until appendicitis has been diagnosed. Anesthesia for surgery is much safer if the stomach is empty. If you are very thirsty, wash your mouth out with water.
- After surgery, a liquid diet is used for a short time. A regular diet may be resumed as the intestinal tract returns to normal.

NOTIFY OUR OFFICE IF

- You or a family member has symptoms of appendicitis.
- The following occur after surgery:
  - Fever of 101.5° F (38.6°C) or higher.
  - Increased redness, swelling, or pain at the incision site or if the site has drainage.
  - Vomiting or diarrhea occurs.

Special notes:

_____

_____

_____

More notes on the back of this page ☐

ARTHRITIS, JUVENILE RHEUMATOID (JRA)

 ## BASIC INFORMATION

DESCRIPTION

A chronic inflammatory disease of the joints that affects children. The joints most often involved are the knees, hands, and feet. Symptoms vary from mild to severe. JRA may start at any age in childhood. Major types are:
- Pauciarticular (limited to a few joints; 40% to 50% of cases.
- Polyarticular (5 or more joints involved; 35% of cases.
- Systemic-onset (involves at least 1 joint and involves inflammation of internal organs; 10% to 20% of cases).

FREQUENT SIGNS AND SYMPTOMS

- The first symptoms are often noticed with physical or emotional stress. Symptoms may occur often or rarely.
- Stiffness in the morning or after a nap.
- Swelling, warm, painful or aching joints. Children may not complain about joint pain.
- Limping. The child may refuse to walk without being able to explain why.
- Clumsiness.
- Fevers that come and go.
- Rashes that come and go.
- Poor appetite and weight loss.
- Swelling of lymph nodes.
- Eye pain and redness.

CAUSES

Unknown. It is probably caused by an autoimmune disorder in which the body's immune system attacks its own normal tissues. Infection may also be a factor.

RISK INCREASES WITH

A family history of JRA.

PREVENTIVE MEASURES

Cannot be prevented at present.

EXPECTED OUTCOMES

Some cases are mild and may disappear at puberty. In other cases, it becomes a progressive, crippling arthritis. Symptoms can usually be controlled with treatment.

POSSIBLE COMPLICATIONS

- Eye complications.
- Permanent joint damage.

 ## DIAGNOSIS & TREATMENT

GENERAL MEASURES

- Your child's health care provider will do a physical exam and ask questions about the symptoms. No one test is available to diagnose JRA. Medical tests may include blood and joint fluid studies and x-rays of the involved joints.

- Treatment involves steps to relieve symptoms, to preserve joint function, to prevent complications, and to help the child live as normal a life as possible.
- Treatment includes drug therapy, physical therapy, occupational therapy, and emotional help. You and your child's health care provider will decide on a treatment plan depending on your child's special needs.
- Occupational therapy helps with activities of daily life
- Help morning stiffness with a warm bath or shower, sleeping in a sleeping bag, doing range-of-motion exercises, or a heating pad or cold pack (if it feels better).
- Learning special techniques to control pain may help.
- Surgery may (rarely) be needed for joint problems.
- Eye exams at least twice a year will help detect any eye complications. Dental exams are also important.
- Children should attend regular school on a daily basis. Where needed, the school system should provide extra services to accommodate the child's needs.
- To learn more: American Juvenile Arthritis Organization, P.O. Box 7669, Atlanta, GA 30357; (800) 283-7800; website: www.arthritis.org.

MEDICATIONS

- Aspirin or other nonsteroidal anti-inflammatory drugs to reduce pain and inflammation will be prescribed.
- Other drugs are usually prescribed to help alter the progress of the disease and delay/prevent joint damage.

ACTIVITY

- Physical therapy exercises will be prescribed. Some the child can do alone. Some the parents will perform for the child. It is important that the child does the exercises because they help control symptoms and prevent complications.
- Splints may be used to support and protect joints.
- In general, contact sports should be avoided. The child should be encouraged to participate in other sports and recreational activities.

DIET

Provide a healthy diet. Maintaining a proper weight for age and height will help protect joints.

 ## NOTIFY OUR OFFICE IF

- Your child has symptoms of juvenile rheumatoid arthritis.
- After diagnosis, new or worsening symptoms occur.

Special notes:

_____

_____

_____

More notes on the back of this page ☐

ARTHRITIS, RHEUMATOID

BASIC INFORMATION

DESCRIPTION
A chronic, inflammatory disease that mainly affects the joints. It often begins between ages 25 and 50, and is more common in women.

FREQUENT SIGNS AND SYMPTOMS
- Redness, pain, warmth, and tenderness in the affected joints. They may be in the hands and wrists (most often), elbows, shoulders, feet, and ankles.
- Morning stiffness.
- Muscle aches, weakness, fever, and weight loss.
- Feeling generally unwell.
- Nodules (bumps) under the skin (sometimes).

CAUSES
Unknown. It is probably caused by an autoimmune disorder in which the body's immune system attacks its own normal tissues. Infection may also be a factor.

RISK INCREASES WITH
- Family history of rheumatoid arthritis or other autoimmune disorders.
- Genetic factors.
- Women.
- Native Americans (occurs more often in this group).

PREVENTIVE MEASURES
No specific preventive measures.

EXPECTED OUTCOMES
The outcome varies. The disease course may be short and limited or progressive and severe. It is presently incurable. Pain relief, prevention of disability, and an active, normal life span are often possible.

POSSIBLE COMPLICATIONS
- About 5% to 10% of patients are eventually disabled.
- Drugs used in treatment can cause adverse affects.
- Heart, lung, blood vessel, or eye problems.
- Anemia.

DIAGNOSIS & TREATMENT

GENERAL MEASURES
- Your health care provider will do a physical exam and ask questions about the symptoms. No one test is available to diagnose arthritis. Medical tests may include blood and joint fluid studies. CT, MRI, or x-rays of the involved joints are usually done.
- Treatment involves steps to relieve symptoms, to preserve joint function, to prevent complications, and help the person live as normal a life as possible.
- Treatment steps include drug therapy, physical therapy, occupational therapy, surgery, and lifestyle changes. A treatment plan is based on your special needs.

- Be sure to educate your-self about the disorder. Avoid arthritis treatment fads.
- Occupational therapy helps with activities of daily life
- Help the morning stiffness with a warm bath or shower, doing range-of-motion exercises, or a heating pad or cold pack (if it feels better).
- Options for treatment (to help symptoms such as pain) include relaxation techniques, counseling, meditation, stress reduction, biofeedback, and support groups. Flare-ups may be triggered by emotional stress.
- Surgery may be recommended for joint problems. It may involve joint replacement, tendon reconstruction, joint realignment, or removing inflamed tissue.
- To learn more: Arthritis Foundation, P.O. Box 7669, Atlanta, GA 30357; (800) 283-7800; website: www.arthritis.org.

MEDICATIONS
- Nonsteroidal anti-inflammatory drugs, including aspirin and others will be prescribed.
- Disease-modifying drugs and biologic response modifiers are two classes of drugs that are often prescribed.

ACTIVITY
- Physical therapy will help maintain strength and joint mobility. Follow instructions for home exercising.
- Exercising in a heated pool is good for stiff joints.
- Activity options include low impact aerobics, flexibility exercises, yoga, tai chi, or hydrotherapy.
- Mobility aids and splints may be recommended.

DIET
Eat a normal, well-balanced diet. Avoid arthritis diet fads, which are common. Lose weight if you are overweight. Being overweight stresses the joints.

NOTIFY OUR OFFICE IF

- You or a family member has symptoms of rheumatoid arthritis.
- The following occur during treatment:
  - Symptoms appear in different joints or other symptoms get worse.
  - New, unexplained symptoms develop. Drugs in treatment may produce side effects.

Special notes:

_____

_____

_____

More notes on the back of this page ☐

ASBESTOSIS

 BASIC INFORMATION

DESCRIPTION

Inflammation of the lung due to breathing asbestos particles. It is a chronic disorder, but is not contagious. Men over age 40 who have been exposed to asbestos are more likely to be affected.

FREQUENT SIGNS AND SYMPTOMS

- Shortness of breath.
- Cough that produces little or no sputum.
- General ill feeling.
- Fitful sleep.
- Appetite loss and weight loss.
- Chest pain.
- Hoarseness.
- Coughing up blood.
- Bluish nails.

CAUSES

Long-term exposure to small particles of asbestos at work or from other sources. The outer part of the lung becomes irritated by the asbestos fibers. This leads to inflammation and to a thickening and scarring of the lung tissue (pulmonary fibrosis). It may take up to 20 years or more between exposure to asbestos and the symptoms of the disease. This period may be shorter after intense exposure.

RISK INCREASES WITH

- Work that involves asbestos.
- Smoking.
- Excess alcohol use.

PREVENTIVE MEASURES

- During exposure to asbestos, wear a protective mask or external-air-supplied hood.
- Follow recommended industrial safety procedures to suppress asbestos dust.
- For workers in asbestos industries, have regularly scheduled x-rays to detect any shadow on the lungs. If a problem develops, the person should stop working with asbestos, even if there are no symptoms.
- Don't smoke.

EXPECTED OUTCOMES

There is no cure. In a few patients, it may remain unchanged, but in most, it is slowly progressive (even without further exposure to asbestos). Symptoms can usually be relieved or controlled.

POSSIBLE COMPLICATIONS

- Chronic obstructive pulmonary disease (COPD).
- Heart failure due to lung disease.
- It may lead to cancer of the lungs (the risk is greatly increased in cigarette smokers).
- Tuberculosis.

 DIAGNOSIS & TREATMENT

GENERAL MEASURES

- Your health care provider will do a physical exam and ask about your symptoms and past exposure to asbestos. Medical tests usually include a CT or x-rays of the lungs and lung function tests. A bronchoscopy may be done (an instrument with a lighted tip is used to view inside the lungs and remove tissue for a biopsy).
- There is no specific treatment for asbestosis. Treatment can help relieve the symptoms and prevent complications.
- Avoid any further contact with asbestos.
- Stop smoking. Find a way to quit that works for you.
- Obtain medical care for any respiratory infection, including the common cold.
- Chest physical therapy techniques will be provided by a respiratory therapist.
- Learn and practice bronchial drainage.
- Use a cool-mist humidifier (if advised) to loosen bronchial secretions so they can be coughed up easily.
- Keep flu and pneumococcal vaccines up-to-date.
- Supplemental oxygen may be required.
- Avoid crowds and persons with infections.
- To learn more: American Lung Association, 61 Broadway, 6th Floor, New York, NY 10006; (800) 586-4872; website: www.lungusa.org.

MEDICATIONS

- Bronchodilators (inhaled or oral) will help open up the bronchial tubes and allow passage of air. This is supervised at first by an inhalation therapist.
- For minor discomfort, use nonprescription drugs, such as acetaminophen or aspirin.

ACTIVITY

Regular exercise in whatever forms possible is important to preserve lung capacity.

DIET

No special diet.

 NOTIFY OUR OFFICE IF

- You or a family member has symptoms of asbestosis.
- New symptoms develop or other symptoms get worse, despite treatment.

Special notes:

_____

_____

_____

More notes on the back of this page ☐

ASTHMA

 BASIC INFORMATION

DESCRIPTION

Asthma involves blockage of normal airflow into and out of the lungs. The blockage develops when certain allergens or irritants are inhaled and cause a reaction in the airways. They become swollen (inflamed), produce excess mucus, and the airway muscles tighten. This leads to the wheezing and other symptoms. Asthma affects all ages but 50% of the cases are in children under age 10. Boys with asthma outnumber girls. In adult-onset asthma, women are more often affected.

FREQUENT SIGNS AND SYMPTOMS
- Chest tightness. Wheezing upon breathing out.
- Coughing, especially at night, may have thick, clear or yellow sputum.
- Rapid, shallow breathing that is easier with sitting up.
- Breathing difficulty that gradually gets worse.
- Neck and chest may be sucked in with each breath.
- Severe symptoms of an asthma attack may include:
  - Cough that sounds tight and dry.
  - Rapid heart-beat and abnormal rapid rate of breathing that becomes more labored.
  - Unable to speak more than a few words without pausing for breath.
  - Sweating, and much anxiety and distress.

CAUSES
The exact cause of asthma remains unclear. It may be due to a combination of genetic factors, certain factors that may sensitize the airways (such as animal dander, and dust mites), and contributing factors (such as childhood respiratory infections).

RISK INCREASES WITH
- Other allergies, such as eczema or hay fever.
- Family history of asthma or allergies.
- Exposure to air pollutants.
- Exposure to allergens (such as pets).
- Smoking and exposure to second-hand smoke.
- For adults, exposure to occupational irritants (fumes, gases, latex products, metals, and others).

PREVENTIVE MEASURES
No specific preventive measures for original disease. Avoiding risk factors where possible may help.

EXPECTED OUTCOMES
- Symptoms can be controlled with treatment.
- Half the children will outgrow asthma.

POSSIBLE COMPLICATIONS
- Missed workdays or school absenteeism.
- Pneumonia, pneumothorax, or respiratory failure.
- Status asthmaticus (a sustained attack that cannot be relieved).
- Poorly controlled asthma and chronic symptoms.

 DIAGNOSIS & TREATMENT

GENERAL MEASURES
- Your health care provider will do a physical exam and ask questions about your symptoms. Medical tests may include x-rays, pulmonary-function tests, an exercise tolerance test, and allergy tests (usually skin testing).
- Treatment will depend on the severity of the symptoms. It may include daily drug therapy, drug therapy for attacks, avoiding triggers, lifestyle changes, self-care, and education. A written treatment plan is usually provided. It should be followed carefully.
- Identify and avoid your particular triggering factors.
- Counseling may help, if asthma is stress-related.
- A peak flow meter may be used at home. It is a small device that measures how well air flows into and out of the airways. You will be instructed on its use.
- Treatment (allergy shots) to desensitize the immune system to specific allergens may be recommended.
- Hospital care may be required for severe attacks.
- To learn more: Asthma & Allergy Foundation of America, 1233 20th St., Suite 402, Washington, DC 20036; (800) 727-8462; website: www.aafa.org.

MEDICATIONS
- Asthma drugs are generally divided into 2 categories:
  - Quick relief. These drugs are prescribed for relief of asthma exacerbations and to prevent exercised-induced asthma (EIA) symptoms.
  - Long-term control. These drugs are prescribed for use on a daily basis to prevent symptoms.

ACTIVITY
- Stay active. Avoid sudden bursts of activity. If an attack follows exercise, sit and rest. Sip warm water.
- Swimming is a good exercise for asthma patients.

DIET
- No special diet. Avoid foods to which you are sensitive to.
- Drink plenty of liquids daily.

 NOTIFY OUR OFFICE IF

- You or a family member has symptoms of asthma.
- Symptoms don't improve, despite treatment.
- Peak flow is in a zone that causes you concern.

Special notes:

_____

_____

_____

More notes on the back of this page ☐

ATELECTASIS

 BASIC INFORMATION

DESCRIPTION
Collapse of lung tissue affecting part or all of one lung. It prevents normal lung function. Atelectasis can affect all ages, but is more common in children under age 10.

FREQUENT SIGNS AND SYMPTOMS
- Sudden, major collapse:
  - Chest pain.
  - Shortness of breath; rapid breathing.
  - Shock (weakness, pale skin, rapid heartbeat).
  - Dizziness.
- Gradual collapse:
  - Cough.
  - Fever.
  - Shortness of breath.
  - Sometimes, no symptoms are noticed.

CAUSES
- Obstructive atelectasis (most common type):
  - Thick mucous plugs from infection or other disease.
  - Inhaled objects, such as small toys or peanuts.
  - Surgery of the chest (thoracic) or abdomen.
- Nonobstructive atelectasis:
  - Pleural effusion (fluid in the lungs).
  - Pneumothorax (air in the area around the lung).
  - Tumors.
  - Lack of surfactant (a substance in the lungs).
  - Scarring of lung tissue (due to disease).
  - Trauma (injury) to the lung.
  - Enlarged lymph glands.

RISK INCREASES WITH
- Chronic obstructive pulmonary disease (COPD).
- Obesity.
- Congenital lung disease, such as cystic fibrosis.
- Neuromuscular disease.
- Smoking.
- Asthma.

PREVENTIVE MEASURES
- Medical care to help prevent postsurgical problems.
- Keep small objects that might be inhaled away from young children (such as peanuts).

EXPECTED OUTCOMES
Outcome is generally good. It usually resolves with treatment. Complications are rare, but will depend on any underlying cause.

POSSIBLE COMPLICATIONS
Infection and chronic lung damage.

 DIAGNOSIS & TREATMENT

GENERAL MEASURES
- Your health care provider will do a physical exam. Medical tests may include blood studies to measure oxygen and carbon dioxide levels, x-rays, or CT of the chest.
- Treatment depends on the cause. It may include drug therapy, chest physical therapy, bronchoscopy, and (rarely) surgery.
- Chest physical therapy may be done to help remove mucous from the lungs. It involves clapping, patting, and massaging the chest and back over the lungs. The lungs may be suctioned with a small plastic tube.
- Bronchoscopy may be done to remove foreign objects or a mucous plug. This involves using an instrument with a lighted tip to see inside the lungs.
- Disabling, chronic atelectasis may have to be treated with surgery to remove the affected part of the lung.
- A tumor may require surgery or radiation therapy.
- To learn more: American Lung Association, 61 Broadway, 6th Floor, New York, NY 10006; (800) 586-4872; website: www.lungusa.org.

MEDICATIONS
- Antibiotics for infection will be prescribed.
- Bronchodilators to assist breathing may be prescribed.
- Pain relievers may be prescribed.

ACTIVITY
Resume your normal activities as soon as symptoms improve. Take frequent showers. Try to avoid low-humidity environments.

DIET
No special diet. Drink plenty of water or other fluids daily to thin lung secretions.

 NOTIFY OUR OFFICE IF

- You or a family member has symptoms of atelectasis.
- Symptoms return after treatment. Atelectasis can recur.

Special notes:

_____

_____

_____

More notes on back of this page ☐

ATHEROSCLEROSIS
(Hardening of the Arteries)

 BASIC INFORMATION

DESCRIPTION

A hardening or narrowing of the arteries. Arteries are blood vessels that carry blood and oxygen to the heart, brain, and other body parts. Atherosclerosis can begin in childhood and progress slowly as people age. In some people, it progresses more rapidly. Up to age 45, it is more common in men. After menopause, women are as equally affected as men are. Atherosclerosis is an underlying medical problem that can lead to:
- Coronary artery disease.
- Stroke.
- Abdominal angina (pain).
- Bowel infarction (blood clot in the intestines).
- Atherosclerosis of the extremities. Legs get reduced blood flow, which leads to intermittent claudication (cramping with or without exercise).
- Other conditions, such as aortic aneurysm.

FREQUENT SIGNS AND SYMPTOMS

- Symptoms often are absent until atherosclerosis reaches advanced stages. Symptoms depend on what part of the body has a decreased blood flow and the extent of disease.
- Muscle cramps if it involves blood vessels in the legs.
- Angina pectoris (chest pain) or a heart attack if it involves blood vessels to the heart.
- Stroke or transient ischemic attack if it involves vessels to the neck and brain.
- Abdominal cramps or pain if blood vessels to the abdomen are involved.

CAUSES

Plaque (made up of cholesterol, muscle cells, fibrous tissue, and calcium) builds up on artery walls that have been damaged in some way. Plaque deposits can grow large enough to reduce blood flow and can also crack or break apart and form clots. Clots can block blood flow or travel to another part of the body and cause serious or fatal problems.

RISK INCREASES WITH

- High blood pressure or diabetes.
- High levels of LDL (the bad cholesterol).
- Low levels of HDL (the good cholesterol).
- Obesity.
- Sedentary lifestyle (lack of physical activity).
- Smoking.
- Family history of atherosclerosis.
- Diet high in saturated fats and trans fatty acids.

PREVENTIVE MEASURES

- Eat a healthy, low-fat, high-fiber diet. Maintain a healthy weight. Exercise regularly. Don't smoke.
- Control diabetes and high blood pressure.
- Control cholesterol levels.

EXPECTED OUTCOMES

There is no cure, but atherosclerosis can be slowed or stopped. If organ damage has developed due to reduced blood flow, the outcome will vary.

POSSIBLE COMPLICATIONS

- Coronary artery disease, which is the number one cause of death in men and women.
- Other disorders as listed in Description.

 DIAGNOSIS & TREATMENT

GENERAL MEASURES

- Your health care provider may do a physical exam. Questions will be asked about your symptoms, smoking, alcohol use, drug use, exercise, and personal and family medical history. Blood pressure and pulse rate are checked. A stethoscope is used to listen for sounds of blood flow in the arteries. Blood studies are done for cholesterol, triglycerides, and blood sugar. Heart function tests (such as exercise stress tests and coronary calcium scores) and blood flow tests may be done.
- Atherosclerosis treatment includes drug therapy and lifestyle changes. Treatment for organ damage caused by atherosclerosis depends on the organ involved.
- Lifestyle changes include diet changes, losing weight, stopping smoking, and increasing exercise.
- Stop smoking. Find a way to quit that works for you.
- To learn more: American Heart Association, local branch listed in telephone directory, or call (800) 242-8721; website: www.americanheart.org.

MEDICATIONS

- Drugs will be prescribed for any diagnosed disorders.
- Cholesterol-lowering drugs are usually prescribed.

ACTIVITY

Activity may depend on state of health. Try to get 20 to 30 minutes of aerobic exercise most days of the week.

DIET

Eat a low-fat, high-fiber diet, that includes fruits and vegetables. Begin a weight-loss diet, if overweight.

 NOTIFY OUR OFFICE IF

You or a family member has symptoms of, or concerns about, atherosclerosis.

Special notes:

_____

_____

_____

More notes on the back of this page ☐

ATHLETE'S FOOT

(Tinea Pedis; Ringworm of the Feet)

 ## BASIC INFORMATION

DESCRIPTION
A common, contagious fungal (tinea) infection of the skin on the feet. It often affects the soles and skin between toes (often the 4th and 5th toes). It usually affects teens and adults (rare in young children).

FREQUENT SIGNS AND SYMPTOMS
· Moist, soft, gray-white or red scales on feet, especially between toes.
· Dead skin between toes.
· Itching in inflamed areas.
· Damp, musty foot odor.
· Small blisters on the feet (sometimes).

CAUSES
Infection by a *Trichophyton* fungus. The germs can be spread by direct contact with an infected person, or by contact with the germs on shoes, socks, shower, or pool surfaces. Animals can also carry the germs and infect a human.

RISK INCREASES WITH
· Infrequent washing of the feet.
· Infrequent changes of shoes or socks.
· Use of locker rooms and public showers.
· Hot, humid weather.
· People who have immune system problems due to illness or medications.
· Persistent moisture around the feet.

PREVENTIVE MEASURES
· Bathe feet daily. Dry completely between the toes and apply drying or dusting powder.
· Wear rubber thongs or wooden sandals in public showers.
· Go barefoot when possible.
· Change socks daily and wear socks made of cotton, wool, or other natural, absorbent fibers. Avoid synthetics.

EXPECTED OUTCOMES
Usually curable in 3 weeks with treatment, but recurrence is common.

POSSIBLE COMPLICATIONS
· A bacterial infection may develop in the affected area.
· A skin rash can sometimes develop on the hands and face (rare).

 ## DIAGNOSIS & TREATMENT

GENERAL MEASURES
· After soaking or bathing, carefully remove scales and material between the toes daily.
· Use a hair dryer to blow warm air on the feet to make sure they are completely dry.
· Keep affected areas cool and dry. Go barefoot or wear sandals during treatment. If socks are worn, keep them dry. If they get wet, change to dry ones.
· See your health care provider if the symptoms are severe. Your health care provider can usually diagnose athlete's foot by looking at the affected skin area. Other skin tests may be done to rule out other skin disorders.

MEDICATIONS
· Use nonprescription antifungal powders, creams, or ointments (such as terbinafine) after each bath.
· For severe cases, you may be prescribed oral, or stronger topical antifungal drugs.

ACTIVITY
No limits. Avoid activities that cause feet to sweat until healing is complete.

DIET
No special diet.

 ## NOTIFY OUR OFFICE IF

· You or a family member has symptoms of athlete's foot that persist, despite self-treatment.
· You develop a fever or the infection seems to be spreading.
· New, unexplained symptoms develop. Drugs used in treatment may produce side effects.

Special notes:

_____

_____

_____

More notes on the back of this page ☐

ATRIAL FIBRILLATION

 ## BASIC INFORMATION

DESCRIPTION

An abnormal heart rhythm. Fibrillation pertains to a "quivering" of muscles. Atrial pertains to the atria, the upper chambers of the heart. The abnormal rhythm reduces the flow of blood through the heart to the brain and other body parts and can cause symptoms. It usually affects older adults and men more than women.

FREQUENT SIGNS AND SYMPTOMS

- There may be no symptoms.
- Irregular and often rapid beating of the heart.
- Weakness, dizziness, shortness of breath, chest pain, or faintness may occur.

CAUSES

The heart has an electrical system that controls the heart rate and the heart's contractions. The average heart beats at a rate of 60 to 100 times per minute. With atrial fibrillation, the electrical system does not function as it should. The atria quiver instead of contracting and heart rate increases (may reach 350 beats a minute). There are different risk factors that can lead to atrial fibrillation and sometimes no cause is found.

RISK INCREASES WITH

- Increased age.
- Coronary heart disease.
- High blood pressure.
- Abnormal heart muscle.
- Mitral valve disease.
- Hyperthyroidism.
- Lung disease (chronic obstructive pulmonary disease, emphysema).
- Pericarditis (heart lining inflammation).
- Pulmonary embolism.
- Congestive heart failure
- Recent heart or lung surgery.
- Use of stimulant drugs (cocaine, decongestants).
- Excessive alcohol use.
- Congenital (present at birth) heart abnormality.
- Lone atrial fibrillation in young, healthy adults.

PREVENTIVE MEASURES

No specific preventive measures. Avoid risk factors where possible.

EXPECTED OUTCOMES

It can often be controlled with treatment. Atrial fibrillation tends to become a chronic condition.

POSSIBLE COMPLICATIONS

- Stroke.
- Arterial thrombosis or embolus (blood clots).
- Congestive heart failure.
- Other heartbeat irregularities can lead to cardiac arrest.

 ## DIAGNOSIS & TREATMENT

GENERAL MEASURES

- Your health care provider will do a physical exam and ask questions about your symptoms. The rapid and irregular heart rate can be heard with a stethoscope (a device for listening to bodily sounds). Medical tests may include blood studies and heart function tests.
- Treatment is aimed at treating the cause of the atrial fibrillation, slowing the heart rate, converting the abnormal rhythm to normal, preventing a recurrence, and preventing complications.
- Treatment steps may include drug therapy, electro-cardioversion, surgery, and other procedures.
- Abnormal heart rhythm may be converted to normal rhythm with drug therapy or with electric shock (electrocardioversion). An electric shock stops the abnormal activity and allows the normal rhythm to take over.
- Recurring atrial fibrillation may be treated with a variety of procedures. These include a pacemaker or atrial defibrillator implantation, AV node ablation, Maze procedure (atrial surgery), and pulmonary vein isolation.
- Some patients may be left in atrial fibrillation long-term if the heart rate is under control.
- To learn more: American Heart Association, local branch listed in telephone directory, or call (800) 242-8721; website: www.americanheart.org.

MEDICATIONS

Drugs may be prescribed for the underlying risk factor, to slow the heart rate, and to prevent blood clots.

ACTIVITY

Aim for 20 to 30 minutes of aerobic exercise 3 or more days a week. Activity may depend on your health status.

DIET

Eat a low-fat, high-fiber diet that includes fruits and vegetables. Begin a weight loss diet, if overweight.

 ## NOTIFY OUR OFFICE IF

- You or a family member has symptoms of atrial fibrillation.
- Any change in heart rate or rhythm, chest pain, sweating, weakness, shortness of breath, or swollen feet and ankles occurs.

Special notes:

_____

_____

_____

More notes on the back of this page ☐

ATTENTION DEFICIT HYPERACTIVITY DISORDER (ADHD)

 ## BASIC INFORMATION

DESCRIPTION

A consistent pattern of behavior that includes inattention, hyperactivity, and impulsivity. Attention deficit hyperactivity disorder (ADHD) is common and affects 3% to 5% of children. It also affects adults.

FREQUENT SIGNS AND SYMPTOMS

· Squirms in seat; fidgets with hands or feet.
· Unable to stay seated when required to do so.
· Easily distracted.
· Blurts out answers before a question is finished.
· Difficulty waiting turn in games and lines.
· Difficulty following instructions.
· Unable to sustain attention in work or play activities.
· Shifts from one uncompleted project to another.
· Difficulty playing quietly.
· Talks excessively.
· Interrupts or intrudes on others.
· Doesn't appear to listen.
· Loses items needed for tasks.
· Often engages in dangerous activities without considering consequences.

CAUSES

Unknown. Many theories have been proposed (but not yet proven). It is thought to have biologic origin. Recent studies suggest that TV watching by young children (age 3 and younger) may be a factor.

RISK INCREASES WITH

Family history of the disorder.

PREVENTIVE MEASURES

No specific preventive measures known.

EXPECTED OUTCOME

Most people don't outgrow ADHD, but do learn to adapt and live fulfilling lives.

POSSIBLE COMPLICATIONS

Later problems may occur, such as school failure, antisocial behavior, and (sometimes) criminal behavior.

 ## DIAGNOSIS & TREATMENT

GENERAL MEASURES

· The child's teacher may be the first to notice the behavior. A school psychologist, your child's doctor, or a special health care provider may diagnose the disorder. Several methods are used to help make the diagnosis. These include observing the child doing activities, mental, social, and intelligence tests, parent's and teacher's evaluation, and rating scales about behaviors.
· Adults are diagnosed based on their performance at work and at home. When possible, their parents rate how the person behaved as a child.

· Treatment for children includes appropriate classroom setting, behavior therapy, drug therapy, and help for parents in managing the child's behavior. A combination of these techniques will have the best outcome.
· Adult patients may have drug therapy and counseling.
· Counseling can help, as can behavior and cognitive therapy. These help child and adult patients focus on ways to change the undesired behavior.
· Help your child at home by providing a structured environment, well-defined behavior limits, and consistent use of parenting techniques.
· Special education classes for all or part of the day may be needed for some children.
· Stay in close contact with the child's teacher. Arrange for extra lessons or tutoring if the child needs help.
· Support groups or parenting skills training are helpful.
· To learn more: Attention Deficit Disorder Association, P.O. Box 543, Pottstown, PA 19464; (800) 487-2282; website: www.add.org.

MEDICATION

· Stimulant drugs (have a calming affect on persons with ADHD) or other drugs approved for ADHD may be prescribed. Some of these drugs have side effects, such as sleep problems, depression, headache, stomach ache, loss of appetite, and stunted growth.
· Antidepressants may be prescribed for adults.

ACTIVITY

Structure your child's activity to the extent possible.

DIET

Most medical research indicates that special diets benefit very few children. Many parents, however, report dramatic changes in behavior after this treatment. This change may result from the extra attention the child receives with preparation of special meals. Discuss any special diets with your child's health care provider.

 ## NOTIFY OUR OFFICE IF

· You believe your child or a family member has symptoms of attention deficit hyperactivity disorder.
· Symptoms become worse after treatment is started.
· New, unexplained symptoms develop. Drugs used in treatment may produce side effects.

Special notes:

_____

_____

_____

More notes on the back of this page ☐

AUTISM

 BASIC INFORMATION

DESCRIPTION

Autism is a disorder that involves the way a child develops. It is usually discovered by the time a child is age 2 and a half, but could be later. Parents may notice that an infant or child is not behaving, talking, playing, or learning new skills as expected for their age group. Asperger's syndrome is like autism, but without the disabilities. It can range from mild to severe.

FREQUENT SIGNS AND SYMPTOMS

• Does not talk or may talk using nonsense words. May use a sing-song voice and repeat what they hear. Unable to carry on a conversation.
• Does not respond to name and avoids eye contact.
• Is over active. Wants to play alone.
• Repeats the same movements over and over such as rocking and flapping or twisting hands.
• Has special routines and does not like change.
• Does not want to be touched, such as being cuddled.
• May injure self by head-banging or biting.
• Is bothered by noises.
• Overly interested in lights or moving objects.

CAUSES

• Unknown. Research continues in hopes of finding the cause. It is known that parents do not cause autism.
• There is no scientific proof to link childhood immunizations to autism.

RISK INCREASES WITH

Unknown. It does affect boys more than girls.

PREVENTIVE MEASURES

None known. Autism cannot currently be detected at birth or through any prenatal tests.

EXPECTED OUTCOMES

• The future is unknown for most autistic children. A child may be mentally retarded, have normal intelligence, or even have a genius-like ability. As they get older, their symptoms may improve, stay about the same, or worsen. Some children will need supervision for life. Some may be able to live independently.

POSSIBLE COMPLICATIONS

• Parents of an autistic child have an increased risk of having another child with the disorder.
• Stress for the family raising an autistic child.
• Autistic children are at a higher risk for seizures.

 DIAGNOSIS & TREATMENT

GENERAL MEASURES

• Diagnosis is difficult, as the signs and symptoms may appear to be caused by another disorder or problem.

There is no specific test for autism. Your health care provider (usually a mental health professional) will perform an exam of your child and ask you about your child's behavior and other signs or symptoms you may have observed. Tests for speech and other skills may be done to see how your child is developing compared to normal levels for their age group.
• Treatment for autism should be started as soon as a child is diagnosed. Speech and behavior therapy and social skills training will help children with autism.
• There is no cure for autism. Treatments can help with many of the symptoms. The treatment plan for each child will depend on how mild or severe their symptoms are. Some children may be able to attend regular public schools. Others may require a special classroom.
• The treatment steps take time and patience. Different treatment methods may need to be tried for a child.
• Parents should join an autism family support group.
• Counseling may help some parents cope with the stress involved with raising an autistic child.
• New treatments for autism are being studied and may be recommended for your child in the future. There are certain treatments that parents or others have tried and found to work for one or a few children. These treatments may or may not work for other autistic children. Always talk to your child's health care provider before you try any new type of treatment.
• To learn more: Autism Society of America, 7910 Woodmount Avenue, Suite 300, Bethesda, MD 20814-3015; (800) 328-8476; www.autism-society.org.

MEDICATIONS

Medicine is usually not needed for this disorder. A drug may be prescribed to help control symptoms that could be a danger to your child, such as self-injury.

ACTIVITY

Help your child to stay as physically active as possible.

DIET

Special diets will not improve the symptoms of autism.

 NOTIFY OUR OFFICE IF

• Your child is not developing as expected for their age.
• After diagnosis, your child develops new symptoms or other symptoms worsen, despite treatment.

Special notes:

_____

_____

_____

More notes on the back of this page ☐

BACK PAIN, LOW

BASIC INFORMATION

DESCRIPTION
Pain in the lower back usually caused by muscle strain. It may also include sciatica (pain that radiates from the back to the buttock and down into the leg). Onset of pain may be immediate or occur some hours after an activity or an injury. The symptoms occur in a cycle, starting with a muscle spasm, the spasm then causes pain, and the pain results in additional muscle spasm.

FREQUENT SIGNS AND SYMPTOMS
Pain and stiffness. It may be ongoing, or only occur when you are in certain positions. The pain may get worse by coughing, sneezing, bending, or twisting.

CAUSES
· Strain or sprain. Muscles, tendons, ligaments of the low back become stretched or torn.
· Bone and joint conditions of the back. These include arthritis, osteoporosis, spinal nerve irritation or inflammation, disk problems, infections, weaker and thinner bones from aging, and others.
· Injury or a fracture.
· Congenital problem (something you were born with).
· Pregnancy, certain illnesses, or infections.

RISK INCREASES WITH
· Exertion or lifting; a severe blow, or a fall.
· Jobs that require a lot of sitting.
· Aging. After age 20, bones start to lose their strength.
· Gardening and other yard work.
· Sports and exercise activities.
· Driving for long periods of time.
· Overweight.
· Smoking.
· Poor body mechanics and poor posture.

PREVENTIVE MEASURES
· Being in good physical condition.
· Exercises to strengthen lower back muscles.
· Learn how to lift heavy objects.
· Use good posture when sitting and standing.
· Lose weight, if overweight.

EXPECTED OUTCOMES
Gradual recovery with time and treatment.

POSSIBLE COMPLICATIONS
Chronic low back pain.

DIAGNOSIS & TREATMENT

GENERAL MEASURES
· Your health care provider will do a physical exam and ask questions about your back pain symptoms. Tests may include blood studies, x-rays of the spine, and other imaging studies. These can help determine the specific cause of the back pain.
· Treatment will depend on the cause of the pain. Usually a combination of drugs and reduced activities for a short period of time is all that is needed.
· Recent medical studies indicate that staying more active is often better for back disorders than prolonged bed rest.
· An ice pack, cold massage, heating pad or hot water bottle applied to the area may help to reduce pain.
· Physical therapy may be prescribed.
· Massage may help. Be sure that the person performing the massage is well-trained, or the massage could cause more harm than help.
· Stop smoking. Find a plan that will help you quit.
· Other options are available depending on degree of injury, such as surgery for disk damage, electrical nerve stimulation, acupuncture, special shoes, etc.
· To learn more: National Institutes of Health, 800-352-9424; website: www.ninds.nih.gov/health_and_medical/pubs/back_pain.htm

MEDICATIONS
· Use mild pain drugs such as aspirin, ibuprofen, or acetaminophen.
· Stronger pain drugs, muscle relaxants and drugs to reduce inflammation may be prescribed.
· Note: Drugs do not hasten healing. They only help to reduce symptoms.

ACTIVITY
· Try to continue with daily schedules to the extent possible. Use care in resuming normal activities.
· Avoid strenuous activity for 6 weeks.
· After healing, an exercise program will help prevent re-injury.

DIET
No special diet. A weight-reduction diet is recommended if being overweight is a problem.

NOTIFY OUR OFFICE IF

· You or a family member has mild, low back pain that persists for 3 or 4 days after self-treatment.
· Back pain is severe or recurrent.
· New or unexplained symptoms develop. Drugs used in treatment may cause side effects.

Special notes:

_____

_____

_____

More notes on the back of this page ☐

BALANITIS

 ## BASIC INFORMATION

DESCRIPTION
Inflammation of the glans (head) of the penis and sometimes the foreskin as well. It is a common condition in males. It occurs more often in males who have a foreskin (have not been circumcised).

FREQUENT SIGNS AND SYMPTOMS
· Tenderness, redness, itching, and swelling of the head of the penis.
· Inflammation of the foreskin.
· Unable to retract foreskin (phimosis).
· Impotence.
· Discharge from the penis.
· Burning during urination (rare).

CAUSES
The inflammation is a reaction to infection (most common cause), injury, or irritation of the penis. Sometimes the cause is unknown.

RISK INCREASES WITH
· Diabetes.
· Poor hygiene.
· Allergy to chemicals in clothing, contraceptive cream, or condom latex.
· Reaction to certain drugs.
· Trauma or minor injury to the foreskin and penis.
· Presence of foreskin.
· Sexual partner affected by vaginitis (rare).
· Being very obese.

PREVENTIVE MEASURES
· Wash daily with soap and water and wash after sexual intercourse. Clean carefully under the foreskin.
· Control diabetes or other medical conditions.
· Weight loss for obese males.
· Use a latex condom during intercourse to help prevent some infections.

EXPECTED OUTCOMES
Usually curable in 1 to 2 weeks with treatment.

POSSIBLE COMPLICATIONS
· Chronic inflammation can cause:
  - Scarring and narrowing of the opening of the penis (urethral stricture).
  - Phimosis (difficult to retract the foreskin).
  - Paraphimosis (unable to replace the foreskin to cover the head of the penis).

 ## DIAGNOSIS & TREATMENT

GENERAL MEASURES
· Your health care provider can usually diagnose the disorder by an exam of the penis. A culture of the discharge from the penis may be done. Tests for other medical disorders such as diabetes may be done.
· Treatment usually involves drugs applied to the penis and practicing good hygiene.
· Use warm-water soaks to relieve pain or discomfort.
· A foreskin that cannot be retracted may be treated with topical steroid drugs, stretching techniques (done 2 to 3 weeks), or by a special slit made in the foreskin.
· Surgery may be recommended to circumcise the penis if balanitis recurs often or scar tissue develops.

MEDICATIONS
· Antibiotics to be applied to the penis are usually prescribed. Rarely, antibiotics to be taken by mouth may be prescribed.
· Steroid skin creams may be prescribed.
· Use acetaminophen or ibuprofen to relieve minor pain.

ACTIVITY
· Avoid sexual intercourse during treatment.
· Resume your normal activities when the infection is cured.

DIET
No special diet.

 ## NOTIFY OUR OFFICE IF

· You or a family member has symptoms of balanitis.
· Symptoms don't improve in 3 days, despite treatment.

Special notes:

_____

_____

_____

More notes on the back of this page ☐

BALDNESS, PATTERN

(Androgenetic Alopecia)

BASIC INFORMATION

DESCRIPTION

Gradual, painless hair loss that occurs in a certain pattern as a person ages. The medical term is androgenetic alopecia. The earlier the hair loss begins, the greater the eventual loss. Some persons have short periods of intense hair loss followed by long, stable periods. In men, hair loss appears as early as the teens; in women, it rarely appears before their 50's.

FREQUENT SIGNS AND SYMPTOMS

- In men, hair thins on top of the head and recedes in the temple and front areas.
- In women, hair tends to thin on top of the head.
- Both sexes may have scattered hair loss.

CAUSES

It is probably due to a combination of hormonal and genetic factors. Male hormones (most often, androgens) are an important factor in balding. Estrogen (a female hormone) may be protective in women, because hair loss rarely begins before menopause. Hair loss that occurs after illness, pregnancy, or as an adverse reaction to drugs is a different form of baldness. Normal everyday stress is not a cause of pattern baldness.

RISK INCREASES WITH

Family history of pattern baldness.

PREVENTIVE MEASURES

Some drug therapies have been shown to slow or reverse baldness to some degree in some men. Other medical treatments are undergoing study.

EXPECTED OUTCOMES

- There is no cure. Balding can range from partial loss to complete baldness.
- In most cases, men let the process run its course. Use of a hairpiece or hair transplant is acceptable to some. Drug therapy may help others.

POSSIBLE COMPLICATIONS

- There are no medical complications.
- Baldness can cause emotional distress, such as anxiety and a negative effect on self-image.

DIAGNOSIS & TREATMENT

GENERAL MEASURES

- There is usually no need for medical care. If you do have concerns about the hair loss, see your health care provider. If it is not a typical hair loss, medical tests may be done to see if there is another cause.
- If you are not comfortable with the hair loss, there are options that you can consider.
  - Wear a hairpiece (toupee or a wig) or get a hair weave (synthetic hair is sewn into existing hair). Be sure to use care in keeping your scalp clean under the hairpiece.
  - Have a hair-transplantation procedure or scalp-reduction surgery. Be sure to seek information about the risks and benefits before undergoing these procedures.
  - Use drug therapy.
- Be cautious about buying and using hair products that claim to thicken or strengthen hair. The often use oils or waxes to give an effect of thickening.

MEDICATIONS

- A nonprescription topical drug, minoxidil, seems to help hair growth in some patients. Its effectiveness varies greatly. If it helps you, you need to continue its use indefinitely to sustain hair growth.
- Finasteride is a drug taken by mouth that can be prescribed for hair loss in men. It is not approved for use in women as it may cause birth defects.

ACTIVITY

No limits.

DIET

No special diet.

NOTIFY OUR OFFICE IF

You or a family member has concerns about hair loss.

Special notes:

_____

_____

_____

More notes on the back of this page ☐

BAROTITIS MEDIA
(Barotrauma)

 BASIC INFORMATION

DESCRIPTION
Damage to the middle ear caused by pressure changes. It affects the middle ear and the eustachian tube (a tube from the ear to the back of the nose and throat).

FREQUENT SIGNS AND SYMPTOMS
- Hearing loss (to varying degrees).
- A plugged feeling in the ear.
- Mild to severe pain in the ears, or over the cheekbones and forehead.
- Dizziness.
- Ringing noises in the ear.
- Crying in infants or young children.

CAUSES
- Damage caused by sudden, increased pressure in the air around you. This occurs in the rapid descent of an airplane or while scuba diving. In these activities, air moves from passages in the nose into the middle ear to maintain equal pressure on both sides of the eardrum. If the tube leading from the nose to the ear doesn't function properly, pressure in the middle ear is less than the outside pressure. The negative pressure in the middle ear sucks the eardrum inward. Blood and mucus may appear later in the middle ear. This damage is more likely if you have a nose or throat infection when scuba diving or traveling by air.
- Injury to external or middle ear (boxing, water skiing, accidents, etc.).

RISK INCREASES WITH
- Recent lung, nose, or throat infection.
- Airplane flight.
- Scuba diving.
- Sky diving.
- High-altitude mountain climbers.
- High-impact sports.

PREVENTIVE MEASURES
- If possible, don't fly when you have a lung, nose, or throat infection. If you must fly anyway, use nonprescription decongestant tablets or sprays. Follow the package instructions.
- During air travel:
  - While taking off or landing, suck on hard candy or chew gum to cause frequent swallowing.
  - Take a moderate-size breath and hold your nose. Try to force air into the eustachian tube by gently puffing out the cheeks with the mouth closed. This is called the Valsalva maneuver.
  - Give an infant a bottle of water or juice while taking off or landing during airplane travel.

EXPECTED OUTCOMES
Most cases of barotitis media heal with self-care.

POSSIBLE COMPLICATIONS
- Permanent hearing loss.
- Ruptured eardrum.
- Middle ear infection.

 DIAGNOSIS & TREATMENT

GENERAL MEASURES
- In most cases, no treatment is necessary and symptoms disappear in hours or days.
- If fluid drains from the ear, place a small piece of cotton in the outer-ear canal to absorb it.
- See your health care provider if symptoms continue. An ear exam usually confirms the diagnosis.
- Rarely, surgery may be required to open the eardrum and release fluid trapped in the middle ear. A plastic tube may be placed in the eardrum to keep it open. The tube falls out on its own in 9 to 12 months.

MEDICATIONS
- For minor pain, you may use nonprescription decongestants and pain relievers, such as acetaminophen.
- Your health care provider may prescribe stronger decongestant or anti-inflammatory nasal sprays or tablets.
- Antibiotics, if infection is present.

ACTIVITY
Resume your normal activities as soon as symptoms improve.

DIET
No special diet.

 NOTIFY OUR OFFICE IF

- You or a family member has symptoms of barotitis media.
- The following occur during treatment: severe headache or other pain, fever and dizziness.
- New, unexplained symptoms develop. Drugs used in treatment may produce side effects.

Special notes:

_____

_____

_____

More notes on the back of this page ☐

BED-WETTING

(Enuresis)

BASIC INFORMATION

DESCRIPTION

Wetting the bed during sleep that occurs more often than once a month in girls over 5 and in boys over 6 years of age. It is more common in boys than in girls. The occurrence of bed-wetting in children is 15% at age 5, 10% at age 6, 7% at age 8, 3% at age 12 and 1% at age 18.

FREQUENT SIGNS AND SYMPTOMS

Bed-wetting at night (occasionally during the day). This is not usually a concern until a child is older than 6.

CAUSES

• In most cases, the cause of bed-wetting is unknown. Most children who wet the bed are quite healthy. The following are other possible causes:
  - Illness, such as diabetes or a urinary-tract infection.
  - A small or weak bladder that cannot hold one night's urine production.
  - Emotional problems caused by stress or separation from the mother.

RISK INCREASES WITH

• Diabetes.
• Urinary-tract infection.
• Family history of bed-wetting (44% chance if one parent was bed-wetter, 77% chance if both parents were bed-wetters).
• First-born child.

PREVENTIVE MEASURES

• No effective preventive methods are known.
• Show your child love, support, and understanding for this problem.

EXPECTED OUTCOMES

Bed-wetting may continue for several years. If there are no medical or emotional problems, children normally outgrow the bed-wetting problem. Consider that your child's bed-wetting means a delay in maturing that will resolve with time.

POSSIBLE COMPLICATIONS

• Psychological and emotional scars that may affect the child's personality for years.
• Urinary-tract infection.

DIAGNOSIS & TREATMENT

GENERAL MEASURES

• Talk to your child's health care provider about the bed-wetting problem. A physical exam will be done and questions asked about the symptoms. Medical tests are sometimes done to rule out infections and diabetes as causes.

• Follow any medical advice. Basic ideas are listed here.
• Prepare the bed and the child:
  - Protect the mattress with a heavy plastic cover.
  - Stop using diapers or plastic pants by age 4. They may make it easy for the child to keep on wetting.
  - Have the child change the sheet on the bed and do the laundry, if he or she is old enough.
• Don't give any liquids to the child for 2 to 3 hours prior to bedtime.
• Have the child urinate at bedtime. You can also wake the child at night to urinate, but this is hard on parents.
• Reward the child for staying dry with praise and hugs. Use gold stars or happy faces to mark dry nights on a calendar.
• Respond gently to accidents. Don't blame, nag, restrict, or punish the child who has wet the bed. This can cause him to give up or lead to other problems.
• Try alarms that are triggered by wetting. These may be used in undergarments, pajamas, or mattresses. They have a high success rate.

MEDICATIONS

The drug vasopressin may be recommended if other methods fail and the family favors medical treatment.

ACTIVITY

No limits.

DIET

No special diet. Encourage your child to drink as much fluid as possible during the day. Limit or discontinue any fluid intake during the 2 to 3 hours before bedtime.

NOTIFY OUR OFFICE IF

• You are concerned about your child's bed-wetting and your child is older than 6.
• The child dribbles urine, has a weak urinary stream, feels pain when urinating, or must strain to urinate.
• New, unexplained symptoms develop. Drugs used in treatment may produce side effects.

Special notes:

_____

_____

_____

More notes on the back of this page ☐

BELL'S PALSY

 ## BASIC INFORMATION

DESCRIPTION

A paralysis or weakness on one side of the face. The onset may be sudden, or may come on over several days. Bell's palsy involves a cranial nerve and the facial muscles that connect to the nerve.

FREQUENT SIGNS AND SYMPTOMS

· Sudden paralysis on one side of the face, including muscles to the eyelid.
· Pain behind the ear on the affected side.
· Flat, expressionless features on one side of the face.
· Distorted smiles and frowns; drooling.
· Changes in taste, saliva, or tear formation.

CAUSES

Unknown. The paralysis is probably caused by swelling of the facial nerve. The swelling may be caused by a viral infection of the facial nerve as it passes through the temporal bone of the skull.

RISK INCREASES WITH

· Common cold, flu, other respiratory infection.
· Pregnancy.
· Diabetes.

PREVENTIVE MEASURES

Cannot be prevented at present.

EXPECTED OUTCOMES

· Bell's palsy causes distress, but it is not dangerous. The amount of nerve damage determines the extent of recovery.
· Improvement is gradual. Recovery time varies, and sometimes requires many months.
· Patients with mild facial paralysis usually recover completely within several months. Those with more severe facial paralysis recover completely in 80% to 90% of cases.
· Surgery may help improve facial appearance and muscle function in patients who do not recover fully.

POSSIBLE COMPLICATIONS

· Eye irritation or injury, because the eye does not close properly and is exposed to dust. If unprotected, the eye may develop ulcers on the cornea.
· Tooth decay and gum disease, due to reduced saliva and difficulty in chewing.
· Emotional and self-esteem problems.

 ## DIAGNOSIS & TREATMENT

GENERAL MEASURES

· Your health care provider will do a physical exam of the affected area. Medical tests such as x-ray may be done to rule out other causes. A nerve study of the facial nerves may be done to determine the extent of nerve damage.
· If you have pain, apply heat to the area twice a day. Use a moist, warm towel and apply for 15 minutes. Cover or close the eye during heat treatments.
· If you cannot wink or close your eye well, you should buy a pair of wrap-around, plastic sports goggles. Wear them to protect your eye from dirt, dust, and dryness.
· At night, apply an eye patch to shut the lid so that the eye stays moist and protected. Sometimes, a patch will be necessary during the daytime.
· As muscle strength returns, use facial massage and exercises. Massage muscles of the forehead, cheek, lips and eyes using cream or oil. Exercise the weak muscles in front of a mirror. Open and close the eye; wink, smile and bare your teeth. Perform the massage and exercises for 15 to 20 minutes several times a day.
· Brush and floss teeth regularly.
· Surgery on the facial nerve may (rarely) be needed.

MEDICATIONS

· Your health care provider may prescribe eye drops for comfort and protection of the exposed eye.
· Cortisone drugs may be prescribed to reduce swelling and inflammation of the affected nerve.

ACTIVITY

Maintain your normal activities. Rest does not help Bell's palsy.

DIET

A soft diet is often necessary.

 ## NOTIFY OUR OFFICE IF

· You or a family member has symptoms of Bell's palsy.
· Eye becomes red or irritated, despite treatment.
· Drooling or pain worsens or fever occurs.
· New, unexplained symptoms develop. Drugs used in treatment may produce side effects.

Special notes:

_____

_____

_____

More notes on the back of this page ☐

BENIGN PAROXYSMAL POSITIONAL VERTIGO (BPPV)

 BASIC INFORMATION

DESCRIPTION

A common, inner ear disorder that causes dizziness or vertigo with certain movements of the head.
- Benign means "not very serious."
- Paroxysmal means "sudden and unpredictable in onset."
- Positional, because it comes about with a change in head position.
- Vertigo, causing a sense of the room-spinning or whirling.

FREQUENT SIGNS AND SYMPTOMS

- A sensation of dizziness or vertigo (spinning). Vertigo begins 5 to 10 seconds after the head moves and lasts less than a minute. Feeling off balance may last longer.
- Most often, only one ear is affected, so symptoms occur when the head is turned that way. Symptoms are brought on when getting out of bed, rolling over in bed, or when looking up for an object on a high shelf.
- Falling, or a feeling of falling.
- Feeling lightheaded or woozy.
- Visual blurring.
- Nausea and vomiting (sometimes).
- Diarrhea, faintness, changes in heart rate and blood pressure, fear, anxiety, or (less often) panic.
- It does not cause hearing loss or noises in the ears (tinnitus).

CAUSES

It is thought to be caused by small crystals of calcium carbonate (also called "ear rocks", otoconia or otoliths) in the ear. Sometimes, these crystals get stuck and do not move normally with changes in position. This disrupts the balance centers in the inner ear and brings on the symptoms. The crystals usually return to normal within several weeks, and no longer cause symptoms.

RISK INCREASES WITH

- Head injury.
- Degeneration of the vestibular system of the inner ear (usually in older people).
- Ear infection or disorder.
- Surgery.
- Central nervous system disease.

PREVENTIVE MEASURES

No specific preventive measures.

EXPECTED OUTCOMES

The condition heals on its own within several weeks. Treatment can hasten healing.

POSSIBLE COMPLICATIONS

BPPV symptoms may come and go, recur after treatment, or become chronic.

 DIAGNOSIS & TREATMENT

GENERAL MEASURES

- Your health care provider will do an exam of the ears and ask questions about your symptoms and activities. When BPPV occurs, there is an involuntary movement of the eyes, which is called nystagmus. To make the diagnosis, the patient's head is put into certain positions and the eye movements are observed. Medical tests may be done to confirm the diagnosis.
- Treatment may involve watchful waiting. No treatment is done at first, in order to see if the problem resolves.
- An office procedure may be done for treatment. It is performed by placing the patient's head in various positions. This will cause the crystals to loosen and return to normal movement. The procedure takes about 5 to 10 minutes. Frequently, only one office procedure is needed. It is painless and has few side effects if any. There may be mild vertigo for a few days afterwards.
- Self-treatment exercises may be recommended. These can be done if symptoms recur, or office procedure was not effective. Instructions will be given on proper techniques for the head maneuvers. They are then done at home several times a day, usually for 2 weeks.
- Rarely, when other treatment is not effective, patients with severe symptoms may require surgery.
- To learn more: Vestibular Disorders Association, PO Box 4467, Portland, OR 97208-4467; (800) 837-8428; website: www.vestibular.org.

MEDICATIONS

Usually not needed for this disorder. Drugs may be prescribed for specific symptoms, such as nausea.

ACTIVITY

Activities may be limited for 24 to 48 hours after the procedure is done. Specific instructions will be given.

DIET

No special diet.

 NOTIFY OUR OFFICE IF

- You or a family member has symptoms of benign paroxysmal positional vertigo.
- Symptoms recur after treatment.

Special notes:

_____

_____

_____

More notes on the back of this page ☐

BIPOLAR DISORDER
(Manic-Depressive Disorder)

BASIC INFORMATION

A condition in which a person has episodes of mania, or cycles of mania and depression. There is usually no relationship between the moods and what is happening in the person's life. Periods of highs can alternate with periods of deep depression. The high periods are called mania. Periods of normal behavior occur in between the mania and the depression. The normal behavior can last for a short time or for years.

FREQUENT SIGNS AND SYMPTOMS
Mania:
- Higher than normal energy levels. Person feels "high."
- Getting up earlier and earlier in the morning. Some people may not sleep at all for 3 to 4 days.
- Easily distracted and restless. Excited to start new projects, but then rarely finish.
- May go on spending sprees.
- May become sexually promiscuous.
- Often irritable. Often have attacks of rage.
- Speech becomes rapid. Speech may not make sense.
- May have very high opinion of one's abilities.
- May forget to eat. May lose weight. Can become exhausted.
- May have delusions of grandeur.

Depression:
- Becomes more and more withdrawn. Sleep may be disturbed. Late rising becomes a habit.
- May stay in one's room. May be afraid to face the world. Often lacks self-esteem.
- Self-neglect.
- Sex drive is lowered.
- Slow speech and movement.
- Imagined problems multiply.
- Worries about imagined illnesses.

CAUSES
There is no single cause. Genetics plays a part. Other factors may include changes in chemicals in the brain and environmental factors, such as stress.

RISK INCREASES WITH
Family history of bipolar disorder.

PREVENTIVE MEASURES
There are no known preventive measures.

EXPECTED OUTCOME
Long-term therapy can help reduce how often and how severe the episodes are.

POSSIBLE COMPLICATIONS
- Relapse, especially if medicine is stopped.
- Problems at work, school or home.
- Failure to get better.
- Alcohol or drug abuse.
- Suicide.

DIAGNOSIS & TREATMENT

GENERAL MEASURES
- Your health care provider will usually do a physical exam and ask questions about your symptoms and activities. Psychological testing may be done. Other medical tests are usually done to rule out infections or disorders that could be causing the symptoms.
- Treatment will depend on the specific symptoms. Follow your health care provider's instructions. Schedule regular office visits. Your health care provider will monitor the effectiveness of the treatment and watch for side effects.
- Hospital care may be required for severe symptoms. A stay at a mental health facility may be recommended.
- Do not stop taking your medicine when you feel better. This may cause a relapse.
- Education and counseling can help you, and your family, cope with the condition. Family members should learn to recognize signs of a coming episode.
- Electroconvulsive therapy (ECT) may be considered if other treatment steps are not successful.
- Seek support groups. Contact social agencies for help. Call a suicide prevention hotline if needed.
- To learn more: Depression and Bipolar Support Alliance, 730 N. Franklin St., Suite 501, Chicago, IL 60610; (800) 826-3632; website: www.dbsalliance.org.

MEDICATION
Drugs will be prescribed to help relieve symptoms of the depression and the manic episodes. Other drugs may be prescribed to help prevent mood swings. Changes in drugs or dosages may be needed at various times to manage the illness more effectively.

ACTIVITY
Maintain daily activities. Exercise on a regular basis.

DIET
Try to eat well even if you have little or no appetite.

NOTIFY OUR OFFICE IF

- You or a family member has symptoms of bipolar disorder.
- You feel suicidal or hopeless. Call 911 if needed.
- Any new symptoms develop that cause concern.

Special notes:

_____

_____

_____

More notes on the back of this page ☐

BLADDER INFECTION, FEMALE
(Cystitis in Women)

BASIC INFORMATION

DESCRIPTION
Inflammation of the urinary tract.

FREQUENT SIGNS AND SYMPTOMS
· Pressure, burning, or stinging during urination.
· Frequent urination, although the amount of urine may be small; increased urge to urinate.
· Sensation of incomplete bladder emptying.
· Pain in the abdomen over the bladder.
· Lower-back pain.
· Blood in the urine; bad-smelling urine.
· Low fever and, possibly, chills.
· Painful sexual intercourse.
· Lack of urinary control (sometimes).
· A need to urinate more often at night.

CAUSES
The inflammation is a reaction to infection (most commonly), injury, or irritation of the bladder lining. It can be brought on by a number of different factors. Sometimes the cause is unknown.

RISK INCREASES WITH
· Infection in other parts of the genitourinary system. Bacteria can reach the bladder from another part of the body through the bloodstream. Bacteria can enter the urinary tract from skin around the genital and anal area.
· Frequent or vigorous sexual activity.
· Pregnancy.
· Poor hygiene.
· Diabetes.
· Certain types of birth control. These can include a diaphragm that fits too-tightly, contraceptive foams or vaginal suppositories that irritate the urethra, or a condom that is not lubricated.
· Urinary tract problems (tumors, calculi, or strictures).
· Urethra (tube from the bladder to the outside) injury.
· Use of a urinary catheter to empty the bladder, such as during childbirth or surgery.
· Incomplete bladder emptying.

PREVENTIVE MEASURES
· Urinate within 15 minutes after intercourse.
· Drink plenty of water every day.
· Get medical care for urinary-tract infections.
· Don't douche, use feminine hygiene sprays, or deodorants. Avoid bubble baths.
· Clean the anal area after bowel movements. Wipe from the front to the rear, rather than rear to front.
· Wear underwear that has a cotton crotch.
· Avoid postponing urination. Be sure to completely empty the bladder with urination.
· In women with frequent recurrence of infection, antibiotics may be prescribed for use before sexual intercourse.

EXPECTED OUTCOME
· Curable in a few days to 2 weeks with treatment.
· Recurrence is common.

POSSIBLE COMPLICATIONS
Inadequate treatment can lead to chronic bladder infections, kidney infection, and (rarely) kidney failure.

DIAGNOSIS & TREATMENT

GENERAL MEASURES
· Your health care provider may do a physical exam. Medical tests will include a urine test.
· Treatment is usually with antibiotic drugs.
· Warm baths may help relieve discomfort.
· Pour a cup of warm water over genital area while urinating. It will help to relieve burning and stinging.

MEDICATION
· Antibiotics for bacterial infection will be prescribed. Antibiotics may reduce the effectiveness of some birth control pills. If you are using birth control pills, discuss this with your health care provider.
· Urinary analgesics may be prescribed for pain. If phenazopyridine (Pyridium) is prescribed, it will turn the urine color to bright orange.

ACTIVITY
Avoid sexual intercourse until you have been free of symptoms for 2 weeks to allow inflammation to heal.

DIET
· Drink plenty of water daily to flush the bladder.
· Avoid caffeine and alcohol during treatment.
· Drink cranberry juice to acidify urine. Some antibiotic drugs have increased effectiveness when the urine is more acidic.

NOTIFY OUR OFFICE IF

· You or a family member has symptoms of cystitis.
· Blood appears in the urine.
· Discomfort and other symptoms don't improve after you have taken the antibiotics for 48 hours.
· New, unexplained symptoms develop. Drugs used in treatment may produce side effects.
· Symptoms recur after treatment.

Special notes:

_____

_____

_____

More notes on the back of this page ☐

BLADDER INFECTION, MALE
(Cystitis in Men)

 BASIC INFORMATION

DESCRIPTION
Inflammation of the urinary bladder. It can occur at any age. After age 50, men are affected more often, due to prostate problems.

FREQUENT SIGNS AND SYMPTOMS
- Burning and stinging when you urinate.
- Urinating more often. The amount of urine may be small.
- Feeling like you need to go even when your bladder is empty.
- Pain in the pubic area.
- Discharge from the penis.
- Low back pain.
- Blood in the urine.
- Low fever.
- Urine that smells bad.
- Not being able to control urination.

CAUSES
Usually a bacterial infection. The infection may start in other parts of the genital or urinary system (such as the kidney or prostate). The bacteria may also enter the bladder from skin around the genitals and anus.

RISK INCREASES WITH
- Blockage in the urinary tract. This may be due to kidney stones or tumor.
- Enlarged prostate gland.
- Lack of circumcision (foreskin can harbor bacteria).
- Injury of the urethra (tube that carries urine from bladder).
- Use of a catheter to empty the bladder, such as following surgery.
- Defects in the urinary tract.
- Certain illnesses, such as diabetes.

PREVENTIVE MEASURES
- Drink at least 8 glasses of fluid a day.
- Use a latex condom during sex. This can help prevent the spread of any infection.
- Avoid the use of catheters, if possible.
- Urinate when you feel the urge, empty the bladder completely, and keep the genital area clean.
- Get medical care for any prostate infection.

EXPECTED OUTCOMES
- Usually curable with treatment.
- Complicated infections in males are sometimes more difficult to treat. The bacteria involved are often resistant to the commonly prescribed drugs.

POSSIBLE COMPLICATIONS
- Recurrent or chronic bladder infections.
- Kidney infection.

 DIAGNOSIS & TREATMENT

GENERAL MEASURES
- Your health care provider will usually do a physical exam and ask questions about your symptoms. Medical tests include urine studies. Additional tests may be done to rule out other disorders.
- Treatment is usually with drugs, or sometimes surgery if a physical defect is the cause.
- Warm baths may provide relief from symptoms.
- To learn more: National Kidney Foundation, 30 E. 33rd St., Suite 1100, New York, NY 10016; (800) 622-9010; website: www.kidney.org.

MEDICATIONS
- Drugs for bacterial infection are usually prescribed. To be sure of a cure, finish the entire prescribed dose even if symptoms improve. If infection recurs, drug therapy for 6 months to 2 years may be recommended.
- Drugs to relieve painful urination symptoms may be prescribed.

ACTIVITY
- Reduce activities as needed until symptoms improve.
- Avoid sexual intercourse until you have been free of symptoms for 2 weeks.

DIET
- Drink at least 8 glasses of fluid daily. Avoid citrus juice, caffeine, and alcohol. They can irritate the bladder.
- Drink cranberry juice if recommended by your health care provider.

 NOTIFY OUR OFFICE IF

- You or a family member has symptoms of a bladder infection.
- Fever develops.
- Blood appears in the urine.
- Symptoms don't improve in one week.
- New, unexplained symptoms develop. Drugs used in treatment may produce side effects.
- Symptoms return after treatment.

Special notes:

_____

_____

_____

More notes on the back of this page ☐

BLADDER TUMOR

 BASIC INFORMATION

DESCRIPTION

An abnormal tissue growth in the bladder. It may be cancerous or noncancerous. If the tumor is cancerous, it may spread to lymph nodes, bones, liver and/or lungs. The tumors are most common in people over age 50 and occur more often in men than women.

FREQUENT SIGNS AND SYMPTOMS

- There are often no symptoms in the early stages.
- Blood in the urine.
- Pain or burning when urinating.
- Needing to urinate more frequently. There may be only small amounts of urine passed.
- Fever.
- Unexplained weight loss.

CAUSES

Unknown in some cases. Exposure to cancer-causing substances in the environment may be the cause in some cases.

RISK INCREASES WITH

- Smoking.
- Family history of bladder tumors.
- Exposure to certain dyes or to chemicals used in the manufacture of rubber.

PREVENTIVE MEASURES

- Avoid exposure to chemical or environmental hazards. Improved methods of protecting workers from chemical hazards have lowered the number of bladder tumors. Regular screening of those who have been exposed in the past is also helpful.
- Don't smoke.

EXPECTED OUTCOMES

When diagnosed early, treatment can be successful. However, it is common for the tumors to return. Regular medical checkups are needed. If cancer has spread, the outcome will depend on many factors.

POSSIBLE COMPLICATIONS

- Spread of cancer to other places in the body.
- Emotional stress about changes in body image.
- Side effects of treatments such as extreme fatigue.
- Treatment can lead to infertility for men and women.

 DIAGNOSIS & TREATMENT

GENERAL MEASURES

- Your health care provider will do a physical exam and ask questions about your symptoms. Medical tests include urine studies. A lighted optical instrument (cystoscope) may be used to see inside the bladder. It can also be used to remove a small piece of tissue, or even a small tumor, for viewing under a microscope. X-ray, MRI, CT or other tests may be done to see if a cancerous tumor has spread (called staging).
- Treatment may include surgery, radiation, chemotherapy (anticancer drugs) and biologic therapy.
- Small tumors may be removed by fulguration. This involves burning off the tumor by high frequency electrical current passed through the cystoscope.
- Larger tumors are removed surgically. This may require removal of part or all of the bladder (cystectomy) and other nearby body organs that may be involved. Various options are available for creation of a new bladder or to divert the urine flow to an external device (ostomy bag) on the outside of the body.
- Radiation and biologic therapy (the body's immune system is used to fight cancer) may be recommended.
- Counseling is helpful in learning to cope with the changes in your body.
- To learn more: American Cancer Society, (800) ACS-2345; website: cancer.org or National Cancer Institute at (800)4-CANCER; website: www.nci.nih.gov.

MEDICATIONS

- Anticancer drugs may be prescribed that are taken by mouth or given through a vein (IV).
- Drugs may be placed inside the bladder (biologic therapy); then a person waits 2 to 3 hours before urinating.

ACTIVITY

Resume your normal activities once your health care provider gives approval. This includes sexual relations.

DIET

No special diet.

 NOTIFY OUR OFFICE IF

- You or a family member has symptoms of a bladder tumor.
- Prescribed drugs produce unexpected side effects.

Special notes:

_____

_____

_____

More notes on the back of this page ☐

BLASTOMYCOSIS

(North American Blastomycosis; Gilchrist's Disease)

 BASIC INFORMATION

DESCRIPTION

An infectious fungal disease that starts in the lungs. It can occasionally spread through the bloodstream to other body parts, especially the skin. Blastomycosis is not spread from person to person, but can be spread through bites from infected dogs. It can involve the lungs, mouth, skin (and tissue below the skin), and the prostate. Higher rates of the disease are found in states bordering the Mississippi and Ohio rivers.

FREQUENT SIGNS AND SYMPTOMS

- Symptoms may begin slowly or infection may be sudden.
- Cough, either wet or dry.
- Chest pain.
- Chills, fever, and sweats.
- Shortness of breath.
- Fatigue, loss of appetite.
- May have bumps or sores on the skin.

CAUSES

Infection with a fungus found in wood and soil. Skin lesions occur most commonly in gardeners or farmers, but the natural source of this fungus is not known.

RISK INCREASES WITH

- Gardening and farming, especially in southeastern states and the Mississippi River valley of the United States.
- Diabetes.
- Use of drugs that suppress the immune system.

PREVENTIVE MEASURES

Cannot be prevented at present.

EXPECTED OUTCOMES

This fungus can cause severe illness that may be fatal without treatment. With treatment, it is usually curable in several weeks.

POSSIBLE COMPLICATIONS

- Spread to other body parts, with serious illness and death. If the infection spreads, the following may appear:
  - Pain in long bones.
  - Skin lesions that begin as small, raised bumps or small, white blisters with pus. They spread slowly. When fully developed, the lesions become open sores with sloping, reddish-purple borders.
  - Swelling and painful, tender lumps in the scrotum.

 DIAGNOSIS & TREATMENT

GENERAL MEASURES

- Your health care provider will do a physical exam and ask questions about your symptoms. Medical tests may include blood tests; culture of the skin lesions, pus, saliva, or lung secretions; x-ray; and biopsy. Biopsy is when a small amount of tissue is removed for viewing under a microscope.
- Treatment is with drugs and other supportive care.
- A hospital stay is usually needed at start of treatment.
- Heat may be helpful for joint pain.
- Weigh yourself daily and keep a weight chart. An unexplained weight loss might indicate that the infection has spread.
- Keep follow-up appointments with your health care provider. It is important to monitor the treatment and watch for side effects or reactions from the medications.

MEDICATIONS

Drugs will be prescribed to kill the underlying fungus.

ACTIVITY

Rest in bed during the worst stage. Resume activities slowly as your strength returns.

DIET

No special diet.

 NOTIFY OUR OFFICE IF

- You or a family member has symptoms of blastomycosis.
- Any of the following occur during treatment:
  - Weight loss.
  - Fever.
  - Diarrhea that cannot be controlled with self-care.
  - Severe headache and stiff neck.
- New, unexplained symptoms develop. Drugs used in treatment may produce side effects.

Special notes:

_____

_____

_____

More notes on the back of this page ☐

50

BLEPHARITIS

BASIC INFORMATION

DESCRIPTION

Inflammation (redness and soreness) of the eyelid edges. It usually involves the eyelids and eyelashes. It can also include the glands that lubricate the lid, and the white area of the eye.

FREQUENT SIGNS AND SYMPTOMS

- Redness and greasy flakes on the eyelid edges.
- Small sores on the eyelid. Crusts may form on the edges of the eyelid.
- Discharge from the lids during sleep. Lids may be stuck together in the morning.
- A feeling that something is in the eye. This can cause itching, burning, redness, and swelling of the lid. May also have tearing and be sensitive to bright light.
- Eye may become irritated if flakes from the lid fall into the eye.
- Eyelashes that fall out.

CAUSES

- Seborrheic blepharitis is caused by a skin condition called seborrhea. It is similar to dandruff.
- Bacterial infection of the eyelash follicles and the glands that lubricate the eye. The infection cannot be spread from one person to another.
- Plugged glands on the eyelid.
- Allergies or lice in the eyelashes.

RISK INCREASES WITH

- Dermatitis (skin infection) of the scalp and other body parts.
- Acne rosacea.
- Exposure to allergens (substances that cause allergic reactions).
- Exposure to chemical or environmental irritants, such as smoke or smog.
- Work that keeps the hands dirty for most of the day.
- Elderly.

PREVENTIVE MEASURES

- Wash hands often, and dry them with clean towels.
- Keep face, eyelids, and scalp clean.
- Avoid places that have lots of dust or other irritating substances.
- Get treatment for any skin disorders.
- Control dandruff with anti-dandruff shampoos.

EXPECTED OUTCOMES

Symptoms can be improved with treatment. The condition is often chronic and the symptoms come and go. If treatment is stopped, it tends to recur. It is usually not a serious condition.

POSSIBLE COMPLICATIONS

- Styes or chalazia (blocked oil gland on the eyelid).
- Conjunctivitis (eye inflammation).
- Loss of eyelashes.
- Ulceration of the cornea (the covering of the eye).
- Scarred eyelids.

DIAGNOSIS & TREATMENT

GENERAL MEASURES

- Your health care provider can diagnose blepharitis by an exam of the affected eyelid area. Other medical tests are not usually needed.
- Treatment will be prescribed for any problem that is causing the disorder or any complications.
- Use warm-water soaks to reduce discomfort and speed healing. Apply soaks for 20 minutes, then rest at least 1 hour. Repeat as often as needed.
- Wash the eyelid edge and eyelashes twice a day. Use a baby shampoo diluted with some water, or a commercial eyelid cleanser. Use a washcloth wrapped around the index finger or cotton swabs. Don't rub too hard as it can lead to irritation. Rinse with warm water and then dry the area.
- Avoid use of eye makeup until symptoms improve. When used, be sure to remove it each night at bedtime.
- Ask your health care provider about using contact lenses while you have the symptoms.

MEDICATIONS

- Eye drops or ointment may be prescribed for use after the eyelid area is cleaned.
- Drugs to be taken by mouth may be prescribed in more severe cases.

ACTIVITY

No limits.

DIET

No special diet.

NOTIFY OUR OFFICE IF

- You or a family member has symptoms of blepharitis.
- You have pain in the eye(s).
- Your vision changes.
- Symptoms recur after treatment.

Special notes:

_____

_____

_____

More notes on the back of this page ☐

BOILS
(Furuncles)

 BASIC INFORMATION

DESCRIPTION

A painful, deep, bacterial infection of a hair follicle. Boils are common and somewhat contagious. They can occur anywhere on the skin, but most often appear on the neck, face, buttocks, and breasts. Carbuncles are clusters of boils that occur when the infection spreads through small tunnels underneath the skin.

FREQUENT SIGNS AND SYMPTOMS

• A domed nodule that is painful, tender, red, and has pus on the surface. Boils can appear suddenly and ripen in 24 hours.
• Fever (rarely).
• Swelling of the closest lymph glands.

CAUSES

Infection, usually from *Staphylococcus* bacteria, that begins in the hair follicle and gets into the skin's deeper layers.

RISK INCREASES WITH

• Poor general health.
• Diabetes.
• Other skin problems (such as acne or skin infection).
• Weak immune system due to illness or drugs.

PREVENTIVE MEASURES

• Keep the skin clean.
• If someone in the household has a boil, don't share towels, washcloths, or clothing with that person.
• If you have a chronic disease (such as diabetes), be sure to follow your medical regimen.

EXPECTED OUTCOMES

Without treatment, a boil will heal in 10 to 20 days. With treatment, the boil should heal in less time, symptoms will be less severe, and new boils should not appear. The pus that drains when a boil opens on its own may infect nearby skin, causing new boils.

POSSIBLE COMPLICATIONS

• The infection may enter the bloodstream and spread to other body parts.
• Scarring.
• Boils may recur.
• Family members may need treatment.

 DIAGNOSIS & TREATMENT

GENERAL MEASURES

• Your health care provider can diagnose boils by looking at the affected skin area. A medical study may be made of the material from the boil.
• Do not burst a boil as this may spread bacteria.
• Taking showers instead of baths reduces the chances of spreading infection.
• Relieve pain with gentle heat from warm-water soaks. Use 3 or 4 times daily for 20 minutes. Wash your hands carefully after touching the boil.
• Prevent the spread of boils by using clean towels only once or using paper towels and discarding them.
• Your health care provider's treatment may include incision and drainage of the boil.

MEDICATIONS

• Antibiotics may be prescribed if infection is severe.
• Don't use nonprescription antibiotic creams or ointments on the boil's surface. They do not work for boils.

ACTIVITY

Decrease activity until the boil heals. Avoid sweating and avoid contact sports (such as wrestling) while lesions are present.

DIET

No special diet.

 NOTIFY OUR OFFICE IF

• You or a family member has a boil.
• The following occur during treatment:
  - Symptoms don't improve in 3 to 4 days, despite treatment.
  - New boils appear.
  - Fever.
  - Other family members develop boils.
• New, unexplained symptoms develop. Drugs used in treatment may produce side effects.

Special notes:

_____

_____

_____

More notes on the back of this page ☐

BONE FRACTURE

 BASIC INFORMATION

DESCRIPTION
A break in a bone often caused by a fall. Different types of fractures can occur depending on the severity. A complete fracture means the bone is broken all the way through. An incomplete fracture means the bone is cracked. An open (or compound fracture) means the fractured bone sticks out through the skin.

FREQUENT SIGNS AND SYMPTOMS
- Pain, swelling, or tenderness near the fracture site.
- Paleness and deformity (sometimes).
- Bleeding or bruising at the site.
- Weakness.
- Cannot bear weight.
- Numbness, tingling, or paralysis below the fracture (rare; this is an emergency).

CAUSES
Injury.

RISK INCREASES WITH
- Activities that carry the risk of injury.
- Reckless behavior that increases the chance of an accident.
- Age. Older adults have bones that are more fragile and also tend to have more falls.
- Osteoporosis and osteopenia.
- Tumors of the bone or bone marrow.

PREVENTIVE MEASURES
- Don't drink alcohol or use mind-altering drugs and drive.
- Use your seat belt in cars.
- Wear protective gear for sports.
- If you have osteoporosis, adhere to your treatment program and avoid situations in which injury is likely.
- Maintain a safe home to prevent falls. No slippery rugs, slick floors, or loose stair railings. Provide mats in bathtubs.

EXPECTED OUTCOMES
- Usually curable with treatment.
- Healing time varies. Recovery is complete when there is no bone motion at the fracture site, and x-rays show complete healing.

POSSIBLE COMPLICATIONS
- Failure to heal (non-union).
- Shock from blood loss.
- Travel of a fat embolus (clump of fat cells) from the injury site to the lungs or brain.
- Obstruction of nearby arteries.

 DIAGNOSIS & TREATMENT

GENERAL MEASURES
- Call 911 for help. Give first-aid treatment for bleeding, cover any open wounds, and move the patient as little as possible. Try to immobilize the area. Don't try to set the bone. Arrange for transport to a hospital or emergency room.
- Your health care provider will do a physical exam of the injured area. X-rays will be done to confirm the bone fracture. In some cases, other tests are needed.
- Bone ends that have been displaced are maneuvered back into place (reduction).
- Most fractures require casts, splints, or a special brace for healing. Crutches or other aids may be used to walk.
- Hospital care may be needed for severe fractures.
- Surgery, if the fracture must be repaired with rods, plates or screws.
- Physical therapy to help in restoring full function to the injured area.

MEDICATIONS
Pain relievers and muscle relaxants, if needed.

ACTIVITY
- Immobility of a bone for a long period of time can cause loss of muscle mass, stiffness in nearby joints, and edema (excess fluid in the tissues). Begin to use the affected part as soon as is safely possible.
- Physical therapy may be prescribed to maintain flexibility of the joint and provide strength to the muscles.
- Resume normal activities as soon as symptoms improve and your health care provider advises you to.

DIET
No special diet. Take vitamin C and zinc supplements to promote bone healing.

 NOTIFY OUR OFFICE IF

- You have symptoms of a bone fracture.
- The following occur after treatment:
  - Swelling above or below the fracture site.
  - Severe, persistent pain.
  - Blue or gray skin below fracture site (such as in the fingernails), or numbness or loss of feeling below the fracture site.

Special notes:

_____

_____

_____

More notes on the back of this page ☐

BOTULISM

 BASIC INFORMATION

DESCRIPTION

· Food-borne botulism is a serious form of food poisoning that is usually caused by eating food contaminated with a toxin. The toxin affects both the central nervous system and the muscular system. The symptoms usually appear suddenly 18 to 36 hours (but the range can be anywhere from 2 hours to 1 week) after eating contaminated food. The disorder can affect all ages.

· Infant botulism is a special type that occurs in children less than 12 months of age.

· Wound botulism occurs when the toxin in a wound spreads to other body parts.

· Adult intestinal colonization botulism occurs in older children and adults with colitis who have had recent bowel surgery or have other intestinal conditions.

FREQUENT SIGNS AND SYMPTOMS

· Blurred or double vision and drooping eyelids.
· Dry mouth.
· Slurred speech.
· Trouble swallowing.
· Vomiting and diarrhea.
· Weakness of the arms and legs. Paralysis.
· No fever.
· No change in mental abilities.

The following symptoms appear in infants:

· Severe constipation.
· Feeble cry.
· Unable to suck.

CAUSES

· A bacteria germ, *Clostridium botulinum* (other types may, rarely, be the cause). The germ may be found in contaminated or incompletely cooked foods. It can also be found in improperly canned foods. The germ generates a strong poison that is absorbed from the digestive tract. The poison spreads to the central nervous system.

· Foods likely to cause botulism include home-canned vegetables and fruits. Also, fish, smoked meats, milk products, and undercooked sausage.

· Honey and corn syrup may cause botulism in infants.

· The bacteria may also contaminate a wound and produce the toxin.

RISK INCREASES WITH

· Infants.
· Home-canned foods.

PREVENTIVE MEASURES

· If a can of food is bulging, don't even open it. If the contents of a can have a strange color or odor, don't even taste the food. Throw it away (safely).

· Don't eat any foods that may not have been properly cooked or canned.

· Don't give infants under age 1 honey or corn syrup, not even a small taste.

· Get proper instructions about canning food.

EXPECTED OUTCOMES

With prompt treatment, the outlook is good.

POSSIBLE COMPLICATIONS

· Long-lasting weakness.
· Nervous system problems that can last up to a year.
· Lung infections, such as pneumonia.
· Respiratory failure caused by weak breathing muscles. It can lead to death.

 DIAGNOSIS & TREATMENT

GENERAL MEASURES

· Diagnosis and treatment involves emergency hospital care. Blood and stool studies can confirm the diagnosis.

· For food-borne infection, vomiting may be induced, enemas given, or a washing out (lavage) of the stomach may be done to help rid the body of the toxin.

· Wound care will be provided for infected wounds.

· Breathing support with a machine (ventilator) may be needed, along with other supportive-care measures.

· Fluids may be given through a vein (IV) or through a tube placed in the nose (nasogastric).

· Health care providers will report the disease to state or federal health authorities. They will arrange to remove any contaminated food from stores.

· If you suspect botulism, refrigerate some of the contaminated food for testing, if possible.

MEDICATIONS

A special drug (antitoxin) may be given by injection. It can prevent the symptoms from getting worse. It may be life-saving, but it has serious side effects.

ACTIVITY

Bed rest during treatment. Resume normal activities as your strength permits.

DIET

After treatment, no special diet is needed.

 NOTIFY OUR OFFICE IF

You or a family member has symptoms of botulism. Call 911 or an ambulance right away. This is an emergency!

Special notes:

_____

_____

_____

More notes on the back of this page ☐

BRAIN OR EPIDURAL ABSCESS

 BASIC INFORMATION

DESCRIPTION

A collection of pus caused by a bacterial infection in the brain. The infection can also be in the membranes that cover the brain and spinal cord. They can affect all ages and are more common in men than in women.

FREQUENT SIGNS AND SYMPTOMS

The following symptoms usually appear gradually over several hours. They resemble symptoms of a brain tumor or stroke:

- Headache, usually severe.
- Fever.
- Stiff neck.
- Confusion or delirium.
- Seizures (convulsions).
- Nausea and vomiting.
- Pain in the back. It may occur if the infection is in the covering of the spinal cord.
- One side of the body may feel numb or weak. The body may be paralyzed on one side.
- Unable to walk normally.
- Trouble speaking.

CAUSES

- An infection that spreads from another part of the head such as sinusitis or a middle ear infection.
- An infection due to a head injury or surgery.
- An infection that spreads through the blood from other infected organs. This includes the lungs, skin, heart valves, or dental infections.
- Infections such as fungal or protozoan, that occur in people with weak immune systems.

RISK INCREASES WITH

- Head injury.
- Chronic illness, such as diabetes.
- Recent infection (in the ears, nose, eyes, or face).
- Weak immune system due to illness or drugs.
- Drug abuse.
- Tongue piercing.

PREVENTIVE MEASURES

- None specific. To reduce risk factors:
  - Seek medical care for infections.
  - Wear protective headgear when you are involved in any activity that could lead to a head injury.

EXPECTED OUTCOMES

Can usually be cured with early diagnosis and treatment.

POSSIBLE COMPLICATIONS

- Seizures, coma, and death (without treatment).
- Rupture of the abscess.
- Brain hemorrhage.

 DIAGNOSIS & TREATMENT

GENERAL MEASURES

- Emergency hospital care is needed.
- Your health care provider will do a physical exam and ask questions about your symptoms and activities. Medical tests may include blood tests, CT, and MRI.
- Medical or surgical treatment will depend on the location of the infection. Usually, surgery is needed to drain the infected area. Drugs will be given for the infection.
- Breathing support with a machine (ventilator) may be needed, along with other supportive-care measures. Fluids may be given through a vein (IV).

MEDICATIONS

- Antibiotic drugs will be given for the infection. They may be continued for several weeks.
- Drugs to prevent seizures may be prescribed.
- Following surgery, you may be given drugs to reduce swelling.

ACTIVITY

While in the hospital, you will need bed rest. After a 2 to 3 week recovery, you should be as active as your strength and feeling of well-being allow.

DIET

While you are in the hospital, essential fluids may be given through a tube in a vein. Following treatment, eat a normal, well-balanced diet.

 NOTIFY OUR OFFICE IF

- You or a family member has any symptoms of a brain abscess.
- New, unexplained symptoms develop. Drugs used in treatment may produce side effects.

Special notes:

_____

_____

_____

More notes on the back of this page ☐

BRAIN TUMOR

 ## BASIC INFORMATION

DESCRIPTION
Abnormal cell growth in the brain. The growth may be benign (noncancerous) or malignant (cancerous). The symptoms can be caused by pressure, as the tumor gets larger, or can be caused by the location, size, and type of tumor. Brain tumors can affect any age group.

FREQUENT SIGNS AND SYMPTOMS
- Headache that is worse when lying down.
- Seizures (convulsions).
- Memory loss, confusion, and loss of concentration.
- Personality and behavior changes.
- Vomiting or nausea.
- Problems with vision. This includes double vision.
- Weakness on one side of the body.
- Lack of balance and dizziness.
- Loss of sense of smell and hearing.

CAUSES
Exact cause is unknown. There are genetic factors and environmental factors involved. Some tumors begin in the brain and are called primary. Other brain tumors are called secondary. They have spread (metastasize) from other cancers in the body. These includes cancers of the breast, lungs, colon, or skin (melanoma).

RISK INCREASES WITH
- Unknown for most brain tumors.
- Radiation to the head for other cancer treatment.
- Rarely, certain types of tumors run in families.

PREVENTIVE MEASURES
No specific preventive measures are known.

EXPECTED OUTCOMES
The outcome depends on several factors. These include type of tumor, its size, location, spread of tumor, other cancer in the body, age and health of the patient. and the patient's response to treatment.

POSSIBLE COMPLICATIONS
- Long-term physical and mental side effects. They may be due to the effect of the tumor or to treatment.
- Tumor may recur after treatment.
- Death.

 ## DIAGNOSIS & TREATMENT

GENERAL MEASURES
- Your health care provider will do a physical exam and ask questions about your symptoms and activities. A variety of medical tests will be done to diagnose the tumor and to see if it has spread to or from other places in the body (called staging).
- The treatment plan will be determined by the stage, size, location and type of tumor, and your age and health status. Because, there are over 120 different types of brain tumors, treatment needs to be specific for each person. Treatment can include surgery, radiation, chemotherapy (anticancer drugs) and immunotherapy.
- Surgery is often needed. It may involve removal of all or part of the tumor and nearby tissue.
- Radiation may be used for certain stages of the tumor. It is normally not used for children under age 3.
- Immunotherapy uses the body's immune system to help fight the cancer.
- Treatment may involve steps to relieve symptoms and make you comfortable, rather than treating the tumor.
- To learn more: American Cancer Society, (800) ACS-2345; website: www.cancer.org or National Cancer Institute, (800) 4-CANCER; website: www.nci.nih.gov.

MEDICATIONS
Your health care provider may prescribe:
- Drugs to reduce swelling of the brain tissue.
- Drugs to control seizures.
- Pain relievers.
- Drugs that kill cancer cells (chemotherapy).

ACTIVITY
Stay as active as your strength allows.

DIET
Eat a normal, well-balanced diet. You may need to take vitamins and minerals if you cannot eat normally.

 ## NOTIFY OUR OFFICE IF

- You or a family member has symptoms of a brain tumor.
- New, unexplained symptoms occur during treatment.

Special notes:

_____

_____

_____

More notes on the back of this page ☐

BREAST ABSCESS

 ## BASIC INFORMATION

DESCRIPTION
An infected area of breast tissue that becomes filled with pus when the body fights the infection. It involves breast tissue, nipple(s), milk glands, and milk ducts. They almost always occur in a breast-feeding woman.

FREQUENT SIGNS AND SYMPTOMS
- Breast pain.
- Breast is tender, red or hard.
- Fever and chills.
- Feeling ill.
- Tenderness in the area under the arm.

CAUSES
Bacteria that enter the breast through the nipple. This can happen if a nipple gets dry and cracked from breast-feeding.

RISK INCREASES WITH
- Breast infection, such as mastitis.
- Pelvic infection after delivery of a baby.
- Previous breast abscess.
- Diabetes.
- Rheumatoid arthritis.
- Use of steroid drugs.
- Heavy cigarette smoking. This is also a risk factor for women who not breast-feeding.
- Lumpectomy with radiation.
- Some breast implants.

PREVENTIVE MEASURES
- Clean the nipples and breasts carefully, before and after nursing.
- Lubricate the nipples after nursing. Use vitamin A & D ointment or an other topical drug if recommended.
- Avoid clothing that irritates the breasts.
- Don't allow a nursing infant to chew nipples.

EXPECTED OUTCOMES
- Usually curable in 8 to 10 days with treatment. Draining the abscess is sometimes needed to speed healing.
- It is rarely required for a patient to stop breast-feeding, even with severe infection. Certain antibiotics and pain relievers will require that breast-feeding be stopped for a short period of time. It will then be necessary to pump the breasts.

POSSIBLE COMPLICATIONS
An abnormal opening (fistula) may develop between the breast and the outside of the body.

 ## DIAGNOSIS & TREATMENT

GENERAL MEASURES
- Your health care provider will do a physical exam of the affected area. This is often all that is needed for diagnosis. Medical tests such as a culture of the pus and ultrasound may be done.
- The abscess may need to be drained. Draining the abscess may be done with a needle inserted into the abscess or with a small incision. This will reduce the pain and help clear up the infection.
- You may or may not be able to keep breast-feeding with the affected breast. Your health care provider will help determine if this is possible. If you can't breast-feed, use a breast pump to remove milk from the infected breast until you can start nursing again on that side.
- Use a warm, moist compress on the breast to relieve pain, hasten healing, and help the flow of milk.

MEDICATIONS
Drugs for pain or antibiotics for infection may be prescribed.

ACTIVITY
After treatment, resume normal activity as soon as symptoms improve.

DIET
No special diet.

 ## NOTIFY OUR OFFICE IF

- You or a family member has symptoms of a breast abscess.
- Any of the following occur during treatment:
  - Fever.
  - Pain becomes more severe.
  - Infection seems to be spreading, despite treatment.
  - Symptoms don't improve in 72 hours.

Special notes:

_____

_____

_____

More notes on the back of this page ☐

BREAST CANCER

 ## BASIC INFORMATION

DESCRIPTION

A malignant growth of breast tissue. It is the most common form of cancer in women. Breast cancer is rare before age 30, and is most common after the age of 50. Men can develop breast cancer also.

FREQUENT SIGNS AND SYMPTOMS

- No symptoms in early stages. It may be detected by a mammogram or by feeling a breast lump.
- Swelling or lump in the breast.
- Vague discomfort in the breast without true pain.
- Inversion of the nipple.
- Distorted breast contour.
- Dimpled or pitted skin in the breast.
- Enlarged nodes under the arm (late stages).
- Bloody discharge from the nipple (rare).

CAUSES

Unknown.

RISK INCREASES WITH

- Women over 50.
- Women who have not had children or who conceived in the late fertile years.
- Family history of breast cancer (especially mother or sister).
- Benign tumors of the breast (fibrocystic disease).
- Early menstruation, late menopause, or first pregnancy after age 30.
- Previous breast cancer in one breast.
- Radiation exposure.
- Patients with endometrial or ovarian cancer.
- Studies of estrogen therapy are not conclusive regarding their role in increasing breast cancer risk.

PREVENTIVE MEASURES

- Monthly self-exam of breasts for signs of cancer.
- Obtain medical breast exams as recommended.
- Mammograms every 1 to 2 years starting at age 40 (or as recommended).
- Eat a well-balanced diet that is low in fat. Studies are unclear about a high-fat diet and breast cancer risk.
- Regular exercise helps reduce breast cancer risk.
- Breast-feeding for at least 6 months (a year is better for mother and baby) will reduce breast cancer risk.
- A drug, such as tamoxifen, may be prescribed for women at high risk for breast cancer.
- A woman with very high risk may choose to have the breasts removed to avoid breast cancer.

EXPECTED OUTCOMES

It is curable with early diagnosis and treatment.

POSSIBLE COMPLICATIONS

- Spread to vital organs if not treated early.
- Complications may occur from treatments.

 ## DIAGNOSIS & TREATMENT

GENERAL MEASURES

- Your health care provider will do a breast exam and ask questions about your symptoms. A number of medical tests will be done. The tests first help diagnose the cancer and then determine if it has spread (staging).
- Treatment varies and depends on location and size of tumor, any spread of the cancer, your health, age, and preferences. Treatment may include chemotherapy (anticancer drugs) and/or radiation therapy, surgery, and biologic therapy.
- Chemotherapy uses drugs and radiation therapy uses radiation to attack the cancer cells. Biologic therapy uses the body's immune system to fight cancer.
- Surgery may be recommended to remove the lump, breast, lymph glands, lymphatic channels, or muscles under the breast.
- The decision for treatment is very complex and often confusing. Be sure all options are explained and that you understand the risks and benefits of each.
- Counseling may help you cope with having cancer.
- To learn more: National Cancer Institute, (800) 422-6347; website: www.nci.nih.gov or Y-Me National Breast Cancer Organization hotline (800) 221-2141; website: www.y-me.org or American Cancer Society, (800) 227-2345; website: www.cancer.org.

MEDICATIONS

- For minor discomfort, use nonprescription drugs such as acetaminophen or ibuprofen.
- Anticancer drugs, hormones, drugs for biologic therapy, or cortisone drugs may be prescribed.

ACTIVITY

- Physical therapy after surgery may be prescribed.
- Start exercising after recovery. It improves survival.

DIET

Eat a well-balanced diet.

 ## NOTIFY OUR OFFICE IF

- You or a family member discovers a lump or other change in the breast.
- New symptoms or concerns develop during or after treatment.

Special notes:

_____

_____

_____

More notes on the back of this page ☐

BRONCHIECTASIS

 ## BASIC INFORMATION

DESCRIPTION

A rare lung disease, in which the bronchial tubes become enlarged and distended (stretched). Pockets form where infections may develop. Bronchiectasis can affect all age groups.

FREQUENT SIGNS AND SYMPTOMS

- Frequent coughing. There may be foul-smelling mucus. The mucus may be green or yellow. Sometimes the mucus is flecked with blood.
- Chest pain and wheezing.
- Repeated lung infections.
- Shortness of breath.
- Feeling tired and weak.
- Weight loss.

CAUSES

The bronchial walls become damaged and weak usually as a result of infections. This damage may develop over years. The cilia (small hairs) that help keep the bronchial tubes clean are destroyed. This allows dust, bacteria and mucus to accumulate.

RISK INCREASES WITH

- Repeated lung infections such as pneumonia.
- Chronic bronchitis.
- Inhaling a foreign object (such as a peanut).
- Tuberculosis, lung cancer, or lung abscess.
- Cystic fibrosis.
- Family history of lung disease.
- Cigarette smoking.
- Weak immune system due to illness or drugs.

PREVENTIVE MEASURES

- None specific. Avoid risk factors where possible:
  - Don't smoke.
  - Obtain medical care for lung infections.
  - Prompt removal of any foreign body that has entered the lungs.
  - Get vaccines for flu and pneumonia.

EXPECTED OUTCOMES

With treatment, many patients can lead nearly normal lives without major problems.

POSSIBLE COMPLICATIONS

- Chronic obstructive pulmonary disease.
- Repeated pneumonia or other infections.
- Cor pulmonale (heart disorder due to lung disease).
- Hospital care and breathing support may be needed for complications.

 ## DIAGNOSIS & TREATMENT

GENERAL MEASURES

- Your health care provider will do a physical exam and ask questions about your symptoms. Medical tests may include blood or sputum (material coughed up from the lung) tests, CT, x-ray, bronchoscopy (looking in the airways with a lighted tube), and pulmonary function tests.
- Treatment includes postural drainage to remove lung secretions, drugs (as needed), treatment for underlying disorder (such as cystic fibrosis), and lifestyle changes.
- Postural drainage involves ridding the lungs of the secretions. You will be taught the proper technique. It is usually done by lying on a bed and hanging your head over the side with the affected lung uppermost. Clapping the chest can help mucus drain. A family member can do this by hand or a mechanical device can be used. This routine is done 1 to 3 times a day.
- Quit smoking. Find a way to stop that works for you.
- Surgery to remove areas of damaged lung tissue may be recommended if other treatments are not effective.
- To learn more: American Lung Association, 61 Broadway, 6th Floor, New York, NY 10006, (800) 586-4872; website: www.lungusa.org.

MEDICATIONS

Your health care provider may prescribe:
- Antibiotic drugs for infections.
- Inhaled beta-agonists to assist breathing.
- Drugs, such as guaifenesin, to loosen mucus in the lungs.
- Drugs to treat any underlying disorder.

ACTIVITY

Remain as active as possible.

DIET

Drink at least 8 glasses of fluid a day.

 ## NOTIFY OUR OFFICE IF

- You or a family member has signs of bronchiectasis.
- Symptoms of lung infection develop or fever occurs.
- Sputum contains blood, changes color, or thickens.
- Chest pain increases or you become short of breath.

Special notes:

_____

_____

_____

More notes on the back of this page ☐

BRONCHIOLITIS

 BASIC INFORMATION

DESCRIPTION

Inflammation and infection of the smallest airways (bronchioles) of the respiratory tract. These airways normally carry air from the large bronchial tubes to tiny air sacs in the lungs. Bronchiolitis mainly affects infants and young children. Boys are affected more often than girls.

FREQUENT SIGNS AND SYMPTOMS

- Often there is a mild common cold and cough before symptoms of bronchiolitis appear.
- Sudden trouble with breathing and wheezing.
- Rapid, shallow breathing.
- Chest and stomach are pulled in and out in seesaw movements with breathing.
- Fever may occur.
- Dehydration.
- Blue skin or nails in severe cases.

CAUSES

Usually a viral infection. Respiratory syncytial virus (RSV) is the most common infection. Other viral infections may sometimes be the cause. Germs are spread by sneezing, coughing, or by contact of hands to nose, mouth, or eyes. Symptoms start 2 to 5 days after the exposure.

RISK INCREASES WITH

- Young children (usually under age 2).
- Winter and early spring seasons.
- Daycare centers.
- Crowded living conditions.
- Exposure to cigarette smoke.
- Children who were born premature, had low birth weight, were born with health problems (neurologic, heart, or lung), or have developed a lung disorder.

PREVENTIVE MEASURES

- No specific preventive measures.
- Wash hands carefully to prevent spread of any germs.
- Avoid exposure to infected persons.
- Don't allow any smoking around a baby or child.
- Children at risk for complications of RSV infections may be given therapy to prevent the infection.

EXPECTED OUTCOMES

The disorder usually heals on its own. Mild cases may last for one or two days. Other cases may take 5 to 12 days for recovery. A few children who have other health problems are more at risk for complications.

POSSIBLE COMPLICATIONS

- Respiratory failure.
- Chronic lung disease.
- Heart disorders.
- Bronchiolitis obliterans (collapse of part of the lung).
- Other infections.

 DIAGNOSIS & TREATMENT

GENERAL MEASURES

- Your health care provider will do a physical exam and ask questions about the symptoms and activities. Medical tests are usually not needed, but may be done to confirm the diagnosis.
- There is no specific treatment for this disorder. Mild cases may be treated at home. Extra rest and drinking plenty of fluids is usually all that is needed.
- Use an ultrasonic, cool-mist humidifier if recommended by your health care provider. Clean the humidifier daily.
- A blocked-up nose may be suctioned with a rubber suction device.
- If the symptoms are more severe, hospital care may be required. Oxygen may be provided through a facemask. Some patients require breathing support with a ventilator (a device to help the lungs). Treatment to help remove lung secretions may be needed.

MEDICATIONS

Hospital care may include drugs to help relieve breathing problems, treat infections, and to prevent complications.

ACTIVITY

Rest until symptoms have improved for 48 hours. Then gradually return to normal activities.

DIET

Offer the child clear fluids often. These include water, tea, or carbonated drinks. Also, lemonade, weak bouillon, fruit juice, or gelatin.

 NOTIFY OUR OFFICE IF

- You or a family member has symptoms of bronchiolitis.
- Cold symptoms become worse.
- Temperature rises to 101°F (38.3°C) or higher.
- Breathing becomes more difficult.
- A cough begins that produces colored mucus.
- The skin, lips, or nails turn bluish in color.
- The child becomes drowsy and lacks energy.

Special notes:

_____

_____

_____

More notes on the back of this page ☐

BRONCHITIS, ACUTE

 BASIC INFORMATION

DESCRIPTION
Inflammation (swelling) of the mucous lining of the bronchi (main air passages) to the lungs. Symptoms of acute bronchitis may start suddenly and last just a few days. It is a common disorder affecting all age groups. Chronic bronchitis persists over a long period of time.

FREQUENT SIGNS AND SYMPTOMS
· A common cold or sore throat may occur prior to bronchitis.
· Cough that produces little or no mucus at first. Later, mucus may be produced.
· Low fever (usually less than 101°F/38.3°C).
· Burning feeling in chest. Feeling of pressure behind the breastbone.
· Wheezing. There may also be trouble breathing.
· Feeling tired.

CAUSES
· Viral infection usually. Most cases begin with a cold virus in the nose and throat. The virus then spreads to the lungs. A bacterial infection may also cause bronchitis. Infection causes the mucous membranes to become inflamed and produce thick, sticky mucus. This narrows the airways and causes the symptoms.
· Irritative bronchitis is caused by allergies, chemicals, and other irritants in the environment.

RISK INCREASES WITH
· Chronic lung disease or chronic sinusitis.
· Smoking or second hand smoke.
· Poor nutrition.
· Allergies.
· Areas with polluted air.
· Elderly and very young age groups.

PREVENTIVE MEASURES
· Avoid close contact with people who have a cold or the flu. Wash hands often to avoid germs.
· Don't smoke.
· If you work around chemicals, dust or other lung irritants, wear a special facemask.

EXPECTED OUTCOMES
Usually curable in 1 week. Cases with complications are usually curable in 2 weeks, with drug therapy. In some people, the cough may continue for several weeks, even after the infection is gone.

POSSIBLE COMPLICATIONS
· Pneumonia.
· Chronic bronchitis.
· Bronchiectasis (bronchial tubes become blocked).
· Pleurisy (swelling of the lining of the lungs).

 DIAGNOSIS & TREATMENT

GENERAL MEASURES
· Your health care provider will do a physical exam and use a stethoscope to listen to your lungs. Medical tests are usually not needed. A chest x-ray may be done if symptoms are more severe.
· Treatment is directed toward relieving the symptoms. Get extra rest and increase fluid intake.
· If you are a smoker, don't smoke during your illness. Smoking makes it harder to recover. Nonsmokers should avoid secondhand smoke.
· Increase air moisture. Take warm showers. Use a cool-mist humidifier if recommended by your health care provider. Clean the humidifier daily.
· To learn more: American Lung Association, 61 Broadway, 6th Floor, New York, NY 10006, (800) 586-4872; website: www.lungusa.org.

MEDICATIONS
· Use acetaminophen for fever and minor pain.
· Nonprescription cough suppressants (to ease coughing) or expectorants (to thin mucus) may be used to relieve symptoms. The mucus should be coughed up, so use cough suppressants with caution.
· Antibiotics may be prescribed for bacterial infection. They will not help a viral infection.
· Drugs may be prescribed for specific symptoms.

ACTIVITY
Get extra rest until symptoms improve. Then return to normal activities, as you feel better.

DIET
No special diet. Drink at least 8 to 10 glasses of fluid each day. This helps makes mucus easier to cough up.

 NOTIFY OUR OFFICE IF

· You or a family member has symptoms of acute bronchitis.
· You develop a high fever and chills.
· You have chest pain.
· You cough up mucus that is thick, colored, or has blood in it.
· You feel short of breath, even when resting.

Special notes:

_____

_____

_____

More notes on the back of this page ☐

BRONCHITIS, CHRONIC

BASIC INFORMATION

DESCRIPTION
Inflammation (swelling) of the mucous lining of the bronchi (main air passages) to the lungs. It often occurs along with emphysema (damaged air sacs in the lungs). Chronic bronchitis usually affects adults over age 45 and women more than men.

FREQUENT SIGNS AND SYMPTOMS
Symptoms don't start suddenly. They develop over time. They include: presence of a mucus-producing cough most days of the month, 3 months of the year for 2 consecutive years.

CAUSES
Repeated irritation or infection in the bronchial tubes. The tubes begin to thicken and become more narrow. They begin to lose their elasticity. The main cause is smoking.

RISK INCREASES WITH
- Smoking.
- History of lung disorders.
- Family history of lung disease.
- Exposure to air pollutants or cigarette smoke.
- Work that involves exposure to high levels of dust and irritating fumes.

PREVENTIVE MEASURES
- Don't smoke. This is the best prevention.
- Avoid fumes in the environment.
- Get prompt medical care for lung infections.

EXPECTED OUTCOMES
There is no cure for this disorder. Treatment can help relieve the symptoms and slow the progress of the disease. Smokers must stop smoking.

POSSIBLE COMPLICATIONS
- Pneumonia.
- Chronic obstructive pulmonary disease (COPD).
- Cor pulmonale (heart disorder).

DIAGNOSIS & TREATMENT

GENERAL MEASURES
- Your health care provider will do a physical exam and ask questions about your symptoms, smoking habits and exposure to pollutants or irritants. Many lung and heart disorders cause symptoms identical to those of chronic bronchitis. Medical tests will be used to make a diagnosis.
- Treatment can help relieve symptoms and help prevent complications. A treatment plan will be developed based on your individual needs.

- Stop smoking. Find a way to quit that works for you.
- Avoid areas with air pollution, dust, or fumes. Consider changing jobs if you need to.
- Install air-conditioning with a filter and humidity control in your home.
- Avoid shouting, laughing loudly, and crying if these make you cough.
- Get a pneumococcal vaccine and annual flu vaccine.
- Your health care provider can teach you exercises to help improve your breathing.
- Lung transplantation may be recommended for advanced cases.
- To learn more: American Lung Association, 61 Broadway, 6th Floor, New York, NY 10006, (800) 586-4872; website: www.lungusa.org.

MEDICATIONS
- Don't take drugs to lessen your cough. They can make this condition worse.
- Antibiotics for infection may be prescribed.
- Oral or inhaled bronchodilator drugs may be prescribed to relax and open the airways in the lungs.
- Oral or inhaled steroids may be prescribed to reduce inflammation.
- Drugs to thin the mucous may be prescribed.

ACTIVITY
- Regular exercise is important. Long periods of being inactive can add to your disability.
- Avoid sudden temperature changes. Avoid cold, wet weather.
- Be careful when exercising or working. Work at a pace that does not make you cough.

DIET
No special diet. Drink plenty of fluids. This can help thin the mucus produced by your lungs.

NOTIFY OUR OFFICE IF

- You or a family member has symptoms of chronic bronchitis.
- You have a fever or vomiting.
- Mucus gets thicker or has blood in it.
- Your chest pain gets worse.
- You feel short of breath even when you are resting or not coughing.

Special notes:

_____

_____

_____

More notes on the back of this page ☐

BRUCELLOSIS
(Undulant Fever; Bang's Disease)

 BASIC INFORMATION

DESCRIPTION
A rare infection passed to humans from infected cows, pigs, sheep, or goats. It cannot be passed from person to person. It affects the bone marrow, lymph glands, liver, and spleen. It is more common in men between ages 20 and 60. The infection may be acute (short lasting) or chronic (persisting over months or years).

FREQUENT SIGNS AND SYMPTOMS
- Sweating, chills, and fever (may come and go).
- Tiredness.
- Upset stomach.
- Tenderness along the spine.
- Headache.
- Muscle and joint aches.
- Constipation.
- Weight loss.
- Depression.
- In later stages of the infection, mental problems and seizures may occur.

CAUSES
Infection from a bacterium, which is passed to humans by ingesting infected food products, direct contact with an infected animal, or breathing in germs in the air. After a person is exposed, symptoms may develop in 1 to 8 weeks.

RISK INCREASES WITH
- Persons who work with animals. This includes farmers, ranchers, meat processors, and veterinarians.
- Travel to some foreign countries.
- Biological warfare.

PREVENTIVE MEASURES
- Don't drink milk from any source that has not been pasteurized.
- Protect yourself when working around animals. Use safety protection (gloves and mask) as needed.
- Farm animals should be immunized.

EXPECTED OUTCOMES
Can usually be cured in 3 to 4 weeks with treatment. Some muscle aches may continue for a period of time.

POSSIBLE COMPLICATIONS
- Endocarditis (heart inflammation).
- The infection may recur.

 DIAGNOSIS & TREATMENT

GENERAL MEASURES
- Your health care provider will do a physical exam and ask questions about your symptoms and activities. Be sure to discuss any contact with animals you have had in the last few months. Medical tests may include studies of blood, urine, and spinal fluid. X-ray, CT, heart tests, and others may be done depending on the symptoms.
- Treatment usually consists of drugs for infection and getting extra rest. If symptoms are more severe, hospital care may be needed.
- It usually is not necessary to keep the ill person away from others.
- Avoid contact with animals that may be the source of the infection.
- Family members who may have been exposed to the same infected food products should see their health care provider.

MEDICATIONS
- Antibiotic drugs will be prescribed for the infection. You usually need to take them for several weeks.
- Drugs to reduce swelling in severe cases and for relief of muscle pain may be prescribed.

ACTIVITY
Get extra rest until fever and other symptoms improve. Return to your normal activities slowly.

DIET
No special diet.

 NOTIFY OUR OFFICE IF

- You or a family member has symptoms of brucellosis.
- Fever or other symptoms return after treatment.
- New, unexplained symptoms develop. Drugs used in treatment may produce side effects.

Special notes:

_____

_____

_____

More notes on the back of this page ☐

BUERGER'S DISEASE
(Thromboangiitis Obliterans)

 BASIC INFORMATION

DESCRIPTION
Blockage of small and medium arteries due to inflammation of blood vessels. The symptoms come on gradually over a period of time. The disease is most common in men between ages 20 and 40 who are heavy cigarette smokers. However, it is now being diagnosed more in women and in people of both sexes over age 50.

FREQUENT SIGNS AND SYMPTOMS
· Numbness and tingling in the legs, feet, arms, and fingers.
· Pain in the feet and legs while walking or during exercise. This pain occurs less often in the hands and fingers. Pain comes from not having enough blood flow to these areas of the body. Pain becomes persistent as disease progresses.
· Raynaud's phenomenon. A condition where the hands, fingers, feet, and toes turn white, blue, or red when exposed to cold.
· Painful sores (ulcers) and gangrene (dead tissue) on the toes and fingertips.

CAUSES
Unknown. The disease is probably triggered by smoking combined with an immune reaction in the body. Most patients are heavy smokers, but some are moderate smokers, and some use smokeless tobacco.

RISK INCREASES WITH
Smoking or using smokeless tobacco.

PREVENTIVE MEASURES
There are no specific preventive measures, except never to smoke.

EXPECTED OUTCOMES
This condition is currently considered incurable. Stopping smoking is the only effective treatment to stop the progress of the disease.

POSSIBLE COMPLICATIONS
· Blood clots in the legs.
· Finger and toe ulcers, gangrene, and amputation.
· Life expectancy is shorter.

 DIAGNOSIS & TREATMENT

GENERAL MEASURES
· Your health care provider will do a physical exam and ask questions about your symptoms and smoking history. This is often enough to make the diagnosis. Medical tests may be done to confirm the diagnosis and check for complications.
· There is no effective drug or specific treatment for the disorder.
· Get treatment for any infection or injury that occurs.
· The disease will get worse if smoking continues, so stop smoking. Join a program to help you stop.
· Avoid exposure to the cold if possible. Cold causes blood vessels to constrict. This deprives your body of a normal blood supply. If you are going out in cold weather, wear warm footwear and gloves.
· Clip nails carefully to avoid injuring the skin.
· Wear shoes that fit well. Wear cotton or wool socks.
· Insert soft pads in your shoes to protect your feet.
· Don't go barefoot outdoors.
· If gangrene develops, amputation of the affected limb, toes, or fingers is likely.
· Counseling may be recommended to help with lifestyle changes required to cope with the disease.

MEDICATIONS
Drugs that open the blood vessels may be prescribed. These drugs will not help if you continue smoking.

ACTIVITY
Stay as active as you can. Begin an exercise program to become as physically fit as possible.

DIET
No special diet.

 NOTIFY OUR OFFICE IF

· You or a family member has symptoms of Buerger's disease.
· You have pain that cannot be controlled.
· Sores develop on your fingers or toes.
· New, unexplained symptoms develop. Drugs used in treatment may produce side effects.

Special notes:

_____

_____

_____

More notes on the back of this page ☐

BULIMIA
(Binge-Eating Syndrome)

BASIC INFORMATION

DESCRIPTION
An eating disorder. It involves bingeing (uncontrolled overeating) and purging (getting rid of unwanted food in the body). Bulimia affects both sexes (women much more than men). It often starts in the teen years.

FREQUENT SIGNS AND SYMPTOMS
Recurrent episodes of binge eating. This is rapid eating of a large amount of food in a short time (usually less than 2 hours), plus at least 3 of the following:
- Preference for high-calorie, convenience foods during a binge.
- Secretive eating during a binge. Patients are aware that the eating pattern is abnormal, and they fear being unable to stop eating.
- Following the eating binge with purging measures, such as laxative use or self-induced vomiting.
- Depression and guilt following an eating binge.
- Repeated attempts to lose weight with severely restrictive diets, self-induced vomiting, and use of laxatives or diuretics.
- Frequent weight changes greater than 10 pounds from first fasting and then extreme overeating.
- There is no underlying physical disorder.

CAUSES
Unknown. It is thought to be largely emotional.

RISK INCREASES WITH
- Strict, compulsive, perfectionistic family.
- Anorexia nervosa (another type of eating disorder).
- Depression.
- Stress, including lifestyle changes, such as moving or starting at a new school or job.
- Personality disorders.
- Excessive concern with being physically attractive.
- Certain occupations (such as ballet dancer, model, or actor).
- Certain activities (such as cheerleading).
- Athletes (such as gymnasts, runners, cyclists, weightlifters, and wrestlers).

PREVENTIVE MEASURES
No specific preventive measures. Early treatment may help keep it from progressing. Encourage a rational attitude about weight in young people.

EXPECTED OUTCOMES
Outcome is variable. Patients, if they desire to change, can often be helped with therapy. For some patients, it may continue long-term. Others just have episodes of bulimia that occur with life events and crisis.

POSSIBLE COMPLICATIONS
- Fluid/electrolyte imbalance, dental disease, stomach and esophagus problems, constipation, and dry skin.
- Malnutrition (not enough nutrients for body's needs).
- Relapse after treatment.

DIAGNOSIS & TREATMENT

GENERAL MEASURES
- Your health care provider can usually diagnose bulimia with a physical exam and by asking questions about your symptoms, eating habits, and weight concerns. There is no one test to diagnose bulimia. Medical tests may be done to check for possible underlying disorder, physical problems, or complications.
- Denial of the severity or even the existence of a problem is common in patients. Most patients resist treatment and behavior change at first. Some want a quick and easy solution that is not feasible.
- The goal of treatment is to establish healthy eating patterns and to maintain normal weight.
- Treatment may include counseling for the patient and the family, nutrition counseling, and drug therapy if needed. Hospital care or care in an eating disorder facility may be required.
- A dental exam is usually recommended.
- Counseling focuses on the misconceptions that patients have of themselves (physically, mentally, emotionally). Support groups may help some patients.
- To learn more: National Eating Disorders Association, 603 Stewart St., Suite 803, Seattle WA 98101; (800) 931-2237; website: www.nationaleatingdisorders.org.

MEDICATIONS
- Antidepressants are usually prescribed.
- Vitamin and mineral supplements may be prescribed.

ACTIVITY
May be limited at first. Then exercise for enjoyment and fitness and not to lose weight.

DIET
A dietitian will help you plan healthy meals that are not rigid, but provide food choices.

NOTIFY OUR OFFICE IF

- You have symptoms of bulimia or you suspect your child has bulimia.
- Treatment does not improve bulimia behavior.

Special notes:

_____

_____

_____

More notes on the back of this page ☐

BUNION

(Hallux Valgus)

 BASIC INFORMATION

DESCRIPTION

A bony swelling or bump that occurs along the side of the big toe joint. Bunions may start in the teenage years, but usually occur in the 20 to 30 age group. Three times as many women as men have bunions.

FREQUENT SIGNS AND SYMPTOMS

· A big toe that points in, toward the other toes. This is called hallux valgus.
· Thickened skin over the bony bump at the base of the big toe.
· Fluid may build up under the thickened skin.
· Foot pain and stiffness.
· The symptoms progress slowly over a period of years.

CAUSES

The big toe has been forced into an incorrect position. This causes the joint to stick out. The big toe may overlap one or more of the other toes.

RISK INCREASES WITH

· Family history of foot problems (inherited weakness in the toe joints).
· Flat feet.
· Arthritis.
· Shoes that have high heels and narrow toes that push the toes together.

PREVENTIVE MEASURES

· Exercise daily to keep muscles of the feet and legs in good condition.
· Wear shoes that have wide toes and fit well. Don't wear high heels or shoes without room for toes in their normal position.

EXPECTED OUTCOMES

A bunion is permanent unless surgery is performed to remove it. Self-care can help improve the symptoms.

POSSIBLE COMPLICATIONS

· Infection of the bunion, especially in persons with diabetes.
· Inflammation and arthritis in other joints caused by difficulty in walking. Arthritis can result from abnormal stress on the foot, hip, and spine.
· Bunion may grow back after surgery.

 DIAGNOSIS & TREATMENT

GENERAL MEASURES

· Your health care provider can diagnose a bunion by its appearance. An x-ray of the toe joint may be done.
· Treatment usually involves self-care steps and surgery, if needed.
· Wear comfortable shoes that fit well.
· If there is swelling, redness, and pain, keep pressure off the affected toe.
· Before bedtime, separate the first toe from the others with a foam-rubber pad.
· Wear a thick, ring-shaped pad around and over the bunion. Use arch supports to relieve pressure on the bunion. These are available in drugstores or shoe-repair shops.
· Custom-made orthotics (shoe inserts) may be prescribed.
· Surgery (bunionectomy) may be recommended when bunion makes walking painful. The bunion is removed and the toe may be straightened. Specific instructions will be provided for self-care after surgery.

MEDICATIONS

Use nonprescription drugs such as aspirin or ibuprofen for pain, swelling, and soreness.

ACTIVITY

If you have surgery, resume your normal activities slowly after surgery. Recovery may take 2 months or more.

DIET

No special diet.

 NOTIFY OUR OFFICE IF

· You or a family member has a bunion that is interfering with normal activities.
· You develop signs of infection after treatment or surgery. Signs of infection include fever, tenderness, or pain.

Special notes:

_____

_____

_____

More notes on the back of this page ☐

BURNS

 ## BASIC INFORMATION

DESCRIPTION

Injury to the skin from contact with heat, radiation, electricity, sunlight, or chemicals. Sometimes internal organs may also be injured. The risk of damage is greatest with infants and young children.

FREQUENT SIGNS AND SYMPTOMS

• Thin or superficial burns (1st-degree burns) are limited to the upper skin layer. They cause redness, tenderness, pain, and swelling.
• Partial thickness burns (2nd-degree burns) affect deeper skin layers. Symptoms are more severe and usually include blisters.
• Full thickness burns (3rd-degree burns) involve all skin layers. Skin is white and appears cooked. There may be no pain in the initial stages.

CAUSES

• Rise in skin temperature from heat sources such as fire, steam, or electricity. Open flame and hot liquid are the most common causes.
• Tissue injury caused by chemicals or radiation, including sunlight.
• Lightning strikes can cause internal burns with few external signs.

RISK INCREASES WITH

• Stress, carelessness, smoking in bed, or excess alcohol use. All of these make accidents more likely.
• Jobs involving exposure to heat or radiation. This includes firefighting, police work, or factory work.
• Faulty electrical wiring.
• Hot water heaters set too high.

PREVENTIVE MEASURES

• Fireproof your home. Install smoke alarms. Plan emergency exits and have regular fire drills.
• Wear protective gear around heat or radiation.
• Don't touch uncovered electric wires.
• Teach children safety rules for matches, fires, electrical outlets, cords, and stoves.
• Use extension cords only when necessary.
• If you have small children, put safety covers on outlets. Get rid of frayed cords.
• Buy flame-resistant sleepwear for children.

EXPECTED OUTCOMES

Most persons recover if the burns affect less than 50% of the body's surface. With less severe burns, skin usually heals in 1 to 3 weeks.

POSSIBLE COMPLICATIONS

• Infection.
• Shock, due to loss of fluids from the body.
• Severe burns can cause serious health problems that can lead to death.

 ## DIAGNOSIS & TREATMENT

GENERAL MEASURES

• For severe burns call 911 for emergency help.
• See your health care provider for burns that aren't severe. The burn area will be examined and treatment given depending on the type of burn and size of the area affected. Special dressings and skin-care products may be prescribed.
• For minor burns treated at home:
  - Place the burned area in cold water, hold it under running water, or use wet compresses on it for 15 minutes (longer for chemical burns). This will reduce pain and swelling. Don't use ice on a burn.
  - Use an aloe vera cream or antibiotic ointment. Wrap the area loosely with sterile gauze dressing. This helps protect the area. Change the dressing each day.
  - Don't break blisters. This can cause infection.
  - Keep the burned area higher than the rest of the body, if possible.
• Emergency care and a hospital stay are usually needed for severe burns. Complications, such as lung damage from smoke, may need treatment. There are special burn centers for the most serious cases. Surgery may be needed to graft skin, and rehabilitation may be needed after burns start healing.

MEDICATIONS

• You may take acetaminophen or ibuprofen for pain.
• Hospital care may include drugs to treat the burns, for pain, and to prevent infection. A tetanus booster is needed if it is not up to date.

ACTIVITY

Resume normal activity as soon as possible. This will help speed recovery.

DIET

No special diet for minor burns. Severe burns may require use of a feeding tube until symptoms improve.

 ## NOTIFY OUR OFFICE IF

• You have a burn that does not heal in 6 days.
• Child under age 2 has a burn, even if it seems minor.
• You develop chills, fever; increased pain, redness, swelling, or pus in the burn area.

Special notes:

_____

_____

_____

More notes on the back of this page ☐

BURSITIS

 ## BASIC INFORMATION

DESCRIPTION
Inflammation (swelling and pain) of a bursa. A bursa is a soft, fluid-filled sac that serves as a cushion between tendons and bones. Areas usually affected are near the shoulders, elbows, knees, pelvis, hips, or Achilles tendons.

FREQUENT SIGNS AND SYMPTOMS
• Pain, swelling, tenderness, and limited movement in the affected joint. Pain may spread into nearby areas of the body.
• A feeling of warmth over the affected joint.

CAUSES
Inflammation can be caused by overuse, injury, disease, or infection. Sometimes no cause is found.

RISK INCREASES WITH
• Injury to a joint.
• Overuse of a joint.
• Exercising more than usual.
• Calcium deposits in shoulder tendons.
• Infection.
• Arthritis.
• Gout.
• People who suddenly increase their activity levels ("weekend warriors").
• Not stretching properly or over-stretching.

PREVENTIVE MEASURES
• Avoid injuries when possible. Don't overuse muscles. Wear protective gear for contact sports.
• Warm-up before exercise. Cool-down after exercise.
• Stay physically fit.

EXPECTED OUTCOMES
This is a common, but not serious problem. Symptoms usually improve in 7-14 days with treatment.

POSSIBLE COMPLICATIONS
• Prolonged healing time if activity is resumed too soon.
• Chronic bursitis may occur due to repeated injuries or recurrent attacks of bursitis.

 ## DIAGNOSIS & TREATMENT

GENERAL MEASURES
• Self-care may be all that is needed.
    - Use RICE therapy (rest, ice, compression, and elevation). Rest the affected joint. Use an ice pack to massage the area several times a day. Use compression by wearing an elastic bandage. Elevate the affected joint by resting it on a pillow.
    - You may use heat, in addition to ice, if it feels better. Apply a hot, wet towel or use a heating pad. A deep-heating ointment may be helpful.
• See your health care provider if self-care does not help or symptoms are severe. Bursitis can be diagnosed by a physical exam. Medical tests are usually not done.
• Your health care provider may sometimes drain fluid from the joint with a needle. Surgery is rarely needed.
• Physical therapy may be recommended to maintain flexibility, mobility, and strength of the joint.

MEDICATIONS
• Use nonprescription acetaminophen or ibuprofen for mild pain.
• Your health care provider may prescribe:
    - Nonsteroidal anti-inflammatory drugs or creams.
    - Antibiotics (if the bursa is infected).
    - Prescription pain relievers for severe pain.
    - Injection with a local anesthetic mixed with a corticosteroid drug.

ACTIVITY
• Rest the affected joint as much as possible. It may help to wear a sling or a brace, or to use crutches until the pain becomes easier to bear. Begin normal, slow joint movement as soon as pain permits.
• Follow directions for any recommended home exercise routines.

DIET
No special diet.

 ## NOTIFY OUR OFFICE IF

• You or a family member has symptoms of bursitis that is severe or self-care methods do not help.
• New symptoms develop after treatment.

Special notes:

_____

_____

_____

More notes on the back of this page ☐

CALCIUM IMBALANCE

BASIC INFORMATION

DESCRIPTION

Calcium is a mineral that helps regulate the heartbeat, transmit nerve impulses, and contract muscles. It also helps form bone and teeth. Too much calcium (hypercalcemia) or too little calcium (hypocalcemia) can cause serious medical problems. The problems can sometimes be life-threatening. Most calcium is stored in the bones, but it is also found in the blood and cells.

FREQUENT SIGNS AND SYMPTOMS

Too little calcium:
- Muscle spasms, twitching, or cramping.
- Arms, hands, legs, and feet may tingle or feel numb.
- Seizures (convulsion).
- Heart-beat is irregular.
- High blood pressure.

Too much calcium (often produces no symptoms):
- Feeling tired and sluggish.
- Loss of appetite.
- Vomiting, diarrhea, dehydration, and thirst.
- Heart-beat is irregular.
- Low blood pressure.
- Depression or mental changes (confused or delirious).
- Seizures or coma (in severe cases).

CAUSES

Too little calcium:
- Parathyroid glands that are underactive. This can be caused by disease or damage to the parathyroid.
- Not getting enough calcium and vitamin D.
- The body does not absorb calcium from the stomach.
- Severe burns or infections.
- Problems with the pancreas.
- Kidney failure.
- Low levels of certain minerals in your blood.

Too much calcium:
- Parathyroid gland that is overactive.
- Broken bones and long periods of bed rest.
- Cancer of the bone marrow.
- Tumors that destroy bone.

RISK INCREASES WITH

Too little calcium:
- Use of certain drugs such as diuretics.
- Injury, cancer, or surgery of the thyroid or parathyroid glands.
- Excess alcohol use.
- Poor nutrition.

Too much calcium:
- Diet that is too high in dairy products or excess use of antacids that contain calcium.
- Kidney disease.
- Being inactive or confined to bed for long periods.

PREVENTIVE MEASURES
- Eat a normal, well-balanced diet.
- Don't drink alcohol, or limit it to 1 to 2 drinks a day.
- Don't use nonprescription antacids on a regular basis.

EXPECTED OUTCOMES

Most cases can be cured with treatment in 1 week.

POSSIBLE COMPLICATIONS
- Heart attack.
- Bones may become weak and break easily.
- Kidney stones from high calcium.
- Ulcer from high calcium.

DIAGNOSIS & TREATMENT

GENERAL MEASURES
- Your health care provider may do a physical exam. Medical tests can include blood studies of calcium levels, x-rays of bones and echocardiogram (a heart study).
- Treatment involves correcting the problem or treating the disorder causing the imbalance. This may be all that is required. In other cases, treatment may be needed to remove excess calcium or replace low calcium levels.

MEDICATIONS
- Drugs may be prescribed to raise or lower your calcium levels, depending on the need. Drugs may be given by mouth or through a needle placed in your vein (IV).
- Other drugs may be prescribed to treat a disorder that is the cause of the calcium imbalance.

ACTIVITY

After treatment, return to your normal activities slowly as symptoms improve.

DIET
- For mild, low calcium level, calcium supplements and vitamin D may be recommended. Get more protein, milk, and milk products in your diet.
- For a mild, high-calcium level, consume fewer dairy products and antacids that contain calcium.

NOTIFY OUR OFFICE IF
- You or a family member has symptoms of calcium imbalance.
- Symptoms get worse or they don't improve with treatment.

Special notes:

_____

_____

_____

More notes on the back of this page ☐

CANDIDIASIS OF SKIN
(Moniliasis)

 BASIC INFORMATION

DESCRIPTION
A yeast infection in skin folds, or in areas of skin that touch other areas of skin. It can affect the underarm area, spaces between fingers and toes, inner thighs, under the breasts, and over the base of the spine. It may affect the skin of the scrotum, vagina, and vaginal lips.

FREQUENT SIGNS AND SYMPTOMS
- Plaques (patches or flat areas) on skin.
- Bright-red patches with poorly defined borders. They are often 2.5 to 5 inches across, but may be larger.
- Patches may weep or ooze.
- Skin appears moist and crusted.
- Itching is usually severe.
- Smaller patches may surround larger patches. They sometimes form small white blisters with pus inside.

CAUSES
Yeast infection of the skin is caused by *Candida*, a type of fungus. *Candida* fungi actually live on the skin and normally cause no harm. If skin is damaged or there is excess moisture and warmth, the fungus germs can grow and cause infection. The infection can be spread from one person to another by direct contact, and less often, by sexual contact. Germs are also spread by sharing damp towels or washcloths.

RISK INCREASES WITH
- Use of oral antibiotics.
- Use of any type of steroids.
- Diabetes.
- The elderly or infants (it causes diaper rash).
- Pregnant women or use of birth control pills.
- Use of plastic pants in infants or pantyhose in women.
- Obesity.
- Existing skin infection or skin disorder.
- Weak immune system because of disease or drugs.
- Work that involves the skin being wet continuously.

PREVENTIVE MEASURES
- Take antibiotics only when prescribed.
- Keep skin cool and dry.
- Avoid risk factors where possible.

EXPECTED OUTCOMES
- Usually curable in 2 weeks with treatment. Without treatment, healing may be slow.
- It is common for these fungal infections to recur.

POSSIBLE COMPLICATIONS
- Nail infection, causing them to thicken or crumble.
- Bacterial infection, in addition to the fungal infection.
- Infection spreading to the whole body (in those with weak immune systems).

 DIAGNOSIS & TREATMENT

GENERAL MEASURES
- Your health care provider can diagnose the infection by an exam of the affected skin area. Medical tests may include a study of a skin scraping or pus.
- Treatment involves drugs and self-care measures. Any skin condition that may have lead to the candidiasis infection should be treated also.
- Keep skin cool and dry. Expose affected skin areas to air as much as possible.
- Wear loose cotton clothing. Avoid synthetic or wool fabrics. Change socks often if feet are affected.
- To avoid spreading germs, don't go barefoot on wet floors where other people may walk. Don't share towels. Clean the bathtub or shower after you use it.
- Protect skin from injury, but don't bandage the affected skin.

MEDICATIONS
Antifungal drugs to be applied to the skin are usually prescribed. Gently massage a small amount into the affected area as directed. Use only enough to cover the affected area. Larger amounts don't help. In more severe cases, an antifungal drug taken by mouth may be prescribed.

ACTIVITY
No limits, except to avoid heat and sweating.

DIET
No special diet. Eating yogurt may or may not help prevent yeast infections (research is unclear).

 NOTIFY OUR OFFICE IF

- You or a family member has symptoms of candidiasis.
- The following occur during treatment:
  - Infection continues to spread despite treatment.
  - Signs of secondary bacterial infection develop. Signs include pain, tenderness, redness, warmth, and oozing.
- New, unexplained symptoms develop. Drugs used in treatment may produce side effects.

Special notes:

_____

_____

_____

More notes on the back of this page ☐

CANKER SORES
(Aphthous Ulcers)

 BASIC INFORMATION

DESCRIPTION
Painful ulcers (sores) that occur in the lining of the mouth. They cannot be spread from one person to another. They may be confused with herpes infections. Canker sores affect both sexes, but are more common in women.

FREQUENT SIGNS AND SYMPTOMS
• Ulcers are small, very painful, shallow, and covered by a gray membrane. Borders are surrounded by an intense red halo.
• Ulcers appear on lips, gums, inner cheeks, tongue, palate, and throat. Usually, 2 or 3 ulcers appear during an attack. As many as 10 to 15 ulcers is not uncommon.
• Ulcers may be so painful during first 2 or 3 days that they interfere with eating or speaking.
• Sometimes there is tingling or burning for 24 hours before the ulcer appears.

CAUSES
Exact cause is unknown.

RISK INCREASES WITH
• Emotional or physical stress; anxiety or premenstrual tension.
• Injury to the mouth lining caused by rough dentures, hot food, toothbrushing, or dental work.
• Irritation from foods, such as chocolate, citrus, acidic foods (e.g., vinegar, pickles), salted nuts, or potato chips.
• Changes in the body's immune system.
• Family history of canker sores.

PREVENTIVE MEASURES
• Brush teeth at least twice a day. Floss regularly to keep the mouth clean and healthy.
• Avoid risk factors where possible.
• Pay attention to your diet and when canker sores develop. Don't eat foods that seem to trigger the sores.

EXPECTED OUTCOMES
Most will heal on their own in 2 weeks. It is common for them to recur. Recurrence can vary from a single canker sore 2 or 3 times a year, to frequent episodes of many sores.

POSSIBLE COMPLICATIONS
Rarely, dehydration may occur if eating and drinking are limited by the pain of the canker sores.

 DIAGNOSIS & TREATMENT

GENERAL MEASURES
• Usually all that is needed for treatment is self-care.
• If you are concerned about the sores, see your health care provider. Canker sores can normally be diagnosed by an exam of the mouth. A culture of the sores may be done to rule out herpes infection.
• Rinse the mouth 3 or more times a day with a salt solution (1/2 teaspoon salt to 8 oz. water) if this isn't painful.
• If a canker sore is caused by a rough tooth, braces, or dentures, consult your dentist. The sore won't heal until the cause is treated.

MEDICATIONS
• A dental paste that contains steroids may be used. If applied as soon as the ulcer begins, it helps reduce pain.
• Aphthasol (amlexanox), a paste used only for canker sores may be prescribed. It helps with pain and hastens healing. Follow instructions on the label on how to use.
• Special mouthwashes may be prescribed.

ACTIVITY
No limits.

DIET
• Avoid foods that irritate the sores. Drink lots of fluids. If possible, eat a well-balanced diet while healing.
• To avoid pain, sip liquids through straws. Foods that cause the least pain are milk, liquid gelatin, yogurt, ice cream, and custard.

 NOTIFY OUR OFFICE IF

• You or a family member has canker sores that don't improve in 2 weeks.
• Other symptoms occur at the same time as canker sores.
• New, unexplained symptoms develop. Drugs used in treatment may produce side effects.

Special notes:

_____

_____

_____

More notes on the back of this page ☐

CARBON MONOXIDE POISONING

BASIC INFORMATION

DESCRIPTION
Breathing in carbon monoxide (CO), a poison gas that has no color or smell. CO is produced when gas or wood is burned. Common sources include smoke from fires, motor vehicle or boat exhaust, space heaters, furnaces, charcoal grills, and gas burning appliances.

FREQUENT SIGNS AND SYMPTOMS
- The first symptoms may be mild and flu-like.
- Headache, feeling dizzy and tired.
- Nausea and vomiting; stomach pain.
- Feeling like you might faint, trouble with walking.
- Difficulty breathing, chest pain, and changes in heartbeat.
- Seizure.
- Vision changes.
- Confusion, depression, and other behavior changes.
- Coma (loss of consciousness).

CAUSES
Carbon monoxide is breathed into the lungs. It gets into the blood system and prevents the flow of oxygen that the body needs for survival. It is the most common form of accidental poisoning in the United States.

RISK INCREASES WITH
- Furnaces or space-heating devices that do not work properly; a fireplace with a clogged chimney.
- Riding in the back of a pickup truck under a closed cover of some type.
- Poor venting (exhaust fumes escape into buildings or homes).
- Use of charcoal grill in enclosed place, such as a tent.
- Faulty motor vehicle exhaust system, or leaving a car running in a garage attached to a house.
- Winter months when heaters are in use and houses are more closed up.

PREVENTIVE MEASURES
- Avoid the risk factors where you are able.
- Install a carbon monoxide alarm in your home. If it goes off, leave the house right away and call 911.
- Make sure the furnace, fireplaces, gas appliances, and heaters in your home work properly. Call your gas company if you think there may be a gas leak.
- Use products that will help prevent fires in your home (such as smoke alarms, fire extinguishers).

EXPECTED OUTCOMES
- In milder cases with quick treatment, recovery is complete and without complications.
- Some patients have delayed symptoms weeks later. They may feel extra tired, have memory problems, feel confused, or have mood and behavior changes.

POSSIBLE COMPLICATIONS
- Poisoning can result in damage to the brain, heart, or lungs; and death. Children, the elderly, and those with lung disease are at high risk for adverse effects.
- Pregnant women may suffer miscarriage, early labor, fetal death, or a child with cerebral palsy.

DIAGNOSIS & TREATMENT

GENERAL MEASURES
- Your health care provider will do a physical exam and test your blood for carbon monoxide. Other medical tests may be done for more severe symptoms.
- This type of poisoning can not be treated at home. Medical care is needed. For mild cases, the symptoms usually disappear after you breathe in pure oxygen through a mask for a few hours.
- Some patients with more severe symptoms will require the use of breathing support in a hospital.
- Rarely, a patient is placed in a sealed chamber where high-pressure oxygen is used for treatment.
- To learn more: Consumer Product Safety Commission, (800) 638-2772, or Medline Plus website: www.nlm.nih.gov/medlineplus/carbonmonoxidepoisoning.html.

MEDICATIONS
Usually not needed. Drugs may be used for seizures if they occur.

ACTIVITY
Limits will depend on how severe the symptoms are.

DIET
No special diet.

NOTIFY OUR OFFICE IF

- You or a family member has symptoms of carbon monoxide poisoning.
- Symptoms get worse, recur, or new symptoms occur after recovery.

Special notes:

_____

_____

_____

More notes on the back of this page ☐

CARCINOID SYNDROME

 BASIC INFORMATION

DESCRIPTION
A group of symptoms caused by tumors (carcinoids). Carcinoids secrete hormones and chemicals that cause the symptoms. The tumors can occur in the small intestine, appendix, rectum, colon, stomach, pancreas, liver, lungs, and (rarely) other organs. Carcinoid syndrome usually affects adults (of both sexes) aged 50 to 70.

FREQUENT SIGNS AND SYMPTOMS
• Carcinoids grow slowly and can be benign or malignant (cancerous). Many persons have no symptoms.
• The primary tumor may cause intestinal obstruction (painful cramps in the middle of the abdomen, vomiting, swelling, and weight loss).
• In a few cases, carcinoid cells spread to other body parts and produce secondary, hormone-producing (serotonin) tumors. Heavy exercise, alcohol use, or eating bananas, tomatoes, plums, avocados, pineapple, or walnuts may trigger symptoms of these secondary tumors. These symptoms include:
  - Flushed skin on the head and neck.
  - Watery eyes.
  - Diarrhea with abdominal cramps.
  - Respiratory symptoms similar to asthma.
  - Irregular heartbeat.
  - Nausea and vomiting.
  - Low blood pressure.
  - Unexplained weight loss.

CAUSES
Unknown.

RISK INCREASES WITH
• Older adults.
• Smoking.
• Family history of multiple endocrine neoplasia, type 1 (a hereditary disorder).

PREVENTIVE MEASURES
Cannot be prevented at present.

EXPECTED OUTCOMES
The outcome will vary. In some, it can be cured with surgery. In others, the problem may progress, recur, or relapse.

POSSIBLE COMPLICATIONS
• Cancer may spread to other body parts.
• Low blood pressure.
• Risk for stroke, blood clots, and similar disorders.
• Bowel obstruction.
• Heart failure.
• Angioedema (hives).
• Renal failure.

 DIAGNOSIS & TREATMENT

GENERAL MEASURES
• Your health care provider will do a physical exam and ask questions about your symptoms. A number of medical tests will be done. The tests help diagnose any cancer and then determine if it has spread (staging).
• Treatment varies and depends on the location and size of the tumor, any spread of a cancer, your health, age, and preferences. Treatment may include surgery, chemotherapy (anticancer drugs), or other drugs.
• Surgery to remove the carcinoid tumor depends on the location. In some cases, surgery can bring about a cure. The entire tumor may be removed, or a portion of the tumor (as large a as possible) will be removed. This relieves symptoms because less of the harmful hormones are produced.
• To learn more: The American Cancer Society, (800) ACS-2345; website: cancer.org or National Cancer Institute, (800)4-CANCER; website: www.nci.nih.gov.

MEDICATIONS
• Your health care provider may prescribe:
  - Antidiarrheal drugs.
  - Anticancer drugs (they do not cure these tumors, but may help symptoms).
  - Drugs to prevent serotonin production.
  - Drugs to prevent flushed skin.
  - Cortisone drugs to reduce inflammation
  - Multivitamins and niacin supplements.

ACTIVITY
Resume your normal activities once symptoms improve. Avoid strenuous exercise.

DIET
• Include at least 2 servings of protein a day (or as advised).
• Avoid foods that trigger symptoms.
• Don't drink alcohol.

 NOTIFY OUR OFFICE IF

• You or a family member has symptoms of carcinoid syndrome.
• Symptoms become worse, despite treatment.

Special notes:

_____

_____

_____

More notes on the back of this page ☐

CARDIAC ARREST

 BASIC INFORMATION

DESCRIPTION
Total loss of heart-pumping action. Delay of treatment for only 3 to 5 minutes may cause death or permanent brain damage. Up to age 45, it is more common in men. After age 45, the incidence is equal in men and women.

FREQUENT SIGNS AND SYMPTOMS
· Brief dizziness, followed by fainting and unconsciousness.
· No pulse. Usually breathing also stops.
· Skin color becomes bluish-white. The pupils of the eye may get bigger.
· Seizures.
· Loss of bowel and bladder control (sometimes). Simple fainting may seem like a cardiac arrest, but heartbeat and breathing continue.

CAUSES
Heart stops beating suddenly. This may be due to a heart that is beating too fast, too slow, or that has an irregular heartbeat. Other causes include electrical shock, drowning, choking, trauma, or respiratory arrest (lungs stop working).

RISK INCREASES WITH
· Heart attack or heart disease.
· Lack of blood circulation and profound shock caused by uncontrolled bleeding or overwhelming infection.
· Loss of oxygen from drowning, choking, or during surgery from the anesthesia.
· Potassium or fluid imbalance in the blood.
· Diabetes.
· Use of certain heart medicines.
· Use of medicines that help with fluid retention. These can cause low potassium in the blood.
· Use of any drug that raises blood pressure in a heart patient. This can include cold capsules, decongestant tablets, and nasal sprays.
· Using drugs of abuse, such as cocaine and intravenous drugs.

PREVENTIVE MEASURES
· Live a healthy lifestyle. Get regular exercise, eat a healthy diet, maintain ideal weight for height, and don't smoke.
· If you have heart disease or other risk factors, follow your treatment instructions carefully.
· Have family members and close friends learn CPR (cardiopulmonary resuscitation).

EXPECTED OUTCOMES
The victim may survive if emergency medical treatment is given in the first few minutes. The outcome depends on what caused the cardiac arrest.

POSSIBLE COMPLICATIONS
Death or permanent brain damage if heart action cannot be resumed in 3 to 5 minutes. Most patients die before reaching an emergency care center.

 DIAGNOSIS & TREATMENT

GENERAL MEASURES
· People who know how to recognize cardiac arrest and can perform CPR can often get the heart beating again. Someone may mistake fainting or other causes of unconsciousness for cardiac arrest. Check for a neck pulse before starting CPR.
· Emergency care involves shocking the heart back into a normal heartbeat. This process is called defibrillation.
· Ensure that you and your family members learn CPR. Call your local Red Cross or hospital for information. You may save a life.
· If you have heart disease or have risk factors, wear a medical alert identification (a bracelet or neck tag).
· Automated external defibrillators (AEDs) are being placed in public places (such as airports). They can be used by anyone to help a person who is having cardiac arrest.

MEDICATIONS
Drugs may be prescribed to treat the cause of cardiac arrest once the crisis is over.

ACTIVITY
After recovery, activities should be resumed gradually. Follow your health care provider's instructions.

DIET
Don't give fluids or foods to anyone with signs of cardiac arrest. He or she could choke.

 CALL FOR EMERGENCY HELP

If the victim is not conscious and not breathing:
· Call 911 (emergency) for an ambulance or medical help.
· Yell for help. Don't leave the victim.
· Begin mouth-to-mouth breathing immediately.
· If there is no heartbeat, give CPR.
· Don't stop CPR until help arrives.

Special notes:

_____

_____

_____

_____

More notes on the back of this page ☐

CARDIOMYOPATHY

 ## BASIC INFORMATION

DESCRIPTION

An inflammatory disorder of the heart muscle. Damage to the heart muscle causes the heart to weaken and not be able to pump enough blood to the body. In addition, blood moves more slowly through an enlarged heart, allowing blood clots to easily form. Cardiomyopathy may affect adults of any age and is more common in males. It can lead to heart failure.

FREQUENT SIGNS AND SYMPTOMS

If the condition is severe enough to cause heart failure, the following symptoms may occur:
- Rapid and abnormal heartbeat.
- Shortness of breath (may be worse when lying down or being physically active).
- Swollen legs, feet, and ankles.
- Feeling tired and weak.
- Chest pain.
- Loss of appetite (a weight gain may, however, occur).
- Dizziness or fainting.
- Cough.

CAUSES

There are different types of cardiomyopathy. They can be caused by a variety of heath problems. Sometimes, no cause is found.

RISK INCREASES WITH

- Viral infection of the heart muscle.
- Severe coronary artery disease.
- High blood pressure and high levels of fats in the blood.
- Alcoholism.
- Heart surgery.
- Family history of heart disease.
- Congenital (being born with) heart disease.
- Certain infections (amyloidosis and sarcoidosis).
- Postpartum (after pregnancy and delivery).
- Smoking.
- Diabetes.
- Stress.
- Being physically inactive (sedentary lifestyle).
- Obesity.

PREVENTIVE MEASURES

Avoid risk factors, where possible.

EXPECTED OUTCOMES

Sometimes, the heart damage cannot be reversed. Improvement can occur. Treatment may help relieve symptoms and prevent further damage. Some patients may be considered for a heart transplant.

POSSIBLE COMPLICATIONS

Congestive heart failure (which can be life-threatening).

 ## DIAGNOSIS & TREATMENT

GENERAL MEASURES

- Your health care provider will do a physical exam and ask questions about your symptoms and activities. Medical tests may include chest x-ray, heart function studies, and blood tests. A tube-like instrument may be inserted into the heart and a biopsy (removal of a sample of heart tissue for testing) may be done.
- The goals of treatment are to help the symptoms and to prevent complications. Treatment steps may involve lifestyle changes, drug therapy, and surgery.
- Lifestyle changes can include stopping the use of alcohol and cigarette smoking, diet changes, weight loss, and limiting physical activity.
- Surgery may include implanting a pacemaker to change the heart rate and pattern. Surgery to remove part of the thickened heart wall or replace heart valves may be needed.
- A heart transplant may be recommended if other treatments are not successful. A long wait for a transplant is normal. A mechanical device may be used to temporarily help the heart's pumping function.

MEDICATIONS

Drugs may be prescribed to improve heart function, to slow and regulate the heart rate, get rid of extra fluid, lower blood pressure, relax blood vessels, and suppress the immune system.

ACTIVITY

Follow medical advice about physical activity limits and when it is safe to resume sexual relations.

DIET

- Eat a diet that is low in salt and fat. Avoid alcohol.
- Begin a weight-loss diet if you weigh more than is healthy for your body type.

 ## NOTIFY OUR OFFICE IF

- You or a family member has symptoms of cardiomyopathy.
- Symptoms return after treatment.
- You have chest pain.
- New, unexplained symptoms develop. Drugs used in treatment may produce side effects.

Special notes:

_____

_____

_____

More notes on the back of this page ☐

CARPAL TUNNEL SYNDROME

 ## BASIC INFORMATION

DESCRIPTION

A nerve disorder that causes pain, loss of feeling, and loss of strength in the hands. It usually affects the thumb and first three fingers. In some cases, it may affect the 4th and 5th fingers only.

FREQUENT SIGNS AND SYMPTOMS

- Tingling or numbness in part of the hand.
- Sharp pains that shoot from the wrist up the arm, especially at night.
- Burning sensations in the fingers.
- Morning stiffness or cramping of hands.
- Thumb weakness.
- Inability to make a fist.

CAUSES

It appears to result from either repetitive hand and wrist movement (repeating the same motion over and over) or an injury. The tendons or ligaments of the wrist become stretched and swollen. This puts pressure on the nerve that goes into the hand and fingers.

RISK INCREASES WITH

- Work that requires repetitive hand or wrist action. This includes factory assembly or packaging work, cashiering, janitors, or cleaning jobs, dental hygienists, butchers and meat cutters, or using a computer mouse.
- Certain medical or physical conditions may increase the risk. These include arthritis, diabetes, untreated hypothyroidism, obesity, menopause, and pregnancy.
- Sports activities, such as racquetball or handball.
- People who smoke, use alcohol, or have high levels of stress may be more at risk.

PREVENTIVE MEASURES

- Take a break at least once an hour if doing repetitive work involving the hands. Stand up, stretch, and/or walk around.
- Learn to use a computer mouse safely. Don't squeeze or grip it too tightly. Use your arm to move it around, not just your wrist in a side-to-side movement.
- Don't wear tight watch bands or bracelets, or clothing that fits tightly at the wrists.
- Ask your health care provider if wrist splints will help you in the work that you do.

EXPECTED OUTCOMES

Symptoms usually improve with treatment.

POSSIBLE COMPLICATIONS

If untreated or treated too late, permanent numbness and a weak thumb or fingers in the affected hand may occur.

 ## DIAGNOSIS & TREATMENT

GENERAL MEASURES

- Your health care provider will examine your hand and wrist and ask questions about your symptoms. Medical tests may be done to study nerve conduction.
- Conservative treatment is usually tried first.
- If you awaken at night with pain in your hand, hang it over the side of the bed, rub it, or shake it.
- Use ice or warm and cold soaks if they help with symptoms.
- Wearing a splint on the affected wrist may be recommended.
- For work at a computer terminal, be sure that the desk, keyboard, and chair are at the proper height. Take a break once an hour.
- Surgery to free the pinched nerve may be needed. The procedure may be done as an outpatient. Allow 2 weeks for healing. Physical therapy will then help rebuild wrist strength.

MEDICATIONS

- You may take aspirin or ibuprofen to reduce pain and inflammation.
- Anti-inflammatory drugs, cortisone injections at the wrist to reduce inflammation, and vitamin B6 injections or tablets may be prescribed.

ACTIVITY

Once symptoms get better, begin a routine of both aerobic and weight-training exercise to improve fitness.

DIET

Eat a normal, well-balanced diet.

 ## NOTIFY OUR OFFICE IF

- You or a family member has symptoms of carpal tunnel syndrome.
- Symptoms of carpal tunnel syndrome don't lessen in 2 weeks after treatment.
- New, unexplained symptoms develop. Drugs used in treatment may produce side effects.

Special notes:

_____

_____

_____

More notes on the back of this page ☐

CATARACT

 BASIC INFORMATION

DESCRIPTION

A clouding of the lens of the eye. The lens is a clear, flexible structure near the front of the eyeball. It helps to keep vision in focus and screens and refracts light. Cataracts may form in one or both eyes. If they form in both eyes, their growth rate may be very different. They can take several months or several years to develop. They do not spread from one eye to the other. Cataracts occur most often in older adults.

FREQUENT SIGNS AND SYMPTOMS

- Blurred vision. It may be worse in bright light. The blurring may first become apparent while driving at night, when lights seem to scatter or have halos.
- Difficulty reading.
- Faded colors.
- Poor night vision.
- Double or multiple vision.
- Opaque, milky-white pupil (advanced stages only).
- Frequent changes in prescription for eyeglasses.

CAUSES

- The lens of the eye is made up of water and protein. The protein is arranged in a certain way that keeps the lens clear and lets light pass through it. A cataract forms when some of the protein clumps together and begin to cloud a small area of the lens. Over time, it grows larger and affects vision.
- Congenital (present at birth) cataracts can occur.

RISK INCREASES WITH

- Natural aging.
- Illnesses with high blood sugar, such as diabetes.
- Prolonged exposure to sunlight.
- Chronic eye disease.
- Exposure to some types of radiation.
- Family history of cataracts.
- Smoking.
- Use of steroid drugs.
- Surgery for other eye problems.
- Injury to the eye (cataract can occur years later).

PREVENTIVE MEASURES

No specific preventive measures. Getting medical care for eye disorders, wearing sunglasses (that filter UV light) outside during the day, and not smoking may help reduce the risk or delay cataract development.

EXPECTED OUTCOMES

Some cataracts never impair vision enough to require surgery. During the time cataracts are forming, frequent eyeglass changes may help vision. Cataracts that cause vision problems can be cured with surgery.

POSSIBLE COMPLICATIONS

- Loss of vision.
- After surgery complications. These include inflammation, infections, bleeding, loss of vision, and light flashes. These can usually be treated successfully.

 DIAGNOSIS & TREATMENT

GENERAL MEASURES

- Cataracts are usually diagnosed with an exam done by an eye doctor (ophthalmologist).
- Treatment depends on amount of vision problems.
- Wear eyeglasses that provide maximum benefit, if vision is not too badly affected.
- Surgery to remove cataracts is recommended if vision loss interferes with daily activities, such as reading, watching television, or driving.
- Surgery may be done on an inpatient or outpatient basis. Usually one eye is operated on at a time (if cataracts are in both eyes). The eye lens is usually removed and replaced with an artificial lens. Different types of surgery are available. Your options will be explained to you. After surgery, you will be given instructions for home care.

MEDICATIONS

Eye drops or drugs taken by mouth may be prescribed after your surgery.

ACTIVITY

No limits. Don't drive at night if your vision is poor.

DIET

No special diet.

 NOTIFY OUR OFFICE IF

(Or notify your eye care provider).
- You or a family member has symptoms of cataracts.
- Any eye symptoms develop after cataract surgery.

Special notes:

_____

_____

_____

More notes on the back of this page ☐

CELIAC DISEASE
(Gluten Enteropathy; Non-Tropical Sprue)

 BASIC INFORMATION

DESCRIPTION
An allergic condition in the small intestine, triggered by gluten. Gluten is a protein found in most grains. It prevents the intestine from absorbing nutrients. Most forms of celiac disease are inherited. It usually begins during infancy or early childhood (2 weeks to 1 year). Symptoms may appear when the child first begins eating food with gluten. In adults, symptoms may develop gradually over months or even years.

FREQUENT SIGNS AND SYMPTOMS
· Weight loss or slowed weight gain in an infant following the introduction of cereal to the diet.
· Poor appetite.
· Loose, pale, bulky, bad-smelling stools; frequent gas.
· Swollen abdomen; stomach pain.
· Mouth ulcers.
· Anemia or vitamin deficiency, with fatigue, pale skin, skin rash, or bone pain.
· Mildly bowed legs in children.
· Vague tiredness and weakness.
· Swollen legs.

CAUSES
Celiac disease is a congenital (present at birth) disorder. It is caused by an intolerance for gluten, a protein present in most grains.

RISK INCREASES WITH
· Family history of celiac disease.
· Pregnancy.
· Other allergies.

PREVENTIVE MEASURES
Cannot be prevented at present.

EXPECTED OUTCOMES
With a strict, gluten-free diet, most persons with celiac disease can expect a normal life. Improvement begins in 2 to 3 weeks.

POSSIBLE COMPLICATIONS
In rare cases, gluten withdrawal does not bring immediate improvement.

 DIAGNOSIS & TREATMENT

GENERAL MEASURES
· Your health care provider may do a physical exam and ask questions about your symptoms. Medical tests may include blood, urine, and stool studies. A biopsy may be done (a small sample of tissue is taken from the small intestine for viewing under a microscope). Sometimes, diagnosis is based on a person going on a gluten-free diet to see if the symptoms stop.
· The only treatment is a gluten-free diet.
· To learn more: Celiac Sprue Association, P.O. Box 31700, Omaha. NE 68131; (877) 272-4272; website: www.csaceliacs.org or Celiac Disease Foundation, 13251 Ventura Blvd., Studio City, CA 91604; (818) 990-2354 (not toll free); website www.celiac.org.

MEDICATIONS
· Iron and folic acid for anemia may be prescribed.
· Calcium and multiple-vitamin supplements for deficiencies may be recommended.
· Cortisone drugs to reduce the body's inflammatory response may be prescribed.

ACTIVITY
No limits.

DIET
Gluten-free diet. Gluten is found in wheat, rye, barley, and possibly oats. It is difficult to exclude gluten from the diet completely. Be patient while becoming familiar with the diet. A dietitian can help you with a diet plan.

 NOTIFY OUR OFFICE IF

· You or your child has symptoms of celiac disease.
· Symptoms don't decrease after 3 weeks of eating a gluten-free diet.
· The child fails to regain lost weight or grow and develop as expected.
· Fever develops.

Special notes:

_____

_____

_____

More notes on the back of this page ☐

CELLULITIS
(Erysipelas)

 BASIC INFORMATION

DESCRIPTION
An inflammation of the skin and the tissues just below the skin (subcutaneous). Cellulitis is most likely to occur on the face, arms, lower legs, and anal area. It can affect all age groups, including children.

FREQUENT SIGNS AND SYMPTOMS
- Tenderness, warmth, swelling, and redness in an area of the skin. A thin red line may extend from the area toward the heart. Fluid or pus may leak out.
- Fever, chills, sweating, and a general ill feeling.
- Lymph glands nearest the area may be swollen.

CAUSES
Infection with bacteria, or, rarely, a fungal infection. It can begin with a minor injury to the skin that is invaded by the bacteria. The infection leads to inflammation, which is the body's response to infection. Cellulitis cannot be passed from one person to another.

RISK INCREASES WITH
- Chronic illness, such as diabetes.
- Weak immune system due to illness or drugs.
- Any injury that breaks the skin.
- Use of drugs by injection.
- Burns.
- Surgical wound infection.
- Skin disorders (eczema or psoriasis) or infections that cause skin symptoms, such as chickenpox.
- Poor blood circulation.

PREVENTIVE MEASURES
- Keep the skin clean.
- Avoid skin damage. Use protective clothing or proper gear for work or sports where injuries may occur.
- Wear shoes that fit well. Avoid going barefoot in areas where there may be risk of injury.
- If the skin is injured, wash the area with soap and water. Check the injured skin for the next few days to make sure it is healing. If not, seek medical care.
- Avoid swimming if you have any sores on your skin.

EXPECTED OUTCOMES
With treatment, symptoms will begin to improve in 2 to 3 days, and complete recovery occurs in 7 to 10 days. Complications are rare, but may develop in those with chronic disease or weak immune systems.

POSSIBLE COMPLICATIONS
- Blood poisoning, if bacteria enter the bloodstream.
- Brain infection, if the condition occurs on the central part of the face.
- Infection of the bone, muscle, and tissue beneath the affected areas.
- Vein or lymph gland inflammation.

 DIAGNOSIS & TREATMENT

GENERAL MEASURES
- Your health care provider can usually diagnose the disorder by a physical exam of the affected area. Medical tests may include blood tests and study of a sample of fluid removed from the affected skin.
- Treatment is with drugs for the infection, rest, and hospital care, if needed.
- Soak the area in warm water to help it heal. This may also reduce pain and swelling.
- Elevate the affected area. Rest the arm or leg on a pillow. Don't move that area of your body unless you have to. This can help reduce swelling.
- If too much fluid is lost from the skin, you may need hospital care. Replacement fluids will be given through a tube into a vein under the skin.

MEDICATIONS
- Antibiotics will be prescribed for infection. They may be taken by mouth or injection. Complete the entire dose prescribed, even if symptoms disappear quickly.
- Use acetaminophen or ibuprofen for minor pain and fever.

ACTIVITY
Get extra rest until symptoms improve. Then return to your normal level of activity.

DIET
No special diet.

 NOTIFY OUR OFFICE IF

- You or a family member has symptoms of cellulitis.
- The following occur during treatment:
  - High fever and chills.
  - Pain, redness, or swelling increases.
  - Red streaks continue to extend, despite treatment.
  - Vomiting.
- New, unexplained symptoms develop. Drugs used in treatment may produce side effects.

Special notes:

_____

_____

_____

More notes on the back of this page ☐

CEREBRAL PALSY (CP)

 BASIC INFORMATION

DESCRIPTION
A group of chronic disorders that affect muscle movement and body coordination. Cerebral refers to the brain and palsy refers to a disorder of movement. It is generally diagnosed in the first 1 to 2 years of life.

FREQUENT SIGNS AND SYMPTOMS
· The number and severity of the following symptoms vary widely among children with cerebral palsy.
· Early sucking difficulty with the breast or bottle.
· Lack of normal muscle tone (early).
· Slow development (walking, talking).
· Unusual body postures.
· Stiffness and muscle spasms (later).
· Uncontrolled body movements.
· Poor coordination or balance.
· Crossed eyes.
· Impaired hearing, vision, or speech.
· Convulsions.
· Normal or above normal intelligence or degrees of mental retardation.

CAUSES
Damage to motor areas of the brain that disrupts its ability to adequately control movement and posture. The reason is often unknown. In most cases, the damage occurs before, during, or shortly after birth, or during infancy. Cerebral palsy is not inherited.

RISK INCREASES WITH
· Birth injury, including severe oxygen shortage.
· Congenital malformation of the nervous system.
· Jaundice in an infant.
· Rh incompatibility (a blood disorder).
· Stroke in a fetus or newborn, or seizures in newborn.
· Low Apgar score (a rating scale done on newborns).
· An infection in the mother during pregnancy, such as rubella (German measles) or toxoplasmosis.
· Prematurity and low birthweight.
· Breech birth, complicated labor and delivery, or maternal bleeding late in pregnancy.
· Mothers that have hyperthyroidism, mental retardation, or seizure disorder.
· Brain disease (meningitis or encephalitis).
· Head injuries during infancy or childhood.

PREVENTIVE MEASURES
Get treatment for, or avoid, preventable risk factors. Get good medical care during pregnancy and don't smoke, use alcohol, or abuse drugs. Protect infants from accidents or injuries.

EXPECTED OUTCOMES
It is not progressive and children will vary widely in the severity of the condition. A child with CP may have high intelligence despite major muscular disability. Those with less-severe impairment can lead relatively normal, productive lives. Children with severe impairments may require special care.

POSSIBLE COMPLICATIONS
Joint deformities; problems with nutrition, speech, vision, or hearing; mental retardation; or seizures.

 DIAGNOSIS & TREATMENT

GENERAL MEASURES
· Your child's health care provider will do a physical exam. Medical tests include testing motor skills and reflexes. Tests are also done to rule out other disorders.
· You and your child's health care team will decide on a program of care based on your child's special needs. The program will change over time as the child matures and the needs change.
· The program can include drug therapy, physical therapy, occupational and speech therapy, behavior therapy, and emotional help. Braces, casts, mechanical aids, hearing aids, and surgery help some specific problems.
· Parents often join a support group to seek help and advice from other parents whose children have CP.
· To learn more: United Cerebral Palsy Foundation, 1660 L St. NW, Suite 700, Washington, DC 20036; (800) 872-5827; website: www.ucp.org.

MEDICATIONS
· Drugs may be prescribed for seizures, to control spasticity, or to reduce abnormal movements. Alcohol "washes" or injections into muscles may be done to reduce spasticity for short periods.
· Stool softeners can be used for constipation.

ACTIVITY
Limits or abilities will depend on degree of impairment.

DIET
Eating and swallowing may be difficult. Special diets and feeding techniques may be needed.

 NOTIFY OUR OFFICE IF

· You are concerned about your child's development or suspect cerebral palsy.
· After diagnosis, you have concerns about your child.

Special notes:

_____

_____

_____

More notes on the back of this page ☐

CERVICAL CANCER

 ## BASIC INFORMATION

DESCRIPTION
Cancer of the cervix. The cervix is the long neck at the end of the uterus where it meets the vagina. While the average age of women at diagnosis is about 45, this cancer can affect women of all ages.

FREQUENT SIGNS AND SYMPTOMS
- In the early stages, there are usually no symptoms.
- Pelvic pain. Pain may occur in the hip and thigh.
- Heavy menstrual periods.
- Spotting or bleeding between menstrual periods.
- Vaginal discharge.
- Pain and bleeding after intercourse.
- Abdominal pain.
- Leaking of feces and urine through the vagina.
- Appetite and weight loss.
- Anemia.
- Weakness.

CAUSES
Unknown. It is probably related to viral infections, specifically human papillomavirus (genital warts).

RISK INCREASES WITH
- Early age of first intercourse (before age 18).
- Multiple sex partners.
- Multiple pregnancies.
- Human papillomavirus infection (genital warts).
- History of abnormal Pap smears.
- Recurrent vaginal infections.
- Smoking.
- Weak immune system due to illness or drugs.
- Sexually transmitted diseases.
- Daughters of mothers who took DES (diethylstilbestrol) to prevent miscarriage between 1938 and 1971.

MEASURES TO REDUCE RISK FACTORS
- Avoid the risks listed above as much as possible.
- Use latex condoms each time you have sexual intercourse. This is important if you or your partner has had multiple previous partners.
- Get regular pelvic exams.
- Get regular Pap smears. It is a test done to detect cancer of the cervix in an early and treatable stage.

EXPECTED OUTCOME
Usually curable with early diagnosis and treatment.

POSSIBLE COMPLICATIONS
- If cervical cancer is not treated early, it can spread to other parts of the body which can be fatal.
- Complications often occur from treatments.

 ## DIAGNOSIS & TREATMENT

GENERAL MEASURES
- Your health care provider will do a physical exam and a pelvic exam. Medical tests will be done, first to diagnose the cancer, and then others to see if it has spread (called staging).
- Surgery is usually done to remove the cancerous area.
- During early cancer stages, this may involve only a small area of the cervix. This will still allow childbearing. The surgery is usually done as an outpatient.
- The cancer cells may be frozen (cryotherapy), cut out with an electrical loop, burned away by laser, or removed in a cone biopsy. Your health care provider will explain these options and any risk factors involved.
- More advanced stages may require removal of the reproductive organs and other affected tissue (radical hysterectomy).
- Chemotherapy and radiation therapy (internal, external, or both) are other treatments for advanced cancer.
- To learn more: The American Cancer Society, (800) ACS-2345; website: cancer.org or National Cancer Institute, (800)4-CANCER; website: www.nci.nih.gov.

MEDICATION
Anticancer drugs (chemotherapy) may be prescribed.

ACTIVITY
- Usually no limits.
- Avoid tampons following surgery.
- You will be advised when you can resume sexual activity.

DIET
Eat a well-balanced diet. Nutritional supplements may be needed if regular food cannot be tolerated.

 ## NOTIFY OUR OFFICE IF

- You or a family member has persistent vaginal bleeding or other symptoms of cervical cancer.
- You have not had a pelvic exam or Pap smear in the past year.
- New symptoms develop after treatment.

Special notes:

_____

_____

_____

More notes on the back of this page ☐

CERVICAL DYSPLASIA

 BASIC INFORMATION

DESCRIPTION

Cervical dysplasia is the growth of abnormal cells on the lining of the cervix. It may be mild, moderate, or severe, depending on the spread and type of the abnormal cells. Dysplasia is not cancer, but can become cancerous. Dysplasia occurs in females age 15 and over, and most often in those age 25 to 35.

FREQUENT SIGNS AND SYMPTOMS

Usually no signs or symptoms occur. The diagnosis results from a routine Pap smear test.

CAUSES

It is believed to be due to human papillomavirus (genital warts) or similar viruses. The human papillomavirus (HPV) is acquired from sexual intercourse, and can, in rare instances, be acquired from skin-to-skin contact.

RISK INCREASES WITH

- History of infection with the human papillomavirus (HPV), which causes genital warts.
- Having a sexually transmitted disease.
- Smoking.
- Weak immune system due to illness or drugs.
- Multiple sexual partners or having sex with a man who has had multiple sexual partners.
- Pregnancy.
- Daughters of mothers who took DES (diethylstilbestrol) to prevent miscarriage between 1938 and 1971.
- Early age of first sexual intercourse (before age 18).
- Lack of folic acid in the diet may play a role.

PREVENTIVE MEASURES

- Sexual monogamy of both partners.
- Yearly Pap smears (will not prevent dysplasia, but will aid in early diagnosis).
- Don't smoke. Avoid second-hand smoke.
- Use of a diaphragm by the female or a condom by the male for sexual intercourse.
- Eat a healthy diet.

EXPECTED OUTCOME

Most dysplasia is the mild form. Many of these cases resolve without treatment. Moderate to severe dysplasia can usually be cured with treatment.

POSSIBLE COMPLICATIONS

- Some moderate or severe dysplasia may progress to cancer of the cervix. It can take years for this to happen.
- Dysplasia may recur after treatment. If a woman has completed childbearing, recurrent dysplasia can be treated with a hysterectomy.
- Rarely, treatment may cause bleeding or infection.

 DIAGNOSIS & TREATMENT

GENERAL MEASURES

- Your health care provider will do a pelvic exam. Medical tests include a Pap smear. A swab of cervical cells may be taken for exam to check for HPV. A colposcopy (exam of the cervix with an instrument with a lighted tip) may be done. It can be combined with a biopsy. A biopsy involves removal of any tissue that appears abnormal for viewing with a microscope. Other tests may be done if further diagnosis is needed. The results of these tests help classify the dysplasia.
- Treatment will vary depending on the degree and extent of the cervical dysplasia. No treatment may be recommended in some cases. Follow up visits will be needed to be sure the dysplasia clears up on its own.
- The abnormal cells may be frozen (cryotherapy), cut out with an electrical loop, burned away by laser, or removed in a cone biopsy. Your health care provider will explain these options and any risk factors involved.
- Follow-up care will depend on the treatment method.
- Follow-up Pap smears every 3 to 6 months, for 1 to 2 years, are usually recommended. This will verify the success of treatment and detect any recurrence. Be sure to schedule annual Pap smears after that time.

MEDICATION

- You may use nonprescription drugs, such as acetaminophen, for minor pain.
- Prescription pain drugs may be prescribed depending on the treatment procedure.

ACTIVITY

- After treatment, resume daily activities, including work, as soon as you are able.
- Delay sexual relations until a follow-up medical exam shows that healing is complete.

DIET

No special diet.

 NOTIFY OUR OFFICE IF

- You or a family member needs to schedule a visit for pelvic exam and Pap test.
- After dysplasia treatment, any new symptoms occur.

Special notes:

_____

_____

_____

More notes on the back of this page ☐

CERVICAL POLYPS

 BASIC INFORMATION

DESCRIPTION

A common disorder that involves a small growth on the cervix. The cervix is the long neck at the end of the uterus where it meets the vagina. Polyps vary in size and look like a bulb on a thin stem. There may be one (usually) or groups of polyps. A polyp can't be seen or felt by a woman. They occur most often in women over age 20 who have had at least one child.

FREQUENT SIGNS AND SYMPTOMS

· No symptoms. They are often found on a routine pelvic exam.
· Bleeding between monthly menstrual periods.
· Heavier bleeding during periods.
· Spotting of blood after sexual intercourse.
· Vaginal discharge.

CAUSES

Exact cause is unknown. Inflammation of the cervix may be involved. This can be from infection, erosion, or other problems. The majority of polyps are benign (not cancerous). In very rare cases, they represent early cancer of the cervix. They are not contagious.

RISK INCREASES WITH

· Women over age 20 who have had one child.
· Recurrent vaginitis or cervicitis (inflammation or infection of the cervix).

PREVENTIVE MEASURES

· No specific preventive measures.
· Get regular pelvic exams and Pap tests. This is the best way to identify cervical polyps.

EXPECTED OUTCOME

Polyps are easily treated and seldom grow back.

POSSIBLE COMPLICATIONS

· Infection can develop following surgery.
· In very rare cases, cancer may first appear as a polyp.
· After treatment, polyps may grow again on another area of the cervix.

 DIAGNOSIS & TREATMENT

GENERAL MEASURES

· Your health care provider will do a pelvic exam. Medical tests are usually not needed.
· Treatment involves surgery to remove the polyps. This can usually be done in a simple office procedure. All tissue removed is examined in a laboratory for any sign of cancer.
· Polyps are usually removed by gently twisting the stem with forceps to break it off.
· A dilation and curettage (D & C) may be done. This involves a scraping procedure.
· You may feel brief, mild pain during the procedure. Mild to moderate cramps may occur for several hours. Spotting of blood may last for a few days.
· If the polyp is large or has a thick stalk, it may require surgery that is more extensive. This may be done in a hospital.
· Don't douche unless it is recommended.
· Use small sanitary pads to protect your clothing from creams or suppositories.

MEDICATION

· Use acetaminophen or ibuprofen for minor pain.
· Antibiotics may be prescribed if signs of an infection are present. Antibiotics can interfere with the effectiveness of some birth control pills. If you are currently taking birth control pills, discuss this with your health care provider.

ACTIVITY

No limits. Delay sexual relations until a follow-up pelvic exam confirms that healing is complete.

DIET

No special diet.

 NOTIFY OUR OFFICE IF

· You or a family member has symptoms of cervical polyps.
· The following occur after treatment:
  - Discomfort persists longer than 1 week.
  - Unexplained vaginal bleeding or swelling develops.

Special notes:

_____

_____

_____

More notes on the back of this page ☐

CERVICAL SPONDYLOSIS

 BASIC INFORMATION

DESCRIPTION
Changes to the spine, at the back of the neck, that occur with aging. These changes can cause problems when they put pressure on the nerves and blood vessels. The disorder is more common in people over age 50, and affects males more often than females.

FREQUENT SIGNS AND SYMPTOMS
· Stiffness and pain in the neck that extends to the shoulder blades, top of the shoulders, upper arms, hands, or back of the head.
· Crunching sounds with movement of the neck or shoulder muscles.
· Numbness and tingling in the arms, hands, and fingers. There is some loss of feeling in the hands, as well as slowing of reflexes.
· Muscle weakness or muscle spasms.
· Headache.
· Dizziness; unsteady walk.
· Feeling extra tired and having disturbed sleep.

CAUSES
With aging, there is wear and tear on the vertebrae (bones of the spine) and the disks between these vertebrae. Bony growths called osteophytes (or spurs) can develop on the vertebrae. Because of these changes, there can be pressure on nerves and blood vessels.

RISK INCREASES WITH
· Adults over age 50.
· Arthritis (inflammation of a joint).
· Previous injuries such as automobile accidents with "whiplash" injury, athletic injuries, or falls.
· Osteoarthritis (wear and tear on joints that comes with aging).
· Smoking may be a risk factor.

PREVENTIVE MEASURES
· There are no specific preventive measures for cervical spondylosis. It comes with aging.
· You can prevent some neck injuries, which might help prevent the risk. Wear protective headgear for contact sports. Use seat belts in vehicles and keep headrests at proper height. Ask your health care provider about neck stretching exercises that you can do on a regular basis.

EXPECTED OUTCOMES
Treatment does not cure the disorder, but does help improve the symptoms and prevent further problems.

POSSIBLE COMPLICATIONS
· Reduced neck flexibility.
· Chronic neck pain.
· Unable to control bowel or urine functions.

 DIAGNOSIS & TREATMENT

GENERAL MEASURES
· Your health care provider will do a physical exam and ask questions about your symptoms. X-rays or MRI scans may be obtained to confirm the diagnosis. Follow any instructions from your health care provider or try the treatment steps listed.
· Wear a cervical collar (neck brace) to prevent unexpected neck-muscle strain.
· Apply moist heat. Take warm showers twice a day and let the water beat on neck and shoulders. Between showers, apply warm soaks to neck. Soak towel or cloth in hot water, wring out, and apply.
· Gentle massage will often help.
· Improve your posture. Pull in the chin and abdomen when sitting or standing. Use a firm chair and sit with buttocks against the back.
· Sleep without a pillow. Instead, use a cervical pillow, wear a soft fabric collar, or put a small rolled towel under the neck.
· If numbness or pain affects the hands or arms, buy or rent a cervical-traction device. To set it up, follow the directions that come with the device.
· Ultrasonic treatments may be recommended.
· Surgery (sometimes) to fuse neck bones, remove a damaged disk. or enlarge the spinal-cord space.

MEDICATIONS
· For minor pain, you may use aspirin or ibuprofen.
· For serious discomfort, stronger pain medicine, muscle relaxants, or antidepressants may be prescribed.

ACTIVITY
Decrease activity or rest in bed for 2 to 3 days. Increase activity as symptoms improve. Swimming and walking are good ways to exercise.

DIET
No special diet.

 NOTIFY OUR OFFICE IF

· You or a family member has symptoms of cervical spondylosis.
· Symptoms persist or worsen despite, treatment.

Special notes:

_____

_____

_____

More notes on the back of this page ☐

CERVICITIS

 ## BASIC INFORMATION

DESCRIPTION

Inflammation of the cervix. The cervix is the long neck at the end of the uterus where it meets the vagina. Cervicitis occurs more often in women under age 25.

FREQUENT SIGNS AND SYMPTOMS

- Often no symptoms occur.
- Vaginal discharge. It may be thick and creamy, foamy and greenish-white, white and curd-like, or thin and grey.
- There may be bleeding after sexual intercourse.

CAUSES

- Infection. Cervicitis is most often caused by an infection (usually a sexually transmitted disease). Bacteria infections, *Neisseria gonorrhoeae* or *Chlamydia trachomatis,* are the most common. Herpes simplex or human papillomavirus (HPV) can also be the cause.
- Allergic reaction (such as to latex).
- Injury or irritation.

RISK INCREASES WITH

- Multiple sexual partners.
- Women who begin having sex at an early age.
- History of sexually transmitted diseases.
- Acute or recurrent vaginitis (vaginal inflammation).

PREVENTIVE MEASURES

- Avoid sexually transmitted diseases. Do not have sexual intercourse with an infected partner. If unsure, have your sexual partner wear a condom during sexual activity.
- Have regular pelvic exams and Pap smear. This is important if you are sexually active.
- Get treatment for any vaginal infections before they spread to the cervix.
- Avoid irritants to the cervix, such as douches or sprays.

EXPECTED OUTCOME

Cervicitis can be cured with treatment.

POSSIBLE COMPLICATIONS

- Pelvic inflammatory disease (PID). The infection spreads to other parts of the reproductive system. PID does not cause symptoms and can lead to infertility.
- Salpingitis (inflammation of the fallopian tubes).
- Endometritis (inflammation of the uterus).
- Cervicitis may recur. This happens more often with an untreated sexual partner.

 ## DIAGNOSIS & TREATMENT

GENERAL MEASURES

- Your health care provider will do a pelvic exam. Medical tests usually include a culture of the vaginal discharge and blood studies and a Pap smear.
- Treatment is with drugs to cure any infection. If a sexually transmitted disease caused the cervicitis, your sexual partner must also be treated.
- Use sanitary pads instead of tampons during treatment.
- Don't douche unless it is recommended.
- Repeated or prolonged cervicitis infections may require other treatment, such as surgery to treat the infected cervix tissue.

MEDICATION

- Oral (or sometimes injected) antibiotics will be prescribed for bacterial infection. Antibiotics may interfere with the effectiveness of some birth control pills.
- Antiviral drugs may be prescribed for viral infection.

ACTIVITY

- Avoid sexual relations until the treatment is complete and the symptoms have gone away—for at least 7 days.
- Do not have sexual relations until your partner is treated.

DIET

No special diet.

 ## NOTIFY OUR OFFICE IF

- You or a family member has symptoms of cervicitis.
- During treatment, discomfort lasts longer than one week or symptoms worsen.
- Vaginal bleeding or swelling develops during or after treatment.

Special notes:

_____

_____

_____

More notes on the back of this page ☐

CHALAZION

 BASIC INFORMATION

DESCRIPTION
A lump (also called a cyst) on the eyelid resulting from chronic inflammation of a gland that lubricates the edges of the eyelid. A chalazion is not a stye.

FREQUENT SIGNS AND SYMPTOMS
A painless swelling on the eyelid. At first, it may seem like a stye. The eyelid may swell, and the eye may feel irritated. After a few days, these early symptoms go away. There is then a painless, slow-growing, firm lump in the eyelid. Skin over the lump can be moved loosely. The upper eyelid is the one usually affected.

CAUSES
Blockage of a type of sweat gland in the eyelid. The blockage may be due to infection.

RISK INCREASES WITH
Skin conditions such as acne or dermatitis.

PREVENTIVE MEASURES
There are no specific measures to prevent chalazions.

EXPECTED OUTCOMES
A chalazion may heal by itself. If not, it can be treated.

POSSIBLE COMPLICATIONS
Some people are prone to chalazions. Once you have one chalazion, you are more likely to get another one.

 DIAGNOSIS & TREATMENT

GENERAL MEASURES
• Self-care is often all that is needed.
• Use warm-water soaks to reduce irritation and swelling. The soaks may also make the area heal faster. Apply soaks for 20 minutes, then rest at least 1 hour. Gently massage the area several times a day. Do not squeeze or try to pop the chalazion.

• See your health care provider if you are concerned about the problem. An exam will be made of the affected eyelid area. Medical tests are not required.
• Treatment may involve drugs to be applied to the eyelid, drugs injected into the chalazion, or surgery to remove it.
• Surgery to remove the chalazion may be recommended. This is usually done in your health care provider's office. The area will be numbed before the lump is removed.
• If you have a tendency to get chalazions, wash your eyelid area every day. Wash with water and baby shampoo that is diluted with water. There is also a commercial product available to clean eyelids. Apply either solution with a cotton swab and rinse with warm water.
• When you first notice that your eyes are getting irritated, use warm compresses and massage the area several times a day. Repeat as often as needed.

MEDICATIONS
• Ointments, drops, or creams that are put on the eye may be prescribed. These drugs help to kill bacteria. Follow instructions provided with the prescription.
• Injection of a drug into the chalazion may be recommended.

ACTIVITY
No limits.

DIET
No special diet.

 NOTIFY OUR OFFICE IF

• You or a family member has symptoms of a chalazion that is not better after 3 to 4 days of self-care.
• Fever, headache, vision changes, eye pain, eye discharge, or swollen eyes occur.

Special notes:

_____

_____

_____

More notes on the back of this page ☐

CHICKENPOX
(Varicella)

 BASIC INFORMATION

DESCRIPTION

A very contagious disease caused by the herpes zoster virus. Symptoms are usually mild in children and may be more severe in adults. Chickenpox can affect all ages, but is most common in children.

FREQUENT SIGNS AND SYMPTOMS

- Fever.
- Abdominal pain or a general ill feeling that lasts 1 to 2 days.
- Skin eruptions that appear almost anywhere on the body, including the scalp, penis, and inside the mouth, nose, throat, or vagina. They may be scattered over large areas, and they occur least on the arms and legs. Blisters collapse within 24 hours and form scabs. New crops of blisters erupt every 3 to 4 days.
- Adults have other symptoms that resemble influenza.

CAUSES

- Infection with the herpes zoster virus. It is spread from person to person by airborne droplets or contact with a skin eruption on an infected person. Symptoms may appear 7 to 21 days after exposure.
- A newborn is protected for several months from chickenpox if the mother had the disease before or during pregnancy. The immunity diminishes in 4 to 12 months.

RISK INCREASES WITH

Weak immune system due to illness or drugs.

PREVENTIVE MEASURES

- Varicella vaccine for healthy children 12 months or older.
- An immune globulin may be used for high-risk persons, such as those who take anticancer or immunosuppressive drugs if they become exposed to the virus.

EXPECTED OUTCOMES

- Children usually recover in 7 to 10 days. Adults may take longer. Adults and persons with weak immune systems are more at risk for complications.
- After recovery, a person has lifelong immunity against a recurrence of chickenpox.
- After chickenpox runs its course, the virus sometimes remains dormant in the body (probably in the roots of nerves near the spinal cord). The same virus may cause shingles many years later.

POSSIBLE COMPLICATIONS

- Bacterial infection of chickenpox blisters. Scarring, if blisters become infected (rare).
- Pneumonia.
- Central nervous system complications (rare).
- Shingles many years later in adulthood (possibly).

 DIAGNOSIS & TREATMENT

GENERAL MEASURES

- Your health care provider can diagnose chickenpox by the appearance of the skin eruptions. Medical tests are usually not needed.
- Treatment is directed toward relieving symptoms. Drug therapy may be prescribed for some patients.
- Use cool-water soaks or cool-water compresses to reduce itching.
- Keep the patient as quiet and cool as possible. Heat and sweat trigger itching.
- Keep the nails short to discourage scratching, which can lead to secondary infection.

MEDICATIONS

- To decrease itching: Topical anesthetics and topical antihistamines provide quick, short-term relief. Preparations containing lidocaine and pramoxine are least likely to cause allergic skin reactions. Lotions that contain phenol, menthol, and camphor (such as calamine lotion) may be recommended. Follow package instructions.
- To reduce fever, use acetaminophen or ibuprofen. Never use aspirin, as it may contribute to the development of Reye's syndrome (a form of encephalitis) when given to children during a viral illness.
- An antiviral drug may be prescribed in some cases.

ACTIVITY

- Bed rest is not needed. Allow quiet activity in a cool environment. A child may play outdoors in the shade during nice weather.
- Keep an ill child away from others, and from school, until all blisters have crusted and no new ones occur.

DIET

Blisters in the mouth may make eating and drinking painful. Fluid intake is needed to prevent dehydration. Try Popsicles, cool drinks, and bland foods.

 NOTIFY OUR OFFICE IF

- You or your child has symptoms of chickenpox.
- Cough, headache, or sensitivity to bright light. develop, fever rises or blisters appear infected.

Special notes:

_____

_____

_____

More notes on the back of this page ☐

CHILD ABUSE

 BASIC INFORMATION

DESCRIPTION

The major types of child abuse (or maltreatment) are:
• *Physical abuse* is physical injury (from minor injury to broken bones, or death). A child may be hit, bitten, shaken, punched, kicked, beaten, burned, or harmed in other ways.
• *Sexual abuse* includes touching a child's genitals, intercourse, forcing a child to watch sexual acts, having a child touch or look at an adult's genitals, watch or be in pornographic films, and any other sexual act.
• *Emotional abuse* harms a child's emotional growth or can destroy a child's confidence. Constant yelling and screaming, name-calling, threats, and not giving love and affection are forms of this abuse.
• *Child neglect* is when the child's basic needs are not met. This can include lack of proper food, clothes, school, hygiene, medical care, or leaving a child alone.

FREQUENT SIGNS AND SYMPTOMS

• All types of abuse will cause both physical and behavioral signs. Parents or other adults who know the child are unlikely to suspect child abuse. A child's injuries or behavior changes can result from other problems also.
• Physical signs. Any type of injury (mild or serious), pain when they urinate, genital bleeding, weight loss or no weight gain (in infants), stomach pain, headaches, or infections. Pregnancy in young adolescents.
• Behavioral signs. Avoiding family and friends, a change in eating habits, sleeping problems, emotional upsets, and poor school performance. Outgrown habits such as bed-wetting or thumb-sucking may recur. There may be inappropriate sexual behavior.
• Older children may abuse drugs or alcohol, talk about suicide, or behave in a reckless and destructive manner.

CAUSES

Abusers are more likely to be someone the child knows, rather than a stranger. Abusers may be parents, relatives, neighbor, babysitters, or other caregivers.

RISK INCREASES WITH

Children:
• A child of any age, sex, race, religion, rich or poor can be a victim of abuse.
• Infants under age one are at a high risk for injury.
• Females are more likely to suffer sexual abuse.
Adult abusers:
• Parents lacking parenting skills, and those with financial, relationship, mental, emotional, or stress problems.
• Adults who were victims of child abuse.

PREVENTIVE MEASURES

• For children, age-appropriate education about abuse.
• If you suspect child abuse, report it without delay.

EXPECTED OUTCOMES

The best hope for the child is early discovery of the problem, and prompt action and treatment.

POSSIBLE COMPLICATIONS

• Physical injuries that could be fatal.
• Serious emotional and mental problems for the child.
• Risk for many different types of problems later in life.

 DIAGNOSIS & TREATMENT

GENERAL MEASURES

• Children are often afraid to tell anyone about abuse. They feel they are at fault and no one will believe them.
• If your child tells you about abuse, stay calm and let the child know that he or she is believed. Take steps to protect the child. Take action to report the abuse. You may want to call the local Child Protective Service. If you are unsure what to do, ask someone you trust.
• Call your child's health care provider if you think your child has been abused. Treatment will be given for any injuries. The child may need hospital care. Health care providers must report any suspected or known cases of child abuse to the proper authorities.
• Mental health counseling for the child and the family can help everyone learn ways to cope better.
• To learn more: Childhelp USA, 15757 N. 78 Ave., Scottsdale, AZ 85260; (480) 922-8212 (not toll free); website: www.childhelpusa.org.
• To report child abuse, call the Local Child Protective Services or the national hotline (800) 422-4453.
• If you have abused a child or think you might, seek help. Call your health care provider or a local help line.

MEDICATIONS

Drugs may be needed to treat or prevent a sexually transmitted disease (STD), or to prevent a pregnancy.

ACTIVITY

No limits unless a child's injuries cause problems.

DIET

No special diet.

 NOTIFY OUR OFFICE IF

• You or another adult suspects child abuse.
• Your child has been abused and needs help coping.

Special notes:

_____

_____

_____

More notes on the back of this page ☐

CHILDHOOD OBESITY

 BASIC INFORMATION

DESCRIPTION
Obesity (or being overweight) means having too much body fat. In children or adolescents, it means they weigh more than normal for their age, height, and sex.

FREQUENT SIGNS AND SYMPTOMS
A health care provider will usually diagnose an overweight child, but a parent may notice that a child:
· Appears heavier than other children of the same age.
· Eats a lot of food, but is always hungry.
· Often feels tired and is not very active physically.

CAUSES
· Usually it is a combination of too little physical activity, being sedentary (sitting for long periods), and poor eating habits (eating too many high-calorie foods).
· A child's genes can play a small part. Genes are what determine a person's height; hair, eye, and skin color.
· A few children may have a hormone problem.

RISK INCREASES WITH
· Not being physically active. Watching television or sitting at a computer for several hours a day.
· Unhealthy eating habits. Eating foods high in fat and sugar. Eating while watching television. Eating when not hungry. Eating too many fast-food meals.
· A child who has obese parents.

PREVENTIVE MEASURES
· Children learn from their parents. If parents practice healthy eating and physical activity habits themselves, their children are more likely to make the right choices.
· Parents should not use food as a reward system.
· Schools need to serve healthful food in school meals.

EXPECTED OUTCOMES
Parents who are concerned and involved can help a child lose weight and increase physical activity levels. It takes time and effort and should be a long-term goal.

POSSIBLE COMPLICATIONS
· Emotional problems, such as being teased by other children, low self-esteem, depression, and anxiety.
· Health risks while still a child and later as an adult. These include type 2 diabetes, problems that can lead to heart disease, orthopedic (bone and muscle) problems, liver disease, asthma, and overweight as an adult.

 DIAGNOSIS & TREATMENT

GENERAL MEASURES
· Health care providers use growth charts as one tool to track children's growth and development. These charts list ideal weights and normal BMI (body mass index) scores for the child's age, height and sex. A BMI score is computed using a child's age, height, and weight. During well-child exams, your child's weight and height are compared to these charts. The results may show the child is overweight. If the child's excess weight is a health concern, a weight loss treatment plan should be worked out.
· A child's treatment plan has five parts. They include goals for pounds to lose, new eating habits, more physical activity, behavior changes, and family involvement.
· Goals for weight loss and physical activity should start low. Your child can see results and not feel stressed.
· Have your child keep a food and activity diary. Write down information about what they eat and do. It helps to see where there is success or a possible problem.
· Reward your child when a certain goal or behavior change is achieved. Don't use food as a reward.
· To learn more: American Obesity Association, 1250 24th St., NW, Suite 300, Washington, DC 20037; (800) 98-obese; website: www.obesity.org. To calculate a child's BMI: www.obesityhelp.com/kidscalc.php. The Centers for Disease Control and Prevention (CDC) has a website to answer children's questions: www.bam.gov.

MEDICATIONS
Drugs used for adult obesity are not used for children.

ACTIVITY
· Establish limits on TV watching and computer time.
· Your child should spend 30 to 60 minutes daily being physically active. This time can include sports, exercise, active games, and doing chores.
· Get the whole family to walk, skate or bike together.

DIET
· Plan healthy meals for the whole family that you sit down and eat together. This way your child won't feel alone in changing eating habits.
· Read food labels. Don't buy foods high in calories, fat and sugar. Look for high fiber food items.
· Limit the number of fast-food meals each week.
· Drink fat-free milk (if the child is over 2).
· Avoid juices and drinks with high sugar content.

 NOTIFY OUR OFFICE IF

· You have concerns about your child's weight.
· You need help in diet planning.

Special notes:

_____

_____

_____

More notes on the back of this page ☐

CHLAMYDIAL INFECTION
(Chamydia)

 BASIC INFORMATION

DESCRIPTION

An infection caused by a bacterium. It causes inflammation of the urethra (the tube that allows urine from the bladder to pass outside the body), vagina, cervix, uterus, fallopian tubes, ovaries, penis, and anus. It is a common sexually transmitted disease in the United States. It can affect anyone who is sexually active. Chlamydial infection may also be transmitted to the eyes or lungs of a newborn infant.

FREQUENT SIGNS AND SYMPTOMS

· Sometimes there are no symptoms during the early stages.
· Women commonly have more symptoms than men.
· Vaginal discharge.
· Urethral discharge (males).
· Anal swelling, pain, or discharge.
· Vagina or tip of the penis becomes reddened.
· Stomach pain.
· Fever.
· Pain when urinating.
· Genital discomfort or pain.

CAUSES

Chlamydia trachomatis bacteria. Symptoms may appear 1 to 3 weeks after exposure. It is spread by:
· Vaginal sexual intercourse.
· Anal sexual intercourse.
· Oral-genital contact.
· Vaginal infection during delivery of a newborn, which may infect the baby.

RISK INCREASES WITH

· Sexually active men and women.
· Unprotected sexual activity, especially in young females.
· Having other sexually transmitted diseases.
· Multiple sex partners.
· Diabetes.
· General poor health.

PREVENTIVE MEASURES

Practice safe sex. Do not have sexual intercourse with an infected partner. If unsure, have your sexual partner wear a condom for sexual activity.

EXPECTED OUTCOME

Complete cure with adequate antibiotic treatment.

POSSIBLE COMPLICATIONS

· Infertility and/or sterility in female.
· Infecting one's sexual partner.
· Infections in pelvic organs, genitals, or rectum.
· Ectopic pregnancy.
· Liver infection (perihepatitis).
· Reiter's syndrome (a type of arthritis).

 DIAGNOSIS & TREATMENT

GENERAL MEASURES

· Your health care provider will do an exam of the genital area. Medical tests may include vaginal smear, rectal smear, and urethral smear for analysis. Testing for other sexually transmitted diseases is recommended.
· Treatment is with antibiotic drugs. All sexual partners must be treated.
· Keep the genital area clean. Use plain unscented soap. Take showers rather than baths.
· Women should wear cotton underpants or pantyhose with a cotton crotch. Avoid those made from non-ventilating materials, such as nylon.
· After urination or bowel movements, cleanse by wiping or washing from front to back (vagina to anus).
· Avoid douches.
· If urinating causes burning, urinate through a tubular device, such as a toilet-paper roll or plastic cup with the bottom cut out, or pour a cup of warm water over the genital area while urinating.
· A follow-up medical exam may be needed after completing the prescribed treatment.

MEDICATION

Oral antibiotics are usually prescribed. Antibiotics may interfere with the effectiveness of some birth control pills. If you are currently taking birth control pills, discuss this with your health care provider.

ACTIVITY

Avoid sexual relations until treatment is completed and symptoms are gone.

DIET

No special diet.

 NOTIFY OUR OFFICE IF

· You or a family member has symptoms of chlamydial infection.
· Symptoms last longer than one week or get worse.
· Unusual vaginal bleeding or swelling develops.
· New, unexplained symptoms develop. Drugs used in treatment may produce side effects.

Special notes:

_____

_____

_____

More notes on the back of this page ☐

90

CHOLECYSTITIS or CHOLANGITIS

 ## BASIC INFORMATION

DESCRIPTION

Cholecystitis is inflammation of the gallbladder. Cholangitis is inflammation of the ducts (tubes) that drain bile from the gallbladder to the small intestine. In both conditions, a bacterial infection may develop. The conditions usually occur in older adults (women more than men). They may rarely occur in children or teens.

FREQUENT SIGNS AND SYMPTOMS

· Cramping pain in the upper right of the abdomen. Pain may also occur in the chest (imitating a heart attack), in the upper back, or the right shoulder. These symptoms frequently follow a meal rich in fats.
· Tenderness in the upper abdomen.
· Nausea and vomiting.
· Belching.
· Slight fever. High fever and chills if there is infection.
· Jaundice (yellow skin and eyes) may occur.
· Pale stools (sometimes).
· Skin itching (sometimes).

CAUSES

· Cholecystitis usually results when a gallstone blocks the outlet of the gallbladder and bile builds up. Chronic cholecystitis results from recurrent inflammation.
· Acalculous cholecystitis is inflammation not caused by gallstones. It may be due to severe illness, surgery, burns, or injury.
· Cholangitis occurs when one or more gallstones pass from the gallbladder into the main bile duct and become lodged. Bile builds up behind the blockage.

RISK INCREASES WITH

· Gallstones.
· Injury or trauma.
· Heart surgery.
· Pregnancy.
· Rapid weight loss, or losing and regaining weight.
· Parasite infection.

PREVENTIVE MEASURES

Avoid risk factors when possible.

EXPECTED OUTCOMES

· Some mild uncomplicated attacks clear up on their own in 1 to 4 days. Most episodes require treatment.
· Recurrences are common. Attacks will stop after surgery to remove the gallbladder.

POSSIBLE COMPLICATIONS

· Gallbladder perforation and peritonitis (inflammation of the lining of the abdomen).
· Blood infection (sepsis).
· Hepatitis (liver inflammation).
· Gallstones may cause intestinal blockage.
· Choledocholithiasis (gallstone in common bile duct).

 ## DIAGNOSIS & TREATMENT

GENERAL MEASURES

· Your health care provider will do a physical exam and ask questions about your symptoms. Medical tests may include blood studies, x-rays, ultrasound, CT, HIDA scans (special x-rays), and gallbladder ejection fraction.
· Specific treatment will depend on degree of severity, infection, size of stones, and your general health.
· Hospital care with emergency treatment may be required for complications.
· In some patients, a tube may be placed through the skin to drain the gallbladder.
· Surgical treatment is usually a cholecystectomy (gallbladder removal) done by laparoscopic technique.
· Nonsurgical treatment methods for gallstones are less often used. They include drugs to dissolve the stones or extracorporeal shock wave lithotripsy to shatter stones.
· To learn more: National Digestive Diseases Information Clearinghouse, 2 Information Way, Bethesda, MD 20892; (800) 891-5389; website: www.niddk.nih.gov.

MEDICATIONS

· Drugs for pain and vomiting may be prescribed.
· A drug to dissolve gallstones may rarely be recommended. It will take about 2 years, works in 50% of patients, and must be taken indefinitely.
· Antibiotics may be prescribed for infection.

ACTIVITY

· Rest in bed until symptoms disappear or recovery from surgery is complete. While in bed, move your legs often to reduce the risk of deep-vein blood clotting.
· Other limits on activity will depend on treatment.

DIET

· Food intake will be limited during hospital care.
· A low-fat diet may be recommended.

 ## NOTIFY OUR OFFICE IF

· You or a family member has symptoms of cholecystitis or cholangitis. If symptoms include shortness of breath, sweating, and nausea, call immediately!
· Fever, jaundice, recurrent vomiting, or severe pain, develops after diagnosis or treatment.

Special notes:

_____

_____

_____

More notes on the back of this page ☐

CHRONIC FATIGUE SYNDROME

 BASIC INFORMATION

DESCRIPTION

Chronic fatigue syndrome (CFS) is a disorder that involves profound fatigue. There is usually an abrupt onset of symptoms that come and go for at least six months. It is unknown whether it represents one or many disorders. It is difficult to diagnose because there is no specific medical test, or a defined set of signs and symptoms. It is seen most often in young adults between 20 and 40. Women outnumber the men about two to one.

FREQUENT SIGNS AND SYMPTOMS

- Fatigue.
- Sore throat.
- Mild fever.
- Lymph node pain.
- Muscle weakness, stiffness, and discomfort.
- Headache.
- Sleep disturbances.
- Mood swings; irritability; depression.
- Confusion; forgetfulness.
- Inability to concentrate.
- Vision changes; sensitivity to light.
- Dry eyes, mouth.
- Diarrhea.
- Loss of appetite.

CAUSES

Unknown. An abnormal immune system response may be involved. Many theories center on an infectious agent, but no such agent has been identified. Epstein-Barr (a virus that causes mononucleosis) and others have been implicated.

RISK INCREASES WITH

Unknown.

PREVENTIVE MEASURES

Unknown.

EXPECTED OUTCOME

Symptoms will usually come and go over a period of time. Generally, there is very slow improvement over months or years.

POSSIBLE COMPLICATIONS

None specific to the disorder. Symptoms are usually most severe during the first 6 months.

 DIAGNOSIS & TREATMENT

GENERAL MEASURES

- Your health care provider will do a physical exam and ask questions about your symptoms. There is no one test to identify CFS. Medical disorders that could be causing the fatigue and symptoms will be ruled out first.

- The guidelines used to help define cases are:
  - Persistence of relapsing fatigue that does not resolve with bed rest and is severe enough to reduce average daily activity by at least 50% for at least 6 months.
  - Other chronic clinical conditions have been satisfactorily excluded, including preexisting psychiatric disease.
- Steps in therapy may include a combination of lifestyle changes, starting a gradual exercise program, counseling, behavior therapy, and drug therapy.
- Lifestyle changes may include finding ways to cut back on work or other activities. This may help reduce physical and emotional stress. Stop smoking (find a way to quit that works for you).
- Counseling and/or behavior therapy may be helpful for coping with the emotional aspects of the disorder and learning how to reduce stress.
- Joining a support group is helpful for some patients.
- Learn more: Chronic Fatigue & Immune Dysfunction Syndrome Association, P.O. Box 220398, Charlotte, NC 28222; (800) 442-3437; website: www.cfids.org.

MEDICATION

- There is no specific drug to treat CFS. Drugs may be prescribed for depression, pain, low blood pressure, allergy-like symptoms, insomnia, or other specific symptoms.
- Other drugs are being studied and may prove to be helpful in treatment. Talk to your health care provider before taking herbal remedies or dietary supplements.

ACTIVITY

- Strenuous exercise should be avoided. Some exercise, however, is important. Begin a gradual program that may be just 3 to 5 minutes a day to start with. Increase the activity by about 20% every 2 to 3 weeks. Setbacks will sometimes occur, so don't be discouraged.
- Get enough sleep at night. Limit daytime napping.

DIET

Eat a healthy diet, drink plenty of fluids, limit caffeine, and avoid alcohol.

 NOTIFY OUR OFFICE IF

- You or a family member has symptoms of chronic fatigue syndrome.
- Symptoms worsen after treatment is started.

Special notes:

_____

_____

_____

_____

More notes on the back of this page ☐

CHRONIC OBSTRUCTIVE PULMONARY DISEASE (COPD)

 BASIC INFORMATION

DESCRIPTION
A term used to describe two related disorders (chronic bronchitis and emphysema) that involve impaired airflow in and out of the lungs. Women are more often affected by chronic bronchitis, while men are more often affected by emphysema.

FREQUENT SIGNS AND SYMPTOMS
Chronic bronchitis:
· Frequent cough or coughing spasm. Mucus is usually present. It is thick and difficult to cough up. The mucus color and thickness may change according to whether infection is present.
· Shortness of breath.
Emphysema:
· Often, no symptoms in the early stages.
· Shortness of breath. It becomes worse over several years.
· Lung infections.
· Weight loss.
· Some wheezing or coughing.
· Little mucus is produced.

CAUSES
Bronchitis is caused by production of excess mucus in the lungs. Emphysema causes tiny air sacs in the lungs to become permanently enlarged. Patients with COPD have features of both conditions.

RISK INCREASES WITH
· Cigarette smoking or secondhand smoke.
· An inherited form of emphysema.
· Chronic exposure to dust, ozone, chemicals, smoke, traffic exhaust fumes, sulfur, and others.
· Frequent lung infections in childhood. They can lead to scarring of lung tissue.
· Aging.
· Personal history of allergies or lung disorders.

PREVENTIVE MEASURES
The most important measure is to avoid smoking. Also, avoid breathing smoke from other people's cigarettes. Secondhand smoke can also lead to this condition.

EXPECTED OUTCOME
Lung function will continue to worsen over time. More and more effort is needed to get air in and out of the lungs. Treatment can help relieve symptoms and help prevent infections. Treatment may help you to lead a more active and productive life. Survival times are very different from person to person. Younger patients may have a better prognosis than older persons.

POSSIBLE COMPLICATIONS
· Frequent infections, anxiety, and depression.
· Other lung diseases, heart failure, and death.

 DIAGNOSIS & TREATMENT

GENERAL MEASURES
· Your health care provider will do a physical exam and ask questions about your symptoms and activities. Medical tests may include blood studies, x-rays and lung function testing.
· Goals of treatment are to relieve symptoms, slow progression of the disorder, and prevent complications.
· Treatment may include drug therapy, lifestyle changes, supplemental oxygen, special exercises, and sometimes, surgery. You and your health care provider will discuss a treatment plan depending on your individual needs. Educate yourself about this disorder.
· Usually, you can be treated at home. Hospital care may be needed for infections or if symptoms get worse.
· If you smoke, stop immediately. This is the most important thing you can do. Avoid secondhand smoke and other lung irritants (air pollution, fumes, dust).
· Get vaccine for pneumonia and yearly flu vaccine.
· Avoid excessive heat, cold, and very high altitudes. Talk to your health care provider about airplane travel.
· Lung surgery or a lung transplant may be an option.
· Joining a support group is helpful for some patients.

MEDICATION
· Drugs may be prescribed to improve the symptoms. They can help open narrowed airways, reduce inflammation, treat or prevent infections, and reduce the amount of mucus in your lungs.
· Drugs may be prescribed for depression or anxiety.

ACTIVITY
· Not being active for long periods of time can make your disability worse. Try to maintain a regular exercise program. Walking is usually a good way to exercise.
· Your health care provider may prescribe physical therapy or special breathing exercises.

DIET
Eat a well-balanced diet. Drink plenty of fluids each day.

 NOTIFY OUR OFFICE IF

· You or a family member has symptoms of COPD.
· Any signs of infection develop (such as fever).
· Symptoms get worse despite treatment.

Special notes:

_____

_____

_____

More notes on the back of this page ☐

CHRONIC PELVIC PAIN

 BASIC INFORMATION

DESCRIPTION

Chronic pelvic pain is any pain in the pelvic area that has lasted for at least 6 months. Pelvic pain is a common problem in women and the pain symptoms will vary for each woman.

FREQUENT SIGNS AND SYMPTOMS

• The main symptom is pain in the pelvic and lower stomach and back area. Other terms women use to describe the problem include discomfort, pressure, aches, tenderness, or a heavy feeling.
• The pain may be mild or severe. It may come and go, or it may be there all the time.
• The pain may occur before or during menstrual periods. Some women may have the pain when they have sex or when they exercise.
• Urination and bowel symptoms may occur, such as diarrhea or constipation.

CAUSES

There are many possible causes for this type of pain and sometimes the exact cause is not found. It may involve health problems that are both physical (such as with menstrual periods) and mental (such as stress).

RISK INCREASES WITH

• Prior health problem such as a pelvic infection or pelvic surgery.
• History of abuse as a child or adult.
• Having family members with chronic pelvic pain.

PREVENTIVE MEASURES

Since there are many causes, there is no sure way to prevent it.

EXPECTED OUTCOME

Pain symptoms can usually be helped with one or more types of treatment.

POSSIBLE COMPLICATIONS

• Depression, sleep problems, poor appetite, and weight loss occur along with the pain.
• Pain limits your normal activities and lifestyle.

 DIAGNOSIS & TREATMENT

GENERAL MEASURES

• Diagnosis begins with a physical exam plus a pelvic exam by your health care provider. You will be asked questions about the pain symptoms you are having. Different tests may be ordered to help find the cause of your pain. These include blood and urine studies, a pregnancy test, and a Pap smear (to check the cells in your cervix). X-rays may be needed. Minor surgery using a laparoscope may be necessary. This is an instrument with a thin, lighted tube. It is inserted into the body through a small incision. It can help diagnose and sometimes treat chronic pelvic pain at the same time.
• Treatment will depend on any health problems diagnosed.
• Your health care provider will talk to you about the treatment options for chronic pain and what may work best for you. Options may include drugs (oral and injections), physical therapy, and possibly surgery. It may be helpful to consult a behavior counselor and learn how to relax and control stress in your life.
• If the cause for the pain is unclear, you may be asked to keep a pain diary for 2 or more months. This can help you and your health care provider see how the pain symptoms relate to what is going on in your life day to day.
• For self-care, apply a heating pad to the painful area. Soak in a bathtub.
• To learn more: National Women's Health Information Center (800) 994-9662; website: www.4woman.gov or the OBGYN.net: The Universe of Women's Health website: www.obgyn.net.

MEDICATION

• You may use nonprescription pain relievers such as ibuprofen or naproxen.
• Drugs to treat any medical problems diagnosed or to help control severe pain symptoms.
• Drugs may be used to stop your menstrual periods for 2 months to see if this helps stop pain.

ACTIVITY

Try to maintain a regular exercise program. It can help with the pain. It will also help you build strength and be more flexible.

DIET

No special diet is usually needed.

 NOTIFY OUR OFFICE IF

• You or a family member has symptoms of chronic pelvic pain.
• Your pelvic pain continues despite treatment.

Special notes:

_____

_____

_____

More notes on the back of this page ☐

CIRRHOSIS OF THE LIVER

 ## BASIC INFORMATION

DESCRIPTION

Damage to the liver that develops gradually over months to years. This can lead to serious health problems because the body depends on the liver for a number of vital functions. Cirrhosis usually occurs in people ages 40 to 60. It is more common in men than women.

FREQUENT SIGNS AND SYMPTOMS

Early stages:
- There may be no symptoms.
- Feeling tired and weak.
- Loss of appetite and weight loss. Nausea may occur.
- Pinhead-sized red spots on the skin.

Later stages:
- Yellow skin and eyes (jaundice).
- Palms of the hands may be reddish and blotchy.
- Urine may be dark yellow or brown.
- Loss of body hair and itchy skin.
- Fluid build-up in the stomach (ascites) and legs.
- In men, testicles may shrink; breasts may be swollen.
- Stool may be black or bloody.
- Bleeding and bruising.
- Mental/personality changes.

CAUSES

Liver damage is due to scar tissue that replaces healthy tissue. This blocks the flow of blood through the liver and decreases liver function. A number of disorders can lead to the liver damage.

RISK INCREASES WITH

- Alcoholism. People are all affected differently by alcohol. An amount that causes cirrhosis in one person may not be a problem for another. Nutrition may be a factor.
- Chronic hepatitis B, C, and D.
- Chronic autoimmune hepatitis.
- Blood vessel disease or chronic heart failure.
- Certain inherited disorders.
- Nonalcoholic steatohepatitis (NASH) - fat in the liver.
- Blocked bile ducts.
- Certain drugs, toxin exposure, and some infections.

PREVENTIVE MEASURES

- Limit alcohol use, or avoid it entirely.
- Avoid other risk factors, where possible.

EXPECTED OUTCOMES

It will vary due to the many causes and possible complications. Stopping alcohol use and treatment of the disorder that lead to cirrhosis may slow or stop the progress of the disease.

POSSIBLE COMPLICATIONS

- Continued alcohol use will lead to more liver damage.
- Cirrhosis can cause serious, sometimes fatal problems in any organ system in the body.

 ## DIAGNOSIS & TREATMENT

GENERAL MEASURES

- Your health care provider will do a physical exam and ask questions about your symptoms, activities and use of alcohol. Medical tests may include blood and urine tests, liver function studies, CT, and ultrasound. A biopsy of your liver may be done. This involves removing a sample of liver tissue for viewing under a microscope.
- Treatment may include drugs, diet and lifestyle changes, prevention or treatment of complications, and liver transplant. Your health care provider will devise a treatment plan based on your individual needs.
- If the condition is caused by alcoholism, stop drinking. Ask for help from family, friends, and community agencies. Contact an Alcoholics Anonymous group.
- Counseling or a support group may be helpful.
- Bleeding (hemorrhage) or excess fluid (ascites) may be treated with drugs or medical procedures.
- Liver transplant may be an option for severe disease.
- To learn more: American Liver Foundation, 75 Maiden Lane, Suite 603, New York, NY 10038; (800) 465-4837; website: www.liverfoundation.org.

MEDICATIONS

- Your health care provider may prescribe:
  - Drugs for the underlying disorder, or to decrease excess fluid in the body, and to prevent bleeding.
  - Supplements, such as vitamins.
  - Drugs to help remove toxins from the body.
  - Drugs for complications, such as infection.
- Don't take any other drugs without medical advice.

ACTIVITY

Stay as active as possible. Rest when you feel tired.

DIET

Eat a well-balanced diet. You will be advised about any limits for fat, salt, or protein in your diet.

 ## NOTIFY OUR OFFICE IF

- You or a family member has symptoms of cirrhosis.
- You have unusual bleeding, bloody vomit, excess fluid build-up, sudden weight gain, yellow skin or eyes, mental changes, fever, pain, or breathing problems.

Special notes:

_____

_____

_____

More notes on the back of this page ☐

CLAUDICATION

 ## BASIC INFORMATION

DESCRIPTION
A feeling of muscle fatigue or cramp-like pain, usually in one or both legs. The discomfort occurs after minimal exercise, such as a short walk, and is normally relieved by resting. The calf is more often affected, but it can occur in the thighs, buttocks, hips, or feet. It is more common in men than in women, particularly men over age 55.

FREQUENT SIGNS AND SYMPTOMS
- Pain, tension, weakness, or cramping in the limb.
- Pain occurs while walking, and pain stops when resting.
- Unable to walk distances.
- Loss of the hair on the toes or lower legs.
- Lameness or limping.

CAUSES
- Blockage or narrowing of the arteries of the legs due to atherosclerosis.
- Rarer cause is spinal stenosis (pressure on nerve roots that pass into either leg).

RISK INCREASES WITH
- Being a male, women after menopause, age over 60.
- Smoking.
- Diabetes.
- Being sedentary (getting little or no exercise).
- High blood pressure.
- Overweight.
- Heart disease.
- High blood cholesterol.

PREVENTIVE MEASURES
- Stop smoking.
- Weight loss, if overweight.
- Routine exercise program.
- Reduce the amount of saturated fats in the diet.

EXPECTED OUTCOMES
Gradual improvement in ability to walk distances without pain. Improvement may take 6 to 12 months. It is important to follow an exercise program.

POSSIBLE COMPLICATIONS
- Pain while resting, as well as when walking.
- Increased risk of falls, due to being unsteady.
- People with diabetes are at highest risk for problems.
- Blood clots, tissue loss, gangrene, and amputation (rare).

 ## DIAGNOSIS & TREATMENT

GENERAL MEASURES
- Your health care provider will do a physical exam and ask questions about your symptoms. A variety of medical tests, including an ultrasound (sometimes done with exercise), may be ordered. These will help confirm the diagnosis and rule out other disorders that have similar symptoms.
- You will be given exercises to do at home, and/or supervised exercises that are done on a treadmill.
- Quit smoking. Find a way to stop that works for you.
- High blood pressure and high cholesterol may be treated with drugs.
- Various surgical procedures, depending on the site of the disease and the health of the patient, are available for more severe cases.

MEDICATIONS
- Low doses of aspirin may be prescribed.
- Drugs to lower blood pressure and reduce cholesterol levels, and special drugs to increase blood flow may be prescribed.
- Taking vitamins C, E, and B has helped some people. Ask your health care provider about taking them.

ACTIVITY
- Begin an exercise program. Walking or riding an exercise bike is recommended. Stop and rest if the pain becomes more severe. Try for 30 to 60 minutes of exercise 3 to 5 days a week.
- Strength training for the arms and legs also helps to improve symptoms.

DIET
Eat a healthy diet (include fruits, vegetables, and fiber). Consider a weight-loss diet, if overweight is a problem.

 ## NOTIFY OUR OFFICE IF

- You or a family member has symptoms of claudication.
- You experience chest pain, shortness of breath, or rapid heart-beat during exercise.
- Drugs used for treatment cause unexpected side effects.

Special notes:

_____

_____

_____

More notes on the back of this page ☐

COCCIDIOIDOMYCOSIS

(Valley Fever; San Joaquin Valley Fever; "Cocci")

BASIC INFORMATION

DESCRIPTION

A lung infection caused by a fungus that lives in soil. Coccidioidomycosis cannot be spread from person to person. It can affect all age groups.

FREQUENT SIGNS AND SYMPTOMS

The infection is usually so mild that it produces no symptoms. People may think they have a mild case of flu. In a few cases the symptoms may include:

- Cough.
- Fatigue.
- Sore throat.
- Chills and fever.
- Chest pain.
- Headache.
- Muscle and joint aches.
- Skin rash.
- General ill feeling.
- Sweating at night.
- Weight loss.
- Stiff neck (sometimes).

CAUSES

Infection by the fungus, *Coccidioides immitis*, which thrives in soil, especially soil that lines rodent burrows. A person becomes infected when they breathe the dust from such soil, and the fungi lodge in the lungs. Symptoms may occur 1 to 4 weeks after exposure.

RISK INCREASES WITH

- Geographic location. The disease is most common in the Southwest: California's San Joaquin Valley, some regions in southern and central Arizona, and southwest Texas.
- Work or environmental exposure to dust, such as farmers, construction workers, landscaping work, an archeology site, dirt biking, and others.
- Risk increases on windy days when the soil is dry and when the soil is disturbed, as with excavation. Outbreaks occur following dust storms or earthquakes. Cases increase during and after rainy seasons.

PREVENTIVE MEASURES

Cannot be prevented at present.

EXPECTED OUTCOMES

Infected persons recover on their own in 3 to 6 weeks. Patients may continue to feel ill for 3 to 6 weeks after signs of infection disappear. Antifungal drugs may be used for persons with severe, widespread infection.

POSSIBLE COMPLICATIONS

- Spread of infection to other parts of the body, which can cause serious complications and could be fatal.
- Pneumonia.
- The disorder may become chronic.
- People with weak immune systems, pregnant women, African Americans, and Filipinos are more at risk for complications.

DIAGNOSIS & TREATMENT

GENERAL MEASURES

- Your health care provider may do a physical exam and ask about your symptoms and activities. Medical tests may include a skin test, blood studies, sputum cultures, chest x-ray and others.
- Treatment usually involves care at home. Get extra rest if needed. Hospital care is required only for severe cases. Very rarely is surgery needed.
- To learn more: Valley Fever Center for Excellence, Mail Stop 1-111INF, 3601 S. 6th Ave., Tucson, AZ 85732; (520) 629-4777 (not toll free); website: www.arl.arizona.edu/vfce.

MEDICATIONS

- Drugs are usually not needed for treatment. You may use nonprescription nonsteroidal anti-inflammatory drugs for pain, and antitussives for cough if needed.
- For infection spread outside the lungs and for certain patients (infants, patients with pneumonia, or immune system problems, diabetes, or pregnancy), antifungal drugs may be prescribed.

ACTIVITY

Stay as active as your strength allows.

DIET

No special diet.

NOTIFY OUR OFFICE IF

- You or a family member has symptoms of coccidioidomycosis.
- Continued weight-loss, fever, diarrhea that cannot be controlled, stiff neck with headache develop.

Special notes: _____

_____

_____

More notes on the back of this page ☐

COLD, COMMON

 BASIC INFORMATION

DESCRIPTION

A contagious viral infection of the upper-respiratory tract. This includes the nose, throat, and sinuses. A cold also affects the ears and lungs. Colds are the most common disease in the world.

FREQUENT SIGNS AND SYMPTOMS

· Stuffy or runny nose. Nasal discharge may be watery at first, becoming thick and yellow.
· Throat feels scratchy or sore.
· Coughing and sneezing.
· Loss of voice.
· Mild headache.
· Fatigue.
· Low-grade fever.
· Watering eyes.
· Cold symptoms start slowly. Flu symptoms are more sudden and include higher fever, major aches, chills, sweats, weakness, possible severe sore throat, cough, and chest discomfort.

CAUSES

Any of at least 100 viruses. Virus particles spread through the air or from person-to-person contact. Colds are often spread with hand-shaking.

RISK INCREASES WITH

· Winter (colds are most frequent in cold weather).
· Children attending school or daycare.
· Household member who has a cold.
· Crowded or unclean living conditions.
· Stress, fatigue, and allergies.

PREVENTIVE MEASURES

· To prevent spreading a cold to others, avoid contact if possible during the contagious phase (first 2 to 4 days).
· Wash hands often, especially after blowing your nose or before handling food.
· Avoid crowded places when possible, especially during the winter.
· Eat a well-balanced, healthy diet. Include plenty of citrus fruits and other sources of vitamin C.

EXPECTED OUTCOMES

Recovery in 7 to 14 days.

POSSIBLE COMPLICATIONS

Bacterial infections of the ears, throat, sinuses, or lungs.

 DIAGNOSIS & TREATMENT

GENERAL MEASURES

· Self-care and time is usually all that is needed for a cold. There is no cure for a cold. There are many remedies for cold symptoms. They include nonprescription

cold preparations, getting extra rest, drinking plenty of fluids, and others that may be suggested by friends and family members. One or more of these may help you feel better until the body's defenses fight off the germs.
· To help relieve nasal congestion, use salt-water drops (1/2 teaspoon of salt to 1 cup of warm water). Put 2 or 3 drops of salt solution into each nostril.
· Don't smoke. It can further irritate the nasal passages.
· For a baby too young to blow his or her nose, use an infant nasal aspirator. If mucus is thick and sticky, loosen it by putting 2 or 3 drops of salt solution (see above) into each nostril. Don't insert cotton swabs into a child's nostrils.

MEDICATIONS

No drugs, including antibiotics, can cure the common cold. To help relieve symptoms, you may use nonprescription drugs, such as acetaminophen, decongestants, nose drops or sprays, cough remedies, and throat lozenges. It is best to get a product that works for one symptom, such as a runny nose, rather than a multi-symptom product. If you take other drugs, talk to your health care provider or pharmacist about possible drug interactions.

ACTIVITY

Bed rest is not needed. Do reduce activity and exercise.

DIET

Regular diet. Drink extra fluids, including water, fruit juice, tea, and carbonated drinks.

 NOTIFY OUR OFFICE IF

· You have increased throat pain, or white or yellow spots on the tonsils or other parts of the throat.
· You have long coughing episodes. Your cough produces thick, yellow-green or gray sputum. You have a cough that lasts longer than 10 days.
· A fever lasts several days, or is over 101°F (38.3°C).
· You have chills, chest pain, or shortness of breath.
· You develop a painful earache or severe headache.
· You develop a skin rash or bruised skin.
· You feel pain in the teeth or over the sinuses.
· You develop enlarged, tender glands in the neck.
· Infant with a cold is unable to bottle-feed or breast-feed.

Special notes:

_____

_____

_____

More notes on the back of this page ☐

COLD SORE

(Fever Blister; Herpes Simplex)

 BASIC INFORMATION

DESCRIPTION

A common viral infection that affects the skin. In most cases, people become infected with the virus in child-hood. The first time a person (usually a child) is infect-ed, symptoms may include mouth sores, sore throat, fever, aching, tiredness, problems with eating, and swollen glands. The virus then stays inactive in the body (sometimes for months or years), until an active infection occurs and cold sores result.

FREQUENT SIGNS AND SYMPTOMS

• Cold sores usually involve the lips. In some cases, they occur on nostrils, cheeks, or fingers. Prior to a cold sore, the skin area may feel itchy, tingly, or sensitive.
• A cluster of small, painful, fluid-filled blisters appear in the affected area. The blisters break and ooze. A yellow crust forms and sloughs off, leaving pink skin and no scarring.

CAUSES

• Herpes simplex virus type 1, or, less often, herpes simplex type 2 (the cause of genital herpes). The virus is spread from person to person by contact with fluid from a cold sore, saliva, contact with an item that has the germs on it, or sharing food or drinks with an infect-ed person. The blisters and open sores can spread the virus until they heal.
• Risk factors (listed below) may trigger an outbreak of cold sores. Cold sores also recur for unknown reasons.

RISK INCREASES WITH

• Physical or emotional stress.
• Illness, including a cold, flu, or fever from any cause.
• Menstrual periods.
• Dental treatment that stretches the mouth.
• Weak immune system due to illness or drugs.
• Exposure to the sun.
• Certain foods or drugs.
• Eczema (a skin infection).
• In daycare settings, sharing toys that children put in their mouths.

PREVENTIVE MEASURES

• Avoid contact (such as kissing or sharing food) with someone who has an active cold sore.
• Wash your hands often when you have a cold sore. This can help prevent spreading the virus.
• Use a sunscreen.

EXPECTED OUTCOMES

Recovery takes a few days to a week. Recurrence will vary for different people. Cold sores may recur often or rarely. Complications are unlikely.

POSSIBLE COMPLICATIONS

Rarely, infection spreads to other places in the body, such as the eyes and brain. Prompt treatment is vital.

 DIAGNOSIS & TREATMENT

GENERAL MEASURES

• Most people will use self-care to treat cold sores:
  - Apply ice to the affected area, or use nonprescrip-tion products for cold sores, to ease discomfort.
  - Don't squeeze or pick at the blisters. Avoid touching them except to apply cream or ointment. Then wash hands carefully. Be careful about touching other places in the body, especially the eyes and genital area, where the infection could spread.
  - Don't share lip products, or cups and other utensils.
• See your health care provider if you are concerned about the symptoms. An exam of the infected area can confirm the diagnosis. Rarely, a medical test may be done of fluid from the sore.
• Medical treatment may include prescription drugs.

MEDICATIONS

• Use aspirin, acetaminophen, or ibuprofen to relieve minor pain. Don't give aspirin to children under 18.
• Nonprescription creams or ointments for cold sores may be used.
• Antiviral drugs may be prescribed. They can be taken by mouth or applied to the skin.

ACTIVITY

No limits on physical activity. Avoid close contact with others, especially newborns and persons who have weak immune systems.

DIET

No special diet.

 NOTIFY OUR OFFICE IF

The following occur with a cold sore:
• The cold sore does not heal in a week.
• Signs of infection, such as fever or pus, instead of clear fluid in the blister. Sores develop on the genitals, or the eyes become infected.
• You have a weak immune system due to illness or drugs.

Special notes:

_____

_____

_____

More notes on the back of this page ☐

COLIC IN INFANTS

 BASIC INFORMATION

DESCRIPTION

Repeated episodes of excessive crying that cannot be explained. The baby is healthy and does not have a specific disorder, such as an ear infection. Colic affects infants up to 5 months old and is more common in a first child and boys. Colic is different in each baby, but is sometimes defined as crying for 3 hours a day at least 3 days a week for 3 consecutive weeks.

FREQUENT SIGNS AND SYMPTOMS

• Crying ranges from being fussy to a high-pitched, loud cry. Crying periods usually occur in late afternoon or evening.
• Colic usually begins at 2 to 4 weeks and can last through 3 or 4 months.
• The infant's stomach may rumble, face may be flushed (red), and the child may draw up the legs as if in pain. There may be passing of gas.
• Colic can cause loss of sleep and feeding problems in infants. In parents, it causes distress, depression, sleep loss, marital problems, and a feeling that parenting ability is lacking.

CAUSES

Unknown. Some possible, but not proven, causes include an immature nervous or digestive system, food allergy or food intolerance, or the baby is extra sensitive to things going on in the home.

RISK INCREASES WITH

No known risk factors.

PREVENTIVE MEASURES

No specific preventive measures.

EXPECTED OUTCOMES

All babies cry, and many have fussy periods. Crying is an important activity and is a way for babies to communicate. Colic is a distressing, but not dangerous, condition. The symptoms can sometimes be relieved. Colic will usually stop after the 3rd or 4th month.

POSSIBLE COMPLICATIONS

None expected.

 DIAGNOSIS & TREATMENT

GENERAL MEASURES

• Be patient and tolerant. Colic is not the parent's fault, so do not blame yourselves.
• Don't feed the baby every time he or she cries. Look for a reason, such as a gas bubble, cramped position, too much heat or cold. Check for a soiled diaper, open diaper pin, or a desire to be cuddled.

• There are many options to try and help soothe the baby. These include:
  - Walking. Carry the baby or put baby in a stroller.
  - Rocking in a rocking chair or swinging in an automatic baby swing.
  - Take baby for a car ride.
  - Massage. Lay baby down on his/her stomach and gently rub the baby's back.
  - Swaddle the baby tightly in a baby blanket.
  - Use noise to help soothe. Run a vacuum or shower. Play soothing music (this may help baby and parents).
  - Vibration. Put the baby in a car seat and place seat on top of a dryer. Watch the baby carefully.
  - Lower lights and reduce excess noise in the home.
  - Some overtired infants may need to cry themselves to sleep. Once you know your baby is not hungry, not soiled, has no fever, no open pins, and you have done all you can, put your baby down for sleep.
  - Colic is distressing, but not harmful.
• Ask someone to take care of the baby in order to give you a break as often as possible. Parents need to get rest and try to avoid becoming too stressed.
• See your baby's health care provider if you are concerned about colic symptoms. A physical exam can be done to make sure there are no health problems. Other medical tests are usually not required.

MEDICATIONS

Drugs are usually not helpful for colic. Don't use any herbs or other supplements without medical approval.

ACTIVITY

No limits.

DIET

• Interrupt bottle feedings after every ounce and burp the baby. Interrupt breast-feedings every 5 minutes.
• Allow at least 20 minutes to feed the baby. Hold the baby in an upright position for 20 minutes after feeding.
• Breast-feeding mothers may try and adjust their diet. Avoid dairy, caffeine, foods that cause gas (beans, cabbage, and others) and spicy foods.
• A change in baby formula may be recommended.

 NOTIFY OUR OFFICE IF

• Your baby has colic and you are concerned about it.
• You fear that you are about to lose emotional control.

Special notes:

_____

_____

_____

More notes on the back of this page ☐

COLITIS, ULCERATIVE
(Granulomatous Colitis)

BASIC INFORMATION

DESCRIPTION
A serious, chronic, inflammatory disease of the colon (large intestine). The inflammation causes small sores or ulcers. It usually affects the rectum (the lower end of the colon), but may affect the entire colon. Rarely, a portion of the small intestine is involved. Ulcerative colitis may occur at any age and in both sexes.

FREQUENT SIGNS AND SYMPTOMS
· Symptoms may be mild, moderate, or severe.
· Pain in the left side of the abdomen. It may improve after bowel movements.
· Episodes of bloody diarrhea with mucus, alternating with symptom-free intervals.
· Severe cramps and pain around the rectum.
· Appetite and weight loss.
· Sweating and nausea.
· Bloated abdomen.
· Fever.
· Symptoms may occur outside the abdomen.

CAUSES
Unknown. Genetic, infectious, immunologic, and psychological factors have all been suggested.

RISK INCREASES WITH
Family history of ulcerative colitis.

PREVENTIVE MEASURES
No specific preventive measures.

EXPECTED OUTCOMES
Symptoms tend to come and go throughout life. Treatment can help. It is curable with surgery.

POSSIBLE COMPLICATIONS
· Life-threatening blood loss, ulceration through the intestinal wall or peritonitis.
· Malnutrition (lack of nutrients).
· Inflammation of joints, eyes, and skin.
· Colon cancer. Risk is greater with ulcerative colitis.
· Life-threatening blood poisoning.

DIAGNOSIS & TREATMENT

GENERAL MEASURES
· Your health care provider will do a physical exam and ask questions about your symptoms. Medical tests may include stool and blood studies and x-ray of the colon (barium enema). A sigmoidoscopy or colonoscopy may be done. In these procedures, a thin tube with a lighted tip is used to view inside the colon and rectum. At the same time, a small piece of tissue can be removed for biopsy.

· Treatment will depend on the severity and extent of the inflammation. Treatment steps may include drug therapy, surgery and, sometimes, diet changes.
· Hospital care may be needed if bleeding or dehydration develops. Fluids may be given through a vein (IV).
· Surgery to remove part of or the entire colon may be needed. This is done for severe symptoms (such as bleeding), rupture of the colon, cancer risk, failure of other treatments, or side effects of steroid drugs. The options for surgery and stool elimination will be explained to you.
· Counseling may help with emotional aspects of the disease or the surgery. Learn relaxation techniques.
· To learn more: Crohn's and Colitis Foundation of America, 386 Park Ave. South, 17th Floor, New York, NY 10016; (800) 932-2423; website: www.ccfa.org.

MEDICATIONS
· Antidiarrheal drugs may be prescribed for diarrhea.
· Sulfa drugs, such as sulfasalazine may be prescribed to help control inflammation.
· Cortisone drugs may be prescribed for more severe symptoms. They may be taken by mouth, injected, given through an enema, or as a suppository.
· Drugs called immunomodulators may be prescribed.
· Antibiotics will be prescribed for infection.
· Vitamin and mineral supplements may be prescribed.
· Iron replacement may be needed.

ACTIVITY
Bed rest may be needed during acute attacks. Resume normal activity as soon as symptoms improve.

DIET
· Eat a healthy diet. Some foods aggravate symptoms in different people. Keep a food diary to learn which foods cause you symptoms so you can avoid them.
· Avoid milk products if you have a lactose intolerance.

NOTIFY OUR OFFICE IF

· You or a family member has symptoms of ulcerative colitis.
· After diagnosis and treatment, fever and chills develop, the frequency of bowel movements or bleeding increases, jaundice (yellow eyes and skin with dark urine) develops, vomiting begins, or pain increases.

Special notes:

_____

_____

_____

More notes on the back of this page ☐

CONGENITAL PYLORIC STENOSIS

(Hypertrophic Pyloric Stenosis)

 ## BASIC INFORMATION

DESCRIPTION

A condition of infancy in which encircling muscles at the end of the stomach enlarge and cause obstruction. It affects the pylorus (a muscular tube that carries food from the stomach to the small intestine). It is more common in firstborn males and usually begins between 2 and 5 weeks of age, but can occur as late as 4 months.

FREQUENT SIGNS AND SYMPTOMS

· Recurrent vomiting after feedings that becomes increasingly forceful.
· Muscular, olive-sized mass in the upper abdomen (sometimes).
· No pain or fever. Infant seems happy, but hungry, after vomiting.
· Constipation.
· Gradual weight loss and dehydration.

CAUSES

The muscular band that encircles the pylorus thickens and eventually closes off the outlet from the stomach.

RISK INCREASES WITH

Family history of pyloric stenosis.

PREVENTIVE MEASURES

Cannot be prevented at present.

EXPECTED OUTCOMES

Curable with surgery. The child usually recovers quickly.

POSSIBLE COMPLICATIONS

Without treatment, weight loss, dehydration, shock, and/or death.

 ## DIAGNOSIS & TREATMENT

GENERAL MEASURES

· Your child's health care provider will do a physical exam. A barium-swallow x-ray or ultrasound may be done to confirm the diagnosis.
· Treatment is with surgery to cut the thickened muscle (pyloromyotomy).
· After surgery:
 - A firm ridge will appear at the incision site. This is a healthy sign and requires no treatment.
 - Wash the incision site gently several times a day.
 - If the baby seems uncomfortable, apply warm compresses to the incision site.

MEDICATIONS

Fluids and electrolytes will be given through a vein (IV) until the baby is ready for surgery. Drugs are usually not needed after surgery.

ACTIVITY

No limits.

DIET

The baby may tolerate small feedings of half-strength formula while awaiting surgery. If not, formula will be given by stomach tube.

 ## NOTIFY OUR OFFICE IF

· Your baby vomits repeatedly.
· The following occur after surgery:
 - Pain, swelling, redness, bleeding, or drainage at the surgical site.
 - Temperature rises to 101°F (38.3°C).

Special notes:

_____

_____

_____

More notes on the back of this page ☐

CONGESTIVE HEART FAILURE

 BASIC INFORMATION

DESCRIPTION

The heart has lost some of its ability to pump blood. The weak pumping causes fluid (congestion) to build up in the lungs and body tissues. Congestive heart failure is more common in older adults, and affects men more than women.

FREQUENT SIGNS AND SYMPTOMS

- Feeling short of breath with activity or after lying down for a while.
- Feeling tired and weak.
- Coughing or wheezing.
- Sleep apnea (disturbed breathing at night).
- Swollen legs, ankles, and stomach.
- Appetite loss. A weight gain is due to retained water.
- Muscle wasting (loss of muscle mass).
- Swollen or protruding neck veins.
- Less urine, and a need to urinate at night.
- Less mentally alert, or unable to concentrate.
- Having to sleep propped up or in a recliner.

CAUSES

Over time, various disorders cause the muscles, valves, and blood vessels of the heart to become damaged and weak. The heart is not able to pump enough blood, oxygen, and nutrients to other organs in the body that they need in order for them to function properly.

RISK INCREASES WITH

- Uncontrolled high blood pressure.
- Disease of the heart valves.
- Damage following a heart attack.
- Coronary artery disease.
- Cardiomyopathy (enlarged heart).
- Congenital (being born with) heart disease.
- Abnormal rhythm or irregular heartbeat.
- Risk factors for heart disease that can lead to heart failure include: Smoking, obesity, high levels of fats in the blood, use of certain drugs, diet high in fat or salt, diabetes, alcohol abuse, and lack of physical activity.

PREVENTIVE MEASURES

If you have a condition that can lead to congestive heart failure, get medical care. Follow your treatment plan. Eat a diet high in fiber, and low in fat and salt. Don't abuse alcohol and don't smoke. Exercise regularly.

EXPECTED OUTCOMES

Symptoms may be relieved with treatment. Long-term outcome depends on each individual patient and the severity of heart failure.

POSSIBLE COMPLICATIONS

Heart attack, cardiac arrest, severe heart rhythm problems, pulmonary edema (fluid in the lungs), side effects of drugs, total heart failure, and death.

 DIAGNOSIS & TREATMENT

GENERAL MEASURES

- Your health care provider will do a physical exam and ask questions about your symptoms and activities. Medical tests may include blood studies and x-rays. Studies may be done of heart activity, function, and size. They help determine if there has been a heart attack and the extent of any heart damage.
- The goal of treatment is to improve the heart's pumping function. This may include drugs, lifestyle changes, and surgery. Your health care provider will devise a treatment plan based on your individual needs.
- Don't smoke. Find a way to quit that works for you.
- Hospital care may be needed for severe cases. Supplemental oxygen may be used to help breathing.
- Surgery may be required for heart valve problems.
- A heart transplant may be recommended for severe cases that do not respond to other treatment. A mechanical device may be used temporarily to help the heart's pumping function.
- Wear or carry identification that says you have this condition. Be sure it lists any drugs that you take.
- To learn more: American Heart Association, local branch listed in telephone directory, or call (800) 242-8721; website: www.americanheart.org.

MEDICATIONS

Drugs may be prescribed to improve heart function, to slow and regulate the heart rate, remove extra fluid, lower blood pressure, relax blood vessels, suppress the immune system, and to treat any underlying disorder.

ACTIVITY

Follow medical advice about physical activity limits and when it is safe to resume driving and sexual relations.

DIET

- Eat a diet that is low in salt and fat. Avoid alcohol.
- Go on a weight loss diet if your weight is a problem.

 NOTIFY OUR OFFICE IF

- You or a family member has symptoms of congestive heart failure.
- After diagnosis, any new symptoms occur that cause concern, or other symptoms become worse.

Special notes:

_____

_____

_____

More notes on the back of this page ☐

CONJUNCTIVITIS

(Pink Eye)

 BASIC INFORMATION

DESCRIPTION

An inflammation (redness and soreness) of the conjunctiva. The conjunctiva is a clear membrane that covers the white part of the eye and the inside of the eyelids. Conjunctivitis is a very common condition in children.

FREQUENT SIGNS AND SYMPTOMS

- Symptoms vary depending on the cause.
- One or both eyes may be affected.
- Eye discomfort or pain.
- Gritty feeling in the eye (like there is a piece of sand in the eye).
- Redness of the eye (leading to the term "pinkeye").
- Clear, green, or yellow discharge from the eye.
- After sleeping, crusts on lashes that cause eyelids to stick together.
- Swollen eyelids.
- Sensitivity to bright light.
- Intense itching (allergic type only).

CAUSES

- Bacterial or viral infection. Conjunctivitis may occur with colds or childhood diseases such as measles. These infections can be spread from one eye to the other. They can also be spread from one person to another.
- Chemical irritation or dust, smoke, chlorine, and other types of air pollution, or home chemicals.
- Allergies caused by cosmetics, pollen, animal dander, or other allergens. (Both eyes are usually affected.)
- A blocked tear duct.

RISK INCREASES WITH

- Children and the elderly.
- Contact lens wearers.
- Contact with an infected person.
- Newborns of mothers who are carriers of gonorrhea or chlamydia.

PREVENTIVE MEASURES

- Wash hands often to avoid spreading germs.
- Avoid exposure to eye irritants.
- Newborns in hospital deliveries are routinely given antibiotic eye drops.
- Do not share eye makeup. Discard mascara after 4 to 6 months.

EXPECTED OUTCOMES

- Most forms will heal on their own in 1 to 2 weeks with no serious harm.
- Allergic conjunctivitis can be cured if the allergen is removed. However, it is likely to recur.

POSSIBLE COMPLICATIONS

Complications are rare, but may include other eye infections or problems of the cornea.

 DIAGNOSIS & TREATMENT

GENERAL MEASURES

- Sometimes, the infection is treated with self-care. See your health care provider if you have any concerns about the symptoms. An exam of the affected eye will confirm the diagnosis.
- Treatment of conjunctivitis varies with the cause.
- Wash hands often with antiseptic soap, and use paper towels to dry. Don't touch the eyes. Gently wipe the discharge from the eye using disposable tissues.
- For infectious conjunctivitis, use warm-water compresses on the eye to reduce discomfort. Cool compresses feel better with allergic conjunctivitis. Apply for 5 to 10 minutes several times a day.
- Do not use eye makeup while symptoms are present.
- Do not wear contact lenses until symptoms are gone.

MEDICATIONS

- You may use nonprescription artificial tears in the eyes to help relieve symptoms.
- Antibiotic eye drops or ointments may be prescribed. Antibiotics taken by mouth may be prescribed for more severe cases.
- Steroid eye drops or ointments may be prescribed. Follow instructions carefully as these products can cause other, more severe eye problems.
- For allergic conjunctivitis, you may use nonprescription anti-allergy eye drops.

ACTIVITY

Return to work or school once symptoms improve.

DIET

No special diet.

 NOTIFY OUR OFFICE IF

- You or a family member has signs of conjunctivitis.
- The infection does not improve in 48 hours, despite treatment.
- Fever occurs or pain increases.
- Vision is affected.

Special notes:

_____

_____

_____

More notes on the back of this page ☐

CONSTIPATION

 BASIC INFORMATION

DESCRIPTION

Having fewer bowel movements than usual and difficulty in passing stools. In most people, constipation is harmless. In some, it can be a sign that something else is wrong with the body. People may think they are constipated when their bowel movements are actually regular. There is no right number of daily or weekly bowel movements. Everyone has different bowel patterns.

FREQUENT SIGNS AND SYMPTOMS

- Hard, dry, or lumpy stools.
- Having to strain to have a bowel movement.
- Fewer than three bowel movements a week.
- Pain or bleeding with bowel movements.
- Feeling bloated or sluggish.
- Feeling like you still need to go after having a bowel movement.

CAUSES

The slow movement of feces (stool) through the large intestine. This results in a dry, hard stool.

RISK INCREASES WITH

- Constipation can be a symptom or a complication of many different medical disorders.
- Emotional factors such as depression or anxiety.
- Not getting enough fluids.
- Not enough fiber in the diet.
- Being inactive.
- Taking certain drugs.
- Problems with the rectum.
- Laxative abuse.
- Travel-related constipation.
- Advancing age.

PREVENTIVE MEASURES

- Eat a well-balanced diet. Include lots of fiber.
- Exercise regularly.
- Drink at least 8 glasses of fluid a day.

EXPECTED OUTCOMES

Usually curable with exercise, diet, and enough fluids.

POSSIBLE COMPLICATIONS

- Hemorrhoids.
- Becoming dependent on laxatives.
- Uterine or rectal problems.
- Colon problems; blocked bowel.
- Chronic constipation.

 DIAGNOSIS & TREATMENT

GENERAL MEASURES

- Self-care may be all that is needed for treatment. If you have any concerns, see your health care provider. A physical exam may be done and questions asked about your symptoms and activities. Medical tests may be done depending on the severity of the symptoms.
- Treatment will be prescribed for any specific cause.
- In most cases, constipation can be helped with changes in diet and lifestyle (such as more exercise). Laxatives are usually not needed for mild constipation.
- Make a regular time each day for bowel movements. The best time is often within 1 hour after breakfast. Don't try to hurry. Sit at least 10 minutes, even if a bowel movement doesn't occur.
- Drinking hot water, tea, or coffee may make you feel the need to have a bowel movement.
- A person dependent on laxatives should slowly stop using them. Normal bowel function will begin again.

MEDICATIONS

For occasional constipation, you may use stool softeners, mild nonprescription laxatives, or enemas. Don't use laxatives or enemas regularly, because you can become dependent on them. Avoid harsh laxatives. Ask your pharmacist or health care provider which laxatives are best to use.

ACTIVITY

Get regular exercise and stay physically fit. This helps stimulate the bowel and can maintain healthy bowels.

DIET

Drink at least 8 glasses of fluid each day. Eat a high-fiber diet (beans, bran cereals, raw fruits, and vegetables). Avoid refined cereals and breads, pastries, and sugar.

 NOTIFY OUR OFFICE IF

- Constipation persists despite self-care, especially if the constipation is a change in your normal bowel patterns. Changes in bowel patterns may be a sign of cancer.
- You have a fever or severe stomach pain.

Special notes:

_____

_____

_____

More notes on the back of this page ☐

COR PULMONALE
(Pulmonary Hypertension)

 ## BASIC INFORMATION

DESCRIPTION
An enlarged heart due to chronic lung disease or lung dysfunction. Cor pulmonale is usually chronic (ongoing), but may be acute (short term). It is more common in adults over 50, and occurs in men more than women.

FREQUENT SIGNS AND SYMPTOMS
Early stages:
- No symptoms (usually).

Later stages:
- Shortness of breath with physical activity.
- Feeling weak and tired.
- Chest pain.
- Fainting or near fainting.
- Rapid heartbeat.
- Cough or wheezing.
- Swelling of the ankles, feet.
- Swelling of the stomach (ascites).
- Bluish color of the skin.
- Neck veins swollen (distended).

CAUSES
Lung disease or dysfunction leads to pulmonary hypertension (high blood pressure in the lungs). This slows or blocks blood flow in the lungs. This in turn causes an extra load on the right side of the heart as it tries to pump enough blood through the lungs. The heart muscle becomes overdeveloped (enlarged) and the load on the heart becomes too great leading to heart failure.

RISK INCREASES WITH
- Chronic lung disease, such as emphysema, chronic bronchitis, silicosis, cystic fibrosis, and others.
- Blood clots in the lungs (pulmonary embolism).
- Extensive loss of lung tissue due to surgery or injury.

PREVENTIVE MEASURES
- Avoid risk factors for lung disease, such as smoking.
- Obtain medical care for any heart or lung disorder.

EXPECTED OUTCOMES
The outcome will depend on the underlying lung disorder. Symptoms can often be relieved or controlled with treatment.

POSSIBLE COMPLICATIONS
Serious, sometimes fatal, heart failure.

 ## DIAGNOSIS & TREATMENT

GENERAL MEASURES
- Your health care provider will do a physical exam and ask questions about your symptoms and activities. Medical tests may include blood studies, x-ray, lung scan, lung function tests, and echocardiogram (heart study).
- Treatment steps usually include drug therapy, supplemental oxygen, and surgery (if needed). Hospital care may be required, especially if a blood clot is diagnosed.
- Supplemental oxygen is usually needed on a continuous basis. An oxygen therapist can arrange for the type of oxygen that allows you to be up and about.
- Surgery may be needed to correct heart defects.
- Lung transplant or heart-lung transplant may be recommended in some cases.

MEDICATIONS
Drugs may be prescribed to improve heart function, to slow and regulate the heart rate, get rid of extra fluid, lower blood pressure, thin the blood, relax blood vessels, and to treat any underlying disorder.

ACTIVITY
Be as active as your condition allows, but don't overexert. Rest between activities.

DIET
You may be advised to follow a low-salt diet and limit your fluid intake.

 ## NOTIFY OUR OFFICE IF

- You or a family member has symptoms of cor pulmonale.
- The following occur during treatment:
  - Temperature of 101°F (38.3°C) or higher.
  - Weight gain of 3 to 4 pounds in 1 or 2 days.
  - Increased shortness of breath.
  - Increased swelling of the ankles or stomach.
  - Cough with mucus that is discolored or bloody.

Special notes:

_____

_____

_____

More notes on the back of this page ☐

CORN or CALLUS

 BASIC INFORMATION

DESCRIPTION

· A corn is a thickening (bump) of the outer skin layer, usually over bony areas such as toe joints. Corns affect toe joints and the skin between toes.

· A callus is a painless thickening of skin caused by repeated pressure or irritation. A callus can appear on any part of the body, especially hands, feet, or knees, that endures repeated pressure or irritation.

FREQUENT SIGNS AND SYMPTOMS

· Corn: A small, tender and painful raised bump on the side or over the joint of a toe. Corns are usually 3 mm to 10 mm in diameter and have a hard center.

· Callus: A rough, thickened area of skin that appears after repeated pressure or irritation.

CAUSES

Corns and calluses form to protect a skin area from injury caused by repeated rubbing or squeezing. Pressure causes cells in the irritated area to grow at a faster rate, leading to overgrowth.

RISK INCREASES WITH

· Shoes that fit poorly. Socks that bunch up.

· Persons with jobs that involve pressure on the hands or knees, such as carpenters, writers, guitar players, or tile layers.

· Foot deformity.

· Athletic activities that put stress on hands or feet.

PREVENTIVE MEASURES

· Don't wear shoes or socks that fit poorly.

· Avoid activities that create constant pressure on specific skin areas.

· When possible, wear protective gear, such as gloves or knee-pads.

· Keep skin moisturized.

EXPECTED OUTCOMES

Usually curable if the problem that caused it can be removed. Allow 3 weeks for recovery. Corns and calluses are likely to recur, even with treatment, if the cause is not removed.

POSSIBLE COMPLICATIONS

Back, hip, knee, or ankle pain caused by a change in the way you walk due to pain in your foot.

 DIAGNOSIS & TREATMENT

GENERAL MEASURES

· Self-care is often all that is needed.

· Remove the source of pressure, if possible. Get rid of shoes that do not fit well.

· Use corn and callus pads to reduce pressure on the irritated areas.

· Peel or rub the thickened area with a pumice stone to remove it. Don't cut it with a razor. Soak the area in warm water to soften it before peeling.

· See your health care provider or a foot care provider if self-care is not effective. Diagnosis is done by an exam of the affected area. Medical tests are usually not needed, but an x-ray may be done.

· Medical care may involve shaving or cutting off the hardened area of skin, removing the corn or callus with a medicine used on the skin, and (rarely) surgery. Surgery does not remove the cause, and scarring from surgery is painful and may complicate healing.

MEDICATIONS

· Peel the upper layers of the corn once or twice a day, and then apply a nonprescription 5% or 10% salicylic ointment. Cover with adhesive tape.

· A corn or callus may sometimes be injected with cortisone medicine to reduce swelling or pain.

· An antibiotic may be prescribed for skin infection.

ACTIVITY

Resume your normal activities as soon as symptoms improve.

DIET

No special diet.

 NOTIFY OUR OFFICE IF

· You or a family member has corns or calluses that do not heal, despite self-treatment.

· You develop signs of infection around a corn or callus. Signs of infection include redness, swelling, pain, heat, or tenderness.

Special notes:

_____

_____

_____

More notes on the back of this page ☐

CORNEAL ABRASION & ULCER

 ## BASIC INFORMATION

DESCRIPTION
The cornea is the thin, clear, front part of the eye that covers the iris (colored part) and the sclera (white part). An abrasion is a worn-off, scratched, or scraped area of the cornea. An ulcer is an open sore of the cornea. They both can affect people of any age.

FREQUENT SIGNS AND SYMPTOMS
- Eye pain that may be severe.
- Eyes are sensitive to bright light.
- Feeling as if a foreign body is in the eye.
- Watering of the eye.
- Blurred vision.
- Redness in the white of the eye.
- Discharge from the eye.
- Clouding of the cornea.

CAUSES
- Corneal abrasion usually occurs from some type of injury to the eye. It may be a direct injury by a pencil, staple, pin, fingernail, or other object. It may be due to particles flying in the air, such as sand, dust, or from woodworking.
- Corneal ulcer usually occurs when the cornea has been injured and germs enter the injured area and cause an infection. The germs may be viral, bacterial, fungal, or may be a parasitic infection.

RISK INCREASES WITH
- Contact lens wear.
- Recent eye infection or injury, or general infection.
- Very dry eyes (lack of tearing).
- Small children playing with pointed objects.
- Athletes playing sports without using eye protection.
- Work or hobbies that use pointed tools or produce dust, and construction or farm workers.
- Weak immune system, such as with HIV.
- Severe allergies.
- Eyelids that do not close completely.

PREVENTIVE MEASURES
- Avoid eye injury. Wear safety goggles or protective eye gear when using power tools or when participating in certain sports activities.
- Don't touch your eyes if you have cold sores.
- Handle contact lenses properly.
- Wash hands often to prevent spread of any germs.

EXPECTED OUTCOMES
Abrasions are usually mild and heal on their own in a few days. Corneal ulcers are a more serious eye problem, but should heal in 2 to 3 weeks with treatment.

POSSIBLE COMPLICATIONS
Scarring of the cornea, which can cause permanent partial or complete blindness.

 ## DIAGNOSIS & TREATMENT

GENERAL MEASURES
- Usually, an eye doctor (ophthalmologist) will examine the eye using a slit lamp (an eye microscope). A yellow dye may be used in the eye to make it easier to see the affected area. Medical tests may include a vision test and a culture study of corneal scraping.
- Treatment will depend on the underlying cause. This may involve removing any foreign object in the eye and drug treatment for the eye. Rarely, hospital care may be needed for severe ulcers.
- An eye patch may be used for a short term with an abrasion.
- Apply cool-water compresses to the eye as often as they feel good.
- Wear sunglasses. They may help relieve pain.
- If corneal ulcers cause scarring that affects vision, a corneal transplant may be needed.

MEDICATIONS
- Eye drops or ointments for an eye infection will be prescribed.
- For minor pain, you may use a nonprescription drug such as acetaminophen. Stronger pain drugs may be prescribed if needed.
- A tetanus shot may be needed if it is not up to date.

ACTIVITY
Resting your eyes will help with healing. Limit your reading. Don't drive until you have medical approval.

DIET
No special diet.

 ## NOTIFY OUR OFFICE IF

- You or a family member has symptoms of a corneal abrasion or corneal ulcer. Seek medical care right away.
- After diagnosis, eye pain becomes more severe, vision changes (blurring or loss of vision), or eye becomes red.

Special notes:

_____

_____

_____

More notes on the back of this page ☐

CORONARY ARTERY DISEASE

(Coronary Atherosclerosis; Ischemic Heart Disease)

 ## BASIC INFORMATION

DESCRIPTION

Heart disease that is due to hardening and narrowing of the coronary arteries that provide the blood supply to the heart. There are three main coronary arteries. When any or all become narrowed, they can no longer provide adequate oxygen for heart cells. The disorder often affects adults of both sexes over age 40. It is less common in women before menopause.

FREQUENT SIGNS AND SYMPTOMS

- Usually no symptoms occur in the early stages.
- Angina pectoris (burning, squeezing, heaviness, or tightness in the chest that may extend to the left arm, neck, jaw, or shoulder blade).
- Irregular heart rate.
- Heart attack.

CAUSES

It usually results from atherosclerosis. This is a build-up of plaque on the artery walls.

RISK INCREASES WITH

- Smoking.
- Hypertension (high blood pressure).
- Family history of coronary artery disease, diabetes, high blood pressure, or atherosclerosis.
- Poor nutrition, especially too much fat in the diet.
- Previous heart attack or stroke.
- Lack of exercise.
- Hostile or impatient personality type.
- Elevated cholesterol or LDL (low density lipoprotein) and/or low level of HDL (high-density lipoprotein).
- Overweight.

PREVENTIVE MEASURES

- Don't smoke.
- Eat a low-fat, low-salt, high-fiber diet.
- Exercise regularly.
- One aspirin a day (if medically advised).
- Reduce stress level when possible.
- If you have diabetes or hypertension, adhere to the treatment plan, including diet limits.
- Maintain ideal body weight.

EXPECTED OUTCOMES

Symptoms can usually be controlled with treatment and prolong life and improve its quality.

POSSIBLE COMPLICATIONS

- Heart attack or stroke.
- Kidney disease.
- Congestive heart failure.
- Heartbeat irregularity problems.
- Sudden death.

 ## DIAGNOSIS & TREATMENT

GENERAL MEASURES

- Your health care provider will do a physical exam. Medical tests may include electrocardiogram (measures electrical activity of the heart), echocardiogram (measures sound waves), exercise-tolerance test, coronary calcium scoring, radionuclide stress test, blood studies, x-rays of the chest, and coronary angiogram (cardiac catheterization).
- Treatment may include drug therapy, lifestyle changes, and surgery.
- Lifestyle changes include diet changes, losing weight, exercising, stopping smoking, and stress control.
- Counseling for stress problems may be helpful.
- Stop smoking. Find a way to quit that works for you.
- Surgical treatment is available in some high-risk patients. Balloon angioplasty can open narrowed vessels. Vein graft bypass can help restore blood to the heart. Large arterial obstructions can be removed by endarterectomy. Entire segments of diseased vessels can be replaced by woven plastic tube grafts.
- End-stage coronary artery disease can still be cured with a heart transplant (in rare cases).
- To learn more: American Heart Association, local branch listed in telephone directory, or call (800) 242-8721; website: www.americanheart.org.

MEDICATIONS

- Nitroglycerin, anticoagulants, drugs for angina pectoris and blood-vessel spasms, and drugs to increase the blood supply to the heart may be prescribed.
- Cholesterol-lowering drugs are usually prescribed.
- Vitamin supplements may be recommended.

ACTIVITY

20 to 30 minutes of aerobic exercise each day (if able).

DIET

Eat a low-fat, high-fiber diet that includes fruits and vegetables. Begin a weight loss diet, if overweight.

 ## NOTIFY OUR OFFICE IF

- You or a family member has symptoms of coronary artery disease
- After diagnosis, new or unexplained symptoms occur.

Special notes:

_____

_____

_____

More notes on the back of this page ☐

COSTOCHONDRITIS
(Tietze's Syndrome)

 BASIC INFORMATION

DESCRIPTION

An inflammation of the cartilage of one or more ribs, most commonly the second or third ribs. The pain that results is often increased by movements that change the position of the ribs, such as lying down, bending over, coughing, or sneezing. Pain may mimic that of heart disease or digestive disorders. It is more common in young adults, but can occur in any age group. The term Tietze syndrome is often used for costochondritis.

FREQUENT SIGNS AND SYMPTOMS

- Pain in the chest wall, usually sharp in nature.
- Pain worsens with movement.
- Pain may occur in more than one location and may radiate into the arm.
- Tightness in the chest.
- Affected area is sensitive to the touch.

CAUSES

Inflammation (soreness and swelling) of the cartilage where the ribs attach to the sternum. The cause of the inflammation is often unknown.

RISK INCREASES WITH

- Trauma, such as a severe blow to the chest.
- Unusual physical activity.
- Upper respiratory infection.

PREVENTIVE MEASURES

Avoid activities that may strain or cause trauma to the rib cage.

EXPECTED OUTCOMES

Complete healing. The disorder is benign and the course is usually of a short duration.

POSSIBLE COMPLICATIONS

None likely.

 DIAGNOSIS & TREATMENT

GENERAL MEASURES

- Your health care provider will do a physical exam and ask questions about your symptoms. There is no specific test that can diagnose costochondritis. An x-ray or bone scan may be done to rule out other disorders.
- Use a heating pad or ice massage on the affected area. Use the one that feels better for you.
- Avoid sudden movements that will intensify the pain.
- Gently stretching the chest muscles several times a day may be helpful.

MEDICATIONS

- Mild pain drugs, such as aspirin or ibuprofen, may help relieve discomfort.
- Stronger pain drugs or steroid injections may be prescribed, but these are rarely needed.

ACTIVITY

Activities may need to be limited until symptoms improve. Get extra rest when you are able to.

DIET

No special diet.

 NOTIFY OUR OFFICE IF

- You or a family member has symptoms of costochondritis.
- Pain continues or gets worse after treatment.

Special notes:

_____

_____

_____

More notes on the back of this page ☐

CROHN'S DISEASE
(Regional Ileitis; Granulomatous Ileitis)

 BASIC INFORMATION

DESCRIPTION
An inflammation (painful swelling) of the digestive tract. It can affect any part of the tract from the mouth to the anus, but most often affects the ileum. The ileum is the lower part of the small intestine. Crohn's is a type of inflammatory bowel disease (IBD). It often starts between ages 15 to 35, and affects men and women equally. Symptoms can come and go. Periods between flare-ups vary from every few months to every few years. Sometimes, symptoms appear only once or twice, and then the disease disappears.

FREQUENT SIGNS AND SYMPTOMS
- Cramps and pain in the abdomen (stomach area). The pain is often in the lower-right part of the abdomen.
- Diarrhea.
- Loss of appetite and weight loss.
- Stools may be bloody or contain mucus.
- General ill feeling with fatigue
- Fever may occur.
- Children with this condition may not grow at a normal rate, and have delayed puberty.

CAUSES
Unknown. The inflammation may result from the body's immune system overreacting to an infection. Genetic and environmental (such as diet) factors may play a role.

RISK INCREASES WITH
- Family history of Crohn's or other bowel disease.
- Smoking.
- History of allergies.
- People of Jewish and European ancestry.
- A diet high in fat or refined foods may be a risk factor.

PREVENTIVE MEASURES
At this time, there is no way to prevent this condition.

EXPECTED OUTCOMES
There is no cure for the disease, but patients can have a reasonable quality of life. Treatment can help relieve symptoms. Over time, the treatment usually becomes less effective, and many patients develop complications that require surgery.

POSSIBLE COMPLICATIONS
- Intestines may become blocked (bowel obstruction).
- An abnormal opening (fistula) may develop between the bowel and nearby areas.
- Abscess (pus-filled sore).
- The bowel may burst or begin to leak.
- Higher risk of colon cancer.
- The body may not be able to absorb nutrients well.
- Bleeding. This can lead to low iron levels in blood.

 DIAGNOSIS & TREATMENT

GENERAL MEASURES
- Your health care provider will do a physical exam and ask questions about your symptoms and activities. Medical tests may include blood and stool studies, special x-rays, CT, MRI, or ultrasound. A colonoscopy (a colon exam using a thin, lighted tube) may be done.
- Treatment steps can include drugs, diet changes, and surgery. Hospital care may be needed for severe symptoms. A feeding tube may be inserted into the stomach.
- For home care, use heat to relieve pain. Apply a heating pad or take warm-water baths. Check stool daily for signs of bleeding.
- Surgery may be required. It may improve the symptoms and delay progress of the disease.
- To learn more: Crohn's and Colitis Foundation of America, 386 Park Ave. South, 17th floor, New York, NY 10016; (800) 932-2423; website: www.ccfa.org.

MEDICATIONS
- Your health care provider may prescribe:
  - Drugs for inflammation (anti-inflammatories, steroids, or anti-TNF [tumor necrosis factor] drugs).
  - Drugs to relieve pain.
  - Antidiarrheals to control diarrhea.
  - Vitamin supplements.
  - Drugs that suppress the immune system.
  - Antibiotics for infection.

ACTIVITY
Remain as active as your symptoms allow.

DIET
- Avoid foods that aggravate the condition. This may include alcohol, milk products, fatty foods, fiber, popcorn, nuts, and spices. Keep a food diary to help find what foods you can and cannot eat.
- Eat small, frequent meals. Take small bites and chew food completely. Drink fluids with meals. Drink liquid nutrient formulas if it is difficult to eat regular food.

 NOTIFY OUR OFFICE IF

- You or a family member has symptoms of Crohn's.
- Symptoms get worse or new ones develop.
- Blood appears in the stools.

Special notes:

_____

_____

_____

More notes on the back of this page ☐

CROUP
(Laryngotracheobronchitis)

BASIC INFORMATION

DESCRIPTION
Infection, redness, and swelling of the larynx (vocal cords). It may extend into the trachea (windpipe) and bronchi (airways in the lungs). Children under age 5 are most often affected.

FREQUENT SIGNS AND SYMPTOMS
- The infection can start gradually with a cold, cough, and low fever. Frequently, symptoms come on suddenly in the middle of the night.
- Barking cough. It may be worse when child cries.
- Trouble breathing, especially at night.
- Noisy breathing or wheezing (called stridor).
- Hoarseness.
- Throat discomfort with difficulty in swallowing.
- More severe symptoms include fast breathing, ribs that seem to pull in when breathing, paleness, and bluish skin around the mouth.

CAUSES
A contagious, viral infection is the usual cause. Croup often occurs in outbreaks in the winter and early spring months. Symptoms may begin 3 to 5 days after exposure, but time will vary depending on the type of virus.

RISK INCREASES WITH
- Repeated colds and lung infections or lung disease.
- Previous croup.
- Allergies.

PREVENTIVE MEASURES
No specific preventive measures. Wash your hands often to prevent the spread of any germs.

EXPECTED OUTCOMES
Croup can be frightening, because attacks usually happen at night and the child has trouble breathing. In almost all cases, croup is not serious and clears up in about a week or less. Complications are rare, but they may occur in children born prematurely or children with lung disease such as asthma.

POSSIBLE COMPLICATIONS
- Recurrence of croup.
- Ear infection.
- Pneumonia.
- Lymph node inflammation.

DIAGNOSIS & TREATMENT

GENERAL MEASURES
- If symptoms are more severe or you are concerned about the symptoms, see your child's health care provider. A physical exam is usually all that is needed for diagnosis.

- A child who has severe breathing problems may need hospital care. Oxygen may be given to help breathing.
- Most children can be treated at home using supportive care. There are no specific drugs to treat croup.
- Turn on the hot water in the bathroom shower and let the room fill with steam. Hold the child in your arms in the bathroom filled with steam for 10 to 15 minutes. Repeat this procedure if another attack occurs.
- Wrapping the child in a blanket and walking around outdoors may help. It is better if outdoor air is cool.
- Keep the child comfortable in a semi-seated position. Use TV, radio, or a story to distract the child so he or she can relax. Crying can aggravate symptoms.
- Use a cool-mist humidifier or vaporizer near the child's bed for several nights during and after an attack even if the child appears well. Simple croup can recur. Clean the humidifier daily.

MEDICATIONS
- Since the cause is usually viral, antibiotics do not help. Cough medicines are also not helpful.
- Acetaminophen may be given to lower fever.
- Injected drugs may be given to a child in the hospital.
- Steroids and/or bronchodilators (to help open the airways) may be prescribed.

ACTIVITY
Rest until symptoms improve.

DIET
Usually, a child with croup is not as hungry as normal. It is important to drink plenty of fluids. Offer frequent small amounts of clear fluids or Popsicles.

NOTIFY OUR OFFICE IF

- Your child is having trouble breathing and cannot swallow saliva or water. This is an emergency! Call 911 or take the child to the nearest emergency room.
- Nails or lips become bluish.
- Mild croup symptoms don't improve with home care.

Special notes:

_____

_____

_____

More notes on the back of this page ☐

CRYPTOCOCCOSIS
(Torulosis)

BASIC INFORMATION

DESCRIPTION
A fungal disease that usually affects the lungs, but may spread to other body parts. Cryptococcosis is more common in men between ages 40 and 60. It is much more serious when there are underlying illnesses or risk factors. This condition has become more common since the emergence of AIDS.

FREQUENT SIGNS AND SYMPTOMS
· Some people may have no symptoms or symptoms are mild and go unnoticed.
· Fever.
· Cough, sometimes with mucus.
· Headache, sometimes severe.
· Shortness of breath.
· Weight loss.
· Tiredness.
· Personality or mental changes if the infection affects the nervous system. This can include confusion or depression or being agitated.
· If the skin is infected, sores or ulcers may occur.
· The infection may cause symptoms in bones, the prostate, and the eyes.

CAUSES
Infection with *Cryptococcus neoformans*. A person gets the infection by breathing in air that contains the germs. The germs are found throughout the world, often in pigeon droppings. The infection is not passed from one person to another. Animals may also get the infection, but do not spread it to humans.

RISK INCREASES WITH
· AIDS.
· Organ transplant.
· Drugs that suppress the immune system.
· Cancer (Hodgkin's disease, leukemia, myeloma, lung cancer, and others).
· Chronic lung disease, diabetes, cirrhosis, rheumatoid arthritis, lupus, and splenectomy (spleen removal).

PREVENTIVE MEASURES
Avoid areas that have pigeon droppings.

EXPECTED OUTCOMES
In those with normal immune systems, the infection usually heals on its own or with treatment. In those with weak immune systems, treatment may control the disease, but not cure it. Lifelong drug therapy may be needed to prevent a relapse.

POSSIBLE COMPLICATIONS
· Infection or inflammation of the brain (encephalitis) or the membranes that surround the brain (meningitis).
· Permanent brain damage, vision loss, and death.

DIAGNOSIS & TREATMENT

GENERAL MEASURES
· Your health care provider will usually do a physical exam and ask questions about your symptoms and activities. Medical tests may include blood, urine, and spinal fluid studies. A brain CT or MRI may be done.
· Some patients require no treatment. Those with underlying disorders are usually treated with drugs.
· Hospital care may be needed for severe symptoms.
· Weigh daily. Keep a weight chart. An unexplained weight loss might mean that the infection has spread.

MEDICATIONS
Antifungal drugs are often prescribed. One drug is usually given by injection at first, followed by another drug that is taken by mouth. People with HIV or AIDS will usually need to take an antifungal drug for life.

ACTIVITY
Get extra rest until the symptoms improve.

DIET
No special diet.

NOTIFY OUR OFFICE IF

· You or a family member has symptoms of cryptococcosis. Especially if you have a severe headache.
· Symptoms recur after treatment.
· New, unexplained symptoms develop. Drugs used in treatment may produce side effects.

Special notes:

_____

_____

_____

More notes on the back of this page ☐

CUSHING'S SYNDROME

 BASIC INFORMATION

DESCRIPTION

A disorder due to excess levels of cortisol, a hormone. Cortisol helps the body respond to stress and change. The adrenal gland (located over the kidney) and pituitary gland (at the base of the brain) are involved in the production of cortisol. Cushing's syndrome most often affects adults ages 20 to 50.

FREQUENT SIGNS AND SYMPTOMS

- Round (moon-like) face and puffy eyes.
- Thin, fragile skin; easy bruising.
- Weakness.
- Weight gain. Fat areas, such as around the torso.
- Growth of facial hair in women.
- Stretch marks (red/blue streaks on the skin).
- Mental, mood, and emotional changes.
- Menstrual changes (increase, irregular, or no period).
- More likely to get infections.
- Sexual and fertility problems.
- High blood pressure.
- Children may have growth retardation, acne, or very early or very late puberty.

CAUSES

- It may result from an overproduction of cortisol by the adrenal glands due to a variety of medical disorders.
- It may result from long-term use of cortisol-like drugs (steroid hormones) to treat medical disorders (such as asthma, arthritis, and inflammatory bowel disease).

RISK INCREASES WITH

- An abnormal growth in the pituitary gland. This causes production of excessive ACTH (adrenocorticotropic hormone). This in turn stimulates the adrenal glands to secrete hormones. This is called Cushing's disease.
- A benign or cancerous tumor in the adrenal gland.
- Tumors in other places in the body produce hormones that in turn cause the adrenal glands to produce excess cortisol.
- Prolonged use of steroid hormone drugs.

PREVENTIVE MEASURES

If steroid hormone drugs are prescribed, take the lowest dose possible for the shortest time.

EXPECTED OUTCOMES

Outcome will depend on the cause of Cushing's syndrome, the degree of excess cortisol, the length of the disease, and the person's basic health. If the cause is treatable, the symptoms may resolve in 2 to 18 months.

POSSIBLE COMPLICATIONS

- Osteoporosis and bone fractures due to osteoporosis.
- Side effects of steroid hormones.
- Diabetes, high blood pressure, infections, kidney stones, or spread of cancerous tumors.

 DIAGNOSIS & TREATMENT

GENERAL MEASURES

- Your health care provider will do a physical exam and ask questions about your symptoms and drug use. Medical tests may include studies of blood and urine to measure hormone levels, pituitary gland and adrenal gland function tests, and CT, MRI, or x-rays.
- Treatment will depend on the cause of the disorder.
- If it is due to steroid hormone use, the dosage may be slowly reduced (depending on the disease being treated). If the steroid hormone needs to be continued, other drugs may be taken to control the side effects.
- Pituitary gland tumors may be treated with surgery or radiation. If the pituitary gland is removed, hormone replacement therapy will be needed for life.
- Adrenal gland adenoma tumors are removed with surgery. The other adrenal gland is left in place and will eventually take over hormone production.
- Adrenal gland cancerous tumors can be cured if diagnosed early. Often, they are not diagnosed until they have spread beyond the adrenal gland. When this happens, they are not curable. Drugs can treat symptoms.
- Tumors in other places in the body may be treated with surgery, radiation, or chemotherapy. This may help improve the Cushing's syndrome.
- Wear a medical alert type bracelet or pendant indicating your medical problem and the drugs you take.

MEDICATIONS

- Drugs to suppress adrenal gland function, cortisone drugs (if adrenal gland removed), or drugs to replace pituitary hormones may be prescribed.
- Drugs to lower blood pressure, to prevent bone loss, and to reduce blood sugar may be prescribed.

ACTIVITY

No limits. Energy will improve once treatment begins.

DIET

No special diet, unless otherwise advised.

 NOTIFY OUR OFFICE IF

- You or a family member has symptoms of Cushing's syndrome.
- Signs of infection occur or other symptoms develop.

Special notes: _____

_____

_____

_____

More notes on the back of this page ☐

CYSTIC FIBROSIS (CF)

 ## BASIC INFORMATION

DESCRIPTION
An inherited disease affecting the body's glands that produce secretions such as mucus, sweat, tears, saliva, and digestive juices. These secretions are normally thin and slippery and act as a lubricant. In cystic fibrosis (CF), the secretions are thick and sticky. This means the lungs, pancreas, intestines, and other organs are clogged up. One in 3,900 newborns is born with CF in the United States.

FREQUENT SIGNS AND SYMPTOMS
- Symptoms will vary in different patients.
- In a newborn, there are thick, sticky stools (meconium). They may cause intestinal obstruction.
- Delayed growth.
- Poor weight gain despite good appetite.
- Bad-smelling, large, fatty stools.
- Sometimes, because the air is chronically trapped in the chest, the child gets a barrel-chested appearance.
- Chronic cough or wheezing.
- Sticky, hard-to-cough-up sputum.
- Salty sweat.
- Polyps in the nose.
- Frequent chest and sinus infections.
- Rounding (clubbing) of the fingertips or toes.
- Rectal prolapse and intussusception (bowel disorder).

CAUSES
A defective gene. People can carry the gene for cystic fibrosis, but not develop it. If both parents are carriers of the defective gene, there is a 25% chance that a child will have the disease, a 50% chance, the child will be a carrier, and 25% chance the child will not have the disease or be a carrier.

RISK INCREASES WITH
Family history of cystic fibrosis.

PREVENTIVE MEASURES
If you have a family history of cystic fibrosis, seek genetic counseling before starting a family.

EXPECTED OUTCOMES
- This condition is currently considered incurable and is often fatal in childhood. Careful long-term care by parents and a medical care team can help children lead reasonably comfortable lives. Children with milder forms are living to adulthood, especially if the disorder is detected early. Median survival age is 33.
- Medical research is ongoing to find a cure.

POSSIBLE COMPLICATIONS
- Repeated respiratory infections.
- CF can cause various other medical problems such as infertility, diabetes, osteoporosis, digestive system problems, and lung and heart disorders.

 ## DIAGNOSIS & TREATMENT

GENERAL MEASURES
- Your child's health care provider will do a physical exam. Medical tests include a sweat test (repeated twice). CF is diagnosed if the sweat contains high amounts of salt. Very young infants may not produce enough sweat for this test, so genetic blood studies may be done to aid with diagnosis. Tests may be done for lung, pancreas, and liver functions.
- Testing of brothers and sisters of a child with CF is usually recommended even if they have no symptoms.
- A medical team (for lung therapy, diet needs, and medical help) will be provided for the child's care.
- Goals of therapy are to prevent and treat infections, keep lungs free of sputum, improve airflow, and provide adequate calories and nutrition.
- Learn as much as possible about CF. Parents may want to join a support group.
- You will be instructed on how to perform daily postural drainage to drain mucus from the lungs. This is done with clapping on the front and back of the chest. Mechanical aids and special vests are available to help.
- Keep your child's vaccines (including flu) up-to-date.
- Transplants for lung, liver, and pancreas are possible.
- To learn more: Cystic Fibrosis Foundation, 6931 Arlington Road, Bethesda, MD 20814, (800) 344-4823; website: www.cff.org.

MEDICATIONS
- Drug therapy may include digestive enzymes to help with digestion, antibiotics for infections, mucus-thinning drugs, and bronchodilators to help open airways.
- Gene therapy is being studied.

ACTIVITY
As much as the condition permits. Encourage your child to lead as normal and active a life as possible.

DIET
High in calories, fat, and protein. Vitamin supplements and supplemental nutrition may be needed.

 ## NOTIFY OUR OFFICE IF

- You suspect your child has cystic fibrosis.
- After diagnosis, symptoms get worse at any time.

Special notes:

_____

_____

_____

More notes on the back of this page ☐

DECOMPRESSION SICKNESS
(Bends)

BASIC INFORMATION

DESCRIPTION
A painful, sometimes life-threatening condition of blood gases that is caused by a sudden drop in environmental pressure.

FREQUENT SIGNS AND SYMPTOMS
The following may occur right away or up to 24 hours after the pressure change:
• Mild-to-severe joint pain, especially in the shoulders, elbows, hips, and knees.
• Chest pain, shortness of breath, and a burning sensation behind the breastbone.
• Chokes. This is severe breathing difficulty experienced by scuba divers and others who go from high to normal air pressure too rapidly. Bubbles of nitrogen develop in the blood stream and obstruct blood supply to vital organs, sometimes resulting in severe injury or death.
• Coughing.
• Weakness, loss of normal sensation, paralysis, loss of consciousness, and coma (rare).
• Unable to speak, blindness, or deafness.
• Abdominal pain.
• Difficult urination.

CAUSES
Formation of nitrogen bubbles in the blood. Nitrogen is a normal blood component. If the pressure around the body drops rapidly, as in surfacing too quickly while scuba diving, or climbing too rapidly in a non-pressurized aircraft, the nitrogen collects in bubbles in the blood vessels. This blocks the normal blood flow and deprives the body of blood and oxygen.

RISK INCREASES WITH
• Commercial diving or recreational scuba diving. Repeated dives in one day increase the risk.
• Some kinds of high-performance aircraft.
• Working in compression chambers.

PREVENTIVE MEASURES
• Obtain certified instruction before scuba diving.
• Don't dive if you are not in good general health. You are at risk if you are obese or have a medical history of: Don't dive if you are not in good general health. You are at risk if you are obese or have a medical history of:
  - Lung conditions, such as asthma.
  - Pneumothorax.
  - Heart disease.
  - Chronic sinusitis.
  - Alcoholism.
• Allow for a slow, gradual change to normal air pressure when scuba diving. (The U.S. Navy has tested and set up guidelines.)
• Avoid air travel for 24 hours after diving.

EXPECTED OUTCOMES
Usually good for patients who receive early treatment. In others, it depends on duration and severity of symptoms prior to treatment.

POSSIBLE COMPLICATIONS
• Permanent brain damage.
• Permanent bone destruction due to blockage of blood supply.

DIAGNOSIS & TREATMENT

GENERAL MEASURES
• Self-care is impossible for this condition. If you observe someone with symptoms of decompression sickness, get emergency medical care immediately.
• Treatment involves time in a decompression chamber to force nitrogen bubbles to dissolve into the blood.
• Treatment is best when it is done early. However, some patients may benefit even at 6 to 9 days after the incident. Medical care is critical even if symptoms resolve because 25% of patients will relapse.
• For assistance in locating the nearest treatment chamber in your area, call the emergency Divers Alert Network (DAN) at any hour (919) 684-8111. For non-emergency information, call (919) 684-2948; website: www.diversalertnetwork.org.

MEDICATIONS
Drugs are usually not needed for this disorder. Don't take pain relievers. These may further decrease normal breathing function.

ACTIVITY
Resume your normal activities as soon as symptoms improve after treatment.

DIET
No special diet.

NOTIFY OUR OFFICE IF

You have symptoms (or observe them in another person) of decompression sickness within 24 hours after scuba diving or rapid ascent without pressurization.

Special notes:

_____

_____

_____

More notes on the back of this page ☐

DEHYDRATION

BASIC INFORMATION

DESCRIPTION

The body is not able to function properly due to excess fluid loss, or not enough fluid intake. Dehydration is most dangerous in newborns, infants, and persons over 60. The dehydration may be mild, moderate, or severe depending on the percentage of body weight lost.

FREQUENT SIGNS AND SYMPTOMS

- Dry mouth and swollen tongue. Severe thirst.
- Decreased or no urination; urine color may be deep yellow. In infants, there may be no wet diapers.
- Sunken eyes and wrinkled skin.
- Inability to sweat.
- Infants may have no tears when crying.
- Fatigue.
- Low blood pressure.
- Increase in heart rate and breathing.
- Dizziness, confusion, coma.

CAUSES

- Severe vomiting or diarrhea from any cause.
- Heavy sweating.
- Too much urine output.
- Not taking in a sufficient amount of food or water.

RISK INCREASES WITH

- Newborns, infants, and adults over 60.
- Illness with high fever.
- Not eating or drinking due to illness or mouth sores.
- Use of drugs, such as diuretics ("water pills").
- Excess exposure to sun or heat.
- Diabetes or kidney disease.
- Injuries to the skin, such as burns, can cause fluid loss through the damaged skin.

PREVENTIVE MEASURES

- If you are vomiting or have diarrhea, take small sips of a fluid replacement product. This is important during an illness with a fever. Children need to be observed for any symptoms of dehydration.
- If you use diuretics, weigh yourself daily.
- Carry water with you to outdoor activities. Drink plenty of water while exercising. Avoid exercising outdoors in very hot weather.
- Avoid drinking alcohol in hot weather.

EXPECTED OUTCOMES

Curable with control of the underlying cause and replacement of necessary fluids.

POSSIBLE COMPLICATIONS

- Depends on any medical problems. Usually with mild to moderate symptoms, no complications are expected.
- Severe dehydration or electrolyte imbalance may lead to seizures, heart problems, brain damage, or death.

DIAGNOSIS & TREATMENT

GENERAL MEASURES

- Your health care provider will do a physical exam and ask questions about your symptoms. Blood tests may be done to check electrolyte levels (these include sodium, potassium, and bicarbonate). Electrolytes are vital for the body to function normally. Other tests may be needed to find the specific cause of the dehydration.
- Treatment will be aimed at restoring body fluids and treating any illness that is diagnosed.
- For mild dehydration, drink frequent small amounts of clear liquids. Large amounts may bring on vomiting.
- Drink electrolyte solutions. For adults, dilute solutions such as Gatorade or Recharge with an equal amount of water. For children, use special products (such as Pedialyte or Ricelyte). Instructions are on the labels.
- If the dehydration is severe, a hospital stay may be needed for fluid replacement.

MEDICATIONS

Usually not needed for dehydration.

ACTIVITY

Rest in bed until symptoms get better.

DIET

A special diet is usually not needed. Resume a normal diet after the diarrhea and vomiting stops. Avoid alcohol and highly seasoned foods for several more days.

NOTIFY OUR OFFICE IF

You or a family member has symptoms of dehydration.

Special notes:

_____

_____

_____

More notes on the back of this page ☐

DELAYED ONSET MUSCLE SORENESS (DOMS)

BASIC INFORMATION

DESCRIPTION

Delayed onset muscle soreness (DOMS) occurs hours after an exercise is over. DOMS is not an injury as such, but can be painful. Nearly every healthy adult has had DOMS no matter what the person's fitness level is. The symptoms of DOMS are a normal response, and are part of the process that leads to improved strength once the muscles recover. You can expect a certain amount of DOMS when getting in shape.

FREQUENT SIGNS AND SYMPTOMS

• Symptoms start about 8 to 24 hours after the activity and end within 3 to 7 days. They may be worse the second day than they are the first day.
• Muscle pain, aches, soreness, stiffness, and swelling.
• The muscles may be less flexible.
• Muscle areas feel tender when touched.

CAUSES

Exact cause is not clear and there may be several factors involved including the buildup of lactic acid. DOMS results from doing any new or changed exercise or activity.

RISK INCREASES WITH

• Too much exercise, or a change in activity from non-impact, such as biking, to high-impact (such as running).
• New or heavy strength exercises. Even if you exercise on a regular basis, any new type of activity may cause delayed soreness.

PREVENTIVE MEASURES

• There are no sure ways to prevent DOMS. Some ways to help reduce the amount of soreness are listed here.
• Most reports show that stretching prevents DOMS. If you do stretch before or after exercising, do so slowly, and only to the point at which you feel slight discomfort. Hold the stretch for anywhere between 10 and 30 seconds.
• Warm-up before you start an activity. Do a few minutes of slow walking or biking.
• Give your muscles time to adjust to an activity. Make changes slowly (over several weeks if needed) to a new exercise program or new or different sports activity.
• Cool down after a workout.
• If you start a new weightlifting program, begin with weights you can lift easily, and then add weight slowly.
• Drink plenty of fluids to help clear lactic acid from the tissues.

EXPECTED OUTCOMES

The soreness is usually gone within 3 to 7 days. Your muscles will not get sore again if you keep doing the exercise or activity on a regular basis.

POSSIBLE COMPLICATIONS

None expected. There is no long-term damage or change in function of the muscles involved.

DIAGNOSIS & TREATMENT

GENERAL MEASURES

• Self-care is often all that is needed. If pain is severe, see your health care provider.
• Use ice massage. Fill a Styrofoam cup with water and freeze it. Tear a small amount of foam from the top so ice sticks out. Rub the ice gently over the painful area in a circle about the size of a softball. Do this for 15 minutes at a time, 3 or 4 times a day, and before workouts.
• After 72 hours, if muscle is still sore, apply heat, such as hot soaks, instead of ice if it feels better.
• Use your hands to massage the muscle gently and often. Massage will provide comfort and reduce swelling, but it won't speed the recovery.

MEDICATIONS

• For minor pain and inflammation, you may try aspirin (not for children) or ibuprofen, but they do not always work for DOMS.
• Some people find that vitamin C supplements help.
• Nonprescription topical products may be used to soothe sore muscles.
• Drugs will not help to prevent DOMS.

ACTIVITY

• Keep on with some exercising. Perform low-impact aerobic exercise to increase blood flow to the muscles.
• If muscle soreness or pain increases after you begin exercising, stop and use ice on the muscles.

DIET

No special diet.

NOTIFY OUR OFFICE IF

You or a family member has delayed onset muscle soreness that is severe or has lasted more than a week.

Special notes:

_____

_____

_____

More notes on the back of this page ☐

DEMENTIA

 ## BASIC INFORMATION

DESCRIPTION

Dementia is a disease that attacks the brain. It is not a normal part of aging. Dementia results in problems with memory, thinking, and behavior. It can interfere with a person's ability to function and take care of everyday tasks. There are many types of dementia. Common types are Alzheimer's disease, multi-infarct, and vascular dementia. Dementia often affects people over age 65.

FREQUENT SIGNS AND SYMPTOMS

· Memory problems. Forgetfulness, such as about recent events or ordinary information such as birth date and address; not able to recognize family and friends.
· Confusion and poor judgment.
· Loss of interest in normal activities.
· Trouble speaking well.
· Disorientation, especially at night.
· Poor personal hygiene and appearance.
· Sleep problems.
· Personality changes.
· Anxiety, depression, being suspicious, agitation, wandering, verbal abuse, or being assaultive.
· Incontinence, hallucinations, delusions (later stage).

CAUSES

Nerve cells in the brain become damaged and die. Once the cells die, they cannot be replaced. The brain shrinks and brain function deteriorates. Most dementias are progressive (get worse with time) and cannot be cured. There are a few causes of dementia that may be potentially reversible, such as with a brain tumor.

RISK INCREASES WITH

· Inadequate blood supply to the brain. It may be due to blood clots, strokes, tumor, high blood pressure, or hardening of the arteries (atherosclerosis).
· Severe, or repeated, head injury (such as in boxing).
· Infections, such as AIDS or syphilis.
· Down syndrome, Parkinson's disease, Huntington's chorea, and some hereditary disorders.
· Metabolic disorders, such as thyroid disease.
· Certain nutritional deficiencies.
· Toxic causes (alcoholism, drugs, heavy metals).

PREVENTIVE MEASURES

Most dementias are not preventable. Reducing risk factors may help. Maintain a healthy lifestyle, protect yourself from head injuries, and control chronic illnesses.

EXPECTED OUTCOMES

Most dementia progress at varying rates, a few stay the same, and a few may reverse with treatment of a cause.

POSSIBLE COMPLICATIONS

Each type of dementia has its own complications. Most have a downward course that leads to death.

 ## DIAGNOSIS & TREATMENT

GENERAL MEASURES

· Family members may notice early behavior changes and seek medical care. The health care provider will do a physical exam and ask questions about the symptoms. There is no specific test to diagnose dementia. Medical tests may include cognitive tests (answering questions), blood, urine, and spinal fluid studies, heart studies, CT, MRI, PET scans, or others. Testing rules out other disorders or find a cause of dementia that can be treated.
· A diagnosis of dementia is overwhelming, both for the patient and the family. Educate yourselves as much as possible about what to expect and how to plan for it. With early diagnosis, the patient can take part in making decisions for the future.
· Treatment will depend on the severity of the symptoms. Different drugs are available that can help slow the progress of some dementias (such as Alzheimer's).
· Drugs to treat the behavior symptoms can help make a patient more comfortable and make their care easier.
· Caring for a family member with dementia is a difficult task. Caregivers need to take care of themselves. Joining a support group for caregivers may be helpful.
· To learn more: Alzheimer's Association, 225 N. Michigan Ave., Fl 17, Chicago. Il 60601; (800) 272-3900; website: www.alz.org.

MEDICATIONS

· Drugs as needed to help control behavior symptoms (insomnia, agitation, wandering, depression, anxiety, and others) will be prescribed.
· Drugs that slow the progress of Alzheimer's disease for a limited time may be prescribed.
· Drugs to treat causes of dementia may be prescribed.

ACTIVITY

Patient activity may require supervision at all times.

DIET

Regular diet. Feeding help will eventually be needed.

 ## NOTIFY OUR OFFICE IF

· Symptoms of dementia appear in a family member.
· Caregivers of dementia patients have any questions.

Special notes:

_____

_____

_____

More notes on the back of this page ☐

DEPRESSION

BASIC INFORMATION

DESCRIPTION
Depression is a mood disorder. The symptoms that occur (emotional and physical) interfere with everyday life for an extended period of time. Symptoms may be mild, moderate, or severe. Depression is common and affects children and adults (women more than men).

FREQUENT SIGNS AND SYMPTOMS
- Loss of interest in life, feeling bored and listless.
- Fatigue and lack of energy.
- Insomnia, excess sleep, or sleeping problems.
- Lack of pleasure, or withdrawal, from usual activities.
- Change in appetite that leads to weight gain or loss.
- Loss of sex drive.
- Difficulty making decisions; concentration difficulty.
- Unexplained crying bouts.
- Inappropriate guilt feelings, self-hate, lack of self-esteem, and feeling unworthy.
- Irritability, anger, and agitation.
- Headache or other aches and pains.

CAUSES
It is not fully known what causes depression. It appears to be a combination of factors. Chemical imbalances in the brain may cause or contribute to depression. Other factors may include biologic, genetic, psychological, environmental, and developmental events.

RISK INCREASES WITH
- Women are more at risk than men.
- Previous episode of depression.
- Family history of depression.
- Advanced age.
- Compulsive, rigid, perfectionistic, or highly dependent personality.
- Other emotional or personality disorder.
- Substance abuse, such as alcoholism or drugs.
- Failure in job, marriage, or a personal relationship.
- Death or loss of a loved one.
- Recent, stressful life experience.
- Living alone, social isolation.
- Surgery, major illness, or disability.
- Passing from one life stage to another (e.g., retiring).
- Use of some drugs, not taking prescribed drugs, or side effect of drugs.
- Some chronic diseases.

PREVENTIVE MEASURES
Depression is often not preventable. Reduce your risks where possible. If you have recurring depression, drugs may be prescribed for prevention.

EXPECTED OUTCOME
Treatment helps most patients. Depression may sometimes recur or it may be a one-time episode.

POSSIBLE COMPLICATIONS
- Alcohol or substance abuse.
- Problems with physical health.
- Failure to improve with treatment.
- Suicide.

DIAGNOSIS & TREATMENT

GENERAL MEASURES
- Your health care provider will do a physical exam and ask questions about your symptoms and activities. Screening tests for depression are helpful in diagnosis. Medical tests may be done to rule out other disorders.
- Therapy consists of treating acute symptoms, avoiding a relapse, and preventing recurrence.
- Psychotherapy or counseling along with drug treatment appears to obtain the best results.
- Types of psychotherapy include cognitive therapy, behavioral therapy, and interpersonal therapy. Therapy may involve 12 to 20 sessions over 12 to 16 weeks.
- Hospital care or inpatient at a special treatment center may be required for severe depression.
- Seek support groups. Contact social agencies for help. Call the National Mental Health Association, (800) 969-6642; website: www.nmha.org.
- Call a suicide-prevention hot line if you feel suicidal.
- Electroconvulsive therapy (use of electric shocks to produce a seizure) may be used in severe cases.

MEDICATION
- Antidepressant drugs will usually be prescribed. Multiple drugs are necessary in some cases. It will take 2 to 4 weeks or longer for improvement.
- Drugs for other symptoms may be prescribed.

ACTIVITY
A regular exercise program can help relieve depression.

DIET
Eat a normal, well-balanced diet.

NOTIFY OUR OFFICE IF

- You or a family member has symptoms of depression.
- Symptoms don't improve with treatment.

Special notes:

_____

_____

_____

More notes on the back of this page ☐

DERMATITIS, ATOPIC
(Eczema)

BASIC INFORMATION

DESCRIPTION
A common, chronic skin disorder. *Dermatitis* means skin inflammation (redness and soreness). *Atopic* refers to hereditary disorders. Atopic dermatitis often affects infants and children, but can occur in all age groups. It affects males and females equally. It cannot be passed from one person to another.

FREQUENT SIGNS AND SYMPTOMS
· Itchy, dry skin. Scaling, redness, swelling, weeping, cracking, and crusting of the skin may occur. It often affects the skin creases of elbows, knees, neck, face, hands, feet, groin, genitals, and around the anus. It may also affect the skin around the eyes.
· Itching is worse during sleep.
· An itch-scratch cycle develops. The itch causes a person to scratch, which in turn worsens the itch.
· An infant may be irritable and restless.

CAUSES
Unknown. It may be a combination of genetic (hereditary) factors and environmental factors.

RISK INCREASES WITH
· Hay fever or asthma or food allergy.
· Family history of atopic dermatitis or other allergic disorders.
· Weak immune system due to illness or drugs.
· People living in dry climates.

PREVENTIVE MEASURES
· No preventive measures for the original outbreak.
· Identify and then avoid the factors that may trigger an outbreak in an individual. These can include:
 - Emotional factors (stress and anger).
 - Irritants (wool, perfumes, fabric softeners, smoke, some soaps, etc.).
 - Allergens (substances that inflame the skin) such as pollen, or cat and dog dander.
 - Temperature or climate.
 - Skin infections.

EXPECTED OUTCOMES
The disorder can come and go throughout life. Symptoms may decrease with age. Treatment and self-care will help relieve symptoms in most people.

POSSIBLE COMPLICATIONS
· Skin infections.
· Skin may become thick and leathery or scarred from scratching.
· Anxiety and depression due to a chronic disorder.
· Eye problems (blepharitis, cataracts, conjunctivitis).
· Herpes simplex infections are more severe in people with atopic dermatitis.

DIAGNOSIS & TREATMENT

GENERAL MEASURES
· Your health care provider will perform a skin exam and ask questions about your symptoms and medical history. There is no test to diagnose atopic dermatitis. Skin tests may be done to rule out other skin problems.
· Treatment steps involve healing the skin, preventing flare-ups, and treating symptoms when they occur.
· Lubricate the skin often, especially after bathing. Use petroleum, or alpha-hydroxy containing lanolin-based ointments.
· Bathe in cool to warm water (not hot) with products other than soap. Use cool-water soaks for crusting, oozing skin. These decrease itching and remove crusts.
· Wear loose fitting, cotton clothing. Avoid fabric softeners and anti-static laundry products.
· Reduce any emotional problems in your life, if possible. The itching often increases during stressful periods.
· To learn more: National Eczema Association, 4460 Redwood Hwy, Suite 16-D, San Rapheal, CA 94903; (800) 818-7546; website: www.nationaleczema.org.

MEDICATIONS
· To relieve minor itching, use nonprescription topical steroids or coal-tar preparations.
· You may be prescribed stronger topical steroids, oral or injected steroid drugs (for short periods only), antihistamines, antibiotics for infections, drugs to suppress the immune system, or other, newer drugs.
· A treatment called PUVA may be helpful. It combines a special light used with a cream applied to the skin.

ACTIVITY
No limits. Avoid prolonged exposure to hot climate.

DIET
If food allergy is suspected, ask your health care provider if a diet change will help.

NOTIFY OUR OFFICE IF

· You or a family member has symptoms of atopic dermatitis.
· A fever and other signs of infection develop, or uncontrolled itching occurs during a flare up.

Special notes:

_____

_____

_____

More notes on the back of this page ☐

DERMATITIS, CONTACT

 BASIC INFORMATION

DESCRIPTION

A common skin disorder caused by substances that irritate the skin or cause an allergic skin reaction. When an irritant causes the dermatitis, the symptoms usually begin right after exposure. With an allergen-caused dermatitis, the symptoms may take several hours or more to develop. Contact dermatitis can not be spread from one person to another. It occurs in people of all ages and affects women more than men.

FREQUENT SIGNS AND SYMPTOMS

- Itching and swelling of the skin.
- Slight redness in milder cases.
- Bright red weeping areas in some cases.
- Blisters that break open and ooze, crust, or scale.
- Swelling of face, eyes, genital area (severe allergy)

CAUSES

- There are many causes of contact dermatitis. It may take time and effort to find the exact cause for each person, and sometimes, the cause is not found. Sometimes the causes may be from a mix of allergens and irritants, especially dermatitis on the hands.
- Irritants include soaps, detergents, bleaches, cleaners; bromine or chlorine used in swimming pools. Also, some oils, tars, a variety of plants including poinsettia, and numerous other items.
- Allergic reaction may come from nickel (found in earrings, rings, and watches); glues; household cleansers; leather; paints; latex (in balloons, rubber bands, elastic waist bands); chemicals (in hair dyes, perfumes, deodorants, and cosmetics); plants such as poison ivy, oak, or sumac; and numerous other possibilities.
- Reaction to topical drugs such as antibiotics or anesthetics.

RISK INCREASES WITH

- Ongoing use of hot water, detergents, or any irritant that changes the moisture content of skin.
- Jobs or hobbies that bring you in contact with substances that irritate or cause an allergic reaction.

PREVENTIVE MEASURES

- Avoid contact with any irritant or allergen that has caused dermatitis in the past.
- Wear appropriate protective clothing.
- Protect skin from sunburn and other burns.

EXPECTED OUTCOMES

Symptoms can usually be controlled with treatment and avoiding the irritant or allergen in the future.

POSSIBLE COMPLICATIONS

- Recurrence is common.
- Bacterial infection or other skin problems may occur.

 DIAGNOSIS & TREATMENT

GENERAL MEASURES

- Treatment most often involves products applied to the skin to relieve the itching, redness, and soreness.
- Reduce water temperature to lukewarm for bathing or other uses. Use Aveeno (a commercial product for soaking). Pat skin dry rather than rubbing it.
- See your health care provider if self-help steps are not working. A skin exam is usually all that is needed for diagnosis. Questions will be asked about any contact with possible irritating and allergic substances to help find the cause. Skin allergy testing may be done.
- Once the cause is known, avoid contact with that substance. Wear protective gloves for wet work. Use petroleum jelly to protect the hands.

MEDICATIONS

- Use nonprescription cream, lotion, or ointment products to help relieve symptoms. These can add moisture to the skin, have an anti-itching effect, and may include a mild topical anesthetic. Use these skin care products for mild cases. For more severe cases, use 0.5% or 1 % hydrocortisone product. Follow label instructions.
- Oral antihistamines may help relieve itching.
- Your health care provider may prescribe:
  - Other topical skin care products. These may include stronger steroid drugs to reduce redness and soreness or lubricants to preserve moisture.
  - Oral (taken by mouth) steroids for severe cases.
  - Antibiotics (topical or oral) for bacterial infections.

ACTIVITY

No limits.

DIET

No special diet.

 NOTIFY OUR OFFICE IF

- You or a family member has contact dermatitis and self-help treatment is not working.
- Signs of infection (swelling, tenderness, redness, warmth) develop at the site of irritation.

Special notes:

_____

_____

_____

More notes on the back of this page ☐

DERMATITIS HERPETIFORMIS

BASIC INFORMATION

DESCRIPTION
A chronic skin inflammation that involves clusters of small itching blisters. The disorder is hereditary, but not contagious or cancerous. It usually affects the skin of the elbows, knees, shoulders, arms, legs, and over the bottom of the spine (sacrum).

FREQUENT SIGNS AND SYMPTOMS
· Small clusters of 5 to 20 blisters.
· Clusters appear at the same time on both sides of the body in the same places.
· They itch, but are not usually painful (if there are no complications).
· May feel a burning or stinging sensation.

CAUSES
Unknown. It may be an autoimmune system disorder.

RISK INCREASES WITH
· Exposure to heat and humidity.
· Gluten sensitivity. This is a protein found in wheat and other foods that cannot be digested by some persons because of genetic disease.
· Family history of dermatitis herpetiformis.

PREVENTIVE MEASURES
Cannot be prevented at present. To prevent a recurrence of symptoms, continue to take drug therapy as directed and prevent injury to normal skin.

EXPECTED OUTCOMES
This is a chronic disease. Treatment can control symptoms (including itching) but it will not cure the disease.

POSSIBLE COMPLICATIONS
People with dermatitis herpetiformis also may have disease of the small bowel (without symptoms), which resembles that of patients who are intolerant to gluten. The only way to diagnose this is with a biopsy.

DIAGNOSIS & TREATMENT

GENERAL MEASURES
· Your health care provider will do a physical exam of the affected skin area. Biopsy of the skin (removal of a small amount of tissue or fluid for viewing under a microscope that aids in diagnosis).
· Soak in cool water or use cool-water compresses to reduce itching.

MEDICATIONS
· For itching, you may use nonprescription drugs such as a low-dose steroid lotion, ointment, or cream. They reduce inflammation and itching in 24 to 48 hours.
· Topical anesthetics and topical antihistamines. These provide quick, short-term relief. Many cause skin sensitivity, but lidocaine and pramoxine usually do not.
· Lotions containing phenol, menthol, and camphor (such as calamine lotion). These are soothing, but use with care. Large amounts may be absorbed through the skin into the bloodstream; they can be toxic.
· To control blistering, one of two oral drugs, sulfapyridine or dapsone, may be prescribed. If either one is needed, it will be required indefinitely.

ACTIVITY
No limits, except to avoid overheating and moisture.

DIET
Restricting gluten in your diet will reduce the amount of drug you will need.

NOTIFY OUR OFFICE IF

· You or a family member has symptoms of dermatitis herpetiformis.
· New, unexplained symptoms develop. Drugs used in treatment may produce side effects.

Special notes:

_____

_____

_____

More notes on the back of this page ☐

BASIC INFORMATION

DESCRIPTION

A skin condition with greasy, or dry, white scales. Dandruff and cradle cap are both forms of seborrheic dermatitis. It can involve the skin of the scalp, eyebrows, forehead, face, folds around the nose, behind ears and external ear canal, or skin of the trunk, especially over the breastbone (sternum), or in skin folds. It can not be spread from person to person.

FREQUENT SIGNS AND SYMPTOMS

Flaking, white scales over reddish patches on the skin. Scales stick to hair shafts. They may itch, but they are usually painless unless complicated by infection.

CAUSES

Unknown. Causes may be different in infants and adults.

RISK INCREASES WITH

- Hot, humid weather, or cold, dry weather.
- Oily skin.
- Other skin disorders, such as acne rosacea, acne, or psoriasis.
- Family history of seborrheic dermatitis.
- Obesity.
- Parkinson's disease, stroke, or head injury.
- Use of drying lotions that contain alcohol.
- People with immune disorders.

PREVENTIVE MEASURES

- Cannot be prevented. To reduce severity or frequency of flare-ups:
  - Shampoo often.
  - Dry skin completely after bathing or showering.
  - Wear loose, ventilating clothing.

EXPECTED OUTCOMES

This is a chronic condition, but it often can come and go. When it does occur, symptoms can be controlled with treatment. It does not cause hair loss.

POSSIBLE COMPLICATIONS

- Embarrassment and social discomfort.
- Bacterial skin infection in affected areas.

 ## DIAGNOSIS & TREATMENT

GENERAL MEASURES

- See your health care provider if self-help steps are not working. A skin exam is usually all that is needed for diagnosis.
- Shampoo once a day. Loosen scales with your fingernails while shampooing. Leave the shampoo on for about 5 minutes and then rinse off.
- For infants, use mild baby shampoo to wash the hair and rinse completely. Brush the hair gently with a soft brush after shampooing and other times during the day.

MEDICATIONS

- For minor dandruff, you may use nonprescription dandruff shampoos. They may contain different types of ingredients, and all are effective.
- For seborrheic skin infections in teens and adults, a nonprescription steroid lotion may be used.
- For more severe problems, shampoos that contain coal tar, or scalp creams that contain cortisone may be prescribed. Follow instructions that are provided with each product on how to apply to hair or skin.

ACTIVITY

No limits.

DIET

No special diet.

 ## NOTIFY OUR OFFICE IF

- You or a family member has symptoms of seborrheic dermatitis that don't respond to self-care.
- Patches of seborrheic dermatitis ooze, form crusts, or drain pus.

Special notes:

_____

_____

_____

More notes on the back of this page ☐

DIABETES FEET & SKIN PROBLEMS

 BASIC INFORMATION

DESCRIPTION

Infections of the skin, often of the feet, are more common in people with diabetes than in nondiabetics. The feet of a diabetic person are more prone to all forms of trauma. The common response is infection.

FREQUENT SIGNS AND SYMPTOMS

- Often there is no pain associated with infection or injury to the foot.
- New sores or ulcers that take a long time to heal.
- Unusual, persistent warmth or coolness.
- Numbness or muscle weakness.

CAUSES

Infections and other foot problems result from blood circulation problems, nerve damage, and an impaired immune system in diabetic patients.

RISK INCREASES WITH

- Ingrown toenail.
- Plantar corn or callus; blisters.
- Poor-fitting shoes.

PREVENTIVE MEASURES

- Wash feet daily with soap and warm (but not hot) water. Dry thoroughly and gently, especially between the toes. Powder the feet once a week with talcum.
- When the feet are thoroughly dry, apply a cream or lanolin lotion into the skin of the feet to keep the skin soft and free from scales and dryness. Do not rub so vigorously that the feet become tender. Do not cut corns or calluses or try to remove them with patent or other medicines.
- Prevent calluses under the balls of the feet by exercise: curl and stretch the toes 20 times a day; finish each step that you take on the toes (not on the balls of the feet).
- If toenails are brittle and dry, apply a cream or lanolin lotion under and around the nails for a few nights after soaking. Clean the nails carefully with clean orangewood sticks. Cut nails carefully and straight across. Do not cut on the sides of the nail or the cuticle. If you go to a foot health care provider (podiatrist, foot specialist, or chiropodist), be sure to tell them that you have diabetes.
- If your toes overlap or are pushed close together, separate them with lamb's wool.
- Remove shoes for short periods when you can.
- Do not wear bedroom slippers when you should wear shoes. Slippers do not give proper support.
- Do not go outside with bare feet.
- Wear shoes of soft leather that fit, but are not tight. Break in new shoes gradually 1 hour a day.
- Use cotton bed socks if you need extra warmth for your feet when you are in bed to sleep, but do not use hot-water bottles or electric heating pads. Don't burn the feet! Electric blankets are satisfactory.
- Do not wear garters or sit with legs crossed. Either will decrease circulation to the feet. (The circulation may already be less than normal because of the effect diabetes may have on your blood vessels.)
- Wear thin socks of cotton (not wool) to prevent moisture, which stimulates germs that cause athlete's foot or other skin infections. Wear clean socks that you change at least once a day. Do not wear loose socks with raised seams.
- Check your feet every day for any changes in the skin. Use a mirror to see the bottom of the feet or back of the heel.

EXPECTED OUTCOMES

Using preventive measures and seeking early treatment of infections should help to avoid serious problems.

POSSIBLE COMPLICATIONS

Serious foot infections, gangrene, and amputation.

 DIAGNOSIS & TREATMENT

GENERAL MEASURES

- See your health care provider if new skin problems occur and don't go away on their own in a day or two.
- To learn more: Contact the local or national office of the American Diabetes Association, Attention: National Call Center, 1701 Beauregard St., Alexandria, VA 22311; (800) 342-2383; website: www.diabetes.org.

MEDICATIONS

Specific drugs for infections may be prescribed.

ACTIVITY

Continue with regular activities unless foot problems interfere.

DIET

Follow prescribed diet.

 NOTIFY OUR OFFICE IF

- Skin on the foot becomes red, itchy, swollen, or is painful.
- Feet are persistently cold.
- Corns or calluses occur despite preventive measures.
- Cramps occur in the legs or feet.

Special notes:

_____

_____

_____

More notes on the back of this page ☐

DIABETES HYPOGLYCEMIA

 BASIC INFORMATION

DESCRIPTION

Hypoglycemia means low blood sugar. When blood sugar drops too far below normal, a group of symptoms develop. Signs and symptoms vary in different people. Get to know your signs and symptoms. Also, your daytime symptoms may vary from those that occur at night.

FREQUENT SIGNS AND SYMPTOMS

Mild:
- Hunger.
- Weakness.
- Nervousness.
- Emotional ups and downs.
- Difficulty in concentrating.
- Sweating.
- Headache.

Moderately severe:
- Increased weakness.
- Excessive perspiration.
- Skin that is cold and clammy to touch.
- Numbness about the mouth, and sometimes, fingers.
- Pounding of heart.
- Loss of memory.
- Double vision.
- Staring expression.
- Difficulty walking.
- Unaware of surroundings.

Severe:
- Twitching of muscles.
- Unconsciousness.
- Convulsions.
- Unaware of passing urine.

CAUSES

Hypoglycemia occurs when there is too much insulin in the body and not enough intake of food. It is more frequent in insulin-dependent type diabetes.

RISK INCREASES WITH

- Eating meals at times other than regular hours.
- Skipping meals or eating only parts of meals.
- Dosing with too much insulin or certain other diabetic drugs.
- More exercise or activity than usual.
- Alcohol use.
- Other, rarer risk factors.

PREVENTIVE MEASURES

- It is important to follow your treatment plan of diet, drugs, and exercise, and do regular blood sugar testing.
- Take prompt action if early symptoms of hypoglycemia occur. Family, friends, and co-workers should know the symptoms and what to do in an emergency.
- Always carry some type of sugar with you.

EXPECTED OUTCOMES

Full recovery is the usual outcome. It depends on quick diagnosis and treatment.

POSSIBLE COMPLICATIONS

- Diabetic shock or seizures.
- Permanent brain damage.

 DIAGNOSIS & TREATMENT

GENERAL MEASURES

- If hypoglycemia symptoms begin, eat or drink something that has sugar in it. This includes hard candy, fruit juice, or glucose tablets that you can buy at a drug store. If there are 30 minutes or more to the next meal, some protein and starch foods should also be eaten. They can help prevent another reaction.
- If the patient passes out, glucagon needs to be injected. Diabetic patients and their families should have glucagon at hand and know how to inject it.
- Check blood sugar about 15 to 20 minutes after treatment for hypoglycemia. Repeat treatment if needed.
- If no glucagon is at hand, get the patient to the nearest emergency center or telephone for emergency help.
- To learn more: Contact the local or national office of the American Diabetes Association, Attn: National Call Center, 1701 Beauregard St., Alexandria, VA 22311; (800) 342-2383; website: www.diabetes.org.

MEDICATIONS

Try to find the cause of the hypoglycemia. The insulin dose may need to be adjusted.

ACTIVITY

Rest until symptoms resolve.

DIET

Maintain your regular diet, unless eating habits are the cause of the hypoglycemia. Changes may need to be made in your diet.

 NOTIFY OUR OFFICE IF

- You or a family member has symptoms of hypoglycemia that are not controlled by simple measures.
- Attacks are recurring.
- Changes need to be made in insulin dosages.

Special notes:

_____

_____

_____

More notes on the back of this page ☐

126

DIABETES INSIPIDUS

 BASIC INFORMATION

DESCRIPTION
A rare disorder of the hormone system, centered in the pituitary gland. It disrupts normal fluid regulation in the body. This condition has nothing to do with blood sugar levels or other types of diabetes. It can affect all ages and occurs equally in men and women.

FREQUENT SIGNS AND SYMPTOMS
· Excessive thirst that is difficult to satisfy.
· Passing large amounts of diluted, colorless urine (up to 15 quarts a day).
· Dry hands.
· Constipation.

CAUSES
In one type (neurogenic or central), the pituitary gland in the brain does not make enough of an antidiuretic hormone (called ADH) needed for the body to function. In another type (nephrogenic), there is enough ADH hormone produced, but the kidneys don't work with the hormone as they should. Two other types involve an abnormal thirst (dipsogenic) and pregnancy (gestagenic). The cause for diabetes insipidus may be known or unknown.

RISK INCREASES WITH
· Tumor of the pituitary gland or other brain tumor.
· Head injury, with damage to the pituitary gland.
· Brain infection, such as encephalitis or meningitis.
· Blockage of the arteries to the brain.
· Aneurysm or other blood vessel problems.
· Granulomas (chronic inflammation).
· Drugs, such as lithium.
· Kidney disorders.
· Family history of diabetes insipidus.

PREVENTIVE MEASURES
No specific preventive measures.

EXPECTED OUTCOMES
The prognosis is generally good depending on the underlying disorder.

POSSIBLE COMPLICATIONS
· Electrolyte imbalance, especially low levels of sodium or potassium. Either of these can cause heartbeat irregularity, fatigue, and congestive heart failure.
· Young children may have growth failure.

 DIAGNOSIS & TREATMENT

GENERAL MEASURES
· Your health care provider will do a physical exam and ask questions about your symptoms. Medical studies may include water-deprivation tests to determine levels of ADH. Blood and urine studies are usually done. If diabetes insipidus is diagnosed, A CT or MRI of the brain may be done to check for any problems.
· Treatment involves controlling fluid balance and preventing dehydration and identifying the cause of the diabetes insipidus.
· Check weight daily and maintain a record.
· Wear a medical identification bracelet or neck pendant that indicates your medical problem and the drugs you take.
· To learn more: Diabetes Insipidus Foundation, 5203 New Prospect Dr., Ellicott City, MD 21043; (706) 323-7576 (not toll free); website: www.diabetesinsipidus.org.

MEDICATIONS
· Desmopressin (DDAVP) may be prescribed. It is a synthetic ADH and may be used in nose drops, by mouth, or in an injection form.
· Drugs may be prescribed to help the body balance salt and water.

ACTIVITY
No limits.

DIET
· Monitor fluid intake as advised by your health care provider.
· A low sodium diet may be prescribed.

 NOTIFY OUR OFFICE IF

· You or a family member has symptoms of diabetes insipidus.
· Symptoms don't improve, despite treatment.
· New, unexplained symptoms develop. Drugs used in treatment may produce side effects.

Special notes:

_____

_____

_____

More notes on the back of this page ☐

DIABETES TYPE 1

 BASIC INFORMATION

DESCRIPTION

Diabetes is a chronic condition in which the body is not able to control the amount of glucose (a form of sugar) in the blood. Glucose is needed by the body to produce energy, but too much glucose leads to serious problems. Glucose levels are normally controlled by the hormone, insulin, which is produced in the pancreas. With diabetes, there is either not enough insulin produced or the body is unable to use the insulin that is produced. There are two main types of diabetes, type 1 and type 2. Type 1 diabetes is also called insulin-dependent diabetes or juvenile diabetes. About 5% to 10% of people with diabetes have type 1. It can develop at any age, but often occurs in children, teenagers, or young adults.

FREQUENT SIGNS AND SYMPTOMS

- Fatigue and excess thirst.
- Increased appetite and weight loss.
- Frequent urination.
- Itching around the genitals.
- General ill feeling.
- Blurred vision.
- Increased risk of infections, such as urinary-tract infections and yeast infections of the skin, mouth, or vagina.

CAUSES

In type 1 diabetes, little or no insulin is made by the pancreas. It is one of a group of autoimmune disorders. In these disorders, the immune system mistakenly attacks the body itself. Why this occurs is unknown. Other possible factors include a viral infection or an injury to the pancreas.

RISK INCREASES WITH

Family history of diabetes. It occasionally skips one generation.

PREVENTIVE MEASURES

Cannot be prevented.

EXPECTED OUTCOMES

There is no cure. Adhering to a treatment plan can improve symptoms and delay progress of the disease. Long-term complications may occur.

POSSIBLE COMPLICATIONS

- Cardiovascular (heart and blood vessel) disease, such as stroke, atherosclerosis, and coronary-artery disease.
- Foot or leg amputation due to poor circulation.
- Kidney damage.
- Blindness.
- Nerve damage (neuropathy).
- Sexual impotence in men.
- Hypoglycemia (low blood sugar).
- Hyperglycemia (high blood sugar).
- Ketoacidosis (very high blood sugar).

 DIAGNOSIS & TREATMENT

GENERAL MEASURES

- Your health care provider will do a physical exam and ask questions about your symptoms. Medical tests include blood glucose and urine studies. A glucose tolerance test may be done. A hemoglobin A1C (HbA1c) may be done as a follow-up. This test measures average blood glucose levels for the past 2 to 3 months.
- Type 1 diabetes is treated with insulin, exercise, diet, and steps to prevent complications. A diabetes educator can help you learn to manage your diabetes.
- Learn all you can about diabetes. Learn the techniques of self-monitoring of blood sugar and monitor regularly. Learn the signs and symptoms of high and low blood glucose levels and what to do. Keep glucose tablets handy for treating low blood sugar, if needed.
- Get regular foot care and regular eye check-ups.
- Stop smoking. Find a way to quit that works for you.
- Wear a medical alert type bracelet or pendant to indicate you have diabetes and that you take insulin.
- Get medical care for any infection.
- To learn more: American Diabetes Association, 1701 North Beauregard St., Alexandria, VA 22311, (800) 342-2383; website www.diabetes.org.

MEDICATIONS

- Insulin will be prescribed. Dosage will be based on your individual needs. It is self-injected, or in some cases, an infusion pump is used. Forms of insulin are classified by how fast they work or how long they last.
- Aspirin (for adults), cholesterol-lowering drugs, and drugs for high blood pressure may also be prescribed.

ACTIVITY

Daily exercise helps control diabetes. Follow your health care provider's advice about an exercise plan.

DIET

A healthy diet is part of treatment. Don't skip meals. A dietitian can help you with meal plans.

 NOTIFY OUR OFFICE IF

- You or a family member has symptoms of diabetes.
- After diagnosis, any symptoms cause you concern or problems occur with glucose control.

Special notes:

_____

_____

_____

More notes on the back of this page ☐

DIABETES TYPE 2

 ## BASIC INFORMATION

DESCRIPTION

Diabetes is a chronic condition in which the body is not able to control the amount of glucose (a form of sugar) in the blood. Glucose is needed by the body to produce energy, but too much glucose leads to serious problems. Glucose levels are normally controlled by the hormone, insulin, which is produced in the pancreas. With diabetes, there is either not enough insulin produced or the body is unable to use the insulin that is produced. There are two main types of diabetes, type 1 and type 2. Type 2 is the most common type (about 90% to 95% of people with diabetes), and is also known as non-insulin dependent diabetes. It often affects people over age 40.

FREQUENT SIGNS AND SYMPTOMS

· Many people don't know they have diabetes. There may be no symptoms or symptoms develop gradually.
· Fatigue and excess thirst.
· General ill feeling, increased appetite, weight loss, and frequent urination.
· Slow healing of cuts and bruises.
· Blurred vision.
· Impotence (erectile dysfunction).
· Increased risk of infections.

CAUSES

The pancreas may produce enough insulin, but, for unknown reasons, the body is unable to use it effectively (insulin resistance). After several years, insulin production decreases and glucose builds up in the blood.

RISK INCREASES WITH

· Family history of diabetes.
· Gestational diabetes (diabetes during pregnancy).
· Overweight, especially with fat around the abdomen.
· High blood pressure; high cholesterol or triglycerides.
· Sedentary lifestyle (lack of physical activity).
· Metabolic syndrome (a set of conditions).
· African Americans, Native Americans, Hispanic Americans, Pacific Islanders, and Asian Americans.

PREVENTIVE MEASURES

Control weight (lose weight if overweight). Exercise regularly. Eat a healthy diet. Control high blood pressure and high cholesterol levels.

EXPECTED OUTCOMES

Good blood glucose control (with lifestyle changes and/or drugs) can help prevent or delay complications.

POSSIBLE COMPLICATIONS

· Type 1 diabetes (insulin-dependent diabetes).
· Cardiovascular (heart and blood vessel) disease.
· Kidney damage; blindness; and nerve damage.
· Hypoglycemia (low blood sugar), hyperglycemia (high blood sugar), or ketoacidosis (severe reaction).

 ## DIAGNOSIS & TREATMENT

GENERAL MEASURES

· Your health care provider will do a physical exam and ask questions about your symptoms. Medical tests include blood glucose and urine studies. A glucose tolerance test may be done. A hemoglobin A1C (HbA1c) may be done as a follow-up. This test measures average blood glucose levels for the past 2 to 3 months.
· Type 2 diabetes is treated with lifestyle changes (exercise and diet) and drug therapy, if needed. A diabetes educator can help you learn to manage your diabetes.
· Learn all you can about diabetes. Learn the techniques of self-monitoring of blood sugar and monitor regularly. Learn the signs and symptoms of high and low blood glucose levels and what to do. Keep glucose tablets handy for treating low blood sugar, if needed.
· Get regular foot care and regular eye check ups.
· Stop smoking. Find a way to quit that works for you.
· Wear a medical alert type bracelet or neck tag to indicate you have diabetes and the drugs you take.
· Get medical care for any infection.
· To learn more: American Diabetes Association, 1701 North Beauregard St., Alexandria, VA 22311, (800) 342-2383; website www.diabetes.org.

MEDICATIONS

· One or more types of oral antidiabetic drugs may be prescribed. Your health care provider will discuss the options, the benefits, and the risks with you. Insulin may be prescribed if oral drugs are not effective.
· Aspirin (for adults), cholesterol-lowering drugs, and drugs for high blood pressure may also be prescribed.

ACTIVITY

Daily exercise helps control diabetes. Follow your health care provider's advice about an exercise plan.

DIET

A healthy diet is part of treatment. Don't skip meals. A dietitian can help you with meal plans.

 ## NOTIFY OUR OFFICE IF

· You or a family member has symptoms of diabetes.
· After diagnosis, any symptoms cause you concern or problems occur with glucose control.

Special notes:

_____

_____

_____

More notes on the back of this page ☐

DIAPER RASH

 BASIC INFORMATION

DESCRIPTION
Skin irritation in infants. It involves the skin in the area covered by diapers. This includes the genitals, rectum, upper thighs, and lower stomach. Diaper rash is very common.

FREQUENT SIGNS AND SYMPTOMS
· Moist, painful, red, spotty, and sometimes itchy skin in the diaper area. The skin may be cracked and split.
· In male infants a red, raw and sometimes bloody area may appear around the opening at the tip of the penis.

CAUSES
· It is most often a form of contact dermatitis. Diaper rash results from the skin being irritated by moisture in the urine or stool.
· Less often, it may be an allergic reaction. This can be from disposable diapers or baby wipes, or soap used for washing cloth diapers.

RISK INCREASES WITH
· Not changing diapers often enough.
· Skin gets rubbed from rough diapers.
· Cloth diapers may not be washed properly.
· Family history of skin allergies.
· Hot, humid weather.

PREVENTIVE MEASURES
· Change diapers often.
· Use diaper products that are breathable. These allow more air to circulate. Breathable disposable diapers, cloth diapers, and diaper covers are available.
· Avoid using plastic pants.
· Leave diaper off for 10 to 30 minutes between diaper changes for air exposure.

EXPECTED OUTCOMES
Curable with treatment. The rash is rarely serious. Recurrence is common.

POSSIBLE COMPLICATIONS
Skin infection in the rash area.

 DIAGNOSIS & TREATMENT

GENERAL MEASURES
· Home care is all that is usually needed. See your child's health care provider if you are concerned about the rash.
· Expose the affected skin area to air as when possible.
· Change diapers often, even at night, if the rash is more severe.
· Clean the skin under the diaper with warm water and mild soap that is not perfumed. Baby wipes may also be used, but they might irritate skin in some babies.
· Don't use talcum powder or cornstarch.
· Apply small amounts of petroleum jelly, lanolin ointment, or zinc oxide ointment to the skin at the first sign of diaper rash, and thereafter 2 or 3 times a day.
· After you launder cloth diapers, put them in boiling water for 15 minutes. This will remove any leftover soap and kill any germs.

MEDICATIONS
Your child's health care provider may recommend medicated ointments or creams to be applied to the skin to help clear up the rash.

ACTIVITY
No limits.

DIET
No special diet. Avoid baby foods that cause diarrhea.

 NOTIFY OUR OFFICE IF

· Home treatment doesn't cure the rash in 1 week.
· The following occur during treatment:
  - Fever.
  - Sores develop in the rash area.

Special notes:

_____

_____

_____

More notes on the back of this page ☐

130

DIARRHEA, ACUTE

 BASIC INFORMATION

DESCRIPTION
An abnormal increase in the liquidity and frequency of stools. This is a symptom, not a disease. Simple diarrhea is common among all age groups.

FREQUENT SIGNS AND SYMPTOMS
- Cramping abdominal pain.
- Loose, watery or unformed bowel movements.
- Lack of bowel control (sometimes).
- Fever (sometimes).

CAUSES
Either the intestines produce too much fluid or not enough fluid is absorbed from the intestines. There are many causes, including infections.

RISK INCREASES WITH
- Viral gastroenteritis (stomach "flu").
- Food intolerance or lactose intolerance.
- Emotional upsets or stress.
- Food poisoning.
- Eating foods, such as prunes or beans.
- Children in daycare.
- Food allergy.
- Malabsorption syndromes.
- Disease or tumor of the pancreas.
- Diverticulitis, appendicitis, or fecal impaction.
- Excess alcohol use.
- Use of drugs, such as laxatives, antacids, antibiotics, quinine, or anticancer drugs.
- Radiation treatments for cancer.
- Recent illness.
- Irritable bowel syndrome.
- Inflammatory bowel disease.
- Crowded or unsanitary living conditions.
- Weak immune system due to illness or drugs.
- Travel to foreign country.
- Drinking contaminated water.

PREVENTIVE MEASURES
- Wash hands often to prevent spread of germs, especially after using the bathroom.
- Avoid undercooked or raw seafood, buffet or picnic foods left out for several hours, and food served by street vendors.

EXPECTED OUTCOMES
It goes away by itself and leaves no lasting effects. Most cases of diarrhea last a short time (24 to 48 hours) and a search for the cause may be unnecessary.

POSSIBLE COMPLICATIONS
Dehydration if diarrhea is prolonged, especially in infants.

 DIAGNOSIS & TREATMENT

GENERAL MEASURES
- In most cases, this disorder will be self-treated at home. Call your health care provider if symptoms are more severe or they cause you any concern.
- Your health care provider may do a physical exam. Medical tests may include studies of blood and stool.
- Treatment usually involves drinking plenty of fluids and rest as needed. There is no specific drug therapy.
- It is not necessary to keep persons with diarrhea away from others in the family or household. Try to avoid close contact if possible. Wash hands often.
- Hospital care may be needed, if dehydration is severe.

MEDICATIONS
- Drugs are usually not needed for treatment. If symptoms are severe or prolonged, you may use drugs for nausea or diarrhea such as loperamide or Pepto-Bismol.
- Some infections may require specific drug treatment.
- If a drug you take is the cause of the problem, you may be advised to change drugs or stop taking the drug.

ACTIVITY
Get extra rest if needed. Be sure to have access to a toilet or bedpan.

DIET
- Suck ice chips or drink small amounts of clear fluids often. Replace lost fluids and electrolytes with products such as Pedialyte or Ricelyte for infants and children, and diluted rehydration fluids (Gatorade) for adults.
- Once the symptoms improve, try a diet of complex carbohydrates (rice, wheat, potatoes, bread, cereal, and lean meat such as chicken). Milk and dairy products usually do not need to be limited.
- Avoid high sugar foods or fatty foods for a few days.

 NOTIFY OUR OFFICE IF

- Diarrhea lasts more than 48 hours.
- Mucus, blood, or worms appear in the stool, or fever or severe pain develops in the abdomen or rectum.
- Dehydration develops. Signs include dry mouth, wrinkled skin, excess thirst, and little or no urination.

Special notes:

_____

_____

_____

More notes on the back of this page ☐

DIARRHEA, CHRONIC, NONSPECIFIC OF CHILDHOOD

 BASIC INFORMATION

DESCRIPTION
Diarrhea is called chronic when it lasts more than three weeks. Most cases of diarrhea in children are acute and last less than 10 days. Nonspecific chronic diarrhea usually affects otherwise healthy children ages 1 to 3.

FREQUENT SIGNS AND SYMPTOMS
- Loose stools, sometimes watery.
- Stools are sometimes normal.
- Stools are more frequent than usual.
- Pain in the stomach area.
- Occasional soreness of the anal area caused by many bowel movements.

CAUSES
Nonspecific means no cause has been found such as infection or food intolerance. It may have to do with some aspect of the diet. Sometimes, the children affected drink excessive amounts of fluid or juices (such as apple juice).

RISK INCREASES WITH
No specific risk factors.

PREVENTIVE MEASURES
Cannot be prevented at present.

EXPECTED OUTCOMES
Despite the chronic diarrhea, affected children grow and develop normally. Diet changes can help resolve the diarrhea symptoms in some children. In others, bowel movements often become normal at about age 4.

POSSIBLE COMPLICATIONS
Usually no complications. Emotional problems such as anxiety may occur with parents and children.

 DIAGNOSIS & TREATMENT

GENERAL MEASURES
- Your child's health care provider will do a physical exam and ask questions about the symptoms. Information about your child's activities, and eating and drinking habits will help with the diagnosis. Medical tests may be done to rule out any specific cause.
- Treatment may include diet changes for your child or lifestyle changes such as being more active.
- Don't blame or criticize your child for this problem. Don't expect toilet training to be successful as soon as with some other children. Treat your child as normal and try to ignore the problem. Avoid tension. If the child becomes anxious about diarrhea, the problem may become worse or emotional problems may arise.

MEDICATIONS
Drugs are usually not needed for this disorder. Your child's health care provider may sometimes prescribe antidiarrheal drugs for a short period of time. Don't give your child herbal products or other dietary supplements without medical approval.

ACTIVITY
Your child should be physically active as appropriate for the age group.

DIET
Your child's health care provider will discuss diet changes with you. The goal is to achieve a healthy diet with regard to fat, fiber, fluids, and fruit juices. High-fiber foods such as beans, fruit, breads, and cereals are important in the diet.

 NOTIFY OUR OFFICE IF

- Your child has diarrhea that lasts over 3 weeks.
- There is blood in the stool.
- Fever occurs.
- Your child becomes listless, refuses to eat, or cries loudly and persistently, even when picked up.
- Your child begins to lose weight or is not growing as expected.

Special notes:

_____

_____

_____

More notes on the back of this page ☐

DIPHTHERIA

 ## BASIC INFORMATION

DESCRIPTION

An acute, highly contagious respiratory infection. It affects the throat, skin, heart, and central nervous system. Incubation period is from 2 to 5 days.

FREQUENT SIGNS AND SYMPTOMS

Early stages:
- Sore throat.
- Low fever.
- Swollen neck glands.

Late stages:
- Airway obstruction and breathing difficulty.
- Shock (low blood pressure, rapid heartbeat, paleness, cold skin, sweating, and anxious appearance).

CAUSES

A bacterial germ, *Corynebacterium diphtheriae*, infects the throat and sometimes the skin. The germ produces poisons that spread to the heart, central nervous system, and other organs.

RISK INCREASES WITH

- Adults over 60 and children under 5.
- Poor nutrition.
- Outbreak in the community.
- Crowded or unclean living conditions.
- Lack of up-to-date immunizations.
- Alcoholism.

PREVENTIVE MEASURES

- Immunization with diphtheria vaccine.
- Improved nutrition and standard of living.
- Notify the local health department of any case of diphtheria. Anyone having contact with the patient must be examined and treated.

EXPECTED OUTCOMES

Usually curable in 1 week if treatment is begun promptly, followed by slow recovery for several weeks. A delay in treatment may result in death or long-term heart disease.

POSSIBLE COMPLICATIONS

- Heart inflammation and heart failure.
- Suffocation.
- Nerve inflammation.
- Misdiagnosis as a less-serious infection, resulting in dangerous delay of treatment.

 ## DIAGNOSIS & TREATMENT

GENERAL MEASURES

- Your health care provider will do a physical exam. Medical tests usually include a throat culture and blood studies.
- Hospital care and isolation of the patient are needed until fully recovered. Protect susceptible individuals (the non-immunized, very young, or elderly) from exposure. Patients may require mechanical assistance in breathing.
- Dispose of all secretions (nose and mouth) and excretions (urine and feces) in an acceptable manner. Call the local health department for instructions.

MEDICATIONS

- Diphtheria antitoxin to neutralize the diphtheria toxin will be given during hospital care.
- Antibiotics to fight remaining diphtheria germs will be prescribed.

ACTIVITY

Prolonged bed rest (3 weeks or until fully recovered), especially if the heart is involved.

DIET

Liquid to soft diet as tolerated.

 ## NOTIFY OUR OFFICE IF

- You or a family member has symptoms of diphtheria or you observe them in someone else.
- Anyone in your family is exposed to diphtheria.
- Your immunizations are not current.
- The following occur during treatment:
  - Temperature rises to 102°F (38.9°C).
  - Increasing difficulty breathing.
  - Increasing shortness of breath.
  - Confusion.

Special notes:

_____

_____

_____

More notes on the back of this page ☐

DISK, RUPTURED
(Herniated Disk; Slipped Disk)

BASIC INFORMATION

DESCRIPTION
A ruptured disk is one that has moved or slipped out of its normal position. Disks are part of the backbone and normally help the back to flex and bend. Disks are pads that are soft and gel-like in children and get harder as a person ages. Disks act as a cushion between each of the hard bones (vertebrae) of the spine.

FREQUENT SIGNS AND SYMPTOMS
· Sharp or shooting pain in the lower back. Pain goes from the buttock down the back of one or both legs (sciatica). Movement can make it worse.
· Unable to bend or straighten the back.
· Back pain may develop over time in some cases. It may be more apparent when getting out of bed or when coughing.
· Numbness or tingling in an arm or leg. There may be some loss of strength in one or both legs.

CAUSES
A disk ruptures due to wear and tear or excess strain. The ruptured, bulging disk can be painless. It becomes painful when it puts pressure on nearby ligaments or nerves. Most disk injuries occur in the lower back. The disks in the upper back are less often affected.

RISK INCREASES WITH
· Heavy lifting.
· Poor physical condition.
· Twisting violently or jumping hard.
· Obesity.
· Elderly.
· Degenerative disk disease (changes that occur in disks as person ages).

PREVENTIVE MEASURES
· Use proper posture when lifting.
· Exercise regularly to maintain good muscle tone and flexibility.

EXPECTED OUTCOMES
Recovery usually takes about 6 weeks and is helped with simple treatment measures. If needed, surgery can relieve serious symptoms.

POSSIBLE COMPLICATIONS
· Loss of bladder and bowel function.
· Muscle loss and weakness.

DIAGNOSIS & TREATMENT

GENERAL MEASURES
· Your health care provider will do a physical exam and ask questions about your symptoms and recent activities. To confirm diagnosis, tests may include x-rays of the neck or lower spine.

· For most patients, treatment with simple measures is all that is needed. This starts with relief for pain and inflammation. Further measures include steps to restore back strength and a return to normal activity.
· Use ice packs to the painful area during the first 72 hours. After that, try using heat. Take warm showers or baths. Use warm compresses or a heating pad.
· In some cases, electrical stimulation, or a neck collar, or a back brace may be prescribed to aid healing.
· Other treatment options that may help include chiropractic care, acupuncture, or massage therapy.
· Learn how to stand, sit, and lift properly so that injury does not recur.
· Surgery is needed if the disk is causing any loss of body function (such as bowel function) or nerve damage. Different procedures are available depending on the individual problem.
· Physical therapy is often needed after surgery to restore full function to the back.

MEDICATIONS
· For minor pain, you may use nonprescription drugs such as acetaminophen or ibuprofen.
· Other drugs may be prescribed:
  - Pain relievers.
  - Muscle relaxants.
  - Drugs to reduce swelling around the rupture.
  - Laxatives or stool softeners to prevent constipation.

ACTIVITY
· A long bed rest is not helpful. Rest for only 1 to 2 days, then begin to resume your normal activities.
· Take short walks. Don't sit for long periods. Follow any exercise routine prescribed by your health care provider or physical therapist.

DIET
No special diet. Increase dietary fiber and drink at least 8 glasses of fluid a day to prevent constipation.

NOTIFY OUR OFFICE IF

· You have symptoms of a ruptured disk.
· The following occur during treatment:
  - Increased pain or weakness in the back or legs.
  - Problems with bladder or bowel control.
  - Fever or stomach pain occurs.
  - Symptoms don't improve with self-care.

Special notes:

_____

_____

_____

More notes on the back of this page ☐

DISLOCATION or SUBLUXATION

 BASIC INFORMATION

DESCRIPTION
A dislocation is a joint injury in which the ends of the bones are forced from their normal position. They are no longer connected. If the bones still have some contact, it is called a subluxation. An injury may also affect the joint capsule, ligaments, and nerves.

FREQUENT SIGNS AND SYMPTOMS
• Sudden joint pain, swelling, or an out-of-place joint after an injury. The shoulder is most often affected, but it may happen to any joint including the elbow, finger, knee, ankle, toe, hip, or jaw.
• Limited or no movement around a joint.

CAUSES
Injury (fall or hit) that puts too much pressure on a joint. Less often, a dislocation may occur as a result of disease that affects the structure of the joint. A joint is where two or more bones come together in the body. Ligaments connect bones to bones.

RISK INCREASES WITH
• Contact sports.
• Sports or activities that require quick motion, twisting, or pivoting.
• Hypermobile (loose) joints that move beyond their normal range with little effort.
• Previous dislocation or subluxation of the joint.

PREVENTIVE MEASURES
• For sports or recreational activities (such as skating), wear proper equipment to protect the joints.
• Use safety measures in the home to prevent falls or other accidents.
• Do weight training to strengthen muscles and joints.

EXPECTED OUTCOMES
Usually curable with prompt treatment. After the dislocation has been treated, the joint may require a cast or sling for 2 to 8 weeks. Full recovery after surgery may take up to 6 months.

POSSIBLE COMPLICATIONS
• Damage to nearby nerves or major blood vessels.
• Soreness and swelling may persist for many months.
• Repeated injuries in the joint may lead to arthritis.

 DIAGNOSIS & TREATMENT

GENERAL MEASURES
• Right after an injury:
  - An untrained person should not try to move the joint back into position. It could cause further injury.
  - Apply ice packs to the involved joint. Elevate it (prop it up) if possible to ease pain and prevent swelling.

- If needed, use a splint or sling to prevent movement while taking the injured person to a medical facility.
• Your health care provider will do an exam of the injured joint and ask questions about the activity that caused the injury. Medical tests usually include x-rays of the joint and nearby bones to check for fractures.
• Treatment to realign the bones after a dislocation or subluxation is called reduction. It may include maneuvers to put the bones back into the normal position. In some cases, surgery may be needed.
• After reduction treatment, the joint may be put into a splint or cast. This allows it to heal. Crutches may be needed while the injury heals. Elevate the injured area on a pillow when you are resting.
• Frequent dislocations in the same joint may need surgery to correct or replace the joint.

MEDICATIONS
• Anesthesia or muscle-relaxing drugs may be used to make the joint realignment possible.
• Use acetaminophen or ibuprofen for mild pain.
• Stronger pain relievers may be prescribed.

ACTIVITY
• Physical therapy may be prescribed to restore normal strength and range of motion to the joint.
• Your health care provider will advise you about returning to sports and other physical activities.

DIET
Do not eat any food before treatment in case a general anesthetic is needed.

 NOTIFY OUR OFFICE IF

• You or a family member has symptoms of a dislocation or subluxation.
• Difficulty moving a joint develops after injury.
• Any joint area becomes numb, pale or cold, after injury. This is an emergency!
• Dislocations occur repeatedly that you can "pop" back into normal position.

Special notes:

_____

_____

_____

More notes on the back of this page ☐

DISSEMINATED INTRAVASCULAR COAGULATION (DIC)

 BASIC INFORMATION

DESCRIPTION
A serious, life-threatening disorder that involves blood clotting factors. This disorder is a complication of a variety of other diseases. It can affect all ages and occurs equally in men and women.

FREQUENT SIGNS AND SYMPTOMS
· Bleeding from any or several body parts, such as the nose or gums. Bleeding may be heavy. Common signs of bleeding include:
 - Vomiting up blood or material that looks like coffee grounds.
 - Red or black stools.
 - Vaginal bleeding.
 - Red or cloudy urine.
 - Bruising, pinpoint red spots on the skin, or bleeding under the skin (purpura).
· Severe stomach or back pain caused by bleeding into body organs.
· Cough, shortness of breath, fever, and confusion.

CAUSES
A decrease in blood-clotting factors which leads to severe bleeding (hemorrhaging).

RISK INCREASES WITH
· Widespread or major infection.
· Cancer.
· Certain types of surgery.
· Diseases such as arthritis, ulcerative colitis, Crohn's disease, sarcoidosis, Raynaud disease, and others.
· Burns or injuries.
· Pregnancy complications such as placental abruption, eclampsia, or retained dead fetus.
· Poisonous snakebite.
· Transfusion or blood disorders.
· Heart attack.
· Prosthetic devices, shunts, or heart assist devices.

PREVENTIVE MEASURES
Obtain prompt medical care for any underlying cause.

EXPECTED OUTCOMES
Outcome depends on the underlying cause, severity of the DIC, age, and health status.

POSSIBLE COMPLICATIONS
· Kidney failure.
· Shock.
· Gangrene and amputation.
· Blood clots and hemorrhage (excess bleeding).
· Hemothorax (blood in the lungs).
· Death.

 DIAGNOSIS & TREATMENT

GENERAL MEASURES
· Patients with this condition are often very ill. Hospital care is needed for diagnosis and treatment.
· Treatment will be provided for the DIC symptoms such as bleeding, and for any underlying disorder.
· Oxygen may be provided through a face-mask. Some patients require breathing support with a ventilator (a device to help the lungs).
· Surgery for the underlying disorder (sometimes).

MEDICATIONS
· Blood transfusions or replacement of blood products may be needed.
· Drugs to prevent blood clots and to help control hemorrhage are usually prescribed.
· Drugs as needed to treat the underlying disorder or medical problem.

ACTIVITY
Bed rest.

DIET
Whatever type of diet is tolerated, depending on patient's condition.

 NOTIFY OUR OFFICE IF

· You or a family member has symptoms of DIC. This is an emergency.
· Symptoms recur after treatment.

Special notes:

_____

_____

_____

More notes on the back of this page ☐

DIVERTICULAR DISEASE

 ## BASIC INFORMATION

DESCRIPTION

· Diverticulosis is the presence of small, shallow, sac-like depressions (diverticula) in the wall of the colon. These diverticula may be present without any symptoms. They occur in 30% to 40% of persons over age 50. They increase with each decade of life.

· Diverticulitis occurs when diverticula become infected or inflamed. It can be a serious and dangerous disorder.

FREQUENT SIGNS AND SYMPTOMS

Diverticulosis symptoms:

· No symptoms (usually).

· Mild cramping that comes and goes. Bloating or tenderness in the abdomen. Passing gas or bowel movements may relieve these symptoms.

· Constipation or diarrhea.

Diverticulitis symptoms:

· Pain in the abdomen that becomes constant. Pain may be disabling from the start or may not become disabling for several days.

· Areas of the abdomen become tender to the touch.

· Fever, chills, nausea, and vomiting.

· Blood in the stool.

CAUSES

Exact cause is unknown. A low-fiber diet is thought to be the main factor in developing diverticula. Why they become infected or inflamed is also unknown. It is possible that stool or bacteria are caught in the diverticula.

RISK INCREASES WITH

· Diet that does not have enough fiber.

· Constipation.

· Age over 50.

· Smoking. It is a risk factor for complications.

PREVENTIVE MEASURES

No specific preventive measures. To reduce risks, eat a high-fiber diet, exercise daily, avoid constipation, and don't smoke.

EXPECTED OUTCOMES

Most cases are mild, respond well to treatment, and have no recurrence. If complications occur, they can usually be treated successfully.

POSSIBLE COMPLICATIONS

· Intestinal bleeding or infections.

· Perforation, tear, or blockage of the intestines.

· Abscess (pus-filled, infected area).

· Peritonitis (colon inflammation).

· Recurrent attacks of diverticulitis.

· Fistula (abnormal opening in the body).

 ## DIAGNOSIS & TREATMENT

GENERAL MEASURES

· Your health care provider may do a physical exam and a digital rectal exam (a gloved, lubricated finger is inserted into the rectum). Questions will be asked about your symptoms and bowel habits. Medical tests may include blood and stool studies, x-ray or CT.

· If there are no symptoms, treatment may not be needed. For mild symptoms, treatment may include a change in diet and the use of stool softeners. For more severe symptoms, bed rest, drugs, hospital care, and surgery may be needed.

· Surgery may be done for complications. These include abscess, fistula, intestinal obstruction, perforation, or peritonitis. A part of the affected colon may be removed (resection) and the remaining sections rejoined. A colostomy involves creating a temporary hole (stoma) in the abdomen to remove stool.

· For self-care:

- Try to have a bowel movement at the same time each day. Allow about 10 minutes, and don't strain.

- Check your stool for bleeding. Ask your health care provider if a sample is to be taken to the medical office.

- To relieve mild pain, use a heating pad.

· To learn more: National Digestive Diseases Information Clearinghouse, 2 Information Way, Bethesda, MD 20892; (800) 891-5389; website: www.digestive.niddk.nih.gov.

MEDICATIONS

· Antibiotics will be prescribed for infections.

· Stool softeners may be recommended.

· Don't take laxatives, unless prescribed for you.

ACTIVITY

If you have fever or severe pain, stay in bed. Resume normal activity as soon as symptoms improve.

DIET

Eat a diet that is high in fiber. Drink plenty of fluids.

 ## NOTIFY OUR OFFICE IF

· You or a family member has symptoms of diverticular disease.

· Symptoms don't improve or they become worse.

Special notes:

_____

_____

_____

More notes on the back of this page ☐

DOMESTIC VIOLENCE
(Battering; Spousal Abuse)

 BASIC INFORMATION

DESCRIPTION
Any violence between current or former partners in an intimate relationship. It may include physical, sexual, emotional, or financial abuse. The victim is usually a woman (95% of abuse cases). Because of shame and guilt, the victim may not report the abuse to police, medical care givers, or talk about it with family or friends. Abuse is common. It may occur in any race, age group, economic or educational level, or nationality.

FREQUENT SIGNS AND SYMPTOMS
In female victims:
• Physical or sexual abuse injuries. These include broken bones, bruises, burns, choking, bites, rape and others. Most injuries are to the head, neck, chest, abdomen and breasts. Arm injuries may result from self defense.
• Other symptoms may include chronic pelvic pain, sexual dysfunction, anxiety, sleep disorders, depression, post-traumatic stress disorder (PTSD), eating disorders, psychological problems, and thoughts of suicide.
In male abusers:
• Angry, suspicious, tense and/or moody behaviors. Sometimes they can be very charming. They go from periods of abuse to periods of affection.
• May display extreme jealousy and be very possessive. May not allow partner's friends/family to visit or call.
• Makes threats of violence or legal threats (such as custody of the children). May play with guns or knives.
• Prohibits access to money or other basic needs.

CAUSES
The abuser's goal is to control the victim by the use of fear and force. It is unclear why some men are abusers and other men with similar risk factors are not.

RISK INCREASES WITH
• A history of abuse in a family. Many male abusers and, often, female victims, witnessed abuse or were victims.
• Male abusers tend to use alcohol or drugs, are often unemployed, and may be less educated. However, many educated, professional men are abusers.
• Males who are dependent on women, have money worries, feelings of inadequacy, and have traditional (or archaic) attitudes (such as about sex).
• Females lacking self-esteem and females who feel dependent and useless.
• Pregnant females.

PREVENTIVE MEASURES
Women should seek help at the first sign of abuse. Don't assume the abuser will change or stop the abuse.

EXPECTED OUTCOME
• For victims, help is available, if they choose to seek it.
• Abusers are unlikely to change their behavior.

POSSIBLE COMPLICATIONS
• Years of emotional and physical abuse.
• Alcohol and drug abuse by a female victim.
• Murder or suicide.

 DIAGNOSIS & TREATMENT

GENERAL MEASURES
• If you are abused:
  - Protect yourself, especially the head and abdomen. Get away from the abuser and get help. Document the abuse with pictures, telling someone, or calling 911.
  - Have a personal safety plan set up. Have a place to stay, a way to get there, transportation, and survival funds. Have clothing and personal essentials packed.
  - Seek legal help. Police departments are improving in responding to the problems of domestic violence.
  - Numerous agencies and shelters for helping abused women and children are available. Call a local crisis line.
• Treatment steps for a victim:
  - Get medical care for any injuries.
  - Counseling is important. The variety of treatment options will help a woman learn to cope, regain self-confidence and her ability to function.
• Treatment for the abuser:
  - Treatment is often resisted by an abuser. Educational and treatment groups have had some success.
  - Abusers must be confronted with the results of the behavior; that they can go to jail if they don't change.
• To learn more: National Domestic Violence Hotline (800) 799-7233; website: www.ndvh.org or National Coalition Against Domestic Violence, P.O. Box 18749, Denver, CO 80218; (303) 839-1852 (not toll free); website: www.ncadv.org.

MEDICATION
Drugs may be prescribed for anxiety or depression.

ACTIVITY
No limits.

DIET
No special diet.

 NOTIFY OUR OFFICE IF

You or a family member is a domestic violence victim.

Special notes:

_____

_____

_____

More notes on the back of this page ☐

DOWN SYNDROME
(Trisomy 21)

 BASIC INFORMATION

DESCRIPTION

A chromosome abnormality that usually results in abnormal physical appearance, mental retardation and other health conditions. It is the single most common cause of birth defects.

FREQUENT SIGNS AND SYMPTOMS

Appearance: (some may have only a few of the recognizable traits, while others may have many).
· Lack of normal muscle tone. The child seems "floppy."
· Head that is not shaped normally, including a small or odd-shaped skull.
· Facial features may include small, flattened nose, small mouth, and large tongue.
· Slanting, almond-shaped eyes. The inner corner of the eyes may have a rounded fold of skin (epicanthal fold). Iris may be abnormal.
· Ears that are not of normal shape.
· Broad hands with large, unusual palm creases. The little finger curves inward (sometimes).
Other conditions:
· Heart and gastrointestinal defects may be diagnosed.
· Slow growth and development. The child never reaches full height.
· Mental retardation.

CAUSES

Genetic. An extra chromosome creates abnormalities. Studies have shown that something goes wrong with the egg itself. It is not yet known why this occurs.

RISK INCREASES WITH

Many risk factors have been studied to see if they increase the risk of having a baby with Down syndrome. The only one that has been proven is the increasing age of the woman.

PREVENTIVE MEASURES

· If you or your partner has a family history of Down syndrome, get genetic counseling prior to starting a family.
· If you are pregnant and over age 40, or you or your partner have a family history of Down syndrome, get a test that can detect if the fetus has Down syndrome.

EXPECTED OUTCOMES

With help, people with Down syndrome can reach their full potential and lead happy, loving, and useful lives.

POSSIBLE COMPLICATIONS

· More risk of infections, leukemia, and thyroid disease.
· Heart failure caused by heart defects.
· Alzheimer's disease in 25% of patients over age 35.
· Death often occurs before age 40, but advances in care are helping patients lead longer lives.

 DIAGNOSIS & TREATMENT

GENERAL MEASURES

· Down syndrome is usually diagnosed at birth by the appearance of the baby. It is an extremely difficult time for new parents, and counseling may be helpful. Some parents blame themselves and need help to cope with feelings of guilt.
· Raising the child to his or her full potential should be the goal for parents of a child with Down syndrome.
· Learn all you can about programs in your city to help children with Down syndrome. Join a support group.
· Learning programs for these children begin in infancy and continue all through their lives. Some children can be taught in regular classrooms (with extra help), while others may need special education. They can take part in, and enjoy, sports, music, art, and other activities.
· Health care is important. Children with Down syndrome are more likely to get infections and other illnesses. Surgery may be needed to correct heart or intestinal disorders.
· As adults, they can hold jobs, live in group-homes, have social lives, and some may even marry.
· To learn more: National Down Syndrome Society, 666 Broadway, New York, NY 10012; (800) 221-4602; website: www.ndss.org or National Down Syndrome Congress, 1370 Center Dr, Suite 102, Atlanta, GA 30338; (800) 232-NDSC; website: www.ndscenter.org.

MEDICATIONS

Drugs are usually not needed unless an illness occurs.

ACTIVITY

Encourage the child to be as active as possible (unless heart disease is present) in a protected environment.

DIET

No special diet. Extra patience may be needed in feeding an infant with Down syndrome. Some have difficulty sucking or are not eager to eat.

 NOTIFY OUR OFFICE IF

· You have a child with Down syndrome and have any questions or concerns.
· A child with Down syndrome develops signs of infection (fever, chills, pain, headache, tiredness, nausea).

Special notes:

_____

_____

_____

More notes on the back of this page ☐

DROWNING, NEAR-

 BASIC INFORMATION

DESCRIPTION
Almost drowning. It results from being submerged in water or other fluid. Children under age 4 and young adults (ages 15 to 24) are often the victims.

FREQUENT SIGNS AND SYMPTOMS
· Difficulty breathing or shortness of breath.
· Fast or slow heartbeat.
· May be unconscious.
· Anxious appearance.
· Skin may be bluish-white, cold, and pale.
· Coughing or vomiting.
· May have breathed foreign material into lungs.

CAUSES
Submersion in water results in the larynx (the tube from the throat to the lungs) relaxing and letting water enter the lungs. Water in the lungs means the lungs can't function properly and transfer oxygen to the blood. The body's organs can become damaged from lack of oxygen.

RISK INCREASES WITH
· Not able to swim or overestimating swimming ability.
· Alcohol or drug use combined with water activity.
· Accidents from diving, surfing, or water skiing.
· Seizure, stroke, or heart problem while swimming.
· Unsupervised children in or near water. This includes bathtubs or pails of water (such as used for mopping).
· Unfenced swimming pools.
· Boating or scuba diving.

PREVENTIVE MEASURES
· Learn cardiopulmonary resuscitation (CPR).
· Have all family members learn to swim.
· Adult supervision of children near water.
· Install a fence around a home swimming pool. Always be sure that pool gates are locked.
· Never swim alone.
· Don't drink alcohol or abuse drugs and swim.
· Wear life jackets in boats.
· Scuba divers should be fully trained, use proper caution when diving, and avoid risky dives.

EXPECTED OUTCOMES
· With mild symptoms, patients are usually sent home after 6 to 8 hours in the emergency room/hospital. Complications are unlikely.
· More severe symptoms require extended time for treatment and could result in complications.

POSSIBLE COMPLICATIONS
· Pulmonary edema (fluid in the lungs).
· Lung infection.
· Permanent brain damage.
· Heart problems, including cardiac arrest and death.

 DIAGNOSIS & TREATMENT

GENERAL MEASURES
· If the victim is unconscious and not breathing, yell for help. Have someone call 911 (emergency) for an ambulance or medical help. Don't leave the victim.
· Try to warm the person with whatever means are at hand (blankets, towels, jackets).
· Begin mouth-to-mouth breathing.
· If there is no pulse, give external cardiac massage.
· Don't stop rescue effort until medical help arrives.
· The near-drowning victim should be taken to the nearest hospital for intensive care even if the victim has become conscious. Complications may occur several hours after the near drowning.
· Emergency care usually includes supplemental oxygen, body temperature control, maintenance of the body's electrolytes and blood sugar levels, and prevention of complications. Treatment for any injuries will be provided.

MEDICATIONS
· Drugs used for treatment may include:
    - Cortisone drugs, to prevent or treat inflammation of the lungs.
    - Antibiotics, to prevent lung infection.
    - Bronchodilators, to enable oxygen to enter the lungs.
    - Anticonvulsants, to prevent seizures.

ACTIVITY
Complete bed rest for at least the first 24 hours.

DIET
Nutrition may be provided through a vein (IV) while in the hospital. After recovery, no special diet is needed.

 NOTIFY OUR OFFICE IF

· Someone appears to have drowned. Call for emergency help immediately!
· Cough, shortness of breath, or fever develop after treatment.

Special notes:

_____

_____

_____

More notes on the back of this page ☐

DRUG HYPERSENSITIVITY

 BASIC INFORMATION

DESCRIPTION
Allergic reaction caused by drugs. The reaction may happen immediately after using the drug or days to weeks later. Drug hypersensitivity can occur in any age group. Females are more often affected than males.

FREQUENT SIGNS AND SYMPTOMS
- Rash (most common), hives (urticaria), itching skin.
- Wheezing.
- Swelling (lips, tongue, and/or face).
- Anaphylaxis (a life-threatening reaction). It can cause difficult breathing with a wheeze, hives, swelling, fainting, lightheadedness, dizziness, confusion, rapid pulse, fast heart rate, diarrhea, nausea or vomiting, and stomach pain or cramping).
- Serum sickness (a delayed type of reaction that occurs a week or more after exposure). It can occur with the first time use of a drug. Symptoms include fever, rash, joint pain, and nerve damage.

CAUSES
Hypersensitivity of the immune system in certain people. It leads to a misdirected response against a substance that does not cause a response in most people. The body becomes sensitized by the first exposure to the drug. The second or subsequent exposure causes an immune response (production of antibodies and release of histamine). Injected drugs are more of a risk than those taken by mouth or applied to the skin.

RISK INCREASES WITH
- Use of almost any drug. The following are more likely:
  - Penicillin and cephalosporin antibiotics.
  - Sulfa drugs.
  - Animal serums.
  - Vaccines.
  - Anesthetics applied to the skin.
  - Allergy extracts.
  - Iodine-containing compounds (used in some x-rays).
- Injected drugs, especially in high doses.
- Personal or family history of other allergies, such as hay fever, asthma, or eczema.
- Serious illness.
- Weak immune system due to illness or drugs.

PREVENTIVE MEASURES
- Tell any health care provider you consult about the drug reactions you have had.
- Learn the name of any drug you are given. If it causes a reaction, avoid it in the future.

EXPECTED OUTCOMES
In many cases, stopping the drug is all that is needed. In other cases, symptoms can be relieved with treatment. Most symptoms should resolve in about 2 weeks.

POSSIBLE COMPLICATIONS
- Asthma.
- Anaphylaxis (can be life-threatening if not treated).

 DIAGNOSIS & TREATMENT

GENERAL MEASURES
- Your health care provider may do a physical exam. Questions will be asked about your symptoms and the drugs you take (including nonprescription, herbals, or other supplements). Usually, a diagnosis can be made based on the type of reaction, the timing of the reaction, and that a drug you used is known to cause reactions. Sometimes, skin tests or blood tests are done.
- The first step of treatment is to stop using the drug that caused a reaction. Usually, another drug can be safely substituted. Symptoms of the drug reaction may be treated with other drugs.
- If there is no substitute drug that can be used, other treatment steps may be taken. There are methods (called desensitizing) that gradually introduce a drug into the body in small doses.
- Wear a medical alert type pendant or bracelet if you have drug hypersensitivity.
- Keep an anaphylaxis kit at home, on your person, nearby at work, and in your car for emergency use if anyone in the family has had a severe drug reaction.

MEDICATIONS
- Cortisone drugs to decrease inflammation, antihistamines for itching symptoms, and bronchodilators for wheezing may be prescribed.
- Epinephrine may be injected to treat anaphylaxis.

ACTIVITY
No limits once symptoms improve.

DIET
No special diet.

 NOTIFY OUR OFFICE IF

- You have symptoms of drug hypersensitivity or observe them in someone else.
- You or a family member has anaphylaxis symptoms. This is an emergency! Call 911. Get help immediately!

Special notes:

_____

_____

_____

More notes on the back of this page ☐

DUMPING SYNDROME

 BASIC INFORMATION

DESCRIPTION

A group of symptoms that are usually a complication of stomach surgery. Most patients experience the problem to a minor degree for 1 to 6 months after surgery. The symptoms are of 2 types: early dumping syndrome and late dumping syndrome. Symptoms of the first begin a few minutes to 45 minutes after every meal. Symptoms of the second begin 2 to 3 hours after eating. Most persons experience late dumping syndrome, and a person cannot have both forms. People with a rare disorder called Zollinger-Ellison syndrome may also have dumping syndrome.

FREQUENT SIGNS AND SYMPTOMS

Early dumping syndrome:
· Weakness and fainting.
· Sweating.
· Irregular or rapid heartbeat.
· Decreased blood pressure.
· Skin gets flushed (reddens).
· Dizziness.
· May become hard to breathe.
· Vomiting.
· Explosive diarrhea and stomach cramps.
Late dumping syndrome:
· Sweating, anxiety, and tremors.
· Exhaustion and faintness.
· Decreased blood pressure.
· Headache.

CAUSES

· Early dumping syndrome: Rapid entry of food and fluids directly into the small intestine, producing decreased blood pressure and increased blood flow to the intestines.
· Late dumping syndrome: Low blood sugar caused by too much insulin being made by the body in response to sudden dumping of food and fluids into the intestine.

RISK INCREASES WITH

The larger the amount of stomach removed, the more severe the dumping syndrome.

PREVENTIVE MEASURES

Cannot be prevented. Recurrence and severity can be reduced with changes in the diet.

EXPECTED OUTCOMES

The problem clears up on its own for most patients. Early dumping syndrome usually lasts 3 to 4 months. Late dumping syndrome usually lasts 1 year, but it may persist for many years.

POSSIBLE COMPLICATIONS

· Poor nutrition and weight loss.
· Anxiety.

 DIAGNOSIS & TREATMENT

GENERAL MEASURES

· Your health care provider will do a physical exam and ask questions about your symptoms. Medical tests may be done to confirm the diagnosis.
· Treatment includes diet changes and sometimes drugs. In ongoing severe cases of dumping syndrome, surgery may be considered.
· Lie down as soon as you finish any meal. This helps reduce the symptoms.
· To learn more: National Digestive Diseases Information Clearinghouse, 2 Information Way, Bethesda, MD 20892, (800) 891-5389; website: www.niddk.nih.gov.

MEDICATIONS

· Your health care provider may prescribe drugs to help with digestion or lower blood sugar.
· Vitamin and mineral supplements to compensate for poor absorption.

ACTIVITY

· Between symptoms, there are no limits.
· With symptoms, rest until they pass.

DIET

Diet control is the most important treatment. Eat a diet low in sugar and other simple carbohydrates. Increase fat and protein food items. Avoid milk and milk products. Avoid foods that are very hot or very cold. Eat 6 small, evenly spaced meals a day. Take meals dry without water or beverages and drink fluids only between meals.

 NOTIFY OUR OFFICE IF

· You or a family member has symptoms of dumping syndrome not relieved by diet changes.
· You vomit blood, have black, tarry stools, or other signs of internal bleeding.
· New, unexplained symptoms develop. Drugs used in treatment may produce side effects.

Special notes:

_____

_____

_____

More notes on the back of this page ☐

DYSENTERY, BACILLARY
(Shigellosis)

 BASIC INFORMATION

DESCRIPTION
A bacterial infection of the intestinal tract that is spread by close person-to-person contact. It often happens in epidemics (affects a large number of people at the same time). It occurs most often in young children.

FREQUENT SIGNS AND SYMPTOMS
- Stomach cramps.
- Fever.
- Diarrhea (up to 20 or 30 watery bowel movements in one day). There may be small amounts of blood, mucus, or pus in the stool.
- Nausea or vomiting.
- Muscle aches or pain.

CAUSES
Bacteria called *Shigella* bacillus that attack the lining of the colon. It spreads from person to person, usually from germs on the hands. The infection is also spread from germs on objects such as toys, in food, or in drinking water (in areas with poor sanitation). Symptoms start 1 to 7 days after being exposed to germs.

RISK INCREASES WITH
- Travel to foreign countries.
- Crowded or unclean living conditions.
- Poor health.

PREVENTIVE MEASURES
- Wash hands after bowel movements and before handling food. Children need to be reminded often.
- Avoid contact with an infected person.
- Put soiled clothes and bedclothes in covered buckets of soap and water until they can be washed.

EXPECTED OUTCOMES
The infection resolves on its own or with treatment in about 5 to 7 days. Most *Shigella* infections are mild.

POSSIBLE COMPLICATIONS
Severe cases may occur in the very young or the elderly. Symptoms include convulsions, severe dehydration, and disorders that cause kidney failure and a type of arthritis.

 DIAGNOSIS & TREATMENT

GENERAL MEASURES
- Your health care provider will do a physical exam and ask questions about the symptoms. Tests and culture of a stool sample may be done to confirm the diagnosis.
- Treatment usually includes fluids (to replace those lost from diarrhea), a bland diet, and drug therapy.
- Watch for signs of dehydration. These include severe thirst, dry mouth and tongue, tiredness, sunken eyes, dry skin, being irritable and less urination.
- Keep the patient away from others if possible.
- Use warm compresses on the stomach to help relieve pain.
- A hospital stay may be needed if patient is severely ill. This may happen with small children with dehydration or severe rectal bleeding.

MEDICATIONS
- Antibiotics are usually prescribed. They help speed recovery and reduce risk of spreading germs. Be sure to take them for as long as prescribed.
- Don't use antidiarrhea drugs, unless they are prescribed. These may extend the illness.

ACTIVITY
Keep the ill person at home and away from others when possible. Return to daycare, school, or work is permitted after taking antibiotics for five days.

DIET
Be sure to drink plenty of liquids. A soft or liquid diet may be recommended. Use special drinks (or popsicles) that replace body fluids quickly.

 NOTIFY OUR OFFICE IF

- You or your child has symptoms of the infection.
- The following occur during treatment:
  - Rectal bleeding or bloody stools.
  - Signs of dehydration appear.
  - Symptoms get worse despite treatment.

Special notes:

_____

_____

_____

More notes on the back of this page ☐

DYSHIDROTIC ECZEMA

(Dyshidrosis; Pompholyx)

 BASIC INFORMATION

DESCRIPTION
A skin condition, with small blisters on the hands or feet. It is a type of eczema (dermatitis).

FREQUENT SIGNS AND SYMPTOMS
· Burning and itching in the hands and feet before the skin breaks out. Small blisters appear. They may be on the tips and sides of fingers, toes, palms, and soles of the feet.
· Blisters are nontransparent and deep; they are either even with the skin, or slightly raised. They don't break easily. Eventually, small blisters come together and form large blisters.
· Hands and feet may be wet with perspiration.
· Blisters may worsen after contact with soap, water, or irritating substances.

CAUSES
Unknown. Excessive sweating is not a cause of this problem, but is often linked with it.

RISK INCREASES WITH
· Women are more often affected than men.
· Periods of anxiety, stress, anger, and frustration seem to play a role.
· Other risk factors are being studied.

PREVENTIVE MEASURES
No specific preventive measures are known.

EXPECTED OUTCOMES
Outcome varies for different patients. Some recover completely with or without treatment. Others may continue to have symptoms even with treatment.

POSSIBLE COMPLICATIONS
· Continued peeling and cracking of the involved skin.
· Bacterial skin infection may occur.

 DIAGNOSIS & TREATMENT

GENERAL MEASURES
· Your health care provider can diagnose the condition by an exam of the affected skin area. Medical tests are usually not needed.
· Treatment involves drugs and self-care measures.
· Keep heat and moisture away from the affected areas whenever possible.
· Wear cotton socks and leather-soled shoes. Don't wear tennis shoes or other footwear made of man-made materials.
· Remove shoes and socks frequently to allow sweat to dry.

· Wear heavy-duty, cotton-lined vinyl gloves when in contact with water, soap, detergent, and other chemicals. Dry insides of gloves after use. Throw away gloves if they develop a hole.
· Wear gloves when you peel or squeeze acid fruits and vegetables.
· Wear leather or heavy-duty fabric gloves for housework or gardening.
· Avoid contact with irritating chemicals, such as paint; paint thinner; and polish for cars, floors, shoes, furniture, and metal.
· Use cool, moist compresses to help soothe the affected skin.
· Use lukewarm water and very little mild soap to shower or bathe.
· If emotional stress is a problem, try to identify the cause and find ways to control it. Counseling or learning stress management techniques may help.

MEDICATIONS
· Steroid creams or ointments are usually prescribed.
· If symptoms worsen, steroids or other drugs taken by mouth may be prescribed.

ACTIVITY
Avoid activities or environments that lead to stress or excessive sweating. Sweating does not cause the disorder, but may aggravate it.

DIET
No special diet.

 NOTIFY OUR OFFICE IF

· You or a family member has symptoms of dyshidrotic eczema.
· Signs of infection (swelling, redness, tenderness, or warmth) appear around blisters.
· Symptoms don't improve after 1 week, even with treatment.
· Symptoms recur after treatment.

Special notes:

_____

_____

_____

More notes on the back of this page ☐

DYSMENORRHEA
(Menstrual Cramps)

 BASIC INFORMATION

DESCRIPTION
Painful menstrual cramps. Primary dysmenorrhea often begins within a year or two of the first menstrual period (puberty). Secondary dysmenorrhea usually occurs after a woman has had normal periods for some time.

FREQUENT SIGNS AND SYMPTOMS
· Severity of symptoms varies from woman to woman, and from one time to the next in the same woman.
· Cramping and, sometimes, sharp pains in the lower abdomen, lower back, and thighs. The pain usually begins with your period and lasts for hours to days. For some women, the pain may begin a week or more before her period and last for a few days after it stops.
· Other symptoms that may occur:
 - Nausea, vomiting, diarrhea, headache, and sweating.
 - Lack of energy.
 - Fainting.
 - Feeling irritable, anxious, or depressed.

CAUSES
Menstrual pain is a result of strong contractions of the muscles of the uterus. In primary dysmenorrhea, this is due to excess prostaglandin (a hormone-like substance) production. In secondary dysmenorrhea, this is due to an abnormality or disease of the uterus, fallopian tubes, or ovaries.

RISK INCREASES WITH
· Pelvic infections.
· Sexually transmitted diseases.
· Endometriosis or endometritis (uterine lining disorders).
· Adenomyosis (benign growth of the uterine lining).
· Fibroids or other conditions of the uterus.
· Congenital (being born with) uterine or vaginal abnormalities.
· Use of an intrauterine device (IUD).
· Smoking or alcohol use.
· Not having given birth.
· Family history of dysmenorrhea.
· Obesity.

PREVENTIVE MEASURES
· Take female hormones that prevent ovulation, such as oral contraceptives.
· Treatment of the underlying cause.

EXPECTED OUTCOME
· Symptoms can be helped with treatment.
· Symptoms improve with age and with childbirth. Symptoms are rare in postmenopausal women.

POSSIBLE COMPLICATIONS
· Severe pain that interferes with normal activity.
· Infertility from underlying cause.

 DIAGNOSIS & TREATMENT

GENERAL MEASURES
· Your health care provider will do a physical exam and a pelvic exam. Questions will be asked about your menstrual history. Medical tests may include blood and urine studies, and an ultrasound.
· Initial treatment aims are to relieve pain. Long-term goals of treatment involve treating any underlying cause with drugs, counseling, or possibly surgery.
· Heat helps relieve pain. Use a heating pad or hot-water bottle on the abdomen or back. Take warm baths. Sit in a tub of hot water for 10 to 15 minutes as often as needed.
· Transcutaneous electrical nerve stimulator (TENS) treatment may help relieve pain.
· Counseling may be helpful, if stress is a problem.
· Hypnosis therapy may help some women.
· Try to stop smoking and decrease alcohol use.
· Surgery may be recommended for women whose pain cannot be controlled by other methods.

MEDICATION
· For minor discomfort, use nonsteroidal anti-inflammatory drugs (NSAIDs) such as ibuprofen, naproxen or aspirin (for those over age 18).
· Antiprostaglandins (for painful menstrual periods) and oral contraceptives, which prohibit ovulation, may be prescribed.
· In severe cases, hormones (e.g., gonadotropin-releasing hormone [Gn-RH]) can stop ovary function to relieve pain.
· You may be prescribed vitamin B or vitamin E supplements. These help relieve symptoms in some persons.

ACTIVITY
Exercise reduces the discomfort of menstrual cramps.

DIET
· Avoid drinking caffeine-containing beverages.
· Herbal teas may help reduce symptoms for some.

 NOTIFY OUR OFFICE IF

· You or a family member has symptoms of dysmenorrhea that cannot be relieved.
· Bleeding becomes excessive.

Special notes:

_____

_____

_____

More notes on the back of this page ☐

DYSPAREUNIA

 BASIC INFORMATION

DESCRIPTION
Pain that occurs with sexual intercourse. Dyspareunia and vaginismus (spasm of the pubic muscles of the lower vagina) may occur together in a woman. Dyspareunia also occurs in men, but less often.

FREQUENT SIGNS AND SYMPTOMS
· Pain in the genital area during sexual activity. It can occur before, during, or after sexual intercourse.
· Women may have pain on entry or during intercourse (with deep thrusts of partner's penis).
· Men may have pain in the penis or testes.
· Pain may be mild or severe, and vary with different intercourse positions.

CAUSES
· Physical and medical problems.
· Emotional, interpersonal, and environmental problems (often referred to as psychosocial problems).
· It may be a combination of factors. Sometimes no cause is found.

RISK INCREASES WITH
Physical:
· Infection, inflammation, or injury of the genitals or the urinary tract.
· A lack of vaginal lubrication. This can be due to illness, drugs, or lack of estrogen (such as at menopause).
· Vaginal scarring from operations or radiation therapy.
· Episiotomy scar (from repair after childbirth).
· Intact hymen (covering of the vaginal opening).
· Allergy to diaphragms, condoms, or contraceptive foams and jellies.
· Endometriosis or pelvic inflammatory disease.
· Muscle spasms of the vagina (vaginismus).
· Vulvodynia (chronic vulva pain).
· Tilted or enlarged uterus.
Emotional:
· Lack of sexual arousal or sexual foreplay, being unhappy with a sexual partner, fatigue, or anxiety.
· Lack of sexual experience or information.
· Past sexual abuse (such as rape) or emotional trauma.
· Fear of pregnancy.

PREVENTIVE MEASURES
· Get medical care for genital infections.
· Don't use perfumed soaps, bubble baths, or toilet paper that is scented or colored. Don't douche.
· Get counseling for depression, stress, or anxiety.

EXPECTED OUTCOME
Physical causes are often curable with treatment. Psychosocial causes may be helped with treatment.

POSSIBLE COMPLICATIONS
Treatment may be long-term and may not always help. An intimate relationship with partner may suffer.

 DIAGNOSIS & TREATMENT

GENERAL MEASURES
· Your health care provider will do a physical exam and a genital exam. You will be asked about your symptoms and sexual history. Medical studies, such as a Pap smear and culture of vaginal discharge may be done to diagnose medical problems that can be treated.
· Treatment will be directed to any physical or emotional cause that is diagnosed.
· In cases of scarring, problems with the hymen, or others, a minor surgical procedure may relieve symptoms.
· Sitz baths often relieve tenderness. Sit in a tub of lukewarm water for 10 to 15 minutes, 3 or 4 times a day.
· Use a nonprescription lubricant, such as K-Y Lubricating Jelly, during sexual intercourse.
· Instructions may be given for exercises or techniques to dilate (widen) the vagina. They involve use of fingers or dilators to condition the body and mind to the sensation of something being inserted into the vagina.
· Try different positions for sexual intercourse to discover new ones that might reduce penile penetration and be pain-free.
· Treatments for emotional causes will vary. They can involve education, counseling, sensate focus exercises, and teaching of appropriate foreplay techniques.
· Discuss the lack of sexual arousal with your partner, including ways to improve foreplay.
· To learn more: American College of Obstetricians and Gynecologists, website: www.acog.org.

MEDICATION
Drugs may be prescribed for infection or inflammation. Steroid creams or estrogen creams may be prescribed.

ACTIVITY
A regular exercise program, while not a treatment for dyspareunia, is helpful for general well-being.

DIET
No special diet.

 NOTIFY OUR OFFICE IF

· You or a family member has symptoms of dyspareunia.
· Pain worsens, despite treatment.
· Symptoms do not improve after 3 months of treatment.

Special notes:

_____

_____

_____

More notes on the back of this page ☐

DYSPHAGIA

BASIC INFORMATION

DESCRIPTION

Difficulty or pain in swallowing. It may involve solid foods, liquids or both. It is a common symptom with a wide variety of causes that can be benign or malignant. Chances of a serious disorder are slight. Dysphagia can affect all ages, but it occurs more often in older adults.

FREQUENT SIGNS AND SYMPTOMS

· Pain that occurs with swallowing. Pain and swallowing difficulty may progress over several weeks.
· Sore throat.
· The feeling that food "gets stuck" on the way down.
· Coughing or choking with eating or drinking. Food may come back out through the nose.
· Drooling, belching, and bad breath.
· Pressure sensation in mid-chest.

CAUSES

The swallowing difficulty may involve the mouth, the throat, and the esophagus. There are numerous risk factors that may be the cause.

RISK INCREASES WITH

· Gastroesophageal reflux disease (GERD) or acid reflux.
· Tumors (benign or cancer).
· Stricture (narrowing of the passage).
· Inflammation (esophagitis).
· Infections.
· Recent head, neck, or throat surgery.
· Laryngitis, pharyngitis, or tonsillitis.
· Foreign object lodging at the back of the throat.
· Scratch in the throat lining caused by a foreign object.
· Insufficient production of saliva.
· Esophageal spasm (loss of normal muscle movement).
· In children, it may be caused by delayed maturation, malformation, cerebral palsy, or muscular dystrophy.
· Hernia of part of the esophagus through a weak area in the surrounding muscle.
· Nervous system disorder (stroke, Alzheimer's disease, myasthenia gravis, Parkinson's disease, and others).
· Pressure on the esophagus (a goiter or aortic aneurysm).
· Emotional disorders (anxiety, fear, and others).
· Anemia.
· Smoking.

PREVENTIVE MEASURES

Avoid risk factors where possible.

EXPECTED OUTCOMES

Many causes are minor and easily treated. Other outcomes will vary depending on the cause.

POSSIBLE COMPLICATIONS

· Dehydration or malnutrition due to not eating or drinking enough to meet the body's needs.
· Aspiration, which is the passage of food or liquid through the vocal folds ("going down the wrong way"). The food, fluid, or vomit may enter the lungs.

DIAGNOSIS & TREATMENT

GENERAL MEASURES

· Your health care provider will do an exam of the mouth, throat, head, and neck. You may be asked to chew and swallow so the action can be observed. Medical tests may be done to find the cause of the dysphagia. These may include blood tests, swallowing studies (endoscopy, esophageal manometry, barium x-ray exam), ultrasound, or CT scan. Any testing will be explained to you before it is done.
· Treatment will be provided for the cause of the dysphagia. Specific treatment for the swallowing difficulty may include diet changes and swallowing therapy.
· Oral hygiene is important. Brush teeth twice a day.
· For dry mouth, chew gum or suck on lozenges.
· Hospital care may be required for severe disorders.
· Devices to dilate (widen) the esophagus or surgery may be needed for some disorders.

MEDICATIONS

Drugs will be prescribed as needed for the cause.

ACTIVITY

· Swallowing therapy may be prescribed. It can include exercises to strengthen the swallowing muscles or exercises that are done while swallowing.
· Posture changes may help swallowing: tilting or turning the head to one side, tucking the chin in, using a head-back position, or lying on one's side or back. You will be given instructions about using these positions.

DIET

· A diet may start with pureed foods, progress to soft food and semi-solids, and then resume a regular diet.
· Hospital care may involve intravenous (IV) feeding, or feeding through a nasal or stomach tube.

NOTIFY OUR OFFICE IF

You or a family member develops swallowing difficulty.

Special notes:

_____

_____

_____

More notes on the back of this page ☐

DYSTHYMIA
(Depression, Low-Grade)

 BASIC INFORMATION

A chronic, mild type of depression. The start of dysthymia often goes unnoticed. Many people are not aware of the change in their lives. Symptoms may begin in childhood or in adolescence and go on for years.

FREQUENT SIGNS AND SYMPTOMS
• The depressed mood has occurred for most of each day, for most days, for two years or more (one year for children/teens). There has been no more than two months without some of the symptoms listed.
• Poor appetite or overeating.
• Sleeping too much or too little.
• Lack of energy; feeling tired all the time.
• Feelings of hopelessness.
• Low self-esteem.
• Trouble with concentration and making decisions.

CAUSES
Probably a combination of genetic, developmental, and social factors (such as job loss or divorce).

RISK INCREASES WITH
• Family history of depressive illnesses.
• Loss of a caregiver in childhood.

PREVENTIVE MEASURES
No specific preventive measures. A healthy lifestyle with good nutrition and exercise, having friends, and a job you enjoy may help reduce the risk.

EXPECTED OUTCOME
Most people are helped by treatment. It may take several months before symptoms improve. Sometimes it isn't until a patient has been treated and is feeling better that they realize how depressed they have been.

POSSIBLE COMPLICATIONS
• Dysthymia recurs after treatment.
• Major depression develops.
• Alcohol abuse.

 DIAGNOSIS & TREATMENT

GENERAL MEASURES
• Your health care provider may do a physical exam, and will ask questions about your symptoms and activities. There is no medical test to diagnose dysthymia. Medical tests may be done to rule out other disorders.
• Treatment may include some form of counseling along with drug therapy.
• Cognitive-behavioral therapy is often recommended. The cognitive part teaches people how to change thoughts, behaviors or attitudes. The behavior part teaches people ways to reduce anxiety, such as with deep breathing and muscle relaxation.
• Interpersonal therapy can help a patient identify personal relationship problems and how to correct them.
• Job counseling may be recommended for some patients to be sure their work suits their temperament.
• Join a support group. They help many people with sharing their problems.
• Avoid alcohol. If you need help stopping, ask your health care provider, or contact an Alcoholics Anonymous group in your area.
• Try to reduce emotional stress in your life. Learn techniques to cope with stress.
• To Learn More: National Institute of Mental Health (NIMH), 9000 Rockville Pike, Bethesda, MD 20892, (800) 232-3472; website: www.nimh.nih.gov.

MEDICATIONS
• An antidepressant may be prescribed. The drug may be needed for several months or several years. If one antidepressant doesn't work, another type may help.
• Thyroid supplements may be prescribed.

ACTIVITY
No limits. A daily exercise program is recommended. It can help improve well-being.

DIET
Eat a normal well-balanced diet.

 NOTIFY OUR OFFICE IF

• You or a family member has symptoms of dysthymia.
• Symptoms worsen or don't improve despite treatment.

Special notes:

_____

_____

_____

More notes on the back of this page ☐

148

EAR INFECTION, MIDDLE
(Otitis Media)

 ## BASIC INFORMATION

DESCRIPTION
Infection and inflammation (redness and soreness) in the middle ear. The medical term is acute otitis media (AOM). The infection is most common in infants and children aged 3 months to 3 years, but can occur in any age. Otitis media with effusion (OME) is fluid in the middle ear, but without the symptoms of infection. It often follows AOM.

FREQUENT SIGNS AND SYMPTOMS
- Earache.
- Feeling of fullness in the ear.
- Hearing may be reduced.
- Child is fussy or irritable.
- Fever.
- Dizziness.
- Discharge or leakage from the ear.
- Diarrhea or vomiting (sometimes).
- Pulling at the ear (small children).

CAUSES
The ear infection is usually caused by bacteria, and less often by a virus. The infection creates a build up of fluid or pus in the middle ear. Middle ear infections often occur after a cold or other illness of the nose or throat.

RISK INCREASES WITH
- Recent illness, such as a cold or sore throat.
- Having asthma, allergies, or previous ear infections.
- Family history of ear infections.
- Being in daycare.
- Winter and spring seasons.
- Being bottle-fed while lying down, and (possibly) use of a pacifier.
- Smoking in the household.
- Use of antibiotic drugs in the past 1 to 3 months.
- Genetic factors. American Indians and Eskimos seem to get more ear infections than is usual.

PREVENTIVE MEASURES
- Bottle-feed or breast-feed infants in a sitting position with head up, never lying down. Breast-feeding reduces chances of child having ear infections.
- No smoking in household.
- Wash hands often to prevent spread of germs that can cause colds, sore throats, or other infections.
- Possibly, a pneumococcal vaccine.

EXPECTED OUTCOMES
The outcome is good in almost all cases.

POSSIBLE COMPLICATIONS
- Middle ear infections often recur.
- Chronic otitis media (infection lasts over 6 weeks).
- Rarely, more serious ear problems, hearing loss, brain infection, and other complications may occur.

 ## DIAGNOSIS & TREATMENT

GENERAL MEASURES
- Your health care provider can diagnose a middle ear infection by an exam of the ear. Other medical tests are normally not needed.
- Treatment may include drugs and other steps to relieve pain. Not all infections need antibiotic treatment.
- Apply heat to the area around the ear to relieve pain. Use a warm washcloth.
- Avoid swimming until the infection clears up.
- Sometimes surgery is done to put in plastic tubes through the eardrum to drain pus or fluid from the middle ear. Surgery may be done to remove the adenoids.
- If the eardrum is bulging, a small cut may be made in it to relieve pressure and pain.

MEDICATIONS
- An oral antibiotic may be prescribed for 7 to 10 days. Take the full dose even if symptoms get better. In severe cases, antibiotic injections may be given.
- Ear drops may be prescribed for pain.
- You may use acetaminophen to reduce pain and fever. Do not give aspirin to children.
- Don't use cold remedies, decongestants, or antihistamines. They won't help an ear infection.

ACTIVITY
Rest in bed or reduce activity until symptoms get better.

DIET
No special diet.

 ## NOTIFY OUR OFFICE IF

- You or your child has symptoms of a middle ear infection.
- The following occur during or after treatment: fever, severe headache, earache that persists longer than 2 days despite treatment, swelling around the ear, twitching of the face muscles, or dizziness.

Special notes:

_____

_____

_____

More notes on the back of this page ☐

EAR INFECTION, OUTER
(Otitis Externa; Swimmer's Ear)

BASIC INFORMATION

DESCRIPTION
Inflammation (redness and soreness), infection or irritation of the ear canal that extends from the eardrum to the outside. The medical term is otitis externa.

FREQUENT SIGNS AND SYMPTOMS
- Ear pain that worsens when the earlobe is pulled.
- Itching in the ear.
- Slight fever (sometimes).
- Discharge of pus from the ear.
- Temporary loss of hearing on the affected side.
- A small, painful lump or boil in the ear canal.

CAUSES
- Bacterial (most common) or fungal infection of the delicate skin lining of the ear canal.
- Injury to the ear canal.

RISK INCREASES WITH
- Swimming in dirty or polluted water.
- Excess moisture in the ear from any cause.
- Irritation from cotton swabs or metal objects, such as bobby pins.
- Previous ear infections.
- Disorders like diabetes that affect the immune system.
- Use of hair spray or hair dye that may enter the ear canal.

PREVENTIVE MEASURES
- Dry ears completely after they have become wet.
- Wear ear-plugs when swimming.
- Don't clean your ears with any object.
- If you have had otitis externa, ask your health care provider about keeping the prescribed ear-drops on hand. If the ear canals get wet for any reason, such as swimming or shampooing, put drops in both ears at bedtime.

EXPECTED OUTCOMES
Usually curable with treatment in 7 to 10 days.

POSSIBLE COMPLICATIONS
- Chronic otitis externa. The infection persists or recurs often.
- Spread of infection to bones or cartilage. This is a rare, yet serious complication.

DIAGNOSIS & TREATMENT

GENERAL MEASURES
- Your health care provider can diagnose an outer ear infection by an exam of the ear. Other medical tests are normally not needed.
- Treatment may involve your health care provider cleaning and draining the ear, drug therapy, and other steps to relieve pain.
- Apply heat to the area around the ear to relieve pain. Use a warm washcloth.
- Avoid swimming until the infection clears up.
- Gentle cleaning of the ear canal; remember that a small amount of ear-wax helps protect against infection.
- Keep the infected ear dry. Wear ear-plugs or shower cap for showering.

MEDICATIONS
- You may use acetaminophen or ibuprofen for minor pain. Don't give aspirin to children.
- Your health care provider may prescribe:
  - Eardrops for bacterial infections and cortisone drugs to help other symptoms. An ear wick may be used that allows the drug to reach the end of the ear canal.
  - Oral antibiotics for severe infection.

ACTIVITY
Resume your normal activities as soon as symptoms improve. Avoid getting water in the ears if possible. If you do, dry ears carefully.

DIET
No special diet.

NOTIFY OUR OFFICE IF

- You or a family member has symptoms of outer ear infection.
- Pain persists, despite treatment.

Special notes:

_____

_____

_____

More notes on the back of this page ☐

EARDRUM, RUPTURED
(Tympanic Membrane Perforation)

 BASIC INFORMATION

DESCRIPTION
A hole or tear in the eardrum. The eardrum is a thin membrane (called the tympanic membrane) that separates the inner ear from the outer ear. The eardrum is involved in hearing.

FREQUENT SIGNS AND SYMPTOMS
- Sudden pain in the ear.
- Some loss of hearing.
- Bleeding or discharge from the ear (sometimes).
- Ringing in the ear.
- Dizziness.

CAUSES
- An infection of the middle ear. Fluid or pus builds up behind the eardrum and causes it to burst.
- Injury or trauma to the eardrum.

RISK INCREASES WITH
- Using a sharp object to clean the ear or relieve an itch. This can be a cotton swab, hairpin, or paperclip.
- Changes in air pressure due to scuba diving or during an airplane flight.
- A loud noise such as a nearby explosion.
- Injury to the head, such as a skull fracture.
- A blow or hit directly to the ear.
- Middle-ear infection (otitis media).

PREVENTIVE MEASURES
- Don't put any object into the ear canal.
- Get prompt medical treatment for ear infections.

EXPECTED OUTCOMES
- The eardrum will usually repair itself in 2 months. If it becomes infected, the infection is curable with treatment. Any hearing loss is usually short term.
- Surgery helps if the eardrum does not heal on its own.

POSSIBLE COMPLICATIONS
- Ear infection, with fever, vomiting, and diarrhea.
- Mastoiditis. This is an infection of the mastoid (bony area just behind the ear).
- Permanent hearing loss (rare).

 DIAGNOSIS & TREATMENT

GENERAL MEASURES
- Your health care provider can diagnose the problem by an exam of the ear. Fluid from the ear may be sent to the lab for a medical test. A hearing test may be performed.
- Treatment may involve drugs to prevent infection and for pain.
- A patch may be used to repair the hole. In this procedure, a chemical is applied to the area to help the healing and a paper patch placed on the eardrum. This may need to be redone a few times until healing is complete.
- Try to avoid blowing your nose. If you must, blow gently.
- Keep the ear as dry as possible. Don't swim. Take baths instead of showers. If you do shower, wear a plastic shower cap and be sure the ear is covered.
- Surgery called tympanoplasty may be done to repair the hole if it doesn't heal within 2 months. This can be done in a medical office. Your health care provider will give you instructions for home care after surgery.

MEDICATIONS
- Antibiotics to prevent or treat infections may be prescribed.
- Pain relievers. For minor pain, you may use nonprescription drugs such as acetaminophen.

ACTIVITY
Resume your normal activities as soon as symptoms improve.

DIET
No special diet.

 NOTIFY OUR OFFICE IF

- You or a family member has symptoms of a ruptured eardrum.
- The following occur during treatment:
  - Fever.
  - Pain that persists, despite treatment.
  - Dizziness that continues longer than 12 to 24 hours.

Special notes:

_____

_____

_____

More notes on the back of this page ☐

EARWAX BLOCKAGE
(Cerumen Impaction)

 BASIC INFORMATION

DESCRIPTION
Overproduction of earwax (cerumen), causing blockage of the external ear canal. Wax is produced by glands in the ear to protect the canal leading from the eardrum to the outside. The amount of wax produced varies from person to person. Some produce so little wax that it never accumulates. Others produce enough to block the canal every few months.

FREQUENT SIGNS AND SYMPTOMS
- Decreased hearing.
- Ear pain.
- Plugged feeling in the ear.
- Ringing in the ear.

CAUSES
Overproduction of wax by glands in the external ear canal.

RISK INCREASES WITH
- Exposure to dust or debris.
- Family history of overproduction of earwax.
- Water in the ear, which can cause the wax to swell.
- Use of cotton swabs in an attempt to clean the ear canal.

PREVENTIVE MEASURES
- Avoid areas where the air is dusty or filled with debris. This stimulates overproduction of earwax. Consider wearing earplugs if you must be in this type of environment.
- Monthly use of 1 to 2 drops of glycerin in the ear may soften the wax and prevent recurrent blockage.

EXPECTED OUTCOMES
Earwax can be removed, but stubborn cases require patience.

POSSIBLE COMPLICATIONS
- Ear infection.
- Eardrum damage.

 DIAGNOSIS & TREATMENT

GENERAL MEASURES
To remove earwax at home:
- Buy wax-softening ear-drops at a drug store.
- Lie down with the affected ear toward the ceiling.
- Pull the top of the ear gently up and back toward the back of the head.
- Instill the ear-drops as directed by the instructions on the package.
- Leave the drops in the ear for 20 minutes or as directed. Continue to lie down, if possible. Plug the ear with cotton.
- Sit up, leaning a little toward the affected side.
- Use a soft, rubber bulb syringe to irrigate the ear canal gently with plain warm water.
- Repeat irrigations until the ear feels clear. If the ear doesn't clear, call our office, so that wax can be removed using other methods.
- Don't try to remove wax with a stick or cotton swab. You may damage the eardrum or cause infection in the ear canal. Caution: If you have a perforated eardrum, don't try to remove wax; call our office.

MEDICATIONS
For minor pain, you may use non-prescription drugs such as acetaminophen.

ACTIVITY
No limits.

DIET
No special diet.

 NOTIFY OUR OFFICE IF

- You or a family member has symptoms of an earwax blockage that does not clear, despite treatment described above.
- A child younger than 4 has an earwax blockage.
- Fever and ear pain accompany an earwax blockage. Do not irrigate the ear in this case.

Special notes:

_____

_____

_____

More notes on the back of this page ☐

152

ECTOPIC PREGNANCY

BASIC INFORMATION

DESCRIPTION

An ectopic pregnancy is one that develops outside the uterus. The most common site is in one of the narrow fallopian tubes that connect each ovary to the uterus. Other sites include the ovary or outside the reproductive organs in the abdominal cavity or the cervix. About 1 in 100 pregnancies is ectopic.

FREQUENT SIGNS AND SYMPTOMS

Early stages:
- Missed or late menstrual period.
- Vaginal spotting or bleeding.
- Pain and cramps in the lower abdomen.
- Pain in the shoulder (rare).

Late stages:
- Sudden, sharp, severe pain in the abdomen.
- Dizziness, fainting, and shock (paleness, rapid heartbeat, drop in blood pressure and cold sweats). These may occur before or along with the pain.

CAUSES

An egg from the ovary is fertilized and becomes implanted outside the uterus. This usually occurs in a fallopian tube that has been damaged (resulting in blockage or narrowing). As the fertilized egg enlarges, the fallopian tube may stretch and rupture. This leads to life-threatening internal bleeding.

RISK INCREASES WITH

- Prior abdominal or pelvic infection.
- Pelvic inflammatory disease (PID).
- Pregnancy after a tubal ligation.
- Assisted reproduction techniques, such as in vitro fertilization.
- Adhesions (scar tissue) from prior abdominal surgery.
- Previous ectopic pregnancy.
- Previous tubal or uterine surgery.
- History of endometritis (inflammation of the endometrium, which is the lining of the uterus).
- Endometriosis (a disorder of the fallopian tube).
- Malformed (abnormal) uterus.
- Use of an intrauterine device (IUD) for contraception that results in a pelvic infection.
- Many women diagnosed with an ectopic pregnancy do not have a risk factor.

PREVENTIVE MEASURES

It cannot be prevented.

EXPECTED OUTCOME

An ectopic pregnancy is always going to be lost. It may resolve on its own before a period is missed. Rupture of an ectopic pregnancy is an emergency. Full recovery is likely with early diagnosis and treatment.

POSSIBLE COMPLICATIONS

- Internal bleeding that can be life-threatening.
- Reduced fertility.
- Repeat ectopic pregnancy.

DIAGNOSIS &TREATMENT

GENERAL MEASURES

- Medical tests may include blood studies, pregnancy, ultrasound, and laparoscopy (a telescope-like tool is used to look inside the abdomen).
- Diagnosis and treatment may be done on an outpatient basis. Hospital care may be needed for surgery and supportive care. A blood transfusion may be required.
- Before rupture of the tube, a diagnosed ectopic pregnancy may be treated using the laparoscope instrument, or with an injected drug.
- Surgery may be needed to remove the developing embryo, placenta, and any damaged tissue. The fallopian tube is removed if it cannot be repaired. Future pregnancy is possible with one fallopian tube.
- Weekly blood tests may be recommended to be sure that treatment is successful. If persistent ectopic is diagnosed, a drug may be prescribed for treatment.
- At home, use heat to relieve pain. Apply a heating pad to the abdomen or back. Warm baths help. Sit in a tub of warm water for 10 to 15 minutes. Repeat as needed.
- Counseling may help you with the emotional aspects.
- To learn more: www.ectopicpregnancy.com.

MEDICATION

- In some ectopic pregnancies, methotrexate may be prescribed for treatment. Specific guidelines and close follow-up care are needed when this drug is used.
- After surgery, pain relievers may be prescribed.

ACTIVITY

Your health care provider will advise you when to resume normal activities, as well as sexual relations.

DIET

No special diet.

NOTIFY OUR OFFICE IF

You or a family member has symptoms of ectopic pregnancy, especially a rupture (this is an emergency).

Special notes:

_____

_____

_____

More notes on the back of this page ☐

ECTROPION & ENTROPION

 BASIC INFORMATION

DESCRIPTION
Ectropion is a disorder of the eyelid in which it turns outward (inside out). Entropion is a disorder of the eyelid (usually the lower) in which it curls inward toward the eye.

FREQUENT SIGNS AND SYMPTOMS
Ectropion:
- Turning out of the eyelid, usually the lower.
- Pain, redness, and swelling in the affected eyelid.
- Poor eye lubrication, caused when lubricating tears run down the cheek instead of into the eye.

Entropion:
- Swelling, redness, pain, and excessive tears of the eye. This is caused by the eyelid turning inward and the lashes rubbing against the cornea.

CAUSES
Ectropion:
- Weakening of the muscles and tissues that normally support the lid against the eye.
- Paralysis of the nerve that supplies the eyelid muscles.
- Shrinking of scar tissue from burns, wounds, or surgery near the eye.

Entropion:
- Relaxation of the eyelid's supporting tissue along with the inward pull of the eyelid muscles.
- Chronic eye inflammation (including allergy), creating scar tissue in the eyelid.

RISK INCREASES WITH
Older adults.

PREVENTIVE MEASURES
Cannot be prevented at present.

EXPECTED OUTCOMES
Usually curable with surgery.

POSSIBLE COMPLICATIONS
- Ectropion: Corneal damage caused by dryness.
- Entropion: Blister of the cornea from eyelash and eyelid irritation.

 DIAGNOSIS & TREATMENT

GENERAL MEASURES
- Your eye care provider can diagnose either disorder by an exam of the affected eye.
- Treatment involves minor surgery.
- Apply warm compresses to the eyelids several times a day for swelling and pain. To prepare compresses:
  - Pour warm water into a clean bowl. Soak a clean cloth in the water. Wring it out until it is almost dry.
  - Apply the warm, moist cloth to the closed eye for 10 to 15 minutes. Remoisten the cloth frequently.
- Wear protective glasses or goggles if you are exposed to wind or pollutants.

MEDICATIONS
- Artificial tears may be recommended until surgery can be performed.
- Antibiotics may be prescribed if infection is present.

ACTIVITY
No limits.

DIET
No special diet.

 NOTIFY OUR OFFICE IF

- You or a family member has symptoms of ectropion or entropion.
- The following occur after surgery:
  - Eye pain, redness, or sensitivity to light.
  - Vision changes in any way.

Special notes:

_____

_____

_____

More notes on the back of this page ☐

EMPHYSEMA

BASIC INFORMATION

DESCRIPTION
A chronic, progressive lung disease that causes decreased lung function. Emphysema and chronic bronchitis together are called chronic obstructive pulmonary disease (COPD).

FREQUENT SIGNS AND SYMPTOMS
- In the early stages, there are often no symptoms.
- Trouble breathing that gets worse over several years.
- Breathing is more difficult after physical activity.
- Wheezing.
- Occasional repeated infections of the lungs or bronchial tubes.
- Blue skin and lips.
- Cough with sputum.
- Finger clubbing (fingertips become large).
- Barrel-chest.

CAUSES
Emphysema is caused by destroyed lung tissue, and inflammation and irritation of the airways in the lungs. Smoking is the main reason the lung damage occurs.

RISK INCREASES WITH
- Many years of cigarette smoking. About 15 to 20 percent of smokers get emphysema.
- Family history of emphysema.
- Air pollution.
- Inherited alpha 1-antitrypsin deficiency. This is a disorder that can damage lungs as smoking does.
- History of asthma or bronchitis.
- Men are affected more than women.
- Older age.

PREVENTIVE MEASURES
- Don't smoke. If you do smoke, quit now.
- Avoid places with polluted air.

EXPECTED OUTCOMES
Cannot be cured. Symptoms can be controlled to slow progress and severity of the disease. The disease shortens life expectancy, but patients live many years with it.

POSSIBLE COMPLICATIONS
- Lung infections, failure, or lung collapse.
- Anxiety, panic disorder, and depression.
- Congestive heart failure.

DIAGNOSIS & TREATMENT

GENERAL MEASURES
- Your health care provider will do a physical exam and ask questions about your symptoms. Medical tests will be done to confirm the diagnosis and determine the extent of the disease. These may include blood tests, x-rays, and lung function tests.

- Treatment is aimed at relieving symptoms, slowing the disease, and preventing complications.
- Don't smoke. Smoking will cause the disease to become worse, despite treatment.
- If you work in an area with severe air pollution, do all you can to reduce exposure. Change jobs, if necessary.
- Stay indoors during air pollution alerts.
- Install air-conditioning with a filter and humidity control in your home.
- Avoid sudden temperature or humidity changes, loud talking, laughing, crying, or exertion, if these trigger coughing episodes.
- Avoid higher altitudes where the air is thin.
- Elevate the foot of the bed with 4-inch or 5-inch blocks.
- Home oxygen use may be needed.
- Get counseling for depression, anxiety, and other emotional problems.
- Surgery for lung reduction or lung transplant may be considered (rarely).
- To learn more: American Lung Association, 61 Broadway, 6th Floor, New York, NY 10006, (800) 586-4872; website: www.lungusa.org.

MEDICATIONS
- You may be prescribed:
  - Drugs to relax spasms of bronchial tubes.
  - Steroids to reduce lung inflammation.
  - Antibiotics to fight or prevent infections.
  - Get vaccines against flu and pneumonia.
  - Drugs for depression, anxiety, or panic disorder.

ACTIVITY
Physical exercises and breathing exercises are usually prescribed. Both are important in improving symptoms.

DIET
Drink plenty of fluids each day. This thins lung secretions so they can be coughed up more easily.

NOTIFY OUR OFFICE IF

- You or a family member has symptoms of emphysema.
- The following occur after diagnosis:
  - Any signs of infection such as fever, chills, or aches.
  - Increased trouble breathing or chest pain.
  - Sputum that increases, thickens, changes color, or is bloody.

Special notes:

_____

_____

_____

More notes on the back of this page ☐

EMPYEMA

 ## BASIC INFORMATION

DESCRIPTION
A collection of pus in a body cavity. It usually occurs in the space around the lungs (pleural cavity). It may rarely occur in the gall bladder or the pelvic cavity.

FREQUENT SIGNS AND SYMPTOMS
• Chest pain. Pain varies from slight discomfort to stabbing pain. It is often worse with coughing or breathing. Pain may extend to the lower chest wall or stomach.
• Rapid, shallow breathing.
• Chills.
• Fever.
• Extreme fatigue.
• Dry cough.
• Bad breath.
• Weight loss.

CAUSES
Usually a complication of pneumonia. Infection causes pus to build up in the pleural cavity. The pus, which can amount to a pint or more, puts pressure on the lungs and causes breathing problems.

RISK INCREASES WITH
• Lung or chest infections.
• Chest injury.
• Infection from elsewhere in the body that has spread to the lungs.
• Medical procedures that involve placement of a chest tube or inserting a needle into the chest to draw off fluid.

PREVENTIVE MEASURES
No specific preventive measures.

EXPECTED OUTCOMES
Outcome will depend on several factors. The severity of the infection, the patient's health, any underlying disease, and how effective the treatment is. In otherwise healthy persons, the outcome is generally good.

POSSIBLE COMPLICATIONS
Complications are more likely in the elderly and very ill.

 ## DIAGNOSIS & TREATMENT

GENERAL MEASURES
• Your health care provider will do a physical exam and ask questions about your symptoms. X-ray, CT, or ultrasound tests may be done of the chest. A sample of the pus may be taken for testing by using a needle inserted through the back into the affected area.
• Treatment is done in a hospital and usually involves giving drugs to treat infection and a procedure to drain the pus (fluid).
• The fluid may be drained by using a chest tube or other type of surgery depending on the extent of the infection. The options will be explained to you by the surgeon.
• Treatment of empyema of the gall bladder involves drugs and surgical removal of the gall bladder.

MEDICATIONS
Antibiotics for infection are given through a vein (IV).

ACTIVITY
Gradually return to normal activity after treatment. Allow 2 months for recovery.

DIET
A special diet may be required while in the hospital. After treatment, resume a normal diet.

 ## NOTIFY OUR OFFICE IF

• You or a family member has symptoms of empyema.
• Following treatment, any signs of infection occur, such as fever, chills, aches, or pain.

Special notes:

_____

_____

_____

More notes on the back of this page ☐

ENCEPHALITIS, VIRAL

 ## BASIC INFORMATION

DESCRIPTION
Inflammation of the brain caused by a viral infection. It may occur in one part of the brain (focal), several parts of the brain (multi-focal), or throughout the brain (diffuse). It can occur at any age, but most often affects the very young or the elderly.

FREQUENT SIGNS AND SYMPTOMS
- No symptoms (sometimes).
- Fever.
- Vomiting.
- In infants, a swelling or bulging of the soft spot of the skull.
- Headache.
- Stiff neck.
- Confusion.
- Seizures.
- Occasional weakness or paralysis of an arm or leg.
- Double vision.
- Trouble speaking.
- Hearing loss.
- Drowsiness.

CAUSES
Encephalitis can be caused by one of several types of viruses. These include arboviruses (which are transmitted by mosquitoes or ticks), viruses of the herpes virus family, and others, such as mumps or measles. In some cases, the viral infection may cause no problem until it enters the bloodstream and is carried to the brain cells. In other cases, the infection may first infect other body tissue and then spread to the brain.

RISK INCREASES WITH
- Newborns and infants.
- Adults over 60.
- Weak immune system due to illness or drugs.
- Living in areas with a large mosquito population.

PREVENTIVE MEASURES
- Get medical care for viral infections.
- Take precautions to prevent mosquito bites.

EXPECTED OUTCOMES
Mild viral encephalitis may go unnoticed. In other cases, symptoms last 3 to 5 days. Complications from encephalitis are more likely in infants and the elderly. People in other age groups usually recover completely, but it may take several months.

POSSIBLE COMPLICATIONS
- Bacterial infections may develop.
- A very small number of people suffer permanent brain damage that impairs mental or muscle functions.
- Coma and death (rare).
- Relapse (recurrence of the disease).

 ## DIAGNOSIS & TREATMENT

GENERAL MEASURES
- Your health care provider will do a physical exam and ask questions about your symptoms and activities. Medical tests may include studies of blood and spinal fluid, CT, MRI, and electroencephalogram (which records brain waves). A brain biopsy (removal of a small amount of tissue for viewing under a microscope) may be done.
- Hospital care is needed for severe symptoms. Supportive care will be provided for breathing or heart problems. Fluid and electrolyte levels will be monitored. Steps will be taken to prevent complications.
- If brain function is affected, physical therapy, speech therapy, and behavioral therapy may be recommended.

MEDICATIONS
- Your health care provider may prescribe:
  - Pain relievers, for headache or fever.
  - Antiviral drugs, for certain viral infections.
  - Antibiotics drugs, for bacterial infection.
  - Drugs to reduce inflammation.
  - Drugs to control seizures if needed.

ACTIVITY
Reduce activity until the pain and fever are gone. Gradually return to normal activity. Allow 2 or more months for complete recovery.

DIET
No special diet. May require fluids given through a vein (IV) while in the hospital.

 ## NOTIFY OUR OFFICE IF

- You or a family member has symptoms of encephalitis.
- New, unexplained symptoms develop. Drugs used in treatment may produce side effects.
- Symptoms recur after treatment.

Special notes:

_____

_____

_____

More notes on the back of this page ☐

ENCOPRESIS

BASIC INFORMATION

DESCRIPTION
A condition in which a child over age four passes bowel movements (stools) on a regular basis into places other than a toilet.

FREQUENT SIGNS AND SYMPTOMS
· Bowel movements in underwear. Sometimes the bowel movements may be on the floor or other places.
· Not able to control bowel movements.
· Hard bowel movements.
· Secretive behavior about bowel movements.
· The child has a bad smell.
· The child may or may not have constipation.

CAUSES
There may be a physical or emotional factor, or both, involved. The child may be able to control the bowel movement, but chooses not to. The child may not be able to control the bowel movement. The child may have a more liquid bowel movement that leaks out.

RISK INCREASES WITH
· Boys are affected more often than girls.
· Constipation or diarrhea.
· A physical or emotional change in the child's life, such as the birth of a sibling or recent illness with diarrhea.
· Resistance to using the toilet because of too much pressure to do so.
· Painful bowel movements.
· Resistance to using toilet facilities at school, on camping trips, or outdoor toilets.
· Eating problems that cause constipation.
· Problems due to mental abilities or a medical illness that affects the colon.

PREVENTIVE MEASURES
· Avoid undue emphasis on toilet training. Approach it calmly, with realistic expectations. Don't shame or blame the child for accidents.
· Be sensitive to stressful situations that your child faces. Talk together about the child's feelings.
· Maintain good diet and nutrition for your child.

EXPECTED OUTCOMES
Usually curable. Parents need to be patient. It may take time for the problem to get better.

POSSIBLE COMPLICATIONS
· Child may suffer from embarrassment, shame, guilt, and low self-esteem.
· Skin rash in rectal area.
· Chronic constipation.
· Stool impaction (hard bowel movement remains in the colon).

DIAGNOSIS & TREATMENT

GENERAL MEASURES
· Your child's health care provider will do a physical exam. Questions will be asked about the child's symptoms and other areas of the child's life. Medical tests may be done to check for illness or a physical problem.
· Treatment usually consists of diet changes, behavior training, and sometimes drugs, such as laxatives or stool softeners. Each child is different and will respond to different treatment steps. Follow any special instructions from your child's health care provider.
· Respond gently to accidents. For children who are old enough, have them clean themselves and change into clean underwear. Don't blame, criticize, restrict, or punish the child for accidents. This may cause the child to give up, as well as lead to other emotional problems.
· After meals, have the child sit on the toilet for about 10 minutes. Praise the child for having bowel movements in the toilet. Give a reward for staying clean all day.
· Ask for the school's help. The child needs quick access to the bathroom at school, especially if shy or new at school.
· Don't make this problem the main focus of the child's or your family's life. Do try to identify stresses in the child's life and make every effort to ease them. Consider counseling for the child if needed.

MEDICATIONS
Lubricant laxatives or other types may be used. Enemas or suppositories may be needed for an impaction.

ACTIVITY
No limits.

DIET
Provide a diet high in fiber with plenty of fruits and vegetables. Use whole-grain products for cereals and breads. Be sure your child drinks enough fluids.

NOTIFY OUR OFFICE IF

· Your child has encopresis, and it persists longer than 2 months, despite your efforts.
· Your child has a fever, diarrhea, hard or bloody bowel movements, or there is blood around the rectum.

Special notes:

_____

_____

_____

More notes on the back of this page ☐

ENDOCARDITIS
(Bacterial Endocarditis; Infective Endocarditis)

 ## BASIC INFORMATION

DESCRIPTION
An infection and inflammation involving the endocardium (the inner lining of the heart chambers) and the heart valves.

FREQUENT SIGNS AND SYMPTOMS
- Fatigue and weakness.
- Recurrent fever, chills, and heavy sweating, especially at night.
- Loss of appetite and weight loss.
- Vague muscle aches and joint pains.
- Headache.
- Cough.
- Shortness of breath.
- Swelling of the feet, legs, and stomach.
- Fast or irregular heartbeat.
- Red spots on the skin.

CAUSES
An infection (usually bacterial, sometimes fungal) that enters the bloodstream and infects the heart valves. The infection may start with a skin disorder or injury, a medical or dental procedure, or a skin prick (as with an IV drug user).

RISK INCREASES WITH
- Rheumatic fever.
- History of endocarditis.
- Congenital (being born with) heart disease.
- IV (intravenous) drug abuse.
- Mitral valve prolapse with a heart murmur.
- Weak immune system due to illness or drugs.
- Artificial heart valves or other artificial devices in the heart, such as a pacemaker wire.

PREVENTIVE MEASURES
- If you have heart-valve damage or a heart murmur, ask about antibiotic use before medical procedures that may bring bacteria into the blood. These include dental work, childbirth, and some surgeries.
- Once you have had endocarditis, follow your health care provider's advice about preventing a relapse.
- Don't abuse IV drugs.

EXPECTED OUTCOMES
Usually curable with early diagnosis and treatment. Recovery can take weeks. If untreated, or if treatment is delayed, heart function declines resulting in serious complications.

POSSIBLE COMPLICATIONS
- Heart problems, including heart attack, congestive heart failure, arrhythmias, and others.
- Blood clots may break off and travel to other places in the body, such as the brain or kidneys.
- Kidney problems.

 ## DIAGNOSIS & TREATMENT

GENERAL MEASURES
- Your health care provider will do a physical exam and ask questions about your symptoms. Medical tests may include blood studies, echocardiogram and electrocardiogram (heart function tests), x-rays, and CT.
- Treatment usually involves drugs for the infection, supportive care for symptoms, and steps to prevent complications.
- Hospital care is normally needed during acute phase. Once stable, some patients can continue with treatment at home.
- Surgery may be done to replace an infected heart valve in some patients.
- Wear a medical alert bracelet or neck tag that states you have had this medical problem.

MEDICATIONS
Antibiotics (for a bacterial infection) will be prescribed. They are normally needed for 2 to 6 weeks. Antibiotic treatment is often given through a vein (IV), but in some cases may be taken orally.

ACTIVITY
- Rest in bed until fully recovered. While in bed, move your legs often to help prevent clots from forming in deep veins.
- Resume your normal activities, including sexual relations, when strength allows or upon medical advice.

DIET
No special diet.

 ## NOTIFY OUR OFFICE IF

- You or a family member has symptoms of endocarditis.
- The following occur during or after treatment:
  - Weight gain without diet changes.
  - Blood in the urine.
  - Chest pain or shortness of breath.
  - Sudden weakness or numbness in muscles of the face, trunk, or limbs.

Special notes:

_____

_____

_____

More notes on the back of this page ☐

ENDOMETRIAL HYPERPLASIA
(Adenomatous Hyperplasia of the Uterus)

BASIC INFORMATION

DESCRIPTION
Endometrial hyperplasia is an excess growth of tissue in the endometrium (inner lining of the uterus). It is not cancerous, but some hyperplasia is known to be pre-cancerous (called atypia). Types of hyperplasia include:
· Simple or complex (adenomatous) hyperplasia without atypia.
· Simple or complex (adenomatous) hyperplasia with atypia.

FREQUENT SIGNS AND SYMPTOMS
· Bleeding after menopause.
· Vaginal discharge, especially after menopause.
· Lower abdominal cramps (sometimes).
· Bleeding between normal menstrual periods.
· Heavy menstrual flow.

CAUSES
Excess estrogen (a female hormone) as compared with the amount of progesterone (another female hormone). This excess is caused internally, or from the use of hormone-containing drugs. Tamoxifen, a drug used for breast cancer, is a risk factor for hyperplasia.

RISK INCREASES WITH
· Estrogen replacement therapy without progestin use.
· Diabetes.
· Obesity (25 or more pounds over normal weight).
· Women in the years around menopause.
· Polycystic ovary syndrome.
· Women who skip menstrual periods, or have none.

PREVENTIVE MEASURES
· If taking estrogen, balance it with progesterone.
· Weight loss, if obesity is a problem.
· Birth control pills (oral contraceptives) contain estrogen, along with a form of progesterone. They may help protect against endometrial hyperplasia in women who do not have regular periods.

EXPECTED OUTCOME
· In most cases, hormonal treatment with progesterone (progestin) will reverse the hyperplasia caused by the excess estrogen.
· In other cases, it is often curable with D & C (dilatation and curettage) or a hysterectomy. If a woman chooses not to have surgery, hormone therapy usually controls symptoms.

POSSIBLE COMPLICATIONS
· Without treatment, women who have hyperplasia with atypia have a higher risk for endometrial cancer.
· Excessive, uncontrolled bleeding.

DIAGNOSIS & TREATMENT

GENERAL MEASURES
· Your health care provider will do a physical exam and a pelvic exam. Medical tests may include blood tests of hormone levels and Pap smear. A vaginal ultrasound, an endometrial biopsy, a D & C (dilatation and curettage) procedure, or a hysteroscopy (use of a telescopic instrument inserted through the vagina to look inside the uterus) may be done. They are used to diagnose the type of hyperplasia and to rule out cancer.
· Treatment will be based on findings from the medical tests, your age, and desires about future pregnancy.
· Drugs are normally the first step in treatment. They will cause the lining to shed and prevent it from building up again. This will show up as vaginal bleeding or a menstrual period.
· Long-term follow-up with your health care provider will be required to help avoid a recurrence. Periodic endometrial biopsies, and possibly other tests, will be used to watch for complications of this condition.
· For some women, a hysterectomy (surgery to remove the uterus) is recommended. It may help when hormone therapy has failed and precancerous cells are discovered.

MEDICATION
Progesterone (progestin), a female hormone, may be prescribed. It may be given by mouth or a skin patch.

ACTIVITY
No limits unless you have surgery. Then resume your activities gradually. You may resume sexual relations once medical approval is given.

DIET
Usually, no special diet is required. If you are overweight, losing weight might help decrease estrogen in the body.

NOTIFY OUR OFFICE IF

· You or a family member has symptoms of endometrial hyperplasia.
· The following symptoms occur during treatment: Excessive bleeding, signs of infection, or new, unexplained symptoms develop.

Special notes:

_____

_____

_____

More notes on the back of this page ☐

160

ENDOMETRIOSIS

 BASIC INFORMATION

DESCRIPTION

The inner lining of the uterus (called the endometrium) is made up of endometrial tissue. This tissue normally builds up during the menstrual cycle. It is then shed each month during the normal menstrual period. Endometriosis occurs when this tissue grows outside the uterus in places such as the fallopian tubes or the ovaries. Rarely, the tissue may grow in other areas of the body. The disorder can affect females between puberty and menopause. It is most common between ages 20 and 30.

FREQUENT SIGNS AND SYMPTOMS

· Symptoms may begin suddenly or develop over years.
· Pelvic pain that may occur at anytime. It may increase during menstrual periods, especially the last days.
· Pain with sexual intercourse.
· Premenstrual spotting, blood in the urine, or blood in the stool (sometimes).
· Back pain.
· Infertility.

CAUSES

Unknown. One theory is that, during menstruation, some of the menstrual tissue backs up through the fallopian tubes into the abdomen, where it implants and grows. Another theory is that endometriosis may be genetic, or that certain families may have risk factors that lead to endometriosis. The body's immune system may also play a role in the cause.

RISK INCREASES IN/WITH

· Women who don't become pregnant or who delay childbirth.
· Women with family history of endometriosis.
· Medical conditions that involve the cervix or vagina.

PREVENTIVE MEASURES

There are no specific preventive steps.

EXPECTED OUTCOME

It is an ongoing, long-term disorder that may get worse over time. Symptoms can often be relieved with treatment. Women with severe disease may have less success with treatment. The ability to become pregnant depends on factors such as severity of the disorder and success of treatment.

POSSIBLE COMPLICATIONS

· Infertility.
· Severe pain that causes depression, stress, and problems with daily living activities.
· Adhesions (scar tissue) of pelvic organs.
· Endometriosis can recur after treatment.
· Cysts and pelvic masses called endometriomas.
· An increased risk of cancer is a possibility.

 DIAGNOSIS & TREATMENT

GENERAL MEASURES

· Your health care provider will do a physical exam and a pelvic exam. Medical tests may include laparoscopy. A thin, lighted tube (called a laparoscope) is inserted through a small incision (cut) in the abdomen to view internal organs and to sometimes remove tissue. Open surgery (laparotomy) may be needed for diagnosis.
· Treatment may include drug therapy, surgery, or both. Alternative treatments (such as acupuncture) may help. Treatment will vary depending on the severity of the disease and the patient's age and desire for pregnancy. A patient may desire pregnancy now, at a later time, or not at all.
· Different procedures are used for treatment. The options will be explained to you. A hysterectomy may be suggested for women who do not desire pregnancy.
· Use a heating pad or take warm baths to relieve pain. Cold therapy may help. Use ice packs on the abdomen.
· Put a pillow under your knees when you rest or sleep. When lying on your side, pull the knees up to the chest.
· To learn more: Endometriosis Association, 8585 N. 76th Place, Milwaukee, WI 53223, (800) 992-3636; website: www.endometriosisassn.org.

MEDICATION

· You may use nonprescription drugs, such as nonsteroidal anti-inflammatory drugs, to relieve minor pain.
· Stronger pain relievers may be prescribed.
· Hormonal drugs to stop ovulation may be prescribed.

ACTIVITY

· Exercise, such as walking, may help to relieve pain.
· You may be taught to do Kegel exercises to help strengthen the pelvic floor muscles.

DIET

Avoid alcohol and caffeine. They can make the pain more severe in some women.

 NOTIFY OUR OFFICE IF

· You or a family member has symptoms of endometriosis.
· Severe pain occurs, or other symptoms recur.
· Pregnancy does not occur after trying for 1 year.

Special notes:

_____

_____

_____

More notes on the back of this page ☐

EPIDIDYMITIS

 BASIC INFORMATION

DESCRIPTION

An inflammation and infection of the epididymis. These are thin-walled tubes at the top of a man's testicles. They carry sperm from the testicles to the vas deferens. The vas deferens is another tube that carries the sperm from the testicle to the prostate before ejaculation. Epididymitis more often affects men ages 19 to 35.

FREQUENT SIGNS AND SYMPTOMS

- Pain, heat, redness, and swelling at the back or top of one testicle (sometimes both).
- Fever and chills.
- Pain or burning with urination.
- Discharge from the penis (sometimes).

CAUSES

- Infection in the urinary tract or the prostate.
- Sexually transmitted diseases (STDs).
- Amiodarone (a heart drug).
- Intense exercise, such as heavy lifting, may be a cause.
- A whole body infection that spreads through the bloodstream to the epididymis.
- Sometimes, no cause is found.

RISK INCREASES WITH

- Recent urethral or urinary tract infection.
- Abnormalities or recent surgery involving the genitals or urinary tract.
- Unsafe sexual practices that lead to STDs.
- Catheter (use of a tube to carry urine from the body).
- Presence of a foreskin (being uncircumcised).

PREVENTIVE MEASURES

- Practice safe sex or abstain from sexual activity.
- Avoid catheters if possible.
- Practice good hygiene, especially if uncircumcised.

EXPECTED OUTCOMES

Usually curable with treatment. Pain often goes away in 1 to 3 days. Complete healing may take several weeks.

POSSIBLE COMPLICATIONS

- Abscess (pus-filled area).
- May become sterile (unable to father children) if untreated.
- The disorder may become chronic.
- Infection of the testicles or infection spreads into the bloodstream, or, rarely, a severe scrotal infection.

 DIAGNOSIS & TREATMENT

GENERAL MEASURES

- Your health care provider will do an exam of the genitals. Medical tests usually include urine or discharge studies to check for bacteria or sexually transmitted diseases. Blood studies or ultrasound may also be done.
- The goal of treatment is to cure the infection and reduce pain and swelling. Treatment can usually be done at home with rest, drugs and self-care.
- Support the weight of the scrotum and tender testicles. Roll a soft bath towel and place it between the legs under the inflamed area.
- Apply an ice bag (wrapped in a cloth) to the inflamed parts to help reduce swelling and relieve pain. Do this for 10 to 15 minutes at a time several times a day. Don't use heat.
- Wear an athletic supporter or two pairs of athletic briefs when you return to normal activity.
- Surgery may be recommended in cases of blockage or narrowing of the urethra, or for an abscess.

MEDICATIONS

- Antibiotics will be prescribed for infection. They may be given by injection or taken orally.
- Use ibuprofen or naproxen for mild pain and inflammation. Stronger drugs may be prescribed for more severe pain.
- Stool softeners may be used to prevent constipation.

ACTIVITY

Rest in bed until fever, pain, and swelling improve. Don't engage in sexual intercourse. Wait at least 1 month (or as advised) after all symptoms disappear before resuming sexual relations.

DIET

Eat natural laxative foods, such as prunes, fresh fruit, whole-grain cereals, and nuts, to prevent constipation.

 NOTIFY OUR OFFICE IF

- You or a family member has symptoms of epididymitis.
- Pain is not relieved by treatment.
- You develop severe scrotal pain, urinary pain or a discharge, fever, chills, or you become constipated.

Special notes:

_____

_____

_____

More notes on the back of this page ☐

EPIGLOTTITIS

 BASIC INFORMATION

DESCRIPTION

A life-threatening inflammation of the epiglottis. The epiglottis is a small flap of tissue in the back of the throat that keeps food from going into the windpipe (trachea). Immediate treatment is needed as swelling of the epiglottis may lead to complete blockage of the airway within 12 hours of onset. It is more common in young children (ages 2 to 4) and boys more than girls. It can occur in adults as well.

FREQUENT SIGNS AND SYMPTOMS

- Muffled voice or cry (with croup, it is more hoarse).
- Minimal cough (with croup, it is a barking cough).
- Sore throat.
- Fever.
- Hoarseness.
- Drooling caused by difficulty swallowing saliva.
- Increased breathing difficulty.
- Noisy, high-pitched, squeaky inhalations.
- Purple skin and nails.
- Odd head posture. The person tilts the neck back and leans forward with the tongue stuck out and the nostrils flared, trying to inhale more air.

CAUSES

Usually a bacterial infection. There may be other, more rare, causes.

RISK INCREASES WITH

Unknown.

PREVENTIVE MEASURES

None specific. If your child has had epiglottitis previously, treat all respiratory infections early and with medical care. Immunize children against *Haemophilus influenza*.

EXPECTED OUTCOMES

Full recovery with prompt diagnosis and treatment.

POSSIBLE COMPLICATIONS

- Pneumonia, meningitis, septic arthritis, pericarditis, or cellulitis.
- Without treatment, complete airway obstruction and death can occur within hours.

 DIAGNOSIS & TREATMENT

GENERAL MEASURES

- Never attempt to look at the back of the child's throat if you suspect epiglottitis.
- Have the child sit up rather than lie down.
- Keep the child calm and still until reaching the hospital. Panic increases breathing difficulty.
- Hospital care is needed. Your health care provider will perform exams under special controls to prevent complications.
- Intensive care will be provided. A tube may be inserted in the throat to assist breathing (intubation). Surgery may be done to make an opening in the windpipe (trachea). Usually the tube is withdrawn or the opening is closed in 1 to 3 days.

MEDICATIONS

- Antibiotics will be prescribed for infection. Continue for a minimum of 10 days or as advised.
- Steroid drugs may be given to reduce inflammation.

ACTIVITY

Bed rest is needed until all symptoms disappear. Activities may then be resumed gradually.

DIET

Fluids only (usually through a vein) until the patient can swallow. Once the patient is home, return to a normal diet.

 NOTIFY OUR OFFICE IF

- Your or a family member has symptoms of epiglottitis, especially signs of breathing difficulty. Or call 911. This is an emergency.
- Your child has had epiglottitis in the past, and symptoms of respiratory infection appear.

Special notes:

_____

_____

_____

More notes on the back of this page ☐

EPILEPSY

(Seizure Disorder)

 BASIC INFORMATION

DESCRIPTION

Epilepsy is a brain disorder involving recurrent seizures of all types. Seizures are episodes of disturbed brain function that cause changes in attention and/or behavior. Epilepsy affects both sexes and all ages. It often begins between ages 2 and 14. The two main categories of seizures are generalized seizures (the whole brain is involved) and partial seizures (a limited area of the brain is involved). Each category has different seizure types.

FREQUENT SIGNS AND SYMPTOMS

Generalized seizures types:
- Tonic-clonic (grand mal)—complete loss of consciousness, falling, jerking movements, urine incontinence.
- Absence (petit mal)—brief loss of consciousness.
- Myoclonic— brief jerking movements.

Partial seizures types:
- Simple partial—stays conscious, and weakness, numbness, unusual smells or tastes, muscle twitching, turning head to side, visual changes, or vertigo may occur.
- Complex partial—altered consciousness, automatic repetitive behavior, uncontrolled laughing, unusual thoughts, hallucinations, fears, or smells odd odors.

CAUSES

Abnormal changes in how the cells in the brain send signals to each other. The causes are often unknown.

RISK INCREASES WITH

- Family history of seizure disorders.
- Brain injury to the fetus during pregnancy.
- Birth injury (such as lack of oxygen).
- Poisoning from substance abuse or environmental toxins (such as lead poisoning).
- Infection of the brain (such as meningitis).
- Head injury (such as from accidents or shaken baby syndrome).
- Blood sugar problem (hypoglycemia).
- Metabolic illness (such as hypocalcemia).
- Brain tumor.
- Stroke.

PREVENTIVE MEASURES

No specific preventive measures.

EXPECTED OUTCOMES

There is no cure. Treatment can prevent most seizures and allow a near-normal life.

POSSIBLE COMPLICATIONS

- Seizures continue despite treatment.
- For some patients, epilepsy carries a stigma. It can lead to emotional problems, difficulty in social and family relationships, and problems in finding employment.
- Status epilepticus (a prolonged seizure state).
- Sudden, unexpected death.

 DIAGNOSIS & TREATMENT

GENERAL MEASURES

- Your health care provider will do a physical exam. Medical tests usually include blood studies; one or more types of brain scans; and electroencephalogram (EEG), a study of the brain's electrical activity.
- Treatment for epilepsy usually involves drug therapy.
- Vagus nerve stimulation may be an option. A device implanted in the neck provides mild electrical stimulation to the vagus nerve to help control seizures.
- Surgery may be helpful in a few cases. An area of the brain causing seizures may be removed, or certain nerve pathways in the brain may be interrupted.
- Seizures may result from too little sleep, stress, not taking your drugs, menstrual periods, or flashing lights.
- Wear a medical-alert type bracelet or pendant that shows you have epilepsy (in case you have a seizure).
- To learn more: Epilepsy Foundation of America, 4351 Garden City Dr., Landover, MD 20785; (800) 332-1000; website: www.efa.org.
- If you observe a seizure in someone, loosen his or her clothing, lay person flat, and protect him or her from injury.

MEDICATIONS

Anticonvulsant drugs will usually be prescribed. Dosage changes are often needed. If a person is seizure-free for 2 or more years, drug withdrawal may be considered.

ACTIVITY

No limits. Most states allow persons with epilepsy to drive a vehicle after being seizure-free for 1 year.

DIET

No special diet. Don't drink alcohol.

 NOTIFY OUR OFFICE IF

- You or a family member has symptoms of epilepsy.
- Drugs used in treatment produce unexpected side effects.
- The pattern of seizure activity changes.
- Call 911 (emergency) if the seizure is prolonged, or other symptoms occur that may require emergency care.

Special notes:

_____

_____

_____

More notes on the back of this page ☐

ERYTHEMA INFECTIOSUM
(Fifth Disease)

 BASIC INFORMATION

DESCRIPTION
An infectious, mild, viral illness that occurs in outbreaks (often during the winter and spring months). It most often affects children ages 5 to 14, and is rare in infants and adults. The word erythema means skin redness, and infectiosum means infectious. The name fifth disease comes from its place on a list made up many years ago of the five most common childhood infections.

FREQUENT SIGNS AND SYMPTOMS
· The illness begins with a headache, stuffy or runny nose, and sometimes, a low-grade fever and feeling of fatigue. These symptoms may get better.
· From 3 to 10 days later, a rash appears. It is called "slapped cheeks appearance" because it starts as a rash on the cheeks. The rash spreads to the trunk, buttocks, and limbs. It has a lace-like pattern, and it may be itchy.
· Rarely, other symptoms may occur such as sore throat, red eyes, diarrhea, and swollen glands.
· In adults, there may be mild joint pain or swelling.
· About 20% of infected people will have no symptoms.

CAUSES
A virus called parvovirus B-19. The germs come from fluids in the nose, mouth, and throat of someone who has the infection. When an infected person coughs or sneezes, the germs are spread into the air. The period of time from exposure to the germs until symptoms begin is 4 to 28 days with an average of 16 to 17 days. Once the rash appears, the germs are no longer being spread.

RISK INCREASES WITH
Children in school and daycare centers.

PREVENTIVE MEASURES
· No specific preventive measures. Outbreaks can last for months, so there is no need to keep a child out of school or daycare.
· A pregnant woman should avoid daycare centers and schools if there is an outbreak.
· Wash hands often to prevent spread of any germs.

EXPECTED OUTCOMES
Complete recovery. The rash usually clears in 10 days to 2 weeks. Once you have had the infection, you are immune (you cannot get it again).

POSSIBLE COMPLICATIONS
· None expected in most cases. In patients with disorders such as sickle-cell anemia or a weak immune (body's germ-fighting) system, the illness can cause a serious anemic reaction.
· In pregnant women there is a small risk of miscarriage if the infection occurs during the first 20 weeks of pregnancy. There is no evidence that it causes birth defects.

 DIAGNOSIS & TREATMENT

GENERAL MEASURES
· Home care is usually all that is needed for treatment. Call your health care provider if you have concerns about the symptoms, or if you or a child has a chronic illness. Pregnant women should call their obstetric provider if they have been exposed or if they have any symptoms of the illness.
· Your health care provider will examine the appearance of the rash to diagnose the infection. In a few cases, a blood test is done to confirm the diagnosis.
· For home care, use Aveeno (an oatmeal bath product) for a cool, soaking bath. This can help with the itching.
· The rash may become redder, or it may come back again after it seemed to clear up, after spending time in the sun, taking a warm bath, getting excited, or exercising. This is no cause for concern.

MEDICATIONS
· There are no drugs for treating the illness. You may use acetaminophen for fever. Don't give a child younger than 18 aspirin for fever.
· If the rash itches, use plain calamine lotion.
· Your health care provider may prescribe other drugs.

ACTIVITY
No limits needed. Get extra rest during the illness if you or your child feels tired.

DIET
No special diet. Drink plenty of fluids.

 NOTIFY OUR OFFICE IF

· If you or your child has symptoms of erythema infectiosum and you have concerns about the illness.
· Symptoms don't improve or worsen after home treatment.
· You are pregnant and have been exposed to erythema infectiosum.

Special notes:

_____

_____

_____

More notes on the back of this page ☐

ERYTHEMA MULTIFORME

 ## BASIC INFORMATION

DESCRIPTION

An inflammatory disorder of the skin and sometimes, the mucous membranes (thin, moist linings of body cavities). The disorder is called erythema multiforme minor (80% of the cases) when only the skin is involved. It is called erythema multiforme major when the mucous membranes are also involved. Erythema multiforme affects children and teens, as well as adults. More severe forms of the disorder are Stevens-Johnson syndrome and toxic epidermal necrolysis.

FREQUENT SIGNS AND SYMPTOMS

• Rash spots that are red and evenly shaped. They often appear in rings like bull's-eyes.
• Rash usually appears on palms, soles, and other areas of arms and legs. It may spread to the face and the rest of the body.
• Rash is itchy, sometimes painful, or has a burning sensation.
• Rash develops into blisters, hives, or becomes ulcerated (open sores).
• With erythema multiforme major, the mucous membranes of the mouth, eyes, and genitals may become inflamed. Fever, headache, sore throat, or diarrhea may also occur.

CAUSES

It is thought to be an immune response. The most common cause is the herpes simplex virus (the same virus that causes cold sores). It is less often caused by drug reactions, cancer, radiation, other viruses, or bacteria. Sometimes, no cause is found.

RISK INCREASES WITH

• Previous history of erythema multiforme.
• Drugs such as sulfonamides, tetracyclines, barbiturates, metronidazole, nonsteroidal anti-inflammatories, oral contraceptives, pseudoephedrine, bupropion, and others. The reaction to the drug may not occur until days or weeks after first using it.
• Cancer.
• Radiation therapy.

PREVENTIVE MEASURES

Therapy to prevent herpes simplex virus outbreaks may be recommended in some cases.

EXPECTED OUTCOMES

Rash develops over 1 to 2 weeks. It usually clears up in 2 to 3 weeks, but it may take 5 to 6 weeks.

POSSIBLE COMPLICATIONS

• May progress from the minor form to the major form of erythema multiforme.
• Recurrence of the disorder.

 ## DIAGNOSIS & TREATMENT

GENERAL MEASURES

• Your health care provider may diagnose the disorder by the appearance of the skin rash. A biopsy may be done (involves removing a small piece of the affected skin for viewing under a microscope). Blood tests may be done.
• Treatment may involve drug therapy. In some cases, no treatment is needed. If a drug is the cause of the disorder, it will normally be discontinued.
• Wet dressings and soaks or lotions may help to soothe the skin. Bathing in lukewarm to cool water three times a day for 30 minutes is also helpful.
• If mouth sores are present, good oral hygiene is important to reduce risk of infection and to relieve discomfort.
• The more severe forms of the disorder may require hospital care.

MEDICATIONS

• Corticosteroids (topical or oral) may be prescribed to reduce inflammation and irritation.
• Antivirals may be prescribed to treat viral infection such as herpes simplex virus.
• Antibiotics will be prescribed for bacterial infection.
• If mouth sores are present, topical drugs or mouthwashes may be prescribed.
• If eyes are involved, eyewashes or other topical drugs may be prescribed.
• Pain remedies, sedatives, or antihistamines may be prescribed to help provide relief of symptoms.

ACTIVITY

As tolerated by the extent of the symptoms.

DIET

• Usually no special diet is needed.
• If mouth sores are present, a soft or liquid diet may be better tolerated.

 ## NOTIFY OUR OFFICE IF

• You or a family member has symptoms of erythema multiforme.
• Symptoms worsen during treatment.

Special notes:

_____

_____

_____

More notes on the back of this page ☐

ERYTHEMA NODOSUM

BASIC INFORMATION

DESCRIPTION

An inflammatory disorder of the skin and the tissue under the skin. It is not contagious. It usually affects the skin of the legs, especially areas over the large bone (shin bone) in the lower leg. It can affect all ages, but is more likely to occur in females (ages 20 to 45).

FREQUENT SIGNS AND SYMPTOMS

· An upper respiratory infection may precede the skin symptoms by 1 to 2 weeks. There may be a period of feeling generally unwell and fever. Joint aches may occur, especially of the knee.

· Red lumps (also called lesions or nodules) appear on the shins or about the knees or ankles. They vary in size from a cherry to a grapefruit. There may be 2 to 50 or more.

· The lumps are raised slightly above the skin. They are hot and painful. The color is bright red to start, then purple, and then fades to a bruise-like color.

· Other, smaller, red lumps may appear on the outer arms, face, and neck.

· Lumps continue to appear for about 10 days or more.

· Conjunctivitis (eye inflammation) may occur.

CAUSES

Exact cause is unknown. Inflammation may be due to infection, use of certain drugs, or other factors.

RISK INCREASES WITH

· Drugs, such as birth-control pills (especially those high in estrogen), sulfonamides, iodides, and bromides.

· A preceding infection, including *Streptococcus* (most common), coccidioidomycosis, histoplasmosis, sarcoidosis, blastomycosis, tuberculosis, and *Yersinia* infections.

· Autoimmune disease.

· Chronic bowel inflammation.

· Dysproteinemia (involves protein in the blood).

· Eating foods with food dyes or preservatives.

· Cancer.

· Pregnancy.

PREVENTIVE MEASURES

Remove or treat the cause if it can be identified.

EXPECTED OUTCOMES

Lumps diminish in size and tenderness and heal in about 3 to 6 weeks. Complete healing may take several months. It does not leave scars.

POSSIBLE COMPLICATIONS

· None expected from erythema nodosum.

· Less than 20% of cases recur.

· Other complications can arise depending on the cause.

DIAGNOSIS & TREATMENT

GENERAL MEASURES

· Your health care provider will do an exam of the affected skin. Medical tests are not needed to diagnose erythema nodosum, but they may be done to diagnose an underlying disorder.

· Erythema nodosum often heals on its own. Symptoms may be treated with drug therapy. Treatment may be provided for an underlying disorder. If a drug is the cause of the disorder, it will normally be discontinued.

· For self-care:
  - Elevate the legs whenever possible.
  - Use elastic wrap or support stockings.
  - Soak the affected areas in water. Warm-water soaks are usually more soothing for pain or inflammation. Cool-water soaks feel better for itching.

MEDICATIONS

· For minor discomfort, use nonprescription drugs such as aspirin (not for children) or other nonsteroidal anti-inflammatory drugs.

· Potassium iodide may be prescribed.

· Corticosteroids may be prescribed in very severe cases.

· Topical drugs for the skin usually do not help.

ACTIVITY

Rest in bed as much as possible with the legs elevated. This may help prevent new lumps from developing. When symptoms improve, resume normal activity.

DIET

No special diet.

 NOTIFY OUR OFFICE IF

· You or a family member has symptoms of erythema nodosum.

· Any new symptoms arise that you think may be due either to the disorder or the drugs prescribed.

Special notes:

_____

_____

_____

More notes on the back of this page ☐

ESOPHAGEAL STRICTURE

 BASIC INFORMATION

DESCRIPTION
Esophageal stricture is a narrowing of the tube (esophagus) that connects the throat to the stomach. The narrowing interferes with swallowing.

FREQUENT SIGNS AND SYMPTOMS
• A gradual decrease in the ability to swallow. At first, it becomes difficult to swallow solid foods. Then it becomes difficult to swallow liquids.
• Uncomfortable feeling when swallowing.
• Food feels like it gets stuck in the throat.
• Stomach acid washing back into mouth.
• Vomiting (sometimes with mucus or blood).

CAUSES
Scarring of the lining of the esophagus. As the scar tissue builds up, it forms a ring that narrows the opening of the esophagus. The scarring most often results from excessive gastric acid in the stomach backing up (called reflux) into the esophagus. This causes repeated inflammation (esophagitis), which damages the lining of the esophagus. Other risk factors may also lead to scarring.

RISK INCREASES WITH
• Gastroesophageal reflux disease (GERD).
• Hiatal hernia (part of the stomach protrudes through the diaphragm).
• Prolonged use of feeding (nasogastric) tubes.
• Swallowing of corrosive (e.g., acid or lye) chemicals.
• Infections of the esophagus.
• Radiation injury to the esophagus.
• Injury from an endoscope (a tube-like device used to examine the internal organs).
• Cancer of the esophagus.

PREVENTIVE MEASURES
• Get medical care for any problems that involve difficulty swallowing or acid reflux.
• Keep dangerous products out of children's reach.
• Don't swallow any substance that may harm the esophagus.

EXPECTED OUTCOMES
Treatment can help relieve the stricture, but treatment may need to be repeated.

POSSIBLE COMPLICATIONS
• Not able to eat and drink enough foods and fluids.
• Perforation (hole) in the damaged esophagus.
• Inflammation that may lead to internal bleeding.
• Stricture recurs after treatment.
• Aspiration, which is the passage of food or liquid through the vocal folds ("going down the wrong way"). The food, fluid, or vomit may enter the lungs.

 DIAGNOSIS & TREATMENT

GENERAL MEASURES
• Your health care provider may do an endoscopy. This is a medical test using an instrument with a lighted tip (endoscope) that is inserted into the esophagus. A small amount of tissue may be removed for testing (biopsy) to make sure the stricture is benign. A special x-ray of the esophagus may be done.
• Treatment will be provided for any underlying disorder, such as gastroesophageal reflux disease.
• Treatment for the stricture usually involves a medical procedure to widen (dilate) the esophagus. Different types of procedures are available. They are normally done with the patient sedated. Your health care provider will explain the options to you.
• Surgery to remove the stricture may be recommended, if other treatments fail.
• Stop smoking. Smoking may make symptoms worse.
• See your dental care provider to be sure dentures and oral prostheses are fit well and are not loose.

MEDICATIONS
Drugs for reflux problems may be prescribed.

ACTIVITY
Usually no limits.

DIET
• Eat a soft or liquid diet after treatment, until normal swallowing is possible. Avoid spicy foods that irritate the esophagus.
• Don't drink alcohol.

 NOTIFY OUR OFFICE IF

• You or a family member has symptoms of esophageal stricture.
• The following occur during treatment:
  - Chest pain or fever.
  - Inability to speak.
  - Swallowing problems do not improve.

Special notes:

_____

_____

_____

More notes on the back of this page ☐

ESOPHAGUS CANCER

BASIC INFORMATION

DESCRIPTION

A malignant (cancerous) tumor of the esophagus. This is the tube connecting the mouth to the stomach. This type of cancer usually affects adults over age 60 and both sexes, but is more common in men.

FREQUENT SIGNS AND SYMPTOMS

- Early cancer does not usually cause symptoms.
- Swallowing difficulty that gradually gets worse.
- Pain when swallowing.
- Rapid weight loss.
- Chronic cough. May cough up blood
- Hoarseness.
- Feeling weak and tired.
- Vomiting.

CAUSES

Unknown. Risk factors for one type of cancer are due to smoking or alcohol use. Risk factors for a second type of cancer are due to esophageal conditions. Most esophagus cancers are primary (they begin there). Some are secondary (they spread from cancer elsewhere in the body).

RISK INCREASES WITH

- Ages over 60 and male.
- Smoking (including cigarettes, pipes, or cigars) or smokeless tobacco.
- Excess alcohol use.
- Barrett's esophagus (a precancerous condition).
- Previous esophagus, head, or neck cancer.
- Hiatal hernia.
- Esophageal stricture.
- Chronic gastric reflux (gastroesophageal reflux disease or GERD).

PREVENTIVE MEASURES

- Don't smoke.
- Don't drink more than 1 or 2 alcoholic drinks, if any, a day.
- Obtain medical care for any gastrointestinal disorders.

EXPECTED OUTCOMES

- Recovery improves if diagnosed at an early stage. The diagnosis often comes too late for effective treatment. However, symptoms can be relieved or controlled.
- Research into causes and treatment continues. There is hope for improved treatment and cure.

POSSIBLE COMPLICATIONS

If treatment is delayed, esophagus cancer can spread rapidly to the lungs, liver, brain, and bones.

DIAGNOSIS & TREATMENT

GENERAL MEASURES

- Your health care provider will do a physical exam and ask questions about any symptoms. A number of medical tests will be done. The tests first help diagnose the cancer and then determine if it has spread (staging).
- Treatment varies and depends on the location and size of the tumor, any spread of the cancer, your health, age, and preferences.
- Treatment may include chemotherapy (anticancer drugs) and/or radiation therapy, surgery, and biologic therapy.
- Chemotherapy uses drugs and radiation therapy uses radiation to attack the cancer cells. Biologic therapy uses the body's immune system to fight cancer.
- Surgery may be performed to remove the tumor if the cancer has not spread in the body. Procedures may be done to allow passage of food and liquids.
- Treatment may involve steps to relieve symptoms and make you comfortable, rather than treating the cancer.
- Stop smoking or the use of any tobacco product.
- Counseling may help you cope with having cancer.
- To learn more: American Cancer Society, (800) ACS-2345; website: www.cancer.org; or National Cancer Institute, (800) 4-CANCER; website: www.nci.nih.gov.

MEDICATIONS

- Your health care provider may prescribe:
  - Pain relievers.
  - Drugs to reduce anxiety.
  - Chemotherapy (anticancer drugs).
  - Anticholinergics or calcium-channel blockers for esophageal spasms.

ACTIVITY

Remain as active as possible.

DIET

Soft to liquid. Prior to surgery, special nutritional support may be required (such as a feeding tube).

NOTIFY OUR OFFICE IF

- You or a family member has symptoms of cancer of the esophagus, especially difficulty swallowing.
- Pain or symptoms get worse despite treatment.

Special notes:

_____

_____

_____

More notes on the back of this page ☐

ESSENTIAL TREMOR

 BASIC INFORMATION

DESCRIPTION

Essential tremor is one type of movement disorder. Movement disorders affect the ability to produce and control movement. Parkinson's disease is a different type of movement disorder. Essential tremor is a common problem in people aged 60 and older. Men and women are affected equally.

FREQUENT SIGNS AND SYMPTOMS

· The main symptom is tremor, which is a trembling or an up-and-down movement of the hands. The tremor may be noticed when doing simple tasks such as holding a glass of water. The tremor may occur in the arms, head, and voice. Rarely, it affects the trunk and legs.

· Walking in an unsteady manner.

· The symptoms start on a gradual basis, usually in mid-to-late life. In a few cases, symptoms begin in childhood, go away for many years, and then start up again.

· Being tired, feeling anxious, or being in hot climates can make the symptoms worse.

· Symptoms usually disappear when you sleep or rest.

CAUSES

· In about half of the cases, the cause is genetic. The genes were passed on by your parents. Familial tremor is the term used when it affects more than one person in a family.

· In the other half of the cases, the cause is unknown.

RISK INCREASES WITH

· Family history of essential tremor.

· Age. Most often, the disorder occurs in older people.

PREVENTIVE MEASURES

None known.

EXPECTED OUTCOMES

· In many people, the disorder may not get worse and the tremor may be mild throughout life.

· Others may have symptoms that get worse as they get older. There are treatments that can help relieve the symptoms.

POSSIBLE COMPLICATIONS

· The tremor makes it difficult to do everyday tasks in the home, perform hobbies, or other activities you may enjoy.

· Tremor may cause difficulty in performing your job.

· Feeling embarrassed about the tremor may lead to an avoidance of social activities.

 DIAGNOSIS & TREATMENT

GENERAL MEASURES

· Your health care provider will do a physical exam, and ask questions about your symptoms and your activities. You may be asked to write, drink from a glass, or hold a piece of paper so that the tremor can be observed. There are a variety of medical problems that can involve similar symptoms. Medical tests on blood and urine are usually done to rule out other disorders.

· Treatment may not be needed if the symptoms are mild and are not causing other problems.

· Treatment steps may include special exercises using weights for your hands and arms. These will be taught to you by a physical therapist. You can then continue doing them at home.

· Counseling may help if you are having emotional problems in coping with the changes in your life brought on by the symptoms.

· Surgery is rare, but may help if symptoms are severe.

· Joining a support group may help some people. Ask your health care provider about groups in your area.

· To learn more: We Move, 204 West 84th St., New York, NY, 10024; (800) 437-MOV2; website: www.wemove.org.

MEDICATIONS

There are several different classes of drugs that are used to treat tremors. Your health care provider will discuss the options with you and decide if they are appropriate.

ACTIVITY

Try to maintain an active lifestyle. Exercise each day.

DIET

· Avoid caffeine in coffee, tea, and soft drinks. It may make the symptoms worse.

· Avoid alcohol, or use it on a limited basis. It may help the tremors short term, but it is not wise to use it as a form of treatment.

NOTIFY OUR OFFICE IF

· You or a family member has symptoms of essential tremor.

· Symptoms get worse despite treatment.

Special notes:

_____

_____

_____

More notes on the back of this page ☐

170

EXERCISE FOR HEALTH

 BASIC INFORMATION

DESCRIPTION

Exercise is a part of a healthy lifestyle at any age. It helps you feel and look better, aids in weight loss, and can lower the risk for many common diseases. Exercise can be fun—even though it may not seem fun at first. Talk to your health care provider about exercising. People who have not been active, have health problems, are pregnant, or elderly may need special advice.

REASONS PEOPLE GIVE FOR NOT EXERCISING

People have many reasons for not exercising. Look for ways to overcome the ones that affect you.

· *Not enough time or exercising is inconvenient:* Find available time slots. Take exercise breaks at work. Walk for 10 to 15 minutes at a time.

· *Lack of energy:* Plan exercise time during the day or week when you do feel more energetic. Convince yourself that exercise will actually boost your energy level.

· *It is not enjoyable, or it is boring:* Watch television while you exercise. Do gardening or mow the lawn. Exercise with a friend. Join an exercise class.

· *Fear of injury, or have had a recent injury:* Learn how to warm up and cool down. Wear proper shoes for the activity. Pick activities that have little risk.

· *Lack of confidence in being able to exercise:* Exercise with friends who have the same skill level. Take a class to learn a new skill. Walking is the easiest exercise.

· *Not able to maintain an exercise routine due to travel for work or other conflicting schedules:* Walk in hotel halls and take stairs instead of elevators. Pack stretch bands and jump rope and use them in your room. Pick places to stay with pools or fitness rooms.

· *Family or friends are not supportive or encouraging:* Ask your family for support. Invite family or friends to exercise with you. Join a fitness class or hiking club.

· *No place to walk nearby, such as a park or sidewalks, or the weather is bad:* Always have activities that you can do indoors. Exercise to a video-tape. Walk in the mall. Ride an exercise bike.

· *Family obligations take too much time:* Exercise with the kids, such as walking or swimming. Plan on exercising when kids are at school, playing, or sleeping.

WHAT TO DO TO GET STARTED

· Plan on making exercise or physical activity a part of your everyday life. Do things you enjoy. Many people are getting their exercise doing things such as biking, skiing and tennis. Others prefer less active recreation such as walking, gardening, or golf.

· Children and adults should try to get at least 30 to 60 minutes of exercise a day. You can break this into shorter periods of 10 or 15 minutes during the day.

PARTS OF AN EXERCISE PLAN

· *Endurance:* Find an activity that makes you breathe harder, on most or all days of the week. That's called "endurance activity," because it builds your stamina.

· *Muscle strength:* Lack of use lets muscles waste away. Start lifting weights and increase the weight slowly. This will build bone mass and help avoid osteoporosis.

· *Balance:* Do things to help your balance. Stand on one foot, then the other, without holding onto anything for support. Walk heel-to-toe (the toes of the foot in back should almost touch the heel of the foot in front when you walk this way).

· *Stretch:* Stretching won't build endurance or muscles, but helps keep you limber and flexible, and reduces injuries.

SUGGESTIONS FOR BEING ACTIVE

· Walk, cycle, jog, or skate to work, school, stores, etc. Walk during breaks at work. Keep a comfortable pair of shoes handy in your office or car.

· Park the car farther away from where you want to go.

· Take the stairs instead of the elevator.

· Play actively with children or pets.

· Garden at home, or do home repair work.

· Exercise while watching television. Ride an exercise bike, walk in place, lift weights, or stretch.

CAUTIONS

· Don't overdo the activity. Listen to your body. A few muscle aches are to be expected, but not pain.

· Start off a new routine at an easy pace. Then increase your time and effort. If you can talk without any trouble at all, your activity is probably too easy. If you can't talk at all, it's too hard.

· Use the correct equipment, especially shoes.

· Take 3 to 5 minutes to warm up. For example, start a walk at a slow pace, and then increase to a brisk pace.

· Be aware of any warning signs of heart problems: Severe sweating, chest and arm pain, and dizziness.

· Drink plenty of water to replace any lost fluids.

 NOTIFY OUR OFFICE IF

You or a family member has questions about exercising.

Special notes:

_____

_____

_____

More notes on the back of this page ☐

EYE CONTUSION or LACERATION

BASIC INFORMATION

DESCRIPTION

Eye injury, including blunt injury (contusion) or cut (laceration). It can involve the eyeball, eyelid, bones around the eyeball (eye socket), and the muscles attached to the eyeball.

FREQUENT SIGNS AND SYMPTOMS

· Swelling, redness, tenderness, pain, bleeding, or bruising ("black eye") in or around the eye. A black eye may take 1 to 2 days to develop.
· Change in ability to see clearly.

CAUSES

A blunt or sharp blow or cut to the eye or the area around the eye.

RISK INCREASES WITH

· Doing work that may risk injury to the eyes. This includes bartending (opening bottles), carpentry, or construction work.
· Paintball, BB guns, rifles, or slingshot usage.
· Sports such as baseball, softball, basketball, soccer, football, or hockey.
· Using a rotary lawn mower.
· Fist fights. Eye injuries may occur in fights. Fights are more likely with alcohol use.

PREVENTIVE MEASURES

When possible, wear appropriate eye protection for any activity that may lead to eye injury. This can include eye coverings or face shields.

EXPECTED OUTCOMES

Some injuries are mild and heal on their own. Others are usually curable with treatment. Allow 2 weeks for complete healing.

POSSIBLE COMPLICATIONS

· Permanent vision loss.
· Infection.
· Cataract.

DIAGNOSIS & TREATMENT

GENERAL MEASURES

· If you have any blurred vision, you must see a health care provider.
· For a minor contusion (black eye) during the first 24 hours, use ice packs to reduce swelling. The next day, make a warm compress by folding a clean cloth in several layers. Dip in warm water, wring out slightly, and put on the eye. Dip the compress often to keep it moist. Apply compress for an hour, rest an hour, and repeat.

· For a minor cut or scrape around the eye, apply pressure to stop any bleeding. Use a clean cloth to clean the wound. Cover with a bandage if a cut or scrape is large.
· For most eye injuries, or if you are unsure if it is serious, see your health care provider. Seek emergency care if the injury is severe.
· Your health care provider can diagnose the problem with an exam of the injured eye area.
· Treatment may involve stitches to repair cuts, or other surgical procedure.
· At home, sleep with the head raised with two pillows until symptoms get better.
· Protect eyes from bright light or sunlight by wearing dark glasses until healing is complete.

MEDICATIONS

· Antibiotic eye-drops to prevent infection may be prescribed.
· Use acetaminophen or ibuprofen for pain relief.
· Eye-drops, to dilate (enlarge) the eye pupil and rest the eye muscles, may be prescribed.

ACTIVITY

For minor injury, resume normal activities after healing. For other injuries, your health care provider will give you specific advice about sports and work activities.

DIET

No special diet.

NOTIFY OUR OFFICE IF

· You have a cut or other eye injury. This may be an emergency.
· The following occur after eye injury: fever, vision changes, or eye pain that persists after treatment.

Special notes:

_____

_____

_____

More notes on the back of this page ☐

EYE, FOREIGN BODY IN

BASIC INFORMATION

DESCRIPTION
A small speck of metal, wood, stone, sand, paint, an eyelash, or other foreign material in the eye.

FREQUENT SIGNS AND SYMPTOMS
- Pain, irritation, watering, and redness in the eye.
- Eye is sensitive to light.
- Foreign body (object) that can be seen when the eye is examined. Sometimes the object is very small, trapped under the eyelid, and cannot be seen except with a medical exam.
- Scratchy feeling when blinking.

CAUSES
Accident.

RISK INCREASES WITH
- Windy weather.
- Jobs or activity, such as carpentry or grinding, in which fine pieces of wood or other materials fly loose in the air.

PREVENTIVE MEASURES
Wear protective eye coverings if your job or hobby involves the risk of eye injury.

EXPECTED OUTCOMES

Most objects can be removed simply with self-care, in a health care provider's office, or emergency room.

POSSIBLE COMPLICATIONS
- Infection, especially if the object is not removed completely.
- Permanent vision damage.

DIAGNOSIS & TREATMENT

GENERAL MEASURES
- For small foreign bodies, be sure not to rub the eye. Try to flush the eye using one of these options:
  - Gently pour warm (not hot) water from a pitcher over the eye. Keep eye open.
  - Stand at a sink with warm water running and cup your hands and put your face in the running water.
  - Use an eye dropper with warm water.
  - If outside, use a garden hose, but don't use high pressure. A water fountain may also be used to flush out the eye.
  - Check the eye often to see if the object is gone.
  - If flushing is not working, you may consider trying to remove the object with the tip of a tissue or cotton-tipped swab. Lift upper or lower eyelid (someone else may need to help you). Be extremely careful to not touch the eye itself with the swab. You could injure the cornea.

- If you removed the object, but it was large, or the patient is a child, a health care provider should be seen for follow-up check.
- Use moist compresses to relieve discomfort after removal of particle. Prepare by folding a clean cloth in several layers. Dip in warm water, wring out slightly and apply to the eye. Dip the compress often to keep it moist. Do this for 1 hour, rest 1 hour, and then repeat.
- Most eye injuries should be seen by your health care provider. Ask someone else to drive you to the medical office or emergency center. Don't try to drive yourself. Keep the eye closed, if possible, until the exam.
- Your health care provider will do an exam of the injured eye. It may include staining the eye with a harmless substance to outline the object, examining the eye through a magnifying lens, and/or use of a special ultraviolet light.
- The procedure to remove the object will be determined by its size and location within the eye.
- An eye patch may be applied to keep the eye closed.
- A follow-up exam should be done in 1 to 2 days.

MEDICATIONS
- Antibiotic eye-drops may be prescribed to prevent infection.
- Pain relievers may be prescribed.

ACTIVITY
Resume your normal activities gradually after removal of the foreign body and the patch, if one is applied.

DIET
No special diet.

NOTIFY OUR OFFICE IF

- You or a family member has a foreign body in the eye that you are concerned about. If it is an emergency, call 911 to get emergency help right away.
- The following occur after removal:
  - Pain increases or does not disappear in 2 days.
  - Fever develops.
  - Vision changes.

Special notes:

_____

_____

_____

More notes on the back of this page ☐

FAILURE TO THRIVE

 BASIC INFORMATION

DESCRIPTION
Failure of infants or young children to grow and develop normally. Failure to thrive is actually a group of symptoms, rather than a specific disorder. It has many possible causes.

FREQUENT SIGNS AND SYMPTOMS
· Height and weight do not progress normally, as measured on standard growth charts.
· Physical skills may be slow to develop. This includes rolling over, sitting, crawling, standing, or walking.
· Mental and social skills may be delayed. This includes talking, social interaction, or self-feeding.
· Child lacks energy, has small muscles, rash or other skin changes, swollen arms or legs, and changes in hair.
· Other symptoms (they may be due to a medical condition).

CAUSES
It may be due to medical conditions (sometimes called organic failure). It may involve psychosocial and environmental causes, such as family concerns or problems in the home (sometimes called nonorganic failure). It may also be a combination of the two.

RISK INCREASES WITH
· Pregnancy problems (such as alcohol use or intrauterine growth restriction) or premature infants or children with chromosomal abnormalities.
· Children who have trouble eating, are unable to suck, have vomiting or reflux problems, or have infections.
· Children who are unable to absorb nutrients or need extra nutrients, due to certain medical disorders.
· Children with chronic illness (cystic fibrosis, asthma).
· Child neglect, abuse, or lack of attention by parents.
· Not providing enough food for a child. Child who refuses to eat, or problems with weaning a child.
· Parents who lack parenting skills.
· Dysfunctional family, difficult parent-child interactions, or lack of support (family or friends).
· Depression, alcohol or drug abuse in a parent.
· Poverty of parents (unable to provide needed foods).

PREVENTIVE MEASURES
· Get instructions on proper nutrition for a new baby.
· Take your child regularly to "well-baby" checkups.
· Arrange for parenting classes if you are new parents.

EXPECTED OUTCOMES
If the problem is short-term and the cause can be corrected, normal growth and development may resume. Recovery may take several months. In other cases, the outcome will depend on the underlying condition.

POSSIBLE COMPLICATIONS
Ongoing mental, emotional, and physical delays.

 DIAGNOSIS & TREATMENT

GENERAL MEASURES
· Your child's health care provider will do a physical exam. The child's height and weight will be compared to standard growth charts to determine if there is delayed growth. Medical tests may include blood and urine studies. To help pinpoint a cause for growth delay, questions may be asked about the pregnancy and birth, the child's behavior and eating habits, other family members, stress problems, and other concerns.
· Treatment will depend on the cause. Organic causes may be treated medically. Nonorganic causes may be treated with counseling, education, and other help for the parents. The main goal of any treatment is to be sure your child has the proper nutrition.
· Hospital care may be needed for some children.
· Home visits from a nurse may be recommended.
· Community programs that help mothers and children are available. Other help can be provided to get financial aid (such as food stamps), medical benefits, parenting classes, or counseling for emotional problems.
· If child neglect or abuse is suspected, child protective services or other authorities may become involved.

MEDICATIONS
Drugs may be prescribed for an underlying disorder.

ACTIVITY
No limits.

DIET
· Changes in your child's diet will be prescribed. They may include special formulas for infants, high-calorie foods for older children, and high-energy shakes (such as Pediasure or Boost). Specific instructions will be provided. Be sure to follow the instructions carefully.
· Tube feedings may be needed for severe cases. These can often be done at home.

 NOTIFY OUR OFFICE IF

· You are concerned that your child is not developing properly or growing as expected.
· You have any questions and concerns about the diet instructions for your child or other symptoms occur.

Special notes:

_____

_____

_____

More notes on the back of this page ☐

FAINTING
(Syncope)

BASIC INFORMATION

DESCRIPTION
A sudden, temporary loss of consciousness due to a decrease in the supply of blood and oxygen to the brain. Fainting may be a symptom of a health problem or a one-time event. Syncope is the medical term for fainting.

FREQUENT SIGNS AND SYMPTOMS
· Paleness and sweating.
· Sudden light-headedness.
· General weakness, followed by a fall.
· Blurred vision (sometimes).
· Nausea (sometimes).
· Rapid heartbeat and rapid breathing.

CAUSES
· The heart can not pump enough blood for the body to function properly. This occurs with heart disease and blood vessel disorders.
· The blood volume (amount of blood) is low. This can be due to bleeding or dehydration.
· Stimulation of the vagus nerve (in the neck, chest, and intestine) may slow the heart. This can happen with pain, fear, distress, vomiting, a large bowel movement, and even urinating can stimulate the nerve.
· Blood flow back to the heart is reduced. This occurs with straining when coughing, passing a stool, or in older men when trying to urinate (called micturition).
· Standing up or sitting down too quickly causes a sudden change in blood pressure. This is called orthostatic hypotension. Standing for long periods on a hot day can cause a similar problem due to lack of leg muscle use.
· Very rapid breathing or hyperventilating due to anxiety. Too much carbon dioxide is exhaled which then causes blood vessels in the brain to narrow.
· Other causes may be due to stroke, anemia, low blood sugar, lung problems, and others.
· In some cases, the cause of fainting is unknown.

RISK INCREASES WITH
· Heart disease or certain other chronic disorders.
· Certain drugs, such as those that slow the heartbeat.
· Being elderly.

PREVENTIVE MEASURES
· Often, fainting can not be prevented. If you feel faint, lie down with feet up or sit in a chair and bend over.
· Avoid the problems that can cause fainting if possible. Try not to get overly anxious. Get treatment for any medical disorder and avoid constipation. Men can urinate while sitting down if standing causes fainting. Avoid sudden changes in physical activity, such as when getting up from a chair or bed (move slowly).

EXPECTED OUTCOMES
A person will recover from simple fainting in 1 or 2 minutes. There are normally no long-term effects.

POSSIBLE COMPLICATIONS
· Injury while fainting, such as from a fall.
· Complications caused by a disorder that lead to the fainting.
· Recurrent fainting can have a major impact on a person's lifestyle. It may prevent driving a motor vehicle.

DIAGNOSIS & TREATMENT

GENERAL MEASURES
· See your health care provider after any fainting event. A physical exam may be done and questions asked about your symptoms and activities. Medical tests may include an ECG (electrocardiogram). It measures the electrical activity of the heart. Other tests may be done depending on the results of the ECG, or if other health disorders are suspected.
· Sometimes, no treatment is needed. In other cases, treatment may be prescribed for a diagnosed problem. Rarely, a patient may need hospital care for a period.
· If you are subject to frequent fainting spells, avoid activities in which fainting may endanger your life or others. This includes climbing ladders, driving motor vehicles, or operating dangerous machinery. Take measures to make your home safe in case you fall during a fainting event.

MEDICATIONS
Drugs are usually not needed for fainting. They may be prescribed for a health problem that is diagnosed.

ACTIVITY
You can usually resume normal activities right away unless advised differently by your health care provider.

DIET
No special diet. Drink adequate fluids. Avoid alcohol.

NOTIFY OUR OFFICE IF

You or a family member has a fainting event even if it seems mild. Fainting may be a symptom of a disorder that requires treatment.

Special notes:

_____

_____

_____

More notes on the back of this page ☐

FATTY LIVER
(Steatosis)

 BASIC INFORMATION

DESCRIPTION
The liver is one of the largest organs in the body and has many functions. Fatty liver is a build-up of fat in the liver cells. Alcohol-related fatty liver occurs in alcohol drinkers. Nonalcoholic fatty liver disease (NAFLD) occurs in people who seldom or never drink alcohol. Fat in the liver may cause no problems by itself. In some cases, it may be a sign of more serious problems.

FREQUENT SIGNS AND SYMPTOMS
• Usually there are no symptoms. The fatty liver condition is often discovered during a routine physical exam, or when medical tests are done for other reasons.
• There may be some pain or tenderness in the upper-right abdomen, behind the ribs. This is where the liver is located.
• Feeling tired.
• Jaundice (yellow skin and eyes).

CAUSES
It is not known what causes fat to build-up in the liver. It is known that fat increases in the liver with a number of conditions or disorders. Eating fatty foods does not cause fatty liver.

RISK INCREASES WITH
• Heavy use of alcohol.
• Obesity.
• Diabetes.
• Use of certain drugs.
• Metabolic syndrome (a group of health problems).
• Malnutrition (poor diet).
• High triglycerides (high fat levels in the blood).
• Intestinal bypass surgery for obesity.
• Tuberculosis.
• Pregnancy. It is a rare complication.
• Other uncommon diseases and some poisons.

PREVENTIVE MEASURES
• There are no specific preventive measures.
• Avoid alcohol.
• Eat a healthy diet. Maintain an ideal body weight.
• Pregnant women should get good prenatal care.

EXPECTED OUTCOMES
• Fatty liver can be partially reversed when the underlying cause is treated or removed.
• In pregnancy, it usually clears up after delivery.

POSSIBLE COMPLICATIONS
• Inflammation of the liver. This is called alcoholic steatohepatitis or nonalcoholic steatohepatitis (NASH).
• Other types of liver problems.
• If untreated in a pregnant woman, it can be life-threatening for the mother and the fetus.

 DIAGNOSIS & TREATMENT

GENERAL MEASURES
• Your health care provider will ask about alcohol and drug use, and do a physical exam. An enlarged liver can often be felt with fingertips during the exam. Blood tests are done to check liver function. Other tests, including a liver biopsy, can confirm fatty liver. In a biopsy, a long needle is used to remove a small bit of liver tissue for viewing with a microscope.
• Simple fatty liver may require no treatment.
• Treatment of any medical condition and lifestyle changes will normally reverse fatty liver.
• Treatment of diabetes includes diet, drugs, or insulin.
• Stop drinking alcohol. For help, join a local support group such as Alcoholics Anonymous.
• For an obesity problem, weight loss is necessary.
• If a pregnancy is far enough along, the recommended treatment is delivery.
• To learn more: American Liver Foundation, 75 Maiden Lane, Suite 603, New York, NY 10038; (800) 443-7872; website: www.liverfoundtion.com.

MEDICATIONS
• Drugs to treat fatty liver are being studied.
• Drugs may be prescribed for specific disorders.
• Certain drugs may be stopped if they are a risk factor.
• Weight loss drugs may be used for a short time.
• Vitamin and mineral supplements may be prescribed.

ACTIVITY
Start a daily exercise routine, such as walking.

DIET
• Eat a healthy diet that is low in calories, low in cholesterol, with plenty of fruits, vegetables, and fiber.
• Start a weight-loss diet if obesity is a problem.

 NOTIFY OUR OFFICE IF

• You or a family member has symptoms of fatty liver.
• You need information about weight-loss diets, avoiding alcohol, or starting an exercise routine.

Special notes:

_____

_____

_____

More notes on the back of this page ☐

FEBRILE SEIZURE

BASIC INFORMATION

DESCRIPTION

A febrile seizure is a convulsion that occurs with a fever in infants or small children. The fever may be from many causes, such as a cold or ear infection. Febrile seizures are common in young children. For many children, a febrile seizure occurs just one time. About one-third of the children will have recurrent febrile seizures. Few children have more than three.

FREQUENT SIGNS AND SYMPTOMS

- Repeated rhythmic jerking or stiffening of your child's arms and legs. The child may cry out initially.
- Eyes rolled back in the child's head.
- Lack of consciousness.
- Twitches in only a part of the body, such as an arm or a leg, or only on the right or the left side.
- Usually occur on the first day of a fever. Parents may not even know the child is ill.
- Rectal temperatures higher than 102°F (38.9°C).
- *Simple febrile seizure* stops by itself within a few seconds to 10 minutes. *Complex febrile seizure* lasts longer than 15 minutes, occurs in one part of the body, or recurs during the same illness.
- Child may be confused or drowsy after a seizure.

CAUSES

Exact cause is unknown. The high fever, and possibly one that rises quickly, may trigger a brain disturbance.

RISK INCREASES WITH

- Children ages 6 months to 6 years.
- Slightly more common in boys than girls.
- Very high fever or a rapidly rising temperature.
- A history of febrile seizures in other family members.
- Rarely, fever and seizure occurs after a vaccination.
- Risk factors for recurrent seizures include:
  - Young age (less than 15 months) for the first seizure.
  - Family members with a history of febrile seizures.
  - Fever was below 102°F (38.9°C) at time of first seizure.

PREVENTIVE MEASURES

- None for a first febrile seizure. There is no way to know for sure if a child is at risk.
- Fever-reducing drugs may help reduce future risk.
- Certain children with recurrent febrile seizures are sometimes given preventive drugs.

EXPECTED OUTCOMES

- Outcome is usually excellent, with no lasting effects.
- The child will not be aware of having had the seizure.
- Most children who have febrile seizures will outgrow them by four to five years of age.
- Febrile seizures do not cause brain damage.

POSSIBLE COMPLICATIONS

- Injury may result from bumping or falling into objects.
- There is a very small risk that certain children who have febrile seizures will develop epilepsy.

DIAGNOSIS & TREATMENT

GENERAL MEASURES

- Medical care may include emergency room treatment or seeing your child's health care provider. Either way, your child will be examined and questions asked about the seizure symptoms. Medical tests may be done to be sure there is not a more serious illness causing the fever.
- Reassurance to parents about the benign nature (not serious) of the seizure should help ease concerns.
- If a febrile seizure recurs, follow these instructions:
  - Stay calm!
  - Do not put anything in your child's mouth.
  - Place your child on his/her side to help drain saliva from the mouth. Don't try to hold your child still.
  - Loosen clothing.
  - Move objects away from your child to avoid injury.
  - Support child's head with a pillow or other soft object.
  - Try to watch a clock so you can time the seizure.

MEDICATIONS

- Drugs may be prescribed for any infection present.
- In rare cases, drugs may be prescribed for prevention.
- Give acetaminophen or ibuprofen at the first sign of fever. Don't give aspirin to children under age 18.

ACTIVITY

Allow your child rest or sleep after a seizure.

DIET

No special diet.

NOTIFY OUR OFFICE IF

- Your child has another febrile seizure.
- Any febrile seizure lasts more than 15 minutes.
- Your child seems to be looking or acting ill, more so than when first examined.
- You have any concerns about your child's symptoms.

Special notes:

_____

_____

_____

More notes on the back of this page ☐

FECAL IMPACTION

 ## BASIC INFORMATION

DESCRIPTION
A large, firm amount of stool that cannot be passed voluntarily. In most cases, the impacted stool is in the rectum, which is the lowest end of the bowels. Sometimes, the impaction may extend further up into the bowels.

FREQUENT SIGNS AND SYMPTOMS
· Lack of normal bowel movements.
· Sense of fullness in the rectum, but unable to pass stool.
· Pain or cramps in the stomach or abdomen area (often after meals).
· Thin, watery discharge from the rectum.
· Headache, nausea, vomiting, loss of appetite.
· General sick feeling.

CAUSES
Irregular bowel function causes dry, hardened feces to remain in the colon or rectum.

RISK INCREASES WITH
· Long term constipation.
· Rectal disorders that make normal bowel movements uncomfortable, such as painful hemorrhoids or fissures.
· Rectal or colon cancer.
· Swallowing substance for x-rays of the intestinal tract.
· Nerve problems in the colon or rectum, as with a spinal-cord injury, stroke, Parkinson's disease, or multiple sclerosis.
· Being elderly or bedridden (such as after surgery).
· Disorders such as hypothyroidism or hypercalcemia.
· Use of some drugs, such as narcotic pain remedies.

PREVENTIVE MEASURES
· Increase the fiber in the diet. Drink adequate amounts of fluid each day. Begin a program of regular exercise.
· Set aside a regular time each day for bowel movement (within an hour after breakfast is best). Don't try to hurry. Sit at least 10 minutes.
· If mild constipation develops, use a stool softener or a suppository.

EXPECTED OUTCOMES
Usually curable with treatment. Impaction may recur, unless the underlying cause is removed.

POSSIBLE COMPLICATIONS
· Injury to the rectum.
· If the impaction is not removed, the problem can worsen and surgery may be required.

 ## DIAGNOSIS & TREATMENT

GENERAL MEASURES
· Your health care provider will do an exam of the abdomen area and a digital rectal exam. The rectal exam is done with a gloved finger inserted into the rectum. Medical tests such as x-ray and others may be done to confirm the diagnosis and check for complications.
· The impacted mass may be removed partially by your health care provider. This is done as with the rectal exam. A gloved finger (sometimes two) is inserted into the rectum and the mass is broken up. The rest of the stool may be removed with the use of a suppository. In some cases, water irrigation with a special instrument inserted into the rectum is used.

MEDICATIONS
After treatment, stool softeners may be prescribed.

ACTIVITY
No limits. Be as active as your health permits. Good physical fitness improves bowel function.

DIET
· Eat a normal, well-balanced diet that is high in fiber.
· Drink at least 8 glasses of fluid each day.

 ## NOTIFY OUR OFFICE IF

· You or a family member has symptoms of a fecal impaction.
· Your normal bowel pattern changes.

Special notes:

_____

_____

_____

More notes on the back of this page ☐

FEMALE ATHLETE TRIAD

 BASIC INFORMATION

DESCRIPTION

Female athlete triad is a result of three related conditions. It can occur in females of any age, or athletic skill level. An athlete may have one, two, or all three of these conditions that make up the triad:
· Disordered eating (harmful eating behavior) combined with excessive exercise.
· Menstrual periods stop (amenorrhea).
· Loss of bone density (osteoporosis).

FREQUENT SIGNS AND SYMPTOMS

· Weight loss
· Fatigue (sometimes).
· Not having monthly periods or periods that are not regular.
· Young females may not start their first period.
· Stress fractures (bones break for no apparent reason).
· Injuries to muscles.
· Eating only small amounts of food. May overeat (binge) and then throw up or use laxatives (purge).

CAUSES

Not eating enough food for the energy being spent. Muscles and bones soon start wearing down. Estrogen hormone levels decrease, causing problems with menstrual periods and loss of bone density.

RISK INCREASES WITH

· Compulsive exercising. Workouts become the most important part of life.
· Overly concerned with reaching goals.
· Pushed by coach(es) or parents to lose weight for improved performance.
· Stress (emotional as well as physical).
· Activities where low body weights and thin body shape seem to be important. These include track and field, swimming, rowing, cycling, basketball, body-building, ballet, and gymnastics.

PREVENTIVE MEASURES

· Eat a healthy, well-balanced diet. Don't skip meals.
· Maintain a healthy body weight for your height.
· Keep track of your menstrual periods.
· Do not over exercise or over train.
· Educate athletes on good eating and exercise habits.

EXPECTED OUTCOMES

Outcome will vary for each athlete. With prompt diagnosis and early treatment, menstrual periods can return to normal, and further bone loss can be halted.

POSSIBLE COMPLICATIONS

· A decrease in athletic performance.
· Permanent bone loss and risk of bone fractures.
· Serious medical problems (can be life-threatening).

 DIAGNOSIS & TREATMENT

GENERAL MEASURES

· Your health care provider will do a physical exam. It may include a pelvic exam. You will be asked about your diet and any weight changes, your exercise routine, and menstrual-cycle history. Blood tests and a bone density test may be done.
· Treatment involves an increase in the amount of food you eat, weight gain, and sometimes reducing physical activity. Small changes may be all that is needed.
· Parents, along with trainers and coaches should be involved in treatment plans. This is important with adolescent (early teens) patients.
· Some may benefit from seeing a mental health provider for any stress or emotional problems.
· The treatment steps are not easy and will take time, but female athletes need to make the changes to improve their overall health now and in the future.

MEDICATIONS

· Hormones may be prescribed to stop bone loss.
· Take calcium pills to help prevent more bone loss.

ACTIVITY

Try for a balance in activity levels that will still allow you to train, compete, and achieve your goals while not harming your health. Ask your health care provider and coach to help you make specific plans.

DIET

It is important to get adequate calories, protein and calcium and eat foods you enjoy. Proper nutrition can enhance athletic performance. Consult an expert in nutrition to help you in making the right choices.

 NOTIFY OUR OFFICE IF

· You or a family member has symptoms of any of the conditions that make up the female athlete triad.
· Symptoms don't improve after a few months of treatment.

Special notes:

_____

_____

_____

More notes on the back of this page ☐

FERTILITY PROBLEMS IN MEN

 BASIC INFORMATION

DESCRIPTION
Infertility is the inability to achieve pregnancy after 1 year of sexual activity without contraception. Infertility occurs in 10% to 15% of all couples. Fertility depends on the production of normal quantities of healthy sperm, ability to achieve an erection, and ejaculation of sperm into the vagina during sexual intercourse. About 30% of infertility causes can be linked to male partners.

FREQUENT SIGNS AND SYMPTOMS
Failure to impregnate a fertile woman.

CAUSES
• Certain physical problems of the penis or testicles, such as undescended testicles.
• Excess alcohol use.
• Urinary-tract infection.
• Hormone problems.
• Endocrine disorders.
• Severe chronic or metabolic disorders (such as uremia or cirrhosis).
• Mumps.
• Use of some drugs, such as antihypertensives, cytotoxic drugs, male hormones, and MAO inhibitors.
• Sexually transmitted disease, such as syphilis and nonspecific urethritis that causes scarring.
• Injury to the genitals.
• Varicose veins in the testicles (varicocele).
• Emotional reasons, such as fear of infertility.
• Overheating of the testicles caused by vigorous, repetitive exercise or underwear that is too tight and holds the testicles too close to the body.
• Intercourse problems (e.g., premature withdrawal, poor timing with menses, too infrequent).
• Ejaculatory dysfunction.
• Exposure to insecticides or industrial chemicals.

RISK INCREASES WITH
• Diabetes.
• Poor nutrition and poor general health.
• Smoking.

PREVENTIVE MEASURES
Specific preventive measures depend on the cause.

EXPECTED OUTCOME
Some fertility problems are minor and reversible. Often, no clear cause for infertility is found. Each patient should approach treatment with optimism.

POSSIBLE COMPLICATIONS
Emotional stress caused by feelings of guilt, inadequacy, and loss of self-esteem.

 DIAGNOSIS & TREATMENT

GENERAL MEASURES
• Diagnosis begins with a detailed medical history and general physical exam. Further testing may include medical tests, such as blood studies of hormones and semen analysis (to determine quality, quantity, form, and motility). Surgical diagnostic procedures such as testicular biopsy and other special tests of sperm function and quality may be done.
• Results of the tests will determine the need for any special treatment such as drug therapy or surgery.
• Some general suggestions include:
 - Counseling for sexual therapy techniques, marriage problems, or alcoholism may be helpful.
 - Heat may decrease sperm production in the testicles. To prevent this, don't wear tight underwear or athletic supporters that hold the testicles too close to the body. Don't take hot baths. Avoid long bicycle rides.
 - Advise your health care provider if you work with environmental chemicals or are exposed to radiation on a routine basis. These can be a risk factor for infertility.
 - Stop smoking. It can reduce sperm counts and impair sperm motility.
 - Avoid alcohol or any drugs of abuse.
 - Have sexual intercourse during the time your partner is ovulating. Don't ejaculate for 3 days prior to intercourse. Intercourse should occur about every 36 hours during fertile period.
• To learn more: American Infertility Association, 666 Fifth Ave., Suite 278, New York, NY 10103; (888) 917-3777; website: www.americaninfertility.org.

MEDICATION
• Drugs may be prescribed to treat a cause of infertility.
• Vitamin supplements may be recommended.

ACTIVITY
Usually no limits.

DIET
Eat a well-balanced diet.

 NOTIFY OUR OFFICE IF

You or a family member has concerns about infertility.

Special notes:

_____

_____

_____

More notes on the back of this page ☐

FERTILITY PROBLEMS IN WOMEN

 ## BASIC INFORMATION

DESCRIPTION
The inability to become pregnant after 1 year of sexual activity without contraception. Infertility occurs in 10% to 15% of all couples. Female fertility depends on normal functioning of the reproductive tract and the production of hormones needed for normal sexual development and functioning. About 30% of all infertility is attributed to the female, 30% to the male, and the rest is a combination or unknown.

FREQUENT SIGNS AND SYMPTOMS
Inability to conceive.

CAUSES
Infertility can be caused by a wide variety of factors, and sometimes the cause is unknown.

RISK INCREASES WITH
- Endometriosis (disorder of the uterine lining).
- Pelvic inflammatory disease.
- Ovulatory problem (unable to ovulate [release eggs]).
- Physical problems of the reproductive system.
- Repeated weight-gain/weight-loss cycles.
- Hormone problems (such as thyroid).
- Vaginitis (inflammation of the vagina).
- Disorders of the cervix, such as infection, laceration or tearing from previous childbirth, or narrowing of the cervical opening for any reason.
- Amenorrhea (no menstrual periods).
- Chemical changes in the cervical mucus.
- Ovarian cysts.
- Smoking.
- Tumors.
- Emotional stress.
- Use of some drugs.
- Intrauterine device (IUD) may be a possible cause.
- Diabetes.
- Compulsive or excessive exercising.
- Marriage problems and infrequent sexual intercourse.
- Age. Female fertility decreases with age.
- Drugs of abuse, such as heroin or cocaine.

PREVENTIVE MEASURES
Obtain medical care for any treatable disorder that causes infertility. Avoid preventable causes of infertility.

EXPECTED OUTCOME
Some fertility problems are minor and reversible. Other problems may be helped with treatment.

POSSIBLE COMPLICATIONS
- Emotional stress, including feelings of guilt, inadequacy, and loss of self-esteem.
- Treatment costs are high and often not covered by insurance.
- Long-term effects of fertility drugs are unknown.

 ## DIAGNOSIS & TREATMENT

GENERAL MEASURES
- The first diagnostic tests may include a health history, blood tests, and a pelvic exam. Further testing may then be done. Multiple tests are available to study specific aspects of reproduction. You may be referred to a fertility specialist. The causes of infertility can be complex.
- Treatment will be based on the findings. Drug therapy or surgery may be recommended.
- General suggestions that may help you conceive:
  - Live a healthy lifestyle. Reduce stress. Eat a well-balanced diet. Exercise in moderation.
  - Give up alcohol, drug abuse, and cigarettes.
  - Get counseling for depression or marital problems.
  - Keep a basal body-temperature chart to become familiar with your ovulation pattern. Have intercourse just before ovulation.
  - Don't use a lubricant during sexual intercourse.
  - Your partner should withdraw his penis quickly from your vagina after ejaculation.
  - After your partner's ejaculation, place pillows under your buttocks to provide easier access for the sperm.
  - Maintain a positive attitude.
- To learn more: American Infertility Association, 666 Fifth Ave., Suite 278, New York, NY 10103; (888) 917-3777; website: www.americaninfertility.org.

MEDICATION
- Drugs may be prescribed to treat a cause of infertility.
- Ovarian stimulating drugs may be prescribed.
- Begin taking folic acid now. This will reduce the risk of birth defects once you become pregnant.

ACTIVITY
Too much exercising may contribute to infertility.

DIET
Eat a well-balanced diet. If overweight, try to lose weight. Avoid caffeine and alcohol.

 ## NOTIFY OUR OFFICE IF

- You or a family member is unable to get pregnant.
- Pregnancy is not achieved after treatment. There are additional options.

Special notes:

_____

_____

_____

More notes on the back of this page ☐

FEVER OF UNKNOWN ORIGIN (FUO)

Information From Your Health Care Provider

 BASIC INFORMATION

DESCRIPTION
Fever of unknown origin is a diagnosis given in cases where a person has had a fever (off and on) for at least 3 weeks, and no cause has been found after a basic medical evaluation.

FREQUENT SIGNS AND SYMPTOMS
Temperature above 101°F (38.3°C) on several occasions over a 3-week period.

CAUSES
In infants and children:
- Infections.
- Collagen or autoimmune diseases.
- Tumors and cancer, especially leukemia.

In adults:
- Infections.
- Collagen or autoimmune diseases.
- Tumors and cancer, especially kidney cancer and leukemia.
- Self-induced (in some emotionally unstable persons).
- Drugs can cause a fever as an adverse reaction.

RISK INCREASES WITH
- Weak immune system due to illness or drugs.
- Chemical or environmental exposure to polluted water or air.
- Travel in areas with unsanitary conditions.
- Exposure to others with infectious diseases.
- Elderly persons.
- Drug abuse.

PREVENTIVE MEASURES
There are no specific preventive measures.

EXPECTED OUTCOMES
Recovery without any treatment occurs in some cases. In other cases, the outcome depends on successful diagnosis and treatment of the underlying disorder.

POSSIBLE COMPLICATIONS
Depends on the underlying condition causing the fever.

 DIAGNOSIS & TREATMENT

GENERAL MEASURES
- Your health care provider will do a physical exam and ask about your symptoms and activities. Because a fever may be the first evidence of a serious condition (in its early stages), careful medical testing may be done. This may include blood studies and a urine culture, x-rays of the chest, CT scan, an ultrasound, echocardiogram (heart function test), thyroid studies, liver function tests, an HIV antibody test, and others.
- Hospital care may be recommended for elderly patients, patients with weak immune systems, and those with a serious chronic illness.
- When at home, keep a daily temperature chart. Rectal temperatures are most accurate.
- Treatment will depend on the underlying cause that is found.

MEDICATIONS
- Acetaminophen or ibuprofen may be prescribed, to lower the fever.
- Until the cause is found, other prescription drugs may be withheld to avoid masking symptoms of the underlying disorder.
- In certain patients, antibiotics, steroids, or other drugs may be prescribed prior to a specific diagnosis.

ACTIVITY
Get extra rest while you have a fever.

DIET
No special diet. Drink extra fluids while you have a fever.

 NOTIFY OUR OFFICE IF

- You or a family member has an unexplained fever that lasts longer than 24 hours.
- New symptoms develop. They may provide a clue about the underlying cause of the fever.

Special notes:

_____

_____

_____

More notes on the back of this page ☐

FIBROCYSTIC BREAST CHANGES

 BASIC INFORMATION

DESCRIPTION

Fibrocystic changes are the most common cause of breast lumps in women. Over 50% of women have these changes at some point in their lives. The changes are not cancerous and are not a threat to health. They can affect females from puberty to around age 50.

FREQUENT SIGNS AND SYMPTOMS

· The changes may affect one or both breasts. Single lumps may occur, but multiple lumps are common.
· Lumps may offer resistance when pressed with finger-tips and they may feel tender. They often enlarge before menstrual periods and shrink afterward.
· Breasts may be swollen and engorged.
· Mild to severe breast pain. It may be constant, on or off, irregular, or occur just before menstrual periods.
· Some women develop cysts, which are fluid-filled sacs that feel smooth and firm.
· Lumps come in different sizes. When the lumps are relatively large and near the surface, they can be moved freely within the breast.

CAUSES

The cause is not unclear. Ovarian hormones appear to play a role. Fibrocystic changes may be caused by abnormal hormone levels or by an increased response of breast tissue to normal hormone levels.

RISK INCREASES WITH

Women who have not had children, have irregular menstrual cycles, or have a family history of fibrocystic breast changes or breast cancer. Studies on caffeine use, high-fat diet, and smoking are inconclusive.

PREVENTIVE MEASURES

Specific preventive measures are unknown. It may help to eat a low-fat diet, avoid smoking, and avoid caffeine.

EXPECTED OUTCOME

Women with fibrocystic breast changes continue to have breast lumps that appear and dissolve. Some remain permanently. Treatment may help relieve symptoms. The condition often disappears after menopause (unless estrogen-replacement therapy is used).

POSSIBLE COMPLICATIONS

Only about 5% of fibrocystic breast changes have atypical cells that are a risk factor for developing cancer.

 DIAGNOSIS & TREATMENT

GENERAL MEASURES

· Your health care provider will do a breast exam and examine the underarm area. Medical tests may include mammogram, ultrasound, and surgical diagnostic procedures, such as cyst aspiration.

· Some cysts can be aspirated (removing the fluid). This is done in a health care provider's office. Removing the fluid should cause the lump to disappear. If the lump does not disappear, further diagnostic testing is done.
· The breast changes may get better without treatment. If symptoms continue, diet changes may help and drug therapy may be an option. Keep a pain diary for 2 to 3 months to determine the pattern of the pain.
· Applying heat to the breasts may help the discomfort.
· Wear a well-fitting, supportive bra (day and night).
· Surgery may sometimes be done to remove a lump.
· Stop smoking. Find a way to quit that works for you.
· Examine your breasts carefully each month. Report new lumps or any changes in lumps that have been diagnosed previously.
· Get routine mammogram studies as advised.
· Visit your health care provider at least every year for a breast exam. If you have a family history of cancer, more frequent follow-up visits may be recommended.
·To learn more: Do an Internet search or visit a library.

MEDICATION

· A mild diuretic to may be prescribed.
· Birth control pills may be prescribed to help control hormone levels. For more severe symptoms, danazol or bromocriptine may be prescribed.
· Use nonprescription pain remedies for the pain.
· Some women take vitamin A, vitamin B-6, vitamin E, or evening primrose oil to relieve symptoms. Ask your health care provider about these supplements.

ACTIVITY

No limits. A regular exercise program is usually recommended. Avoid activities that cause breast discomfort.

DIET

· Avoiding beverages that contain caffeine (coffee, tea, and some soft drinks) may help relieve symptoms.
· Eat a low-fat diet. Reducing salt and sugar may help.

 NOTIFY OUR OFFICE IF

· You or a family member has undiagnosed lumps in the breast.
· You detect a change in a lump, or new lumps appear.

Special notes:

_____

_____

_____

More notes on the back of this page ☐

FIBROID TUMORS OF THE UTERUS
(Myomas; Leiomyomas)

 ## BASIC INFORMATION

DESCRIPTION
An abnormal growth of cells in the muscular wall (myometrium) of the uterus. The term *fibroid* is misleading. The cells are not fibrous. They are composed of abnormal muscle cells. Uterine fibroids are common, and almost always benign (not cancerous). Fibroid size can be very tiny to the size of a cantaloupe or larger. Rarely, fibroids can involve the cervix. Major types of fibroids include:
- Subserous, which appear on the outside of the uterus.
- Intramural, which are confined to the wall of the uterus.
- Submucous, which appear inside the uterus.
- Pedunculated myomas, which are attached to the uterine wall by stalks.

FREQUENT SIGNS AND SYMPTOMS
- Often, no symptoms occur. The fibroids may be diagnosed during a pelvic exam.
- Menstruation is more frequent, with (possibly) heavy bleeding, and (sometimes) passing clots.
- Bleeding between periods.
- Feelings of pressure on the bladder, rectum, or spine.
- Anemia (weakness, fatigue and paleness).
- Increased vaginal discharge (rare).
- Painful sexual intercourse, or bleeding after intercourse (rare).

CAUSES
Exact cause is unknown. May involve excess estrogen.

RISK INCREASES WITH
- Use of certain oral contraceptives and estrogen replacement therapy, as these stimulate fibroid growth.
- Genetic factors. They occur 3 to 5 times more often in African American women than in white women.
- Family history of fibroids.
- Diet high in fat and/or obesity may be a risk factor.

PREVENTIVE MEASURES
Cannot be prevented at present. Routine pelvic exams can help with early diagnosis and treatment.

EXPECTED OUTCOME
- Treatment is usually not needed when there are no symptoms or the symptoms are mild.
- Drugs can help relieve some symptoms, but will not cure fibroids. Fibroids can be removed with surgery.
- Fibroids may decrease in size after menopause.

POSSIBLE COMPLICATIONS
- Heavy bleeding and anemia.
- Complications can sometimes occur in a pregnancy.
- Fibroids may return after surgical treatment.
- Fibroids may affect fertility.
- Fibroids may become cancerous (about 1 in 1000).

 ## DIAGNOSIS & TREATMENT

GENERAL MEASURES
- Your health care provider will do a physical exam and a pelvic exam. Medical tests may include blood studies and an ultrasound. More specialized tests (laparoscopy, hysteroscopy, hysterosalpingogram, or biopsy) may be done to verify the type of fibroid.
- Treatment will vary depending on symptoms and diagnostic tests, location and size of the fibroids, general health, and desire for future pregnancies.
- No treatment may be needed in cases of mild symptoms. You will be re-examined every 3 to 12 months.
- Hormone therapy, to suppress natural estrogen, is often the first step in treatment or before surgery.
- Surgery may be recommended. Several different surgical procedures are possible. Be sure you understand all aspects of your choices, and the risks and benefits involved. Hysterectomy is surgery to remove the uterus. A myomectomy removes the fibroids.
- Uterine fibroid embolization (UFE), also called uterine artery embolization (UAE), is a nonsurgical procedure. It treats fibroids by cutting off their blood flow.
- Radiofrequency ablation (RFA) or myomacoagulation (called myolysis) uses electric current to treat fibroids.
- Cryomyolysis uses a probe that freezes the fibroid.
- Blood transfusions may be needed for severe anemia.

MEDICATION
- A combination of nonsteroidal anti-inflammatories, birth control pills, or progestins may be prescribed.
- Iron supplements may be prescribed for anemia.
- A gonadotropin-releasing hormone may be prescribed. It will induce an abrupt, artificial menopause that stops the bleeding and reduces size of the fibroid.

ACTIVITY
No limits, unless surgery is performed.

DIET
No special diet.

 ## NOTIFY OUR OFFICE IF

- You or a family member has symptoms of fibroids.
- Symptoms become more severe after treatment.

Special notes:

_____

_____

_____

More notes on the back of this page ☐

FIBROMYALGIA
(FIBROSITIS)

 BASIC INFORMATION

DESCRIPTION
Fibromyalgia is a painful condition that involves muscles, tendons, and joints. It may affect the muscle areas of the low back, neck, shoulder, chest, arms, hips, and thighs. It is a chronic problem that can come and go for years. Symptoms may be brought on by a change in the weather, being in cold or damp places, stress, hormone changes, or in response to activity. It is a common condition that occurs in both men and women in all age groups, including children. It most often affects women ages 20 to 50.

FREQUENT SIGNS AND SYMPTOMS
- Pain and aches in the muscles, often described as "hurting all over all the time."
- Fatigue and sleep problems.
- Areas of the body are tender to the touch (tender points). Common tender points are the front of the knees, the elbows, the hip joints, and around the neck.
- Feeling stiffness in mornings; having swollen joints, and the hands and feet may be numb and tingly.
- Headache, anxiety, and depression.
- Other symptoms may also occur, such as digestion, bowel, and urinary problems; vision changes; emotional or mental changes; allergies; dry eyes and mouth; and painful menstrual periods.

CAUSES
The cause is unknown and there are many theories. Research is ongoing into finding possible causes.

RISK INCREASES WITH
- Females ages 20 to 50.
- Having a relative with the condition. It appears to run in families.

PREVENTIVE MEASURES
There are no steps that will prevent fibromyalgia.

EXPECTED OUTCOMES
The symptoms vary and may improve on their own or can be helped with treatment. The condition does not lead to more serious illness, nor is it life-threatening.

POSSIBLE COMPLICATIONS
Stress or other problems may cause the pain symptoms to worsen or flare up, usually only for a short time.

 DIAGNOSIS & TREATMENT

GENERAL MEASURES
- There is no special test to diagnose fibromyalgia. Your health care provider will do a physical exam, check the tender points in your body, and ask about all the symptoms you have. These same symptoms occur in other health problems. Tests such as blood work and x-rays may be done to be sure of the diagnosis.
- There is no cure for fibromyalgia. Taking steps to reduce the symptoms is the main goal.
- Treatment steps vary. They may include prescribed drugs and injections, exercise, physical therapy, acupuncture, chiropractic care, or massage therapy. Counseling can help reduce stress and anxiety and promote well-being.
- Make changes in your life that may be needed to help you cope day-to-day. Maintain your social life and contact with friends.
- Join a local support group so you can talk with others about self-help ideas that work.
- Keep your activity levels about the same each day.
- Get as much sleep as you need.
- Don't smoke. Find a way to quit that works for you.
- To learn more: National Fibromyalgia Association, 2200 N. Glassell St., Suite A, Orange, CA 92865, (714) 921-0150 (not toll-free); website: www.fmaware.org.

MEDICATIONS
- For minor pain, use nonprescription drugs such as acetaminophen or ibuprofen.
- Drugs may be prescribed for symptoms of pain, depression, anxiety, and sleep problems. They will take a few weeks to work and side effects are common.

ACTIVITY
A daily exercise program is important. It will improve your fitness level, help reduce muscle pain, and let you sleep better. Talk to your health care provider about an exercise routine that will suit your needs.

DIET
- Avoid caffeine and alcohol.
- Eat a healthy diet. Your health care provider or a dietician can help you plan a diet.

 NOTIFY OUR OFFICE IF

- You or a family member has some of the symptoms of fibromyalgia.
- Symptoms continue or worsen despite treatment.
- New symptoms develop. Drugs used in treatment may cause side effects.

Special notes:

_____

_____

_____

More notes on the back of this page ☐

FLUID & ELECTROLYTE DISORDERS

 BASIC INFORMATION

DESCRIPTION
An imbalance of the fluids and electrolytes in the body. Electrolytes are minerals found in the body that maintain many important body functions. The major electrolytes are sodium, calcium, potassium, magnesium, bicarbonate, phosphate, and chloride. An imbalance problem can affect any age group.

FREQUENT SIGNS AND SYMPTOMS
· Dry mouth and wrinkled skin.
· Increased, decreased, or no urination.
· Fatigue.
· Muscle weakness, cramping, or twitching.
· Puffy legs, hands, face, or stomach.
· Lung congestion. Problems with breathing.
· Changes in mental status, depression, irritability.
· Fast or slow heartbeat.
· Constipation, nausea, and vomiting.
· Seizures or coma.

CAUSES
A variety of diseases and medical problems can lead to an imbalance. When the body loses fluids (such as with diarrhea) or retains fluids (such as with heart failure), the electrolyte balance is affected. Electrolytes may be too low (hypo-) or too high (hyper-).

RISK INCREASES WITH
· Diarrhea and/or vomiting.
· Heavy sweating.
· Serious burns, wounds, or other injuries.
· Heart or kidney disorders.
· Excess fluid intake.
· Use of diuretics (water pills).
· Laxative abuse.
· Certain types of prescription drugs.
· Diabetes.
· Endocrine diseases.
· Bone disorders.
· Milk-alkali syndrome (excess calcium intake).
· Fever.
· Unusual or extreme diets, or eating disorders.
· Alcoholism.
· Infants, young children, and people over 60. These people lose fluids very quickly when sick.

PREVENTIVE MEASURES
· Avoid risk factors, where possible.
· Get medical care for chronic medical problems.

EXPECTED OUTCOMES
Treatment of electrolyte imbalance is usually effective. A long-term outlook depends on the underlying cause.

POSSIBLE COMPLICATIONS
Severe imbalances can cause serious and fatal disorders.

 DIAGNOSIS & TREATMENT

GENERAL MEASURES
· Your health care provider may do a physical exam and ask questions about your symptoms and activities. Medical tests include blood studies of electrolyte levels.
· Treatment will depend on the underlying cause. This may include changes in diet or fluid intake, changes in drugs that may have caused the problem, prescribing new drugs, or other therapies as needed.
· Treatment steps include correcting the fluid and electrolyte imbalance. Electrolytes that are too low will be replaced. Electrolytes that are too high will be reduced. Hospital care may be needed for some patients to provide IV (intravenous) treatment. Patients with milder symptoms may be cared for at home.
· Dialysis (use of a machine to filter wastes) may be needed for some patients with kidney disorders.

MEDICATIONS
· Electrolyte replacements may be prescribed. They may be given through a vein (IV) or taken orally.
· Drugs to reduce high electrolyte levels may be prescribed.
· Drugs to treat an underlying disorder may be prescribed.

ACTIVITY
Rest in bed until treatment is complete. Resume normal activities gradually.

DIET
· For a severe imbalance, solid food may be withheld until fluids and electrolytes return to normal.
· Diet changes may be recommended by your health care provider to help prevent problems in the future.

 NOTIFY OUR OFFICE IF

· You or a family member has symptoms of a fluid and electrolyte imbalance or dehydration.
· Your weight increases or decreases several pounds in one day.

Special notes:

_____

_____

_____

More notes on the back of this page ☐

FOLLICULITIS

 BASIC INFORMATION

DESCRIPTION

An inflammation of the hair follicles. Follicles are where the roots of body hair grow. Folliculitis can involve the hair on the skin anywhere on the body. It usually affects the face (such as the beard area in men), scalp, legs, armpits, and groin area. A stye is folliculitis on an eyelid. Folliculitis can affect any age group.

FREQUENT SIGNS AND SYMPTOMS

· Small groups of bumps (called papules or pustules) develop, usually with a hair in the middle of each bump. The bumps are small, and yellow-white in color, with a red area around them.
· Pain, redness, and swelling of the skin may occur.

CAUSES

Most often it is an infection of the hair follicles with *Staphylococcus or Pseudomonas* bacteria. It may also be caused by a fungal infection or irritation. Folliculitis may be superficial (on the surface of the skin) or deep in the hair follicle.

RISK INCREASES WITH

· Recent illness such as a nasal infection.
· Diabetes.
· Weak immune system due to illness or drugs.
· Excess sweating (hyperhidrosis).
· Eczema or dermatitis.
· Skin injuries, abrasions, surgical wounds, or draining abscess.
· Shaving, waxing, or plucking hairs.
· Tight clothing.
· Poor hygiene.
· Obesity.
· Use of hot tubs or saunas.
· Use of certain skin care products or overuse of topical steroids.

PREVENTIVE MEASURES

· Wash hands often to prevent spread of any germs.
· Frequent bathing. Keep fingernails short and clean.
· Wash towels and linens often to prevent spread of germs.
· Avoid risk factors where possible.

EXPECTED OUTCOMES

Most cases clear up within 2 weeks. Some may take longer.

POSSIBLE COMPLICATIONS

· May progress to other types of skin problems.
· Scarring may occur.
· Folliculitis may recur or become chronic.

 DIAGNOSIS & TREATMENT

GENERAL MEASURES

· Self-care is often all that is needed. See your health care provider if you have concerns about the disorder.
· Your health care provider can diagnose folliculitis by an exam of the affected area. A culture of fluid from the pustule or other tests may be done.
· Treatment involves supportive care of the skin and drug therapy if needed.
· Don't scratch the affected area. The germs can be transferred from under the fingernails to other parts of the body.
· Use warm-water soaks to relieve itching and help healing.
· Clean area with antibacterial soap. Shampoo daily if the scalp is involved.
· Avoid using oils or greasy-type ointments on the skin.
· If you shave, change razor blades daily or use an electric razor.
· If folliculitis recurs or becomes chronic, shaving may need to be discontinued for a period of time.

MEDICATIONS

· If there are only a few bumps, you may use nonprescription, topical antibiotics (such as mupirocin). Apply as directed.
· Oral antibiotics may be prescribed.
· A topical antibiotic drug applied into the front of the nose may be prescribed. The nostrils are a source of bacteria that can be spread to other parts of the body.
· Other drugs may be prescribed if a cause other than bacteria is diagnosed.

ACTIVITY

No limits.

DIET

No special diet. A weight-loss diet may be recommended for obese patients.

 NOTIFY OUR OFFICE IF

· You or a family member has symptoms of folliculitis.
· You develop a boil or signs of spreading infection.
· Folliculitis recurs after treatment.

Special notes:

_____

_____

_____

More notes on the back of this page ☐

FOOD ALLERGY

 BASIC INFORMATION

DESCRIPTION

Food allergy is a reaction of the body's immune system to some foods. Many people think they have a food allergy when it is food intolerance. Intolerance is caused by digestion problems, such as lactose or milk intolerance. A food allergy can cause severe symptoms. Food intolerance symptoms are rarely serious. It is important to know which one you have. Your health care provider can help you with the diagnosis.

FREQUENT SIGNS AND SYMPTOMS

· Diarrhea, stomach pains, nausea, or vomiting.
· Skin hives, rash (called eczema), itching, redness, and swelling of hands, feet, face, and lips.
· Cough, wheezing, or sneezing; runny nose.
· Infants may have blood in the stool or colic.

CAUSES

· The immune system reacts to certain proteins found in foods. It treats them as harmful to the body and tries to fight them off by releasing chemicals and histamines. This is what starts the allergic symptoms. Why it occurs in some people is unknown.
· Just about any food can cause an allergic reaction. Most common are milk, eggs, wheat, soy, peanut, tree nuts (walnuts and pecans), fish, and shellfish. Chocolate is not a common cause.

RISK INCREASES WITH

· People who have other allergy problems.
· Having family members who have a food allergy.
· Young children. Food allergy is more common.

PREVENTIVE MEASURES

· Food allergy cannot be prevented. A reaction can be prevented once the food causing it is known.
· It has not been proven that breast-feeding an infant prevents food allergies later in life. It does help delay the baby's exposure to foods that can cause allergies. Start solid foods at about age six months.

EXPECTED OUTCOMES

· Infants will often outgrow food allergy by 2 to 4 years.
· Adults with food allergy (particularly to milk, fish, shellfish, or nuts) are more likely to have their allergy for many years.
· Research is ongoing so new methods for treatment and prevention may become available.

POSSIBLE COMPLICATIONS

None expected as long as the foods are avoided. Rarely, anaphylaxis (a severe, life-threatening reaction) occurs. Symptoms come on very quickly. They can include those listed above plus trouble breathing, fast heart rate, and loss of consciousness. Seek emergency help if it happens.

 DIAGNOSIS & TREATMENT

GENERAL MEASURES

· For diagnosis, your health care provider will ask questions about your symptoms and your diet, and may include a physical exam. Testing might involve skin and blood allergy tests, a food challenge test, or an elimination diet that you do at home.
· Once you know for sure that you have a food allergy, the treatment is to avoid the food or foods involved.
· Often, the food allergy is in a young child. Parents will need to discuss the allergy with any people who will be caring for, teaching, or working with the child. They need to know what foods are involved and how to handle a severe reaction if one occurs. Once a child is older, parents can begin to teach the child how to take control of the allergy.
· To learn more: Food Allergy & Anaphylaxis Network, 10400 Eaton Place, Suite 107, Fairfax, VA 22030; (800) 929-4040; website: www.foodallergy.org.

MEDICATIONS

· Drugs will not cure a food allergy. Drugs may be prescribed to relieve some of the symptoms such as an antihistamine for itching or rash.
· If your food allergy is severe, you should carry a kit with a self-injecting device that contains the drug epinephrine. It can be used if the food is eaten by mistake and a reaction occurs. Know how to use the device. In addition, your family or others need to know how to give the injection if you are unable to do so.

ACTIVITY

No limits.

DIET

· Read the food labels carefully on all food products.
· Use a food allergy cookbook to help prepare meals.
· Ask waiters in restaurants for details about foods and other items on the menu.

 NOTIFY OUR OFFICE IF

You or a family member has symptoms of food allergy or food intolerance.

Special notes:

_____

_____

_____

More notes on the back of this page ☐

FOOD POISONING

 ## BASIC INFORMATION

DESCRIPTION

A term used to describe illnesses suspected of being caused by contaminated food (or beverages). Food poisoning can affect all ages. Outbreaks can affect several members of a household, customers who dined at the same restaurant, nursing home patients, cruise ship passengers, university students, children in daycare, or shoppers who bought contaminated food in a store.

FREQUENT SIGNS AND SYMPTOMS

• Symptoms can begin within hours to days after eating the food. It depends on the cause of the contamination and how much food was ingested (eaten).
• Nausea and vomiting.
• Abdominal cramps or pain.
• Diarrhea.
• Bloody stools.
• Fever, chills, headache, and weakness may occur.
• In severe cases, shock and collapse.

CAUSES

• Certain bacteria such as *Campylobacter, Escherichia coli, Salmonella,* and others. Botulism is a rare, life-threatening food poisoning.
• Virus infection such as Norwalk virus (a common contaminant of shellfish), adenovirus, and rotavirus.
• Chemical causes such as contamination with insecticide or food served in lead-glazed pottery.
• Eating plants or animals that contain a naturally occurring poison, such as mushrooms or toadstools. Shellfish may contain a toxin that is not destroyed by cooking.

RISK INCREASES WITH

• Eating food that is improperly prepared.
• Lack of good hygiene when preparing food.
• Drinking water or eating raw foods when traveling in a foreign country.

PREVENTIVE MEASURES

• Avoid raw seafood or meat.
• Avoid unpasteurized food products.
• Properly cook and store foods.
• Keep food preparation areas and utensils clean.
• Throw food items away that are old, have an "off" smell, or those in bulging tin cans.
• Always wash hands before preparing food.

EXPECTED OUTCOMES

Most cases are mild and clear up within a few days.

POSSIBLE COMPLICATIONS

Dehydration is the most common complication. More serious complications are rare but can be life-threatening, especially in very young or elderly patients or persons with weak immune systems.

 ## DIAGNOSIS & TREATMENT

GENERAL MEASURES

• In mild cases, self-care may be all that is needed. See a health care provider if symptoms are other than mild.
• Your health care provider may do a physical exam. Questions will be asked about your symptoms and recent foods you have eaten, and whether other people have eaten the same foods. Cultures may be made from a stool sample. If some of the food that made you sick is available, you may be asked to bring it in for testing.
• The main treatment is to replace fluid and electrolytes (salts and minerals) lost through vomiting or diarrhea.
• Hospital care may be required if symptoms are severe. Fluids may be given through a vein (IV).
• If several persons are affected, contact the local health department. They can interview patients and food handlers and take samples of suspected contaminated food.

MEDICATIONS

• Usually, drugs are not needed to treat food poisoning. They may be prescribed for certain symptoms.
• Antibiotics may be prescribed.
• Don't take drugs for diarrhea unless they are prescribed. They may prolong the symptoms.

ACTIVITY

Get extra rest until diarrhea, vomiting, and fever are improved. Be sure to have access to a toilet or bedpan.

DIET

• Suck ice chips or drink small amounts of clear fluids often. Replace lost fluids and electrolytes with products such as Pedialyte or Ricelyte for infants and children, and diluted rehydration fluids (Gatorade) for adults.
• Once the symptoms improve, try a diet of complex carbohydrates (rice, wheat, potatoes, bread, cereal, and lean meat such as chicken). Milk and dairy products usually do not need to be limited.
• Avoid high-sugar foods or fatty foods for a few days.

 ## NOTIFY OUR OFFICE IF

You or a family member has signs or symptoms of food poisoning that cause concern or are not improving.

Special notes:

_____

_____

_____

More notes on the back of this page ☐

FROSTBITE

BASIC INFORMATION

DESCRIPTION
• Frostbite is the destruction of body tissue from exposure to temperatures or wind chill below freezing. Arms, legs, fingers, toes, face, nose, and ears are areas of the body that are usually affected. It can occur at any age, but is more common in males ages 30 to 49.
• Nonfreezing cold injuries include frostnip, chilblains, and immersion foot (cold and wet exposure).

FREQUENT SIGNS AND SYMPTOMS
• In milder cases, there may be burning, numbness, tingling, itching, or coldness in the affected area. Skin may be white and frozen in appearance, and may have some resistance when pressed.
• In more severe cases of frostbite, there may be no sensations in the affected area. Swelling and blood-filled blisters may appear. Skin may be white or yellow, look waxy, and turn purple as it is rewarmed. The area is hard when it is pressed. The affected area can look blackened and dead.
• Hypothermia (low body temperature) can cause uncontrolled shivering, weakness, and confusion.

CAUSES
Frostbite occurs when ice crystals form in skin and blood vessels, which leads to destruction of the cells. Further damage can occur upon rewarming when blood flow resumes into the damaged blood vessels.

RISK INCREASES WITH
• Car accidents or car breakdowns in bad weather (especially in remote areas).
• Drinking too much alcohol or abusing drugs.
• Elderly persons.
• Diabetes, blood-vessel diseases, or smoking.
• Persons with mental disorders.
• Homeless persons.
• High-altitude travel or activities.
• Poor conditioning, inadequate clothing, clothing that is wet and tight, dehydration, malnutrition, and fatigue.

PREVENTIVE MEASURES
• Dress for the cold weather. Dress in layers. Carry extra gear such as a jacket, gloves, socks, hat, and blankets.
• Avoid smoking and alcohol.
• Travel with someone, in case help is needed.

EXPECTED OUTCOMES
For milder cold injuries, complete recovery is expected. More severe frostbite may have complications. Full recovery can take months.

POSSIBLE COMPLICATIONS
• Minor complications, such as pain, changes in sensitivity of the affected area, and skin color changes.
• Major complications, such as amputation.

DIAGNOSIS & TREATMENT

GENERAL MEASURES
• Emergency care for frostbite:
  - Call for help. Arrange for transport to a hospital.
  - Move patient to a warm area. Keep the affected area elevated. Keep the person warm to prevent hypothermia. Remove tight clothing or jewelry (they may block blood flow).
  - Don't rewarm the affected area if there is a chance it may freeze again. Don't rewarm it using an open fire or dry heat. Put the affected area in warm (not hot) water.
  - Give warm fluids to drink (no alcohol or caffeine).
  - Never massage (rub) the affected areas.
  - Cover the area with soft, cloth bandages. Place cloth or cotton between toes/fingers to prevent rubbing.
• Medical care:
  - An exam by a health care provider is done to check for life-threatening problems and to diagnose frostbite or other type of cold injury, such as frostnip.
  - Rewarming for frostbite is usually done in a warm bath until the thaw is complete. It can be a painful process. Fluids are often given through a vein (IV). Supplemental oxygen may be needed.
  - Hospital care may be required to treat skin damage, assess the extent of injury, and to prevent infection. Whirlpool bath therapy may be done to remove dead tissue. The affected area may be elevated and splinted.
  - It may take months to see if the affected tissue will be healthy or permanently damaged. Surgery may be done to remove damaged tissue, including amputation.

MEDICATIONS
You may be prescribed drugs for pain relief, antibiotics to prevent infection, and/or a tetanus booster.

ACTIVITY
Will depend on extent of damage. Physical therapy may be needed.

DIET
Warm fluids to start with, as tolerated thereafter.

NOTIFY OUR OFFICE IF

You or a family member has symptoms of frostbite or cold injury, or you observe them in someone else.

Special notes:

_____

_____

_____

More notes on the back of this page ☐

190

GALLSTONES

(Cholelithiasis)

 BASIC INFORMATION

DESCRIPTION

Stones in the gallbladder. The gallbladder is an organ in the body that stores bile. Gallstones can affect young people and adults, and are more common in women.

FREQUENT SIGNS AND SYMPTOMS

· No symptoms in about 40% of cases.
· Sharp pain in the upper-right stomach area or between the shoulder blades.
· Nausea and vomiting.
· Bloating or belching.
· Fatty foods cause indigestion.
· Jaundice, which causes yellow skin and eyes.

CAUSES

Bile is a liquid made by the liver and stored in the gallbladder. Its use in the body is to help with digestion. Gallstones form when substances in the bile liquid harden. This may be due to too much cholesterol or bilirubin, or not enough bile salts, or the gallbladder not emptying as it should. Stones may be small like a grain of sand or as large as a golf ball. There may be one or hundreds of tiny stones.

RISK INCREASES WITH

· People over age 60.
· Women get gallstones twice as often as men.
· Disorders such as cirrhosis of the liver, blood disorders, Crohn's disease, cystic fibrosis, sickle-cell anemia, or biliary tract infection.
· Stomach reduction surgery.
· Genetic factors. Some ethnic groups are more likely to have gallstones.
· Overweight.
· Diabetes.
· Too much estrogen in the body. It may be from pregnancy, birth control pills, or hormone replacement.
· Rapid weight loss or fasting.
· Drugs that lower cholesterol can actually increase the cholesterol in the bile, which can lead to gallstones.

PREVENTIVE MEASURES

There are no specific preventive measures.

EXPECTED OUTCOMES

Gallstones that cause no symptoms can safely be left alone. They are unlikely to cause problems. For those who do have symptoms, treatment is available.

POSSIBLE COMPLICATIONS

· A stone becomes lodged in a duct. Ducts are tubes that carry bile to and from the gallbladder. A lodged stone can cause serious problems with the gallbladder, pancreas, or liver.
· Gallstones may recur if treatment does not include removing the gallbladder.

 DIAGNOSIS & TREATMENT

GENERAL MEASURES

· Your health care provider will do a physical exam and ask questions about your symptoms. Medical tests may include blood tests and an ultrasound, which can detect the stones by sound waves. Other tests may be done to confirm the diagnosis or check for complications.
· There are several ways to treat gallstones that are causing symptoms. They include surgery, shockwave treatment, drugs, and sometimes diet changes.
· Some people try diet changes and drugs to help symptoms. This may work for a while, but not permanently.
· Surgery to remove the gallbladder. For most people, this will relieve the symptoms. Surgery options include:
 - Laparoscopic procedure. This procedure uses tiny incisions through the skin and a special instrument to remove the gallbladder.
 - Open surgery. A more serious procedure that requires a longer incision to remove the gallbladder.
· Shockwave (lithotripsy) treatment to break up (shatter) the stones may be an option for some patients.
· To learn more: National Digestive Diseases Information Clearinghouse, 2 Information Way, Bethesda, MD 20892; (800) 891-5389; website: www.digestive.niddk.nih.gov.

MEDICATIONS

Drugs can be taken by mouth to dissolve stones. This treatment is used for certain types of stones and can require up to 2 years to be effective.

ACTIVITY

You will be advised of limits depending on the type of treatment. Get extra rest while you recover.

DIET

No special diet unless advised differently by your health care provider.

 NOTIFY OUR OFFICE IF

· You or a family member has symptoms of gallstones.
· Fever rises to 101°F (38.3°C).
· Pain occurs that lasts for more than 3 hours.

Special notes:

_____

_____

_____

More notes on the back of this page ☐

GANGRENE

 ## BASIC INFORMATION

DESCRIPTION

Gangrene is dead tissue. It forms when a wound becomes infected or tissue is destroyed by an accident. It can happen to any body part, including internal organs. The most common areas are toes, feet, legs, fingers, hands, and arms. The most dangerous areas are stomach organs.

FREQUENT SIGNS AND SYMPTOMS

• Skin may be pale at first, then turn red or bronze, and finally, a purple or blue-black color.
• Crackling of the skin. This feels like pressing on air bubbles under the skin.
• Swelling of the skin tissue.
• Pain or loss of sensation in affected area.
• Bad-smelling discharge from the dead tissues.
• Fever, sweating, and fast heartbeat.

CAUSES

Gangrene occurs when blood flow to a section of the body is blocked or reduced. There are two types. Dry gangrene is when there is no infection and is often caused by a blood clot or frostbite. Wet (gas) gangrene occurs when a wound becomes infected with bacteria.

RISK INCREASES WITH

• Infection with bacteria.
• Body injury caused by accidents, surgery, or deep puncture wounds.
• Crush injury that cuts off blood supply.
• Blood clot in an artery.
• Hardening of the arteries.
• Prolonged frostbite.
• Diabetes.
• Smoking.
• Excess alcohol use.
• Poor blood circulation.
• Old age.

PREVENTIVE MEASURES

• Avoid any risk factors where possible.
• If you have diabetes, stick closely to your program to control diabetes. Check your feet often for signs of unhealthy tissue.
• Seek medical advice for signs of infection (warmth, swelling, redness, pain, or tenderness) in a skin injury.

EXPECTED OUTCOMES

Can be cured in the early stages with drugs and treatment to remove dead tissue.

POSSIBLE COMPLICATIONS

• Liver damage, kidney failure, shock, and coma.
• Limb removal (amputation).
• Gangrene can be fatal, even with treatment.

 ## DIAGNOSIS & TREATMENT

GENERAL MEASURES

• Hospital care is needed for treatment. Your health care provider will do an exam of the affected area. Medical tests will be done to determine the extent of the problem. These may include blood studies and a culture of the fluid from the wound. Imaging tests such as x-ray, CT, or MRI may help with diagnosis.
• Treatment for gangrene will involve drugs and surgery to remove dead tissue. Removal of the dead tissue may need to be repeated over several days.
• Treatment will be given for any medical problem that is causing the gangrene, and to help restore blood flow to the affected area.
• You may need oxygen supplied through a mask or into the nose to help you breathe.
• You may be placed in a sealed chamber (hyperbaric) where high-pressure oxygen is used for treatment.
• Amputation of an infected body part may be needed to keep the infection from spreading. This often involves part of an arm or leg. Instructions will be provided for ongoing home care and physical therapy following surgery.

MEDICATIONS

In the hospital, you will be given antibiotics, pain relievers, and usually blood thinners to prevent blood clotting. Additional drugs may be needed to treat other disorders diagnosed.

ACTIVITY

• Rest in bed until healing begins. Your health care provider will advise you of any limits to your activities.
• Physical therapy may be needed after an amputation.

DIET

Eat a high-protein, high-calorie diet while your body is repairing damaged tissue. Take vitamin and mineral supplements. Drink fluids (6 to 8 glasses daily).

 ## NOTIFY OUR OFFICE IF

• You or a family member has symptoms of gangrene.
• Pain continues, despite drugs and treatment.
• Fever or infection develops during recovery.

Special notes:

_____

_____

_____

More notes on the back of this page ☐

192

GASTRIC EROSION

 ## BASIC INFORMATION

DESCRIPTION

A sore or raw area on the inner lining (mucosa) of the stomach. Gastric erosions can affect all ages. They are more common in men than in women.

FREQUENT SIGNS AND SYMPTOMS

· Vomiting blood. Blood may be bright red or look like black coffee grounds.
· Blood in the stool. Blood will appear black or "tarry."
· Often there are no symptoms. A person may be unaware of the bleeding.

CAUSES

The stomach's lining is delicate and can easily be damaged by too much stomach acid or other irritants. The damage can result in erosions or ulcers that may cause bleeding. Erosions can be shallow or deep and are often in the shape of a circle.

RISK INCREASES WITH

· Drugs that irritate the stomach lining. These include aspirin and other nonsteroidal anti-inflammatory drugs.
· Tobacco use. It increases stomach acid.
· Excess alcohol intake. It irritates the stomach lining.
· Bacteria infection.
· Physical stress such as from burns or surgery.
· Rarely, in children, a swallowed coin that contains zinc can cause erosion.
· Emotional stress was once considered the main risk factor. Medical experts are now unsure of its role and research is ongoing.
· No specific food (or diet) has been identified as a risk factor. A person should avoid any foods that cause an upset stomach.

PREVENTIVE MEASURES

· If possible, take pills that have a protective coating.
· Don't smoke or drink alcohol.

EXPECTED OUTCOMES

Usually curable in 2 weeks.

POSSIBLE COMPLICATIONS

· Perforation, in which the erosion opens a hole through the stomach wall. Surgery is sometimes needed to correct the problem.
· Anemia due to blood loss.

 ## DIAGNOSIS & TREATMENT

GENERAL MEASURES

· Your health care provider will do a physical exam and ask questions about your symptoms. Medical tests may include studies of the stool and blood, and x-rays of the stomach.
· Treatment usually involves taking drugs to reduce stomach acid. This helps relieve symptoms and promote healing.
· Your health care provider may have you check your stool daily for any signs of bleeding. You will be given instructions on how to do this.
· Stop smoking. Your health care provider can help with suggestions for a cease smoking program.

MEDICATIONS

· Drugs to reduce stomach acid may be recommended. These may be prescription drugs or others that are non-prescription.
· An antibiotic may be prescribed for bacteria infection.
· If a drug you are currently taking is a cause of erosion, a change in dosage or a different drug may be prescribed.
· For minor pain, you may use acetaminophen.

ACTIVITY

Resume normal activities as soon as symptoms improve.

DIET

Eat small, frequent meals for 1 to 2 weeks. No specific foods need to be avoided. Don't drink alcohol.

 ## NOTIFY OUR OFFICE IF

· You or a family member has signs of bleeding described in Frequent Signs and Symptoms.
· You develop diarrhea. This may represent a reaction to drugs used in treatment.
· You have severe pain that is not helped by treatment.
· You are unusually weak, pale, or lightheaded.
· Symptoms of gastric erosion recur after treatment.

Special notes:

_____

_____

_____

More notes on the back of this page ☐

GASTRITIS

 BASIC INFORMATION

DESCRIPTION
Inflammation of the stomach lining. Inflammation causes pain, swelling, redness, and heat. Gastritis may start as a sudden attack, or develop slowly over a period of time.

FREQUENT SIGNS AND SYMPTOMS
- Stomach pain and cramps.
- Black stool or bloody vomit due to stomach bleeding.
- Appetite loss.
- Fever.
- Weakness.
- Swollen stomach.
- Sharp, dull, or annoying pain in the chest.
- Acid taste in the mouth.
- Mild nausea and diarrhea (rare).
- Belching or gas.

CAUSES
The inflammation is a reaction to injury, infection, or irritation of the stomach lining. It can be brought on by a number of different factors. Sometimes the cause is unknown.

RISK INCREASES WITH
- Drinking too much alcohol.
- Use of nonsteroidal anti-inflammatory drugs such as aspirin or ibuprofen.
- Illness that has weakened the body.
- Surgery and being in the hospital for other problems.
- Serious injury or severe burns.
- Smoking.
- The presence of a bacteria in the stomach.
- Pernicious anemia, immune problems, and chronic bile reflux.

PREVENTIVE MEASURES
- Eat and drink moderately.
- Don't skip meals or eat irregularly.
- Avoid foods you find hard to digest.
- Don't smoke.
- Avoid drugs that irritate your stomach, if possible.

EXPECTED OUTCOMES
Usually can be cured in several days with treatment, and if the cause is taken away.

POSSIBLE COMPLICATIONS
Bleeding is an uncommon but dangerous complication, especially in the elderly.

 DIAGNOSIS & TREATMENT

GENERAL MEASURES
- Your health care provider will do a physical exam and ask questions about your symptoms. Diagnosis is made by examining the stomach through a tube passed down the throat to the stomach. A small amount of tissue may be taken for a test. Blood and stool tests may be done.
- Goals of treatment are to relieve the symptoms and get rid of the gastric irritant or other cause.
- Smoking and alcohol drinking should be stopped. Your health care provider can help you find the plan that will work for you.
- A hospital stay may be necessary if extreme bleeding occurs.

MEDICATIONS
- Drugs are usually prescribed to reduce stomach acid. Acid irritates the stomach lining.
- Take acetaminophen for minor pain. Don't use aspirin.
- Other drugs, such as antibiotics for infection, may be prescribed.
- A drug you take may be causing the problem. Your health care provider may stop the drug, change the dose, or prescribe a new drug.

ACTIVITY
Resume normal activities as soon as symptoms improve.

DIET
Don't eat solid food on the first day of the attack. Drink liquids often, preferably milk or water. Resume a normal diet slowly. Avoid hot and spicy foods, alcohol, coffee, and acidic foods until symptoms are gone.

 NOTIFY OUR OFFICE IF

- You or a family member has symptoms of gastritis.
- You vomit blood.
- Bowel movements become black or tarry.
- Pain becomes severe.
- Signs of dehydration, such as a dry mouth, wrinkled skin, excess thirst, or decreased urination, develop.

Special notes:

_____

_____

_____

More notes on the back of this page ☐

194

GASTROENTERITIS
(Stomach Flu)

BASIC INFORMATION

DESCRIPTION
Irritation and inflammation of the stomach and intestines. Gastroenteritis is a general term and is often used when there is a nonspecific, uncertain, or unknown cause. The disorder can affect all ages, but is most severe in young children (1 to 5 years). Adults usually have mild cases, sometimes with no symptoms.

FREQUENT SIGNS AND SYMPTOMS
· Diarrhea is the main symptom, and sometimes, the only one. Diarrhea may range from 2 or 3 loose stools to many watery stools.
· Nausea and vomiting.
· Stomach cramps, pain, or tenderness.
· Fever or chills.
· Appetite loss.
· Weakness.
· Dehydration.

CAUSES
· Viral infections are the most common cause. They are spread by contact with an infected person or by touching an object that has germs on it. Contaminated food or water is another source for infection.
· Other causes are bacterial or parasitic infections, food-borne toxins, shellfish and marine animal poisoning, food intolerance, drug-caused diarrhea, and colitis.

RISK INCREASES WITH
· Children in daycare centers.
· Crowded living or working conditions.
· Older adults in nursing homes.
· Schools, dormitories, camps, or cruise ships
· Weak immune system due to illness or drugs.
· Use of drugs, such as antibiotics, laxatives, or antacids.
· Contaminated food or water.
· Travel to foreign countries.

PREVENTIVE MEASURES
· No specific preventive measures.
· Wash hands often to prevent spread of any germs.
· Don't share eating utensils or towels.
· Use safety precautions in storing and cooking foods.
· When traveling in foreign countries, take care to eat food and drink water that is known to be safe.
· Vaccines against some viruses are being studied.

EXPECTED OUTCOMES
The prognosis is excellent. Diarrhea and other symptoms usually clear up in 2 to 5 days. Adults may feel somewhat weak and fatigued for about a week.

POSSIBLE COMPLICATIONS
Serious dehydration that requires special treatment. Other complications are rare.

DIAGNOSIS & TREATMENT

GENERAL MEASURES
· In most cases, this disorder will be self-treated at home. Call your health care provider if symptoms are severe or if they cause you any concern.
· Your health care provider may do a physical exam. Medical tests may include studies of blood and stool.
· Treatment usually involves rest and fluids. There is no specific drug for viral infections.
· It is not necessary to keep persons with gastroenteritis away from others in the family or household. Try to avoid close contact if possible.
· Hospital care may be needed, if dehydration is severe.

MEDICATIONS
· Drugs are usually not needed for treatment. If symptoms are severe or prolonged, you may take antinausea and antidiarrhea drugs such as Pepto-Bismol or loperamide.
· Some infections may require specific drug treatment.
· If a drug you take is the cause of the problem, you may be advised to change drugs or stop taking the drug.

ACTIVITY
Get extra rest until diarrhea, nausea, vomiting, and fever are improved. Be sure to have access to a toilet or bedpan.

DIET
· Suck ice chips or drink small amounts of clear fluids often. Replace lost fluids and electrolytes with products such as Pedialyte or Ricelyte for infants and children, and diluted rehydration fluids (Gatorade) for adults.
· Once the symptoms improve, try a diet of complex carbohydrates (rice, wheat, potatoes, bread, cereal, and lean meat such as chicken). Milk and dairy products usually do not need to be limited.
· Avoid high-sugar foods or fatty foods for a few days.

NOTIFY OUR OFFICE IF

· Symptoms of gastroenteritis last longer than 2 days.
· Symptoms continue or worsen after treatment.
· Blood or mucus appears in the stool.

Special notes:

_____

_____

_____

More notes on the back of this page ☐

GASTROESOPHAGEAL REFLUX DISEASE (GERD)

 BASIC INFORMATION

DESCRIPTION

A condition that occurs when acids from the stomach move backward (reflux) into the esophagus (the food pipe that carries food from the mouth to the stomach).

FREQUENT SIGNS AND SYMPTOMS

· Persistent heartburn (stomach acid touches the lining of the esophagus and causes a burning sensation in the chest). You can have GERD without having heartburn.
· Regurgitation (acid can be tasted in the back of the mouth).
· Hoarseness in the morning.
· Difficulty swallowing.
· Feels like you have food stuck in your throat, like you are choking, or your throat is tight.
· Dry cough and bad breath.
· Excessive clearing of the throat.
· Burning in the mouth.
· Infants and children may have repeated vomiting, coughing, and other respiratory (lung) problems. Most babies grow out of GERD by their first birthday.

CAUSES

The problem occurs when the lower esophageal sphincter (LES) does not close properly. This allows stomach contents to leak back, or reflux, into the esophagus. The LES is a ring of muscle at the bottom of the esophagus. It acts like a valve between the esophagus and stomach. It is unknown why people get GERD.

RISK INCREASES WITH

· Hiatal hernia may contribute. It occurs when part of the stomach protrudes into the diaphragm (the muscle wall that separates the stomach from the chest).
· Alcohol use.
· Overweight.
· Pregnancy.
· Smoking.
· Certain foods can trigger symptoms (chocolate, caffeine, fatty and fried foods, garlic, onions, mint, spicy foods, spaghetti, chili, pizza, and citrus fruits).

PREVENTIVE MEASURES

Follow steps listed in treatment section.

EXPECTED OUTCOMES

Symptoms can be improved with treatment. GERD may come and go for weeks or months, or it may persist.

POSSIBLE COMPLICATIONS

· Inflammation of the esophagus (esophagitis).
· Ulcers.
· Scars from tissue damage narrow the esophagus.
· Barrett's esophagus (disorder that can lead to cancer).
· Erosion or weakening of the teeth.
· Asthma, chronic cough, and pulmonary fibrosis may be aggravated or even caused by GERD.

 DIAGNOSIS & TREATMENT

GENERAL MEASURES

· Your health care provider will do a physical exam and ask questions about your symptoms, diet, and activities. Medical tests may be done at this time or after simple treatment measures are tried.
· Treatment will depend on how severe your GERD is. It may involve lifestyle changes, drugs, further medical testing, or surgery.
· Lifestyle changes:
  - If you smoke, stop. Find a plan that works for you.
  - Make changes in your diet.
  - Wear loose-fitting clothes.
  - Avoid lying down for 3 hours after a meal.
  - Raise the head of your bed 6 to 8 inches by putting blocks of wood under the bedposts.
· If lifestyle changes and drugs don't help, one or more medical tests may be done to check for other problems:
  - Barium swallow (a type of x-ray).
  - Endoscopy. A thin, flexible plastic tube with a tiny camera is used to see inside the esophagus.
  - A device may be inserted into the esophagus that measures acid reflux. The device remains for 24 or 48 hours while you go about your regular activities.
· Surgery is a treatment option when drugs and lifestyle changes do not work. Surgery may also be a reasonable alternative to a lifetime of drugs and discomfort.

MEDICATIONS

Nonprescription antacids, or drugs that stop acid production or help the muscles that empty your stomach may be prescribed. Combinations of these drugs may help control symptoms. Your health care provider will help you decide which ones will work best for you.

ACTIVITY

No limits.

DIET

Do not drink alcohol. Lose weight, if needed. Eat small meals. Avoid the foods that trigger symptoms.

 NOTIFY OUR OFFICE IF

· You or a family member has symptoms of GERD.
· Symptoms continue despite treatment.

Special notes:

_____

_____

_____

More notes on the back of this page ☐

196

GESTATIONAL DIABETES

(GDM; Gestational Carbohydrate Intolerance)

BASIC INFORMATION

DESCRIPTION
A type of diabetes that occurs only in pregnant women. Gestational diabetes mellitus (GDM) affects 2% to 5% of all pregnancies.

FREQUENT SIGNS AND SYMPTOMS
· Usually no symptoms are apparent. A prenatal exam may find that the fetus is larger than normal for the stage of pregnancy.
· Diagnosis is based on glucose testing done during the 24th to 28th week of pregnancy for nondiabetic mothers. Earlier testing is often done for patients diagnosed with GDM in a previous pregnancy, a birth weight over 9 pounds in a previous infant, or for other risk factors.

CAUSES
Your body isn't able to use the sugar (glucose) in your blood as well as it should, so the level of sugar in your blood becomes higher than normal.

RISK INCREASES WITH
· Previous pregnancy with GDM.
· Obesity (especially if excess fat is around the waist).
· Mother over age 30.
· Polycystic ovarian syndrome (PCOS).
· Family history of diabetes.
· Excess weight gain in pregnancy.
· Previous birth of an infant weighing over 9 pounds.
· Four or more previous pregnancies.
· History of an unexplained fetal death or stillbirth.
· Some population groups, such as Native Americans, Mexican-Americans, Asians, and East Indians.

PREVENTIVE MEASURES
There are no specific preventive measures. Weight loss in overweight women prior to pregnancy may help. Careful attention to diet and exercise in pregnant women with risk factors may help.

EXPECTED OUTCOME
· Successful treatment and a healthy baby often depend on the mother's motivation and ability to change her lifestyle. For some, dietary control is sufficient. Others may require drug therapy.
· In most cases, labor occurs naturally, and the birth is usually vaginal. Cesarean section may be required if the fetus is considered too large for vaginal birth.
· Gestational diabetes usually clears up with delivery.

POSSIBLE COMPLICATIONS
· Excess amniotic fluid (polyhydramnios).
· Premature labor.
· May need to have labor induced.
· Preeclampsia.
· Miscarriage (rare).
· Risk for mother of diabetes in the future.

DIAGNOSIS & TREATMENT

GENERAL MEASURES
· Your obstetric provider will do a glucose test.
· Treatment will include diet changes, moderate exercise program, and drug therapy, if needed.
· You will learn how to monitor your glucose levels. At first, glucose checks may need to be done up to 4-6 times daily. Once glucose levels are in the desired range and diet changes are made, glucose checks may be reduced with your obstetric provider's approval.
· To learn more: Contact the local or national office of the American Diabetes Association, Attention: National Call Center, 1701 Beauregard St., Alexandria, VA 22311; (800) 342-2383; website: www.diabetes.org.

MEDICATION
· Drugs are usually not needed if glucose control is achieved with diet and exercise.
· Insulin injections or oral antidiabetic drugs may be prescribed for some patients.

ACTIVITY
A program of moderate, non–weight-bearing exercise is usually recommended. Exercising for even small time periods can have major benefits. Follow any prescribed exercise program carefully.

DIET
· Diet changes are an important part of the treatment. Specific diet instructions will be provided. Following this diet will decrease the risks to the mother and her unborn child.
· The diet changes will involve increased fiber intake, fat limits, avoiding sweets, and monitoring caloric intake to prevent excess weight gain.

NOTIFY OUR OFFICE IF

· You are 24 to 28 weeks pregnant and have not had a screening test for gestational diabetes.
· After diagnosis, you develop any new signs or symptoms that cause you concern.

Special notes:

_____

_____

_____

More notes on the back of this page ☐

GIARDIASIS

 BASIC INFORMATION

DESCRIPTION
An intestinal infection caused by a parasite. Giardiasis is a frequent cause of diarrhea. It may occur in clusters or outbreaks, affecting many persons at a time. It can affect any age, but is more common in young children.

FREQUENT SIGNS AND SYMPTOMS
- Often, there are no symptoms.
- Symptoms can be mild and recurrent, persisting for months, or longer.
- Sudden diarrhea and stomach cramping. Some persons have only mild diarrhea and upset stomach.
- Stools may have a foul smell and be greasy.
- Nausea and vomiting.
- Slight fever (rare).

CAUSES
A parasite, *Giardia lamblia*. The germs may be spread in food or water contaminated by feces from infected animals or humans. Germs can be spread from one person to another due to poor hygiene. Symptoms begin in 1 to 3 weeks after being infected.

RISK INCREASES WITH
- Drinking from a water supply that is contaminated.
- Drinking unsafe water while camping or hiking.
- Swimmers who swallow contaminated water.
- Weak immune system due to illness or drugs.
- Children or workers at preschool or daycare center.
- Foreign travel.
- Oral or anal sex.

PREVENTIVE MEASURES
- Don't drink unsafe water. Boil or treat it first.
- Avoid uncooked foods that may have been rinsed in contaminated water.
- Wash hands often to prevent spread of any germs.
- Keep children with diarrhea away from others.
- To avoid spreading the germs, don't swim if you have diarrhea.
- When traveling in foreign countries, take care to eat food and drink water that is known to be safe.

EXPECTED OUTCOMES
Complete recovery is expected within 1 to 2 weeks with treatment. Symptoms may go away even without treatment, but a person can carry the germs for weeks or months.

POSSIBLE COMPLICATIONS
- Dehydration.
- Chronic giardiasis.
- Malabsorption (unable to absorb nutrients from food) and weight loss.

 DIAGNOSIS & TREATMENT

GENERAL MEASURES
- Your health care provider may do a physical exam. Questions will be asked about your symptoms and activities. Health providers are often aware if there is an outbreak of giardiasis in the community. Medical tests may include stool studies to detect the parasites.
- Giardiasis responds well to drugs. Treatment is usually done at home. Drug treatment for family members who are infected, but have no symptoms, may be recommended. Pregnant women may require special treatment.
- Hospital care to replace lost fluids may be required for patients with severe diarrhea and dehydration.
- Prevention is the best treatment. Be cautious when away from normal drinking-water supplies.
- Practice careful personal hygiene if you, or others around you, have diarrhea.

MEDICATIONS
Antiparasitic drugs such as metronidazole (Flagyl) and others may be prescribed. Alcohol interacts with metronidazole to cause stomach cramps and nausea, so don't drink alcohol during this treatment.

ACTIVITY
No limits.

DIET
- Maintain an adequate fluid intake (at least 8 glasses of water or liquid a day).
- Some persons develop lactose intolerance. A lactose-free diet may be recommended.

 NOTIFY OUR OFFICE IF

- You or a family member has symptoms of giardiasis.
- New, unexplained symptoms develop. Drugs used in treatment may produce side effects.

Special notes:

_____

_____

_____

More notes on the back of this page ☐

GILBERT SYNDROME

 BASIC INFORMATION

DESCRIPTION

A disorder that causes increased blood levels of bilirubin. Bilirubin is a yellow chemical that results from red-blood-cell breakdown. Gilbert syndrome is usually a chance finding of routine testing. It affects both sexes, but is most common in men. It is present from birth, but symptoms may not appear until ages 20 to 40.

FREQUENT SIGNS AND SYMPTOMS

• Usually there are no symptoms.
• Mild jaundice (yellow skin and eyes) may occur in some patients. It may come and go.
• Some patients have symptoms that are nonspecific. These include stomach cramps, tiredness, and general ill feeling. They may be related to anxiety in some cases.

CAUSES

A dysfunction of the liver in processing bile. This leaves above-normal levels of bilirubin in the blood. If blood levels are high enough, jaundice may appear.

RISK INCREASES WITH

The signs of jaundice may be brought on by dehydration, fasting, illness, menstrual periods, and stress (trauma or overexertion).

PREVENTIVE MEASURES

No specific measures to prevent Gilbert syndrome.

EXPECTED OUTCOMES

The condition is harmless.

POSSIBLE COMPLICATIONS

No known complications.

 DIAGNOSIS & TREATMENT

GENERAL MEASURES

• Your health care provider will usually do a physical exam. Blood tests of bilirubin and liver function will be done to help confirm the diagnosis.
• No treatment is necessary. Your health care provider will explain that the syndrome is benign and will not cause health problems or affect lifestyle.

MEDICATIONS

Drugs are not necessary for this disorder.

ACTIVITY

No limits.

DIET

No special diet.

 NOTIFY OUR OFFICE IF

You or a family member has symptoms of Gilbert syndrome. This usually involves skin that looks a bit yellow.

Special notes:

_____

_____

_____

More notes on the back of this page ☐

GINGIVITIS

 BASIC INFORMATION

DESCRIPTION
Inflammation (redness, soreness, swelling) or infection of the gums. This is a mild form of gum disease, but it can lead to more serious problems.

FREQUENT SIGNS AND SYMPTOMS
· Gums that have become swollen, tender, red, and soft around the teeth. Gums may bleed easily.
· Bad breath.
· No pain.
· Fever (rarely).

CAUSES
Plaque. It is a sticky substance made up of food particles, germs, and mucus that builds up on the teeth.

RISK INCREASES WITH
· Poor dental hygiene, other tooth problems, and mouth infections.
· Poor nutrition. This can include eating too much sugar or vitamin deficiencies.
· Adverse reactions to drugs, such as phenytoin and barbiturates.
· People with diabetes, gastroesophageal reflux disease (GERD), or osteoporosis.
· Disorders that affect the immune system such as arthritis, lupus, and AIDS.
· Smoking.
· Pregnancy.
· Female hormones can affect the gums.

PREVENTIVE MEASURES
· Practice good oral hygiene to prevent plaque formation.
· Brush teeth and your tongue twice a day. Brush your teeth properly. A soft brush is less likely to damage teeth and gums than a hard brush. Scrub clear, sticky plaque off the teeth daily with a soft toothbrush. Place the brush at the gum line and gently rotate it, pointing bristles toward the gum. Brush one section of teeth at a time.
· Floss your teeth at least once a day. Use waxed or unwaxed dental floss. Wind most of it around the middle finger of each hand. Use index fingers as guides to force the floss between the teeth gently. Gently clean adjacent tooth surfaces with a back-and-forth, sawing motion at the gum line. Floss between all lower teeth. Loosen floss and place it on the tops of the thumbs. Floss between all upper teeth, using thumbs as guides.
· Make regular appointments with your dental health care provider for cleaning and treatment of cavities.
· Have regular dental checkups twice a year.
· Eat a well-balanced diet. Take vitamin supplements if you are unable to eat well-balanced meals.
· Quit smoking. Find a plan that will work for you.

EXPECTED OUTCOMES
With treatment and preventive steps, outlook is good.

POSSIBLE COMPLICATIONS
Without treatment, gingivitis can lead to more serious gum disease, infections, and tooth loss.

 DIAGNOSIS & TREATMENT

GENERAL MEASURES
· Your dental health care provider can diagnose gingivitis with an exam of your teeth and gums. A special tool is used to check the depth of pockets in the gums. X-rays of the teeth help reveal any bone loss.
· Treatment usually includes cleaning the teeth by a dental hygienist or other dental health care provider. There are different techniques depending on the degree of plaque build-up.
· Other dental work may be needed. Teeth may need straightening, cavities filled, or missing teeth replaced.
· Surgery may be needed to remove infected gum tissue, if other treatment fails.
· To learn more: American Dental Association, 211 E. Chicago Avenue, Chicago, IL 60611, (312) 440-2500(not toll free); website: www.ada.org.

MEDICATIONS
· Antibiotics may be prescribed to fight infection. They may be taken by mouth (orally) or applied to the gums with special devices.
· Fluoride mouthwash may be recommended.

ACTIVITY
No limits.

DIET
No special diet. Avoid candy, sweet drinks, or sweet snacks. Sugar stimulates the production of acid, which attacks normal teeth.

 NOTIFY OUR OFFICE IF

OR CALL YOUR DENTIST
· You or a family member has symptoms of gingivitis.
· The following occur after treatment:
  - Bleeding increases or there is more pain.
  - Fever of 101°F (38.3°C) or higher.
  - Neck or face is swollen, or it is hard to swallow.

Special notes:

_____

_____

_____

More notes on the back of this page ☐

GLAUCOMA, ANGLE-CLOSURE

BASIC INFORMATION

DESCRIPTION

Glaucoma is a progressive disease of the optic nerve that can lead to loss of vision. It is usually due to increased intraocular pressure (IOP), but it can be due to other causes. Angle-closure glaucoma is one of the two main types of glaucoma, and it is the less common type. Open-angle glaucoma is the more common type. The disease process, the treatment, and the prognosis are different for each type. Angle-closure glaucoma symptoms can occur suddenly (acute), or develop over time (chronic). It occurs more often in people over 55 and in women more than in men.

FREQUENT SIGNS AND SYMPTOMS

- Acute angle-closure glaucoma (symptoms are sudden, and often occur in a darkened room, such as a movie theater, or during periods of stress):
    - Severe, throbbing eye pain. Eye becomes red.
    - Blurred vision.
    - May see halos around lights.
    - Nausea, vomiting, and headache.
- Chronic angle-closure glaucoma (not acute):
    - There may be no symptoms.
    - Slightly blurred vision, mild eye pain, or seeing halos around lights. These symptoms may come and go.

CAUSES

Normal eye pressure is maintained by a balance of fluid (aqueous) that flows into the front of the eye and then drains out. The angle of the eye (where the iris and cornea meet) is where the drains (called trabecular meshwork) are located. With angle-closure glaucoma, the angle of the eye is not as wide (or open) as it should be. When the pupil dilates (gets larger), it pushes the iris forward and narrows the angle even more so that the drain is blocked or covered over. In acute cases, this happens suddenly. In chronic cases, it occurs over time. The blocked drain causes a buildup of fluid and pressure in the eye. The pressure can damage the optic nerve, sometimes within hours, and lead to vision loss.

RISK INCREASES WITH

- Adults over 55. Females more than males.
- Family history of glaucoma.
- Farsightedness.
- Asian or Eskimo descent.
- Use of certain drugs with cholinergic inhibition.

PREVENTIVE MEASURES

- Regular eye exams:
    - Under age 45, have an exam every 4 years if there are no risk factors and every 2 years with risk factors.
    - Over age 45, have an exam every 2 years if there are no risk factors and every year with risk factors.
- Get medical care for any changes in your vision.

EXPECTED OUTCOMES

Symptoms can usually be controlled with treatment.

POSSIBLE COMPLICATIONS

With acute glaucoma, blindness in the affected eye is possible, if treatment is delayed or unsuccessful.

DIAGNOSIS & TREATMENT

GENERAL MEASURES

- An acute attack is an emergency situation. In the hospital, drugs are given to constrict the pupil and to reduce the fluid production of the eye.
- A gonioscopy test may be done. This test is a way to view the trabecular meshwork in angle-closure glaucoma. (It is not visible in other types of eye tests.) The test involves placing a contact lens on the front of the eye. Topical anesthetic is used to prevent discomfort. The contact lens allows the person doing the exam to check the trabecular meshwork for signs of glaucoma.
- Surgery (iridectomy with a laser beam) to prevent further attacks is often performed. A small opening is made in the iris so that the aqueous humor (fluid in the eye) can drain. It is usually done in the other eye as a preventive measure.
- To learn more: Glaucoma Foundation, 116 John St, Suite 1605, New York, NY 10038; (800) 452-8266; website: www.glaucomafoundation.org.

MEDICATIONS

Eye drops may be prescribed to lower pressure inside the eye. Follow the instructions and schedule carefully.

ACTIVITY

No limits after treatment, unless advised otherwise.

DIET

No special diet.

NOTIFY OUR OFFICE IF

- You or a family member has symptoms of acute angle-closure glaucoma. This is an emergency!
- Other vision or eye problems develop.
- New, unexplained symptoms develop. Drugs used in treatment may produce side effects.

Special notes:

_____

_____

_____

More notes on the back of this page ☐

GLAUCOMA, OPEN-ANGLE

 BASIC INFORMATION

DESCRIPTION

Glaucoma is a progressive disease of the optic nerve that can lead to loss of vision. It is usually due to increased intraocular pressure (IOP), but it can be due to other causes. Open-angle glaucoma (or primary open-angle glaucoma [POAG]) is one of the two main types of glaucoma, and it is more common. The other type, angle-closure glaucoma, is less common. The disease process, the treatment, and the prognosis are different for each type. Open-angle glaucoma affects all ages, but it occurs more often in people over 40.

FREQUENT SIGNS AND SYMPTOMS

· Usually, there are no warning symptoms.
· Later stages of the disease include loss of peripheral vision in small areas, blurred vision, halos around lights, blind spots, and poor night vision.

CAUSES

· Normal eye pressure is maintained by a balance of fluid (aqueous) that flows into the front of the eye and then drains out. The angle of the eye (where the iris and cornea meet) is where the drains (called trabecular meshwork) are located. For unknown reasons, the drains become clogged. The fluid builds up over time and eye pressure increases. This causes damage to the optic nerve, which leads to vision loss.
· Restricted blood supply to the optic nerve is another cause. People with normal eye pressure and open-angle glaucoma have what is called normal-tension glaucoma.

RISK INCREASES WITH

· Glaucoma suspect (IOP without optic nerve damage).
· Adults over 45.
· Family history of glaucoma.
· Diabetes.
· Myopia (nearsightedness).
· Previous eye injury.
· Regular, long-term steroid use.
· African Americans (have a greater tendency).
· Low blood pressure.

PREVENTIVE MEASURES

· Regular eye exams:
  - Under age 45, have an exam every 4 years if there are no risk factors and every 2 years with risk factors.
  - Over age 45, have an exam every 2 years if there are no risk factors and every year with risk factors.
· Get medical care for any changes in your vision.

EXPECTED OUTCOMES

The disorder can usually be controlled with treatment to prevent further vision loss.

POSSIBLE COMPLICATIONS

Optic nerve damage that cannot be reversed. A permanent vision loss can occur.

 DIAGNOSIS & TREATMENT

GENERAL MEASURES

· An eye exam is usually done by an eye doctor (ophthalmologist). It includes a tonometry exam (measures pressure within the eyeball) and visual field test (to see how your vision is affected). An ophthalmoscope is used to see into the eye to view the optic nerve. A person has glaucoma if their eye exam shows changes to the optic nerve and blind spots.
· There is no cure. The goal is to protect the optic nerve from future damage and possible loss of vision. Treatment may include drug therapy, laser surgery, eye operations, or a combination of methods.
· Laser surgery can help improve the draining of the excess fluid. Other eye surgery may be done to open up the draining area and relieve pressure.
· To learn more: Glaucoma Foundation, 116 John St, Suite 1605, New York, NY 10038; (800) 452-8266; website: www.glaucomafoundation.org.

MEDICATIONS

One or more types of eye drops to lower pressure inside the eye will be prescribed. Follow the instructions and schedule carefully, even if symptoms improve. If eye drops do not control the pressure, oral drugs (taken by mouth) will usually be prescribed.

ACTIVITY

No limits.

DIET

No special diet.

 NOTIFY OUR OFFICE IF

· You or a family member has symptoms of chronic glaucoma.
· Any sign of eye infection develops.
· Pain begins in the eye.
· Redness occurs in the eye.
· Vision changes suddenly.

Special notes:

_____

_____

_____

More notes on the back of this page ☐

GLOMERULONEPHRITIS

 ## BASIC INFORMATION

DESCRIPTION
A group of disorders that cause inflammation of the glomeruli. These are filtering units in the kidneys that help filter out waste products and water and salt from the blood. Over time, the inflammation can lead to loss of kidney function. It is more common in children 5 to 15 years old, and occurs in males more than females.

FREQUENT SIGNS AND SYMPTOMS
- Mild inflammation produces no symptoms. Diagnosis is possible only with urine studies.
- Dark-colored urine (color of tea or a cola drink).
- Reduced urine.
- Urine may be bloody.
- Puffy eyelids.
- Swelling of the face, hands, feet, and stomach.
- Side pain.
- Weakness.
- Headache, fever, nausea, or vomiting.
- High blood pressure. It causes no symptoms, but may be measured with home blood pressure monitors.
- Shortness of breath.
- Loss of appetite.

CAUSES
- Postinfectious type (more common). This type develops after a *streptococcus* (often referred to as strep) infection. It may be a strep infection such as a sore throat or a skin infection.
- Other types (less common). These may be caused by other types of infections, whole body (systemic) diseases, IV drug abuse, kidney (renal) disease, and other medical problems. Sometimes the cause is unknown.

RISK INCREASES WITH
- Strep infection, such as scarlet fever.
- Persons diagnosed with any of the possible causes.

PREVENTIVE MEASURES
No specific preventive measures. Get treatment for any strep infection to help reduce risk.

EXPECTED OUTCOMES
- Outlook is excellent for most post-streptococcal cases in children. Mild cases may recover on their own. Some may be helped with treatment. Symptoms usually improve in 2 weeks to several months.
- In those cases caused by other medical problems, the outcome will vary depending on the underlying cause.

POSSIBLE COMPLICATIONS
- Kidney failure. It may lead to dialysis (use of a machine to filter body waste) and a kidney transplant.
- Chronic glomerulonephritis.
- Complications may occur in patients who have other health problems such as severe high blood pressure.

 ## DIAGNOSIS & TREATMENT

GENERAL MEASURES
- Your health care provider will do a physical exam and ask questions about your symptoms and recent illnesses. Medical tests may include blood, urine studies, and x-rays. A kidney biopsy may be done. This involves removal of a small amount of kidney tissue for viewing under a microscope.
- The goals of treatment are to relieve symptoms and to treat and prevent complications. Treatment may involve drugs, diet changes, and extra rest.
- Hospital care may be needed for severe symptoms.
- To learn more: National Kidney Foundation, 30 E. 33rd St., Suite 1100, New York, NY 10016; (800) 622-9010; website: www.kidney.org.

MEDICATIONS
- You may be prescribed:
  - Antibiotics for strep infection.
  - Drugs for high blood pressure.
  - Diuretics, to help remove excess fluid.
  - Steroids, to reduce inflammation.
  - Drugs, to suppress the immune system.
  - Drugs for other types of infection, or to treat an underlying disorder.

ACTIVITY
Stay in bed, except to go to the bathroom, until symptoms have improved. Bed rest ensures an adequate blood flow to the kidney. Blood flow is best when lying down. Resume normal activities gradually.

DIET
Diet changes may be recommended to help reduce the work of the kidneys. These may include eating less salt, potassium, and protein.

 ## NOTIFY OUR OFFICE IF

- You or a family member has symptoms of glomerulonephritis.
- Urine changes color or urine output is decreased.
- New symptoms occur during treatment.

Special notes:

_____

_____

_____

More notes on the back of this page ☐

GONORRHEA

BASIC INFORMATION

DESCRIPTION

An infection caused by a sexually transmitted disease (STD). In males, it usually involves the urethra (urine canal). In females, it usually involves the cervix and, sometimes, the urethra. In both sexes, the rectum, throat and other body parts may be involved. Gonorrhea can affect anyone (even young children) who has sexual contact with an infected person. It most often occurs in younger persons (ages 15 to 29), and in men more than in women.

FREQUENT SIGNS AND SYMPTOMS

· Symptoms usually begin 2 to 5 days, or up to 30 days after being exposed. Females have few or no symptoms. Males usually have symptoms.
· Burning sensation when urinating.
· White to yellow-green discharge from the urethra.
· Rectal discomfort and discharge (sometimes).
· Sore throat (mild).
· Females may have abdominal cramps.
· Conjunctivitis (eye inflammation). This occurs when the person touches infected genitals and then the eyes.
· If the infection spreads to other body parts: joint pain, low fever, rash, headache, neck pain, and stiffness.

CAUSES

Infection from *Neisseria gonorrhoeae*, a bacteria. It grows easily on delicate, moist tissue. The bacteria is transmitted sexually (vaginal, anal, or oral sex). It can be spread from mother to child during birth.

RISK INCREASES WITH

· Any sexually active persons.
· Having sex with an infected person.
· Multiple sexual partners, whether heterosexual or homosexual.
· Child sexual abuse.
· Passage of newborn through the infected birth canal of the mother.

PREVENTIVE MEASURES

· Abstain from sexual activity.
· Avoid sexual partners whose health practices and status are uncertain.
· Use a latex condom during sexual intercourse.

EXPECTED OUTCOMES

Usually curable in 1 to 2 weeks with treatment.

POSSIBLE COMPLICATIONS

· Persons who have no symptoms are at risk for complications and can unknowingly spread the infection.
· Spread from mother to child during birth. This can cause serious complications in the newborn.
· Blood poisoning (gonococcal septicemia).
· Infectious arthritis.

· Pelvic inflammatory disease in females (PID), which can lead to infertility.
· Heart inflammation or infection around the liver.
· Epididymitis (which can lead to infertility), prostate problems, and urethral scarring in males.
· Risk of getting HIV is higher.

DIAGNOSIS & TREATMENT

GENERAL MEASURES

· Your health care provider will do a physical exam and a pelvic exam. Medical tests may include blood and urine studies and studies of the discharge from the vagina, urethra, rectum, throat, or eyes. Tests for other sexually transmitted diseases are usually done. Other tests may be done if complications are suspected.
· Treatment is with antibiotic drugs. Follow-up tests may be done to confirm a cure. If the eyes are involved, an eye doctor (ophthalmologist) should be consulted. Hospital care may be needed for severe symptoms.
· Inform all sexual contacts so they can seek treatment.
· For self-care:
 - Use separate towels, washcloths, and disposable eating utensils during treatment.
 - Wash hands often, especially after using the bathroom.
 - Don't touch your eyes with your hands.
· To learn more: Centers for Disease Control & Prevention (CDC) National STD Hotline (800) 227-8922; website: www.cdc.gov/std.

MEDICATIONS

· Antibiotics will be prescribed. Take complete dosage.
· You may take nonprescription drugs, such as acetaminophen or aspirin (for adults), to reduce discomfort.

ACTIVITY

No limits on physical activity. Don't resume sexual activity until treatment is complete.

DIET

No special diet.

NOTIFY OUR OFFICE IF

· You or a family member has symptoms of gonorrhea.
· Symptoms don't improve with treatment.

Special notes:

_____

_____

_____

More notes on the back of this page ☐

GOUT

BASIC INFORMATION

DESCRIPTION
Recurrent attacks of joint inflammation, especially the base of the big toe. Gout may also involve the foot, ankle, knee, elbow, hand, arm, or shoulder. It affects adults of both sexes but is more common in men than women, until after menopause.

FREQUENT SIGNS AND SYMPTOMS
• Sudden onset of severe pain (usually at night) in the inflamed joint. This is often at the base of the big toe.
• Involved joints may be hot, swollen, and very tender. Skin over the joint is red and shiny.
• Fever, chills, or fatigue (sometimes).

CAUSES
A high level of uric acid in the blood. This may be due to increased production of uric acid or decreased elimination of uric acid by the kidneys.

RISK INCREASES WITH
• Men over 60.
• Family history of gout.
• Obesity.
• Excess alcohol use.
• Thyroid disorders.
• Use of certain drugs, such as diuretic drugs (water pills), high blood pressure drugs, aspirin, drugs that treat gout, and others.
• High blood pressure.
• Starvation or dehydration.
• Eating large amounts foods that contain purines. These include anchovies, sardines, sweetbreads, kidney, liver, tongue, and large amounts of red meat, shellfish, peas, lentils, and beans.

PREVENTIVE MEASURES
Avoid risk factors, where possible.

EXPECTED OUTCOMES
The first attack may last a few days. Recurrent attacks are common unless the uric acid level in the blood is reduced. Symptoms can be relieved with treatment.

POSSIBLE COMPLICATIONS
• Crippled, deformed joints.
• Kidney stones.
• Continued gout attacks (if untreated).

DIAGNOSIS & TREATMENT

GENERAL MEASURES
• Your health care provider will do an exam of the joints. Medical tests may include blood and urine levels of uric acid and studies of fluid removed from the joint. An x-ray or a bone scan may be done.

• Goals of treatment are to control the symptoms, prevent a recurrence, and to lower uric acid levels. Treatment usually involves drug therapy, lifestyle changes, and rarely, surgery.
• Lifestyle changes may include diet changes and weight loss (if overweight).
• Surgery is rare, but may be recommended if the disorder was untreated or treated late.
• For home care: Use warm or cold compresses on painful joints. Keep the weight of bedclothes off any painful joint by making a frame that raises sheets off the feet.

MEDICATIONS
• Nonsteroidal anti-inflammatory drugs to control inflammation and pain are usually prescribed.
• Other drugs for an attack of gout may be prescribed.
• Lifelong treatment with drugs to decrease uric acid production or to increase the kidneys' excretion of uric acid may be needed. These drugs have side effects and adverse reactions. Obtain as much information as possible regarding their use.

ACTIVITY
• During an attack, rest and elevate the foot. Take care to avoid joint injury. Wear shoes that fit properly.
• When able, exercise daily.

DIET
• Limit foods that contain purines (see Risk Factors). Note: all protein foods contain purine, so no one should avoid all purines.
• Drink plenty of water and other liquids daily. Fluids keeps the urine diluted, which helps prevent kidney stones.
• Don't drink alcoholic beverages, especially beer or red wine. They can worsen or trigger an attack.
• If you are overweight, begin a medically approved weight-loss diet. Do not go on a crash diet, as rapid weight loss may bring on a gout attack.

NOTIFY OUR OFFICE IF

• You or a family member has symptoms of gout.
• Pain gets worse, or fever and chills occur.
• New, unexplained symptoms develop. They may indicate an adverse reaction of drugs, or interactions between drugs.

Special notes:

_____

_____

_____

More notes on the back of this page ☐

GRANULOMA ANNULARE

 BASIC INFORMATION

DESCRIPTION
A common benign skin disorder. It can involve the skin on the bottoms of feet and backs of fingers, hands, arms, elbows, legs, and knees. It can affect all ages but is common in children and young adults. Females are more often affected than males.

FREQUENT SIGNS AND SYMPTOMS
· Small, raised bumps (called papules) on the skin.
· Bumps have a domed or slightly flat shape. Their color may vary on different people. Bumps may be skin-colored, reddish, bluish, or yellowish.
· They don't hurt, and usually don't itch.
· The bumps cluster in a ring. Bumps around the ring border are close, but don't grow completely together. This gives the border a beaded appearance. The ring's center is often darker than the edge.
· The appearance may change in size and shape over a few weeks to 6 months.
· The area affected may be small (localized) or wide-spread (generalized) over the body.

CAUSES
Unknown.

RISK INCREASES WITH
· Diabetes.
· Damage to the skin such as from injury, sunburn, or insect bite.

PREVENTIVE MEASURES
No specific preventive measures. Avoid injury to the skin. Protect skin from sunburn with sunscreen or clothing.

EXPECTED OUTCOMES
The disorder will heal on its own, but it usually takes months to years. The disorder may also recur with no apparent cause or timing.

POSSIBLE COMPLICATIONS
No complications are expected.

 DIAGNOSIS & TREATMENT

GENERAL MEASURES
· Your health care provider can diagnose the disorder by an exam of the affected skin area. In some cases, other medical tests are done to confirm the diagnosis.
· Treatment is usually not needed, and currently, there is no effective drug treatment that works for everyone. Your health care provider will discuss options with you.
· You may use cosmetics or fake-tan products to help hide the affected skin areas.

MEDICATIONS
· Steroid creams or ointments to be applied to the skin may be prescribed.
· Your health care provider may inject steroids directly into the bumps.
· A treatment called PUVA may be recommended. It combines a special light, used with a cream applied to the skin.

ACTIVITY
No limits.

DIET
No special diet.

 NOTIFY OUR OFFICE IF

· You or a family member has symptoms of granuloma annulare.
· The disorder recurs.

Special notes:

_____

_____

_____

More notes on the back of this page ☐

GRANULOMA, PYOGENIC

 BASIC INFORMATION

DESCRIPTION
A fairly common skin growth. It is not contagious or cancerous. Pyogenic granuloma can involve skin anywhere on the body. It often affects the head, neck, upper trunk, and fingers. It can also affect the gums and other mucous membranes of the mouth. It occurs most often in children of both sexes (ages 5 to 15) and pregnant women.

FREQUENT SIGNS AND SYMPTOMS
• Papule (small, raised bump on the skin). Usually, a single one is present, but in rare cases, there may be multiple papules.
• It first appears as pinhead-sized, but it grows rapidly over a period of a few weeks to about a half inch in size.
• The color is scarlet, brown, or blue-black.
• Will bleed easily when injured.
• They don't hurt or itch.
• May ulcerate (become an open sore) and form a crust.

CAUSES
Unknown. Pyogenic refers to an infectious process, but these lesions are misnamed. Because they frequently appear in late childhood or pregnancy, hormonal changes may be a factor in their development.

RISK INCREASES WITH
• Pregnancy.
• Recent injury (they may develop at the injured site).
• Use of certain drugs (such as oral contraceptives, retinoids, or protease inhibitors).

PREVENTIVE MEASURES
• Cannot be prevented at present.
• Because pyogenic granuloma resembles melanoma (skin cancer), medical diagnosis can be important.

EXPECTED OUTCOMES
Some heal on their own (such as in pregnancy). Others can be successfully treated.

POSSIBLE COMPLICATIONS
Recurrence is common.

 DIAGNOSIS & TREATMENT

GENERAL MEASURES
• Your health care provider will do an exam of the affected skin area. Medical tests usually include a skin biopsy (removal of a small amount of tissue for viewing under a microscope).
• The growths can be removed by several different methods.
• Often, they are scraped off with an instrument called a curette and then cauterized (using heat to heal tissue). This helps to decrease the chance that they will regrow.
• Laser surgery can be used to destroy the growth.
• In some cases, it may be treated with chemicals (such as silver nitrate).
• The growth may be removed by surgery excision and closed with stitches.
• If a drug is the cause of the pyogenic granuloma, stopping the drug often leads to healing.

MEDICATIONS
• For minor pain, you may use nonprescription drugs such as acetaminophen or aspirin. Don't give aspirin to children under age 18.
• If the scab cracks or oozes, apply a nonprescription antibiotic ointment several times a day.

ACTIVITY
No limits, except to avoid injury to the area while it is healing.

DIET
No special diet.

 NOTIFY OUR OFFICE IF

• You or a family member has symptoms of pyogenic granuloma.
• The wound bleeds after surgery, and applying pressure for 10 minutes cannot stop it.
• The wound shows signs of infection, such as redness, swelling, pain, or increased tenderness.

Special notes:

_____

_____

_____

More notes on the back of this page ☐

GRIEF
(Bereavement)

 BASIC INFORMATION

The emotional reaction following the death of a loved person, a divorce, loss of a body part or its function, loss of self-esteem (such as losing a job), or other significant loss. Grief is a normal, appropriate reaction to loss. It comes in many forms. Grieving people gradually adjust to their loss and begin to make positive plans for the future. There are no guidelines for the normal time for grieving. Sometimes, grief is serious or long-lasting enough that medical help is needed.

FREQUENT SIGNS AND SYMPTOMS
- Feelings of sadness, numbness, pain, anger, despair, or guilt. These feelings can come and go for months, and may be overwhelming at times.
- Sudden crying spells.
- Hallucinations (such as a sense of having seen or heard the dead person).
- Anxiety and depression.
- Being unwilling to accept the loss; for example, keeping the dead person's room or clothing as if he or she is expected to return.
- Unable to sleep.
- Nervousness and being overactive.
- Stomach problems.
- Tiredness, agitation, tearfulness.
- Increased use of alcohol and other drugs.

CAUSES
Grief naturally follows a loss.

RISK INCREASES WITH
Existing emotional problems can affect how a person responds to loss. This includes depression, social aloneness, strong feelings of guilt, self-blame, or anger due to one's relationship with the dead person.

PREVENTIVE MEASURES
Grieving should not be prevented or denied. It is a normal and expected response to a loss.

EXPECTED OUTCOME
With time, the grief lessens and adjustment begins. Your mind, body, and spirit will begin to heal. The feelings of grief may come and go, and will probably recur occasionally for years.

POSSIBLE COMPLICATIONS
- Difficulty maintaining relationships and jobs.
- Excess use of alcohol or other drugs.
- Chronic anxiety and depression.
- Symptoms that may need medical help include:
  - Severe depression, panic attacks, chronic anxiety.
  - Strong feelings of guilt, bitterness, or remorse.
  - Grief continues for 2 years or more. A person may build a life around the grief and never accept the loss.
  - Talk about or threats of suicide.

 DIAGNOSIS & TREATMENT

GENERAL MEASURES
- Express your feelings following the loss. Don't keep them "bottled up" inside. Look to family and friends for help and support.
- Religious or spiritual help may be of benefit to some people. Talk to your pastor or other religious professional about your feelings.
- Join a grief support group. They are available in most areas. People often find comfort in sharing their feelings with others who have had similar experiences.
- Slowly begin to rebuild your life. Interest yourself in things you have enjoyed in the past or try some new activities.
- Avoid the overuse of alcohol or drugs to suppress the emotions that you are feeling.
- See your health care provider if the feelings of grief are severe, or continue interfering with your daily life and/or work. A physical exam may be done and questions asked about your symptoms and feelings.
- Grief counseling may be recommended. It can help bring about a healthy resolution of grief.
- Don't expect your feelings of grief to follow any pattern or a particular timetable.

MEDICATIONS
Your health care provider may prescribe drugs, such as sedatives or antidepressants, for a short time. In most cases, drugs are not needed.

ACTIVITY
Normally, no limits. Try to do some physical activity daily.

DIET
Eat a normal, well-balanced diet.

 NOTIFY OUR OFFICE IF

- You or a family member has symptoms of grief that are getting worse or not getting better with time.
- Any of the Possible Complications occur.

Special notes:

_____

_____

_____

More notes on the back of this page ☐

GUILLAIN-BARRÉ SYNDROME
(Infectious Polyneuropathy)

BASIC INFORMATION

DESCRIPTION
A rare, inflammatory condition involving the peripheral nerves. These are nerves outside the brain and spinal column. It causes rapid weakness and loss of sensation. Guillain-Barré can affect all ages but is more common in young adults and the elderly.

FREQUENT SIGNS AND SYMPTOMS
· Muscle weakness starting in the lower limbs (feet and legs) and ascending (moving up) to the abdomen and chest, and to the arms and hands. The weakness spreads over days to weeks.
· Facial weakness and drooping, double vision, difficulty in speaking, and in swallowing.
· Pain, often in the back and legs; muscle cramps and tenderness; numbness, tingling, or burning sensations.
· Irregular heart beat, high or low blood pressure.
· Shortness of breath.
· Complete paralysis (sometimes) for weeks or months.

CAUSES
Unknown. It may be an autoimmune disorder. It sometimes follows a bacterial or viral infection.

RISK INCREASES WITH
Recent illness, such as a respiratory infection or gastroenteritis (stomach flu).

PREVENTIVE MEASURES
Cannot be prevented at present.

EXPECTED OUTCOMES
· Complete recovery without any lasting effects in many cases. Adults recover better than children. For some persons, symptoms clear in 15 to 20 days. Others require a year or more. Many mechanical devices can aid mobility until the person recovers.
· Some patients will have moderate lasting effects, and a few will have severe disabilities.

POSSIBLE COMPLICATIONS
· A relapse may occur after initial improvement.
· Respiratory failure.
· Permanent muscle weakness or numbness.
· Permanent total or partial paralysis (rare).
· Pneumonia.
· Deep vein thrombosis.
· Contractures of joints.

DIAGNOSIS & TREATMENT

GENERAL MEASURES
· Your health care provider may be able to diagnose the disorder by the symptoms and with a physical exam. Medical tests may be done, such as lumbar puncture for spinal fluid analysis, electromyography (studying nerve and muscle disorders by recording electrical activity of muscles), and lung function tests.
· Hospital care is needed in an intensive care unit so the condition can be closely monitored. There is no specific treatment for the disorder. Care involves supportive measures and methods to help speed recovery.
· A respirator (breathing machine) may be needed if muscles of respiration become greatly weakened. A tracheotomy (opening in the throat for breathing) may be required.
· Immunotherapy may be used to help shorten the duration and severity of the disease. It involves either plasmapheresis or IV immune globulin (injections).
· Plasmapheresis is a procedure where blood plasma is withdrawn from the patient, treated to remove antibodies, and then returned to the body by transfusion.
· Rehabilitation will begin as soon as it is feasible. It may involve physical therapy, occupational therapy (to promote self-care), speech therapy (to help with speaking and swallowing problems), and recreational therapy (helps the patient adjust to any disability).
· To learn more: Guillain-Barré Foundation, P.O. Box 262, Wynnewood, PA 19096; (610) 667-0131 (not toll free); website: www.guillain-barre.com.

MEDICATIONS
· IVIG (IV immune globulin) may be prescribed.
· Drugs as needed for symptoms, such as pain.

ACTIVITY
· Remain as active as muscle strength permits. Have a family member or physical therapist passively move and stretch muscles.
· Ongoing physical therapy will be needed to rebuild strength.

DIET
A feeding tube may be needed for patient with severe swallowing problem.

NOTIFY OUR OFFICE IF

· You or a family member has symptoms of Guillain-Barré syndrome.
· New symptoms occur after a patient returns home.

Special notes:

_____

_____

_____

More notes on the back of this page ☐

HAND, FOOT, & MOUTH DISEASE

 BASIC INFORMATION

DESCRIPTION

A common childhood infection with symptoms that begin in the mouth and throat. Hand, foot, and mouth disease most often affects children under the age of 10. Adults may get the infection, but it is less common.

FREQUENT SIGNS AND SYMPTOMS

· Sore throat with blisters and sores in the mouth and throat lining.
· Sudden fever that is usually mild.
· Rash with blisters on the hands, feet, and groin.
· Refusal to eat.
· Stomach pain or headache (sometimes).

CAUSES

Viral infection commonly caused by coxsackieviruses. The germs are spread from person to person or by touching an object (such as a toy) that has the germs on it. It takes about 3 to 6 days after exposure for the symptoms to start. Outbreaks may occur in nursery schools or child-care centers.

RISK INCREASES WITH

Summer and fall seasons.

PREVENTIVE MEASURES

· No specific preventive measures.
· Try to prevent exposure of infants and young children to anyone with an infection. Wash hands often to prevent spread of germs.
· Pregnant women should consult their obstetric provider if they are exposed to an infected person.

EXPECTED OUTCOMES

The infection is usually mild and complete recovery occurs in about a week. It rarely recurs once someone has had the infection.

POSSIBLE COMPLICATIONS

· The infection may be more serious in some infants and dehydration can occur.
· Other complications are rare.

 DIAGNOSIS & TREATMENT

GENERAL MEASURES

· Home care is usually all that is required for this infection. See your health care provider if you are concerned about the symptoms.
· Your health care provider can diagnose the infection by an exam of the affected mouth and skin area. Other medical tests are normally not needed.
· There is no specific treatment for the infection, but treatment may help relieve pain and fever symptoms.
· Rinse the mouth with salt water (1/2 teaspoon salt to 1 cup water) after eating, if the child is old enough to rinse without swallowing.
· Use separate dishes or disposable plates and cups to help avoid spreading the infection to other children in the family.

MEDICATIONS

To reduce high fever or for pain, you may use nonprescription drugs such as acetaminophen. Don't use aspirin in young children. Antibiotics are not effective for this infection.

ACTIVITY

Have the child get extra rest at home until any fever is gone. Children may return to school or daycare while they still have the rash.

DIET

Encourage the child to increase their fluid and soft food intake. This may include milk, liquid gelatin, ice cream, custard, or special products that you can buy at grocery or drug stores.

 NOTIFY OUR OFFICE IF

· Your child has symptoms of hand, foot and mouth disease.
· Symptoms get worse or do not improve.

Special notes:

_____

_____

_____

More notes on the back of this page ☐

HANTAVIRUS

 ## BASIC INFORMATION

DESCRIPTION

Hantavirus (named after a place in Korea) causes an illness called hantavirus pulmonary syndrome (HPS). Hantavirus has probably caused people to get sick for years in the United States, but it was not known about until recent years.

FREQUENT SIGNS AND SYMPTOMS

Early symptoms are flu-like:
- Chills.
- Fever.
- Muscle aches.
- Cough.
- General ill feeling.
- Feeling tired; lack of energy.
- Somewhat short of breath.

Later symptoms:
- Extreme difficulty in breathing.

CAUSES

Several types of mice can carry the hantavirus without getting ill. Where they nest, they leave the germs in their urine, feces (droppings), and saliva. If the nests are disturbed, the germs can get into the air as dust. When humans breathe in the air containing the germs, they can become infected. Infection may also come from a mouse bite, or from germs in food, water, or on something you touched. It may take a few days to 6 weeks for symptoms to appear once a person is exposed to the germs. The germs are not passed between humans.

RISK INCREASES WITH

No known risk factors.

PREVENTIVE MEASURES

- Avoid exposure to rodent urine and feces.
- Use caution in cleaning areas where mice nests might be located.
- Keep a clean home. This includes clearing out potential nesting sites and maintaining a clean kitchen.

EXPECTED OUTCOMES

The outcome will vary for each patient. To date, there is no treatment to stop the infection once it sets in. But steps can be taken to help control the symptoms while your body fights off the infection.

POSSIBLE COMPLICATIONS

Hantavirus pulmonary syndrome is a serious infection, and is fatal in about one-third of cases.

 ## DIAGNOSIS & TREATMENT

GENERAL MEASURES

- The breathing problems progress very quickly and treatment must occur in the hospital. Usually this is in an intensive care unit. Your health care provider will do a physical exam and discuss the possible exposure to rodents. A number of medical tests will be done to confirm the diagnosis.
- The main treatment is to help with any breathing problems.
- Supplemental oxygen is used to help the breathing. In severe cases, a machine may be needed to assist with the breathing.
- The family should maintain a hopeful outlook, and be as supportive as possible.

MEDICATIONS

Your healthcare provider will prescribe drugs as needed to help control any bleeding and improve lung function.

ACTIVITY

Resume your normal activities slowly once the symptoms are improved.

DIET

May require feeding through a vein (IV) while in the hospital. Then return to a regular diet with recovery.

 ## NOTIFY OUR OFFICE IF

You or a family member has symptoms of hantavirus pulmonary syndrome, especially if you live in an area, or have traveled to an area, where the virus is present.

Special notes:

_____

_____

_____

More notes on the back of this page ☐

HAY FEVER
(Allergic Rhinitis)

 BASIC INFORMATION

DESCRIPTION
An allergic response to an allergen in the air. Hay fever affects the eyes, nose, sinuses, throat, and bronchial tubes in the lungs. The name is confusing since hay does not cause an allergic reaction and there is no fever. Attacks flare up in pollen season.

FREQUENT SIGNS AND SYMPTOMS
- Itching, watery eyes.
- Frequent sneezing; stuffy nose with a clear discharge.
- Itching in the roof of the mouth.
- Wheezing (sometimes).
- Burning in the throat.

CAUSES
- The body's immune system produces antibodies that release a chemical called histamine. Histamine in turn produces swelling and irritation in certain areas (nose, sinuses, eyes).
- Allergens in the air that cause an allergic sensitivity include: Pollen (from weeds, flowers, grasses, and trees), mold, dust, mites, tobacco smoke, and other air pollutants.

RISK INCREASES WITH
- Having other allergic reactions, such as eczema or asthma.
- Smoking.
- Spring and autumn. Most plants produce pollen during these seasons.
- Family history of allergies.
- Weak immune system due to drugs or illness.

PREVENTIVE MEASURES
There is no way to prevent having allergies. You can take steps to help prevent having symptoms.

EXPECTED OUTCOMES
Symptoms can be controlled with treatment, but the condition persists over a lifetime. It is usually more troublesome than disabling.

POSSIBLE COMPLICATIONS
- Difficulty in sleeping and chronic fatigue.
- Increased risk for other infections.

 DIAGNOSIS & TREATMENT

GENERAL MEASURES
- Your health care provider will do a physical exam and ask questions about your symptoms. Medical tests such as blood and allergy skin tests may be recommended, but are usually not required for diagnosis.
- Try to remove as many allergens from your home or the surrounding property area as possible.

- Prepare your bedroom as follows:
  - Empty the room of furniture, rugs or carpet, and drapes or curtains. Clean the walls, woodwork, and floors with a damp mop. Wax the floor.
  - Cover box springs, mattress, and pillows with plastic covers. Use bedclothes that can be washed often.
  - Use throw rugs that can be washed easily.
  - Use wood or plastic chairs, not stuffed chairs.
  - Use window shades or blinds, not drapes/curtains.
  - Use a vacuum cleaner, damp rags, and a damp or oiled mop to clean the bedroom once a week.
- Other preventive measures:
  - Keep windows and doors closed, where possible.
  - Don't handle objects that are very dusty, such as books or stored clothing.
  - Don't keep stuffed animals or toys in the house.
  - Remove all pets (except fish) from the house.
  - Wear a filter face-mask during exposure to allergens, including during housecleaning.
  - Install an air-purification unit in your home's heating and air-conditioning system, preferably a high-efficiency particulate (HEPA) filter.
  - Drive an air-conditioned car.
  - Have someone else mow the lawn.

MEDICATIONS
- You may be prescribed:
  - Antihistamines; decongestants; cortisone eyedrops or nasal spray; cortisone tablets (severe cases only); cromolyn nasal spray; or cromolyn nose drops. These drugs relieve symptoms, but they don't cure hay fever.
  - Desensitization injections for known allergens for severe or year-round cases. Once allergens are known (through skin or blood tests), small amounts are injected over a period of time. This helps block the immune system from releasing the histamine. This process may take months or years for effective results.

ACTIVITY
No limits. Avoid areas with known allergens.

DIET
No special diet.

 NOTIFY OUR OFFICE IF

You or a family member has severe symptoms of hay fever that are interfering with normal activities.

Special notes:

_____

_____

_____

More notes on the back of this page ☐

HEAD INJURY
(Traumatic Brain Injury)

BASIC INFORMATION

DESCRIPTION
Injury to the head. It involves the scalp, skull, or brain. Head injuries may be external (closed) or internal (penetrating). Head injuries can cause physical problems, cognitive (thinking) dysfunction, or emotional changes. Most head injuries are minor (such as a small bump or "goose egg" on the head), but some can be life-threatening or cause permanent brain damage. Young children, teens, and the elderly are more often affected.

FREQUENT SIGNS AND SYMPTOMS
· Head injury symptoms may occur right away, or hours or days later. Signs and symptoms can include one or more of the following effects.
· Swelling bleeding at the site of the injury.
· Fracture of the skull.
· Loss of consciousness (short time or for long period).
· Abnormal breathing.
· Clear or bloody fluid from the nose, mouth, or ear.
· Drowsiness, confusion, irritability, or loss of memory.
· Unable to feel or control muscle function.
· Black-and-blue color around the eyes.
· Vomiting and nausea.
· Changes in vision or speech.
· Pupils of different sizes.
· Dizziness.
· Pain, such as headache or stiff neck.
· Seizure.

CAUSES
· Accidents (motor vehicle, work-related, sports, falls, physical assault, outdoor activities, and in the home).
· Child abuse or shaken baby syndrome.

RISK INCREASES WITH
· Alcohol or substance abuse.
· Contact sports, such as football, soccer, or boxing.
· Prior head injury.
· Illnesses that affect balance or walking ability.
· Not using seat belts or not wearing helmets.

PREVENTIVE MEASURES
· Don't drink or use mind-altering drugs and drive.
· Wear protective headgear when head injury is a risk.
· Use your auto seat belt always. Place young children in approved safety car seats.

EXPECTED OUTCOMES
The outcome will vary depending on a variety of factors (e.g., age, type of injury, severity of symptoms, and treatment). Many head injuries are mild and heal on their own with no lasting effects. Others can be treated successfully. Some may require extended hospital care and long-term rehabilitation.

POSSIBLE COMPLICATIONS
Permanent physical or mental disabilities, and social and economic problems (such as loss of job).

DIAGNOSIS & TREATMENT

GENERAL MEASURES
· Self-care is sometimes done for mild injuries. Get medical help right away if any of the symptoms listed occur or other head injury symptoms cause concern. Give first aid if needed. Call 911 for emergency help.
· Medical care starts with checking the person's ABCs (airway, breathing, and circulation). Any visible head injuries will be treated. Medical tests usually include testing the person's alertness. Other tests, such as x-ray, CT, or MRI are often done to check for brain damage.
· A person with a mild head injury can be sent home after initial medical care. Someone must stay with the person and watch for serious symptoms over the next 24 hours. Instructions may include waking the patient every 2 to 3 hours to check for alertness. Get medical help if you cannot awaken or arouse the person.
· In other head injuries, the treatment will depend on the severity. Hospital care may be needed for a period of time, and then rehabilitation care may be required.
· To learn more: Brain Injury Association, 1776 Massachusetts Ave, NW, Washington, DC 20036; (800) 444-6443; website: www.biausa.org.

MEDICATIONS
For self-care, you may use acetaminophen for pain or discomfort. Avoid aspirin. It can increase bleeding risk.

ACTIVITY
After treatment, rest as needed. Follow your health care provider's instructions about resuming physical activity.

DIET
Food intake will depend on the extent of injury.

NOTIFY OUR OFFICE IF

· You or a family member has symptoms of a head injury or observe them in someone else. Get emergency help if needed!
· After a head injury, you observe any new, changed, or worsening symptoms.

Special notes:

_____

_____

_____

More notes on the back of this page ☐

HEADACHE, CLUSTER

 ## BASIC INFORMATION

DESCRIPTION

A very severe headache that typically causes pain on one side of the head, behind the head, or around one eye. The headaches tend to recur at the same time each day for several days or weeks, separated by attack-free weeks or months. They affect adults over age 30, and men much more than women.

FREQUENT SIGNS AND SYMPTOMS

- Sudden onset of headache. It often occurs at night while sleeping.
- Headache reaches a peak within 15 minutes and lasts about 2 to 3 hours.
- Pain around the eye.
- Severe, piercing, or boring pain.
- Teary eyes.
- Swollen and droopy eyelid.
- Stuffy or runny nose.
- Slow heartbeat.
- Nausea.
- Sweating.

CAUSES

The cause is unknown. It may be a combination of factors, such as dilating blood vessels in the head, disturbance of the trigeminal nerve, or abnormal activity in part of the brain.

RISK INCREASES WITH

- Male, age over 30.
- Smoker.
- Previous head injury.
- Sleep apnea (periods of not breathing at night).
- Persons who are in stressful jobs, are self-employed, sociable, active, and responsible.
- Possibly a genetic factor (unproven as yet).

PREVENTIVE MEASURES

Since the cause is unknown, no specific measures to prevent first episode.

EXPECTED OUTCOMES

The cluster headache attacks may come and go, or be ongoing. Many people are headache-free for a year or more, but then they may start up again. Various drug therapies are available that can help control attacks.

POSSIBLE COMPLICATIONS

Cluster headaches do not cause complications or lead to other disorders. They are debilitating and can interfere with daily activities.

 ## DIAGNOSIS & TREATMENT

GENERAL MEASURES

- Your health care provider can usually diagnose the disorder based on the history of the headache patterns and symptoms. Medical tests are normally not required.
- Treatment goals are to treat the symptoms and prevent or abort future attacks. It may involve drug therapy, use of oxygen, and lifestyle changes.
- During cluster periods, avoid bright light or glare, alcohol, excessive anger, stressful activity, or excitement. These can trigger attacks. Keeping a headache diary may be useful to help identify other triggers.
- Don't smoke. It may interfere with drug therapy.
- Some patients also have sleep apnea. Treating the apnea (with a mechanical device) helps headaches also.
- Surgical treatments may be considered when drug therapy is not helpful. Surgery has limited effectiveness.
- To learn more: National Headache Foundation, 428 West St. James Pl., 2nd Flr., Chicago, IL 60614; (888) 643-5552; website: www.headaches.org.

MEDICATIONS

- Your health care provider may prescribe one or more drugs to treat the headache and for prevention:
  - Drugs called triptans (by mouth or by injection).
  - Dihydroergotamine (Migranal) by injection.
  - Ergotamine tartrate, in a tablet, suppository, aerosol, or injection form.
  - Oxygen therapy for home use.
  - Lidocaine nasal spray or nasal drops.
  - Phenylephrine (can be used for nasal stuffiness).
  - Other drugs to help treat/prevent cluster headaches.

ACTIVITY

Vigorous physical activity at first symptoms may abort attack.

DIET

Avoid alcohol and foods containing nitrates (such as smoked meat).

 ## NOTIFY OUR OFFICE IF

- You or a family member has symptoms of cluster headache.
- Attacks continue after treatment is started.

Special notes:

_____

_____

_____

More notes on the back of this page ☐

HEADACHE, MIGRAINE

 ## BASIC INFORMATION

DESCRIPTION

A severe type of headache that involves more than just the headache pain. There are five stages that may occur with a migraine. Prodrome (warning signs), aura (beginning symptoms), headache itself, resolution (pain stops), and postdrome (tiredness and other symptoms). Migraines may start occurring before age 20, affect both sexes, and are more common in females.

FREQUENT SIGNS AND SYMPTOMS

- The nature of attacks varies between persons and from time to time in the same person.
- Prodrome (hours/days before attack). It can include changes in mood, behavior, energy, and appetite.
- Aura (minutes or an hour before attack). It affects vision, hearing, or smell.
  - The most common symptoms are the inability to see clearly and seeing bright spots and zig-zag patterns.
  - Visual disturbances may last several minutes or several hours. They stop once the headache begins.
- Headache. Dull, boring pain in the temple that spreads to the entire side of the head.
  - Pain becomes more intense and throbs. Nausea, vomiting, and/or sensitivity to light and sound.
  - Headaches can last from 4 to 72 hours.
- Postdrome (may occur after an attack and last for hours or days). It includes exhaustion, weakness, lethargy, and elation (in some cases).

CAUSES

Exact cause is unknown. It may be due to a central nervous system disturbance that sets off a chain of events in the body. Genetic factors are involved also.

RISK INCREASES WITH

- Females.
- Family history of migraines.
- Other disorders (such as asthma, allergies, *H. pylori* infection, epilepsy, and fibromyalgia).

PREVENTIVE MEASURES

No preventive steps for first attack. After diagnosis, take steps to help prevent future attacks. Try to avoid the triggers of migraines (such as some foods and drugs, bright lights, weather changes, high altitudes, and stress). Keep a diary to learn your own specific triggers.

EXPECTED OUTCOMES

People with migraines tend to have them over many years. They can often be controlled with treatment. Migraines may end when a person gets older.

POSSIBLE COMPLICATIONS

- Interferes with day-to-day life (work, family, or social).
- Status migraine (lasts over 72 hours) or stroke (rare).

 ## DIAGNOSIS & TREATMENT

GENERAL MEASURES

- Your health care provider can usually diagnose the disorder based on the history of the headache pattern and symptoms. Medical tests are normally not required.
- Treatment is usually with drug therapy and self-care.
- Hospital care may be needed for a severe attack.
- Counseling, behavior therapy, or stress reduction techniques may be recommended.
- For self-care at the first sign of a migraine attack:
  - Apply a cold cloth to your head and lie down in a quiet, dark room. Relax and sleep if possible.
  - Minimize noise, light, and odors (such as cooking odors and tobacco smoke). Don't read.
- To learn more: National Headache Foundation, 428 West St. James Pl., 2nd Flr., Chicago, IL 60614; (888) 643-5552; website: www.headaches.org.

MEDICATIONS

- No single drug works best for everyone. A variety of drugs can be prescribed for symptoms and prevention.
- Triptans in self-administered by subcutaneous (under the skin) injection, oral tablet, or nasal spray.
- Ergot preparations in a tablet, suppository, aerosol, or injection form.
- Use nonprescription drugs such as ibuprofen, or aspirin (if over age 18), or acetaminophen.
- Narcotics or butalbital (alone or with other drugs).
- Antihistamines to expand blood vessels.
- Antiemetics to decrease nausea and vomiting.
- Vasoconstrictors to narrow blood vessels.
- Beta-adrenergic, calcium channel blockers, or antidepressants to prevent attacks.
- Note: Overuse of drugs can cause a "rebound" into another headache.

ACTIVITY

Exercise daily to maintain fitness. Rest during headache.

DIET

Keep a diary to see if any foods trigger your migraines.

 ## NOTIFY OUR OFFICE IF

- You or a family member has migraine symptoms.
- Treatment is not helping the migraines.

Special notes:

_____

_____

_____

More notes on the back of this page ☐

HEADACHE, TENSION

 ## BASIC INFORMATION

DESCRIPTION
Tension headaches are the most common type of headache. These headaches may occur on 15 days out of a month (chronic) or less often (episodic).

FREQUENT SIGNS AND SYMPTOMS
· Dull, steady pain on both sides of the head. The pain may be mild to severe. It usually comes on gradually.
· Tight feeling or tenderness in the muscles of the head, neck or scalp. "Like a band around the head."
· Some people may clench their teeth.
· Tension headaches are different from migraines, which cause intense pain, usually on one side of the head. Migraines also cause nausea and light sensitivity.

CAUSES
The cause is not clearly understood. It now appears that it is caused by a problem of the central nervous system and changes in brain chemicals. It has been thought the cause was stress and tension that puts strain on the muscles of the neck, scalp, face, and jaw. There are other possible causes being studied also.

RISK INCREASES WITH
People who might get tension headaches:
· Women (more often affected than men).
· Those who are overworked on a continuous basis.
· Persons with chronic poor posture.
· Persons with sleep disorders.
· Those who suffer from depression, stress, or anxiety.
· Certain chronic medical problems.
· Abuse of alcohol or other substances.
Things that might bring on (trigger) a tension headaches include:
· A stressful event.
· Eating certain foods.
· Not eating on time; caffeine withdrawal.
· Intense physical exercise.
· Taking certain drugs.
· Hormone changes in women.
· Eyestrain.
· Fatigue.
· Having a cold or the flu.

PREVENTIVE MEASURES
Avoid any of the risk factors when possible.

EXPECTED OUTCOMES
Most tension headaches can be relieved with treatment, and do not disrupt home or work activities.

POSSIBLE COMPLICATIONS
· None expected for a simple headache.
· Chronic tension headaches may require trying several types of treatment. The headaches may continue if the risk factors are not changed or treated.

 ## DIAGNOSIS & TREATMENT

GENERAL MEASURES
· Self-care can includes mild pain relievers. If possible, stop what you are doing and try to relax. Take a hot bath or shower. Lie down. Place a warm or cold cloth, whichever feels better, over the aching area.
· Self-care is often effective for handling the headache. If that doesn't work, or the pain gets worse, or headaches occur often, see your health care provider.
· Your health care provider will do a physical exam, and ask questions about your symptoms and your lifestyle. Medical tests and blood studies may be done to make sure there is no other medical problem involved.
· Chronic tension headaches may be treated with different methods for stress reduction and relaxation techniques, and prescribed drugs. Drugs that have been overused for headache pain may need to be withdrawn.
· There are more treatment options that you and your health care provider may discuss. These may include physical therapy, hypnosis, massage therapy, and others.
· To learn more: National Headache Foundation, 820 N. Orleans, Suite 217, Chicago, IL 60610, (888) 643-5552; website: www.headache.org.

MEDICATIONS
· You may take nonprescription pain relievers such as ibuprofen, naproxen, aspirin (if over age 18), or acetaminophen.
· Stronger drugs, for pain, and drugs to prevent chronic tension headaches may be prescribed.

ACTIVITY
Exercise on a regular basis and get enough sleep.

DIET
Eat a healthy diet high in fiber, fruits, and vegetables.

 ## NOTIFY OUR OFFICE IF

· You or a family member has tension headaches and self-treatment steps are not working.
· Headaches recur or get worse despite treatment.
· New symptoms are caused by adverse drug reaction.

Special notes:

_____

_____

_____

More notes on the back of this page ☐

HEALTH RECORD, PERSONAL

 BASIC INFORMATION

DESCRIPTION

It is important to maintain a health and sickness history for yourself and for your children. This information can be helpful for future reference. Any health care provider you visit will ask about past medical experiences and about your health in general. Don't rely on memory. Write things down in a medical journal. It can be as simple as a spiral notebook. The information can be kept on a computer file or on specially designed health-history forms. The items listed below suggest what information to include in the personal medical record.

ITEMS TO INCLUDE IN YOUR HEALTH RECORD:
• Birth date, details about the delivery and birth, and any problems that took place.
• Serious illnesses and treatments.
• Chronic illnesses and treatments.
• Minor illnesses, problems or infections that recur such as ear infections, repeated colds, skin problems, headaches, or others.
• Drugs prescribed and any side effects or adverse reactions to them. List the generic name as well as the brand name of each drug. If unsure, ask the pharmacist or your health care provider.
• List any nonprescription drugs or supplements taken on a regular basis (vitamins, laxatives, aspirin, and others). Make note of any reaction to them, and whether they helped the problem being treated.
• Allergies to food, air pollutants, chemicals, latex, or other substances or products.
• Food intolerances, such as lactose intolerance.
• Immunizations (child and adult vaccination history).
• Medical tests and results. This can include such items as weight, height, and blood pressure when taken in the health care provider's office.
• Operations and hospital stays. Ask for copies of operation reports, discharge summaries, and for tests done while in the hospital.
• Keep a record of your exercise habits.
• Note down any special weight-loss diets tried, and their results.
• Note dates and results of any self-testing performed, such as breast exam or skin exam.
• Sexual problems for both male and female partners. If sexually active with more than one partner, write down information about the sexual encounters, and whether protection was used.
• Ongoing use of alcohol and amount consumed.
• Cigarette smoking and number smoked or other use of other tobacco products.

• Make a note of emotional disorders such as stress, depression, feelings of sadness, or other problems that can affect emotional well-being.
• Reproductive history (date of first menstrual period, length of menstrual cycles, contraceptive methods used, and pregnancy history).
• Note down any other facts about health matters, no matter how minor, that you think may be useful to the health care provider.
• Write down medical history of parents, brothers and sisters, and grandparents. This includes any serious illnesses or other medical, mental, or emotional problems. Find out about cause of death for deceased family members. List information about asthma and allergies, breast cancer, diabetes, glaucoma, Alzheimer's disease, alcoholism, and any information known about inherited disorders.
• Keep copies of prescriptions, test results, and immunization records in the same file.
• Take this medical record with you when a visit to a health care provider is scheduled. It will assist you in answering questions correctly and completely when a medical history is taken.

BE SURE TO INCLUDE:
• Personal information such as your name, birth date, and social security number.
• People to contact in case of emergency.
• Name, addresses, and phone numbers of your personal physician, dentist, and other health care providers.
• Health insurance information.
• Living wills and advanced directives information.
• Organ donor authorization.

 NOTIFY OUR OFFICE IF

You or a family member has questions or concerns about medical history information.

Special notes:

_____

_____

_____

More notes on the back of this page ☐

HEARING IMPAIRMENT or LOSS

BASIC INFORMATION

DESCRIPTION
Hearing loss may be partial or total. It may develop gradually or suddenly. It may occur at any age. There are two types of hearing loss:
• Conductive loss. It is caused by anything that blocks the conduction of sound from the outer ear through to the inner ear.
• Sensorineural loss. It results from damage to the inner ear such as to the auditory nerve or hair cells of the cochlea. This type includes the gradual hearing loss that occurs with aging called presbycusis.
• A mixed loss involves both types of hearing loss.

FREQUENT SIGNS AND SYMPTOMS
• In an infant, there is a lack of response to sounds.
• Trouble understanding speech. Misunderstanding others and responding inappropriately.
• Difficulty in hearing a phone ring, or problem hearing over the phone.
• Difficulty hearing in a group of people or when there is background noise.
• Avoiding social activities (may feel embarrassed).
• Turning up the volume of the radio or television.
• Asking others to repeat themselves.
• Ringing in the ears, dizziness, or pain.

CAUSES
Hearing loss occurs when any part of the hearing system is unable to function. A wide variety of conditions can cause hearing loss. Sometimes, no cause is found.

RISK INCREASES WITH
Conductive:
• Middle ear infection (otitis media).
• Collection of fluid in middle ear (glue ear).
• Blockage of the outer ear by wax.
• Damage to the eardrum from infection or injury.
• Otosclerosis (growth of spongy tissue in the ear).
• Rarely, rheumatoid arthritis affects joints in the ear.
Sensorineural:
• Aging (hearing starts decreasing in the 30s and 40s).
• Noise exposure (repeated and continuous).
• Viral infection such as mumps.
• Ménière's disease.
• Certain drugs (aspirin, quinine, some antibiotics).
• Acoustic neuroma (benign tumor).
• Brain infection, inflammation or tumor.
• Multiple sclerosis.
• Stroke.
• Congenital (present at birth). A family history of hearing loss is also a risk factor.

PREVENTIVE MEASURES
Avoid the risk factors where possible. Get medical care for any infections or any symptoms of hearing loss.

EXPECTED OUTCOMES
The outcome depends on the cause. The hearing loss may be temporary, treatable, or manageable.

POSSIBLE COMPLICATIONS
• Complete loss of hearing (deafness).
• Language delay or learning problems in a child.
• Emotional, social, and work-associated problems.

DIAGNOSIS & TREATMENT

GENERAL MEASURES
• Your health care provider will do an exam of the ears and ask questions about your symptoms. Hearing tests may include tests done with a tuning fork and an audiogram (to measure hearing levels). Other hearing studies and speech testing may be done. Tests help determine the extent of hearing loss and whether it is conductive or sensorineural.
• Treatment will depend on the cause. It may involve simple procedures (like earwax removal), drug therapy, surgical treatments, and sound amplification (hearing aids). You may be asked to consult a health care provider who specializes in hearing problems.
• If the hearing loss is related to drugs, changes in dosage or stopping the drug may help.
• To learn more: National Institute on Deafness and Other Communication Disorders, 31 Center Dr., MSC 2320, Bethesda, MD 20892, (800) 241-1044; website: www.nidcd.nih.gov/health/hearing.

MEDICATIONS
Drugs may be prescribed for any treatable disorder that is diagnosed.

ACTIVITY
No limits.

DIET
No special diet.

NOTIFY OUR OFFICE IF

• You suspect you have a hearing loss, especially if you must ask others often to repeat themselves or family members frequently ask you if your hearing is all right.
• A family member shows signs of hearing loss.

Special notes:

_____

_____

_____

More notes on the back of this page ☐

HEART ATTACK
(Myocardial Infarction)

BASIC INFORMATION

DESCRIPTION
A sudden instance of abnormal heart function. A heart attack is a life-threatening event. It most often affects adults over 40. It is more common in men, but the incidence is rising for women.

FREQUENT SIGNS AND SYMPTOMS
- Chest pain or "heavy, squeezing, or crushing" feeling in the chest.
- Pain that radiates from the midchest over the breast bone to the jaw, neck, either arm, the area between the shoulder blades, or upper abdomen (sometimes).
- Feeling of impending doom.
- Shortness of breath.
- Nausea and vomiting.
- Sweating.
- Dizziness and/or weakness.
- Choking sensation.

CAUSES
A heart attack occurs when the supply of blood and oxygen to an area of heart muscle is blocked. This is usually due to a blood clot in a coronary artery. The blockage leads to an irregular heartbeat or rhythm that causes a severe decrease in heart function. When the heart actually stops, it is called cardiac arrest.

RISK INCREASES WITH
- Men over age 45 and women over age 55.
- Family history of early heart disease.
- Personal history of coronary artery disease (CAD).
- Smoking.
- Obesity.
- High LDL cholesterol levels or low HDL cholesterol.
- High blood pressure.
- Diabetes.
- Sedentary lifestyle (lack of physical activity).

PREVENTIVE MEASURES
Exercise daily. Maintain a healthy weight. Eat a healthy diet. Don't smoke. Get medical care for diabetes, high blood pressure, and high cholesterol. A daily, low-dose aspirin may be prescribed by your health care provider.

EXPECTED OUTCOMES
The amount of damage from a heart attack depends on how much of the heart is affected, how soon treatment begins, and other factors. Survivors should allow 4 to 8 weeks for recovery. Repeat heart attacks are common.

POSSIBLE COMPLICATIONS
- Irregular heart rhythms.
- Shock.
- Congestive heart failure.
- Pericarditis (heart lining inflammation).
- Blood clots in other parts of the body.

DIAGNOSIS & TREATMENT

GENERAL MEASURES
- If you have any symptoms of a heart attack, seek medical help right away. Don't drive yourself.
- If you suspect heart attack symptoms in someone, call 911 for help.
- Diagnosis and treatment of a heart attack begins when emergency medical personnel arrive after you call 911. In the hospital emergency room, health care providers will work fast to find out if you are having or have had a heart attack and to give you treatment.
- If you are having a heart attack, treatment is done to restore the blood flow to the heart, and to monitor your vital signs to detect and treat complications.
- Long-term treatment after a heart attack may include cardiac rehabilitation, checkups and tests, lifestyle changes (such as stopping smoking or weight loss), and drug therapy.
- To learn more: American Heart Association, 7272 Greenville Ave., Dallas, TX 75231; (800) 242-8721; website: www.americanheart.org.

MEDICATIONS
- Drugs to dissolve and/or prevent blood clots may be used for emergency care.
- After a heart attack, drugs may be prescribed to help the heart function, treat high blood pressure, prevent clots, or to lower cholesterol levels.

ACTIVITY
- Resume your normal activities gradually during recovery. An exercise program will usually be recommended.
- You will be advised about when to return to work, resume sexual relations, or drive a car.

DIET
- After a heart attack, eat a low-fat, high-fiber diet.
- Maintain ideal weight. Start a reducing diet if overweight.

NOTIFY OUR OFFICE IF

- You or a family member has symptoms of a heart attack. This is a life-threatening emergency!
- New symptoms occur during recovery.

Special notes:

_____

_____

_____

More notes on the back of this page ☐

HEART RHYTHM IRREGULARITY
(Arrhythmia)

 BASIC INFORMATION

DESCRIPTION

A change in the regular beat of the heart. Arrhythmias are common, and many are mild and require no treatment. Almost all adults have some amount of irregular heartbeats. They can affect all ages, but they are most likely to occur in people over age 65.

FREQUENT SIGNS AND SYMPTOMS

- A fluttering in the chest; the heart seems to skip a beat, or beat irregularly, or beat very fast or slowly.
- Shortness of breath and/or mild chest pains.
- Faintness, dizziness, or weakness.
- Feeling anxious.
- No symptoms (frequently).

CAUSES

The heart has an electrical system that controls its rate and contractions. The average heart beats at a rate of 60 to 100 times per minute. With arrhythmias, the electrical system does not function as it should. There are different types of arrhythmias depending on what part of the heart is involved. They can be due to a number of causes. In some cases, no cause is found.

RISK INCREASES WITH

- Heart diseases. This includes rheumatic fever, congenital heart disease, cardiomyopathy, previous heart attack, or heart-muscle inflammation.
- Endocrine disorders, such as thyroid and adrenal gland diseases.
- Fluid and electrolyte imbalance, such as too little or too much potassium.
- Side effects of certain drugs, such as digitalis, beta-adrenergic blockers, stimulants, and diuretics.
- Use of certain drugs, such as caffeine, alcohol, amphetamines, and many nonprescription cough and cold remedies.
- Overdose of certain drugs, including antidepressants, marijuana, and cocaine.
- Postoperative effects following chest or heart surgery.
- Chronic kidney disease.
- High blood pressure.
- Smoking.
- Stress.
- Sleep deprivation (lack of sleep).

PREVENTIVE MEASURES

Avoid risk factors where possible and get treatment for those that are treatable.

EXPECTED OUTCOMES

Irregular heartbeats that occur only occasionally are typically harmless and require no treatment. Other arrhythmias can usually be controlled with treatment.

POSSIBLE COMPLICATIONS

- Complications may arise from the heart disease that is causing the arrhythmia.
- Some arrhythmias can lead to complications if they are untreated.

 DIAGNOSIS & TREATMENT

GENERAL MEASURES

- Your health care provider will do a physical exam and listen to the heart with a stethoscope. Medical tests usually include an electrocardiogram (ECG) or you may be asked to wear a Holter monitor (a portable ECG) for 1 to 5 days. These aid in diagnosing heart diseases by measuring the electrical activity of the heart. Other tests may be done to see if the cause is a heart disease.
- Treatment, if needed, will depend on the cause.
- You may require cardioversion (brief electric shock to the heart) to restore normal rhythm.
- Surgery may be needed to correct some heart problems (coronary-artery bypass, to replace damaged heart valve, or insertion of a pacemaker or atrial defibrillator).
- Counseling may be helpful if stress is a major factor.
- Wear a medical alert bracelet or pendant showing the name of your condition.
- To learn more: American Heart Association, 7272 Greenville Ave., Dallas, TX 75231; (800) 242-8721; website: www.americanheart.org.

MEDICATIONS

Antiarrhythmic drugs may be prescribed. You may need to try several of them to find the most effective one. Certain arrhythmias may also require anticoagulant drug therapy.

ACTIVITY

Your health care provider will advise you if there are any limits.

DIET

Avoid caffeine-containing beverages and alcohol.

 NOTIFY OUR OFFICE IF

- You or a family member has symptoms of heart-rhythm irregularity.
- New, unexplained symptoms develop.

Special notes:

_____

_____

_____

More notes on the back of this page ☐

HEARTBEAT, RAPID
(Tachycardia)

 BASIC INFORMATION

DESCRIPTION

A heart rate (or heartbeat) that is faster than normal. In adults, the resting heart rate is normally between 60 and 100 beats per minute. Tachycardia is the medical term for rapid heart rate. Bradycardia is a slow heart rate.

FREQUENT SIGNS AND SYMPTOMS

- Some people may have no symptoms.
- Heart pounding or palpitations. The pulse at the wrist or neck will be 100 to 180 beats per minute, which is much faster than normal.
- Faintness; a feeling of doom or anxiety.
- Chest pain.
- Cough.
- Being short of breath.
- Dizziness.
- Heavy sweating.

CAUSES

An electrical system in the heart normally controls the heart rate so that it remains at 60 to 100 beats per minute. This allows the heart to provide the body with the blood and oxygen it needs to function. When something causes the heart to beat too fast, it may not be able to supply all the blood and oxygen needed by the body.

RISK INCREASES WITH

- Heart attack, heart disease, or surgery.
- Thyroid disease.
- Fever.
- Anemia.
- Stress, anxiety, fear, anger, or being nervous.
- Smoking.
- Dehydration.
- Infections.
- Sleep deprivation (not getting enough sleep).
- Too much caffeine.
- Use of some drugs, such as albuterol, cocaine, ephedrine, or others, and some herbal remedies.

PREVENTIVE MEASURES

- Often, the problem cannot be prevented.
- Avoid the risk factors where possible.
- Regular exercise.

EXPECTED OUTCOMES

Most heartbeat problems are temporary and harmless. If the rapid heartbeat is ongoing, it can usually be controlled with treatment.

POSSIBLE COMPLICATIONS

An ongoing rapid heartbeat can lead to life-threatening heart problems.

 DIAGNOSIS & TREATMENT

GENERAL MEASURES

- Your health care provider will do a physical exam and ask questions about your symptoms and activities. Tests may be done to measure the heart's electrical activity. Other tests may be done to check for medical problems that could cause rapid heart rate.
- A few patients may require immediate treatment, including electrical shock (cardioversion), to stop the rapid heart rate. In milder cases, no treatment may be required. Other treatment may depend on the cause.
- If the rapid heart rate occurs often, a small electrical device called implantable cardioverter-defibrillator (ICD) may be implanted under the skin. It can detect irregular heartbeats and shock the heart back into normal rhythm, when needed.
- Surgery may (rarely) be recommended.
- Ask your health care provider about ways to reduce stress in your life, and to stop smoking, if you smoke.
- The following steps sometimes slows the heartbeat:
  - Hold your breath briefly.
  - Pinch the skin on your arm enough to cause pain.
  - Bathe your face in cold water or put your head briefly in a sink of cool water.
  - Hold your nostrils closed and blow gently through the nose, making the eardrums pop.
- To learn more: American Heart Association, 7272 Greenville Ave., Dallas, TX 75231; (800) 242-8721; website: www.americanheart.org.

MEDICATIONS

For repeated attacks, one or more drugs to control heart rhythm may be prescribed.

ACTIVITY

Exercise regularly for 20 to 30 minutes a day (with medical approval). Being fit will improve heart health.

DIET

Avoid caffeine and alcohol.

 NOTIFY OUR OFFICE IF

- You or a family member has an episode of rapid, irregular heartbeat that does not end in 4 or 5 minutes.
- Shortness of breath or chest pain develops.

Special notes:

_____

_____

_____

More notes on the back of this page ☐

HEARTBURN

 ## BASIC INFORMATION

DESCRIPTION

Heartburn (also known as acid indigestion) is a symptom, not a disease, and has nothing to do with the heart. It can affect all ages, but is most common in adults over 60. The symptoms are sometimes mistaken for a heart attack. When heartburn occurs often or complications develop, the problem is known as GERD (gastroesophageal reflux disease).

FREQUENT SIGNS AND SYMPTOMS

- Belching or backward flow of stomach contents into the mouth and throat. This produces an acid taste.
- Heavy burning, discomfort, or pain in the chest.
- It may be difficult to swallow.
- Mild stomach pain or bloated feeling.

CAUSES

Heartburn is caused by a backflow of acid from the stomach into the esophagus. The esophagus is the tube that goes from the mouth to the stomach. The muscles that close off the upper stomach become lax (loose). This allows stomach juices to enter the esophagus and irritate its lining.

RISK INCREASES WITH

- Hiatal hernia (part of the stomach bulges into the chest).
- Ulcers (open sores) of the esophagus.
- Stress.
- Improper diet or overeating.
- Overweight.
- Smoking.
- Excess alcohol use.
- Use of certain drugs.
- Eating spicy or acidic (citrus, tomatoes) foods.
- Drinking carbonated beverages.
- Exercise, lying down, bending over, or straining too soon after a meal.
- Disorders of the gastrointestinal tract.

PREVENTIVE MEASURES

- Avoid smoking.
- Don't overeat or use an excess amount of alcohol.
- Reduce the amount of fats, deep-fried foods, spices, coffee, tea, and tomato products in your diet.
- Don't bend over or lie down right after eating.
- Don't wear tight clothes that restrict your body.
- Elevate the head of the bed 4 to 6 inches with blocks.
- Lose weight if you are overweight.

EXPECTED OUTCOMES

Symptoms usually clear up on their own. In other cases, symptoms can be relieved with treatment.

POSSIBLE COMPLICATIONS

Gastroesophageal reflux disease (GERD).

 ## DIAGNOSIS & TREATMENT

GENERAL MEASURES

- Heartburn usually begins within about an hour after eating and may continue for several hours. Self-care involves taking preventive measures and heartburn drugs, if needed, to control the symptoms.
- If the problem gets worse or self-care is not working, see your health care provider. A physical exam will be done and questions asked about your symptoms. Medical tests are usually not needed, but may be done to help diagnose any complications.
- Stop smoking. Find a way that will work for you.
- Rarely, surgery may be recommended when other treatment steps are not helping the symptoms.
- To learn more: National Heartburn Alliance, 303 East Wacker Drive, Suite 440, Chicago, IL 60601; (877) 471-2081; website: www.heartburnalliance.org.

MEDICATIONS

- For minor discomfort, you may use any of the heartburn preventive drugs available without a prescription. Different ones work for different people. If one type does not work for you, a different type may help.
- A stronger type of heartburn drug may be prescribed.
- If a drug you take is causing heartburn, a change in dosage or a new drug may be prescribed.

ACTIVITY

Resume normal activities as soon as symptoms improve.

DIET

- Avoid foods and beverages that cause excess stomach acid, such as spicy dishes, coffee, acidic fruit juice, or alcohol. Avoid chocolate, and eat less high-fat foods.
- Eat small, frequent meals.

 ## NOTIFY OUR OFFICE IF

- If you or a family member has heartburn that continues or worsens despite self-care.
- The following symptoms occur with heartburn could mean a heart attack. Seek emergency help:
  - Shortness of breath; pain in the jaw, neck, and arm.
  - Sweating, cold, clammy feeling, nausea or vomiting.

Special notes:

_____

_____

_____

More notes on the back of this page ☐

HEARTBURN DURING PREGNANCY

 BASIC INFORMATION

DESCRIPTION

Heartburn is the term used to describe a burning pain in the chest and upper abdomen. It is common for pregnant women to have the symptoms of heartburn. It usually comes and goes until delivery. Although it can cause you some discomfort, heartburn will not hurt your baby.

FREQUENT SIGNS AND SYMPTOMS

· Burning pain in the center of the chest and upper abdomen. It is often causes an unpleasant taste in the mouth.
· Belching (burping).

CAUSES

· Heartburn is not a heart disorder. It is caused by a backflow of acid from the stomach into the esophagus. The esophagus is the tube that goes from the mouth to the stomach. The muscles that close off the upper stomach become lax (loose), allowing stomach juices to enter the esophagus and irritate its lining.
· Changes caused by pregnancy include an increase in the amount of stomach acid. It also takes longer for the stomach to empty.
· During late pregnancy, the enlarged womb presses on the stomach and may increase the symptoms.

RISK INCREASES WITH

· Overeating or eating and then lying down.
· Smoking.
· Excess use of alcohol.

PREVENTIVE MEASURES

Avoid risk factors listed above.

EXPECTED OUTCOME

The heartburn goes away after the baby is born unless the cause is not related to pregnancy. There are normally no complications.

POSSIBLE COMPLICATIONS

Heartburn may affect your ability to eat a healthy diet. Low food and fluid intake might cause problems for the mother and the baby.

 DIAGNOSIS & TREATMENT

GENERAL MEASURES

· Heartburn is usually self-diagnosed. Your obstetric provider may make the diagnosis from the symptoms you describe, and rarely, may recommend other medical tests.

· General treatment suggestions:
 - Avoid bending over or lying down right after eating.
 - Don't wear tight girdles or belts.
 - Place books or blocks under the head of your bed to raise it about 4 inches, or sleep propped up with several pillows.
 - Don't smoke.

MEDICATION

· While medicine is not usually needed for this disorder, in some cases it may be of benefit. Simple antacid mixtures or tablets, such as magnesium trisilicate, may be helpful. These drugs should be used only with your obstetric provider's approval. Other drugs may be prescribed if simple measures don't help the symptoms.
· Don't take any herbal remedies without asking your obstetric provider.
· If you can live with the symptoms, try to avoid use of drugs.

ACTIVITY

Stay active. Avoid exercises that require bending over.

DIET

· Eat small, frequent meals.
· Don't rush through your meals; eat slowly.
· Avoid drinking large quantities of fluids during meals.
· Don't eat before bedtime.
· Avoid highly seasoned food.
· Don't drink alcohol.
· Avoid very hot or very cold beverages.
· Avoid eating while lying down.
· Chewing gum may be helpful for some women.

 NOTIFY OUR OFFICE IF

· You or a family member has symptoms of heartburn during pregnancy. This should be diagnosed.
· The following occur after diagnosis:
 - Simple measures don't bring relief.
 - You begin vomiting late in pregnancy.
 - You vomit material that has blood in it or looks like coffee grounds.
 - You have black or tarry stools.

Special notes:

_____

_____

_____

More notes on the back of this page ☐

HEATSTROKE or HEAT EXHAUSTION
(Sunstroke)

BASIC INFORMATION

DESCRIPTION
Illness caused by excess exposure to heat, not enough fluid intake, or a failure of the body's ability to regulate its temperature. It can affect all ages, but is more common in the elderly.

FREQUENT SIGNS AND SYMPTOMS
Heat exhaustion:
- Dizziness, fatigue, faintness, headache.
- Skin that is pale and clammy.
- Pulse rapid and weak.
- Breathing is fast and shallow.
- Muscle cramps.
- Intense thirst.

Heatstroke:
- Often preceded by heat exhaustion and its symptoms.
- Skin that is hot, dry, and flushed.
- No sweating.
- High body temperature.
- Rapid heartbeat.
- Confusion.
- Loss of consciousness.

CAUSES
- Heat exhaustion is caused by a lack of fluid intake, a lack of salt intake, and a problem with the body's production of sweat. Sweat is what helps to cool the body.
- Heat stroke is caused by overexposure to extreme heat and a breakdown in the body's temperature regulation system. The body becomes overheated to a dangerous degree. The body's temperature can reach 107°F (41.7°C).

RISK INCREASES WITH
- Elderly persons.
- Excess alcohol use or drug abuse.
- Poor health or chronic illness, such as diabetes, high blood pressure, or heart disease.
- Exercise or work in a hot, humid location. This can be indoors or outdoors.
- Loss of body fluids, from sweating and failure to drink enough fluids.
- Heavy, tight clothing.
- High fever.

PREVENTIVE MEASURES
- Wear light, loose-fitting clothing in hot weather.
- Drink water often; don't wait until you are thirsty.
- Drink extra water if you sweat a lot. If urine output decreases, increase your water intake.
- If you become overheated, open a window or use a fan or air conditioner. This helps sweat dry up, which cools the skin.
- Take precautions when going outside in hot weather.

EXPECTED OUTCOMES
Fast treatment usually brings full recovery in 1 to 2 days.

POSSIBLE COMPLICATIONS
- Can involve any major organ system (heart, lungs, kidneys, brain).
- Related to duration and amount of heat and to speed of treatment.

DIAGNOSIS & TREATMENT

GENERAL MEASURES
- If someone with symptoms is very hot and not sweating: Cool the person rapidly. Remove their clothing, use a cold-water bath, or wrap in wet sheets. Get them to the nearest hospital. This is an emergency!
- If someone is faint but sweating: Lie the person down in a cool place. Give them cool water (not iced) to sip or a sports drink containing electrolytes. Get medical advice for proper care.
- Your health care provider will do a physical exam and ask questions about the symptoms and activities. Usually no medical tests are needed for diagnosis.
- Medical treatment will depend on how severe the symptoms are. Fluids may be given through a vein (IV).

MEDICATIONS
Drugs are usually not needed for these disorders. Drugs may be needed for complications that develop.

ACTIVITY
- Rest with legs elevated while symptoms are present.
- Activity may be resumed after symptoms improve.

DIET
No special diet.

NOTIFY OUR OFFICE IF

You or a family member has symptoms of heatstroke or heat exhaustion, or observe them in someone else. Call immediately! These conditions may be serious or fatal.

Special notes:

_____

_____

_____

More notes on the back of this page ☐

HEEL PAIN

(Heel Contusion; Heel Spur; Heel Bursitis)

 BASIC INFORMATION

DESCRIPTION

Heel pain or discomfort caused by several conditions.

• Contusion or bruise of the heel bone. This causes inflammation of the tissue (periosteum) that covers the heel bone (calcaneus).

• Heel spur. A hard, bony sliver or needle that develops on the heel. It can cause inflammation and other problems in tendons and ligaments in the foot.

• Heel bursitis. This is inflammation of the connective tissue that surrounds a joint.

FREQUENT SIGNS AND SYMPTOMS

Pain and tenderness in the heel and sole of the foot under the heel bone. Pain often occurs after resting or after rising in the morning. There may be no pain when sitting. One or both feet can be affected.

CAUSES

Heel pain is usually a result of putting too much stress on the heel bone and the soft connective tissues (called the fascia) that attach to it.

RISK INCREASES WITH

• Running, jogging, or fast walking.
• Previous, or recent, foot or leg injury.
• Poorly cushioned shoes; lack of arch support.
• Prolonged standing; sciatica (leg nerve pain).
• Overweight.

PREVENTIVE MEASURES

• Avoid activities that put constant strain on the foot. Switch to swimming or cycling.
• Wear a shoe with inserts.
• Wear athletic shoes with good shock support in the heels, good flexibility, and good support to control side-to-side motion.
• No more than 1.5-inch heels on everyday shoes.

EXPECTED OUTCOMES

Usually curable with treatment. Different types of treatment work for different people.

POSSIBLE COMPLICATIONS

Soreness and arthritic changes in the heel that place extra stress on joints, such as those in the knee, hip, and spine.

 DIAGNOSIS & TREATMENT

GENERAL MEASURES

• Most people try self-care first. See your health care provider if the pain continues. A physical exam of the foot and ankle will be done. Questions will be asked about your symptoms and activities.

• Medical care may include physical therapy, casts, taping, night splints, injections, ultrasound, orthotics, or surgery. Treatment steps will depend on the symptoms.

• Use ice massage, or soak the heel in ice water. Do this for 15 minutes at a time, 3 or 4 times a day.

• Lightly massage the heel and calf before getting out of bed. Apply heat with a heating pad if it feels good.

• Taping helps some people. Apply athletic tape as directed on the product's instructions.

• Try heel cushions or lifts, arch supports, or medial wedge supports (available at sporting-goods stores and drug stores). Use products in both shoes so that other problems don't develop. Custom orthotics (inserts designed for an individual) may be helpful.

• Purchase shoes that fit well. Sandals help some people. Break in new shoes slowly by wearing them a few minutes per day to start.

• Stretching exercises will help.

MEDICATIONS

• To relieve minor pain, you may use ibuprofen or aspirin (adults only).

• Stronger anti-inflammatory drugs or injections of a steroid drug into the heel to reduce inflammation may be prescribed.

ACTIVITY

Stay off your feet as much as possible, especially at the beginning of treatment.

DIET

No special diet, unless you are overweight. If so, lose weight to reduce stress on the foot.

 NOTIFY OUR OFFICE IF

You or a family member has heel pain that isn't helped by self-care.

Special notes: _____

_____

_____

_____

More notes on the back of this page ☐

225

HEMOPHILIA

 BASIC INFORMATION

DESCRIPTION
An inherited bleeding problem that causes dangerous bleeding. It affects 1 in 10,000 males and appears early in childhood. The two main types of hemophilia occur only in boys. Hemophilia is passed via a gene from mother to son. Most mothers who pass the gene on are carriers of hemophilia and have no symptoms of it.

FREQUENT SIGNS AND SYMPTOMS
· Symptoms often don't occur until the baby starts to crawl or walk. Sometimes, a circumcision procedure causes excess bleeding and is the first symptom.
· Painful, swollen joints or swelling in the leg or arm when bleeding occurs.
· Bruising. Bruises may be large and deep.
· Heavy bleeding from small cuts.
· Nosebleeds.
· Blood in the urine or stool.

CAUSES
Lack of a blood-clotting (coagulation) factor. Clotting is the process by which blood changes from a liquid to a solid substance in order to stop bleeding. There are 13 clotting factors in the body. Hemophilia occurs in three of them. Hemophilia A lacks enough clotting factor VIII. Hemophilia B lacks enough clotting factor IX. Hemophilia C (rare in the United States) lacks enough clotting factor XI.

RISK INCREASES WITH
Family history of the disorder.

PREVENTIVE MEASURES
· Cannot be prevented at present. If your family has a history of this disorder, get genetic counseling before having children. If you are pregnant, talk to your obstetric provider about testing to see if the baby has inherited hemophilia.
· Testing for a female to check her hemophilia carrier status is done with a blood study. Blood studies of other family members are usually needed also.

EXPECTED OUTCOMES
· The disorder is not curable, but it is not fatal. With treatment, patients can have a near-normal life span.
· The disorder may be mild, moderate or severe. It depends on amount of the clotting factor produced.
· Studies looking into causes and treatment continues. There is some hope for better treatment and/or a cure.

POSSIBLE COMPLICATIONS
· Bleeding events needing emergency treatment.
· Joint damage and problems caused by bleeding.
· Adverse reaction to clotting-factor treatment.
· Risk of getting other diseases through donated blood. Risk is less with genetically produced clotting products.

 DIAGNOSIS & TREATMENT

GENERAL MEASURES
· Your child's health care provider will do a physical exam and ask questions about the symptoms and activities. Blood tests can diagnose blood-clotting problems.
· Family education about the disorder is the first step. Parents need to learn how to recognize signs and symptoms of bleeding and how to provide therapy. They need to learn ways to keep a child safe and about appropriate physical activities. Vaccines need to be current.
· Parents need to make sure that anyone (sitters, relatives, teachers) who takes care of a child with hemophilia knows what to do in an emergency.
· Practice good dental hygiene. This helps avoid problems that can cause bleeding, such as pulling a tooth.
· Hospital care to control bleeding may be needed when the bleeding is heavy or unusual.
· A person should wear a medical alert type of identification showing that they have hemophilia.
· To learn more: National Hemophilia Foundation, 116 West 32nd St., 11 Floor, New York, NY 10001, (800) 424-2634; website: www.hemophilia.org.

MEDICATIONS
· Bleeding can be controlled by injections of clotting factor. It can be taken as a preventive measure. Patients can be trained to give themselves the treatment.
· Desmopressin (DDAVP) may be injected into veins or given as a nasal drug. It can help to stimulate a release of the body's own clotting factor.
· Drugs to reduce joint pain may be prescribed.
· Avoid aspirin and other nonsteroidal anti-inflammatory drugs. They can increase bleeding.

ACTIVITY
Exercise daily. Avoid activities that can cause injury, such as contact sports. Swim, bicycle, or walk instead.

DIET
No special diet.

 NOTIFY OUR OFFICE IF

· You or a family member has symptoms of hemophilia.
· Bleeding or other symptoms cause any concern.

Special notes:

_____

_____

_____

More notes on the back of this page ☐

HEMORRHOIDS

 ## BASIC INFORMATION

DESCRIPTION

Swollen veins of the rectum or anus. Hemorrhoids may be located inside of the anal canal, or at the anal opening. Hemorrhoids may be present for years, but go unnoticed until bleeding occurs.

FREQUENT SIGNS AND SYMPTOMS

· Rectal bleeding. Bright-red blood may show as streaks on toilet paper or be a part of a bowel movement. Blood may be a slow trickle for a short while following bowel movements. It almost always colors the toilet water.
· Pain, itching, or discharge after bowel movements.
· A lump or swelling that can be felt in the anus.
· A feeling that the rectum has not emptied completely after a bowel movement.

CAUSES

Repeated pressure on the anal or rectal veins, which causes them to stretch.

RISK INCREASES WITH

· A diet that lacks fiber.
· Prolonged sitting or standing.
· Overweight people.
· Pregnancy.
· Chronic constipation or diarrhea.
· Loss of muscle tone in older adults.
· Rectal surgery or episiotomy.
· Liver disease.
· Anal sex.
· Colon cancer.

PREVENTIVE MEASURES

· Don't try to hurry bowel movements, but do try to avoid straining and prolonged sitting on the toilet.
· Lose weight if you are overweight.
· Include plenty of fiber in your diet.
· Drink 8 to 10 glasses of fluid per day.
· Exercise regularly.

EXPECTED OUTCOMES

Hemorrhoids usually clear up with proper care, but symptoms may come and go. Stubborn cases may require surgery.

POSSIBLE COMPLICATIONS

· Anemia, if there is a lot of blood loss.
· Severe pain caused by a blood clot in a hemorrhoid.
· Infection or inflammation of a hemorrhoid.

 ## DIAGNOSIS & TREATMENT

GENERAL MEASURES

· Your health care provider can diagnose hemorrhoids by a physical exam of the rectal area. Medical tests may be done to check for complications.
· Treatment is aimed at easing the symptoms.
· Never strain to push your stool out.
· When sitting on the toilet, place feet on a low footstool to aid bowel movement.
· Clean the anal area gently with soft, moist paper after each bowel movement.
· To relieve pain, sit in 8 to 10 inches of warm water for 10 to 20 minutes several times a day.
· To reduce pain and swelling of a blood clot or swollen hemorrhoid, stay in bed for 1 day and apply ice packs to the anal area.
· Surgery may be recommended when simple treatment measures are not helping the symptoms.

MEDICATIONS

· For minor pain, itching, or to reduce swelling, you may use drug products to relieve symptoms of hemorrhoids. If these symptoms occur during pregnancy, ask your obstetric provider which drugs are safe to use.
· Use a stool softener, if a laxative is needed.
· Other drugs may be prescribed for complications.

ACTIVITY

Get 30 minutes of exercise on a daily basis. Bowel function improves with good physical fitness.

DIET

· To prevent constipation, eat a well-balanced diet that contains many high-fiber foods.
· Drink 8 to 10 glasses of fluid daily.
· Go on a weight loss diet if you are overweight.

 ## NOTIFY OUR OFFICE IF

· You or a family member has symptoms of hemorrhoids
· Hemorrhoids continue to cause severe pain.
· A hard lump develops where a hemorrhoid has been.
· Rectal bleeding is heavy. Rectal bleeding can be an early sign of cancer.

Special notes:

_____

_____

_____

More notes on the back of this page ☐

HEPATITIS, VIRAL

BASIC INFORMATION

DESCRIPTION
Inflammation of the liver caused by a virus. Viral hepatitis has several types. The most common are type A, type B, and type C. Other types are type D and type E.

FREQUENT SIGNS AND SYMPTOMS
· After an infection occurs, there may be no symptoms, or symptoms may take weeks to months to appear. A person may first have flu-like symptoms, such as fever, fatigue, nausea, vomiting, diarrhea, and loss of appetite.
· Jaundice (yellow eyes and skin) caused by a buildup of bile in the blood.
· Dark urine and light, "clay-colored", or whitish stools.
· Pain in the upper-right abdomen.

CAUSES
· Types A and E: The virus usually enters the body through water or food (especially raw shellfish) that has been contaminated by sewage (fecal-oral contact).
· Type B: Usually sexually transmitted (contact with body fluids of an infected person), or by blood transfusions contaminated with the virus, or from injections with non-sterile needles or syringes. An infected mother can pass it to her newborn. Cause may be unknown.
· Type C: Usually spread through intravenous (IV) drug use, blood transfusions, and other exposures to contaminated blood or its products. Cause may be unknown.
· Type D: Occurs with infection of hepatitis type B.

RISK INCREASES WITH
· Alcoholism, blood transfusions, kidney disease, blood-clotting disorders, organ transplants, having prior sexually transmitted diseases.
· Daycare centers (children and workers, especially those who change diapers).
· Infants born to mothers with hepatitis B or C.
· Health care workers.
· Jobs or work that involves contact with body fluids.
· Close contact with an infected person.
· Getting a tattoo or body piercing.
· People who engage in anal sex, and persons who have multiple sexual partners.
· IV drug abuse or intranasal cocaine use.
· Travel to countries where hepatitis is common.

PREVENTIVE MEASURES
· Avoid the risk factors listed above if possible.
· If exposed to someone with hepatitis, seek medical advice about receiving gamma-globulin injections to prevent or decrease the risk of some types of hepatitis.
· Persons at risk for hepatitis should get hepatitis A and B vaccines (other vaccines are being studied) and immune globulin in addition to vaccine. Your health care provider can advise you if you are in a risk group.
· Routine hepatitis B vaccine for all newborns.

EXPECTED OUTCOMES
Most people recover fully in 1 to 4 months.

POSSIBLE COMPLICATIONS
· Liver disorders that could be fatal. This includes liver cancer.
· Chronic hepatitis. Some patients look and feel well and do not know they are infected. They can still pass the infection on to others. Some patients have symptoms that lead to liver damage (this can take 20 years).

DIAGNOSIS & TREATMENT

GENERAL MEASURES
· Your health care provider will do a physical exam. Medical tests may include blood and urine studies and liver function tests. A liver biopsy may be done by using a needle to remove liver tissue for microscopic exam.
· Acute (short term) hepatitis usually requires little or no treatment. Chronic hepatitis is treated with drugs. Hospital care may be needed for severe symptoms.
· Most patients can be cared for at home. Keeping apart from others is not needed. If you have hepatitis or are caring for someone with it, wash your hands often.
· To learn more: Centers for Disease Control & Prevention (CDC) hotline: (888) 443-7232; website: www.cdc.gov/ncidod/diseases/hepatitis/index.htm.

MEDICATIONS
Interferon, steroids, or antivirals may be prescribed.

ACTIVITY
· Extra rest may be helpful. People differ widely in the rate at which they can return to normal activity.
· Avoid contact sports until blood tests show no virus.
· Food handlers will be advised when to resume work.

DIET
Small, nutritious meals help promote recovery. Drink at least 8 glasses of water a day. Don't drink alcohol.

NOTIFY OUR OFFICE IF

· You or a family member has symptoms of hepatitis or have been exposed to someone who has it.
· Extreme drowsiness, confusion, ongoing vomiting, jaundice lasts over 3 weeks, unusual bleeding or bruising occurs during recovery.

Special notes:

More notes on the back of this page ☐

HEPATOMA

(Liver Cancer; Hepatocellular Carcinoma)

 ## BASIC INFORMATION

DESCRIPTION

A malignant tumor that begins in the liver. This is a primary liver cancer. Cancers that develop elsewhere in the body (such as the breast) and spread to the liver are secondary liver cancers. Hepatoma is more common in men and in those over the age of 40.

FREQUENT SIGNS AND SYMPTOMS

· Hard lump in the right upper abdomen.
· Weight and appetite loss.
· Jaundice (yellow skin and eyes).
· Abdominal pain that feels like a pulled muscle.
· Low blood sugar (weakness, sweating, hunger, tremor, and headache).
· Fever.
· Fluid in the abdomen; enlarged spleen.
· Unusual bleeding.

CAUSES

Exact cause is unknown. There are certain known risk factors.

RISK INCREASES WITH

· Cirrhosis of the liver.
· Alcoholic liver disease.
· Hepatitis types B, C, D, and G infection.
· Family history of liver cancer.
· Alcoholism.
· Misuse of anabolic steroids.
· Geographic locations. This is especially common in South Africa and Southeast Asia.

PREVENTIVE MEASURES

· No specific preventive measures. Steps can be taken to reduce a person's risk factors.
· Avoid alcohol or drink no more than 1 or 2 alcoholic drinks a day.
· Vaccine to prevent hepatitis B in high-risk persons.
· Screening tests for high-risk persons to diagnose and treat cancer at an early stage.

EXPECTED OUTCOMES

· This condition is considered incurable. Only a small number of patients survive 5 years after diagnosis. However, symptoms can sometimes be relieved.
· Research into causes and treatment continues, so there is hope for effective treatment.

POSSIBLE COMPLICATIONS

· Liver failure.
· Internal bleeding.
· Spread to other organs, especially the lungs, adrenal glands, and bones.

 ## DIAGNOSIS & TREATMENT

GENERAL MEASURES

· Your health care provider will do a physical exam and ask questions about your symptoms. Medical tests may include blood studies and liver-function tests. Other tests are usually done to confirm the diagnosis and to determine if cancer has spread (called staging).
· Treatment will depend on the stage of the cancer, your health, and your preferences. The treatments involve surgery, chemotherapy (anticancer drugs), and radiation (less often used). Since most hepatomas cannot be removed by surgery, alternate treatment forms are evolving. These include embolization, radiofrequency ablation, cryotherapy, and injections of alcohol. Your health care provider will discuss the options.
· Surgery is done only for cancer in an early stage. The cancer can still recur, because cancer cells may have spread before surgery.
· Liver transplants have been done in a few select patients.
· Counseling may help in coping with this disorder.
· To learn more: American Cancer Society, (800) ACS-2345; website: www.cancer.org; or National Cancer Institute, (800) -4-CANCER; website: www.nci.nih.gov.

MEDICATIONS

· For minor discomfort, you may use nonprescription drugs such as acetaminophen. Stronger pain relievers will be prescribed as needed.
· Anticancer drugs may be prescribed.

ACTIVITY

Stay as active as your strength allows.

DIET

No special diet. Don't drink alcohol.

 ## NOTIFY OUR OFFICE IF

· You or a family member has symptoms of hepatoma.
· Signs of bleeding develop, especially from the gastrointestinal tract. Signs include bloody vomit or vomit that contains black material resembling coffee grounds, blood in the stool, or black, tarry stools.

Special notes:

_____

_____

_____

More notes on the back of this page ☐

HERNIA

 BASIC INFORMATION

DESCRIPTION

A part of a body organ or tissue protrudes (pokes out) through the muscle wall that normally holds it in place. The most common types involve the lower torso (abdominal wall area). They include:
- Inguinal hernia and femoral hernia (both involve muscles in the groin).
- Incisional hernia (involves muscles at the site of a prior surgery).
- Umbilical hernia (in newborns, involves muscles around the navel).
- Epigastric hernia (occurs in the upper abdomen, between the breastbone and the navel).
- Periumbilical hernia (develops around the navel, more common in women).

FREQUENT SIGNS AND SYMPTOMS
- A swelling, lump, or bulge in the abdomen. It may be more apparent when standing or coughing. It may reduce in size when pushed back into the abdomen or when lying down.
- Heavy feeling, discomfort, or pain may occur in the abdomen, especially when bending over or lifting.
- Constipation.

CAUSES
Weakness in muscle wall or connective tissue (called fascia). The weakness may be present at birth or acquired later in life. Incisional hernias result from previous surgery.

RISK INCREASES WITH
- Premature infants.
- Adults over 60.
- Chronic cough or chronic lung disease.
- Obesity or overweight.
- Pregnancy.
- Straining, as with chronic constipation.
- Family history of hernias.
- Heavy lifting.

PREVENTIVE MEASURES
- Most hernias cannot be avoided. Maintaining proper weight and regular exercise to keep muscles toned may help prevent some types of hernias.
- Seek medical help if constipation or a chronic cough are problems.

EXPECTED OUTCOMES
Umbilical hernias usually heal on their own by age 4 and rarely require surgery. Other hernias are usually curable with surgery.

POSSIBLE COMPLICATIONS
- Strangulated hernia (loses its blood supply). It may cause serious complications, sometimes fatal.
- Hernia may recur after surgery.
- Surgery complications may develop.

 DIAGNOSIS & TREATMENT

GENERAL MEASURES
- Your health care provider will usually diagnose the hernia by means of a physical exam. An x-ray or ultrasound may be done if any complications are suspected.
- Surgery is usually advised to repair the hernia (called a herniorrhaphy). Many hernia repairs can now be done by laparoscopy. Surgery is usually done on an outpatient basis. In most cases, the surgery is elective (performed by choice), but there may be an emergency if the hernia is strangulated.
- If the hernia is causing only mild discomfort and can readily be pushed back, a supportive garment or truss may be used for treatment. This may be done if surgery is not possible or surgery needs to be delayed. See your health care provider for periodic exams of the hernia.

MEDICATIONS
For minor discomfort, you may use nonprescription drugs such as acetaminophen or ibuprofen.

ACTIVITY
- Speed of recovery will depend on general heath and the type of hernia repaired. Work and regular activities can usually be resumed in a week (or as advised). Complete recovery can take 4 to 6 weeks. Avoid heavy lifting for about 3 months.
- Your health care provider will advise you about returning to sports or exercise activities.

DIET
- Eat a diet high in fiber to avoid constipation.
- Maintain ideal weight.

 NOTIFY OUR OFFICE IF

- You or a family member has symptoms of a hernia.
- If you have vomiting, fever, severe pain, or are unable to have a bowel movement. Call immediately! This can be an emergency.

Special notes:

_____

_____

_____

More notes on the back of this page ☐

HERPANGINA

 ## BASIC INFORMATION

DESCRIPTION
A virus of the mouth and throat. It may be mistaken for canker sores, strep throat, or herpes. It most often affects young children (1 to 10 years).

FREQUENT SIGNS AND SYMPTOMS
· Fever.
· Sudden sore throat, with redness, swelling, and painful swallowing.
· Tiny blisters in the affected areas. The blisters become small ulcers (open sores).
· General ill feeling.
· Vomiting and stomach pain (sometimes).

CAUSES
Infection from a virus (usually coxsackie) that is spread from person-to-person. Symptoms appear from 2 to 14 days (average time is 3 to 5 days) after being exposed. If blisters appear on the palms or soles, it is a different disorder called hand, foot and mouth disease.

RISK INCREASES WITH
· Summer and early fall seasons.
· Children in daycare or school where the infection is occurring.

PREVENTIVE MEASURES
· Cannot be prevented at present.
· Wash hands carefully to prevent its spread.
· Avoid close personal contact with infected persons, such as kissing or sharing food.

EXPECTED OUTCOMES
Rapid recovery in a few days to a week.

POSSIBLE COMPLICATIONS
There are usually no complications.

 ## DIAGNOSIS & TREATMENT

GENERAL MEASURES
· Your health care provider usually diagnoses the disorder by an exam of the blisters in the mouth and throat.
· Usually no treatment is needed other than simple pain relievers.
· Careful handwashing is important to help prevent the infection from being spread to other children.

MEDICATIONS
· You may use nonprescription drugs, such as acetaminophen or ibuprofen, to relieve pain and fever. Don't give aspirin to children under age 18.
· Antibiotics do not help a viral infection such as this.

ACTIVITY
· Extra rest until the fever and sore throat disappear.
· A child may be kept at home from daycare or school for a few days if symptoms are present.

DIET
No special diet. Drink extra fluids, such as water, fruit ices, ice chips, or cool-gelatin solutions. Avoid acidic fruit juices, which irritate inflamed tissues.

 ## NOTIFY OUR OFFICE IF

Your child has symptoms of herpangina.

Special notes:

_____

_____

_____

More notes on the back of this page ☐

HERPES, GENITAL

 ## BASIC INFORMATION

DESCRIPTION
An infection caused by one of two types of herpes simplex virus (HSV). Herpes type 2 virus (HSV-2) is the usual cause of genital herpes. Herpes type 1 virus (HSV-1) causes common cold sores around the mouth, but can also cause genital herpes. Genital herpes can affect any sexually active male or female.

FREQUENT SIGNS AND SYMPTOMS
• No symptoms may occur or they may not be noticed. A person may not realize they are infected.
• Early symptoms may include itching or burning in the genital or anal area. This may be followed by pain. Women may have vaginal discharge.
• Within a few days, sores appear in the vaginal area, on the penis, around the anal opening, on the buttocks, thighs, or the mouth. The sores start as red bumps, then turn into a cluster of blisters, that open and cause pain. They then crust over and heal. There is no scarring.
• First episode may include a general ill feeling, difficult and painful urination, swollen lymph glands, and fever.
• Symptoms can recur since the virus permanently remains in the body. Future outbreaks may be milder. They may occur several times a year in some, but others may have only one or two outbreaks in a lifetime.

CAUSES
Having sex (intercourse or oral sex) with someone who is having a herpes outbreak. An outbreak means that HSV is active and usually causes visible sores in the genital area. The sores shed the virus that can infect another person. In some cases, a person may have an outbreak with no visible sores. They can still shed the virus and infect the other person.

RISK INCREASES WITH
Anyone who is sexually active.

PREVENTIVE MEASURES
Avoid sexual intercourse, oral or anal sex, or skin-to-skin contact if either partner has blisters or sores. Use a latex (rubber) condom during intercourse if either sex partner has inactive genital herpes.

EXPECTED OUTCOMES
Genital herpes cannot be cured. During symptom-free periods, the virus returns to its dormant (inactive) state. Symptoms recur when the virus is reactivated. The symptoms vary from person to person and from time to time in the same person. Symptoms and recurrence can be relieved with treatment.

POSSIBLE COMPLICATIONS
Complications are rare in otherwise healthy persons. A person with a weak immune system may have more severe and prolonged outbreaks.

 ## DIAGNOSIS & TREATMENT

GENERAL MEASURES
• Your health care provider can usually diagnose the disorder by an exam of the affected area. Medical tests may include blood studies or studies of fluid taken from the sores.
• Treatment goals are to relieve the symptoms and prevent recurrences. Treatment steps may include drugs and self-care.
• For self-care, keep the affected area clean and dry. Avoid touching the sores, but if you do, wash your hands right away. Warm baths with a tablespoon of salt added can ease some of the discomfort.
• Certain "triggers" can lead to outbreaks. They include skin friction, sex, stress, sunlight/sunburn, wind, fever, surgery, menstruation, infection, and some drugs. A person will begin to recognize their triggers and take steps to avoid them.
• Consider counseling for problems of emotional stress.
• If you are pregnant and have herpes, be sure to advise your obstetric provider so any safeguards can be taken.
• Women should have an annual pelvic exam and Pap smear.
• To learn more: Herpes Resource Center, P.O. Box 13827, Research Triangle Park, NC 27709; hotline (919) 361-8488 (not toll-free); website: www.ashastd.org/hrc.

MEDICATIONS
Antiviral drugs in oral form are often prescribed for treatment and prevention of outbreaks. A topical form is available, but it is not as effective.

ACTIVITY
• No limits on daily activities.
• Avoid sexual relations until symptoms disappear.

DIET
No special diet.

 ## NOTIFY OUR OFFICE IF

• You or a family member has symptoms of genital herpes.
• Symptoms don't improve in 1 week, despite treatment.

Special notes:

_____

_____

_____

More notes on the back of this page ☐

HERPES ZOSTER

(Shingles)

BASIC INFORMATION

DESCRIPTION

A condition that causes pain, a rash, and blisters on the skin. You can get it only if you have had chickenpox in the past. It can affect all ages, including children, but is most common in adults over age 50.

FREQUENT SIGNS AND SYMPTOMS

· It starts with pain, tingling, or burning on the skin.
· A rash appears a few days after the first symptoms begin. It appears as a band of reddened skin on one side of the chest, neck, or face. The rash turns into fluid-filled blisters. These may itch or be very painful. The blisters then begin to dry out and crust over within several days.
· Mild chills and fever.
· General ill feeling.
· Mild nausea, stomach ache cramps, or diarrhea.
· Chest pain, face pain, or burning pain in the skin of the stomach, depending on the affected area.

CAUSES

Herpes zoster is caused by the varicella-zoster virus, the same virus that causes chickenpox. After a chickenpox infection, the virus remains inactive in nerve cells in the body. In some people, the virus becomes active again and causes zoster. Why this happens is unknown.

RISK INCREASES WITH

· Anyone who has had chickenpox.
· Adults over 50.
· Cancer.
· High stress situations.
· People who have a weak immune system due to drugs or illness.

PREVENTIVE MEASURES

Cannot be prevented at present. Vaccines being tested for chickenpox have not helped prevent zoster.

EXPECTED OUTCOMES

The rash usually clears in 14 to 21 days. The nerve pain may last for a month or longer. One attack usually provides immunity against herpes zoster, but a few persons have had more than one attack.

POSSIBLE COMPLICATIONS

· Skin infection may occur in the herpes zoster blisters.
· Chronic pain, especially in the elderly. It lasts for months or years in the nerves where the blisters have been. This is called post-herpetic neuralgia.
· Spread of zoster over the body or to internal organs.
· If the face is affected, eye complications can occur.
· When blisters are present, herpes zoster patients can spread the virus and cause chickenpox in people who have never had it. Avoid physical contact with pregnant women, infants, and those with weak immune systems.

DIAGNOSIS & TREATMENT

GENERAL MEASURES

· Your health care provider can usually diagnose the disorder by a skin exam of the affected area and asking questions about your pain symptoms. If the rash has not appeared, it is more difficult to diagnose. Medical tests may be done to confirm the diagnosis.
· Goals of treatment are to relieve the itching and the pain as much as possible. This is usually done with topical and oral drugs. The nerve pain that remains after the skin clears up is the most difficult to treat.
· For self-care:
  - When bathing, wash blisters gently.
  - Don't bandage the blistered area.
  - Try applying cool, moist compresses to help decrease the pain.
  - Soak in a tub of water to which cornstarch or an oatmeal product (such as Aveeno) has been added.

MEDICATIONS

· Use calamine lotion or capsaicin ointment for the blisters. For minor pain and discomfort, you may use drugs such as aspirin (not for children), acetaminophen, or ibuprofen.
· You may be prescribed one or more drugs to help treat the symptoms. Antiviral drugs can help if the disorder is diagnosed early. Injections of a nerve block may be recommended in severe cases.
· Other drugs for pain may be prescribed. Different ones may need to be tried, as they are not always effective for every person.

ACTIVITY

No limit, except those caused by the symptoms.

DIET

Maintain a healthy diet.

NOTIFY OUR OFFICE IF

· You or a family member has symptoms of herpes zoster.
· Pain gets worse, despite treatment.
· New symptoms develop. Drugs may have side effects.

Special notes:

_____

_____

_____

More notes on the back of this page ☐

HIATAL HERNIA

 BASIC INFORMATION

DESCRIPTION

A part of the stomach protrudes (pokes) through the diaphragm into the chest. The diaphragm is a thin muscle between the chest and the stomach. The esophagus (the tube from the mouth) connects to the stomach through an opening in the diaphragm called the hiatus. A hiatus may become weak and allow part of the stomach to push up through the weak area and into the chest. This becomes a hiatal hernia. It is a common problem, and it often affects older persons, especially women.

FREQUENT SIGNS AND SYMPTOMS

Hiatal hernias do not usually cause symptoms. A person with a hiatal hernia may be more likely to have reflux or it may make existing reflux worse. Reflux occurs when stomach acid backs up into the esophagus. This can lead to heartburn symptoms such as burning in the chest after a meal.

CAUSES

A person may be born with a hiatal hernia or develop one as they get older. An injury or surgery may lead to the problem also.

RISK INCREASES WITH

- Muscle weakness and loss of elasticity (ability of muscles to stretch and regain shape) due to aging.
- Injury or surgery of the diaphragm.
- Obesity.
- Lifting or straining.
- Pregnancy (it increases pressure in the abdomen).
- Ascites (excess fluid in the abdomen).
- Smoking.

PREVENTIVE MEASURES

There are no specific preventive measures.

EXPECTED OUTCOMES

Reflux and heartburn symptoms can usually be relieved with treatment.

POSSIBLE COMPLICATIONS

- Esophageal complications.
- Gastroesophageal reflux disease (GERD).

 DIAGNOSIS & TREATMENT

GENERAL MEASURES

- Your health care provider will usually do a physical exam and ask about your symptoms and eating habits. Medical tests may include x-rays of the esophagus and stomach. An endoscopy (the passing of a tube with a camera on the end into the esophagus) may be done.

- The goals of treatment are to relieve any reflux symptoms and to manage and prevent complications.
- Raise the head of your bed 4 to 6 inches. This allows gravity to keep stomach acid away from the hernia.
- Don't smoke. Find a way to stop that works for you.
- Don't wear tight pantyhose, girdles, belts, or pants.
- Don't strain with bowel movements or urination.
- Surgery to repair the hernia may be recommended for certain patients with complications of GERD or other health problems, such as chronic lung disease. Some repairs can now be done by laparoscopy.

MEDICATIONS

- Antacids in table or liquid form. These are most effective for some persons when they take them 1 hour before meals and at bedtime. Others find them more helpful 1 to 2 hours after meals and at bedtime. Try both ways to find the best schedule for you.
- Use stool softeners to prevent constipation.
- Nonprescription or prescription drugs called H2-receptor blockers or proton pump inhibitors are often prescribed for symptoms.
- Drugs that help the stomach empty more quickly may be prescribed.

ACTIVITY

Don't bend over or lie down right after a meal.

DIET

- Avoid large meals. Eat 6 small meals a day instead. Eat slowly. Don't eat anything 1 to 2 hours before bedtime.
- A diet with more fiber may help prevent constipation.
- Lose weight, if you are overweight.
- Avoid alcohol, caffeine-containing drinks (coffee, tea, cocoa, cola drinks), and any other food, juice, or spice that may cause symptoms.

 NOTIFY OUR OFFICE IF

- You or a family member has symptoms of heartburn.
- Call immediately if pain occurs along with shortness of breath, sweating, or nausea.
- You vomit blood or have recurrent vomiting.
- Fever occurs.
- Symptoms don't improve in 1 month with treatment.

Special notes:

_____

_____

_____

More notes on the back of this page ☐

HICCUP
(Hiccough, Singultus)

 BASIC INFORMATION

DESCRIPTION
Hiccups are a symptom, not a disease. Hiccups involve the diaphragm (the large, thin muscle that separates the chest from the abdomen) and the phrenic nerve (the nerve that connects the diaphragm to the brain). Almost everybody gets hiccups, even unborn babies.

FREQUENT SIGNS AND SYMPTOMS
A sharp, quick sound produced from the mouth by a spasm of the diaphragm. The spasm closes muscles in the back of the throat.

CAUSES
Irritation of nerves that control breathing muscles, especially the diaphragm. The cause of short hiccup episodes is usually unknown. Prolonged or recurrent hiccup episodes may be caused by many different medical problems.

RISK INCREASES WITH
- Swallowing hot or irritating substances.
- Diseases of the pleura (thin membrane layers that cover the lung).
- Pneumonia.
- Uremia (a blood infection).
- Alcoholism.
- Disorders of the stomach, esophagus, bowel, or pancreas.
- Pregnancy.
- Bladder irritation.
- Hepatitis of the liver.
- Spread of cancer from another part of the body to the liver or part of the pleura.
- Recent surgery, especially abdominal surgery.
- Emotional causes.
- Use of drugs, such as those that irritate the stomach.
- Full stomach.
- Laughter or intense emotions.
- Changes in temperature.
- Alcohol use.
- Noxious fumes (bad smells in the air).

PREVENTIVE MEASURES
Cannot be prevented at present.

EXPECTED OUTCOMES
Short hiccup episodes usually don't indicate disease. They will go away on their own or with treatment. Continued hiccups can be a problem and require medical care to find and treat the cause.

POSSIBLE COMPLICATIONS
None, unless hiccups are prolonged, which may indicate a medical problem.

 DIAGNOSIS & TREATMENT

GENERAL MEASURES
- These instructions are for short hiccup episodes. Prolonged hiccups require medical care. Try one or more methods to see which works best for you.
  - Hold your breath and count to 10.
  - Breathe into a paper bag, and rebreathe air in the bag. Don't use a plastic bag because it may cling to nostrils.
  - Insert your thumb between your teeth and upper lip; press the upper lip with your index finger just below the right nostril.
  - Press a forefinger into each ear for about 20 seconds.
  - Drink a glass of water rapidly.
  - Swallow dry bread or crushed ice.
  - Pull gently on the tongue.
  - Close eyelids and apply gentle pressure to the eyeballs.
  - Swallow a teaspoon of dry sugar.
- See your health care provider if hiccups continue or recur often. A physical exam will be done and questions asked about your symptoms and activities. Medical tests are usually not needed, but may be done to check for a suspected medical problem.
- In rare cases, drugs or nerve surgery may be needed for severe, persistent hiccups.

MEDICATIONS
Usually no drugs are needed for this disorder. In some severe or prolonged cases, drugs may be prescribed to help control the hiccups.

ACTIVITY
No limits.

DIET
Avoid overeating or drinking carbonated drinks.

 NOTIFY OUR OFFICE IF

- Hiccups persist longer than 8 hours.
- You suspect a prescription drug may be the cause of hiccups.

Special notes:

_____

_____

_____

More notes on the back of this page ☐

HIDRADENITIS SUPPURATIVA

 BASIC INFORMATION

DESCRIPTION
Hydradenitis means inflammation of the sweat glands. Suppurative means there is pus. The armpits are usually affected, but it can occur on the buttocks, groin, or under the breasts in females. It can affect both sexes, but is more common in young females.

FREQUENT SIGNS AND SYMPTOMS
Nodular lesions (sores) with the following features:
- They are firm, tender, and domed.
- Larger ones soften in the center and become painful.
- When pressed, they feel like an overfilled inner tube.
- They open, and often drain pus.
- Individual lesions (with or without drainage) heal slowly over 10 to 30 days.
- Scars are left on the skin after healing.
- Severity of the disorder varies from a few lesions per year to several lesions that form as old ones heal. They often show up at the same place on the skin.

CAUSES
Exact cause is unknown. The apocrine glands (a form of sweat glands) in the body seem to cause the problem. Substances in these glands enlarge the gland. The outlets become blocked, probably by heat, sweat, or incomplete gland development. The substances that are in the glands force sweat and bacteria into skin tissue, which then becomes infected.

RISK INCREASES WITH
- Exposure to heat and moisture.
- Family history. This disorder is most common in black females.
- Smoking may be a risk factor.
- Obesity does not cause the disorder, but may make it worse.

PREVENTIVE MEASURES
No specific preventive measures.

EXPECTED OUTCOMES
This disorder may last many years, from puberty through the following 10 to 20 years. Symptoms can often be controlled with treatment. There is no cure for this disorder.

POSSIBLE COMPLICATIONS
- Extensive lesions that do not respond to treatment.
- Scarring may restrict movement of arm.
- Other medical problems due to infection or inflammation.

 DIAGNOSIS & TREATMENT

GENERAL MEASURES
- Your health care provider can usually diagnose the disorder by an exam of the affected area. Medical tests may be done to check for infection or other problems.
- Treatment usually involves self-care measures, drug therapy, and sometimes surgery.
- Avoid getting overheated and sweating.
- Avoid tight clothing or clothes that irritate the skin.
- Wash with antibacterial soap. A liquid form may be used for washing, and then applied as a lotion. It may help reduce odor.
- Don't shave the infected area.
- Avoid stress if you can. It may make symptoms worse.
- Use soaks to relieve itching and hasten healing. Warm-water soaks are usually more soothing for pain or inflammation. Cool-water soaks feel better for itching.
- Surgery to open and drain abscesses or to remove involved skin may be recommended.

MEDICATIONS
- You may be prescribed:
  - Injection of cortisone drugs directly into the lesions.
  - Antibiotics to fight infection.
  - Hormones to help subdue inflammation.
  - Isotretinoin has been effective in some patients. This is a potent drug, and must be given under medical supervision.
- For minor discomfort, you may use drugs such as acetaminophen.

ACTIVITY
Restrict your activity in hot weather. Avoid working in the heat, if possible. Swimming is an excellent activity.

DIET
No special diet, unless you need to lose weight. Losing weight may help ease the symptoms.

 NOTIFY OUR OFFICE IF

- You or a family member has symptoms of hidradenitis suppurativa.
- Lesions don't improve after 5 days of treatment, or new symptoms develop.

Special notes:

_____

_____

_____

More notes on the back of this page ☐

HIGH CHOLESTEROL

(Hypercholesterolemia)

BASIC INFORMATION

DESCRIPTION

A total cholesterol level that is higher than the healthy range. The medical term is hypercholesterolemia. Cholesterol is a lipid (similar to fat) carried in the blood. It has several important functions in the body, but too much of it can cause problems. The liver makes all the cholesterol the body needs. More cholesterol comes from foods, such as meat, dairy products, and eggs.

FREQUENT SIGNS AND SYMPTOMS

High cholesterol in itself does not cause any symptoms.

CAUSES

Total cholesterol is made up LDL cholesterol and HDL cholesterol. A high level of LDL causes a fatty buildup in the walls of the arteries (blood vessels). That means less blood and oxygen get to the heart. This can lead to heart disease or stroke. LDL is called the "bad" cholesterol. HDL, the "good" cholesterol seems to have a protective effect against heart disease. Triglycerides are another form of fat in the blood. High levels of triglycerides may increase the risk of disease.

RISK INCREASES WITH

· Too much saturated fat and cholesterol in the diet.
· Being overweight.
· Not being physically active.
· Heredity. High cholesterol can run in families.
· Age. As people get older, cholesterol levels rise. For women, LDL levels tend to rise after menopause.

PREVENTIVE MEASURES

· Eat a low-fat, healthy diet.
· Exercise on a routine basis.
· Maintain the proper body weight.
· Cholesterol and triglyceride testing every 3 to 5 years.

EXPECTED OUTCOMES

High cholesterol can be lowered to desired levels with changes in lifestyle, or drugs, if needed.

POSSIBLE COMPLICATIONS

· Heart disease and stroke. Other factors that can increase their risk include:
  - Smoking.
  - Stress.
  - Medical problems, such as diabetes.
  - Use of some drugs.
  - High blood pressure.
  - Age (men over 45, women over 55).
  - Family history of early heart disease.
· Atherosclerosis, which is hardening of the arteries.
· There may be some decrease of kidney function.
· Poor circulation.

DIAGNOSIS & TREATMENT

GENERAL MEASURES

· Your health care provider will have your blood tested for cholesterol levels. The blood test will check for levels of total cholesterol, LDL, HDL, and triglycerides.
· The test results must be looked at on an individual basis, and take into account your other risk factors for heart disease. Cholesterol levels are measured in milligrams per deciliter (mg/dL).
  - Desired level for total cholesterol is less than 200; 200 to 239 is borderline high risk; over 240 is high risk.
  - LDL below 130 is the recommended level; below 100 is ideal; over 160 is high risk.
  - HDL of 60 and above is good; under 40 is high risk.
  - Triglyceride of 150 is borderline high; 200 is high.
· You and your health care provider can decide on an action plan to reduce your risks of heart disease and stroke. This may include changes in diet, more exercise, weight loss, quitting smoking, and drug therapy.
· Diet and lifestyle changes do not mean you have to give up all the good things you enjoy.
· To learn more: American Heart Association, 7272 Greenville Ave., Dallas, TX 75231; (800) 242-8721; website: www.americanheart.org.

MEDICATIONS

Cholesterol-lowering drugs may be prescribed if diet and exercise changes are not effective, or if you are at high risk for heart disease.

ACTIVITY

Increase physical activity. Try to get at least 30 minutes of aerobic exercise (such as walking) every day.

DIET

· Limit foods that contain saturated fats and high amounts of cholesterol. Read food labels carefully.
· Eat a diet that is high in fiber with lots of fruits and vegetables.
· Begin a weight-reduction diet if you are overweight.

NOTIFY OUR OFFICE IF

You or a family member wants to learn your cholesterol levels or needs help with diet and exercise planning.

Special notes:

_____

_____

_____

More notes on the back of this page ☐

HIP FRACTURE

 ## BASIC INFORMATION

DESCRIPTION

A complete or partial break (fracture) in the femur. The femur is the major bone in the hip joint. Breaks from common injuries affect both sexes and all ages. Spontaneous (occurs without an injury) breaks, and breaks from minor injuries, affect mostly older people. Nine out of 10 hip fractures occur in persons over 65, and 3 out of 4 occur in women.

FREQUENT SIGNS AND SYMPTOMS

· Severe pain when trying to walk.
· Pain may occur in the groin or thigh.
· Swelling, tenderness, and bruising in the hip area.
· Deformed hip appearance.

CAUSES

Hip fractures are usually caused by injuries (trauma) such as falls, other types of accidents, and sports injuries. Weakened bones are more at risk of a fracture.

RISK INCREASES WITH

· Female, over age 65, and white.
· Osteoporosis, especially in women after menopause.
· Decreased bone mineral density.
· Falls. Risk of falls increases with muscle weakness, problems with walking or balance, use of certain drugs, disorders such as Parkinson's and stroke, poor eyesight, foot problems, arthritis, previous falls, and home risks.
· Self-reported poor health.
· Family history of hip fracture.
· Sedentary (lack of physical activity) lifestyle.
· Previous fractures of any kind.
· Previous hyperthyroidism.
· Motor vehicle accidents and physical activities such as contact sports for younger hip fracture patients.

PREVENTIVE MEASURES

· Protect against falls, especially in the home.
· Drug therapies to improve bone density.
· Daily exercise program to improve bone strength and to maintain muscle strength and balance.

EXPECTED OUTCOMES

Outcome depends on the age and health of the patient and the location of the fracture. In older persons, there is often a loss of ability to function as they did before the fracture. The function loss may be mild to severe.

POSSIBLE COMPLICATIONS

· Surgical-wound infection, incomplete healing, and other surgery complications.
· Being immobile for a prolonged period can lead to blood clots, pulmonary embolism, pneumonia, and weakened muscles.
· Loss of mobility (may require wheelchair use), loss of independence, reduced quality of life, and depression.

 ## DIAGNOSIS & TREATMENT

GENERAL MEASURES

· Self-care is not appropriate. Hospital care with surgery is the main treatment. The surgeon reattaches fractured bone parts and secures them with surgical steel pins; the surgeon may replace body parts with a medical device (complete hip or parts of a hip) in people whose bones can no longer grow back together. Unlike most fractures, hip fractures usually don't require casts.
· After surgery, time is usually spent in a rehabilitation center for therapy to help regain mobility and functions of daily living.
· Ongoing physical therapy may be needed to continue to rehabilitate the muscles, bones, and joints.

MEDICATIONS

· Pain relievers as needed may be prescribed.
· Antibiotics for infection and blood thinners to prevent blood clots may be prescribed after surgery.
· Stool softeners to prevent constipation.
· Drugs to increase bone mass and to prevent bone loss may be prescribed.

ACTIVITY

· After surgery, move the unaffected leg often to decrease the risk of deep-vein blood clots. Most patients are urged to get up and move about as soon as possible.
· A physical therapist will be needed for rehabilitation, which can take several months. A walker or crutches will be used at first. Swimming and riding an exercise bike are good forms of therapy.
· Resume your normal activities to the extent possible as healing progresses.

DIET

Clear liquids for the 1st day after surgery, then no special diet. Increased calcium may be recommended.

 ## NOTIFY OUR OFFICE IF

· You or a family member has symptoms of a hip fracture. Call immediately if you have numbness or loss of feeling below the fracture site. This is an emergency!
· Any new symptoms develop after surgery.

Special notes:

_____

_____

_____

More notes on the back of this page ☐

HIRSUTISM

BASIC INFORMATION

DESCRIPTION

Hirsutism is increased growth of hair on the face and body that occurs in women. It usually occurs gradually over an extended period of time. It may begin with puberty. Hirsutism is a benign condition and is mostly a cosmetic problem. When it occurs along with signs of masculinity (maleness), a more serious disorder may be involved.

FREQUENT SIGNS AND SYMPTOMS

• Excessive growth of thick, dark hair in body areas of women where hair growth is normally absent or minimal. It grows in a male pattern (beard, moustache, chest, around the nipples, genitals, and other places).
• Hair growth may occur along with irregular or absent menstrual periods, acne, deepening of the voice, and infertility problems.

CAUSES

It may be due to genetic (hereditary) factors, hormonal dysfunction, certain drugs, and some medical disorders. In some cases, no cause is found.

RISK INCREASES WITH

• Family history of hirsutism.
• Dark-haired persons, especially those of Hispanic, African-American, Mediterranean, or Indian ancestry.
• Use of drugs such as testosterone, steroids, and others.
• Adrenal disorders.
• Adrenal or ovarian tumor.
• Polycystic ovarian syndrome.
• Anorexia, acromegaly, hypothyroidism, or porphyria.

PREVENTIVE MEASURES

There are no specific preventive measures.

EXPECTED OUTCOME

Diagnosis and treatment of the cause can often halt further hair growth. Treatment may take 6 to 12 months. Excess hair may be removed by various methods.

POSSIBLE COMPLICATIONS

• Poor self-image. May feel unattractive, stressed, anxious, and find social activities with other people difficult.
• Complications may occur from underlying disorder.

DIAGNOSIS & TREATMENT

GENERAL MEASURES

• Your health care provider will do a physical exam. A variety of medical tests may be done to help diagnose any disorder that could be the cause of the hair growth.

• The treatment depends on the cause of the hirsutism. A mild case of hirsutism with no menstrual problems may not require treatment. For others, treatment sometimes depends on the patient's desire for pregnancy.
• Treatment may involve drugs, surgery, and hair removal techniques.
• Tumors may be treated with surgery.
• Cosmetic treatments of hirsutism include covering up with makeup, bleaching, and removal with physical methods. These include rubbing, cutting, shaving, plucking, or waxing. Chemical depilatories are designed to use on specific body locations. Home hair-removal devices are available. All of these methods are temporary; their effects lasting from hours to days.
• Permanent hair removal may be done with electrolysis or thermolysis. These use an electric current to remove hair. Multiple treatments are needed. It is time-consuming, can be costly, and cause some discomfort.
• Permanent hair removal may be done with a laser. Larger areas can be treated quickly and with minimal discomfort. Multiple treatments are needed. It is costly.
• Newer forms of hair removal include pulsed light and photodynamic (use of a topical drug and special light).
• The various forms of hair removal can cause skin irritation, folliculitis (inflamed hair follicles), skin color changes, and, rarely, scarring.

MEDICATION

• There are a variety of drugs used to treat the underlying cause of hirsutism. They may take 3 to 6 months for results. They can help decrease new hair growth. They will not change the amount of hair you already have.
• Eflornithine (Vaniqa), a topical drug, may be prescribed for reducing facial hair.
• If skin gets irritated, use nonprescription 1% hydrocortisone cream.
• If a drug is causing hirsutism, it is usually stopped.

ACTIVITY

Usually no limits.

DIET

No special diet. If overweight, losing weight may help.

NOTIFY OUR OFFICE IF

• You or a family member has symptoms of hirsutism.
• Hair growth continues despite treatment.

Special notes:

_____

_____

_____

_____

More notes on the back of this page ☐

HISTOPLASMOSIS

 BASIC INFORMATION

DESCRIPTION
A fungus infection that normally affects people who live in eastern and Midwestern parts of the United States. Most cases are minor and go undiagnosed. It can involve the lungs, central nervous system, and gastrointestinal system.

FREQUENT SIGNS AND SYMPTOMS
· Frequently, no symptoms are present.
· Persistent cough and other symptoms, similar to a cold.
· Loss of appetite, diarrhea, and weight loss.
· Fever; headache.
· Irritability.
· Paleness.
· Abdominal swelling.
· Breathing difficulty (rare).

CAUSES
Infection by the fungus, *Histoplasma capsulatum*. People become infected by breathing dust that contains fungus spores. The fungus is found in soil contaminated by feces of birds and bats that carry the fungus. This soil is most often found in pigeon lofts, barns, chicken houses, and in damp areas under bridges, along streams, and in caves.

RISK INCREASES WITH
· Geographic location. The disease is normally found in the western Appalachian slopes and the Mississippi, Missouri, and Ohio River valleys. Millions of people living in these areas have been infected, but never have symptoms or they are so mild that they go unnoticed.
· Working in construction-related activities that disturb contaminated soil (e.g., bulldozing or demolition).
· Spelunking (cave exploring).

PREVENTIVE MEASURES
No specific preventive measures. Wear protective masks for work in areas that might be contaminated.

EXPECTED OUTCOMES
· Mild cases usually resolve on their own. Most people only feel tired or "bad" for several weeks.
· Severe cases are treatable with antifungal drugs.

POSSIBLE COMPLICATIONS
· People with weak immune systems or middle-aged smokers are more at risk for complications.
· Spread of infection to other organs. This is rare, but it can be fatal.
· Histoplasmosis often recurs in AIDS patients.
· Eye problems if infection spreads.

 DIAGNOSIS & TREATMENT

GENERAL MEASURES
· Your health care provider will do a physical exam and ask about your symptoms and activities. Medical tests may include sputum culture, blood studies, skin tests, and chest x-ray.
· Treatment is usually with drugs and supportive care.
· Don't smoke.
· Use warm compresses or a heating pad on the chest to relieve pain.

MEDICATIONS
· For mild cases, no medicine is usually necessary.
· For more-severe cases, antifungal drugs will be prescribed. Some may be given intravenously (IV).
· For AIDS patients, chronic therapy with antifungal drugs will be necessary.
· You may use nonprescription drugs, such as acetaminophen or aspirin (not for children), to relieve pain.

ACTIVITY
Stay in bed until fever, pain, and shortness of breath disappear for at least 48 hours. Then resume your normal activities gradually. Many people are tired and weak after recovery. Don't expect too much too soon.

DIET
No special diet.

 NOTIFY OUR OFFICE IF

· You or a family member has symptoms of histoplasmosis.
· The following occur during treatment:
  - Weight loss continues.
  - Fever rises to 101°F (38.3°C) orally.
  - Diarrhea is severe.
  - Severe headache and stiff neck occur.

Special notes:

_____

_____

_____

More notes on the back of this page ☐

HIV & AIDS (Human Immunodeficiency Virus; Acquired Immunodeficiency Syndrome)

BASIC INFORMATION

DESCRIPTION

Human immunodeficiency virus (HIV) is a virus that gradually destroys the body's ability to fight infection and certain cancers. Acquired immunodeficiency syndrome (AIDS) is a secondary immunodeficiency syndrome resulting from HIV infection.

FREQUENT SIGNS AND SYMPTOMS

- Initial infection with HIV may produce no symptoms.
- Fatigue and unexplained weight loss.
- Recurrent respiratory and skin infections and fever.
- Swollen lymph glands throughout the body.
- Genital changes.
- Diarrhea.
- Mouth sores.
- Night sweats.

CAUSES

HIV is a virus (retrovirus) that invades and destroys cells of the body's immune system.

RISK INCREASES WITH

- Sexual contact with infected persons. Homosexual men are at the greatest risk.
- Multiple sexual partners (particularly anal intercourse).
- Contaminated needles used by IV drug abusers.
- Transfusions of blood or blood products from a person with acquired immunodeficiency syndrome (rare).
- Children born to an HIV infected mother.
- Exposure of hospital workers and laboratory technicians to blood, feces, and urine of HIV-positive patients. Greatest risk is with an accidental needle injury.
- Note: Nonsexual contact does not transmit the disease. A person with HIV infection is not a risk to the general population.

PREVENTIVE MEASURES

- Avoid sexual contact with HIV-affected persons or known IV drug users. Limit sexual activity to partners whose sexual histories are known.
- Use condoms for vaginal and anal intercourse. Their consistent use may reduce transmission.
- The risk of oral sex is not fully known. Ejaculation into the mouth should be avoided.
- Avoid IV drugs. Do not share unsterilized needles.
- Avoid unscreened blood products. Some of the foreign countries may not test the blood as the United States does.
- Infected people or those in risk groups are advised not to donate blood, sperm, organs, or tissue.
- Early diagnosis is helpful. If you are at risk, obtain a medical test even if you feel well. If you plan to be, or are pregnant, HIV testing can be helpful.

EXPECTED OUTCOME

This condition is currently considered incurable. Symptoms can be relieved or controlled. AIDS may not develop for years following a positive HIV test. Once ill, survival averages vary.

POSSIBLE COMPLICATIONS

Serious infections; cancer; death.

DIAGNOSIS & TREATMENT

GENERAL MEASURES

- Your health care provider will do a physical exam and ask questions about your sexual history. Medical tests may include blood studies and an HIV antibody test. It may not become positive for 6 months after exposure to HIV. Tests for other sexually transmitted diseases and infections are usually done.
- Treatment incudes drug therapy and self-care. Hospital care may be needed for complications.
- Advise past/present sexual partners to get HIV tests.
- Counseling helps a person cope with having HIV.
- Get regular medical and dental check-ups. Tell any health care provider you consult that you have HIV.
- Avoid exposure to people with infections.
- Join a support group.
- To learn more: National AIDS Hotline: (800) 342-2437; website: www.cdc.gov/hiv/dhap.htm.

MEDICATION

Drugs to treat HIV and AIDS, and drugs to treat infections or complications will be prescribed.

ACTIVITY

Fatigue or infections can limit some activities. Get the rest you need, but try to exercise to the extent possible.

DIET

Try to maintain good nutrition. Poor eating habits, changes in metabolism, and weight loss are common.

NOTIFY OUR OFFICE IF

- You or a family member has symptoms of HIV.
- Any infections occur after diagnosis. Symptoms include fever, cough, and diarrhea.
- Other new symptoms develop. Drugs used in treatment have many side effects.

Special notes:

_____

_____

_____

More notes on the back of this page ☐

HIVES
(Urticaria; Giant Urticaria)

 BASIC INFORMATION

DESCRIPTION
An allergic reaction that involves the skin. Hives may occur anywhere on the body, but the arms, legs, and trunk are most often affected. Urticaria is the medical name for hives. Hives are very common and can affect any age group.

FREQUENT SIGNS AND SYMPTOMS
• Raised, red areas on the skin. They may be referred to as wheals or welts. They usually itch, but they may also burn or sting. The size may range from small spots to the size of a dinner plate. They can sometimes cause the whole lip or eyelid to swell.
• Wheals can join together quickly and form large, flat plaques. These are raised, skin-colored areas.
• Wheals and plaques change shape, go away, and come back in minutes or hours.

CAUSES
Release of histamines. These are chemicals in the cells of the human body that are released during an allergic reaction. They may be released due to a specific reaction or in some cases for unknown reasons.

RISK INCREASES WITH
• Drugs. Nearly all drugs cause hives in some persons.
• Insect bites; viral infections; some chronic medical disorders.
• Exposure to cold, heat, water, or sunlight.
• Exposure to animals, especially cats.
• Eating eggs, fruits, nuts, and shellfish. Other foods sometimes cause hives in infants but not in adults.
• Food dyes and preservatives (possibly).
• Infection (bacterial, viral, fungal).
• Cancer, especially leukemia.
• Other factors include: physical and emotional stress, other allergies, or a family history of allergies.

PREVENTIVE MEASURES
• There are no specific preventive measures to stop the first outbreak of hives. Once you have had hives and know the cause, you need to avoid it in the future.
• Your health care provider may advise you to keep an emergency kit handy if you have had severe reactions.

EXPECTED OUTCOMES
Hives usually clear up within hours or days (even if the cause is unknown). They can be uncomfortable, but normally they cause no complications. A few cases become chronic and may last for weeks.

POSSIBLE COMPLICATIONS
• Other allergic reactions may occur with hives:
  - Angioedema (face, throat, and tongue swelling).
  - Anaphylaxis (severe reaction that causes shock and difficulty in breathing).

 DIAGNOSIS & TREATMENT

GENERAL MEASURES
• Most persons will treat hives at home. Try to identify the cause of the hives. See your health care provider if the hives are more severe or cause concern. Your health care provider will do a physical exam of the affected skin. Questions will be asked to help identify the cause. Medical tests are usually not needed.
• Treatment usually involves antihistamines, stopping the cause of the hives when known (such as a drug, cosmetic, or soap), and self-care measures. If the reaction is severe, hospital care may be needed.
• Don't wear tight underwear or foundation garments. Any skin irritation may trigger new outbreaks.
• Don't take hot baths or showers.
• Apply cold-water compresses or soaks.
• Try to relax and not become over-stressed.

MEDICATIONS
• Use nonprescription antihistamines for the itching.
• Prescription antihistamines, steroids, or other drugs to relieve itching and rash may be prescribed.
• Epinephrine by injection for severe symptoms.

ACTIVITY
Decrease activities until several days after hives disappear. Avoid getting hot, sweaty, or overly excited.

DIET
• If foods are suspected as a cause, keep a food diary to help identify the offending food.
• Avoid alcohol and coffee or other caffeine-containing beverages if they appear to trigger outbreaks.

 NOTIFY OUR OFFICE IF

• You or a family member has hives that aren't helped by self-care or last for more than 2 days.
• The following occur during an episode of hives:
  - Swollen lips, tongue, or face.
  - Shortness of breath or wheezing.
  - Stomach pain, vomiting, or diarrhea.
  - Any feeling of weakness or faintness.
• New, unexplained symptoms develop. Drugs used in treatment may produce side effects.

Special notes:

_____

_____

_____

More notes on the back of this page ☐

HODGKIN'S DISEASE

 ## BASIC INFORMATION

DESCRIPTION
Malignant cancer of the lymph glands. This is a form of lymphoma. It involves the lymphocytes (white blood cells), lymph glands (glands that check infection and produce immune substances), and spleen (a large lymph gland). Hodgkin's disease can affect all ages, but is most common in young adults and older persons. It is rare in children under 10.

FREQUENT SIGNS AND SYMPTOMS
· Swollen, non-tender, rubbery, distinct lymph glands anywhere in the body, but most commonly in the neck, armpit, or groin.
· Intermittent fever and night sweats.
· Itching all over the body.
· Weight loss.
· Jaundice (yellow skin and eyes).
· General ill feeling.
· Cough.

CAUSES
Unknown, but research suggests a viral infection may be a factor.

RISK INCREASES WITH
People with weak immune systems due to illness or drugs.

PREVENTIVE MEASURES
No specific preventive measures.

EXPECTED OUTCOMES
Usually curable with radiation therapy and anticancer drugs, if diagnosed and treated early. With treatment, the 10-year survival rate is about 80%.

POSSIBLE COMPLICATIONS
· Spread of cancer to other places in the body.
· Infertility in males and females.
· Heart or lung disorders, anemia, hypothyroidism, and infections.
· Cancer may return.

 ## DIAGNOSIS & TREATMENT

GENERAL MEASURES
· Your health care provider will do a physical exam and ask questions about your symptoms and activities. Different medical tests are done to verify the diagnosis and to determine if the cancer has spread to other places in the body (called staging).
· Treatment may be radiation alone, chemotherapy alone, or the two in combination. Treatment will depend on the stage of the disease, your health, and your preferences.
· Radiation therapy may consist of daily treatments, Monday through Friday, for about four weeks. Side effects that occur will stop once treatment is complete.
· Good oral hygiene is important to prevent mouth sores, if receiving chemotherapy.
· Males receiving therapy may want to consider sperm-banking in case of sterility. Females may want to store fertilized eggs.
· Counseling may help you to cope with having cancer.
· To learn more: American Cancer Society, (800) ACS-2345; website: www.cancer.org or National Cancer Institute, (800) 4-CANCER; website: www.nci.nih.gov.

MEDICATIONS
· Anticancer drugs. These may cause side effects or adverse reactions in some people. They may be given as an outpatient or require a hospital stay.
· Steroid drugs may be prescribed for short periods.

ACTIVITY
Remain as active as your strength allows. Regular exercise can help both physical and emotional health.

DIET
No special diet.

 ## NOTIFY OUR OFFICE IF

· You or a family member has symptoms of Hodgkin's disease.
· Any new symptoms develop or other symptoms get worse during treatment.

Special notes:

_____

_____

_____

More notes on the back of this page ☐

HYPERALDOSTERONISM

(Aldosteronism; Conn's Syndrome)

 BASIC INFORMATION

DESCRIPTION

An endocrine disease caused by too much aldosterone, a hormone made by the adrenal gland. Excess aldosterone causes the kidneys to take in too much sodium and water, and eliminate too much potassium. It can affect both sexes (females more than males) and is more common in adults between ages 30 and 50.

FREQUENT SIGNS AND SYMPTOMS

- Fatigue and weakness.
- Temporary paralysis (sometimes).
- Tingling sensations in the arms, legs, hands, and feet.
- Urinary frequency, especially at night.
- Thirst.
- Severe muscle spasms.
- Vision problems.

The following may show up in medical tests:

- Low blood levels of potassium.
- High blood levels of sodium.
- High blood pressure.

CAUSES

- It involves the adrenal glands, which are attached to the upper part of the kidneys. The increased adrenal secretion of aldosterone is caused by:
  - A tumor of the adrenal gland.
  - High blood pressure or kidney disease, causing increased production in the kidneys of a hormone (renin) that controls aldosterone levels.

RISK INCREASES WITH

- Kidney disease.
- Congestive heart failure.
- Cirrhosis of the liver.
- Use of oral contraceptives.
- Use of drugs that cause potassium loss.
- Pregnancy.

PREVENTIVE MEASURES

If you have kidney disease or high blood pressure, remain under medical care, and adhere to your treatment program even if you have no symptoms.

EXPECTED OUTCOMES

If the disorder is caused by an adrenal tumor, it is often curable with surgery. If it is caused by kidney disease or high blood pressure, medical treatment for these disorders will control the symptoms.

POSSIBLE COMPLICATIONS

- Congestive heart failure.
- Atherosclerosis.
- Kidney failure.

 DIAGNOSIS & TREATMENT

GENERAL MEASURES

- Your health care provider will do a physical exam and ask questions about your symptoms. Medical tests may include blood studies of electrolyte levels and CT or MRI scan of the kidneys and adrenal glands.
- Treatment usually involves drugs and a sodium-restricted diet.
- Weigh yourself daily and keep a record. Report a gain of 3 or more pounds in a 24-hour period.
- Surgery to remove adrenal gland in some patients.
- Wear a medical alert bracelet to identify your medical condition and any drugs that you take.

MEDICATIONS

- Drugs to decrease the aldosterone effect may be prescribed. This drug may cause breast enlargement and sexual impotence in men. Other drug options are available.
- Drugs for high blood pressure may be prescribed.

ACTIVITY

No limits, if surgery is not necessary. If it is, resume your normal activities gradually.

DIET

Eat a diet that is low in sodium and high in potassium. Foods rich in potassium include dried apricots and peaches, raisins, citrus fruits, lentils, and whole-grain cereals.

 NOTIFY OUR OFFICE IF

- You or a family member has symptoms of hyperaldosteronism.
- New, unexplained symptoms develop. Drugs used in treatment may produce side effects.

Special notes:

_____

_____

_____

More notes on the back of this page ☐

HYPEREMESIS GRAVIDARUM

Information From Your Health Care Provider

 ## BASIC INFORMATION

DESCRIPTION

Severe nausea and vomiting in a pregnant woman. This is more serious than the typical nausea and vomiting in pregnancy (or morning sickness). Hyperemesis gravidarum usually occurs before the 20th week of pregnancy; often between the fourth and twelfth week.

FREQUENT SIGNS AND SYMPTOMS

· Severe and frequent nausea and vomiting. Symptoms may increase over a few weeks or, sometimes, months.
· Dehydration (less urine, skin may be pale and dry).
· Failure to gain weight, or there is weight loss.
· Unable to eat and maintain proper nutrition.
· Some affected women may have a distinct odor to their breath (ketonic odor).
· Often unable to work, perform daily household tasks and routines, or care for young children.
· Fast heartbeat (sometimes).
· Symptoms may subside and recur (wax and wane).

CAUSES

Unknown. The most common theories involve:
· Changes in hormones.
· Liver or stomach problems.
· Nutrition problems.
· Psychological factors, such as depression or a poor response to stress.
· Thyroid disorder or endocrine imbalance.
· *Helicobacter pylori* (a bacteria that can cause ulcers) may be a factor.

RISK INCREASES WITH

· Younger maternal age.
· First pregnancy.
· Being overweight.
· Multiple-pregnancy (more than one fetus).
· Single marital status.
· Diet high in fat.
· Women with eating disorders.
· Hyperemesis gravidarum in a previous pregnancy.
· Emotional stress.

PREVENTIVE MEASURES

There is no known prevention. To reduce risk, maintain a healthy diet, get adequate sleep, and control stress.

EXPECTED OUTCOME

Usually curable with time and treatment. Pregnancy can continue to the successful delivery of a healthy baby.

POSSIBLE COMPLICATIONS

· Emotional and physical complications may occur.
· May increase the risk of the baby having a lower than normal birth weight.

 ## DIAGNOSIS & TREATMENT

GENERAL MEASURES

· Your obstetric provider will usually do a physical exam and ask questions about your symptoms. Medical tests may be done to check for other health problems.
· Hospital care is often needed to replace lost fluids and electrolytes (substances needed for body function). Fluids are given through a vein (IV) to provide nutrition and relieve dehydration.
· If symptoms are not too severe, home care with diet instructions and rest may be recommended.
· Reduce stress whenever possible. Counseling is often helpful for emotional problems.
· You and your obstetric provider may discuss alternate treatments for nausea and vomiting. These include acupressure wristbands or nerve stimulation device (which have been used to help motion sickness) or hypnosis.
· Weigh daily. Report unusual changes to your obstetric provider.
· To learn more: Hyperemesis Education and Research Organization, P.O. Box 452443, Garland TX, 75045; website: www.hyperemesis.org.

MEDICATION

· Intravenous (IV) fluid, vitamins, and electrolyte replacement may be required.
· Other drugs may be prescribed for nausea.
· Don't use any nonprescription drugs or herbal products to prevent vomiting without medical advice.

ACTIVITY

Increased rest benefits most patients.

DIET

· Avoid those foods or smells that trigger symptoms.
· Drink fluids one half hour before or after meals.
· Eat dry toast or crackers before you get out of bed.
· Eat small, frequent meals. High-protein meals may help nausea. Sit upright for 45 minutes after eating.

 ## NOTIFY OUR OFFICE IF

· You or a family member has symptoms of hyperemesis gravidarum.
· You are unable to keep any food or fluids down for 24 hours.

Special notes:

_____

_____

_____

More notes on the back of this page ☐

HYPERHIDROSIS

 BASIC INFORMATION

DESCRIPTION
A condition of excessive sweating that affects both men and women, and sometimes, children. The excessive sweating may occur for no apparent reason.

FREQUENT SIGNS AND SYMPTOMS
• Heavy sweat from underarm area, soles, palms, and other body parts.
• Sweating occurs without warning or cause.
• The amount of sweating, body parts involved, and when it occurs differs in different people.
• An odor, which is caused by bacteria in sweat.

CAUSES
• Primary hyperhidrosis is the term used when there is no physical cause for the excessive sweating. Sweating is normally regulated by the body's sympathetic nervous system. In some people, this system becomes overactive. Why this occurs is unknown.
• Secondary hyperhidrosis results from a specific factor such as diabetes.

RISK INCREASES WITH
• Secondary hyperhidrosis may be caused by:
  - Diabetes.
  - Hyperthyroidism.
  - Menopause.
  - Some cancers.
  - Some drugs, such as narcotics.
  - Obesity.
  - Certain psychiatric conditions.

PREVENTIVE MEASURES
No specific measures to prevent hyperhidrosis. Steps may be taken to help control the sweating.

EXPECTED OUTCOMES
Secondary hyperhidrosis can often be controlled with treatment of the underlying condition. Primary hyperhidrosis can be helped using a variety of treatment options. No single treatment works for everyone.

POSSIBLE COMPLICATIONS
• Emotional distress caused by social embarrassment.
• Rashes from deodorants or antiperspirants.

 DIAGNOSIS & TREATMENT

GENERAL MEASURES
• Your health care provider will do a physical exam and ask questions about your symptoms and activities. Medical tests may be done to identify any disorder that is causing the excessive sweating.

• Medical care:
  - Treatment will be given for an underlying condition.
  - Counseling, if stress is a major factor.
  - Drugs may be recommended.
  - Electrical devices that temporarily reduce sweating of palms or feet may be recommended.
  - Surgery to remove sweat glands or sever nerves to major sweat areas, in more serious cases.
• Self-care:
  - Bathe often, using a deodorizing soap.
  - Change clothes often.
  - Wear loose-fitting clothes made of natural fibers, such as cotton.
  - Use underarm sweat shields.
  - Use antiperspirants and deodorants. Use an unscented product that contains aluminum chloride.
  - Use drying powders.
  - Wear cotton socks.
  - Wear leather shoes or sandals. Don't wear shoes of man-made materials.
  - Shave underarm hair.

MEDICATIONS
• Drugs to reduce activity of the central nervous system may be prescribed. Side effects can be a problem.
• Prescription antiperspirants may be prescribed.
• Botulinum toxin (Botox) injections may be prescribed. It helps reduce or stop the sweating for 3 to 6 months.
• Other drugs may be prescribed to be taken by mouth or applied to the skin.

ACTIVITY
No limits.

DIET
No special diet. Drink at least 8 glasses of fluid a day.

 NOTIFY OUR OFFICE IF

• Excessive sweating is causing you problems at work or in social situations.
• Treatment for excessive sweating is not working.

Special notes:

More notes on the back of this page ☐

HYPERLIPIDEMIA

BASIC INFORMATION

DESCRIPTION

Hyperlipidemia is the medical term used to describe having high amounts of lipids in the blood. Lipids, such as cholesterol and triglycerides, are fat or fat-like substances that maintain important body functions. They travel in the bloodstream attached to proteins. The lipid-protein combinations are called lipoproteins. Lipoproteins help the lipids get absorbed by the body's cells. Hyperlipidemia is called primary if it is inherited and secondary if it is caused by illness or other health problem. Subcategories of hyperlipidemia include:
- Hypercholesterolemia (high levels of cholesterol).
- Hypertriglyceridemia (high levels of triglycerides).
- Hyperlipoproteinemia (high levels of lipoproteins).

FREQUENT SIGNS AND SYMPTOMS
- There are usually no symptoms. It may be discovered on routine blood studies.
- There may be pinkish-yellow deposits of fat in the skin beneath eyes, elbows, and knees, and in tendons.

CAUSES
- There are five types of lipoproteins—defined by size and density. Two types carry cholesterol and the other three types carry triglycerides.
  - Cholesterol is carried through the blood by high-density lipoproteins (HDL) and low-density lipoproteins (LDL). High levels of LDL and/or low levels of HDL can increase the risk of heart disease and stroke.
  - Triglycerides are carried by three lipoproteins. These are very low-density lipoprotein (VLDL), intermediate density lipoproteins (IDL), and chylomicrons. High triglyceride levels may increase the risk of heart disease and stroke.
- Guidelines suggest that to reduce risks, HDL should be above 40, LDL should be below 130, and triglycerides should be below 150, for most people.

RISK INCREASES WITH
- Hereditary factors.
- A diet that is high in fat and cholesterol.
- Illness or medical problems, such as diabetes, hypothyroidism, nephrotic syndrome, alcoholism, or obstructive liver disease.
- Sedentary lifestyle (lack of physical activity).
- Age. Males over 40 and females over 55.

PREVENTIVE MEASURES
- Exercise daily. Maintain a healthy weight. Eat a healthy diet.
- Don't smoke or use excess amounts of alcohol.
- Get a medical test to check your blood levels of cholesterol and triglycerides.

EXPECTED OUTCOMES
Usually treatable or controllable with diet and drugs.

POSSIBLE COMPLICATIONS
Atherosclerosis (fatty deposits on artery walls). This is a major cause of coronary heart disease and stroke.

DIAGNOSIS & TREATMENT

GENERAL MEASURES
- Your health care provider may do a physical exam and ask questions about any symptoms. For diagnosis, a blood study will be done to measure blood lipids.
- Treatment will depend on the results of your blood studies, your health risks, and other medical problems.
- For some patients, an altered diet and lifestyle changes may be sufficient for treatment. Others may require drugs to reduce blood lipids.
- Emotional stress can increase the risk of heart disease. Look for ways to reduce stress in your life. Learn relaxation methods.
- Quit smoking. Find a way to stop that works for you.

MEDICATIONS
- Many different drugs are now prescribed to control blood lipids. Your health care provider will discuss the options, and their risks and benefits with you.
- Drugs to treat diseases, such as high blood pressure, diabetes, or thyroid conditions may be prescribed.

ACTIVITY
Regular exercise is helpful for reducing weight, staying fit, and controlling stress. It might help in increasing the body's ability to clear fat from the blood after meals.

DIET
- Eat a diet that is low in fat (particularly saturated fat). Eat a high fiber diet with plenty of fruits and vegetables. Medical advice on a proper diet may be helpful.
- Lose weight, if you are overweight. The more overweight you are, the more lipids your body produces.
- Reduce alcohol intake.

NOTIFY OUR OFFICE IF

- You or a family member has symptoms or a family history of hyperlipidemia.
- New, unexplained symptoms develop.

Special notes:

_____

_____

_____

More notes on the back of this page ☐

HYPERPARATHYROIDISM

 BASIC INFORMATION

DESCRIPTION
The parathyroids are four pea-sized glands located within the thyroid gland in the neck. They produce a hormone (PTH) that helps maintain the body's mineral levels. Hyperparathyroidism occurs when these glands become overactive and produce too much PTH. This triggers an imbalance of minerals (calcium and phosphorous) that affects the body's bones and muscles. Hyperparathyroidism can affect both sexes and all ages. It is more common in women ages 30 to 50.

FREQUENT SIGNS AND SYMPTOMS
· There may be no symptoms, or the symptoms may be mild to severe. This disorder comes on over years, so symptoms may not get noticed at first. Many cases are first diagnosed on a routine blood test.
· Loss of appetite, thirst, frequent urination, weight loss, or constipation.
· Feeling tired, depressed, or anxious.
· Muscle weakness, bone and joint pain.
· Nausea, vomiting.
· Severe side (flank) pain caused by kidney stones.
· Easy bone fractures due to reduced calcium in the bones.
· High blood pressure.
· Pain in the upper abdomen caused by a peptic ulcer or pancreatitis (inflammation of the pancreas).

CAUSES
· Benign tumors (adenomas) that grow in one or two of the parathyroid glands. Why the tumors occur is unknown.
· Sometimes caused by an enlargement of the glands (hyperplasia); the cause for this is unknown.
· Very rarely is a cancer involved.

RISK INCREASES WITH
Females over age 50.

PREVENTIVE MEASURES
No specific preventive measures.

EXPECTED OUTCOMES
Outcome is favorable in almost all cases.

POSSIBLE COMPLICATIONS
· Weak bones (osteopenia and osteoporosis).
· Kidney damage.
· Peptic ulcer.
· Pancreatitis.
· Nervous system problems.
· Hypoparathyroidism (too little PTH) caused by removal of too much parathyroid tissue during surgery.

 DIAGNOSIS & TREATMENT

GENERAL MEASURES
· Your health care provider usually will do a physical exam and ask questions about your symptoms. Medical tests may include studies of blood and urine, x-rays of bones, and other tests to confirm the diagnosis.
· Surgery is usually the best form of treatment. The parathyroid gland or glands that are producing the excess hormones are removed. There are different types of operations that are done. Your health care provider will explain them to you.
· In mild cases, or when there are no symptoms, watchful waiting may be an option. This means monitoring the patient for a time to see if the disorder shows signs of getting worse. A follow-up exam may be done every 6 months for 1 to 3 years, and then less often, if tests are normal.

MEDICATIONS
· Don't take antacids that contain calcium without medical approval.
· Estrogen or bone-building drugs for postmenopausal females may be prescribed.

ACTIVITY
· Follow medical advice about returning to normal activities following surgery.
· Exercise daily to maintain good health.

DIET
· Drink extra water to prevent complications.
· Your health care provider will discuss the amount of calcium intake that is recommended. This is usually about 1000 mg/day.

 NOTIFY OUR OFFICE IF

· You or a family member has symptoms of hyperparathyroidism.
· Any new symptoms occur after surgery.
· You did not have surgery and you need to schedule appointment for follow-up studies.

Special notes:

_____

_____

_____

More notes on the back of this page ☐

HYPERTENSION
(High Blood Pressure)

 ## BASIC INFORMATION

DESCRIPTION

Blood pressure measures the force of blood as it flows through the arteries. Adult blood pressure is considered normal at 120/80. The first number is systolic pressure, which measures pressure as the heart contracts (pumps). The second number is diastolic, which measures pressure when the heart is relaxed (between beats). If blood pressure stays high over time (140/90 or above), it is called high blood pressure or hypertension. It is a common disorder and often affects adults over 60. Prehypertension is when the blood pressure is between 120/80 and 140/90. The risk of stroke and heart attack begins to rise as the blood pressure goes above 115/75.

FREQUENT SIGNS AND SYMPTOMS

· Usually no symptoms occur. It is often discovered when blood pressure is measured.
· Vague, mild symptoms such as headache, dizziness, blurred vision, or nausea may occur.

CAUSES

Mostly unknown (called primary hypertension). In some cases, it results from certain medical problems (called secondary hypertension).

RISK INCREASES WITH

· Aging and hardening of the arteries.
· Prehypertension.
· Chronic kidney disease or thyroid dysfunction.
· Narrowing of the aorta (major artery of the heart).
· Adrenal gland disorders.
· Alcoholism.
· Hormone problems of adrenals or pituitary glands.
· Overweight; smoking; stress.
· Sedentary (lack of physical activity) lifestyle.
· Sensitivity to sodium (salt).
· Genetic factors (it is common in African Americans).
· Family history of hypertension.
· Use of certain drugs. These include birth-control pills, steroids, diet pills, and decongestants.

PREVENTIVE MEASURES

No specific preventive measures. Avoid risk factors where possible. Maintain a healthy weight, be physically active, eat a healthy diet (limit salt), drink little or no alcohol, and don't smoke. If you have a family history of hypertension, have frequent blood-pressure checks.

EXPECTED OUTCOMES

Outlook is good if blood pressure can be controlled.

POSSIBLE COMPLICATIONS

Without treatment, high blood pressure can lead to heart attack, stroke, congestive heart failure, pulmonary edema, and kidney failure. High blood pressure is called the "silent killer."

 ## DIAGNOSIS & TREATMENT

GENERAL MEASURES

· Your health care provider will do a physical exam, measure your blood pressure, and ask questions about your lifestyle and family medical history. Medical tests may include blood and urine studies. Other tests may be done to find a cause for the high blood pressure or to determine if there are any complications.
· Treatment steps will depend on each individual. You and your health care provider will decide on a treatment plan. Steps may involve diet changes, weight loss, stopping smoking, increasing exercise, limiting alcohol use, reducing stress, and taking drugs.
· Take your blood pressure at home each day. Write down the results. Have your blood pressure checked regularly by a health professional.
· Counseling, meditation, biofeedback, relaxation techniques, or other therapies can help you reduce stress.
· Talk to your health care provider before trying alternate forms of treatment such as acupuncture, diet supplements, and others.

MEDICATIONS

· One or more antihypertensive drugs to reduce blood pressure may be prescribed. Do not stop taking them unless advised by your health care provider.
· Avoid nonprescription cold, allergy, and sinus decongestant drugs. They may raise blood pressure.

ACTIVITY

Increase physical activity. Exercise moderately hard for 30 minutes, most, if not all, days of the week. It helps reduce stress, control body weight, and lowers blood pressure. Get medical advice about an exercise plan.

DIET

Eat a healthy diet, high in fiber, fruits and vegetables. Limit fat and salt use. If overweight, limit calories.

 ## NOTIFY OUR OFFICE IF

· You or a family member has blood pressure concerns.
· Blood pressure increases or drugs used for treatment cause unexpected side effects.
· Call 911 if symptoms of a heart attack or stroke occur.

Special notes:

_____

_____

_____

More notes on the back of this page ☐

HYPERTHYROIDISM

(Thyrotoxicosis, Toxic Goiter)

 BASIC INFORMATION

DESCRIPTION

Hyperthyroidism means the thyroid gland is overactive and produces too much thyroid hormone. The most common form of hyperthyroidism is called Graves' disease. The thyroid hormone is used by the body for metabolism (producing energy). Hyperthyroidism often affects adults between ages 20 and 50, mostly women.

FREQUENT SIGNS AND SYMPTOMS

- Anxiety, nervousness, and restlessness.
- Feeling warm or hot all the time.
- Sweating.
- Heart palpitations.
- Weight loss, even though appetite increases.
- Sleeplessness.
- Fatigue and weakness.
- Frequent bowel movements.
- Women may have less menstrual flow.
- Eyes appear to bulge out, there is swelling around the eyes, and vision changes may occur.
- Goiter (visibly enlarged thyroid) may occur.
- Hair loss.
- Tremor of the hands.

CAUSES

Graves' disease is an autoimmune disorder. In these disorders, the immune system by mistake attacks the body itself in different ways. In Graves' disease, abnormal antibodies from the immune system cause the thyroid to produce more hormone. Other causes of hyperthyroidism may be due to disorders of the thyroid.

RISK INCREASES WITH

- Thyroid nodules or tumors.
- Thyroiditis (inflammation of thyroid gland).
- Personal or family history of thyroid or autoimmune diseases.
- Radiation treatment.
- Females more than males.
- Excess iodine intake.
- Stress may be a contributing factor.

PREVENTIVE MEASURES

No specific preventive measures.

EXPECTED OUTCOMES

Treatment is effective in controlling the disorder. It may take 6 months for the thyroid levels to return to normal.

POSSIBLE COMPLICATIONS

- Thyroid eye disease. This includes blurred and double vision, difficulty in seeing, tearing, and light sensitivity.
- Heart problems.
- Dermopathy (a skin disorder).
- Hypothyroidism (low thyroid hormone levels).
- Surgery complications such as infection or bleeding.

 DIAGNOSIS & TREATMENT

GENERAL MEASURES

- Your health care provider will do a physical exam. Medical tests include blood studies for thyroid levels. Radioactive iodine studies may be done.
- Treatment usually involves drugs to reduce thyroid hormone levels. Permanent treatment involves use of radioactive iodine or surgery. With these two treatments, thyroid hormone production is decreased. Sometimes, hypothyroidism (too little thyroid hormone) occurs, which will need to be treated.
- Radioactive iodine treatment is usually done as an outpatient. The iodine (taken by mouth) causes the thyroid gland to shrink over a period of months.
- Surgery to remove part of the thyroid (called a thyroidectomy) may be recommended in some cases. This is usually done in a hospital with a general anesthetic.
- For eye symptoms, an exam and follow-up by an eye specialist (ophthalmologist) may be recommended.

MEDICATIONS

- Antithyroid drugs to depress thyroid activity are usually prescribed. Follow-up blood tests are done to adjust the dosage until thyroid hormone levels are normal.
- Beta blockers to treat the heart and nervous system symptoms may be prescribed.
- Thyroid replacement drugs may be prescribed if the thyroid gland becomes underactive due to treatment.
- Avoid any drugs or supplements that contain iodide. Iodide may interfere with drugs used in treatment.

ACTIVITY

Usually no limits in otherwise healthy persons. In older persons or those with heart problems, decrease activity until thyroid levels are normal.

DIET

No special diet.

 NOTIFY OUR OFFICE IF

- You or a family member has symptoms of hyperthyroidism.
- Symptoms worsen suddenly, especially after surgery.
- New, unexplained symptoms develop.

Special notes:

_____

_____

_____

More notes on the back of this page ☐

HYPOCHONDRIASIS

 ## BASIC INFORMATION

DESCRIPTION

A disorder that causes a person to feel that he or she has a serious or fatal disease, even though there is no medical evidence of this. It occurs equally in men and women. It may begin at any age, but is most common in early adulthood.

FREQUENT SIGNS AND SYMPTOMS

- Preoccupied for over 6 months with the fear of having a serious disease. There may be constant thought about the possibility of heart disease or cancer.
- Anxiety and reports of symptoms involving any body part. Symptoms may be vague or specific.
- Symptoms may change, but the person's belief that a serious condition exists does not.

CAUSES

The cause is uncertain. It is based on misinterpreting normal body sensations. There are a number of risk factors that have been identified. A person with the disorder may be aware that the fear of having a serious disease is unfounded, excessive, or unreasonable.

RISK INCREASES WITH

- Other mental health problems, such as anxiety.
- Recent stressful event or major life change.
- Having a need for attention. (A person may be unaware of this.)
- Having personal relationship problems. (A person may be looking for care and concern.)
- Family history of hypochondriasis.
- People who had a serious illness or experience of adversity in childhood. Parents may have rewarded illness by giving a child special privileges and attention for being sick, or they may have neglected the child.

PREVENTIVE MEASURES

No specific measures known.

EXPECTED OUTCOME

Patients may have periods of hypochondriasis for months and years, and then go months and years without hypochondriasis. Some patients recover from the disorder. For others, it may be a lifelong problem.

POSSIBLE COMPLICATIONS

- Can affect all aspects of a person's life. This includes work, social, and personal relationships.
- A real illness may be overlooked.
- Becoming dependent on pain relievers or sedatives.
- Patients tend to "doctor shop." They feel rejected if they aren't believed about the symptoms.
- Taking unnecessary medical tests that are dangerous or could result in complications.

 ## DIAGNOSIS & TREATMENT

GENERAL MEASURES

- Your health care provider will do a physical exam and ask questions about your symptoms. Medical tests may include a blood study. A mental (emotional) health exam may be done also.
- Your health care provider will assure you that the diagnosis of the symptoms shows there is no threat to life or risk of disability. Regular follow-up medical appointments may be scheduled for further assurance.
- Having the diagnosis of hypochondriasis is hard for anyone to accept. Feelings of anger, sadness, or frustration are normal. Education about the disorder for you and your family may help you cope. Your health care provider is the first source. Then learn what you can from books or researching on the Internet.
- Behavior therapy can help a patient understand what generates the symptoms and how to overcome worrisome thoughts.
- Interpersonal therapy can help a patient identify personal relationship problems and how to correct them.
- Group therapy may help some patients.
- Patients should depend on one health care provider for their treatment. Avoid going to different health care providers and having repeat medical tests.

MEDICATIONS

- Antidepressants may be prescribed for anxiety or depressive symptoms.
- Other drugs may be prescribed for symptoms such as mood disorders or stress.

ACTIVITY

Exercise daily. This can improve physical fitness as well as having a positive affect on mental health. It helps improve mood, reduce tension, and improve sleep.

DIET

Eat three regular, healthy meals daily. Avoid alcohol or caffeine.

 ## NOTIFY OUR OFFICE IF

You or a family member has symptoms of this disorder and wants help with the problem.

Special notes: _____

_____

_____

More notes on the back of this page ☐

HYPOGLYCEMIA, FUNCTIONAL

 ## BASIC INFORMATION

DESCRIPTION
A low level of blood sugar (glucose) in the body. Functional (or reactive) hypoglycemia is usually a reaction to eating. It is not a disease in itself and is not a common medical condition as many persons would believe. Symptoms vary greatly among people in frequency and severity.

FREQUENT SIGNS AND SYMPTOMS
- Headache.
- Nervousness or anxiety.
- Sweating.
- Dizziness.
- Fast heartbeat.
- Weakness or faintness.
- Shaking muscles.
- Hunger.
- More severe symptoms are less likely. They may include being forgetful, poor concentration, confusion, poor coordination, or slurred speech.

CAUSES
The amount of sugar (glucose) in the blood normally increases for one to two hours after a meal, especially a high-carbohydrate meal (sugars and starches). In many people, instead of increasing, the glucose level may drop to a level that is lower than before the meal. It will then rise back again to normal levels. Most of these people do not have any symptoms from the drop in glucose levels. In a few, the symptoms of hypoglycemia occur.

RISK INCREASES WITH
- Improper diet.
- Obesity.
- Smoking, alcohol, stress, or other emotional or mental problems may contribute.

PREVENTIVE MEASURES
- Follow instructions under Diet.
- Get treatment for emotional problems such as stress.
- Don't smoke.
- Don't drink alcohol.
- Recognize early symptoms and drink or eat something that contains sugar.

EXPECTED OUTCOMES
The symptoms usually clear up on their own or with glucose in a very short period of time. A change in diet may help prevent symptoms from occurring in the future.

POSSIBLE COMPLICATIONS
None expected.

 ## DIAGNOSIS & TREATMENT

GENERAL MEASURES
- Your health care provider may do a physical exam. Medical tests may include blood-sugar and glucose-tolerance studies to rule out other medical problems.
- Long-term treatment usually involves diet changes.
- Short-term treatment during an episode can raise blood sugar more quickly. This includes drinking juice or a soft drink or eating candy to raise the glucose level. Take a protein food, such as milk or cheese, at the same time. This helps the body slowly absorb the glucose and avoid a "seesaw" effect of glucose levels.
- Counseling or other therapy may help you learn to cope with stress or emotional problems.

MEDICATIONS
Drugs are not usually needed for treatment.

ACTIVITY
Regular exercise may improve blood-sugar control. It can help to reduce stress and build self-esteem. It helps to control and maintain an ideal weight. It also helps improve heart and lung function, lower blood pressure, improve blood circulation, and lower cholesterol levels.

DIET
- Eat several smaller meals a day that are low in simple carbohydrates, moderate in fats, and high in protein.
- Don't skip meals.
- Between-meal snacks should include protein, such as chicken, eggs, cheese, nuts, or skim milk, rather than carbohydrates.
- Avoid sugar and foods containing sugar (especially on an empty stomach).
- Weight-loss diet will help if being overweight is a problem.
- Limit or avoid alcohol.
- Avoid caffeine (coffee, tea, or soft drinks).

 ## NOTIFY OUR OFFICE IF

You or a family member has symptoms of functional hypoglycemia.

Special notes:
_____

_____

_____

More notes on the back of this page ☐

HYPOPARATHYROIDISM

 ## BASIC INFORMATION

DESCRIPTION

The parathyroid glands lie within the thyroid glands in the neck. They produce parathyroid hormones, which along with vitamin D and calcitonin (a hormone produced by the thyroid gland), regulates the calcium level in the body. With hypoparathyroidism, there is a decreased production of hormones by the parathyroid glands causing a low level of calcium in the blood. The disorder is rare and affects children more often than adults.

FREQUENT SIGNS AND SYMPTOMS

Acute phase:
· Tetany (painful cramp-like spasms of the face, hands, arms, and sometimes feet).
· Tingling and numbness in feet or hands.
Chronic phase:
· Scaling skin.
· Splitting nails.
· Poor tooth development.
· Seizures.
· Mental retardation in children.
· Psychosis in adults.

CAUSES

· Complication of surgery on the parathyroid glands, the thyroid glands, or other neck tissues.
· Genetic autoimmune disorder (possibly).
· Radiation of the thyroid gland.
· Hemochromatosis (disease in which excessive iron accumulates in the liver).
· No apparent reason (sometimes).
· Occasionally the parathyroids are absent from birth.

RISK INCREASES WITH

Neck surgery or trauma.

PREVENTIVE MEASURES

There are no specific preventive measures.

EXPECTED OUTCOMES

· This condition is currently considered incurable. It requires lifelong replacement therapy to control symptoms. Without treatment, it is fatal.
· Scientific research into causes and treatment continues, so there is hope for increasingly effective treatments and a cure.

POSSIBLE COMPLICATIONS

· Cataracts.
· Brain damage.
· Heartbeat abnormalities and congestive heart failure.
· Difficulty breathing.
· Malformation of teeth.
· Seizures.

 ## DIAGNOSIS & TREATMENT

GENERAL MEASURES

· Your health care provider may do a physical exam. Medical tests may include blood and urine studies, ECG (electrocardiogram—method of diagnosing heart diseases by measuring electrical activity of the heart), CT, and x-rays of bones to detect increased bone density.
· If you are suffering an acute attack of tetany (see Symptoms), you may need hospital care for calcium injections to provide quick relief.
· For self-care, if muscle cramps start, place a paper bag over your mouth. Blow into it and rebreathe your breath. This will raise carbon-dioxide levels in the blood and decrease muscle spasms.
· Apply lubricating creams or ointments to dry, scaling skin.
· Keep nails trimmed to prevent splitting.
· Get periodic medical tests to check calcium levels in your blood. It is important to remember to have these tests done on time.

MEDICATIONS

· Vitamin D and calcium supplements are normally prescribed. A lifelong course of these drugs is necessary.
· Intravenous (IV) calcium may be given for severe muscle spasms.
· Other drugs for treating muscle spasms may be prescribed.

ACTIVITY

No limits.

DIET

A high-calcium, low-phosphorus diet may be helpful. Your health care provider will advise you of special diet needs.

 ## NOTIFY OUR OFFICE IF

· You or a family member has unexplained muscle spasms of the hands, feet, or throat, or numbness, or tingling in the hands or feet.
· Muscle spasms do not decrease in 1 week, despite treatment.

Special notes:

_____

_____

_____

More notes on the back of this page ☐

HYPOTHERMIA

 BASIC INFORMATION

DESCRIPTION

A drop in body temperature to below normal because of exposure to cold. It can occur indoors due to lack of heat, outside in cold weather, or from being in water. Hypothermia can take several hours or even several days to develop. It affects all the major organ systems in the body.

FREQUENT SIGNS AND SYMPTOMS

Early symptoms (it can start slowly):
- Poor muscle coordination.
- Mental confusion.
- Shivering.
- Low body temperature that is below 96°F (35.5°C). Normal body temperature is around 98.6°F (37°C).
- Slow pulse.
- Weakness, drowsiness.

Late symptoms:
- Rigid muscles.
- Temperature drops even lower.
- Purple fingers, toes, and nail beds.
- Loss of consciousness.

CAUSES

The exposure to cold temperatures starts affecting different functions of the body. The brain and nerves work more slowly. The heart rate becomes irregular. Muscles don't work normally.

RISK INCREASES WITH

- Adults over 60 or infants.
- Mentally impaired.
- Poorly heated homes.
- Outdoor work.
- Chronic disease (heart, lung, and other disorders that prevent moving around).
- Homeless persons.
- Excess alcohol use.

PREVENTIVE MEASURES

- Be sure the home is heated adequately.
- In cold weather, wear windproof clothing in many loose layers, including a scarf, hat, and mittens. In the rain, change to dry clothing as soon as possible.
- Avoid alcohol use if you are going out into the cold.
- Don't skate or fish on ice unless you know that it's safe.
- If camping, walking, or hiking in a cold climate, carry emergency gear for use if stranded or injured. Travel with a partner.
- Persons who are unable to care for themselves fully, such as the elderly, the mentally impaired, or the alcoholic, should be visited or supervised during cold weather.

EXPECTED OUTCOMES

The outcome is usually good if the patient is otherwise healthy and treatment is started quickly. Some children have been revived despite being in ice water for an hour or more.

POSSIBLE COMPLICATIONS

Many complications can occur depending on the patient's health and the length of the exposure to cold.

 DIAGNOSIS & TREATMENT

GENERAL MEASURES

- Urgent medical care is needed. Arrange transport to the nearest emergency center right away.
- The following may be helpful while waiting for emergency help: Dry the person if wet. Keep the person lying down and cover them with blankets. If the person is outdoors, move them inside. If unable to do so, cover with a blankets and protect them from the weather. Try to warm the main body area first, then the arms and legs. In wilderness conditions, if help is not near, undress the victim and yourself and establish skin-to-skin contact.
- In the hospital or emergency center, the process of rewarming will be started. The patient will be treated until the temperature returns to normal. Medical tests are often needed to check for any complications.

MEDICATIONS

Drugs will be provided as needed for any complications.

ACTIVITY

After treatment, normal activity should be resumed gradually.

DIET

Don't give alcohol to a person with hypothermia. Warm fluids may be given if the patient is able to swallow.

 NOTIFY OUR OFFICE IF

You or a family member has symptoms of hypothermia or you observe the symptoms in someone. This may be an emergency.

Special notes:

_____

_____

_____

More notes on the back of this page ☐

HYPOTHYROIDISM

 BASIC INFORMATION

DESCRIPTION

Hypothyroidism means the thyroid gland is underactive and produces too little thyroid hormone. The thyroid is a small butterfly-shaped gland in the neck. Just about all chemical reactions in the body are affected by the thyroid hormone. Hypothyroidism most often affects older adults, and women more than men.

FREQUENT SIGNS AND SYMPTOMS

- A person will have some, but not all of the symptoms.
- Feeling cold (especially hands and feet).
- Decrease in sweating.
- Dry, itchy skin; paleness.
- Loss of appetite, but a weight gain occurs.
- Constipation.
- Loss of energy, feeling tired or sluggish.
- Coarse, dry, brittle hair, or hair loss.
- Muscle aches.
- Blurred vision; hearing loss.
- Sleepiness or insomnia.
- Emotional or mental changes and mood swings.
- Puffy skin around the eyes.
- Decreased sex drive.
- Changes in menstrual cycle.
- Deepened or hoarse voice.

CAUSES

A variety of medical disorders or health problems can damage, inflame, enlarge, shrink or otherwise affect the thyroid gland and cause it to be underactive.

RISK INCREASES WITH

- Autoimmune disorder such as Hashimoto's thyroiditis. The body's immune system functions abnormally and attacks the thyroid gland.
- Treatment for hyperthyroidism (e.g., surgery, iodine).
- Drugs (e.g., lithium) that cause thyroid dysfunction.
- Radiation or surgery of head, neck, or chest.
- Congenital (being born with hypothyroidism).
- Adults over 60. Women more than men.
- Personal or family history of thyroid disease.
- Rarely, disorders of the pituitary or hypothalamus.
- Too little iodine (rare in the United States).

PREVENTIVE MEASURES

No known preventive measures. Screening tests for those at risk may help with early diagnosis.

EXPECTED OUTCOME

Normal thyroid levels can be achieved with treatment. Most people will need to take thyroid hormones for life.

POSSIBLE COMPLICATIONS

- Risk of infections, heart disease, and pituitary tumors.
- Infertility and risk of miscarriage in pregnant women.
- Myxedema coma (rare life-threatening complication).

 DIAGNOSIS & TREATMENT

GENERAL MEASURES

- Your health care provider will do a physical exam and ask questions about your symptoms. Blood tests will be done for thyroid hormone and TSH (thyroid-stimulating hormone) levels. Blood tests may result in a diagnosis of pronounced hypothyroidism or subclinical (mild) hypothyroidism.
- Treatment for pronounced hypothyroidism involves restoring thyroid blood levels to normal with synthetic thyroid hormone. Follow-up is usually needed for several months to be sure of the correct dose of thyroid replacement. Then the follow-ups may be less frequent but still done on a regular basis.
- Treatment may be recommended for mild hypothyroidism, depending on symptoms and other factors.
- Rarely, hospital care may be needed if emergencies occur, such as myxedema coma.
- Pregnancy will require careful monitoring and additional thyroid replacement as the pregnancy advances.
- To learn more: American Thyroid Association, (800) 849-7643; website: www.thyroid.org.

MEDICATION

Thyroid hormone replacement is often prescribed. Dosage will depend on age, weight, capacity of thyroid function, other drugs you take, and intestinal function. Don't switch brand names of your thyroid drug without consulting your health care provider.

ACTIVITY

No limits. Stay as active as possible.

DIET

No special diet for hypothyroidism. Avoid constipation by eating a high-fiber diet. A weight-loss diet is recommended if you are overweight.

 NOTIFY OUR OFFICE IF

- You or a family member has hypothyroidism symptoms.
- Symptoms don't improve after 3 weeks of treatment, or new, unexplained symptoms develop.
- Coma or seizures occur. Call for emergency help immediately!

Special notes:

_____

_____

_____

More notes on the back of this page ☐

ID REACTION
(Autoeczematization; Autosensitization)

 BASIC INFORMATION

DESCRIPTION
An allergic response to a skin condition that occurs somewhere else on the body.

FREQUENT SIGNS AND SYMPTOMS
· Itching (often severe).
· Vesicles (small, fluid-filled blisters) of varying size on the skin.
· It most often occurs on the sides of the fingers, but can be all over the body.

CAUSES
Unknown. An id reaction may be a disorder of the body's immune response to the original skin problem. It may occur with a fungal infection, such as athlete's feet, or other type of skin condition.

RISK INCREASES WITH
· Recent skin rash (such as diaper dermatitis, stasis dermatitis, external otitis, hand eczema, or foot eczema).
· History of allergies.
· Stress may play a role.

PREVENTIVE MEASURES
Treat all skin infections until they are cured.

EXPECTED OUTCOMES
Usually curable in 2 weeks. It may recur again if treatment is stopped before the id reaction and original condition are gone.

POSSIBLE COMPLICATIONS
A bacterial infection may develop.

 DIAGNOSIS & TREATMENT

GENERAL MEASURES
· Your health care provider will do a physical exam of the affected skin and ask questions about your symptoms. A medical test may be done to check for the type of infection that caused the original skin problem.
· Treatment of the first skin condition should also cure the id reaction.
· Id reaction does not respond well to simple measures such as soaks.

MEDICATIONS
· Topical or oral steroid drugs may be prescribed.
· An anti-itching cream for skin can help control the itching.
· Drugs (such as an antifungal) may be prescribed for other skin problems diagnosed.

ACTIVITY
No limits.

DIET
No special diet.

 NOTIFY OUR OFFICE IF

· You or a family member has symptoms of an id reaction.
· The following occur during treatment:
  - Fever higher than 101°F (38.3°C).
  - Infection develops (heat, redness, pain, or tenderness in any of the lesions).

Special notes:

_____

_____

_____

More notes on the back of this page ☐

256

IDIOPATHIC HYPERTROPHIC SUBAORTIC STENOSIS (IHSS; Hypertrophic Cardiomyopathy)

 BASIC INFORMATION

DESCRIPTION

A chronic heart condition that produces an enlarged heart muscle. This restricts the amount of blood the heart pumps. Cardiac output may be low, normal, or high depending on whether stenosis (a narrowing) is obstructive or nonobstructive. If output is normal, idiopathic hypertrophic subaortic stenosis (IHSS) could go undetected for years. It affects all ages, but young people usually have more severe symptoms.

FREQUENT SIGNS AND SYMPTOMS

- Many patients have no symptoms.
- Chest pain (called angina pectoris).
- Strong, rapid heartbeat.
- Fainting from exertion.
- Shortness of breath.
- Swollen feet and ankles.
- Distended (sticking out) neck veins.
- Fatigue.

CAUSES

Thickening of the walls of the heart. This is caused by a defect in the genes and often runs in families. The thickened walls obstruct the flow of blood, and the heart may be unable to pump enough blood for the needs of the body.

RISK INCREASES WITH

Family history of IHSS.

PREVENTIVE MEASURES

If you have a family history of IHSS, obtain genetic counseling before starting a family.

EXPECTED OUTCOMES

Symptoms can often be controlled with treatment. Lifestyle changes may be required.

POSSIBLE COMPLICATIONS

- Abnormal heart rhythm.
- Sudden death.

 DIAGNOSIS & TREATMENT

GENERAL MEASURES

- Your health care provider will do a physical exam. Medical tests may include cardiac catheterization to measure blood flow through heart chambers, CT, MRI, and x-rays of the heart. An ECG (electrocardiogram) and echocardiogram, which are studies to check heart function, and other tests may be done.

- Treatment may include drugs, lifestyle changes, pacemaker or defibrillator insertion, or surgery.
- Lifestyle changes involve reducing activity levels.
- An electronic cardiac pacemaker may be inserted. It helps relieve symptoms by changing the pattern of the heartbeat.
- An implantable-cardioverter defibrillator may be inserted. It can help prevent sudden death.
- A procedure that uses alcohol injected into an artery may be recommended. It can help to reduce obstruction and improve symptoms.
- Surgery may be recommended to reduce the obstruction, if other treatments do not control the problem.
- Counseling may be helpful in adjusting to emotional effects of chronic illness.
- Wear a medical alert type bracelet or pendant to indicate you have this disorder.

MEDICATIONS

Beta-adrenergic blockers or calcium-channel blockers to prevent heartbeat irregularities will be prescribed.

ACTIVITY

- Instructions will be provided about how much physical activity is ideal. Your ability to increase activity is dependent on your response to therapy. Don't regard yourself as an invalid.
- Avoid strenuous activities and sports because of the high risk of sudden death.

DIET

Usually no special diet. A low-salt diet may be recommended if you have fluid buildup. This is a possible sign of congestive heart failure.

 NOTIFY OUR OFFICE IF

- You or a family member has symptoms of IHSS.
- Symptoms worsen during treatment.
- New, unexplained symptoms develop. Drugs used in treatment may produce side effects.

Special notes:

_____

_____

_____

More notes on the back of this page ☐

IMMUNODEFICIENCY DISEASE

BASIC INFORMATION

DESCRIPTION

· Defects in the body's immune system, which means a person is more likely to develop infections and cancer. A healthy immune system protects the body against germs (bacteria, viruses, and fungi), cancer (partial protection), and any foreign material that enters the body.
· Primary immunodeficiency is inherited. Nearly 100 forms have been recognized. One form is common variable immunodeficiency (CVID). A rare form is severe combined immune deficiency (SCID).
· Secondary immunodeficiency is acquired. It occurs in persons who previously had a normal immune system. A form of this type (not discussed here) is the acquired immunodeficiency syndrome (AIDS).

FREQUENT SIGNS AND SYMPTOMS

· Repeated, severe, and hard to cure infections, illnesses, and other health problems. Some are listed here.
· Ear infections (otitis media), and sinus or other respiratory infections, such as pneumonia. Yeast infections, such as candidiasis and eczema (a skin disorder).
· Cancer, especially leukemia and lymphoma.
· Bleeding disorders.
· Other immune disorders (anemia, arthritis).
· Meningitis or encephalitis (brain infections).
· Heart, digestive tract, or nervous system disorders.

CAUSES

· Primary: Being born with a faulty immune system. One or more or all of the essential parts of the immune system are missing due to a genetic defect.
· Secondary: Caused by diseases or other health problems that affect the immune system.

RISK INCREASES WITH

· Surgical removal of the spleen before age 2.
· Use of drugs that suppress the immune system.
· Radiation treatment or severe burns.
· Some cancers, such as leukemia.
· Viral infections, such as measles or influenza.
· Malnutrition (severe nutrient deficiency).
· Blood transfusions or intravenous (IV) drug use.
· Family history of immunodeficiency disease.

PREVENTIVE MEASURES

· No preventive measures for primary type. If you have a family history, get genetic counseling before starting a family.
· Prevention of secondary type may or may not be possible. It depends on the cause.

EXPECTED OUTCOMES

Advances in treatment have improved outlook for many of the patients. Lifelong treatments may be needed.

POSSIBLE COMPLICATIONS

· Infections and other diseases that may not respond to treatment.
· Complications can occur due to specific deficiency.

DIAGNOSIS & TREATMENT

GENERAL MEASURES

· Your health care provider will do a physical exam. Medical tests may include blood studies of antibodies, microscopic exams of blood and tissue cells, skin tests, chest x-rays of the thymus gland, and radioactive studies of immune function.
· Specific treatment will depend on the type of immune deficiency. General treatment involves preventing and treating infections. Your health care provider will discuss your individual treatment steps.
· Surgery to transplant bone marrow or the thymus gland may be recommended.
· Hospital care for treatment of serious infection may be required.
· Avoid exposure to persons with infections. Don't get any type of vaccine without medical advice. Wear a medical alert bracelet or neck tag to identify your medical condition and any drugs you take.
· To learn more: Immune Deficiency Foundation, 40 W. Chesapeake Ave., Suite 308, Towson, MD 21204; (800) 296-4433; website: www.primaryimmune.org.

MEDICATIONS

Antibiotics for infection, transfusion of blood components, and gamma globulin injections may be prescribed.

ACTIVITY

Activity will depend on the type of deficiency. A risk of bleeding will limit activities in some cases.

DIET

Eat a healthy diet. During illness, modify diet if needed.

NOTIFY OUR OFFICE IF

· You or a family member has symptoms of immunodeficiency disease.
· After diagnosis, you have any signs of infection or illness or injury, or unexplained symptoms occur.

Special notes:

_____

_____

_____

More notes on the back of this page ☐

258

IMPETIGO
(Pyoderma)

 ## BASIC INFORMATION

DESCRIPTION
A common bacterial skin infection that affects the top layers of the skin. It usually involves the skin of the face, arms, and legs. Impetigo can affect all ages, but it is most common in infants and children.

FREQUENT SIGNS AND SYMPTOMS
· A localized (not spreading) red rash with many small blisters. Some blisters contain pus, and yellow crusts form when they break. The blisters don't hurt, but they may itch.
· Slight fever (sometimes).

CAUSES
Staphylococcal or streptococcal (or both) bacteria growing in the upper skin layers. It is usually spread from person-to-person, or from germs on something an infected person has touched. The time from exposure to the germs and the start of symptoms is 1 to 3 days. A person is contagious when the rash is crusting or oozing pus.

RISK INCREASES WITH
· Contact with an infected person.
· Skin that is sensitive to sun and irritants, such as soap and makeup.
· Other skin problems, such as bites, burns, infections, sores, or injuries.
· Poor general health.
· Warm, moist weather.
· Children in daycare.
· Poor hygiene.

PREVENTIVE MEASURES
· No specific preventive measures.
· Maintain good general health and good hygiene.

EXPECTED OUTCOMES
Curable in 7 to 10 days with treatment. It may recur in children.

POSSIBLE COMPLICATIONS
· Can lead to other skin conditions and scarring (rare).
· Kidney disorder (rare).

 ## DIAGNOSIS & TREATMENT

GENERAL MEASURES
· Your health care provider can diagnose impetigo by an exam of the infected skin. Medical skin tests are usually not needed.
· Treatment is with drugs used for bacterial infection.
· Self-care steps include:
  - Keep fingernails short. Don't scratch the blisters.
  - If there is an outbreak in the family, urge all members to use antibacterial soap. Wash hands carefully.
  - Use separate towels for each family member, or substitute paper towels temporarily.
  - Don't share razors with other people.
  - Scrub sores with gauze and antiseptic soap. Break any pustules. Remove all crusts, and expose and cleanse all lesions. If crusts are difficult to remove, soak them in warm, soapy water and scrub gently.
  - Cover impetigo sores with gauze and tape to keep hands away from them.
  - Men should shave around sores on the face, not over them. Use an aerosol shaving cream and change razor blades each day. Don't use a shaving brush; it may have germs on it.

MEDICATIONS
· Antibiotic ointments may be prescribed.
· Oral antibiotics may be prescribed.

ACTIVITY
No limits.

DIET
No special diet.

 ## NOTIFY OUR OFFICE IF

· You or your child has symptoms of impetigo.
· Fever occurs.
· The sores continue to spread or don't begin to heal in 3 days, despite treatment.

Special notes:

_____

_____

_____

More notes on the back of this page ☐

IMPOTENCE
(Erectile Dysfunction)

 BASIC INFORMATION

DESCRIPTION
A consistent inability to sustain an erection as needed for sexual intercourse. Impotence can occur at any age. It is not a normal part of aging (though arousal may normally take longer). Impotence affects millions of men.

FREQUENT SIGNS AND SYMPTOMS
· Total inability to achieve an erection, an inconsistent ability to do so, or ability to achieve only brief erections.
· Sexual drive and the ability to have an orgasm may not be affected.

CAUSES
An erection requires a sequence of events. It starts with sexual stimulation in the brain, which sends nerve signals to the arteries and muscles of the penis. The penis fills with blood and grows firm and erect. After the stimulation ends, or ejaculation occurs, the blood leaves the penis, and it softens again. With erectile dysfunction, this sequence of events is disrupted. This can be due to physical (most often) or psychological (mental or emotional) factors.

RISK INCREASES WITH
Physical factors may include:
· Diabetes, endocrine disorder, liver or kidney disease.
· Atherosclerosis (hardening of the arteries), heart or blood vessel disease, or high blood pressure.
· Use of some drugs, such as for high blood pressure.
· Disorders or injuries of the central nervous system.
· Alcoholism, smoking, or drugs of abuse.
· Decreased blood flow to the penis from any cause.
· Surgery (such as for heart or blood vessels).
· Prostate cancer treatment.
· Hormone imbalance.
Psychological factors may include:
· Fear of sexual failure or performance anxiety, low self-esteem, or lack of interest in sex.
· Decrease in sexuality in long-term relationship.
· Depression, anxiety, stress, anger, and guilt.
· Fear of disease (such as sexual) or heart attack.
· Other people are around (such as mother-in-law).

PREVENTIVE MEASURES
· No specific measures. Some general advice is listed.
· Maintain good health and proper weight.
· Avoid any of the risk factors where possible.
· Control any medical conditions such as diabetes.
· Ask about side effects before taking any new drug.
· Have open communication with your sexual partner.
· Try to avoid worrying about sexual performance.

EXPECTED OUTCOMES
Impotence is treatable in all age groups. Near normal sexual activity can often be achieved with treatment.

POSSIBLE COMPLICATIONS
· Reduced quality of life for the man and his partner.
· Depression, anxiety, and low self-esteem.

 DIAGNOSIS & TREATMENT

GENERAL MEASURES
· Your health care provider will do a physical exam and ask questions about your sexual history. Medical tests may be done to diagnose any underlying disorder.
· Treatment steps may involve lifestyle changes, therapy for any illness diagnosed, erectile dysfunction drugs or devices, counseling, and surgery. A treatment plan will be based on your individual case.
· Lifestyle changes may include cutting back on alcohol, smoking, or drug abuse. Reducing stress, diet changes, and increased exercise may be recommended.
· Counseling can help. It may be for emotional problems (such as stress, anxiety, or guilt). Counseling may involve a sex therapist for you and your partner.
· Use of a vacuum inflation device is an option.
· Surgery for an inflatable or non-inflatable penile implant may be helpful if other methods fail.
· Surgery to improve blood flow to the penis may be recommended if there are blood vessel problems.
· To learn more: Erectile Dysfunction Institute, 10949 Bren Road East, Minnetonka, MN 55343; (866) 563-2432; website: www.erectile-dysfunction-impotence.org.

MEDICATIONS
· Drugs for erectile dysfunction (taken by mouth, self-injected, or by suppository) are often prescribed. For proper and safe use, follow all instructions provided.
· If a drug you take is the cause of impotence, a change in drugs or a change in dosage amounts may be made.
· Drugs may be prescribed for an underlying disorder.

ACTIVITY
No limits. Exercise on a regular basis.

DIET
Eat a well-balanced diet and take vitamins.

 NOTIFY OUR OFFICE IF

· You or a family member has symptoms of impotence.
· Erectile dysfunction continues despite treatment.

Special notes:

_____

_____

_____

More notes on the back of this page ☐

INCONTINENCE, STRESS

 BASIC INFORMATION

DESCRIPTION
An involuntary leaking of urine that occurs with sudden increased pressure in the abdomen. It can affect both sexes (males rarely) and all ages. It is most common in older women.

FREQUENT SIGNS AND SYMPTOMS
Leaking of urine. This may happen with lifting, sneezing, singing, coughing, laughing, exercising, sports activity, crying, or straining to have a bowel movement. It may also occur with small movements such as rolling over in bed or standing up from a sitting position.

CAUSES
It is usually due to pelvic floor muscle or sphincter muscle problems. Pelvic floor muscles support the bladder. Sphincter muscles keep the opening of the bladder closed until it is time to urinate, and then they relax. When these muscles become weak or don't function properly, urine can leak out from the bladder.

RISK INCREASES WITH
- Repeated vaginal childbirth.
- Vaginal birth of large children.
- Adults over 60.
- Obesity.
- Surgery or radiation of the genitals or urinary tract.
- Chronic lung disease with a cough.

PREVENTIVE MEASURES
- Maintain good health.
- Get physical exams to detect early problems.
- Urinate regularly.
- Strengthen pelvic floor muscles with Kegel exercises.
  - First step is to identify pelvic floor muscles. When urinating, stop the flow by squeezing the pelvic floor muscles. Another way is to insert a finger into vagina (women) or rectum (men), then tighten the muscles around the finger. Repeat each method until you are sure you can feel which muscles are involved.
  - The exercises can be done any time and any place, lying down or sitting up. Start by emptying the bladder.
  - Tighten the pelvic floor muscles and hold for a count of 10.
  - Relax the muscles completely for a count of 10.
  - Perform 10 exercises, 3 times a day (morning, afternoon, and night). Don't do more than this.
  - It may take 6 weeks to 3 months for improvement.

EXPECTED OUTCOME
Kegel exercises can be effective for mild stress incontinence. With more severe incontinence, other treatment steps may cure the problem or help reduce symptoms.

POSSIBLE COMPLICATIONS
Physical problems are rare. It can affect quality of life.

 DIAGNOSIS & TREATMENT

GENERAL MEASURES
- Your health care provider will do a physical exam and ask questions about your incontinence symptoms. Medical tests of blood and urine may be done to check for other conditions. Additional tests may be done to help diagnose specific urinary-tract problems. You may be asked to keep a diary about your urination patterns.
- Treatment may involve weight loss, smoking cessation, cough suppression, Kegel exercises, drugs, pessary, other types of therapy, or surgery.
- Other therapies include biofeedback, electrical stimulation, bladder training, magnetic innervation, or special weights to strengthen pelvic muscles. These options will be explained to you.
- Learn and practice Kegel exercises. Try to use the squeezing technique just before any sneeze or a cough.
- Wear absorbent underpants or incontinence pads.
- A pessary (support device) to fit inside the vagina to support the uterus is helpful for some women. Other types of devices include urethral plugging or stenting.
- If other methods fail, surgery to tighten relaxed or damaged muscles that support the bladder helps some. Even with surgery, some leakage may continue.
- To learn more: National Association for Continence, (800) 252-3337; website: www.nafc.org or Simon Foundation for Continence, (800) 237-4666; website: www.simonfoundation.org.

MEDICATION
- Drugs to help sphincter muscles may be prescribed.
- Estrogen therapy may be prescribed for women.

ACTIVITY
No limits. Exercise on a regular basis to improve health.

DIET
- Start a weight loss program if you are overweight.
- Decrease your intake of caffeine and alcohol.

NOTIFY OUR OFFICE IF

- You or a family member has symptoms of stress incontinence and self-treatment isn't helping.
- Symptoms don't improve with treatment.

Special notes:

_____

_____

_____

More notes on the back of this page ☐

INCONTINENCE, URGE

 BASIC INFORMATION

DESCRIPTION

Feeling the need or urge to urinate and then being unable to control the bladder until you can get to a toilet. Urge incontinence increases with age and affects women more often than it does men.

FREQUENT SIGNS AND SYMPTOMS

- Loss of urine right after feeling an urge to urinate. It may be a few drops to complete bladder emptying.
- Symptoms may occur with sudden change in position or activity, hearing or touching running water, drinking a small amount of liquid, and during sleep.
- Key-in-lock syndrome may occur. This happens when you rush home, put a key in the door lock, and experience a sudden bladder contraction and urine leakage.

CAUSES

The usual cause is a spasm or contraction of the bladder muscle. It squeezes at the wrong time, earlier than it should, and causes the leakage. The spasm may result from bladder nerve damage, other nerve problems, or problems of the bladder muscles. The bladder may be described as spastic, overactive, or unstable.

RISK INCREASES WITH

- Repeated vaginal childbirth.
- Adults over 60. Women more than men.
- Hormonal changes in women after menopause.
- Obesity.
- Surgery or radiation of the genitals or urinary tract.
- Urinary-tract infection, stone, cancer, or obstruction.
- Certain neurological (nervous system) disorders.

PREVENTIVE MEASURES

- Maintain good health. Urinate regularly.
- Get physical exams to detect early problems.
- Strengthen pelvic floor muscles with Kegel exercises:
  - The first step is to identify pelvic floor muscles. When urinating, stop the flow by squeezing the pelvic floor muscles. Another way is to insert a finger into vagina (women) or rectum (men), then tighten the muscles around the finger. Repeat each method until you are sure you can feel which muscles are involved.
  - The exercises can be done any time and any place, lying down or sitting up. Start by emptying the bladder.
  - Tighten pelvic floor muscles. Hold for a count of 10.
  - Relax the muscles completely for a count of 10.
  - Perform 10 exercises, 3 times a day (morning, afternoon, and night). Don't do more than this.
  - It may take 6 weeks to 3 months for improvement.

EXPECTED OUTCOME

Treatment can help reduce symptoms.

POSSIBLE COMPLICATIONS

Physical problems are rare. It can affect quality of life.

 DIAGNOSIS & TREATMENT

GENERAL MEASURES

- Your health care provider will do a physical exam and ask questions about your incontinence symptoms. Medical tests of blood and urine may be done to check for other conditions. Additional tests may be done to help diagnose specific urinary-tract problems. You may be asked to keep a diary about your urination patterns.
- Treatment may involve drugs for bladder spasms or infection, weight loss, smoking cessation, Kegel exercises, pessary, other types of therapy, or surgery.
- Other therapies include biofeedback, electrical stimulation, bladder training, magnetic innervation, or special weights to strengthen pelvic muscles.
- Have quick access to a toilet. Urinate on schedule.
- Learn and practice Kegel exercises. Try to use the squeezing technique just before any activity that brings on the urinary urge (running water or drinking water).
- Wear absorbent underpants or incontinence pads.
- A pessary (support device) to fit inside the vagina to support the uterus or other types of devices including urethral plugging or stenting may help.
- If other methods fail, surgery to tighten relaxed or damaged muscles that support the bladder helps some. Even with surgery, some leakage may continue.
- To learn more: National Association for Continence, (800) 252-3337; website: www.nafc.org or Simon Foundation for Continence, (800) 237-4666; website: www.simonfoundation.org.

MEDICATION

- Drugs to control bladder spasms may be prescribed.
- Estrogen therapy may be prescribed for women.
- Drugs for infection if needed.

ACTIVITY

No limits. Exercise on a regular basis to improve health.

DIET

- Start a weight-loss program if you are overweight.
- Limit caffeine and alcohol. Reduce overall fluid intake.

 NOTIFY OUR OFFICE IF

You or a family member has symptoms of urge incontinence and self-treatment isn't helping.

Special notes:

_____

_____

_____

More notes on the back of this page ☐

INDIGESTION
(Dyspepsia)

 ## BASIC INFORMATION

DESCRIPTION

Indigestion is the term used to describe chest or abdominal discomfort following meals. The medical term is dyspepsia. Almost everyone will experience indigestion at one time or another. Some people have it every day, others may have it occasionally.

FREQUENT SIGNS AND SYMPTOMS

- Mild nausea.
- Upset stomach.
- Upper abdominal discomfort.
- Gas or belching.
- Bloated or full feeling.
- Stomach may feel full soon after starting a meal.
- Acid taste in the mouth.

CAUSES

There may be excess stomach acid produced, problems with motility (movement of food through the digestive system), irritation of the stomach lining, or an increase in gas. A bacterial infection with *Helicobacter pylori* may also be involved. A number of risk factors are known to lead to indigestion.

RISK INCREASES WITH

- Eating too much and eating too quickly.
- Eating food with a high fat content.
- Poor digestion of gas-forming foods such as beans, cucumbers, cabbage, turnips, and onions.
- Smoking.
- Drinking too much alcohol.
- Lactose intolerance.
- Stress or anxiety.
- Some drugs can irritate the stomach lining. These include nonsteroidal anti-inflammatories (such as aspirin or ibuprofen), iron supplements, antibiotics, and others.
- Swallowing too much air when chewing.
- Exercising right after eating.
- Food allergy.
- Pregnancy.
- Overweight.

PREVENTIVE MEASURES

- Follow guidelines listed under Treatment.
- Avoid risk factors where possible.

EXPECTED OUTCOMES

Indigestion is very common and is usually nothing to worry about. Symptoms can be controlled, but recurrence is likely.

POSSIBLE COMPLICATIONS

Indigestion usually does not cause complications. It can occasionally be a symptom of another disorder that could be more serious.

 ## DIAGNOSIS & TREATMENT

GENERAL MEASURES

- Most people will self-treat this disorder. If symptoms persist or cause concern, see your health care provider. A physical exam may be done and questions asked about your symptoms. Medical tests may sometimes be needed to check for other disorders.
- Treatment and prevention are similar. Follow the steps listed here to help relieve the symptoms.
  - Eat slowly. Chew food carefully and completely.
  - Don't smoke right before or during a meal.
  - Relax after meals, but don't lie down.
  - Avoid excitement or exercise right after a meal.
  - Avoid situations that make you swallow air, such as chewing gum, or drinking carbonated drinks.
  - Avoid tight clothing.
  - Avoid foods you don't digest well.
  - Avoid emotional problems during meals.
  - Place blocks under the head of your bed to raise it a few inches.
  - Avoid nonsteroidal anti-inflammatory drugs. Ask your health care provider about other options.

MEDICATIONS

- You may use nonprescription antacids to neutralize the stomach acid. Use H2 antagonists (such as cimetidine or ranitidine) or proton pump inhibitors (such as omeprazole) to reduce stomach acid.
- Stronger drugs may be prescribed if needed.

ACTIVITY

No limits. Daily exercise (such as 30 minute walk) helps promote good health. Don't exercise right after a meal.

DIET

Eat small meals. Don't eat near bedtime. Avoid foods that cause discomfort. Eat slowly; don't gulp food. Avoid alcohol or caffeine on an empty stomach. Lose weight, if you are overweight.

 ## NOTIFY OUR OFFICE IF

- You or a family member has symptoms of indigestion that persist, are severe, or cause concern.
- Other symptoms occur along with indigestion, such as chest pain, shortness of breath, or rapid weight loss.

Special notes:

_____

_____

_____

More notes on the back of this page ☐

INFLUENZA
(Flu)

 BASIC INFORMATION

DESCRIPTION

A contagious infection caused by viruses that affect the nose, throat, and lungs. Influenza (flu) outbreaks occur in the late fall and winter with varying degrees of severity. The disease spreads through communities creating an epidemic. Influenza affects both sexes and all ages.

FREQUENT SIGNS AND SYMPTOMS

- Chills and moderate-to-high fever.
- Headache.
- Muscle aches, including backache.
- Dry cough.
- Sore throat.
- Runny or stuffy nose.
- Fatigue.

CAUSES

The virus germs are spread when an infected person coughs, sneezes, or speaks. The germs get into the air, and nearby persons breathe in the germs. Flu can also be spread by touching a surface that has the germs on it and then touching your nose or mouth. Adults are contagious 1 day before symptoms and up to 7 days after getting sick. Children may be contagious for longer than 7 days. Symptoms start 1 to 5 days after exposure.

RISK INCREASES WITH

- Crowded places during an epidemic.
- Students in schools.
- Children and the elderly.
- Nursing homes or long-term care centers.
- Recent illness that has lowered resistance.
- Smokers.
- Chronic illness, such as chronic lung or heart disease.
- Weak immune system due to illness or drugs.

PREVENTIVE MEASURES

- Have a yearly influenza vaccine injection or a nasal spray flu vaccine. A different vaccine is made every year because strains of the virus change from year to year. Sometimes, an unpredicted new strain appears and you may still get the flu, but it is usually a milder case. Talk to your health care provider if you have any questions.
- Some antiviral drugs may also help in preventing flu.
- Wash hands often to prevent the spread of any germs.

EXPECTED OUTCOMES

Most people who get the flu get better in a week. A cough or tired feeling may last a little longer. Elderly persons, children 6 months to 23 months, pregnant women, and people with chronic illnesses are more at risk for complications.

POSSIBLE COMPLICATIONS

Pneumonia, dehydration, or worsening of a chronic illness. Children may get sinus problems or ear infections.

 DIAGNOSIS & TREATMENT

GENERAL MEASURES

- Most people who get the flu will use self-care methods at home. See your health care provider if symptoms are more severe, cause any concern, or you are at risk for complications.
- Your health care provider may do a physical exam. A diagnosis of flu can usually be made based on the symptoms. Medical tests are not always needed, but may be done to verify the diagnosis or check for complications.
- Treatment steps may include extra rest, drinking plenty of fluids, and using flu remedies or other drugs.
- To relieve nasal congestion, use salt-water drops (one-quarter teaspoon of salt in four ounces of water).
- To relieve a sore throat, gargle often with warm or cold double-strength tea or salt water (mix one-half teaspoon of salt in one cup of water).
- Use a cool-mist humidifier (if advised) to increase air moisture. Clean humidifier daily.
- Avoid spreading germs. Wash your hands often.
- Use a warm heating pad for aching muscles.

MEDICATIONS

- For minor discomfort, use nonprescription drugs, such as acetaminophen, aspirin, cough syrups, nasal sprays, or decongestants. Do not give aspirin to children under age 18.
- Antiviral drugs may be prescribed.

ACTIVITY

Get extra rest. Rest helps your body fight the virus.

DIET

You may just want liquids at first. Then progress to small meals of bland starchy foods (e.g., dry toast, rice, pudding, cooked cereal, baked potatoes).

 NOTIFY OUR OFFICE IF

- You or a family member has symptoms of influenza that seem more severe or cause concern.
- Symptoms get worse, such as higher fever, shaking chills, chest pain with breathing, coughing that produces a yellow mucus, ear ache, sinus pain, neck pain or stiffness, nausea, or vomiting.

Special notes:

_____

_____

_____

More notes on the back of this page ☐

264

INSECT BITES & STINGS

 BASIC INFORMATION

DESCRIPTION

Skin eruptions and other symptoms caused by insect bites or stings from mosquitoes, fleas, chiggers, bedbugs, ants, spiders, bees, wasps, hornets, scorpions, and other insects. The victim often doesn't remember being bitten or stung.

FREQUENT SIGNS AND SYMPTOMS

• Red lumps in the skin. The lumps usually appear within minutes after the bite or sting. Some don't appear for 6 to 12 hours. Skin reactions fall into 2 kinds:

  - A toxic reaction with pain and sometimes fever, such as from bee stings.

  - A toxic reaction with itching due to the body's release of histamine at the site of the bite, such as from mosquitoes.

CAUSES

The insect bite or sting causes an injection of venom into the skin. This starts a reaction from the body's immune system. The reaction may be mild to severe, depending on how sensitive a person is to the toxin.

RISK INCREASES WITH

• Areas with heavy insect infestations.
• Warm weather in spring and summer.
• Lack of protective measures.
• Perfumes, colognes.

PREVENTIVE MEASURES

• If you cannot avoid exposure, apply insect repellents with diethyltoluamide (DEET) to the skin.
• Wear protective clothing. Apply permethrin to clothing to repel insects and ticks.

EXPECTED OUTCOMES

Most of the symptoms are mild and go away in 2 to 3 days. Scratching may occur for several weeks. Treatment helps, but it doesn't cure quickly.

POSSIBLE COMPLICATIONS

• A bacterial infection at the site of the bite.
• Anaphylaxis (life-threatening allergic reaction) for certain super-sensitive persons.
• Scarring on the skin.
• Disorders caused by certain insects. These include Lyme disease, Rocky Mountain spotted fever, West Nile virus, malaria, and others.

 DIAGNOSIS & TREATMENT

GENERAL MEASURES

• For severe reactions to a bite or sting, get emergency help right away. They can be life-threatening. For most bites and stings, self-care is usually all that is needed.

• Remove stinger. Scrape it out. Don't use tweezers.
• For bee, wasp, yellow-jacket, or hornet stings, rub a paste of meat tenderizer and water into the site.
• For ant bites rub the bite with ammonia; repeat as often as necessary.
• For spider or scorpion bites, capture the insect, if possible, and seek medical help.
• For a tick, use a tweezer to remove it. Put it in a jar with alcohol to kill it. Save it in case more medical problems develop.
• Clean the wound. Apply an ice pack.
• Elevate and rest the affected body part.
• Warm-water soaks help soothe minor pain. Cool-water soaks feel better for itching.
• If you have had anaphylaxis (severe allergic reaction) following an insect bite, carry a special kit to treat it in the future.

MEDICATIONS

• For minor discomfort, you may use:
  - Nonprescription oral antihistamines to decrease itching.
  - Nonprescription topical steroid drugs to reduce redness and soreness and to decrease itching. For face and groin, use only low-potency steroid products without fluorine.
• For serious symptoms, you may be prescribed:
  - Stronger topical steroids or oral steroids if the reaction is severe.
  - Injection of drugs may be needed to prevent or reduce symptoms of anaphylaxis.
• A tetanus shot if needed for some patients.

ACTIVITY

No limits.

DIET

No special diet.

 NOTIFY OUR OFFICE IF

• You or a family member has an insect bite or sting and has a severe reaction. This is an emergency!
• Self-care does not relieve symptoms, or symptoms don't improve after 2 to 3 days of treatment.
• Fever occurs and bitten area becomes red, swollen, warm, and tender. This could mean an infection.

Special notes:

_____

_____

_____

More notes on the back of this page ☐

INSOMNIA

 BASIC INFORMATION

DESCRIPTION
Problems falling asleep, staying asleep, waking early, or a combination of these. Insomnia affects all age groups, but is more common in the elderly. Insomnia is often described by how long it has gone on. Transient is a few days, short-term is less than 3 weeks, and chronic is more than 3 weeks.

FREQUENT SIGNS AND SYMPTOMS
· Difficulty falling asleep.
· A brief period of sleep is followed by wakefulness.
· Normal sleep until very early in the morning, then wakefulness (often with frightening thoughts).
· Daytime fatigue and tiredness.
· Lack of sleep causes problems with social, work, family, and other areas of one's life.

CAUSES
Insomnia is a symptom, not a disease. It can be caused by physical, mental, and environmental problems.

RISK INCREASES WITH
· Depression, anxiety, tension, or stress.
· Daytime napping.
· Noise (including a snoring partner).
· Allergies and early-morning wheezing.
· Heart or lung problems that cause shortness of breath when lying down.
· Painful disorders, such as arthritis.
· Frequent need to urinate at night.
· Night sweats, or disorders that cause excess itching.
· Sexual problems.
· Drinking caffeine drinks such as coffee, tea, or cola.
· Use of some drugs.
· Odd work hours, such as swing shifts.
· A new environment or location.
· Jet lag after travel.
· Lack of exercise.
· Smoking, alcoholism, or drug abuse, including overuse of sleep-inducing drugs.
· Withdrawal from addictive substances.
· Sleep apnea.

PREVENTIVE MEASURES
· Avoid lengthy daytime napping.
· Avoid risk factors, where possible.
· For general good health, eat a healthy diet, exercise daily, maintain weight for height, and don't smoke.

EXPECTED OUTCOMES
Insomnia can usually be relieved by treating the cause, using self-care steps, or with other medical treatment.

POSSIBLE COMPLICATIONS
Insomnia can cause impaired thinking, and health and emotional problems that affect all aspects of life.

 DIAGNOSIS & TREATMENT

GENERAL MEASURES
· You may use self-care steps first. These include:
  - Try to reduce tension, stress, or anxiety in your life.
  - Don't turn your bedroom into an office or a den.
  - Create a comfortable sleep setting.
  - Relax in a warm bath before bedtime.
  - After 15 to 20 minutes of trying to sleep, get up and do some relaxing activity. Don't watch television.
  - Turn off your mind. Focus on peaceful and relaxing thoughts. Play soft music or relaxation tapes.
  - Set a strict sleep schedule and keep to it.
  - Use ear plugs, eye shades, or an electric blanket.
· See your health care provider if self-care doesn't help. A physical exam may be done and questions asked about your symptoms and activities. Medical tests may be done to check for any physical disorders. A sleep study may be prescribed. Medical steps may include:
  - Counseling for problems such as depression.
  - Treatment for any medical order diagnosed.

MEDICATIONS
· Sleep-inducing drugs may be prescribed for a short time if: short-term insomnia is interfering with daily activities; you have a disorder that disturbs sleep; you need to establish regular sleep patterns.
· Long-term use of sleep inducers may be counter-productive or addictive. Don't use sleeping pills unless they are prescribed.

ACTIVITY
· Exercise daily to create healthy fatigue, but not within 2 hours of going to bed.
· Have sexual relations, if they are satisfying and fulfilling before going to sleep.

DIET
Avoid alcohol, caffeine, or a heavy meal within 3 hours of bedtime. Try a light snack with milk at bedtime.

 NOTIFY OUR OFFICE IF

· You or a family member has had insomnia for over 4 weeks or it is interfering with your ability to function.
· Drugs used in treatment produce any side effects.

Special notes:

_____

_____

_____

More notes on the back of this page ☐

INTERSTITIAL CYSTITIS

BASIC INFORMATION

DESCRIPTION
Interstitial cystitis (IC) is a chronic bladder disorder. Symptoms are similar to cystitis (an infection of the urinary tract), but no infection is found. Hunner's ulcer is a rare, and more severe, form of IC.

FREQUENT SIGNS AND SYMPTOMS
- Symptoms vary greatly for each person.
- Pelvic pain and a feeling of pressure.
- Urgent need to urinate day and night (up to 40 times a day). This also causes sleep problems.
- Bladder does not feel like it empties completely when you urinate.
- Pain during sexual intercourse.
- Burning when urinating.
- Vaginal and rectal pain.

CAUSES
The lining (or wall) of the bladder breaks down. Urine stored in the bladder irritates the damaged lining and it becomes red and sore. Why the lining breaks down is not known. Medical tests find no bacteria or virus infection. There actually may be several causes, or there may be different disorders, rather than just one.

RISK INCREASES WITH
- Having allergies (such as to drugs or food).
- Hay fever or asthma.
- Rheumatoid arthritis, lupus (immune disorders).
- Certain bowel or urinary problems.

PREVENTIVE MEASURES
None known.

EXPECTED OUTCOMES
Treatments can help control or relieve the symptoms, but they do not cure the disorder. It may take time to find the treatments that work best for you.

POSSIBLE COMPLICATIONS
- The symptoms may come and go over days, weeks, or months, sometimes years, even with treatment.
- Chronic symptoms can lead to problems with your work, friends, family, and sexual activity.

DIAGNOSIS & TREATMENT

GENERAL MEASURES
- There are a number of medical problems that cause similar symptoms. They include kidney stones, urinary or vaginal infection, cancer, and others. Your health care provider will perform tests to rule out these other causes of the symptoms.
- A physical exam will be performed and urine tests are needed to check for infection. A cystoscopy can con-

firm the diagnosis. In this test, a thin, tube-like device with a light is used to see inside the bladder. The test can be uncomfortable because the bladder is stretched. A drug (anesthetic) will be used to stop pain. A stretched bladder holds more urine so this test helps symptoms also.
- There are a variety of treatment options. It is important to find out what works for you.
- Bladder instillation (a bladder wash or bath) is done at the medical office. It involves stretching the bladder by filling it with a solution for about 15 minutes.
- Bladder training involves teaching yourself to urinate at certain times.
- Counseling or behavior training. Learn how to relax and cope with stress, anxiety, or depression.
- A TENS (transcutaneous electrical nerve stimulation) device uses mild electric pulses to help block pain.
- Surgery is rarely needed. It may be done as a last resort when other methods have failed.
- Don't smoke. Smoking makes symptoms worse.
- Learn about the disorder. Consider a support group.
- To learn more: The Interstitial Cystitis Association (ICA), 51 Monroe St, Suite 1402, Rockville, MD 20850; (800) 435-7422; website: www.ichelp.org.

MEDICATIONS
- You may use nonprescription pain relievers.
- Pentosan polysulfate, brand name Elmiron, may be prescribed. It is used for treating interstitial cystitis.
- Other drugs may be prescribed for depression, anxiety, sleep problems, and severe pain.

ACTIVITY
- No limits other than those caused by the symptoms.
- Regular exercise helps some patients feel better.

DIET
Diet changes help some patients. Avoid drinks with caffeine, alcohol, or artificial sweeteners; spicy foods, chocolate, soda/carbonated beverages, citrus fruits, and tomatoes.

NOTIFY OUR OFFICE IF

- You or a family member has symptoms of interstitial cystitis.
- Treatment is not helping the pain or other symptoms.
- New symptoms occur. Drugs may cause side effects.

Special notes: _____

_____

_____

_____

More notes on the back of this page ☐

INTUSSUSCEPTION

 ## BASIC INFORMATION

DESCRIPTION

An intestinal obstruction in which the bowel telescopes (folds into itself), forming a tube within a tube. It can affect all ages, but it is most common in infants and children between 2 months and 6 years. It is more common in boys.

FREQUENT SIGNS AND SYMPTOMS

• Cramping pain in the abdomen. Infants cry out, bring the legs up to the abdomen. They become pale and sweaty during an attack. Attacks of pain may occur 10 to 20 minutes apart.
• Vomiting.
• Rectal bleeding. This may be dark red material that resembles red current jelly.
• Weakness and lack of energy.
• Swollen abdomen.
• Mass in the abdomen that can be felt.
• Later symptoms: increased weakness, fever, shock (rapid heartbeat, weak pulse, rapid breathing).

CAUSES

• Unknown for infants. The disorder may be caused by a virus infection, but this is unproven.
• In older children (usually over age 3) or in adults, it may be due to an intestinal problem.

RISK INCREASES WITH

• Recent upper-respiratory infection.
• Recent diarrhea illness.
• Cystic fibrosis.
• Blunt injury to the abdomen.
• Lymph nodes that are enlarged; tumor or polyp in the intestine.
• Season of the year (for unknown reasons). It is most common in late spring, early summer, and midwinter.

PREVENTIVE MEASURES

No specific preventive measures.

EXPECTED OUTCOMES

Outcome for most children is very good. With early diagnosis and treatment, complications are unlikely to develop.

POSSIBLE COMPLICATIONS

• Dehydration and shock.
• Intestinal perforation.
• Tissue damage that cannot be reversed.
• An infection may occur after surgery.
• The disorder may recur after barium treatment.
• Without treatment, complications are life-threatening.

 ## DIAGNOSIS & TREATMENT

GENERAL MEASURES

• Your child's health care provider will do a physical exam with careful attention to the abdomen. Medical tests may include blood studies, x-rays, and ultrasound.
• A barium or air enema may be done for diagnosis and treatment. In this procedure, a liquid containing barium is given with a tube into the rectum and special x-rays are taken. The barium helps show the intussusception on the x-ray. In many cases, the pressure of the barium unfolds the bowel and cures the problem. An air enema can work in the same way.
• Surgery to correct the problem may be needed. This is done if the child is too ill for the enema procedure or it was done and did not provide a cure. Surgery involves pushing out the telescoped portion of the intestine. In a few cases, a part of the bowel must be cut out.

MEDICATIONS

• Drugs are usually not needed for this disorder unless infection develops. Then antibiotics may be prescribed.
• Don't use home remedies or nonprescription drugs, such as laxatives, for this condition. They may be dangerous.

ACTIVITY

The child should rest in bed until the obstruction is cleared. Activities may then be resumed gradually.

DIET

Don't feed a child who has signs of intestinal obstruction. Intravenous (through a vein) fluids are given in the hospital until the child can eat again.

 ## NOTIFY OUR OFFICE IF

• Your child has signs or symptoms of intestinal obstruction. This condition changes quickly from a curable one to a life-threatening one.
• Any new symptoms develop after treatment.

Special notes:

_____

_____

_____

More notes on the back of this page ☐

IRITIS
(Uveitis)

BASIC INFORMATION

DESCRIPTION

Redness and soreness (inflammation) of the iris. The iris is the colored part of the eye. The disorder is also called uveitis.

FREQUENT SIGNS AND SYMPTOMS

May start suddenly:
- Severe eye pain.
- Photophobia (sensitivity to light).
- Eye redness.
- Smaller pupil in the affected eye (sometimes).
- Tears.
- Blurred vision.

Gradual onset:
- Eye pain.
- Photophobia.
- Floating spots in the field of vision.
- Blurred vision.

CAUSES

The cause is unknown for most people. It is sometimes one of the symptoms of a disease that affects other parts of the body, such as arthritis. Iritis may sometimes be confused with pink eye (conjunctivitis).

RISK INCREASES WITH
- Ankylosing spondylitis.
- Inflammatory bowel disease.
- Reiter's syndrome.
- Arthritis.
- Behçet syndrome.
- Herpes infections.
- Lyme disease.
- Injuries.
- Sarcoidosis.
- Candidal infection.
- Syphilis.
- Histoplasmosis.
- Toxoplasmosis.
- Tuberculosis.

PREVENTIVE MEASURES

Cannot be prevented at present.

EXPECTED OUTCOMES

Vision can usually be preserved with prompt treatment. Recovery takes 6 to 8 weeks. It sometimes depends on the disorder that is associated with iritis.

POSSIBLE COMPLICATIONS
- Glaucoma.
- Cataracts.
- Permanent or partial vision loss.

DIAGNOSIS & TREATMENT

GENERAL MEASURES

- Iritis can be diagnosed by your eye care provider using special equipment to look into the eye. Other medical tests may be needed to help diagnose any health problem that is associated with iritis.
- Treatment goals are to reduce pain and redness, prevent complications, and treat other health problems that are diagnosed.
- Wear dark glasses, including indoors, until treatment is complete.

MEDICATIONS

- Eyedrops (mydriatics) that dilate the pupil and prevent scarring. You may need to use eyedrops for a long time.
- Oral cortisone drugs or cortisone eyedrops to reduce inflammation may be prescribed.
- Drugs for other medical problems may be prescribed.

ACTIVITY

No limits.

DIET

No special diet.

NOTIFY OUR OFFICE IF

- You or a family member has symptoms of iritis, either sudden or gradual. Call immediately.
- Vision changes in any way.
- New, unexplained symptoms develop. Drugs used in treatment may produce side effects.

Special notes:

_____

_____

_____

More notes on the back of this page ☐

IRRITABLE BOWEL SYNDROME
(Spastic Colon; Mucous Colitis)

BASIC INFORMATION

DESCRIPTION
A functional disorder of the large intestine (bowel). It is not a disease. "Functional disorder" means the bowel doesn't work properly. Irritable bowel syndrome (IBS) can cause a variety of symptoms. Episodes may last for days, weeks, or months. It is not contagious, inherited, or cancerous. It is very common and affects women more than men.

FREQUENT SIGNS AND SYMPTOMS
· Cramp-like pain in the middle or to one side of the lower abdomen. Pain is usually relieved with bowel movements.
· Diarrhea or constipation; usually alternating.
· Swollen or bloated (distended) abdomen and gas.
· Mucus in the stools.
· Straining to have bowel movement.
· Urgency to have bowel movement.
· Feeling that the bowels still have to be emptied after having a bowel movement.

CAUSES
Exact cause is unknown. The nerves and muscles in the bowel seem to be extra-sensitive in people with IBS. Nerves can cause pain and discomfort if they become irritated. Muscles that contract to pass food through the intestines may contract too much and cause cramping and diarrhea. The bowel can overreact to food, stress, exercise, and hormones. Stress may trigger symptoms if you have IBS, but it doesn't cause IBS.

RISK INCREASES WITH
· Under age 35.
· Women more than with men.
· Other family members with similar bowel problems.
· People who have panic disorder, or similar disorders.
· People who have had a history of sexual, physical, or emotional abuse.

PREVENTIVE MEASURES
No specific measures to prevent IBS. After it is diagnosed, you can find ways to help prevent symptoms.

EXPECTED OUTCOMES
The condition is usually recurrent throughout life. Symptoms may be mild to severe and may come and go. Most people can be helped with treatment. No specific treatment works best for everybody. You may need to try more than one to see what works for you.

POSSIBLE COMPLICATIONS
· IBS can affect all aspects of life. It can interfere with work schedules, limit physical activities, disrupt personal relationships, and cause a restricted social life.
· IBS does not cause physical damage to the bowel. It does not lead to bleeding, serious disease, or cancer.

DIAGNOSIS & TREATMENT

GENERAL MEASURES
· Your health care provider may do a physical exam and ask questions about your symptoms and activities. Medical tests may include blood and stool studies, as well as others tests to exclude more serious disorders. A mental health exam may be done also.
· Treatment may involve a combination of diet changes, drugs if needed, and coping with stress.
· Reduce stress in your life. Try various techniques that can help you relax. Meditation, self-hypnosis, or biofeedback may help. Keep a stress and symptom diary so you know who or what may trigger an episode.
· Get counseling for emotional or personal problems.
· Quit smoking. Nicotine may add to the problem.
· Join a support group. This can be reassuring for some.
· To learn more: National Digestive Diseases Information Clearinghouse, 2 Information Way, Bethesda, MD 20892, (800) 891-5389; website: www.niddk.nih.gov/health/digest.

MEDICATIONS
· Antispasmodics to relieve severe cramps and drugs to treat the constipation form of IBS may be prescribed.
· Drugs for depression or anxiety may be prescribed.
· Antidiarrheals or laxatives need to be used with caution. Get medical advice before using them.

ACTIVITY
No limits. Daily physical exercise improves bowel function, keeps you fit, and helps reduce stress.

DIET
· Increase fiber in the diet to promote good bowel function. Add fiber to your diet slowly to give the body time to adjust. Too much fiber can cause gas.
· Avoid foods or drinks that can worsen symptoms. These include fatty foods, milk products, chocolate, alcohol, caffeine, and carbonated drinks. Keep a food diary to help find the foods that cause you problems.
· Avoid large meals, but eat regularly.

NOTIFY OUR OFFICE IF

· If you or a family member has symptoms of IBS.
· Symptoms don't improve despite treatment.

Special notes:

_____

_____

_____

More notes on the back of this page ☐

270

KAPOSI SARCOMA

 ## BASIC INFORMATION

DESCRIPTION

A form of skin cancer that is a found most often in patients with advanced HIV (human immunodeficiency virus) infection. A second form of Kaposi's sarcoma is associated with some immunosuppressive drugs. A third form, referred to as classic, is found in elderly men of Mediterranean and Eastern European ancestry. A fourth form is found in young men in Africa.

FREQUENT SIGNS AND SYMPTOMS

• Skin lesions (sores) usually on the face, arms, and trunk. They may also be found in the mouth, lymph nodes, and other areas.
• The color may be brown, reddish-purple, or purple-black. They usually don't itch or cause pain.
• Lesions in the mouth may interfere with eating or swallowing.
• Lesions on the feet may interfere with walking.
• Swelling of the face, scrotum, and lower extremities if the lymph nodes are affected.
• May cause internal bleeding if the stomach is affected.
• May cause breathing problems if the lungs are affected.

CAUSES

The exact cause is unknown. Multiple causes are probably involved. It is known to be caused, in part, by a type of human herpesvirus called HHV-8.

RISK INCREASES WITH

• Weak immune system due to HIV-AIDS infection.
• Elderly men of Mediterranean and Eastern European descent.
• People with weak immune system, due to drugs taken for organ transplantation.

PREVENTIVE MEASURES

If you have AIDS, using strong anti-HIV drugs can boost the immune system and help prevent Kaposi's sarcoma.

EXPECTED OUTCOMES

• There is no cure. It is a lifelong condition.
• For HIV-AIDS associated infection, the outcome depends on the extent and location of the lesions and the degree of immune system impairment. Treatment can help shrink the lesions, but they often recur.
• For Kaposi's due to an immune-suppressing drug, it often improves if drug is changed or dosage reduced.
• For classic type, patients may develop another form of cancer or die from other causes.

POSSIBLE COMPLICATIONS

• Lesions spread to other parts of the body.
• Other infections.
• Internal bleeding.
• Anemia.

 ## DIAGNOSIS & TREATMENT

GENERAL MEASURES

• Your health care provider will do an exam of the affected skin areas. Medical tests may be done to confirm the diagnosis and to see if the disorder has spread to other places in the body (staging).
• If there are only a few skin lesions, they may be followed up for a period of time rather than being treated.
• More widespread skin lesions can be treated in several ways. They can be frozen (cryotherapy), treated with radiation, cut out surgically, or treated with drugs that are injected into the skin or used on the skin. Your health care provider will discuss your options.
• Cosmetic cover up products can be used on the skin to camouflage the lesions.
• If lesions have spread to the inside (internal organs) of the body, drugs are used for treatment.

MEDICATIONS

• Drugs (antiretrovirals) for AIDS treatment are usually prescribed if they are not being taken already.
• Anticancer drugs may be given.
• Topical retinoic acid may be used for skin lesions.
• New drugs are being studied such as antivirals that can treat the herpesvirus.

ACTIVITY

As tolerated.

DIET

You may need a special diet if the mouth is affected.

 ## NOTIFY OUR OFFICE IF

• You or a household member has symptoms of Kaposi sarcoma.
• New or unexplained symptoms develop. Drugs used in treatment may cause side effects.

Special notes:

_____

_____

_____

More notes on the back of this page ☐

KELOIDS

 BASIC INFORMATION

DESCRIPTION
An overgrowth of fibrous tissue (scar) on the skin. Keloids can appear anywhere on the skin, but most commonly appear on the earlobes, chest, upper back, and shoulders. Keloids are more frequent in black people than in white people and occur more often in young women.

FREQUENT SIGNS AND SYMPTOMS
· Keloids begin as a small bump. The lump grows and turns into firm, raised, hard scars that are slightly pink.
· Scars may continue to grow over a period of time.
· May itch or cause burning sensation.
· They may become a cosmetic problem.
· Scars may become irritated from rubbing on clothing.

CAUSES
Keloids probably occur due to a defective healing process. An excess of collagen forms at the site of a healing scar. Keloids usually arise in an area of injury (such as after a burn or from severe acne), but sometimes arise from a very minor scratch. Why they occur in certain people is unknown.

RISK INCREASES WITH
· Family history of keloids.
· Dark skin pigment.
· Surgical wound.
· Acne.
· Burn injury.
· Ear piercing.
· Vaccination.
· Insect bite.
· Folliculitis barbae (inflammation of a hair follicle).

PREVENTIVE MEASURES
· Avoid injuries to the skin.
· For patients with known tendency to keloid formation, elective surgery should be avoided. If a procedure is necessary, special precautions should be implemented.

EXPECTED OUTCOMES
Scars gradually diminish with treatment. Sometimes, keloids heal on their own. Keloids are generally considered harmless and noncancerous.

POSSIBLE COMPLICATIONS
They may recur, despite treatment.

 DIAGNOSIS & TREATMENT

GENERAL MEASURES
· Your health care provider can diagnose keloids by their appearance on the skin. Other medical tests are usually not needed, but may be done to rule out any other skin problem.
· There are a variety of treatment options. Your health care provider will discuss them with you.
· Treatment may include injections into the scars. This may be combined with surgery to help remove the scars.
· Surgery may also be done in combination with radiation therapy.
· Cryotherapy involves freezing the affected area with liquid nitrogen.
· Special gel sheeting can be used to flatten the scars. It is applied to the area and changed about every week or 10 days for as long as a year.
· Other new therapies are currently undergoing study.

MEDICATIONS
Injection of corticosteroid drugs directly into the keloid. May be repeated every 3 to 4 weeks until desired degree of flattening and softening has been achieved.

ACTIVITY
No limits.

DIET
No special diet.

 NOTIFY OUR OFFICE IF

· You or a family member has signs of keloids.
· Keloids recur after treatment.

Special notes:

_____

_____

_____

More notes on the back of this page ☐

KERATITIS

 ## BASIC INFORMATION

DESCRIPTION

A term used to describe a variety of conditions where there is inflammation, infection, or irritation of the cornea. The cornea is the clear membrane on the front of the eye that covers the iris and the pupil.

FREQUENT SIGNS AND SYMPTOMS

- Symptoms may be mild to severe.
- Eye pain.
- Redness and itching of the eye.
- Feeling that there is something in the eye.
- Photophobia (sensitivity to light).
- Tearing or discharge of the eye.
- Blurry vision.

CAUSES

There are many causes and types of keratitis. In many cases, an injury to the cornea has allowed an infection to occur. Prompt treatment is important.

RISK INCREASES WITH

- Viral, bacterial, or fungal infection. The most common is the same virus that causes cold sores.
- Drying of the eye, caused by an eyelid disorder or insufficient tear formation.
- Foreign object in the eye.
- Intense light, such as from welding arcs or the reflection of intense sunlight from snow or water. Symptoms may not appear for 24 hours after exposure.
- Vitamin A deficiency (rare in normal diet).
- Allergy or sensitivity to eye cosmetics, air pollution, airborne particles (pollen, dust, mold, or yeasts), and other allergens.

PREVENTIVE MEASURES

- Wear protective glasses or goggles if work or sports activity involves eye hazards.
- Eat a well-balanced diet that contains sufficient vitamin A, or take a multiple-vitamin containing vitamin A.
- For dry-eyes, use eye drops recommended by your health care provider.
- Don't share eye makeup.
- Avoid rubbing the eyes when you have cold sores.
- Follow instructions provided with contact lenses for cleaning and length of wearing time.

EXPECTED OUTCOMES

Depends on the cause. With early treatment, most types of keratitis are curable. It may take several months.

POSSIBLE COMPLICATIONS

- Glaucoma.
- Ulceration of the cornea.
- Permanent scarring in the eye.
- Vision loss.

 ## DIAGNOSIS & TREATMENT

GENERAL MEASURES

- A special eye exam can diagnose keratitis. A vision test and other medical tests may be done. You may be referred to an eye care provider (ophthalmologist).
- Treatment usually involves eye medication.
- Cool compresses applied to the closed eye may help.
- Surgery to replace the cornea (severe cases only).

MEDICATIONS

- Antibiotic, antifungal, or antiviral eyedrops or ointments are prescribed depending on the infection.
- Steroid eyedrops may be prescribed.
- Don't treat any eye inflammation without medical advice. Don't use nonprescription eyedrops containing topical corticosteroids. These may worsen the condition or cause eyeball perforation.

ACTIVITY

No limits.

DIET

No special diet.

 ## NOTIFY OUR OFFICE IF

- You or a family member has symptoms of keratitis. Get treatment right away.
- Your vision changes in any way.

Special notes:

_____

_____

_____

More notes on the back of this page ☐

KERATOSES, SEBORRHEIC

 BASIC INFORMATION

DESCRIPTION
Growths on the outer layer of the skin. They may involve the chest, back, face, and/or arms. They can affect adults of both sexes. By age 60, almost everyone has a few seborrheic keratoses. They are not related to skin cancer.

FREQUENT SIGNS AND SYMPTOMS
· Growths are raised, thick bumps. They are flat-topped with well-defined borders.
· Newer growths are relatively flat and light brown. Older ones are dark brown or black.
· Growths are wider than tall. They appear "stuck on."
· They may itch or bleed if they get irritated. They do not cause any pain.
· There may be only 1 or 2 growths, or there may be as many as 100.

CAUSES
Unknown. They are not caused by sunlight. They can not be spread from one person to another.

RISK INCREASES WITH
· Aging.
· Family history of the disorder.

PREVENTIVE MEASURES
They can not be prevented.

EXPECTED OUTCOMES
The number of growths usually increases with age. Each growth is permanent unless removed. Seborrheic keratoses are harmless and require no treatment. People may want them removed (especially if they are unsightly or irritated by clothing).

POSSIBLE COMPLICATIONS
None expected.

 DIAGNOSIS & TREATMENT

GENERAL MEASURES
· Usually, no treatment is needed. If you are concerned, see your health care provider. The growths can be diagnosed with a skin exam. In some cases, a growth may be removed for viewing under a microscope to confirm the diagnosis.
· The growths can be removed if they are unsightly, are irritated by clothing, or cause problems with shaving. Removal methods include cryosurgery (freezing), chemocautery, light electrosurgery, or shave biopsy. Your health care provider will discuss the treatment options with you.
· After removal, a blister (sometimes with blood) will develop at the treatment site. The top of the blister will come off spontaneously in about 2 weeks. You should have little or no scarring. Wash and use makeup or cosmetics as usual. If clothing irritates the blister, cover it with a small adhesive bandage.
· Seborrheic keratoses on the eyelid borders may require special treatment.

MEDICATIONS
Drugs are usually not needed for this disorder.

ACTIVITY
No limits.

DIET
No special diet.

 NOTIFY OUR OFFICE IF

· You or a family member has symptoms of seborrheic keratoses and are concerned.
· You want unsightly seborrheic keratoses removed.
· Treated areas become infected (sore, red, feels warm).

Special notes:

_____

_____

_____

More notes on the back of this page ☐

KERATOSIS, ACTINIC

 BASIC INFORMATION

DESCRIPTION

An area of sun-damaged skin. Actinic keratosis can be a problem for people who spend a lot of time in the sun. It is the most common sun-related skin growth. It is considered a precancerous condition. The skin on exposed areas, such as the scalp, face, ears, lips, arms, and hands are most often affected.

FREQUENT SIGNS AND SYMPTOMS

- Sharply outlined, scaly, or crusted areas on exposed areas of skin.
- There may be single or multiple areas (patches).
- May be red, brown, or skin colored; flat or elevated.
- The patches are usually painless, but may sometimes itch.

CAUSES

- Prolonged exposure to the sun's radiation is the most common cause. It may develop years after the person's most intense sun exposure.
- Exposure to tanning devices, or rarely, to x-rays or certain industrial chemicals may be a cause.

RISK INCREASES WITH

- Outdoor athletic activities and sports.
- Outdoor occupations, such as farming.
- Light (fair) complexion and blue, gray, or green eyes.
- Weak immune system due to illness or drugs.

PREVENTIVE MEASURES

- Protect yourself against direct sun exposure. When outdoors, wear a hat and protective clothing. Use sunscreen lotions and creams with SPF ratings of 15 or more. Avoid sun between 10 AM and 4 PM if possible.
- Do skin self-exams on a regular basis (each month).

EXPECTED OUTCOMES

There are several types of effective treatment, and outcome is usually excellent. New outbreaks do sometimes occur following treatment.

POSSIBLE COMPLICATIONS

- Skin damage.
- Some risk of skin cancer if untreated. This is usually squamous cell carcinoma, which is curable when treated early.

 DIAGNOSIS & TREATMENT

GENERAL MEASURES

- Your health care provider can diagnose the condition by an exam of the skin. Medical tests are usually not needed.
- Several treatment options are available. Your health care provider will discuss which one will work best for you, depending on the extent of the condition, your health, and your age.
- Cryosurgery (the most common treatment) is the application of liquid nitrogen to the skin.
- Curettage is the scraping away of the lesions with a sharp instrument.
- Excisional (cutting) surgery removes the lesions.
- Laser surgery may be used to destroy the cells.
- Dermabrasion is a treatment where the top layers of the skin are ground away.
- Photodynamic therapy. Medicine is applied to the affected skin, and then it is exposed to a special light.
- Chemical peels may be used for facial lesions.
- Get follow-up skin checkups every 6 months to ensure early detection and treatment of skin cancers.

MEDICATIONS

- Applications of 5-fluorouracil or masoprocol to the affected area may be used for a large affected area. These can cause irritation or an allergic reaction.
- Vitamin A and other drugs are being studied.

ACTIVITY

No limits. Reduce direct sun exposure.

DIET

No special diet.

 NOTIFY OUR OFFICE IF

You or a family member has signs of an actinic keratosis. Even though this causes no symptoms, it can be a risk for cancer.

Special notes:

_____

_____

_____

More notes on the back of this page ☐

KERATOSIS PILARIS

 ## BASIC INFORMATION

DESCRIPTION

A common skin disorder in which the openings of the hair follicles become filled with hard plugs. It usually involves the skin on the backs of upper arms, fronts of thighs, or buttocks. It may start in childhood, around age 2 or 3, affects many teenagers, and some adults.

FREQUENT SIGNS AND SYMPTOMS

• Skin bumps that are small, firm, and skin-color or pink, or sometimes red. They have a dry "sandpaper" or "goosebumps" texture.
• They are located at the openings of hair follicles.
• The condition is usually worse in winter months when a person's skin is dryer.
• Bumps usually don't itch and they do not cause pain.

CAUSES

Unknown. It does run in families. It often occurs along with other skin disorders such as ichthyosis (an inherited dry skin condition). The condition cannot be spread from one person to another.

RISK INCREASES WITH

• Family history of keratosis pilaris.
• Ichthyosis (dry and scaly skin disorder).

PREVENTIVE MEASURES

Cannot be prevented at present.

EXPECTED OUTCOMES

Keratosis pilaris is a chronic, harmless skin problem with no permanent cure. The bumps may come and go over a period of time. Many cases clear up on their own as a person gets older. Cosmetic appearance and rough skin texture are often bothersome to patients.

POSSIBLE COMPLICATIONS

Complications are unlikely. A skin infection may occur if the affected area is scratched or overly treated with abrasive methods.

 ## DIAGNOSIS & TREATMENT

GENERAL MEASURES

• If you are concerned about the skin rash, see your health care provider. The condition can be diagnosed by an exam of the affected area.
• Usually, no treatment is needed, but self-care measures may help the appearance.
• Use mild, unscented soap when bathing.
• Apply lubricating ointments or creams to the affected areas 2 or 3 times a day. The most useful time is immediately after bathing to help the skin retain moisture. There is no advantage to using expensive skin products or vitamin creams.
• Go over the affected skin area with a pumice stone, loofah sponge, or washcloth to gently loosen the plugs.

MEDICATIONS

Drugs are usually not needed for this condition. Your health care provider may prescribe a product to be applied to the skin if the condition is more severe.

ACTIVITY

No limits.

DIET

No special diet.

 ## NOTIFY OUR OFFICE IF

• You or a family member has signs of keratosis pilaris and are concerned about them.
• Appearance of the affected area changes. There may be a skin infection.

Special notes:

_____

_____

_____

More notes on the back of this page ☐

KIDNEY INFECTION, ACUTE

(Pyelonephritis, Acute)

BASIC INFORMATION

DESCRIPTION
Infection and inflammation of one, or sometimes both, kidneys. The kidneys filter waste material from the blood and produce urine. Kidney infections affect all ages and both sexes, but they are more common in females.

FREQUENT SIGNS AND SYMPTOMS
- Symptoms often come on suddenly.
- Fever and shaking chills.
- Burning, frequent urination.
- Cloudy urine or blood in the urine.
- Aching (may be severe) in one or both sides of the lower back.
- Pain in the abdomen.
- Fatigue.
- Nausea and vomiting.

CAUSES
Most often, a bacteria called *Escherichia coli*. The infection begins in the bladder (cystitis) and the infected urine moves back up the tubes (ureters) that connect the bladder to the kidneys. This is called reflux.

RISK INCREASES WITH
- Sexual activity in women. Bacteria enters the urethra (tube from bladder to outside) and bladder.
- Blockage or abnormality of the urinary system. This can be caused by stones, obstructions, nerve diseases, tumors, or congenital (being born with) deformity.
- Prostatitis (prostate inflammation).
- Catheters, tubes, or certain surgical procedures.
- Diabetes.
- Chronic bladder infection or tumor.
- Spinal-cord injury or tumor.
- Pregnancy.
- Bubble bath use in young girls.

PREVENTIVE MEASURES
- Women and girls should wipe from front to back (not back to front) after going to the bathroom.
- Avoid sitting around in wet clothing (wet swimsuits).
- Urinate within 15 minutes after sexual intercourse.
- Don't hold urine. If you have the urge to void, do so.
- Drink plenty of fluids every day.

EXPECTED OUTCOMES
With early diagnosis and treatment, an uncomplicated kidney infection is usually curable in 10 to 14 days.

POSSIBLE COMPLICATIONS
- Chronic kidney infection.
- Scarring of kidneys and permanent kidney damage.
- Blood infection.
- Hypertension (high blood pressure).

DIAGNOSIS & TREATMENT

GENERAL MEASURES
- Your health care provider will do a physical exam along with a pelvic exam in females and a rectal exam (for prostate problems) in males. Questions will be asked about your symptoms. Medical tests may include urinalysis, urine culture, and blood studies. Other tests may be done to diagnose kidney stones or obstructions.
- Treatment usually involves antibiotic drugs, or, in some cases surgery or hospital care may be needed.
- Surgery may be needed for an obstruction or kidney stones, or for an abnormality diagnosed in a child.
- Hospital care may be required for severe symptoms or for people with other medical disorders.
- Be sure to see your health care provider for follow-up urine tests to verify that the infection is cured.
- To learn more: National Kidney & Urologic Diseases Information Clearinghouse, 3 Information Way, Bethesda, MD 20892, (800) 891-5390; website: www.kidney.niddk.nih.gov.

MEDICATIONS
- Oral antibiotics. Take all the antibiotics prescribed, even if symptoms clear up.
- Antibiotics (intravenous or by injection), if oral antibiotics don't cure the infection.
- Take nonprescription drugs such as ibuprofen for pain symptoms.
- Urinary analgesics to relieve pain may be prescribed.

ACTIVITY
Rest in bed until any fever and discomfort are gone. Resume sexual relations when advised by your health care provider.

DIET
No special diet. Drink plenty of fluids each day. Drink cranberry juice or vitamin C to acidify the urine.

NOTIFY OUR OFFICE IF

- You or a family member has symptoms of a kidney infection.
- Symptoms and fever persist after 48 hours of antibiotic treatment. A different antibiotic may be needed.
- Symptoms return after treatment is completed.

Special notes:

_____

_____

_____

More notes on the back of this page ☐

KIDNEY INFECTION, CHRONIC
(Pyelonephritis, Chronic)

 BASIC INFORMATION

DESCRIPTION
Infection and inflammation of the kidneys that develops slowly and lasts for months or years. It leads to scarring and eventual loss of kidney function. Kidneys filter waste material from the blood and produce urine. This disorder can affect adults of both sexes, but it is more common in women.

FREQUENT SIGNS AND SYMPTOMS
Usually there are no signs or symptoms, unlike acute kidney infection. The following symptoms occur if chronic kidney failure develops:
- Anemia (paleness and fatigue).
- Weakness.
- Loss of appetite, nausea.
- High blood pressure and buildup of fluid in the body.
- Pain in one or both sides of the lower back.
- Blood in the urine.
- Numbness and tingling of the hands and feet.

CAUSES
The kidneys have been scarred or damaged by a variety of diseases. They begin to lose their ability to function as they normally would in removing waste products from the blood.

RISK INCREASES WITH
- Frequent, acute, bacterial kidney infections.
- Untreated lower urinary-tract infections.
- Diabetes.
- Urinary obstruction, such as stones or tumors.
- Long-term use of catheters.

PREVENTIVE MEASURES
In many cases, there are no preventive measures. Controlling diabetes and getting treatment for urinary-tract infections can help reduce risks.

EXPECTED OUTCOMES
There is no cure. The disease progresses until dialysis or kidney transplant is required. If symptoms occur, they may be relieved with treatment.

POSSIBLE COMPLICATIONS
Chronic kidney failure, which can be fatal.

 DIAGNOSIS & TREATMENT

GENERAL MEASURES
- Your health care provider will do a physical exam. Medical tests include urine studies and urine culture. X-ray, ultrasound, and cystoscopy (use of a tube with a camera on the end to see inside the urinary tract) may be done.
- Treatment may include drugs, surgery, dialysis, and kidney transplant. Follow your treatment plan carefully. This may not be easy for an illness that causes few symptoms in the early stages.
- Surgery may be needed to relieve obstruction or correct any structural problem in the urinary tract.
- If chronic kidney failure develops, a kidney transplant or kidney dialysis can be lifesaving.
- To learn more: National Kidney & Urologic Diseases Information Clearinghouse, 3 Information Way, Bethesda, MD 20892, (800) 891-5390; website: www.kidney.niddk.nih.gov.

MEDICATIONS
- Antibiotics may be prescribed. They are usually taken for months or years.
- Drugs to keep the urine slightly acidic may be prescribed.

ACTIVITY
No limits.

DIET
No special diet. Drink plenty of fluids each day. Drink cranberry juice to acidify the urine.

 NOTIFY OUR OFFICE IF

- You or a family member has symptoms of chronic kidney infection.
- You or a family member has symptoms of an acute kidney infection, such as urgent, frequent, or burning urination; fever and chills; fatigue; and cloudy urine.

Special notes:

_____

_____

_____

More notes on the back of this page ☐

KIDNEY, POLYCYSTIC

 ## BASIC INFORMATION

DESCRIPTION

An inherited kidney disorder in which cysts develop in the kidneys. The cysts replace normal kidney tissue and reduce kidney function. Most people show no symptoms until adulthood. Then symptoms progress slowly for up to 20 years. It is a common hereditary disease in the United States.

FREQUENT SIGNS AND SYMPTOMS

Early stages:
- Blood in the urine that may be visible only by microscope exam.
- Repeated kidney infections.
- A mass in the abdomen.
- High blood pressure.
- No symptoms (often) until the cysts replace so much normal kidney structure that kidney failure occurs.

Symptoms of kidney failure:
- Pain in the lower back.
- Frequent urination.
- Increasing fatigue and weakness.
- Headache.
- Bad breath.
- Nausea, vomiting, or diarrhea.
- Fluid build-up (swelling around the ankles or eyes).
- Shortness of breath.
- Chest pain.
- Itching skin.
- Menstruation stops in women of childbearing age.

CAUSES

This disease is inherited. The cause is unknown.

RISK INCREASES WITH

Family history of polycystic disease.

PREVENTIVE MEASURES

Cannot be prevented at present. If polycystic kidney disease runs in your family, get medical advice about tests to discover if you have kidney cysts. Even if you feel well and don't have the disease, get regular checkups. If you have a family history of polycystic kidney, seek genetic counseling before starting a family.

EXPECTED OUTCOMES

There is no cure for polycystic kidney disease. Medical care may slow the progressive kidney damage by treating complications as they arise.

POSSIBLE COMPLICATIONS

- Kidney failure and end-stage renal disease (ESRD).
- High blood pressure.
- Aneurysms (ballooning of weak places in arteries).
- Infection or rupture of cysts.
- Cysts in the liver and other organs.

 ## DIAGNOSIS & TREATMENT

GENERAL MEASURES

- Your health care provider will do a physical exam and ask questions about your family medical history. Medical tests may include blood studies, CT scan, ultrasound, and others.
- There is no specific treatment for the disorder. Treatment is aimed at preventing complications or treating them if they occur.
- Check your blood pressure each day and keep a record.
- Surgical procedures may be needed if kidney cysts rupture, large cysts cause pain, or if cysts in the liver cause problems.
- If kidney failure develops, dialysis or surgery to perform a kidney transplant may be recommended.
- To learn more: National Kidney & Urologic Diseases Information Clearinghouse, 3 Information Way, Bethesda, MD 20892, (800) 891-5390; website: www.kidney.niddk.nih.gov.

MEDICATIONS

- Antibiotics for infection or antihypertensives to control high blood pressure may be prescribed.
- Most drugs are excreted by the kidney. If you have chronic kidney failure and take prescription drugs, the dose may need adjustment because of this disorder.
- Vitamins and supplements may be recommended.

ACTIVITY

- Take short, frequent rest periods during the day. Otherwise, stay as active as your strength allows.
- Avoid contact sports to reduce any risk of injury to the kidneys.

DIET

Usually, no special diet. A low-salt diet may be recommended if high blood pressure or kidney failure develops. Drink at least 8 glasses of fluid every day.

 ## NOTIFY OUR OFFICE IF

- You or a family member has symptoms of polycystic kidney.
- You have symptoms of kidney failure, signs of infection, urination decreases, or blood appears in urine.

Special notes:

_____

_____

_____

More notes on the back of this page ☐

KIDNEY STONES
(Renal Calculi; Urinary Calculi)

 BASIC INFORMATION

DESCRIPTION

Small, solid particles that form in one or both kidneys. They sometimes travel into the ureter (slender muscular tubes that carry urine from the kidneys to the urinary bladder). Stones vary from the size of a grain of sand to a golf ball, and there may be one or several. Kidney stones usually affect adults of both sexes over age 30, but they occur more often in men.

FREQUENT SIGNS AND SYMPTOMS

- Episodes of severe, off and on pain every few minutes. The pain usually appears first in the back, just below the ribs. Over several hours or days, the pain follows the stone's course through the ureter toward the groin. Pain stops when the stone passes.
- Frequent nausea.
- Cloudy or dark urine or blood in urine.

CAUSES

Stones are made up of crystals that form in the urine. Normally, the urine contains chemicals that stop crystals from forming. These chemicals do not seem to work for everyone, and some people form stones. Why this occurs is unknown. Kidney stones contain various chemicals. They may be made up of calcium (most common), struvite, uric acid, or cystine.

RISK INCREASES WITH

- Family history of kidney stones.
- Hyperparathyroidism (excess parathyroid hormone).
- Urinary-tract infections (UTI) or blockage.
- Gout (uric-acid stones).
- Kidney disorders.
- Certain inherited disorders.
- Excess vitamin C or D intake.
- Drugs such as diuretics (water pills), calcium-based antacids, or protease inhibitors (used for AIDS).
- Chronic bowel inflammation or bowel surgery.
- Bed rest for a long period of time.
- Too little fluid intake.

PREVENTIVE MEASURES

No specific measures to prevent a first kidney stone. If you have had one kidney stone, you are more likely to have another and should take preventive measures. These will depend on the type of stone formed.

EXPECTED OUTCOMES

Most kidney stones will pass out of the body on their own. Stones that cause symptoms or complications can be treated successfully. Stones often recur.

POSSIBLE COMPLICATIONS

- Urinary-tract infection.
- Kidney damage or scarring.
- Kidney function may be lost or reduced.

 DIAGNOSIS & TREATMENT

GENERAL MEASURES

- Your health care provider will do a physical exam and ask about your symptoms and activities. Medical tests may include urinalysis, urine culture, x-rays, and other tests to confirm the diagnosis.
- Small stones may need no specific treatment. They usually pass within 72 hours. Strain all urine and save the stone for analysis of type of stone.
- Treatment may be done to remove larger stones if they don't pass on their own and are causing complications, infection, or severe pain. Options include chemical dissolution, endourologic stone extraction, percutaneous nephrolithotomy, extracorporeal shock wave lithotripsy, and rarely, open surgery. Other, new approaches are also being studied. Your health care provider will discuss these options with you.
- Stones due to excess calcium in the body may require surgical removal of abnormal parathyroid tissue.
- To learn more: National Kidney & Urologic Diseases Information Clearinghouse, 3 Information Way, Bethesda, MD 20892, (800) 891-5390; website: www.kidney.niddk.nih.gov.

MEDICATIONS

- Pain relievers may be prescribed.
- Antispasmodics to relax the ureter muscles and help the stone pass may be prescribed.
- Drugs may be prescribed that will stop the growth of new or existing stones.

ACTIVITY

During a kidney-stone episode, stay as active as possible. Activity may help the stone pass.

DIET

Drink lots of fluids (water is best). Eating less red meat may be helpful. You may be advised to make other diet changes to help prevent more stones.

 NOTIFY OUR OFFICE IF

- You or a family member has symptoms of a kidney stone.
- Symptoms of a kidney infection develop (stinging, burning on urination, or a frequent urge to urinate).

Special notes:

_____

_____

_____

More notes on the back of this page ☐

LABYRINTHITIS

 ## BASIC INFORMATION

DESCRIPTION

Inflammation of the labyrinth (fluid-filled canals and sacs) in the inner ear. The labyrinth contains the vestibular system, which controls a person's balance and eye movement. It also contains the cochlea, which controls hearing. Labyrinthitis may affect one or both ears. It can affect all ages, including children.

FREQUENT SIGNS AND SYMPTOMS

- Vertigo. A sensation that you or your surroundings are spinning around. Head movements make it worse.
- Hearing loss (one or both ears; may be mild or severe).
- Involuntary eye movement.
- Nausea and vomiting.
- Loss of balance (may fall toward the affected side).
- Ringing in the ear (tinnitus).
- Feeling of fullness in the ears.

CAUSES

The exact cause of the inflammation is sometimes unknown or unclear. It may result from an infection or trauma. The whole inner ear is about the size of a dime, so inflammation often affects both hearing and balance.

RISK INCREASES WITH

- Bacterial infection in the middle ear.
- Upper respiratory viral infection.
- Cholesteatoma (a type of cyst in the middle ear).
- Head injury.
- Stress or fatigue.
- Allergies or family history of allergies.
- Smoking.
- Excess alcohol use.
- Use of some prescription or nonprescription drugs.
- Heart, brain, or blood-vessel disease.

PREVENTIVE MEASURES

- Obtain prompt medical care for ear infections.
- Don't take drugs that have caused dizziness symptoms for you in the past.

EXPECTED OUTCOMES

The disorder usually resolves on its own in 1 to 6 weeks. Treatment can help relieve symptoms. Some mild vertigo symptoms may continue for several months.

POSSIBLE COMPLICATIONS

- Injuries from falls that occur due to vertigo.
- Permanent hearing loss on the affected side (rare).

 ## DIAGNOSIS & TREATMENT

GENERAL MEASURES

- Your health care provider will do an exam of the ears and your eye movements. Your head and body may be placed or moved in different positions to help determine what movements bring on the symptoms. You may be asked to walk so your balance can be checked. Medical tests may include hearing tests and others as needed to determine any underlying disorder.
- Treatment includes steps to treat any underlying disorder, rest, and drugs for symptoms if needed.
- Surgical removal of cholesteatoma (an infected collection of debris in the middle ear) and drainage of infected areas may be needed.

MEDICATIONS

- Your health care provider may prescribe:
  - Antinausea drugs (oral or suppositories).
  - Tranquilizers to reduce dizziness.
  - Diuretics to decrease excess fluid in the inner ear.
  - Antibiotics for bacterial infection.
  - Antivirals for virus infection.
  - Antihistamines to relieve symptoms.

ACTIVITY

Keep the head as still as possible. Rest in bed until vertigo stops. Then resume your normal activities gradually. Avoid activities, such as driving, climbing, or working around dangerous machinery until symptoms clear up.

DIET

No special diet is needed. Nausea and vomiting symptoms may make eating difficult. Drink clear liquids and eat bland foods until symptoms improve.

 ## NOTIFY OUR OFFICE IF

- You or a family member has symptoms of labyrinthitis.
- The following occur during treatment:
  - Decreased hearing in either ear.
  - Persistent vomiting.
  - Convulsions or fainting.
  - Fever of 101°F (38.3°C) or higher.
- New, unexplained symptoms develop. Drugs used in treatment may produce side effects.

Special notes:

_____

_____

_____

More notes on the back of this page ☐

LACTOSE INTOLERANCE
(Milk Intolerance; Lactase Deficiency)

BASIC INFORMATION

DESCRIPTION
Difficulty digesting cow's milk. Lactose is the primary sugar in milk. Lactose intolerance occurs in 75% of the black population, 90% of Asians or American Indians, and less than 20% of Caucasians of northwest European origin. It can affect any age group.

FREQUENT SIGNS AND SYMPTOMS
• Symptoms will vary depending on the amount of lactose each person can tolerate. Symptoms occur about 30 minutes to 2 hours after eating or drinking foods that contain lactose. They may be mild to more severe.
In children:
• Foamy diarrhea with diaper rash.
• Vomiting (sometimes).
• Slow weight gain, growth, and development.
In adults:
• Rumbling stomach sounds, stomach cramps, and diarrhea.
• Gas and bloating.
• Nausea.

CAUSES
• Deficiency or absence of the enzyme lactase. Lactase is needed to digest all milk except mother's milk. Without it, sugars in milk absorb fluid and cause diarrhea. Some infants are born with the disorder, but lactose intolerance usually develops in adulthood.
• Temporary lactose intolerance can occur in an infant after a severe case of gastroenteritis (stomach flu) that irritates the intestinal lining.

RISK INCREASES WITH
Family history of lactase enzyme deficiency.

PREVENTIVE MEASURES
Cannot be prevented at present. If you are pregnant and there is a history of lactose intolerance in your family, consider breast-feeding your baby. If not, you may need a non-milk formula.

EXPECTED OUTCOMES
There is no cure for this disorder, but it does not cause a threat to good health. Symptoms can be controlled with diet changes. Symptoms may worsen at times for unknown reasons.

POSSIBLE COMPLICATIONS
Calcium deficiency and weak bones (rare).

DIAGNOSIS & TREATMENT

GENERAL MEASURES
• Your health care provider may do a physical exam. A trial period of no dairy products is usually recommended to see if symptoms stop.

• Medical tests may be done. For older children or adults, a hydrogen breath test or lactose absorption test indicate whether lactose is not being absorbed in the digestive tract. A stool acidity exam may be done. It can be used for infants or young children.
• Treatment involves diet changes. Using lactase enzymes is also an option.
• To learn more: National Digestive Diseases Clearinghouse, 2 Information Way, Bethesda, MD 20892; (800) 891-5389; website: www.digestive.nddic.nih.gov.

MEDICATIONS
• The enzyme lactase is available without a prescription. It can be taken as a tablet or as a liquid that is added to milk and milk products. It acts in much the same way as the naturally occurring enzyme does.
• Calcium supplements may be recommended.
• Some prescription and nonprescription drugs contain lactose as an ingredient. These include some birth-control pills and antacids. They may affect people who have severe lactose intolerance.

ACTIVITY
No limits.

DIET
• If the condition is present at birth, an infant formula that contains little or no lactose, such as a soybean-based formula, will be recommended.
• If the lactose intolerance is short-term and caused by gastroenteritis, a substitute formula is needed for a short time. Cow's milk can be introduced again later.
• Older persons with lactose intolerance should reduce or restrict milk and milk products, such as cheese and ice cream. Lactose-free milk is available.
• Yogurt and fermented products such as hard cheese are often tolerated better than milk.
• Read food labels with care. Avoid products that contain milk, lactose, milk sugar, whey, curds, milk by-products, dry milk solids, and nonfat dry milk powder.

NOTIFY OUR OFFICE IF

• You or your child has symptoms of lactose intolerance.
• Infant fails to gain weight or refuses food or formula.
• Vomiting or diarrhea occurs.
• A milk-free diet doesn't relieve symptoms.

Special notes:

_____

_____

_____

More notes on the back of this page ☐

LARGE INTESTINE CANCER
(Colon Cancer; Colorectal Cancer)

BASIC INFORMATION

DESCRIPTION
Growth of cancer cells in the rectum or colon (large intestine). It may involve the large intestine, including the cecum, ascending colon, transverse colon, descending colon and sigmoid colon, and rectum. This type of cancer often affects adults over age 50.

FREQUENT SIGNS AND SYMPTOMS
- No symptoms in the early stages (frequently).
- Bloody or black, tarry stools or rectal bleeding.
- Cramping stomach pain and feeling of fullness.
- Change in bowel habits, such as diarrhea, constipation, or narrow stools.
- Unexplained weight loss.
- Anemia (pale skin and fatigue).
- Loss of bowel control (sometimes).
- Pain in the rectum (sometimes).

CAUSES
Exact cause is unknown. Genetic and environmental factors may contribute. There are known risk factors.

RISK INCREASES WITH
- Family history of colorectal cancer or colon polyps.
- Inherited genetic abnormality. Two types are familial adenomatous polyposis (FAP) including an attenuated form (AFAP), and hereditary nonpolyposis colorectal cancer (HNPCC).
- Inflammatory bowel disease (ulcerative colitis).
- Intestinal polyps (benign growths).
- Previous colorectal cancer.
- Age over 50.
- Diabetes.
- Diet high in fat and meat (both red and white).
- Obesity.
- Sedentary (not physically active) lifestyle.
- Smoking and alcohol use.

PREVENTIVE MEASURES
- To reduce risk: Exercise daily; eat a low-fat, high-fiber diet; control weight; don't smoke; and limit alcohol.
- Colon cancer screening tests for adults over age 50 and adults over age 40 (or younger) with risk factors.
- Genetic tests for family members at risk.
- Precancerous conditions should be treated.
- Vitamins, calcium, folic acid, nonsteroidal anti-inflammatory drugs, or female hormones may be recommended for some patients as preventive therapies.

EXPECTED OUTCOMES
Outlook varies. The earlier the cancer is diagnosed and treated, the greater the chances for recovery.

POSSIBLE COMPLICATIONS
- Spread to other body parts, which can be fatal.
- Complications may occur due to treatments.

DIAGNOSIS & TREATMENT

GENERAL MEASURES
- Your health care provider will do a physical exam and ask questions about your symptoms. A number of medical tests will be done. The tests help diagnose the cancer and then determine if it has spread (staging).
- Treatment varies and depends on location and size of tumor, any spread of the cancer, your health, age, and preferences. Treatment may include surgery, anticancer drugs (chemotherapy) and/or radiation therapy, and biologic therapy.
- Chemotherapy uses drugs and radiation therapy uses radiation to attack the cancer cells. Biologic therapy uses the body's immune system to fight cancer.
- The goal of surgery is to remove as much of the cancer as possible. Part, or all, of the colon, rectum, and nearby organs may be removed. A colostomy to collect stool or an urostomy to collect urine may be needed to help the body get rid of these wastes.
- Treatment may involve steps to relieve symptoms and make you comfortable, rather than treating the cancer.
- Counseling may help you cope with having cancer.
- To learn more: American Cancer Society, (800) ACS-2345; website: www.cancer.org; or National Cancer Institute, (800) 4-CANCER; website: www.nci.nih.gov.

MEDICATIONS
Your health care provider may prescribe anticancer drugs (chemotherapy), drugs to stimulate the immune system (biologics), and pain relievers.

ACTIVITY
- Avoid sports or activities that might injure the stoma (surgical bowel opening).
- You will be advised when to resume normal activities, including sexual relations.

DIET
Eat a low-fat, high-fiber diet.

NOTIFY OUR OFFICE IF

- You or a family member has symptoms of cancer of the large intestine, especially rectal bleeding or a significant change in bowel habits lasting longer than 7 days.
- New symptoms occur during or after treatment.

Special notes:

_____

_____

_____

More notes on the back of this page ☐

LARGE INTESTINE POLYP

 BASIC INFORMATION

DESCRIPTION
A growth that occurs on the lining of the colon or rectum. A polyp may grow with or without a stalk. Polyps occur singly or in groups. They are a health concern, because most colon cancers arise from polyps. Polyps occur more often as people age.

FREQUENT SIGNS AND SYMPTOMS
- No symptoms (usually).
- Rectal bleeding (sometimes).
- Mucous discharge from the rectum (sometimes).
- Cramps or stomach pain.

CAUSES
Unknown.

RISK INCREASES WITH
- Family history of intestinal polyps.
- Polyposis syndromes. These are genetic abnormalities that are passed down in families. Some syndromes may cause large numbers of polyps in the colon (such as familial adenomatous polyposis [FAP]).

PREVENTIVE MEASURES
- No specific measures to prevent polyps.
- If you have had polyps in the past, you should have regular follow-up exams.
- Patients with a family history of polyps, colon cancer, or polyposis syndromes should have polyp screening tests starting at a young age, or as recommended.
- All adults starting at age 50 should have colon cancer screening tests.

EXPECTED OUTCOMES
Usually curable with treatment. Most polyps are benign (noncancerous). Polyps may recur after treatment.

POSSIBLE COMPLICATIONS
Risk of colorectal cancer. It develops slowly over several years.

 DIAGNOSIS & TREATMENT

GENERAL MEASURES
- Your health care provider will do a physical exam and a digital rectal exam (a gloved, lubricated finger is inserted into the rectum). Medical tests may include blood studies, stool studies, barium x-ray, or virtual colonoscopy (CT scan of the colon). A sigmoidoscopy (exam of rectum and lower end of the colon) or conventional colonoscopy (exam of entire length of colon) may be done. Both of these tests use a lighted tube with a camera on the end to see inside the body. A biopsy is done during a colonoscopy. This involves removal of a small amount of tissue for viewing under a microscope.
- Treatment to remove polyps is usually recommended.
- Polyps can be removed during the colonoscopy procedure. Polyps are snipped off or destroyed by electric cauterization. If the removed polyp is diagnosed as cancer, this may be all the treatment that is needed.
- Surgery (laparotomy) is performed to remove some types of polyps. This is done through an incision made in the abdomen. Part of the colon may be removed and then the two cut ends are rejoined.

MEDICATIONS
Drugs are not usually needed for this disorder. Nonsteroidal anti-inflammatory drugs are being researched to see if they decrease the number and size of polyps.

ACTIVITY
No limits.

DIET
No special diet (unless advised otherwise).

 NOTIFY OUR OFFICE IF

- You or a family member has bleeding or mucous discharge from the rectum.
- Other members of your family have polyps or colorectal cancer. You should have regular exams.
- The following occur after surgery:
  - Increased rectal bleeding.
  - Fever, chills, or aches. This may indicate an infection.

Special notes:

_____

_____

_____

More notes on the back of this page ☐

LARVA MIGRANS, CUTANEOUS

(Creeping Eruptions; Hookworms)

 ## BASIC INFORMATION

DESCRIPTION
A skin infection caused by hookworms. Hookworms are parasites that infest animals, particularly dogs and cats. Humans pick up the infection by coming in contact with sand or soil where an infected animal has passed feces. It is more common in warm, humid areas, such as the southeastern United States.

FREQUENT SIGNS AND SYMPTOMS
First, there may be a tingling or prickling of the skin area. Then it begins to itch. This is followed by a rash or small blisters on the skin. They often form thin, raised tracks (or lines) on the skin leading from the parasite's entry point. The tracks can get longer each day. There are usually several tracks at the same time, each of different length and pattern.

CAUSES
An animal that has hookworms leaves feces on the ground that contains the hookworm eggs. The eggs hatch into larvae that infest the soil around the droppings. When a human comes in contact with the soil, the larvae are able to penetrate the skin and cause the symptoms. The infection cannot be spread from one person to another.

RISK INCREASES WITH
• Working or playing in warm, moist sand in which cats or dogs have defecated. They can be found in a child's sandbox.
• Walking barefoot in sand or dirt.
• Work that requires crawling in confined spaces and contact with infected soil (e.g., plumbers working under houses).

PREVENTIVE MEASURES
• Handle cat litter carefully. Avoid touching soil.
• Don't work or play in soil used by cats and dogs for elimination.
• Have pets treated for worms.

EXPECTED OUTCOMES
The outcome is good. The infection may heal on its own over several weeks or months. Treatment with drugs can hasten the healing process.

POSSIBLE COMPLICATIONS
If the blisters are scratched and opened, a bacterial infection may occur.

 ## DIAGNOSIS & TREATMENT

GENERAL MEASURES
• Your health care provider can usually diagnose the problem by an exam of the affected skin area. Other medical tests may be done to confirm the diagnosis.
• Apply cool, moist compresses to the affected area to help relieve itching.

MEDICATIONS
Your health care provider may prescribe an anti-parasitic drug to be applied to the skin, or taken by mouth (if the infection more severe).

ACTIVITY
No limits.

DIET
No special diet.

 ## NOTIFY OUR OFFICE IF

• You or a family member has symptoms of larva migrans.
• Skin symptoms become worse or new symptoms.
• You take an oral anti-parasitic drug, and new, unexplained symptoms develop.

Special notes:

_____

_____

_____

More notes on the back of this page ☐

LARYNGITIS

 ## BASIC INFORMATION

DESCRIPTION

A minor inflammation of the larynx (voice box) and surrounding tissues. Inflammation causes swelling and pain and is a reaction to injury, infection or irritation. The disorder is common, affects all ages, and occurs more often in late fall, winter, and early spring.

FREQUENT SIGNS AND SYMPTOMS

- Hoarseness, weak voice, or loss of voice.
- Sore throat; tickling in the back of the throat.
- Feeling like you have a lump in your throat.
- Slight fever (sometimes).
- Swallowing difficulty (rare).

CAUSES

There are many factors that can lead to the inflammation of the larynx. The most common is a viral infection.

RISK INCREASES WITH

- Viral infection from a recent cold or flu-like illness.
- Excessive use of the voice (such as singers, politicians, cheerleaders, or young children who cry or yell strenuously).
- Exposure to irritants such as mold, pollen and pollutants, or irritating chemicals.
- Allergies.
- Smoking or being around second-hand smoke.
- Gastroesophageal reflux disease (GERD).
- Rarely, it may be a bacterial infection, or be caused by disorders such as tuberculosis, syphilis, fungal infection, or tumor.

PREVENTIVE MEASURES

- Most cases are caused by a virus. Taking steps to prevent viral infections such as hand washing may help.
- Take care to not overuse the voice.

EXPECTED OUTCOMES

Laryngitis usually clears up on its own in 10 to 14 days.

POSSIBLE COMPLICATIONS

Chronic hoarseness.

 ## DIAGNOSIS & TREATMENT

GENERAL MEASURES

- Most people will self-treat this disorder. If symptoms persist, are severe, or cause concern, see your health care provider. An exam of the throat, ears and nose, can usually confirm the diagnosis. Medical tests are normally not needed.
- Home care is the main form of treatment.
- Avoid using your voice as much as possible. Don't whisper (it can irritate the throat). Write notes to communicate. For most cases, resting the voice for a few days is all that is needed.
- Suck on throat lozenges, cough drops, or hard candy.
- To help relieve minor pain, gargle often with double-strength tea or warm salt water (one-half teaspoon of salt to 8 oz. of water).
- Hot, steamy showers also help.
- Avoid smoking and second-hand cigarette smoke.

MEDICATIONS

For minor discomfort, you may use nonprescription drugs, such as acetaminophen or ibuprofen.

ACTIVITY

Usually no limits.

DIET

No special diet. Increased fluid intake may be helpful.

 ## NOTIFY OUR OFFICE IF

- You or a family member has hoarseness or other symptoms of laryngitis that last longer than 2 weeks.
- You feel very ill, are vomiting, have a high fever, or difficulty breathing. If these symptoms develop in a child, call immediately.

Special notes:

_____

_____

_____

More notes on the back of this page ☐

LARYNX CANCER
(Laryngeal Cancer)

BASIC INFORMATION

DESCRIPTION
Growth of malignant cells in the larynx (voice box). The larynx is about 2 inches long and 2 inches wide and located at the back of the throat. It plays a role in helping a person breathe, swallow, and talk. This type of cancer affects adults, usually over age 40, and it is more common in men than in women.

FREQUENT SIGNS AND SYMPTOMS
- Few or no symptoms in early stages.
- Hoarseness, scratchy, or weak voice.
- "Lump-in-the-throat" feeling.
- Painful or difficult swallowing.
- Trouble breathing.
- Hard, swollen lymph glands in the neck.
- Weight loss.
- Ear pain.
- Chronic cough.

CAUSES
Exact cause is unknown. Smoking or alcohol abuse are known major risk factors.

RISK INCREASES WITH
- Age over 55. Men more than women.
- African-Americans more than whites.
- Smoking.
- Excess alcohol use.
- Having had head or neck cancer.
- Exposure to certain chemicals, toxins, or asbestos.
- Gastroesophageal reflux disease (GERD).

PREVENTIVE MEASURES
- Don't smoke. Don't drink more than 1 or 2 alcoholic drinks, if any, a day.
- Avoid exposure to known toxins.

EXPECTED OUTCOMES
Early diagnosis and treatment offer the best outcome. Later diagnosis or spread of cancer has poorer outlook.

POSSIBLE COMPLICATIONS
- Complications arise from treatments (chemotherapy, radiation, and surgery) that may affect the voice, breathing, swallowing, and eating.
- Spread of cancer in the body, which can be fatal.
- Cancer may recur after treatment.

DIAGNOSIS & TREATMENT

GENERAL MEASURES
- Your health care provider will do a physical exam and ask questions about your symptoms. A variety of medical tests will be done to verify the exact type of cancer cells, the grade (fast or slow growing), and if the cancer has spread (called staging) to other places in the body.

- Treatment will depend on the cancer type, grade and location, its stage, your health, age, and preferences. Preserving a good voice quality is a goal of treatment. Your health care provider will discuss your specific diagnosis and treatment recommendations with you.
- Surgery, radiation, and/or chemotherapy (anticancer drugs) are the usual treatment steps. Other treatments being studied include photodynamic therapy (drugs plus light), biologic therapy (using the immune system to fight the cancer), or gene therapy.
- Advanced cancer often requires surgery. Part or all of the larynx may be removed (laryngectomy). A tracheostomy is performed. This is an opening (stoma) in the throat for breathing. It may be temporary or permanent. A "trach" tube or stoma button keeps it open.
- After larynx removal, therapy will help patients learn to breathe, swallow, eat, and talk. Talking will involve learning esophageal speech or use of a mechanical device.
- Stop smoking. Find a way to quit that works for you.
- Good mouth care helps keep teeth and gums healthy.
- Consider joining a self-help or cancer support group.
- To learn more: American Cancer Society, (800) ACS-2345; website: www.cancer.org or National Cancer Institute, (800) 4-CANCER; website: www.cancer.gov.

MEDICATIONS
Anticancer (chemotherapy) drugs may be prescribed.

ACTIVITY
Following larynx removal surgery, you should be able to do almost all the activities you did before. Straining and heavy lifting may be difficult since you cannot hold your breath. You can shower by using a shield over the stoma. Avoid swimming and water activities unless special instructions and equipment are used.

DIET
Diet changes depend on the treatment. Surgery may require a liquid diet at first, then a soft diet. Learning to swallow again will take practice. Several small meals and snacks during the day may make eating easier.

NOTIFY OUR OFFICE IF

- You or a family member has symptoms of larynx (laryngeal) cancer.
- New symptoms occur during or after treatment.

Special notes:

_____

_____

_____

More notes on the back of this page ☐

LATEX ALLERGY

 ## BASIC INFORMATION

DESCRIPTION
Latex allergy involves reactions of the body to natural rubber latex. Latex is a milky fluid produced by rubber trees and is used in thousands of products. Rubber gloves are the main source of allergic reactions. There are three types of reactions: irritant dermatitis, allergic contact dermatitis, and immediate-type latex allergy.

FREQUENT SIGNS AND SYMPTOMS
Irritant contact dermatitis:
- Dry, crusty, itchy, sore areas on the skin.
- Usually affects the hands.

Allergic contact dermatitis (chemical sensitive):
- Rash that starts 6 to 48 hours after exposure.
- Skin is dry and crusty. Blisters and sores occur.
- Usually affects the hands, but may spread.

Immediate type latex allergy:
- Normally occurs right away, but could take hours.
- Skin is red and itchy; may have hives.
- Eyes are red and watery.
- Runny nose, coughing, or sneezing.
- Chest feels tight; may be short of breath.
- Shock or a life-threatening reaction (rare).

CAUSES
- Irritant dermatitis is due to the skin being irritated.
- Allergic contact dermatitis is due to a chemical in the product, not latex. (This is like a poison ivy reaction.)
- In immediate-type latex allergy, the body's immune system reacts to repeated exposure to latex products.

RISK INCREASES WITH
- Health care workers or others who use latex gloves often, or are exposed to them.
- Having had many operations (where you were exposed to latex gloves).
- Other allergies, such as hay fever, asthma, and eczema.
- Food allergies, including avocado and banana.
- Rubber industry and latex manufacturing workers.
- Certain disorders present at birth, such as spina bifida.

PREVENTIVE MEASURES
For those diagnosed with the allergy, avoid latex.

EXPECTED OUTCOMES
There is no cure for latex allergy. Repeated exposure to latex can worsen the immune system response. Avoiding latex is the best action. Many products are made from latex, so this is not always easy to do.

POSSIBLE COMPLICATIONS
- Some people may need to change jobs due to latex exposure in their workplace.
- Rarely, anaphylaxis, a severe, life-threatening reaction occurs. Seek emergency help if this happens.

 ## DIAGNOSIS & TREATMENT

GENERAL MEASURES
- Your health care provider will do a physical exam and may confirm the diagnosis with a blood test. Skin testing is rarely done, as it may result in a severe reaction.
- There is no treatment, except to avoid latex products.
- Find out which products in your home and work contain latex. Find substitutes you can use for those products. Read labels, or ask, before buying a product.
- Health care workers and others should wear powder-free latex gloves or non-latex gloves. Powder can get in the air, and if breathed in can cause a reaction.
- Most male condoms, as well as diaphragms and cervical caps, are latex. If you use them, ask your health care provider about options for birth control and safe sex.
- Wear a medical alert type tag or ID that lets others know you have this allergy.
- Advise any health care provider you consult that you have a latex allergy.
- Discuss your latex allergy with your employer to find ways to avoid latex exposure in your workplace.
- If your allergy is severe, carry a kit with a self-injecting device that contains the drug epinephrine. Know how to use the device. Instruct your family or others as to how to give the injection if you are unable to.
- To learn more: Asthma and Allergy Foundation of America, 1125 15th Street, NW, Suite 502, Washington, DC 20005; (800) 7-ASTHMA; website: www.aafa.org or Latex Allergy Links website: www.latexallergylinks.org.

MEDICATIONS
Drugs may be prescribed for allergy symptoms.

ACTIVITY
No limits.

DIET
No special diet.

 ## NOTIFY OUR OFFICE IF

You or a family member has latex allergy symptoms.

Special notes:

_____

_____

_____

More notes on the back of this page ☐

LAXATIVE ABUSE

BASIC INFORMATION

DESCRIPTION

Laxative abuse occurs when someone misuses or overuses laxatives. Laxative abuse is defined as (1) use of laxative for weight control, or (2) frequent use of laxatives over an extended period of time. It may result from a false belief that frequent bowel movements are necessary. Patients with eating disorders or binge eaters may abuse laxatives to get rid of large meals. Many individuals unintentionally develop the laxative habit.

FREQUENT SIGNS AND SYMPTOMS

- Chronic constipation or chronic diarrhea.
- Gas and bloating.
- Laxative dependence (need laxatives to produce bowel movements).
- Dehydration due to excess loss of fluid.
- Electrolyte imbalance (minerals needed for body function), which causes tremors, muscle cramps, and spasms.
- Blood in the stools.
- Nausea or vomiting.
- Colon infection.

CAUSES

Short-term or long-term, laxatives create and perpetuate the very problem they were intended to correct. Laxatives induce constipation as the tissues become dried out, muscles become weak, and the delicate nerves lining the colon become damaged. Because of the damage that laxatives cause, ever-increasing dosages of laxatives may be required in order to achieve the desired effect. Where one laxative dose produced results, now two, then three doses a day are required. People who abuse laxatives for a long period of time may end up taking as many as 6 to 8 laxatives a day.

RISK INCREASES WITH

- Patients with eating disorders or binge eaters. They believe they are losing weight and that they are thinner. What is lost is water weight. It comes back on within 48 hours.
- The false belief that frequent bowel movements are necessary.
- Preparation for competitions (sports, pageants, etc.).

PREVENTIVE MEASURES

- Don't use laxatives regularly.
- Avoid constipation. Drink plenty of water with each meal and during the day. Eat more fresh fruits, vegetables, and whole grains to increase dietary fiber. Go to the bathroom when you feel the urge.
- Exercise regularly to stimulate bowel activity.
- Recognize and get treatment for eating disorders (anorexia or bulimia) or disordered eating (abnormal change in eating patterns).

EXPECTED OUTCOMES

Will depend on the extent of the abuse and the motivation of the person. Withdrawal from laxatives can take days, weeks, or even months. Body functions should return to normal with no permanent damage.

POSSIBLE COMPLICATIONS

It depends on the type of laxatives abused, the amount abused, and how long they have been abused. Severe harm to the body, including death, could occur.

DIAGNOSIS & TREATMENT

GENERAL MEASURES

- Ask you health care provider about how to recover normal bowel function and what steps to use to begin to reverse the laxative habit.
- Stopping laxatives may be done gradually or by going "cold turkey" (stopping in one day).
- Changing to products containing psyllium may help if you gradually withdraw from laxatives.
- Withdrawal symptoms may include nausea, constipation, bloating, and gas. They will stop as your body recovers and learns how to regulate itself again.
- Counseling help may be useful for patients who are chronically abusing laxatives. This type of therapy is important for people with eating disorders.

MEDICATIONS

No drugs are usually needed. If a drug you take causes constipation, a change in drug or dosage may help.

ACTIVITY

Exercise daily. Being fit helps maintain bowel function.

DIET

- Be sure to eat enough food to promote regular bowel movements. High-fiber items like fruits, vegetables, and whole grains. Be careful, as some foods may cause intestinal gas, and if you are experiencing discomfort already, this may add to it.
- Drinking lots of water is important. Try to drink 8 to 10 glasses per day if possible. If you are constipated, warm/hot beverages can help.

NOTIFY OUR OFFICE IF

You or a family member has a laxative abuse problem.

Special notes:

_____

_____

_____

More notes on the back of this page ☐

LEAD POISONING

 BASIC INFORMATION

DESCRIPTION
A high level of lead in the body. Lead is all around us. It is found in paint, batteries, drinking water, and pottery or other ceramic dishes. A little bit of lead finds its way into everyone and usually causes no problems. Too much lead in the body can cause serious problems, especially in infants and young children.

FREQUENT SIGNS AND SYMPTOMS
- Often no symptoms or they may be delayed.
- Pale skin, fatigue, feeling sluggish, sleeping problems.
- Behavior changes (such as being irritable).
- Child may be overly active.
- Stomach discomfort and poor appetite.
- Difficulty in concentrating.
- Headache; vomiting; weight loss.
- Constipation.
- Higher lead levels: severe stomach cramps; rigid abdomen, muscle weakness, seizures, or coma.

CAUSES
Breathing in of lead dust or fumes, or taking lead in by mouth (ingestion). Lead in the body interferes with normal body functions. It affects red blood cells and the nerve cells in the brain.

RISK INCREASES WITH
- Children under 3. Their brain and nervous systems are still developing and are more affected by lead.
- Childhood behaviors such as hand-to-mouth activity and pica (repeated eating of nonfood products) increase the risk of taking in lead.
- Homes with lead-based paint (its use stopped in the mid-1970s). Children eat, chew, or suck on the paint. During remodeling, lead paint dust can get into the air.
- Lead plumbing (its use stopped in 1986).
- Using lead-glazed ceramics for food or drink.
- Colored ink in newspapers, magazines, and plastic bags.
- Some candies from Mexico have had high lead levels.
- Hobbies such as glazed pottery making, lead soldering, painting, preparing lead shot, stained-glass making, car or boat repair, and others.
- Work or job exposure. Over 900 occupations have been connected with lead poisoning.
- Some cosmetics and folk remedies.
- Retained bullets or shrapnel.

PREVENTIVE MEASURES
- Have children age 6 months to 6 years tested regularly for lead levels. Talk to your child's health care provider.
- Avoid risk factors where possible.
- Routine blood-lead tests for workers exposed to lead.
- Education about lead and ways to decrease lead exposure. Call (800) 424-LEAD; website: www.epa.gov/lead.

EXPECTED OUTCOME
Lead poisoning without any apparent brain damage generally improves with treatment. Some problems may be long-lasting or permanent.

POSSIBLE COMPLICATIONS
- Damage to the nervous system, kidneys, liver, heart, and other body organ systems.
- Children may have mental retardation, behavior problems, learning disorders, aggressiveness, or delayed or slower growth. Seizures, coma, and death could occur.
- Adults may have loss of sex drive, impotence, or infertility. High lead levels in a pregnant woman can harm her unborn child.

 DIAGNOSIS & TREATMENT

GENERAL MEASURES
- Your health care provider may do a physical exam. Medical tests include blood studies to measure lead levels. Kidney and liver function testing and x-rays of the abdomen may be done.
- Treatment involves avoiding any further exposure to the lead. For some patients, medical therapy will help the body excrete (get rid of) the lead. Hospital care may be needed for severe symptoms.
- A report should be made to the local health department. An inspection of the home or workplace can be done to find the source of lead. Lead-level blood tests should be done for all family members.
- If the source is in the home, the patient needs to live elsewhere until the lead source is removed.

MEDICATIONS
Chelating agents to excrete lead may be prescribed.

ACTIVITY
No limits.

DIET
To reduce lead levels, eat a diet that has plenty of iron, calcium, and zinc; avoid excess fat. Eat lean meat, eggs, raisins, greens, dairy, fruit, and potatoes.

 NOTIFY OUR OFFICE IF

You or a family member has symptoms of lead poisoning or you want lead levels tested.

Special notes:

_____

_____

_____

More notes on the back of this page ☐

290

LEGG-CALVÉ-PERTHES DISEASE
(Slipped Femoral Epiphysis; Coxa Plana)

 ## BASIC INFORMATION

DESCRIPTION
A hip disorder of childhood. It involves gradual weakening of the head of the thigh bone where it meets the pelvis. It can involve either leg at the hip joint. It affects children ages 2 to 12 years (most often 4 to 8) of both sexes, but it is more common in boys (85% of the patients).

FREQUENT SIGNS AND SYMPTOMS
· Pain and stiffness in the hip and thigh. Sometimes both sides are involved.
· Pain in the leg and often in the knee, even though the disorder is in the hip.
· Limping or other problems with walking.
· Symptoms usually begin slowly over time.

CAUSES
The bone becomes weak due to lack of a blood supply to the top of the bone. The weak bone is not able to handle weight. Why this occurs is unknown. It may involve growth hormones in the body or blood clotting problems. Injury is usually not a factor.

RISK INCREASES WITH
· Boys more than girls.
· Use of cortisone drugs for other disorders.
· Overweight persons.
· Periods of rapid growth.
· Children with low birth-weight and delayed development may be more at risk.

PREVENTIVE MEASURES
No specific preventive measures.

EXPECTED OUTCOMES
Often curable in 2 to 3 years with early treatment. The blood supply to the bone becomes normal, and new bone cells start growing to replace the old bone.

POSSIBLE COMPLICATIONS
· Delayed treatment may cause permanent bone injury.
· Osteoarthritis may develop later in life.

 ## DIAGNOSIS & TREATMENT

GENERAL MEASURES
· Your child's health care provider will do a physical exam and ask questions about the symptoms. Medical tests usually include x-rays or other tests to determine how far the problem has progressed.

· Treatment may not be needed for about half of the patients with the disorder. These children will be watched to see if any problems develop. This can include children younger than 6 with no hip motion problems, or older children who maintain good range of motion.
· Other treatment steps are aimed at maintaining the range of motion and keeping the hip-bone in the hip socket. They may include a cast, brace, physical therapy, or surgery.
· Youngsters often have difficulty accepting the need for rest, casts, braces, or other treatment. Help your child find activities and interests that don't involve a lot of movement or athletics.
· Use heat to relieve pain. Warm compresses, heating pads, or other methods are effective.
· Surgery to reinforce the bone's attachment to the joint and prevent further problems (sometimes).
· A hospital stay may be needed for traction (a steady pull on the leg).

MEDICATIONS
For minor discomfort, you may use nonprescription drugs, such as acetaminophen or ibuprofen. Don't give aspirin to children.

ACTIVITY
Bed rest may be necessary for 6 months to 1 year until the condition improves, or until after surgery. When the bones can bear weight, crutches, braces, or casts are usually necessary. After that, activities may be resumed gradually.

DIET
No special diet, unless the child is overweight.

 ## NOTIFY OUR OFFICE IF

· Your child has hip or knee pain, stiffness, or a limp.
· The following occur during treatment:
  - Symptoms don't improve in 4 weeks, despite treatment.
  - Pain increases.

Special notes:

_____

_____

_____

More notes on the back of this page ☐

LEGIONNAIRE'S DISEASE

(Legionella pneumophila Bronchopneumonia*)*

 ## BASIC INFORMATION

DESCRIPTION
A form of lung infection named after an epidemic that affected people attending an American Legion convention in 1976. The disease was probably around long before that, but was not recognized. It can affect all ages, but is more common in middle-aged persons.

FREQUENT SIGNS AND SYMPTOMS
- General ill feeling.
- Headache and muscle aches.
- Chills and fever up to 105°F (40.6°C).
- Cough without sputum that progresses to one with gray or blood-streaked sputum.
- Nausea, vomiting, diarrhea, and tiredness.
- Mental changes such as disorientation or confusion.

CAUSES
- Infection from *Legionella* bacteria. The germs also cause a milder illness called Pontiac fever. The germs are breathed into the lungs. Symptoms begin 2 to 10 days after exposure. The germs are not known to spread from one person to another, or from drinking water. The risk of getting the infection is quite low, especially in healthy persons.
- The bacteria are found in wet or moist environments. They have been found in hot water tanks, in water from shower-heads or faucets, cooling towers, air conditioners, whirlpool spas, soil, potting soil, and other locations.

RISK INCREASES WITH
- Chronic illness, including diabetes, kidney failure, or emphysema.
- Weak immune system due to illness or drugs.
- Smoking. This increases the risk 3 to 4 times over.
- Drinking alcohol to excess.

PREVENTIVE MEASURES
- No specific preventive measures. Take steps to reduce risk factors where possible.
- Though home cooling and heating systems don't usually carry the germs, it is important to keep them clean.
- Don't smoke.
- Avoid alcohol or limit it to 1 to 2 drinks a day.

EXPECTED OUTCOMES
Usually curable with prompt diagnosis and treatment.

POSSIBLE COMPLICATIONS
- Shock or delirium.
- Congestive heart failure.
- Kidney failure.
- Heart-rhythm disturbances.
- If untreated, 15% of cases are fatal.

 ## DIAGNOSIS & TREATMENT

GENERAL MEASURES
- Your health care provider will do a physical exam and ask about your symptoms and activities. Medical tests may include blood studies, sputum culture, and other testing to confirm the diagnosis.
- Treatment is with antibiotics and supportive care.
- Hospital care may be needed for severe cases.
- The following apply to mild cases or to care after a hospital stay:
  - Use a cool-mist humidifier to increase air moisture and thin lung secretions so that they can be coughed up more easily. Clean humidifier daily.
  - Use warm compresses or a heating pad on the chest to relieve chest pain.
  - Practice deep-breathing exercises as often as your strength allows.
  - Avoid talking loudly, laughing, or singing. They may trigger excessive coughing.

MEDICATIONS
- Antibiotics. Be sure to finish all the dosage prescribed.
- If the cough is painful and doesn't produce sputum, you may use nonprescription drugs to suppress it. If the cough produces sputum, don't suppress it.
- You may take aspirin (not for children) or acetaminophen to reduce fever.

ACTIVITY
Rest in bed until completely well. Allow 2 to 4 weeks for recovery.

DIET
No special diet. Drink 6 to 8 glasses of fluid daily.

 ## NOTIFY OUR OFFICE IF

- You or a family member has symptoms of Legionnaire's disease.
- The following occur during or after treatment:
  - Higher fever occurs.
  - Severe chest pain, despite treatment.
  - Increased shortness of breath.
  - Dark or bluish nails, lips, or skin.
  - Blood in the sputum.

Special notes:

_____

_____

_____

More notes on the back of this page ☐

LEUKEMIA, ACUTE

 BASIC INFORMATION

DESCRIPTION

Leukemia is cancer of blood cells. Three types of blood cells are formed in bone marrow. White blood cells fight infections, red blood cells carry oxygen, and platelets help control bleeding. Bone marrow is the soft material in the center of bones. With leukemia, the cancerous (abnormal) cells replace normal cells. The body then develops infections, anemia, or bleeds easily. Acute leukemia usually has a sudden onset and symptoms progress rapidly. Forms of acute leukemia include:
• Acute lymphocytic leukemia (ALL). It affects all ages, but is more common in children.
• Acute myeloid (myelogenous) leukemia (AML). It affects both children and adults (usually older adults).

FREQUENT SIGNS AND SYMPTOMS
• Low fever, chills, and sweating.
• Tiredness and weakness.
• Anemia (pale skin, fatigue).
• General ill feeling.
• Easy bruising or bleeding or cuts that heal slowly.
• Pin-head size spots on the skin.
• Repeated infections.
• Bone or joint pain.
• Loss of appetite and/or weight.
• Other symptoms if cancer cells collect in organs such as brain, lungs, genitals, digestive tract, or kidneys.

CAUSES
Exact cause unknown. It is believed to develop from a combination of genetic and environmental factors.

RISK INCREASES WITH
• Family history of leukemia (such as brother or sister).
• Men more than women; whites and Hispanics.
• Excess exposure to x-rays (radiation).
• Genetic disorder, such as Down syndrome.
• Exposure to benzenes and other toxic chemicals.
• Weak immune system due to illness or drugs.
• AML risks: smoking, history of blood disorder, or previous treatment for childhood ALL.

PREVENTIVE MEASURES
Cannot be prevented. If you have a family history of leukemia, get genetic counseling before starting a family.

EXPECTED OUTCOMES
Depends on the type of leukemia, the patient's health and response to treatment. Remission occurs when there is no evidence of leukemia in the blood or bone marrow. Remission over 5 years often indicates a cure.

POSSIBLE COMPLICATIONS
• Hemorrhage or uncontrolled infection (can be fatal).
• Failure of leukemia to respond to chemotherapy.
• Relapse (leukemia recurs after remission).

 DIAGNOSIS & TREATMENT

GENERAL MEASURES
• Your health care provider will do a physical exam and ask questions about your symptoms. Medical tests include blood studies. Samples of bone marrow (liquid and solid) will be taken for viewing with a microscope. Other tests are done to see if the cancer has spread.
• Treatment depends on the leukemia type and other factors and involves 3 steps. Induction (remission), then consolidation (prevent relapse), and then maintenance. Treatment may include anticancer drugs (chemotherapy), radiation therapy, bone marrow transplant, stem cell transplant, surgery, and biologic therapy.
• Chemotherapy uses drugs, and radiation therapy uses radiation to attack the cancer cells. Biologic therapy uses the body's immune system to fight cancer.
• Bone marrow transplant involves replacing the leukemia-affected marrow with healthy bone marrow.
• Stem cell transplant replaces blood cells destroyed in treatment with stem cells (immature blood cells).
• Blood and platelet transfusions may be needed.
• Surgery may be done to remove the spleen.
• Counseling may help you cope with having cancer.
• Get good dental care to avoid infections and bleeding.
• Avoid crowds and people with infections.
• To learn more: National Cancer Institute, 6116 Executive Blvd., MSC8322, Bethesda, MD 20892; (800) 422-6237; website: www.cancer.gov.

MEDICATIONS
• You will usually be prescribed anticancer drugs. They may be taken by mouth or given through a vein (IV).
• Antibiotics may be prescribed for infections.
• Biologic therapy drugs may be prescribed.

ACTIVITY
As tolerated. Avoid strenuous activities (such as lifting).

DIET
A healthy diet helps you feel better. Ask for medical advice and help if you are having problems with eating.

 NOTIFY OUR OFFICE IF

• You or your child has symptoms of leukemia.
• After diagnosis, symptoms cause you any concern.

Special notes:

_____

_____

_____

More notes on the back of this page ☐

LEUKEMIA, CHRONIC

BASIC INFORMATION

DESCRIPTION

Leukemia is cancer of blood cells in the bone marrow. Three types of blood cells are formed in bone marrow. White blood cells fight infections, red blood cells carry oxygen, and platelets help control bleeding. Bone marrow is the soft material in the center of bones. With chronic leukemia, the cancer (abnormal) cells do not fight infection as well as normal white blood cells do. Chronic leukemia develops over a long period of time. Forms of chronic leukemia include:

- Chronic lymphocytic leukemia (CLL). It affects adults only and is twice as common as CML.
- Chronic myeloid (myelogenous) leukemia (CML). It is rare in children and mostly affects adults.

FREQUENT SIGNS AND SYMPTOMS

- Sometimes, no symptoms occur.
- Low fever, chills, and sweating.
- Tiredness and weakness.
- Anemia (pale skin, fatigue).
- General ill feeling.
- Easy bruising or bleeding or cuts that heal slowly.
- Pin-head size spots on the skin.
- Repeated infections.
- Bone or joint pain.
- Appetite and/or weight loss. Fullness in the stomach.
- Other symptoms if cancer cells collect in organs, such as brain, lungs, genitals, digestive tract, or kidneys.

CAUSES

Exact cause unknown. It is believed to develop from a combination of genetic and environmental factors.

RISK INCREASES WITH

- Family history of leukemia (such as brother or sister).
- Men more than women; whites and Hispanics.
- Excess exposure to radiation.
- Exposure to benzenes and other toxic chemicals.
- Weak immune system due to illness or drugs.
- Smoking.

PREVENTIVE MEASURES

Cannot be prevented. If you have a family history of leukemia, get genetic counseling before starting a family.

EXPECTED OUTCOMES

Depends on the type of leukemia, the patient's health, and response to treatment. Remission occurs when there is no evidence of leukemia in the blood or bone marrow. Remission over 5 years often indicates a cure.

POSSIBLE COMPLICATIONS

- Hemorrhage or uncontrolled infection (can be fatal).
- Failure of leukemia to respond to chemotherapy.
- Relapse (leukemia recurs after remission).

DIAGNOSIS & TREATMENT

GENERAL MEASURES

- Your health care provider will do a physical exam and ask questions about your symptoms. Medical tests include blood studies. Samples of bone marrow (liquid and solid) will be taken for viewing with a microscope. Other tests are done to see if the cancer has spread.
- Treatment depends on the leukemia type and other factors. Treatment for CML may include anticancer drugs (chemotherapy), radiation therapy, bone marrow transplant, stem cell transplant, surgery, and biologic therapy. CLL patients may not need any immediate treatment. Follow-up exams are done. If disease progresses, then chemotherapy may be recommended.
- Chemotherapy uses drugs, and radiation therapy uses radiation to attack the cancer cells. Biologic therapy uses the body's immune system to fight cancer.
- Bone marrow transplant involves replacing the leukemia-affected marrow with healthy bone marrow.
- Stem cell transplant replaces blood cells destroyed in treatment with stem cells (immature blood cells).
- Blood and platelet transfusions may be needed.
- Surgery may be done to remove the spleen.
- Counseling may help you cope with having cancer.
- Get good dental care to avoid infections and bleeding.
- To learn more: National Cancer Institute, 6116 Executive Blvd., MSC8322, Bethesda, MD 20892; (800) 422-6237; website: www.cancer.gov.

MEDICATIONS

- You will usually be prescribed anticancer drugs. They can be taken by mouth or given through a vein (IV).
- Antibiotics may be prescribed for infections.
- Biologic therapy drugs may be prescribed.

ACTIVITY

As tolerated. Avoid strenuous activities (such as lifting).

DIET

A healthy diet helps you feel better. Ask for medical advice and help if you are having problems with eating.

NOTIFY OUR OFFICE IF

- You or your child has symptoms of leukemia.
- After diagnosis, symptoms cause you any concern.

Special notes:

_____

_____

_____

More notes on the back of this page ☐

LEUKOPLAKIA, ORAL

 BASIC INFORMATION

DESCRIPTION

Oral leukoplakia is a general term to describe a white patch on the mouth. It affects all ages, but it is most common in adults over 60, and in men more than in women. Hairy leukoplakia is a different disorder, and it occurs in people who have a weak immune system due to drugs or illness. Another form of leukoplakia occurs in the genitals of women.

FREQUENT SIGNS AND SYMPTOMS

· A white or off-white patch in the membranes of the mouth. The patch may be tiny or the size of a quarter. It can involve the lips, inside of the cheek, floor and roof of the mouth, tongue, or gums. It is not painful.
· The patch feels firm, rough and stiff. It can not be rubbed off.
· The area may be more sensitive when touched or when eating hot or spicy foods.
· It is sometimes first noticed by a dentist when doing a dental exam.

CAUSES

In some cases, the cause is unknown. Certain risk factors, such as smoking, may cause the disorder. It can not be spread from one person to another.

RISK INCREASES WITH

· Use of tobacco products, including cigarettes, chewing tobacco, snuff, pipes, or cigars.
· Repeated trauma to the mouth or tongue such as from a sharp or broken tooth or from dentures.
· Excess alcohol use.
· Infections such as candidiasis, syphilis, or Epstein-Barr virus.

PREVENTIVE MEASURES

· No specific preventive measures.
· For many health reasons, don't smoke or use tobacco products, and avoid alcohol.

EXPECTED OUTCOMES

Leukoplakia by itself does not cause any problems and does not require treatment. The concern is that it may be pre-cancerous, and that makes it important to have it diagnosed. In the majority of cases, cancer will not develop.

POSSIBLE COMPLICATIONS

· In a small percent of cases, cancer may develop.
· Leukoplakia may recur if the problem causing it (such as tobacco use) is not stopped.

 DIAGNOSIS & TREATMENT

GENERAL MEASURES

· Your health care provider can diagnose the disorder with a physical exam of the mouth and tongue. A biopsy is usually done if a pre-cancerous risk is suspected. The biopsy involves the removal of a small amount of skin tissue to be viewed under a microscope.
· Follow-up care may involve a wait-and-watch plan to see if any changes occur in the affected area. Drugs may be prescribed, or surgery may be recommended. Your health care provider will discuss the options with you.
· Stop any tobacco use and/or alcohol use (including alcoholic mouthwashes).
· Get treatment for any tooth problems or have any denture problems fixed.

MEDICATIONS

· Topical or oral forms of vitamin A may be prescribed.
· Other forms of treatment are currently undergoing study.

ACTIVITY

No limits.

DIET

No special diet.

 NOTIFY OUR OFFICE IF

You or a family member has symptoms of leukoplakia.

Special notes:

_____

_____

_____

More notes on the back of this page ☐

LICE

(Pediculosis; Head Lice; Body Lice; Crab Lice)

 BASIC INFORMATION

DESCRIPTION

Lice are tiny parasites that live on the body or in clothing. Pediculosis (lice infestation) is the medical term. Three types of lice affect humans: head lice, body lice, and crab (or pubic) lice. Head lice are common in school children.

FREQUENT SIGNS AND SYMPTOMS

• Itching and scratching of the head or other body parts. It may take 2 to 3 weeks or longer after being infected before itching symptoms start. The itching is more common at night.
• You may see eggs ("nits") on hair shafts.
• Scalp may be red and sore. The hair may be matted.

CAUSES

Tiny parasites that bite through skin to obtain nourishment (blood). The bites cause itching, redness, and soreness.

RISK INCREASES WITH

• Contact with an infected person.
• Contact with an infected object such as combs, hats, helmets, clothing, sheets, or pillowcases.
• Crowded living conditions.
• For crab lice, sexual intercourse with an infected person.
• Body lice are not common. They occur in the homeless, and those who can't bathe or change clothes often.

PREVENTIVE MEASURES

• Bathe and shampoo hair often. However, good hygiene alone will not prevent head lice.
• Don't share combs, brushes, or hats with others. Wash combs and brushes carefully.
• Careful follow-up in schools and daycare centers where head lice have occurred.
• If head lice or nits are found on your child, notify the child's school or daycare.

EXPECTED OUTCOMES

Usually curable with treatment. Allow 5 days after treatment for symptoms to disappear. Lice often recur.

POSSIBLE COMPLICATIONS

Infection at the site of scratching.

 DIAGNOSIS & TREATMENT

GENERAL MEASURES

• Self-diagnosis and self-treatment are sometimes all that is needed for head lice.
• When unsure if hair lice are the problem, or if body or crab lice are the cause, see your health care provider.

Lice are diagnosed with a physical exam of the affected area. A sample of the lice or nit may be removed for viewing under a microscope. Other medical tests may be done in some cases.
• Treatment may be done with a product to kill the lice and eggs. Manual removal may be the best option. It should be done even when an anti-lice product is used. If the lice infect eyelashes, they should be removed by your health care provider.
• Uninfected family members do not need treatment.
• For manual removal, use a special nit comb. A magnifying glass may help you see the nits and lice. Live lice are hard to see as they move quickly. Part the hair in sections and examine each part carefully.
• Wash articles such as combs, curlers, hairbrushes, and barrettes in hot water.
• Vacuuming floors, furniture, car seats or other items may help remove any hairs with nits on them. Special lice sprays may sometimes be recommended.
• Machine-wash clothing and bedding in hot water. Dry in the dryer's hot-air cycle. Putting unwashable items in plastic bags for 2 weeks has been recommended in the past, but is probably not needed. Lice can't live longer than 24 hours unless they have blood for food.
• For more information, contact the National Pediculosis Association., 50 Kearney Rd., Needham, MA 02494; (781) 449-NITS; website: www.headlice.org.

MEDICATIONS

• Nonprescription anti-lice (pediculicide) products are available. One type is Nix which contains permethrin. Follow label instructions for use and follow-up care. Use a special nit comb to help rid the hair of nits. Repeat the treatment in 7 to 10 days.
• Your health care provider may prescribe, and give directions for using, other anti-lice products.

ACTIVITY

No limits.

DIET

No special diet.

 NOTIFY OUR OFFICE IF

• You or a family member has symptoms of lice that you are concerned about.
• Self-treatment for lice has not worked.

Special notes:

_____

_____

_____

More notes on the back of this page ☐

LICHEN PLANUS

 ## BASIC INFORMATION

DESCRIPTION

A chronic skin condition that is not cancerous or contagious. It may involve the skin of the legs, trunk, arms, wrists, scalp or penis. The lining of the mouth or vagina, toenails, and fingernails (around or under the nailbed) may also be involved. It affects all ages, but is most common in adults over 40.

FREQUENT SIGNS AND SYMPTOMS

· Small, slightly raised bumps that itch. The bumps are purplish or reddish-purple with a whitish surface.
· An uneven, whitish line inside the mouth or vagina.
· Sudden hair loss in patches on the head.
· Bumps in the mouth may make it hard to eat.
· If the vagina is involved, it may cause a discharge, bleeding, or pain with intercourse.

CAUSES

Unknown. It may be a problem with the body's immune system.

RISK INCREASES WITH

· Stress (may make it worse).
· Adverse reaction to certain drugs.
· Hepatitis C.

PREVENTIVE MEASURES

Cannot be prevented at present.

EXPECTED OUTCOMES

There is no cure. Symptoms can be helped with treatment. Be patient and keep up with your treatment, even if results are slow. The bumps often go away on their own within a year. Once the bumps are gone, a brown area may remain on the skin. It will fade in time.

POSSIBLE COMPLICATIONS

· Chronic condition where new bumps appear as old bumps clear up.
· Rarely, hair or nail problems, which can include permanent loss.
· Lichen planus in the mouth may slightly increase the risk of oral cancer. Your health care provider will follow-up on a regular basis to watch for any problems.

 ## DIAGNOSIS & TREATMENT

GENERAL MEASURES

· Your health care provider can usually diagnose the condition with an exam of the affected area. Medical skin tests or a biopsy may be done to confirm the diagnosis. A biopsy involves the removal of a small amount of skin tissue to be viewed under a microscope.
· The goal of treatment is to relieve the symptoms; mainly the itching.
· Use cool-water soaks to relieve itching.
· Reducing stress in your life may help with the symptoms as well as prevent a recurrence. Learn ways to help yourself relax.
· If lichen planus is related to a drug you take, your health care provider may change the dose or prescribe a different drug.
· A special treatment called PUVA using ultraviolet light combined with drugs may help some people.
· To learn more: American Academy of Dermatology, 930 E. Woodfield Rd., Schaumburg, IL, 60173-4927; website: www.aad.org.

MEDICATIONS

· You may use nonprescription antihistamines taken by mouth to help·control itching.
· Nonprescription cortisone creams or ointments can help to reduce pain and itching. Follow directions on the label.
· Stronger drugs may be prescribed.

ACTIVITY

No limits.

DIET

No special diet.

 ## NOTIFY OUR OFFICE IF

· You or a family member has symptoms of lichen planus.
· New, unexplained symptoms develop. Drugs used in treatment may produce side effects.

Special notes:

_____

_____

_____

More notes on the back of this page ☐

LIPOMAS

 ## BASIC INFORMATION

DESCRIPTION

Benign, slow-growing tumors of fat cells. Lipomas grow under the skin (subcutaneous). They may involve the trunk, neck, back, upper thighs, or arms. They affect both sexes, and all ages, but are more common in adults. In a few cases, lipomas may grow in deeper body tissues or in the body's organs.

FREQUENT SIGNS AND SYMPTOMS

- Lumps are dome-shaped, and may be small or large.
- Lumps feel "doughy," smooth, and easily movable.
- One or many lipomas may occur on a person.
- Skin over the lump is normal in appearance.
- Most often, they cause no symptoms, such as itching or pain. However, a form of lipoma that contains blood vessels can cause pain.

CAUSES

Unknown, but the tendency is probably inherited. Minor injury may trigger their growth.

RISK INCREASES WITH

Family history of lipomas.

PREVENTIVE MEASURES

Cannot be prevented at present.

EXPECTED OUTCOMES

These lumps are benign and require no treatment. They may be removed if they cause symptoms, are large and/or unattractive, or for medical testing.

POSSIBLE COMPLICATIONS

For the majority of people, there are no complications. In rare cases, certain forms of lipomas may cause complications.

 ## DIAGNOSIS & TREATMENT

GENERAL MEASURES

- Your health care provider can usually diagnose lipomas with an exam of the affected area. In a few cases, medical tests may be done to confirm the diagnosis or check for complications.
- No treatment is needed for lumps that are stable in size.
- Surgical removal (if recommended) is usually done in a medical office. Lipomas can be removed with small incisions or removed by liposuction. Instructions for home care after surgery will be provided.

MEDICATIONS

Drugs are not needed for this disorder.

ACTIVITY

No limits.

DIET

No special diet.

 ## NOTIFY OUR OFFICE IF

- You or a family member is concerned about skin growths.
- The following occur after lipoma surgery:
  - Fever.
  - Bleeding that does not respond to moderate pressure.
  - Signs of infection (warmth, swelling or redness), at the surgical site.

Special notes:

_____

_____

_____

More notes on the back of this page ☐

LIVER CANCER

 BASIC INFORMATION

DESCRIPTION

Growth of malignant cells in the liver. The liver is the largest internal organ in the body. It is located behind the ribs on the right side. Liver cancer can affect all ages, but is most common in men over 60.

FREQUENT SIGNS AND SYMPTOMS

- The early stages may produce no symptoms.
- Loss of appetite and weight loss.
- Tender mass in the right upper abdomen.
- Pain in the upper abdomen.
- Low fever, usually less than 101°F (38.3°C).
- Yellow eyes and skin (from jaundice).
- Swollen abdomen from fluid retention.
- Nausea and vomiting.
- Feeling tired or weak.

CAUSES

- Unknown. People with certain risk factors are more likely to develop liver cancer than others.
- A primary cancer is when it begins in the liver.
- A secondary cancer is when it results from the spread (metastases) of cancer from another place in the body. The most common sources are cancers of the rectum, colon, lung, breast, pancreas, esophagus, or skin (malignant melanoma).

RISK INCREASES WITH

- Chronic viral hepatitis B or hepatitis C infection.
- Liver disease, such as cirrhosis of the liver.
- Long-term exposure to aflatoxin (a substance in fungus that grows on peanuts, corn, other nuts and grains).
- Age over 60; males more than females.
- Family history of liver cancer.
- Tobacco use.
- Certain inherited metabolic disorders.
- Anabolic steroid (male hormone) use.

PREVENTIVE MEASURES

- Cancer screening and hepatitis B vaccine for high-risk persons.
- Avoid excess alcohol use (it can lead to cirrhosis).
- Avoid risk factors such as smoking and steroid use.

EXPECTED OUTCOMES

- This condition can be cured only if it is caught early, has not spread, and surgery is successful. In other cases, it cannot be cured, but treatment can help relieve symptoms and help a person live longer.
- Scientific research into causes and treatment continues, so there is hope for effective treatment and cure.

POSSIBLE COMPLICATIONS

- Kidney failure.
- Spread of cancer to other organs.
- Death from loss of liver function.

 DIAGNOSIS & TREATMENT

GENERAL MEASURES

- Your health care provider will do a physical exam and ask questions about your symptoms. Medical tests may include blood studies and liver function tests. Other tests are usually done in order to confirm the diagnosis and to determine if cancer has spread (called staging).
- Treatment will depend on the stage of the cancer, your health and your preferences. The main treatments involve surgery, chemotherapy (anticancer drugs), and radiation (used less often). Since many liver tumors cannot be removed by surgery, other treatment forms are evolving. These include embolization, radiofrequency ablation, cryotherapy, and alcohol injections. Your health care provider will discuss the options with you.
- Surgery is done only for cancer found in an early stage. The cancer can still recur because cancer cells may have spread before surgery.
- Liver transplants have been done in a few select cases.
- Treatment may involve steps to relieve symptoms and make you comfortable, rather than treating the cancer.
- Counseling may help in coping with this disorder.
- To learn more: American Cancer Society, (800) ACS-2345; website: www.cancer.org or National Cancer Institute, (800) 4-CANCER; website: www.nci.nih.gov.

MEDICATIONS

- For minor discomfort, you may use nonprescription drugs such as acetaminophen. Stronger pain relievers will be prescribed as needed.
- Anticancer drugs may be given.

ACTIVITY

Stay as active as your strength allows.

DIET

No special diet. Don't drink alcohol.

 NOTIFY OUR OFFICE IF

- You or a family member has symptoms of liver cancer, especially unexplained weight loss, low fever, or a mass is felt in the abdomen.
- New or unexpected symptoms develop during treatment.

Special notes:

_____

_____

_____

More notes on the back of this page ☐

LUNG ABSCESS

 BASIC INFORMATION

DESCRIPTION
An infected area of lung tissue, surrounded by lung inflammation. The infected lung tissue dies and is replaced with pus. The infection is not contagious from person to person.

FREQUENT SIGNS AND SYMPTOMS
- Cough with sputum. The sputum is pus-like, often blood-streaked, and sometimes smells bad.
- Bad breath.
- Sweating.
- Fever up to 101°F (38.3°C) or higher.
- Chills.
- Weight loss.
- Chest pain (sometimes).

CAUSES
Lung abscesses are generally caused by a bacterial infection. They are usually a complication of pneumonia. A lung abscess may occur when an unconscious or sedated person inhales infected material from the upper-breathing passages. The patient may be unconscious from a head injury, or heavily sedated.

RISK INCREASES WITH
- Recent illness or disease, such as cancer.
- Alcoholism or substance abuse.
- Recent general anesthesia or injury causing unconsciousness.
- Poor dental hygiene.

PREVENTIVE MEASURES
No specific preventive measures. Be sure to seek prompt medical treatment for lung infections, especially pneumonia.

EXPECTED OUTCOMES
Usually curable with antibiotic treatment (may last for 4 to 6 weeks or for several months).

POSSIBLE COMPLICATIONS
- Abscess may not respond well to antibiotic treatment.
- Rupture of the abscess, causing empyema or massive bleeding in the lung.
- Spread of infection to other body parts, especially the brain.

 DIAGNOSIS & TREATMENT

GENERAL MEASURES
- Your health care provider will do a physical exam. Medical tests may include blood tests, a culture of pus from the abscess, and x-rays of the lung. A bronchoscopy may be done if a foreign body is suspected. This test uses an optical instrument with a lighted tip that is passed into the windpipe, and then into the bronchi.
- Hospital care is usually required.
- Treatment is with antibiotic drugs. Surgery may be needed if antibiotics are not helping the abscess heal.
- Other care in the hospital may involve breathing support with oxygen and procedures to help loosen secretions. Physical therapy can help strengthen the breathing muscles.
- Surgery (sometimes) to remove pus from the abscess or to remove the abscess and part of the lung, if the abscess does not heal.

MEDICATIONS
Antibiotics for prolonged periods to fight infection and prevent a recurrence. They are given through a vein (IV) at first, and then given by mouth.

ACTIVITY
Reduced activity until tests show a healed abscess.

DIET
No special diet. Increase your fluid intake. By drinking extra liquids, the body is forced to eliminate part of the fluid through the lungs. This makes thick lung secretions thinner, so they can be coughed up more easily.

 NOTIFY OUR OFFICE IF

- You or a family member has symptoms of a lung abscess.
- Symptoms of a lung infection recur after treatment, especially a sputum-producing cough, fever, or general ill feeling.

Special notes:

_____

_____

_____

More notes on the back of this page ☐

LUNG CANCER
(Bronchogenic Carcinoma)

 BASIC INFORMATION

DESCRIPTION
Malignant cell growth in the lungs. There are two major types, non-small cell (more common) and small cell. Lung cancer affects adults of both sexes, usually between ages 40 and 70. Lung cancer causes more deaths than any other form of cancer, and the number is increasing. It is related almost exclusively to smoking.

FREQUENT SIGNS AND SYMPTOMS
- Usually there are no symptoms in the early stages.
- Persistent cough.
- Wheezing.
- Chest pain.
- Fatigue and weakness.
- Weight loss.
- Shoulder, arm, or bone pain.
- Coughing up blood.

CAUSES
Abnormal cells grow and destroy healthy lung tissue. Primary lung cancer is one that begins in the lungs. It can spread (metastasize) to other places in the body. Secondary lung cancer is when cancer from another place in the body spreads to the lungs.

RISK INCREASES WITH
- Adults over 60.
- Smoking. Cigarettes (highest risk), pipes, and cigars.
- Secondhand smoke.
- Radon gas.
- Lung diseases.
- Environmental exposure to asbestos, uranium ore, nickel, chromates, bischloromethyl ether, or air pollution.

PREVENTIVE MEASURES
- Don't smoke. Because tumors don't develop for a long time, smokers can quit at any time and greatly reduce the risk of developing lung cancer.
- Obtain regular health checkups that may include a chest x-ray or CT scan if you are a heavy smoker.
- Check your house for radon gas.

EXPECTED OUTCOMES
Outcome depends on the type of cancer, whether it has spread, patient's general health, and response to treatment. The outcome is more favorable with early diagnosis compared to diagnosis of advanced disease. Early diagnosis improves the success rate of treatment.

POSSIBLE COMPLICATIONS
- Spinal cord compression (decreased feeling in lower half of the body).
- Complications from treatments.
- Hypercalcemia (excess calcium in the body).
- Spread to other body parts, which can be fatal.

 DIAGNOSIS & TREATMENT

GENERAL MEASURES
- Your health care provider will do a physical exam and ask questions about your symptoms. A number of medical tests will be done. The tests first help diagnose the cancer and then determine if it has spread (staging).
- Treatment varies and depends on location and size of tumor, any spread of the cancer, your health, age, and preferences. Treatment may include surgery, anticancer drugs (chemotherapy) and/or radiation therapy, and biologic therapy.
- Chemotherapy uses drugs and radiation therapy uses radiation to attack the cancer cells. Biologic therapy uses the body's immune system to fight cancer.
- Surgery to remove all of the lung (pneumonectomy) or part of the lung (lobectomy) may be recommended if cancer is at an early stage.
- Treatment may involve steps to relieve symptoms and make you comfortable, rather than treating the cancer.
- Counseling may help you cope with having cancer.
- To learn more: American Cancer Society, (800) ACS-2345; website: www.cancer.org or National Cancer Institute, (800) 4-CANCER; website: www.nci.nih.gov.

MEDICATIONS
- For minor pain, use nonprescription drugs such as acetaminophen or aspirin (not for children).
- Stronger pain drugs and nausea or anti-anxiety drugs may be prescribed.
- Anticancer drugs or biologic therapy drugs may be prescribed.

ACTIVITY
Be as active as possible. Following treatments, follow medical advice about resuming activities.

DIET
No special diet.

 NOTIFY OUR OFFICE IF

- You or a family member has symptoms of lung cancer.
- After diagnosis, any symptoms occur that cause you concern.

Special notes:

_____

_____

_____

More notes on the back of this page ☐

LUPUS ERYTHEMATOSUS, DISCOID (DLE)

 BASIC INFORMATION

DESCRIPTION

Discoid lupus erythematosus (DLE) is a chronic skin disorder. Localized DLE (the more common form) involves the skin on the face, scalp, ears, and neck. Generalized DLE involves the skin on the arms and chest. DLE is different from systemic lupus erythematosus (SLE), which affects many different internal organs. DLE can affect all ages and both sexes. It typically occurs in women in their 30s.

FREQUENT SIGNS AND SYMPTOMS

• Coin-shaped (discoid), red, raised, scaly skin patches (they may be referred to as rashes, plaques or lesions). Erythematosus means reddening of the skin.
• The centers are lighter in color than the outside ring.
• Patches may appear anywhere on the face. The cheeks and jawline are the most common sites. Some people describe them as "butterfly" rash when they appear on both sides of the nose.
• The patches may sometimes appear on the scalp with patches of hair loss.
• Mucous membranes of the mouth may be affected.
• The affected skin is usually not itchy or painful.
• Scarring occurs as the rash heals.

CAUSES

Unknown. Both genetic (hereditary) and environmental factors may contribute. It is thought to be an autoimmune disorder. In these disorders, the immune system by mistake attacks the body itself. It cannot be spread from one person to another.

RISK INCREASES WITH

Family history of DLE.

PREVENTIVE MEASURES

No specific preventive measures.

EXPECTED OUTCOMES

Outcome is generally good. Symptoms of the disorder may come and go over years, but they are not life-threatening. Treatment can help improve the cosmetic appearance of the rash.

POSSIBLE COMPLICATIONS

• Scarring of the face.
• Systemic lupus erythematosus (about 10% of patients). If it does occur, it is usually not severe.

 DIAGNOSIS & TREATMENT

GENERAL MEASURES

• Your health care provider may do a physical exam and an exam of the affected skin. Medical tests may include blood studies and a skin biopsy. A biopsy involves removal of a sample of the affected skin for viewing under a microscope.
• Treatment involves drug therapy and sunscreens.
• Sun exposure is a trigger for a flare-up. Don't go outdoors between 10 a.m. and 2 p.m., when the sun's ultraviolet light is strongest. If you can't avoid exposure to bright sunlight, wear protective clothing and maximum-protection sunscreen products.
• Regular checkups with your health care provider are important, even when in remission.
• To learn more: Lupus Foundation of America, 2000 L St., NW, Suite 710, Washington, DC 20036; (800) 558-0121; website: www.lupus.org.

MEDICATIONS

• Steroid skin creams or ointments are usually prescribed. Follow instructions carefully about their use.
• Plastic tape coated with steroid, injections of steroid into affected skin, or rarely, oral steroids may be prescribed (with more severe symptoms).
• Antimalaria drugs may be prescribed. They are taken by mouth and often help the symptoms of this disorder.
• Use sunscreens for sun protection.

ACTIVITY

No limits.

DIET

No special diet.

 NOTIFY OUR OFFICE IF

• You or a family member has symptoms of discoid lupus erythematosus.
• The following occur during treatment:
  - New skin symptoms.
  - Swelling, redness, or pain in joints.

Special notes:

_____

_____

_____

More notes on the back of this page ☐

LUPUS ERYTHEMATOSUS, SYSTEMIC (SLE)

 ## BASIC INFORMATION

DESCRIPTION

An inflammatory disease that affects various parts of the body. It can involve the joints, skin, kidneys, brain, heart, and lungs. Systemic lupus erythematosus (SLE) can affect all ages and both sexes, but 90% of cases occur in women between ages of 30 and 50.

FREQUENT SIGNS AND SYMPTOMS

- Lupus symptoms often flare up and then subside.
- Joint aches or pain, with redness and swelling.
- Fever and fatigue.
- Skin rash. Butterfly-like rash on the cheeks.
- Anemia (pale skin and feeling weak).
- Chest pain (with deep breathing).
- Increased sensitivity to the sun.
- Hair loss.
- Ulcers (sores) in the mouth or the nose.
- Seizures.

CAUSES

Unknown. Both genetic (hereditary) and environmental factors may contribute. It is thought to be an autoimmune disorder. In these disorders, the immune system attacks the body itself by mistake. The disease cannot be spread from one person to another.

RISK INCREASES WITH

- Females.
- Family history of lupus.
- Having other autoimmune disorders.
- Smoking.
- Genetic factors. It occurs more often among African Americans, Hispanic Americans, Native Americans, and Asians.

PREVENTIVE MEASURES

Cannot be prevented at present.

EXPECTED OUTCOMES

SLE is currently considered incurable. 20% to 30% of the cases are mild and may have only a skin rash. The majority of cases have continued remissions, flares, and relapses. The flares or relapses may occur 2 to 3 times a year. Many patients lead a normal lifestyle while in remission. Symptoms can often be relieved or controlled with treatment.

POSSIBLE COMPLICATIONS

- Anemia (often due to iron deficiency).
- Blood disorders and blood vessel disorders.
- Complications may occur in the heart, lung, gastrointestinal system, kidneys, joint/muscle/bone, nervous system, and eyes.
- Unable to continue regular job; changes are needed in working conditions.
- Pregnancies in SLE patients are considered high-risk.

 ## DIAGNOSIS & TREATMENT

GENERAL MEASURES

- Your health care provider will do a physical exam and ask questions about your symptoms and activities. Medical tests include samples of blood to measure specific antibodies. Patients with vague, recurrent symptoms may require long-term observation and repeated testing before a final diagnosis can be made.
- Treatment steps depend on the extent and severity of the disorder. Drugs are usually prescribed to treat the condition, as well as the symptoms and complications.
- Obtain prompt medical treatment for any infection.
- Avoid sun exposure or use protection of hats, sunglasses, sunscreens, and long-sleeved clothing.
- Apply heat or ice to relieve joint pain.
- Control the stress in your life. Learn relaxation techniques or obtain counseling if needed.
- Talk to your health care provider if you are thinking about becoming pregnant.
- Get regular medical and dental check-ups.
- To learn more: Lupus Foundation of America, 2000 L St., NW, Suite 710, Washington, DC 20036; (800) 558-0121; website: www.lupus.org.

MEDICATIONS

Drugs to suppress the immune system, steroid and non-steroidal anti-inflammatory drugs, hormones, or anti-malarial drugs may be prescribed. These relieve symptoms but don't cure the disease. Other drugs may be prescribed depending on specific complications.

ACTIVITY

- Remain as active as possible. Extra rest may be needed. Exercises can help to retain range-of-motion. Exercise does not improve joint aches or fatigue.
- Physical therapy may be recommended.

DIET

Eat a healthy diet. Reduce salt intake.

 ## NOTIFY OUR OFFICE IF

- You or a family member has symptoms of systemic lupus erythematosus.
- After diagnosis, any new symptoms occur, other symptoms get worse, or drugs cause side effects.

Special notes:

_____

_____

_____

More notes on the back of this page ☐

LYME DISEASE

BASIC INFORMATION

DESCRIPTION

A disorder caused by a tick bite. Most people who get Lyme disease do not become seriously ill. It is named for Lyme, Connecticut, where it was first described. It has now occurred in 48 of the 50 states.

FREQUENT SIGNS AND SYMPTOMS

Stage 1:
• A rash (called erythema migrans) that starts as a small red spot. The spot expands and becomes round or oval in shape with a clear center. It resembles a bulls-eye.
• Mild flu-like symptoms may occur (fever, headache, stiff neck, fatigue, muscle and joint pain).
Stage 2:
• Rash develops on other places of the body.
• Single-joint pain or body pain.
• Central nervous system symptoms that may range from headache to loss of consciousness.
Stage 3 (may occur months to years after first stage):
• The nerves, joints, heart, and brain may be seriously affected causing a number of new symptoms.

CAUSES

Infection with a spirochete (a specific type of germ), *Borrelia burgdorferi*, transmitted by an infected deer tick bite. The tick bite may occur 3 to 30 days prior to the rash. The infection cannot be spread from one person to another.

RISK INCREASES WITH

Work, play, or recreational activities in states and locations at high risk for ticks. States include those in the northeast, mid-Atlantic, upper north-central United States, and some California counties. Locations include grassy, brushy, or wooded areas.

PREVENTIVE MEASURES

• Wear protective clothing with tight collars and cuffs.
• Use effective insect repellents, such as DEET, in areas with ticks.
• Have dogs and cats wear tick-repellent collars.
• Careful skin check and removal of any ticks. If the tick is removed from the skin within 36 hours, there is usually no infection.
• A vaccine is not currently available.

EXPECTED OUTCOMES

The severity differs from one person to another. Mild cases clear up on their own, without treatment. Most other cases can be treated successfully with antibiotics. In a few cases, symptoms may not respond to antibiotics. Additional treatment may help or be ineffective.

POSSIBLE COMPLICATIONS

• Various degrees of persistent joint or nervous system pain, fatigue, memory problems, and other symptoms.
• Rarely, death may occur.

DIAGNOSIS & TREATMENT

GENERAL MEASURES

• Your health care provider will do a physical exam and ask questions about your symptoms and activities. Medical tests may include blood studies and others to help confirm the diagnosis.
• Early treatment with antibiotic drugs is important to prevent symptoms from getting worse.
• Use crutches to keep weight off affected joints, if necessary.
• Heat relieves joint pain. Take warm baths or showers, or use heating pads.
• To learn more: Lyme Disease Association, PO Box 1438, Jackson, NJ 08527; (888) 366-6611; website: www.lymediseaseassociation.org or American Lyme Disease Foundation, 293 Route 100, Suite 204, Somers, NY 10589; (914) 277-6970 (not toll free); website: www.aldf.com.

MEDICATIONS

• You may be prescribed:
   - An oral antibiotic (usually for 14 to 21 days) for early stage of the disease.
   - Antibiotics given through a vein (IV) for later stages.
   - Nonsteroidal anti-inflammatory drugs.
   - Steroid drugs to reduce the inflammatory response in the heart or central nervous system.

ACTIVITY

Rest in bed until symptoms get better. Then resume normal activities gradually.

DIET

No special diet.

NOTIFY OUR OFFICE IF

• You or a family member has symptoms of Lyme disease.
• New, unexplained symptoms develop. Drugs used in treatment may produce side effects.

Special notes:

_____

_____

_____

More notes on the back of this page ☐

LYMPHOGRANULOMA VENEREUM
(LGV; Lymphogranuloma Inguinale)

BASIC INFORMATION

DESCRIPTION
Lymphogranuloma venereum is a contagious venereal disease that involves the genitals and lymph glands. This disease is found mostly in tropical and subtropical areas. It is rare in the United States. It usually occurs in adults (20s and 30s); in men more than women.

FREQUENT SIGNS AND SYMPTOMS
· The following symptoms begin 1 to 4 weeks after exposure and progress in order.
· A painless blister on the genitals which ulcerates (becomes an open and runny sore) and then heals quickly.
· Enlarged lymph glands in the groin that form large, red, tender masses. These are called buboes.
· Multiple areas of deep infection that discharge thick pus and blood-stained material.
· Other symptoms include:
  - Fever.
  - Muscle aches and pain, including backache.
  - Headaches.
  - Joint pain.
  - Appetite loss.
  - Vomiting.

CAUSES
A bacteria, *Chlamydia*, which is transmitted by sexual activity. This includes direct sexual contact with the genitals, rectum, or mouth.

RISK INCREASES WITH
· Travel to and sexual activity in a country where the disorder occurs frequently.
· Anal intercourse.
· Unprotected sexual activity with new partners.

PREVENTIVE MEASURES
· Use latex condoms during sexual intercourse with new partners.
· Don't engage in sexual activity with an infected person.

EXPECTED OUTCOME
Usually curable with appropriate treatment.

POSSIBLE COMPLICATIONS
· Relapse or reinfection.
· Tissue damage, scarring, rectal or intestinal blockages, and extreme swelling of the genitals.
· In severe cases, it attacks the central nervous system.
· Newborns can contract the disease from infected mothers during birth.

DIAGNOSIS & TREATMENT

GENERAL MEASURES
· Your health care provider will do a physical exam including the genital and rectal areas. Medical tests may include blood studies, a culture of the discharge from the lesions and antibody tests for *Chlamydia*. Tests for other sexually transmitted diseases are often done.
· Treatment may include drugs, surgery, and self-care.
· Surgery may be needed for some complications. Affected lymph glands (buboes) may be drained. An abscess (a pus-filled sore) may be drained. Fistulas (an abnormal passage between two organs or from an internal organ to the body surface) may be repaired.
· Your sexual contacts should be examined also.
· Heat applied to affected area may help discomfort.
· To learn more: Centers for Disease Control & Prevention (CDC) National STD & AIDS Hotlines (800) 227-8922; website: www.cdc.gov/std.

MEDICATION
· Antibiotics for infection will be prescribed.
· For minor discomfort, you may use nonprescription drugs such as acetaminophen.
· Stronger pain relievers may be prescribed.

ACTIVITY
After treatment, resume normal activity as soon as symptoms improve. Don't resume sexual relations until completely healed.

DIET
No special diet.

NOTIFY OUR OFFICE IF

· You or a family member has symptoms of lymphogranuloma venereum.
· The following occur during treatment:
  - Temperature rises to 101°F (38.3°C) or higher.
  - Pain cannot be relieved with simple pain drugs.
· New, unexplained symptoms develop. Drugs used in treatment may produce side effects.

Special notes:

_____

_____

_____

More notes on the back of this page ☐

LYMPHOMAS, NON-HODGKIN'S

(Lymphosarcoma; Reticulum Cell Sarcoma)

 BASIC INFORMATION

DESCRIPTION

Non-Hodgkin's lymphomas are a group of closely related cancers that affect the lymphatic system. Hodgkin's disease is another related, yet different type, of lymphoma. Lymphoma is a term that describes cancer of the body's lymphatic system. The lymphatic system is a part of the body's immune system that fights infections and diseases. Non-Hodgkin's lymphomas tend to occur more often in older adults.

FREQUENT SIGNS AND SYMPTOMS

- Swollen, non-tender, rubbery, distinct lymph glands anywhere in the body, but most often in the armpit, neck, or groin.
- Weight loss.
- General ill feeling.
- Anemia.
- Bleeding from the gastrointestinal tract.
- Jaundice (yellow skin and eyes).

CAUSES

Generally unknown. There is an association with two types of viruses: Epstein-Barr virus (EBV), and human T-cell lymphoma/leukemia virus (HTLV-1). Genetics may be a factor. Other possible causes are being researched and studied.

RISK INCREASES WITH

- Adults over 40. Males more than females.
- Weak immune system due to illness or drugs.
- Previous treatment with radiation, chemotherapy, or immune suppressing, or antispasmodic drugs.
- Work that involves exposure to carcinogens (a substance known to cause cancer).

PREVENTIVE MEASURES

No specific preventive measures.

EXPECTED OUTCOMES

The outcome varies according to the cancer cell type, if it is slow or fast growing, if it has spread, and the individual's age and response to treatment. If one treatment is not working, there may be other options that can be tried. Treatments are constantly improving, so there is hope for cure or remission.

POSSIBLE COMPLICATIONS

- Cancer spreads to other parts of the body.
- Cancer treatments can weaken the body's immune system, which increases the risk for infections.
- Anemia.
- Recurrence of tumors after treatment.
- Any of the complications could be fatal.

 DIAGNOSIS & TREATMENT

GENERAL MEASURES

- Your health care provider will do a physical exam and ask questions about your symptoms. A variety of medical tests will be done to verify the exact type of cancer cells, the grade (fast or slow growing), and if the cancer has spread (called staging) to other places in the body.
- Treatment will depend on the cancer type, grade and location, its stage, your health, age and preferences. Your health care provider will discuss your specific diagnosis and treatment recommendations with you.
- Watchful waiting may be an option. This means monitoring the cancer cells for a period of time before deciding on treatment.
- Radiotherapy and/or chemotherapy (anticancer drugs) are often the first treatment steps.
- Bone marrow or stem cell transplantation may be considered if other methods fail.
- Other treatment options include phototherapy (using ultraviolet light), biologic therapy (using the immune system) to treat the cancer, and possibly new approaches now being studied.
- Surgery is less often used as a treatment.
- To learn more: American Cancer Society, (800) ACS-2345; website: www.cancer.org or National Cancer Institute, (800) 4-CANCER; website: www.cancer.gov.

MEDICATIONS

- Chemotherapy (anticancer drugs) may be prescribed. Side effects from chemotherapy may improve once the body adjusts to the drug.
- Other drugs, such as steroids, may be prescribed.

ACTIVITY

Stay as active as possible.

DIET

No special diet.

 NOTIFY OUR OFFICE IF

- You or a family member has symptoms of non-Hodgkin's lymphoma.
- Any new symptoms develop during treatment or other symptoms worsen.

Special notes:

_____

_____

_____

More notes on the back of this page ☐

MALABSORPTION
(Malabsorptive Syndrome)

 BASIC INFORMATION

DESCRIPTION
The body is not properly absorbing nutrients (vitamins, minerals, proteins, sugars, fats, etc.) from foods. Most nutrients are absorbed through the small intestine. Malabsorption is not a disease in itself. It is a result of some other condition. It can affect all ages.

FREQUENT SIGNS AND SYMPTOMS
- Diarrhea.
- Weakness.
- Weight loss.
- Gas with stomach discomfort and swelling.
- Bad-smelling, bulky stools, often with mucus.
- Mild anemia (pale skin and feeling weak and tired).
- Bone pain.
- Swollen hands and feet.

CAUSES
A variety of health problems can cause malabsorption. The small intestine can be affected by infections, inflammation, irritation, structural defects, injury, surgery, faults in the digestive process, congenital defects, and others.

RISK INCREASES WITH
- Lactose intolerance.
- Celiac disease.
- Crohn's disease, ulcerative colitis, or chronic diarrhea.
- Chronic pancreatitis.
- Cystic fibrosis.
- Small intestine disorders such as diverticulosis, strictures, and partial obstruction.
- Bacteria or parasite infection.
- Short bowel syndrome (due to surgery that removed half or more of the small intestine).
- Stomach or bowel surgery or radiation.
- Liver disease.
- Excess use of laxatives or antacids.
- HIV infection.
- Imbalance of minerals in the body.

PREVENTIVE MEASURES
No specific preventive measures. Avoid risk factors where possible.

EXPECTED OUTCOMES
The degree to which symptoms can be controlled depends on the cause, but many things are common to all malabsorptive disorders. The onset is usually slow and difficult to diagnose. Disorders may be present for months or years before being recognized. Treatment is long, complicated, and may need to be changed often. Patience and a positive attitude are important steps in becoming cured.

POSSIBLE COMPLICATIONS
- Prolonged illness.
- Failure to thrive in infants.
- Additional illness caused by nutritional, vitamin, or mineral deficiency.
- Anemia.

 DIAGNOSIS & TREATMENT

GENERAL MEASURES
- Your health care provider will do a physical exam and ask questions about your symptoms and activities. Medical tests may include blood, stool, and urine studies and x-rays of the intestinal tract. Other tests may be done to help diagnose the cause.
- Treatment depends on the underlying cause and the needs of each patient. Steps may include special feeding methods, diet changes, or drugs.
- Some patients may need feeding through a vein (IV). This is called total parenteral nutrition (TPN).
- Some patients may need tube feeding. A tube is inserted into the stomach or the bowel for feeding.

MEDICATIONS
You may be prescribed enzymes to aid digestion, antidiarrheals, antibiotics, anti-inflammatory drugs, intestinal hormones, medium chain triglycerides, vitamins and other supplements, and antacids.

ACTIVITY
As tolerated by symptoms and physical condition.

DIET
Diet changes may be prescribed. They can be milk-free, gluten-free, low-fat, no-fat, or others restrictions. You will be provided specific diet instructions.

 NOTIFY OUR OFFICE IF

- You or a family member has symptoms of malabsorption.
- Any of the following occur during treatment:
  - Black, tarry bowel movements.
  - Fever of 101°F (38.3°C) or higher.
  - Severe abdominal pain.
  - Muscle cramps.

Special notes:

_____

_____

_____

More notes on the back of this page ☐

MALARIA

 BASIC INFORMATION

DESCRIPTION
A serious infection caused by malarial parasites. Malaria is transmitted by a mosquito bite. Most cases of malaria in the United States are in immigrants and travelers returning from malaria-risk areas. A few cases are transmitted by blood transfusion, from mother to fetus during pregnancy, or by mosquito bite that occurred in the United States. Malaria can occur in all age groups.

FREQUENT SIGNS AND SYMPTOMS
- Symptoms usually occur about 10 to 28 days after infection (though it can be up to a year).
- Fatigue and general ill feeling.
- Muscle and joint pain.
- Symptoms may include headache, nausea, vomiting, and diarrhea.
- Shaking chills, with a fever. This is followed by heavy sweating, along with a drop in temperature.

CAUSES
The mosquito becomes infected with malaria after biting a person with the disease. The parasites multiply in the mosquito for a week, then enter the bloodstream of the next person the mosquito bites. Once in a person's bloodstream, the parasites travel to the liver, where they thrive and multiply rapidly. After several days, thousands re-enter the bloodstream and destroy red blood cells. Some parasites remain in the liver, continue to multiply, and are released again at intervals into the bloodstream.

RISK INCREASES WITH
Living in, or travel to, any country where malaria is a risk. It is most prevalent in rural tropical areas such as found in Latin America, Asia, and Africa.

PREVENTIVE MEASURES
- Take antimalaria drugs before visiting an area where malaria is a risk. Continue to take the drugs after you return. A travel health clinic or your health care provider can give you instructions.
- In mosquito-infested areas, wear long-sleeved shirts and pants, especially from dusk to dawn. Use a DEET insect repellent on exposed skin. Sleep under a bednet that has been dipped in permethrin insecticide.
- Contact Centers for Disease Control (CDC) traveler information about malaria risks and prevention. Toll free voice (877) FYI-TRIP or toll free to get fax information (888) 232-3299, or website: www.cdc.gov/travel.

EXPECTED OUTCOMES
Curable with treatment. Symptoms usually improve in about 48 hours and fever is gone in about 4 days. Children, persons with weak immune systems, and pregnant women are more at risk for complications.

POSSIBLE COMPLICATIONS
- Anemia, jaundice, or brain or kidney damage.
- Bleeding, seizures, or coma.
- Severe hypoglycemia (low blood sugar).
- Pulmonary edema (fluid in the lungs).
- Hemoglobinuria (hemoglobin in the urine).

 DIAGNOSIS & TREATMENT

GENERAL MEASURES
- Your health care provider will do a physical exam and ask questions about your symptoms and recent travels. Medical tests will include blood studies. Other tests may be done if complications are a concern.
- Treatment is with drugs. Hospital care may be needed with severe symptoms.
- All cases of malaria are reported to the local health department.

MEDICATIONS
- One or more antimalaria drugs to kill the parasite will be prescribed. It will depend on the type of malaria diagnosed.
- Take nonprescription acetaminophen for fever.

ACTIVITY
Rest in bed until fever and chills subside. Resume your normal activities gradually as symptoms improve.

DIET
No special diet.

 NOTIFY OUR OFFICE IF

- You or a family member has symptoms of malaria. Symptoms may begin up to one year after returning from travel in a malaria-risk area. During your travels, you should have the name of a medical person or center to contact if symptoms develop.
- After diagnosis, weakness lasts for a prolonged time. This may indicate anemia.
- Symptoms of malaria recur after treatment.
- New, unexplained symptoms develop. Drugs used in treatment may produce side effects.

Special notes:

_____

_____

_____

More notes on the back of this page ☐

MARFAN SYNDROME

 ## BASIC INFORMATION

DESCRIPTION

A rare, inherited connective tissue disorder. Connective tissue supports and adds strength to other body tissue and body parts such as tendons and ligaments and heart valves. The severity of the symptoms varies greatly among patients. It affects males and females equally.

FREQUENT SIGNS AND SYMPTOMS

- Tall and thin body shape.
- Long arms and legs.
- Long, thin fingers (arachnodactyly).
- Chest deformity (may be sunken in or protrude out).
- Curved spine (scoliosis).
- High palate in the mouth and overcrowded teeth.
- "Double jointed;" joint weakness or looseness.
- Dislocation of eye lens, usually upward.
- Myopia (nearsighted).
- Symptoms of heart problems (eg., shortness of breath, tiredness, irregular or rapid heart beat).
- Stretch marks on the shoulders, hips and lower back.
- Easy bruising or bleeding (uncommon).

CAUSES

Inherited disorder in about 85% of cases. Other cases occur with no known cause. The disorder is present from birth and diagnosis can sometimes be made in newborns. However, signs or symptoms are often not seen until adolescence or young adulthood.

RISK INCREASES WITH

- Advanced paternal age may be a risk in those cases that are not clearly inherited.
- Family history of Marfan syndrome.

PREVENTIVE MEASURES

- No preventive measures. Prenatal diagnosis is possible in some cases.
- Each child has a 50% chance of inheriting the disorder from an affected parent. Children may be more or less severely affected.
- Get genetic counseling if you have Marfan syndrome or there is a family history of the disorder.

EXPECTED OUTCOMES

Early diagnosis and steps to prevent and treat complications have helped to improve the outlook for patients. Lifespan is about the same as an average person.

POSSIBLE COMPLICATIONS

- Cardiovascular problems can be life-threatening.
- Bacterial endocarditis (heart inflammation).
- Complications of the aorta (heart artery).
- Heart and lung problems (due to chest deformity).
- Depression and anxiety.
- Retinal detachment (rare).

 ## DIAGNOSIS & TREATMENT

GENERAL MEASURES

- Your health care provider will do a physical exam and ask questions about family medical history. There is no one test to diagnose Marfan syndrome. Medical tests include echocardiogram (for diagnosing heart problems) and an eye exam. Genetic testing may be done.
- Treatment will involve a team approach that involves eye, cardiac, orthopedic, and dental care. Drugs are often used to help prevent complications.
- Annual screening echocardiograms are recommended beginning in adolescence in order to detect the start of any complications. X-rays of spine are needed during growth years to detect scoliosis.
- Have annual eye exams. Special lenses and eye drops or surgery may be needed for lens dislocation.
- Surgery may be needed for cardiovascular problems.
- Scoliosis may require use of a brace or surgery.
- Surgery may be needed if chest bones are sunken in.
- Pregnant women with Marfan syndrome are managed as high-risk patients. Outcome is usually excellent.
- To learn more: National Marfan Foundation, 22 Manhasset Ave., Port Washington, NY 11050; (800) 862-7326; website: www.marfan.org.

MEDICATIONS

- Beta-blockers are often prescribed for heart problems.
- Hormone therapy may be given prior to puberty.
- Antibiotic therapy may be prescribed.

ACTIVITY

- Fully active unless limited by symptoms. Exercise helps physical and emotional well-being. Get medical advice before starting any exercise or sports activity.
- You may be advised to avoid contact sports, activities that risk head injury, rapid decompression (scuba diving), isometric exercises (weightlifting, pull-ups, etc.).

DIET

No special diet.

 ## NOTIFY OUR OFFICE IF

- You believe your child has signs or symptoms of Marfan syndrome.
- After diagnosis, symptoms change or worsen.

Special notes:

_____

_____

_____

More notes on the back of this page ☐

MASTITIS
(Breast Infection)

 BASIC INFORMATION

DESCRIPTION
Mastitis is a breast disorder that usually occurs in a woman who has recently given birth. It develops in about 1 to 2% of new mothers and is more likely in women who are breast-feeding. However, it can occur even in women who are not breast-feeding or pregnant.

FREQUENT SIGNS AND SYMPTOMS
· Symptoms may occur anytime while nursing, but usually begin 1 to 5 weeks after delivery.
· Tender or painful, swollen, hard, hot area of the breast(s).
· Redness of the breasts.
· General feeling of weakness, lack of well-being.
· Fever and chills.

CAUSES
Infection from bacteria germs that enter the mother's breast. Most mastitis occurs only on one side. It is unknown exactly why some women get mastitis and others do not. Germs may gain access to the breast through a crack in the nipple, but women without sore nipples also get mastitis.

RISK INCREASES WITH
· Major risks are breast-feeding and cracked nipples.
· Women with a very abundant milk supply may be more prone to getting mastitis.
· Women who are not breast-feeding but have diabetes, chronic illness, or weak immune system.

PREVENTIVE MEASURES
· There are no specific preventive measures.
· Wash nipples before nursing. Wash hands before touching breasts.
· Regular emptying of the breasts. Breast-feed equally from both breasts.
· If a nipple becomes sore, apply lanolin cream or other skin care products as recommended.

EXPECTED OUTCOME
Usually curable in 10 days with treatment. Symptoms will get better in 1 to 2 days.

POSSIBLE COMPLICATIONS
· Without proper treatment, or with incomplete treatment, mastitis may lead to breast abscess. This is a pus-filled infection in the breast.
· Chronic mastitis may rarely occur in women who are breast-feeding.

 DIAGNOSIS & TREATMENT

GENERAL MEASURES
· Your health care provider will do a physical exam of the breasts. Medical tests may be done to be sure that there are no other problems that may be causing symptoms.
· Treatment includes adequate breast emptying, rest, drinking plenty of fluids, and drug therapy, if needed.
· Apply a warm compress or an ice pack (whichever feels better) to the engorged breast after feeding. Don't use ice packs within 1 hour of nursing; instead use warm compresses.
· Wear a good support bra during treatment.
· Most often, you can continue to breast-feed, even though breasts are infected. Offer the affected breast first to promote complete emptying. If needed, use a breast pump to completely empty the breast.
· Take your temperature 1 to 3 times a day at first, to check for any fever.
· Massage nipples with cocoa butter or a cream, if recommended.

MEDICATION
· Pain relievers. For minor discomfort, you may use nonprescription drugs, such as acetaminophen or ibuprofen.
· Antibiotics for infection may be prescribed. Complete the entire dosage prescribed even if symptoms improve. Breast-feeding can usually be continued while taking the drug.

ACTIVITY
Get extra rest whenever you can.

DIET
No special diet. Eat regularly and drink extra fluids.

 NOTIFY OUR OFFICE IF

· You or a family member has symptoms of mastitis.
· During treatment, a fever occurs, you have nausea or vomiting, feel dizzy, or faint.
· You have signs of a breast abscess. An area with redness, pain, tenderness, and fluctuance (feels like pushing on an inflated inner tube).

Special notes:

_____

_____

_____

More notes on the back of this page ☐

MEASLES
(Red Measles; Rubeola)

BASIC INFORMATION

DESCRIPTION
A viral illness that infects the respiratory tract (lungs, throat, and nasal passages) and skin. Measles is one of the most easily spread diseases. It can occur in all ages, but usually affects children. Measles was once very common, but it is now rare in the United States due to immunization. It is still common in certain other countries in the world. Cases that occur in the United States are often in people who have become infected in other countries.

FREQUENT SIGNS AND SYMPTOMS
Measles symptoms usually occur in the following sequence:
· Fever, often high.
· Fatigue.
· Appetite loss.
· Sneezing and runny nose.
· Harsh, hacking cough.
· Red eyes and sensitivity to light.
· Tiny white spots in the mouth and throat.
· Rash on the forehead and around ears that spreads to the body.

CAUSES
Measles is caused by a virus. Germs are spread by contact with an infected person, breathing in germs in the air, or touching an object with germs on it. Symptoms first appear 7 to 14 days after exposure. An infected person can spread the germs to others 4 to 5 days prior to the start of the rash and 4 to 5 days after it starts.

RISK INCREASES WITH
· People who are not immunized.
· Areas of the world that don't offer immunizations.
· Reduced protective affect of the vaccine over time. A teenager or young adult could become infected with measles if exposed.

PREVENTIVE MEASURES
· Immunize children against measles. Prevention is important because measles can have rare, but serious, complications.
· Careful hand washing helps prevent spread of any type of germs.

EXPECTED OUTCOMES
Symptoms usually clear up after about 3 days.

POSSIBLE COMPLICATIONS
· Ear and chest infections.
· Pneumonia.
· Encephalitis or meningitis.
· Complications can be life-threatening.

DIAGNOSIS & TREATMENT

GENERAL MEASURES
· Your health care provider will do a physical exam and ask questions about your symptoms and vaccine history. Measles is usually diagnosed by the symptoms. A blood test may be done to confirm the diagnosis.
· There is no specific treatment for measles. Home care involves rest, relief of symptoms, and keeping the patient away from other persons that are not immune to measles.
· The eyes are more sensitive to light. Avoid reading books or watching TV for a few days.
· Use a cool-mist humidifier (if advised) to ease the cough and thin lung secretions so they can be coughed up more easily. Clean the humidifier daily.
· Children who are old enough can suck on throat lozenges, cough drops, or hard candy to help ease throat discomfort.
· If fever is 101°F (38.3°C) or higher, take steps to lower it, if the child is uncomfortable, unable to sleep, or vomiting. Use drug therapy as advised by your child's health care provider. A lukewarm bath or sponge bath may help cool a febrile child.

MEDICATIONS
· Use acetaminophen or ibuprofen to relieve discomfort and reduce fever. Don't give aspirin if under age 18.
· An antihistamine or calamine lotion may help relieve the itchy rash. Follow instructions on label and be sure the product is approved for the age group.

ACTIVITY
Rest may help until the fever and rash get better. Children should not return to school or daycare until 4 to 5 days after the fever and rash disappear.

DIET
No special diet. Drink extra fluids, including water, tea, lemonade, and fruit juice.

NOTIFY OUR OFFICE IF

· You or your child has symptoms of measles.
· Breathing difficulty, wheezing, chest or stomach pain, earache, or vision problems occur.

Special notes:

_____

_____

_____

More notes on the back of this page ☐

MELANOMA

BASIC INFORMATION

DESCRIPTION
A skin cancer that can occur on any skin or mucosal surface of the body. Melanoma can spread to other areas of the body, such as the lymph nodes, liver, lungs, and central nervous system. It can affect any age, usually older adults, and is rare in children. It is the most common cancer in women age 25 to 29, and second to breast cancer in women ages 30 to 34.

FREQUENT SIGNS AND SYMPTOMS
• A changing mole is the most common symptom.
• Flat or slightly raised skin lesion. It can be black, brown, blue, red, white, or a mixture of colors. Borders are often irregular. Some may bleed, itch, or cause pain.

CAUSES
Cells (melanocytes) that give skin its brownish color change into melanoma cells. It is unclear why this occurs. Melanomas may appear on normal skin or arise from a mole (nevus) or other abnormal skin area that has changed in appearance. They tend to occur at sites of sun exposure. When the cells grow down into deep skin layers, they invade blood vessels and lymph vessels and are spread to other body areas.

RISK INCREASES WITH
• Moles (more so with large numbers of moles).
• Occupations or activities involving excessive sun exposure, such as farming, athletics, or sunbathing.
• Excess sun exposure and sunburns in childhood.
• Having atypical moles (dysplastic nevi).
• Increased age.
• Genetic factors. This is most common in fair-skin, blond people. It is rare in black people.
• Weak immune system due to illness or drugs.
• Personal or family history of melanoma.
• Sunny or high altitude climates.

PREVENTIVE MEASURES
• Wear sunglasses, broad-rimmed hats, and protective clothing. Always use a sunscreen (15 SPF or higher).
• Examine your skin regularly for changes in pigmented areas (such as moles). Ask a family member to examine your back, scalp, and soles of the feet. Get medical advice about any skin lesion (especially brown or black) that becomes multicolored, develops irregular edges or surfaces, and bleeds or changes in any way.

EXPECTED OUTCOMES
Varies greatly. Early melanomas that have not spread are curable with surgical removal. Once the tumor has spread to distant organs, the prognosis is poor. However, symptoms can be relieved or controlled.

POSSIBLE COMPLICATIONS
• Cancer spreads (metastasis) to other places in the body, which can be fatal.
• Melanoma recurs. It can be the same site or new site.

DIAGNOSIS & TREATMENT

GENERAL MEASURES
• Your health care provider will do an exam of the affected skin area. Biopsy (removal of a small amount of affected skin for viewing under a microscope) aids in diagnosis. Other tests may be done to see if the cancer has spread (staging).
• Treatment varies and depends on location and size of affected area, stage of the cancer, your health, age, and preferences. Treatment may include surgery (most often), anticancer drugs (chemotherapy) and/or radiation therapy, and biologic therapy.
• Goal of surgery is to remove as much of the skin cancer as possible. Skin graft may be done if large areas of tissue are removed. Lymph nodes may also be removed.
• Chemotherapy uses drugs, and radiation therapy uses radiation to attack the cancer cells. Biologic therapy uses the body's immune system to fight cancer.
• Since there is a risk of melanoma recurring, be sure to have regular follow-up medical exams.
• To learn more: American Cancer Society, (800) ACS-2345; website: www.cancer.org or National Cancer Institute, (800) 4-CANCER; website: www.cancer.gov.

MEDICATIONS
• Anticancer (chemotherapy) drugs may be prescribed.
• Biologic therapy drugs may be prescribed.

ACTIVITY
No limits except those involving sun exposure.

DIET
No special diet.

NOTIFY OUR OFFICE IF

• You or a family member has symptoms of melanoma.
• During or after treatment, changes occur in the same or another skin area.

Special notes:

_____

_____

_____

More notes on the back of this page ☐

MENIERE'S DISEASE

BASIC INFORMATION

DESCRIPTION
A disorder of the inner ear that causes a variety of symptoms. In most cases, only one ear is involved. It usually affects adults between ages 30 and 60, and it is slightly more common in women than men. Meniere's is named for the French doctor who described it in 1861.

FREQUENT SIGNS AND SYMPTOMS
• Original symptoms often start suddenly, and recurrent attacks may come on with no warning. Attacks may occur daily, or in some persons, just once a year. Attacks may last 30 minutes to 2 hours, or longer. Symptoms may be mild to severe.
• Vertigo (feeling that you are spinning or everything around you is spinning).
• Noises in the affected ear (tinnitus), such as roaring, ringing, or buzzing.
• Hearing loss that comes and goes and often increases over time.
• Feeling pressure or pain in the affected ear.
• Nausea, vomiting, and sweating may occur with the vertigo. Stomach discomfort, headache, and diarrhea may occur also.

CAUSES
The exact cause is unknown. There is a variety of suggested causes, and research continues.

RISK INCREASES WITH
Unknown (mostly). Salty diets, exposure to excessive noise, stress, recent viral illness, allergies, immune disorders, ear infections, or genetic factors may play a role.

PREVENTIVE MEASURES
No specific preventive measures.

EXPECTED OUTCOMES
There is no cure. Attacks of Meniere's disease recur and worsen over many years. Symptoms can often be relieved with one or more types of treatment. The disorder is frustrating, but not life-threatening.

POSSIBLE COMPLICATIONS
• Permanent hearing loss.
• Chronic tinnitus.
• The symptoms can affect all aspects of a person's life.

DIAGNOSIS & TREATMENT

GENERAL MEASURES
• Your health care provider will do a physical exam and and an exam of the ear. Medical tests may include blood studies, balance studies, various hearing tests, and other tests to rule out other disorders with similar symptoms.
• Treatment usually consists of lifestyle changes (such as with your diet) and drugs, or sometimes surgery, to relieve the symptoms.
• During an attack, lie flat on a surface that does not move. Avoid bright lights. Focus eyes on an object that does not move. Don't eat or drink (to avoid nausea). Once the attack passes, get up slowly. You may feel sleepy and want to sleep for awhile.
• Learn techniques to control stress in your life. This helps some people with Meniere's.
• Avoid noisy places or situations.
• Quit smoking. Find a way to stop that works for you.
• Various treatments may be tried for the tinnitus.
• Different types of surgery may be recommended for severe symptoms or to prevent further hearing loss.
• To learn more: Ear Foundation/Meniere's Network, 1817 Patterson St., Nashville. TN 37203; (800) 545-4327; website: www.earfoundation.com.

MEDICATIONS
• Your health care provider may prescribe:
  - Antinausea drugs, to reduce nausea and vomiting.
  - Scopolamine patches, to treat nausea.
  - Tranquilizers, to reduce dizziness.
  - Antihistamines, to help lessen symptoms.
  - Diuretics, to decrease fluid in the inner ear.
  - Antibiotics placed in the middle ear.
  - Drugs, to suppress an overactive immune system.

ACTIVITY
• Don't drive, climb ladders, or work around dangerous machinery.

DIET
• Salt causes the body to retain fluid. By decreasing salt in your diet, it will help to reduce the amount of fluid in the inner ear.
• Limit the use of caffeine and alcohol.

NOTIFY OUR OFFICE IF

• You or a family member has symptoms of Meniere's disease.
• The following occur during treatment: decreased hearing in either ear, persistent vomiting, fever of 101°F (38.3°C) or higher.
• New, unexplained symptoms develop. Drugs used in treatment may produce side effects.

Special notes:

_____

_____

_____

More notes on the back of this page ☐

MENINGITIS, ASEPTIC
(Viral Meningitis)

 BASIC INFORMATION

DESCRIPTION
An infection of the thin membranes that cover the brain and the spinal cord. Aseptic means it is nonbacterial. This infection can be spread from one person to another. It is more common in group settings such as young children in daycare, football team members, college students, and people who live in group care facilities.

FREQUENT SIGNS AND SYMPTOMS
- Fever.
- Headache, sometimes severe.
- Irritability.
- Eyes become more sensitive to light.
- Stiff neck.
- Vomiting.
- Confusion, lethargy, and drowsiness.

CAUSES
- While this disorder is most often caused by a virus, other types of germs can be the cause. The most common cause is a group of viruses called enteroviruses. Less often, herpes virus, mumps virus, HIV, and other viruses may be the cause. Germs are spread by contact with an infected person, or touching an object with germs on it and then touching the mouth, nose, or eyes.
- Other causes include tuberculosis, various fungi, certain diseases, parasites, exposure to certain chemicals, and some drugs.

RISK INCREASES WITH
- Weak immune system due to illness or drugs.
- Group homes, daycare, or schools where outbreaks may occur.

PREVENTIVE MEASURES
- Keep immunizations up-to-date against viruses such as mumps, measles, and chickenpox. Currently, there is no vaccine for the enteroviruses.
- Wash hands carefully to prevent the spread of any type of germs.

EXPECTED OUTCOMES
Most patients recover fully in 5 to 14 days. In some people, symptoms such as fatigue or lightheadedness may persist longer.

POSSIBLE COMPLICATIONS
Complications are rare. They may occur in those with weak immune systems or the very young.

 DIAGNOSIS & TREATMENT

GENERAL MEASURES
- Your health care provider will do a physical exam and ask about your symptoms and activities. Medical tests may include blood studies, a stool culture, and others to confirm the diagnosis.
- No specific drugs exist to treat aseptic meningitis caused by enteroviruses. The body defenses will normally cure the disorder. Treatment involves getting extra bed rest, treating symptoms such as fever, and drinking fluids.
- If symptoms are severe, hospital care may be needed.

MEDICATIONS
- Nonprescription drugs for fever, nausea, or minor pain may be used.
- Antibiotics may be given if there is a possibility the meningitis is caused by a bacterial infection.
- Drugs may be prescribed for other causes of the meningitis once they are identified.

ACTIVITY
- Rest in bed in a darkened room. Resume your normal activities as soon as symptoms improve.
- Children should stay home from school or daycare until symptoms improve.

DIET
No special diet. Drink 6 to 8 glasses of fluid daily.

 NOTIFY OUR OFFICE IF

- You or a family member has symptoms of aseptic meningitis.
- Symptoms don't improve in a week.

Special notes:

_____

_____

_____

More notes on the back of this page ☐

314

MENINGITIS, BACTERIAL

 BASIC INFORMATION

DESCRIPTION

Bacterial infection or inflammation of the thin membranes (meninges) and fluid surrounding the brain and spinal cord. It is a life-threatening disorder, and prompt treatment is vital. It can affect all ages, but is more severe in persons under age 2 or over age 60.

FREQUENT SIGNS AND SYMPTOMS

- Fever, chills, and sweating.
- Headache.
- Irritability.
- Eyes sensitive to light; pupils may be of different sizes.
- Stiff neck.
- Vomiting.
- Red or purple skin rash (associated with one kind of bacteria).
- Confusion, lethargy, drowsiness, or unconsciousness.
- Sore throat or other signs of respiratory (nose, throat, and lungs) illness may occur before other symptoms.
- Poor feeding in infants.
- Seizures.

CAUSES

An infection usually caused by one of three types of bacteria. *Haemophilus influenzae type b* (Hib), *Neisseria meningitidis,* or *Streptococcus pneumoniae.* (Routine vaccines for children have lowered the risk of Hib infection.) Bacterial germs are spread by close contact with an infected person. The infection may start in another body part, such as the lung, ear, nose, throat, or sinus that spreads to the meninges.

RISK INCREASES WITH

- Newborns, infants, young people, and adults over 60.
- Ear, sinus, respiratory, or tooth infections.
- Weak immune system due to illness or drugs.
- Head injury.
- Close contact with a person with meningitis.
- People with cochlear implants (hearing devices).

PREVENTIVE MEASURES

- Get all the recommended vaccines for infants and adults. Other vaccines may be recommended depending on an individual's health condition.
- Vaccine against *Neisseria meningitidis* (meningococcal vaccine) may be recommended for students going to college and for travelers to certain areas of the world.
- Avoid contact with anyone who has meningitis (depending on bacterial type). If contact occurs, preventive treatment may be recommended.

EXPECTED OUTCOMES

Full recovery is likely in 2 to 3 weeks with prompt treatment and if no complications arise.

POSSIBLE COMPLICATIONS

Death or permanent brain damage including paralysis, hearing loss, speech difficulty, seizures, and mental impairment.

 DIAGNOSIS & TREATMENT

GENERAL MEASURES

- Your health care provider will do a physical exam and ask questions about the symptoms. Medical tests may include blood studies, culture of cerebrospinal fluid, x-rays, CT, and others to confirm the diagnosis.
- Hospital care is usually needed, sometimes in an intensive care unit.
- Treatment involves antibiotics, supportive care for symptoms, and steps to prevent complications.

MEDICATIONS

- Antibiotics will be give through a vein (IV).
- Steroids may be prescribed. They help prevent the risk of hearing loss.
- Anticonvulsants may be used to treat or prevent seizures.

ACTIVITY

After a 2 to 3-week period of recovery, you should be as active as your strength allows.

DIET

You may be given intravenous nutrients in the hospital. At home, eat a normal, well-balanced diet.

 NOTIFY OUR OFFICE IF

- You or a family member has symptoms of bacterial meningitis. Get emergency help if needed.
- You have had contact with someone who has meningitis.

Special notes:

_____

_____

_____

More notes on the back of this page ☐

MENOPAUSE

BASIC INFORMATION

DESCRIPTION

Menopause is the permanent cessation of menstruation. It can occur as early as age 40 or as late as early 60s. It usually spans 1 to 2 years. Menopause is only one event in the "climacteric." This is a biological change in all body tissue and body systems that occurs in both sexes between the mid-40s and mid-60s. Menopause that occurs before age 40 is termed premature. Menopause does not occur suddenly. Perimenopause usually begins a few years before the last menstrual cycle.

FREQUENT SIGNS AND SYMPTOMS

· Some women may go through menopause without having symptoms. In most women, both physical and emotional symptoms usually occur.
· Irregular menstrual periods.
· Hot flashes or flushes and night sweats. These are sensations of heat spreading from the waist or chest toward the neck, face, and upper arms. The medical term is vasomotor symptoms.
· Headaches.
· Dizziness.
· Rapid or irregular heartbeat.
· Vaginal itching, burning, or pain with intercourse.
· Bloating in the upper abdomen.
· Irritable bladder (urge to urinate).
· Tender breasts.
· Mood changes, including tension and anxiety.
· Sleeping difficulty.
· Changes in sex drive.
· Depression, feeling sad or down, and fatigue.

CAUSES

· A normal decline in ovary function. This results in decreased levels of the female hormones, estrogen and progesterone.
· Surgical removal of both ovaries.
· Medical treatment of endometriosis or cancer.

RISK INCREASES WITH

Menopause is a natural part of the aging process for women. Smoking and hysterectomy are risks for premature menopause.

PREVENTIVE MEASURES

No preventive measures needed.

EXPECTED OUTCOME

Menopause is a normal process, not an illness. Most women adapt without major problems or concerns.

POSSIBLE COMPLICATIONS

· Reduced skin elasticity and vaginal moisture.
· Higher risk of hardening of the arteries, heart disease, stroke, and osteoporosis after menopause.
· Changes in feelings of self-worth.

DIAGNOSIS & TREATMENT

GENERAL MEASURES

· Your health care provider can determine if it is menopause by your age and symptoms. It is often diagnosed in females after 1 year of no menstrual periods.
· No specific treatment is usually needed.
· Counseling may be helpful if emotional changes interfere with personal relationships or work.
· Continue to use birth-control measures until 12 months after your last menstrual period.
· Reduce stress in your life as much as possible. Acupuncture, meditation, and relaxation techniques are all helpful ways to reduce any stress of menopause.
· Women who smoke start menopause about two years earlier than nonsmokers do. If you smoke, talk to your health care provider about programs to help you quit.
· To learn more: The North American Menopause Society, P.O. Box 94527, Cleveland, OH 44101; (800) 774-5342; website: www.menopause.org.

MEDICATION

· Estrogen therapy alone or combination with progestogen are options for treating hot flashes. Hormone therapy has benefits as well as risks. The decision is made by a woman and her health care provider.
· Antidepressants may be prescribed for hot flashes.
· Herbal (or those termed natural remedies) help some women. Discuss these with your health care provider.
· Drugs to prevent and/or treat loss of bone density may be prescribed.
· Take calcium supplements and vitamin D if needed.
· For vaginal dryness, use moisturizers and non-estrogen lubricants, such as KY Jelly or Replens.

ACTIVITY

No limits. Exercise helps your well-being. Weight-bearing activities (such as walking) help bone strength.

DIET

Eat a well-balanced diet.

NOTIFY OUR OFFICE IF

· You or a family member has menopause symptoms that cause concern.
· Bleeding occurs 6 months or more after last period.

Special notes:

_____

_____

_____

More notes on the back of this page ☐

MENORRHAGIA

 ## BASIC INFORMATION

DESCRIPTION

Menorrhagia is a common disorder that involves heavy blood loss during menstruation. The average amount of blood loss during a normal menstrual period is about two ounces. With menorrhagia, a woman may lose three ounces or more. Menorrhagia is more a symptom of a disease or condition rather than a disorder in itself. It can affect any woman who has begun menstruation.

FREQUENT SIGNS AND SYMPTOMS

· Menstrual periods have been extra heavy for several months in a row.
· Menstrual periods last for more than 7 days.
· Passing of large clots of blood.
· Paleness and fatigue (anemia).

CAUSES

The menstrual cycle is a process (series of events) that occurs in a woman's body each month. Different factors can disrupt the process and lead to menorrhagia.

RISK INCREASES WITH

· Women near menopause or young women who have not established a regular menstrual cycle.
· Hormone imbalance (estrogen and progesterone).
· Infections of the genitals or urinary tract. This includes sexually transmitted diseases.
· Kidney, liver, or thyroid disease.
· Pituitary tumors, polycystic ovarian syndrome, or blood vessel problems.
· Ectopic pregnancy or a miscarriage.
· Ovarian dysfunction (ovaries do not produce eggs).
· Fibroids (benign uterine tumors).
· Endometriosis or endometrial hyperplasia.
· Cervical or uterine polyps.
· Intrauterine device (IUD).
· Bleeding disorders.
· Drugs (steroids, blood thinners and anticancer).
· Obesity or being overweight.
· Rarely, cancer of the uterus or cervix.

PREVENTIVE MEASURES

No specific preventive measures.

EXPECTED OUTCOME

Varies with cause of the bleeding. Treatment helps reduce the bleeding in most women.

POSSIBLE COMPLICATIONS

· Anemia due to excess blood loss. Menorrhagia is a common cause of anemia in premenopausal women.
· Surgery may be required.
· Sometimes, bleeding is so severe that it interrupts normal daily routines like work, school, and social life.
· Other complications are related to the causes.

 ## DIAGNOSIS & TREATMENT

GENERAL MEASURES

· Your health care provider will do a physical exam and a pelvic exam and ask about your symptoms. Medical tests may include Pap smear, pregnancy test, blood test, ultrasound, and hysteroscopy (using an instrument to see inside the uterus). Liver, kidney, and thyroid function tests, and endometrial biopsy (removal of a small amount of tissue for microscope exam) may be done.
· Treatment usually depends on the age of the woman, her desires for fertility, and any other medical disorder. Treatment steps may include drugs or surgery.
· Stop using an IUD. Use another birth control method.
· Surgery options may include endometrial ablation or endometrial resection, dilatation and curettage (D & C), uterine fibroid embolization, or hysterectomy. The options, risks, and benefits will be explained to you.
· For self-care, wear extra sanitary pads during heavy flow. If a tampon is used, change tampon every 4 to 6 hours. Avoid scented pads and tampons. Don't douche.

MEDICATION

· Use nonsteroidal anti-inflammatory drugs, such as naproxen or ibuprofen, to relieve pain and possibly reduce bleeding. Avoid aspirin (may prolong bleeding).
· One or more types of hormones to control the bleeding may be prescribed.
· If hormones cannot be taken for some reason, other drugs to control the bleeding may be recommended.
· Iron replacement may be prescribed for anemia.
· If a drug you take is the cause, a change in drug or a change in dosage amounts may be recommended.

ACTIVITY

Resting with feet up may help during heavy periods.

DIET

No special diet.

 ## NOTIFY OUR OFFICE IF

· You or a family member has signs or symptoms of menorrhagia.
· Symptoms worsen or new symptoms develop after treatment begins.

Special notes:

_____

_____

_____

More notes on the back of this page ☐

MENTAL RETARDATION

BASIC INFORMATION

DESCRIPTION
Below average, general intellectual functioning along with an inability to adapt to the normal aspects of daily life in a person under age 18. Intellectual functioning is typically measured by an intelligence quotient (IQ) test (if the person can take an IQ test). Those with mental retardation score 70 to 75 or below. The normal range is 80 to 130 (100 is average). Retardation is classified as mild (IQ 50 to 70), moderate (IQ 35 to 49), severe (20 to 34), or profound (IQ less than 20). Mild retardation is the most common form (over 80% of cases). Mildly retarded children may not be identified until they start school. Profoundly and severely retarded children are often diagnosed at birth. Males are affected more than females.

FREQUENT SIGNS AND SYMPTOMS
- Failure to meet developmental milestones. These are physical and behavioral signs of development or maturation of infants and children.
- Persistence of infantile behavior.
- Lack of curiosity.
- Decreased learning ability.
- Inability to meet educational demands of school.
- Behaviors may include: being aggressive, dependent, passive, stubborn; having low self-esteem, injures self; frustrates easily; mood disorders; attention difficulties.
- Physical traits may include: shortness in size, malformed ears and eyes, seizures, and birthmarks.

CAUSES
- Genetic—Inborn errors of metabolism or chromosome disorders. Down syndrome is the most frequent genetic disorder causing mental retardation.
- Intrauterine—Congenital infections, placental-fetal malfunction, complications of pregnancy (infections, preeclampsia, eclampsia, maternal alcohol or drug abuse or poor diet).
- Perinatal (just before the birth)—Prematurity, postmaturity, birth injury, and metabolic disorders.
- Postnatal (after birth)—Endocrine or metabolic disorders, infection, trauma, toxic, and other causes of brain damage, or abuse.

RISK INCREASES WITH
Risk factors are related to the causes.

PREVENTIVE MEASURES
- Genetic counseling and prenatal genetic testing for families with a history of mental retardation.
- During pregnancy, get good prenatal care; eat healthy; avoid smoking, alcohol, or other drugs of abuse.
- Screening of newborns for metabolic disorders.
- Protect children from injury, poisoning, or abuse.

EXPECTED OUTCOME
- Mildly retarded people can learn to lead independent, productive lives.
- Moderately retarded people are trainable. They often require protective care (such as a group home).
- More severely and profoundly retarded people usually require continuous care.

POSSIBLE COMPLICATIONS
- Emotional and behavioral problems in the child.
- Stresses placed on the family.

DIAGNOSIS & TREATMENT

GENERAL MEASURES
- Your child's health care provider will do a physical exam and certain mental tests (if the child is old enough) to help with the diagnosis. You will be asked about your own observation of signs in your child.
- Goals are to develop the child's potential to the fullest. Retardation cannot be reversed, but much can be done to help the child function as normally as possible. Beginning in infancy, special education with social and behavioral training can enhance the child's skills.
- The diagnosis has a profound effect on the family. It will affect every aspect of their lives. Counseling and/or spiritual support are both helpful for parents to learn to accept and cope. Joining a support group for families of children with mental retardation can help also.
- To learn more: The Arc of the United States, 1010 Wayne Ave., Suite 650, Silver Springs, MD 20910; (800) 433-5255; website: www.thearc.org.

MEDICATION
Drugs for medical problems such as seizures may be prescribed. In general, care of a retarded person is educational, not medical.

ACTIVITY
As fully active as child's physical condition permits.

DIET
No special diet.

NOTIFY OUR OFFICE IF

- You are concerned with your child's development.
- New symptoms occur or you feel unable to cope.

Special notes:

_____

_____

_____

More notes on the back of this page ☐

METABOLIC SYNDROME

(Insulin Resistance Syndrome; Syndrome X)

 BASIC INFORMATION

DESCRIPTION

Metabolic syndrome is not just a specific disorder. Rather it is a group (or cluster) of five health risks. Having any three of these five health risks would mean that you have the syndrome. A person with metabolic syndrome is more likely to have heart disease, stroke, and diabetes in the future. The health risks include:
- Abdominal obesity.
- Elevated fasting blood triglycerides (a type of fat).
- Low levels of HDL, or "good" cholesterol.
- High fasting blood sugar (glucose) or high insulin.
- High blood pressure.

FREQUENT SIGNS AND SYMPTOMS

Usually, there are no physical symptoms.

CAUSES

The exact cause of the syndrome is not known. It may be due to a combination of genetic makeup (that you inherit from your parents) and lifestyle choices of diet and physical activity.

RISK INCREASES WITH

Studies are ongoing to see who may be at risk for metabolic syndrome. It does occur more often in Hispanics than in whites or African Americans.

PREVENTIVE MEASURES

- Eat a healthy diet.
- Exercise routinely.
- Don't use tobacco in any form.
- Maintain a healthy body weight.

EXPECTED OUTCOMES

Lifestyle changes involving your diet, weight loss, exercise, and drugs (if needed) can usually reverse the risk factors.

POSSIBLE COMPLICATIONS

If not treated, the syndrome often leads to early heart disease, stroke, and other vascular (blood vessel) problems, as well as diabetes. The more risk factors you have, the more likely you are to have complications.

 DIAGNOSIS & TREATMENT

GENERAL MEASURES

- Your health care provider will order the medical tests and go over the results with you. Metabolic syndrome is diagnosed if you have three or more of the following:

    1. Waistline of 40 inches or more for men and 35 inches or more for women (measured across the belly).

    2. Blood pressure of 130/85 mm Hg or higher.

    3. Triglyceride level above 150 mg/dL.

    4. Fasting blood glucose (sugar) level greater than 100 mg/dL.

    5. HDL, the "good" cholesterol, less than 40 mg/dL (men) or under 50 mg/dL (women).

- You and your health care provider can decide on an action plan to reduce your risks of heart disease and stroke. This may include changes in diet, getting more exercise, weight loss, stopping smoking, and perhaps drug therapy.
- Diet and life-style changes do not mean you have to give up all the good things you enjoy. Even moderate changes can have a big impact on your risk factors.
- To learn more: American Heart Association, 7272 Greenville Ave., Dallas, TX 75231; (800) 242-8721; website: www.americanheart.org.

MEDICATIONS

- Drugs may be prescribed to lower cholesterol and lower high blood pressure.
- Weight loss drugs may be prescribed for a short time.

ACTIVITY

Increase physical activity. Try to get at least 30 minutes of aerobic exercise (such as walking) every day.

DIET

- Limit foods that contain saturated fats and high amounts of cholesterol. Read food labels carefully.
- Eat plenty of fruits/vegetables and high-fiber foods.
- Begin a weight-reduction diet if you are overweight.

 NOTIFY OUR OFFICE IF

- You or a family member wants more information about the metabolic syndrome.
- You need help with diet and exercise planning.

Special notes:

_____

_____

_____

More notes on the back of this page ☐

METATARSALGIA

 BASIC INFORMATION

DESCRIPTION
Metatarsalgia is a general term for pain under the ball of the foot. The ball is the bottom, front part of the foot behind the toes. It is a common problem that can be very painful, but is usually not serious.

FREQUENT SIGNS AND SYMPTOMS
· Pain, dull ache, or burning feeling in the ball of one or both feet.
· It hurts when walking and feels better when you rest.
· It is described as feeling like "have a stone in your shoe" or "walking on pebbles."
· Toes may be painful, or feel numb and tingly.
· Foot may be swollen.

CAUSES
There are five metatarsal bones in the foot that run from the arch to the toe joint. These bones take a lot of pressure when you walk, jump, or run. Anything that puts extra pressure on the front of the foot can cause metatarsalgia.

RISK INCREASES WITH
· High-impact sports that involve running or jumping.
· Wearing shoes that do not fit correctly, are poorly made, or are worn-out.
· For women, wearing high heels, and shoes that are too tight across the ball of the foot.
· Certain foot shapes (such as high arches) or other foot problems.
· With aging, the fat pad in the foot tends to thin out.
· Certain medical problems, such as diabetes.
· Obesity.

PREVENTIVE MEASURES
· Wear good shoes that fit well and are right for the activity.
· Start slowly with any new exercise or sports routines.
· Weight loss may help if overweight.

EXPECTED OUTCOMES
· Treatment can often relieve symptoms in 10 to 14 days depending on what the cause is.
· In some cases, recovery may depend on treatment of any other medical disorder.

POSSIBLE COMPLICATIONS
Without treatment, the foot joint may be less flexible and grow stiff. Pain may increase.

 DIAGNOSIS & TREATMENT

GENERAL MEASURES
· Rest with your feet elevated (raised up) after periods of standing or walking.
· Rub an ice pack over the painful area for about 15 minutes at a time, several times a day.
· Switch to heat after a day or two if it feels better. Use a heating pad or soak your feet in warm water.
· Do simple stretches while seated:
  - Place heels on floor, swing toes in and then out.
  - Lift one leg straight and flex ankle by pointing toes up and then toward the floor; repeat with other leg.
· Wear adhesive felt, gel, or foam padding around toe area. Cushioned insoles, metatarsal pads, or arch supports may help. These can be found at most drug stores.
· Wear shoes that fit well and have plenty of toe room.
· Consult your health care provider if self-treatment does not help to improve the symptoms. Your health care provider will examine the foot, and ask questions about symptoms, your activities, and the that shoes you wear. An x-ray may be taken to make sure there is no bone fracture.
· Special shoes, or special shoe inserts (called orthotics), may be prescribed.
· Surgery may help if there is a problem such as bunions, hammertoes, or a pinched nerve.

MEDICATIONS
For minor pain, you may use nonprescription pain drugs, such as ibuprofen.

ACTIVITY
· Limit activities until the symptoms improve.
· Try swimming or bicycling instead of running or walking while you have the symptoms.

DIET
No special diet.

 NOTIFY OUR OFFICE IF

· You or a family member has metatarsalgia symptoms that have lasted several days or are very painful.
· Pain or discomfort gets worse despite treatment.

Special notes:

_____

_____

_____

More notes on the back of this page ☐

MISCARRIAGE
(Spontaneous Abortion)

BASIC INFORMATION

DESCRIPTION

Loss of a pregnancy prior to the 20th week is generally considered a miscarriage. It happens in about 20% to 30% of first pregnancies. It may occur so early that the woman is unaware that she is pregnant. Many miscarriages are only "threatened." The pregnancy continues to term.

FREQUENT SIGNS AND SYMPTOMS

- Uterine cramps.
- Vaginal bleeding (from slight to heavy).

CAUSES

There are many reasons a pregnancy ends in miscarriage. Most miscarriages occur because a pregnancy is not developing normally. Sometimes, no cause is found. Work, exercise, and having sex do not increase the risk.

RISK INCREASES WITH

The first trimester (first 12 weeks of pregnancy):
- Genetic defect (chromosomal disorder such as Down syndrome) or structural abnormalities of the fetus.
- Uterine abnormalities that prevent the fertilized egg from growing normally.
- Smoking.

The second trimester (13 to 28 weeks of pregnancy):
- Uterine abnormalities that cause detachment of the fetus and placenta.
- Severe stress (physical or emotional).

Anytime:
- Use of substance that harms fetus (cocaine, tobacco).
- Infections, such as viral infections.
- Trauma or severe medical conditions.
- Having certain chronic disorders.

PREVENTIVE MEASURES

- Cannot always be prevented. To reduce risk factors:
  - Obtain regular medical checkups.
  - Eat a normal, well-balanced diet.
  - Avoid alcohol, smoking, or substances of abuse.
  - Don't use nonprescription drugs or herbal products without medical advice.

EXPECTED OUTCOME

- With treatment, a miscarriage is not life-threatening. It usually does not affect a woman's ability to carry a healthy baby to term in the future.
- Feelings of loss and grief are common. Feelings of guilt may also be present.

POSSIBLE COMPLICATIONS

- Uterine infection (fever, chills, and aching).
- Hemorrhaging (bleeding) from other body parts.
- "Incomplete" abortion, in which some placenta or fetal tissue remains in the uterus, or missed abortion, in which the fetus dies but remains in the uterus.

DIAGNOSIS & TREATMENT

GENERAL MEASURES

- Ultrasound exam may be needed for diagnosis. If a fetal heartbeat can be seen, this means that there is a good chance that the pregnancy will proceed normally. When the ultrasound scan shows certain problems or abnormalities with the fetus, then nothing can be done to save the pregnancy.
- For a threatened miscarriage, follow your obstetric provider's orders. Bed rest at home may help stabilize the pregnancy. Bleeding may be severe, requiring hospital care and blood transfusion.
- Following a miscarriage:
  - Expect a small amount of vaginal bleeding or spotting for 8 to 10 days. Avoid tampons for 2 to 4 weeks.
  - Wait through 2 or 3 normal menstrual cycles (or as advised) before attempting to become pregnant again.
- Surgery may be done to remove any remaining tissue or a dead fetus. D & C (dilatation and curettage), or D & E (dilatation and evacuation) may be needed.
- Counseling for patient and partner may be helpful.

MEDICATION

- Oxytocin to control bleeding may be given.
- Pain relievers may be prescribed.
- Antibiotics may be prescribed for an infection.
- An Rh-negative female may be given RhoD (immune globulin).

ACTIVITY

- For a threatened miscarriage: Rest in bed until symptoms disappear. Avoid sexual intercourse.
- After a miscarriage: Reduce activity and rest often during the next 48 hours.

DIET

- For a threatened miscarriage: Drink fluids only, if bleeding and cramping are severe.
- After a miscarriage: No special diet.

NOTIFY OUR OFFICE IF

- You or a family member has vaginal bleeding during pregnancy.
- Bleeding and cramps worsen or you pass tissue or fever and chills occur.

Special notes:

_____

_____

_____

More notes on the back of this page ☐

MITRAL VALVE PROLAPSE

 BASIC INFORMATION

DESCRIPTION

A disorder in which a slight deformity of the mitral valve can produce a degree of leakage of blood. The mitral valve is located in the left side of the heart. Mitral valve prolapse (MVP) causes a heart "click" or murmur that may be heard through a stethoscope (an instrument used for listening to body sounds). In the past, more women than men were diagnosed. Recent studies show that it may affect men and women equally.

FREQUENT SIGNS AND SYMPTOMS

· Often no symptoms are present (about 60% of cases) and the condition may be discovered on a routine physical exam. When symptoms do occur, they may vary from a few that are mild to having many symptoms. The symptoms are sometimes referred to as mitral valve prolapse syndrome (MVPS).
· Chest pain (sharp, dull, or pressing).
· Fatigue, shortness of breath.
· Dizziness.
· Lightheadedness when getting up from a chair or bed.
· Heart palpitations.
· Anxiety and panic attacks.
· Migraines.

CAUSES

The mitral valve is one of four heart valves that keep blood flowing in one direction. Prolapse means that openings (called leaflets) in the valve don't close as firmly as they should. This allows a small amount of blood to leak and cause the murmur. Why MVP occurs is unknown. The condition may be inherited or due to another disease.

RISK INCREASES WITH

· Family history of heart valve disorders.
· Connective tissue disorders (e.g., systemic lupus erythematosus, Marfan syndrome, and others).
· Other heart conditions and some muscle disorders.

PREVENTIVE MEASURES

None known.

EXPECTED OUTCOMES

MVP is usually a benign disorder that needs no treatment and does not prevent a normal active life. Complications are rare.

POSSIBLE COMPLICATIONS

· Excess blood may leak backward through the mitral valve (called mitral regurgitation).
· Endocarditis (inflammation of the heart valves and heart lining).
· Stroke.
· Sudden death.

 DIAGNOSIS & TREATMENT

GENERAL MEASURES

· Your health care provider may do a physical exam and listen to the sounds of the heart. Medical tests may include an echocardiogram (heart function test) to confirm the diagnosis.
· Treatment is usually not needed. A medical follow-up may be done every few years to check for proper heart function.
· In some cases where there is more leakage, drugs and lifestyle changes may be recommended for treatment.
· Surgery for valve replacement may be recommended in a few cases.
· If other symptoms such as fatigue, anxiety, or panic attacks occur, your health care provider can discuss treatment options.

MEDICATIONS

· Antibiotics may be recommended for some patients prior to any dental work or certain types of surgery.
· Other drugs may be prescribed depending on specific symptoms or to prevent complications.

ACTIVITY

· Daily aerobic exercise is helpful for most patients.
· Athletes with MVP who have many symptoms may be restricted from some types of sports.

DIET

· Weight-loss diet is suggested for overweight patients.
· Cutting out caffeine and alcohol may be helpful.

 NOTIFY OUR OFFICE IF

· You or a family member has signs or symptoms of mitral valve prolapse.
· Symptoms worsen or new symptoms occur after diagnosis.

Special notes:

_____

_____

_____

More notes on the back of this page ☐

322

MOLLUSCUM CONTAGIOSUM

 ## BASIC INFORMATION

DESCRIPTION

A contagious, viral infection of the skin. It usually occurs on the face in children. In adults, it usually occurs on the inner thighs, abdomen, or genitals.

FREQUENT SIGNS AND SYMPTOMS

- Small, raised bumps on the skin.
- Bumps are firm, smooth, domed with a central pit, and skin-colored or white. The skin over the bumps is transparent and thin.
- Bumps cause eye irritation if they are on the eyelids.
- They don't hurt or itch.

CAUSES

A virus of the pox group. The germs are spread by person-to-person contact. This virus may be spread sexually. The time period from being exposed to having symptoms is usually 2 to 7 weeks. It may also be spread by touching objects that have the germs on them, such as shared clothing, towels, wash cloths, and sports equipment.

RISK INCREASES WITH

- Other allergies or a family history of allergy.
- Use of drugs that cause a weak immune system.
- Outbreaks have been reported among children using swimming pools.

PREVENTIVE MEASURES

- To prevent spread to other parts of the body or to other people, don't scratch bumps.
- Practice good personal hygiene.
- Avoid sexual contact with infected people. It is unclear if condoms are effective in preventing spread.

EXPECTED OUTCOME

Outcome is good. They heal on their own without treatment in otherwise healthy people. It will take about 10 to 24 months. Treatment helps to prevent their spread to other persons and to speed up the healing time.

POSSIBLE COMPLICATIONS

- Some scarring can occur.
- The bumps can become irritated, inflamed, and infected by bacteria.
- The problem may recur.

 ## DIAGNOSIS & TREATMENT

GENERAL MEASURES

- The health care provider can diagnose the disorder by a skin exam of the affected area. If needed, the diagnosis can be confirmed with a skin scraping and microscopic study.
- Treatment is not always needed. In some cases, drugs may be recommended for treatment.
- Bumps may be removed with surgery. Options include cutting, burning electrically or chemically, or by freezing.

MEDICATION

- Painless, medicated drops may be applied by your health care provider.
- Other drugs may be prescribed that you can apply to the bumps yourself.

ACTIVITY

No limits, except to avoid sexual relations until the bumps disappear.

DIET

No special diet.

 ## NOTIFY OUR OFFICE IF

- You or a family member has symptoms of molluscum contagiosum.
- A reinfection occurs after treatment.
- New unexplained symptoms develop. Drugs used in treatment may produce side effects.

Special notes:

_____

_____

_____

More notes on the back of this page ☐

MONONUCLEOSIS, INFECTIOUS

 BASIC INFORMATION

DESCRIPTION
An infectious viral disease that affects the lungs, liver and lymphatic system. It usually affects children and young adults (from 12 to 40 years of age).

FREQUENT SIGNS AND SYMPTOMS
- Fever.
- Sore throat (sometimes severe).
- Appetite loss.
- Fatigue.
- Swollen lymph glands, usually in the neck, underarms, or groin.
- Enlarged spleen.
- Enlarged liver.
- Jaundice with yellow skin and eyes (sometimes).
- Headache.
- General aching.

CAUSES
A contagious virus (Epstein-Barr virus). It is passed from person to person by close contact, such as kissing, shared food or coughing.

RISK INCREASES WITH
- Stress.
- Recent illness.
- Fatigue or overwork. The high rate among college students and military recruits may result from too little rest and crowded living conditions.
- High school or college students.

PREVENTIVE MEASURES
Avoid close contact with persons having infectious mononucleosis.

EXPECTED OUTCOMES
It usually clears up on its own in 10 days to 6 months. Fatigue usually lasts for 3 to 6 weeks after other symptoms get better. A few patients have a chronic form in which symptoms last for months or years.

POSSIBLE COMPLICATIONS
- Ruptured spleen, resulting in emergency surgery.
- Anemia.
- In rare cases, the heart, lungs, or central nervous system could become involved. The disease can prove serious, even fatal.

 DIAGNOSIS & TREATMENT

GENERAL MEASURES
- Your health care provider will do a physical exam and ask questions about your symptoms. Medical tests may include blood studies.

- No specific cure or treatment is available. Extra rest and healthy diet are important. There is no need to keep away from other people. Do avoid close contact so the germs aren't spread.
- To relieve the sore throat, gargle frequently with warm or cold double-strength tea or warm salt water (mix one-half teaspoon of salt in one cup of water).
- Don't strain hard for bowel movements. This may injure an enlarged spleen.

MEDICATIONS
- For minor pain, you may use nonprescription drugs such as acetaminophen. Don't use aspirin in children under age 18.
- If symptoms are severe, you may be prescribed a short course of cortisone drugs.

ACTIVITY
- Rest in bed while you have fever. Resume activity gradually. Rest when you are tired.
- Don't join in contact sports until at least 1 month after complete recovery.

DIET
No special diet. You may not feel like eating while you are ill. Eat soft foods or drink milk shakes. Drink at least 8 glasses of fluids a day (or more) during periods of fever.

 NOTIFY OUR OFFICE IF

- You or a family member has symptoms of infectious mononucleosis.
- The following occur during treatment:
  - Fever over 102°F (38.9°C).
  - Constipation, which may cause straining.
  - Severe pain in the upper left abdomen (rupture of the spleen is a medical emergency!).
  - Yellowing of the skin.
  - Difficulty swallowing or breathing due to severe sore throat.

Special notes:

_____

_____

_____

More notes on the back of this page ☐

MOTION SICKNESS

 BASIC INFORMATION

DESCRIPTION
An unpleasant, temporary disorder that often occurs while traveling. The semicircular canals in the inner ear are affected. These fluid-filled canals normally maintain a person's sense of balance.

FREQUENT SIGNS AND SYMPTOMS
- Loss of appetite, nausea, and vomiting.
- Spinning sensation.
- Weakness and being unsteady.
- Confusion; anxiety; sweating.
- Paleness.
- Yawning.

CAUSES
Motion that may be from a plane, boat, car; amusement park ride, or swinging. The body, the inner ear, and the eyes send conflicting messages to the brain. The ears may sense motion that the eyes can not see, or the eyes may see movement that the body does not feel. People who suffer from motion sickness may have the symptoms just thinking about movement (such as when sitting on a plane waiting for take-off).

RISK INCREASES WITH
- Travel.
- Ear disorders such as with allergies or infections.
- Smoky environment or poor ventilation.
- Drinking too much alcohol.
- Visual stimuli (moving horizon).

PREVENTIVE MEASURES
- Avoid large meals and alcohol before and during trips.
- Sit in areas of the airplane (usually over the wings) or boat with the least motion.
- Recline in your seat, if possible.
- Breathe slowly and deeply. Don't read.
- Avoid areas where others are smoking, if possible.
- In a car, airplane, or bus, turn on the air vent to improve air movement.
- Take drugs to prevent motion sickness before a trip.
- There are behavior-modification techniques for those who are afraid to fly or have motion sickness. Contact the airline or your travel agent for information.
- Mental and emotional factors can add to motion sickness. Try to resolve concerns about travel before leaving home. Maintain a positive attitude.
- Consider preventive therapy. One technique involves special training for using your eyes that may help avoid the symptoms of motion sickness.

EXPECTED OUTCOMES
Recovery once the trip is over or soon thereafter.

POSSIBLE COMPLICATIONS
No serious complications are expected.

 DIAGNOSIS & TREATMENT

GENERAL MEASURES
- Self-care is usually all that is needed. If your symptoms persist or cause concern, see your health care provider. A physical exam may be done and medical tests may be recommended to rule out other disorders.
- Once you have the symptoms, try to rest in a dark room with a cool cloth over the eyes and forehead.
- Allowing yourself to vomit can help the nausea. However, don't make yourself vomit.
- Acupressure may help. This is done by placing pressure on a point three finger-widths above the wrist on the inner arm. Elastic wristband products can be purchased to put pressure on this area.
- A battery-operated wristband product is available that will apply a mild, electrical pulse to the area. It can be used for prevention and treatment.
- Counseling may help if your work or lifestyle requires travel and you suffer from motion sickness.

MEDICATIONS
- For minor discomfort, you may use nonprescription drugs, such as dimenhydrinate (Dramamine), or meclizine (Bonine) before and during travel. These can cause drowsiness.
- A scopolamine patch to control symptoms may be prescribed.
- Other drugs may be prescribed if simple treatment methods are not effective.

ACTIVITY
Limited only by the symptoms.

DIET
- Eat lightly or not at all before and during brief trips. For longer trips, sip frequently on beverages (tea and juices) to maintain your fluid intake. Avoid alcohol, carbonated drinks, and extra-cold beverages.
- Ginger helps some people. Take it on an empty stomach. It is available in a tea, capsules, or candied pieces.

 NOTIFY OUR OFFICE IF

You or a family member plans to travel and has had disabling motion sickness in the past.

Special notes:

_____

_____

_____

More notes on the back of this page ☐

MOUTH OR TONGUE TUMOR, BENIGN

 BASIC INFORMATION

DESCRIPTION

Abnormal new growth in the mouth or tongue that is unlikely to spread to other body parts. Benign mouth and tongue tumors usually occur alone and grow very slowly over a period of 2 to 6 years. They can involve the lips, gums, roof or floor of the mouth, or tongue.

FREQUENT SIGNS AND SYMPTOMS

· A lump in any part of the mouth or tongue.
· It may become sore and bleed.
· It may interfere with the way dentures fit.
· It may interfere with speech or swallowing.

CAUSES

Unknown. It is most common in people who smoke cigarettes, cigars, or pipes, or use chewing tobacco or snuff. Benign tumors do not spread to other areas.

RISK INCREASES WITH

· Use of tobacco.
· Dentures that fit poorly.

PREVENTIVE MEASURES

· Don't smoke or use tobacco products.
· See your dentist for annual dental exams and for problems with denture fit.

EXPECTED OUTCOMES

Curable with surgical removal. They are not likely to recur.

POSSIBLE COMPLICATIONS

· Bleeding from the tumor.
· Infection in the tumor.

 DIAGNOSIS & TREATMENT

GENERAL MEASURES

· Your health care provider will do a physical exam of the affected area. A biopsy may be done to confirm the diagnosis. A biopsy involves the removal of a small amount of skin tissue to be viewed under a microscope.
· Surgery to remove the tumor may be recommended.
· After surgery, cleanse the mouth 3 to 4 times a day with a soothing salt water solution (mix one-half teaspoon of salt in one cup of warm water).

MEDICATIONS

· For minor discomfort, you may use nonprescription drugs such as acetaminophen or ibuprofen.
· Antibiotics will be prescribed if infection exists.

ACTIVITY

No limits.

DIET

No special diet after recovery. A liquid diet may be necessary for a day or two after surgery.

 NOTIFY OUR OFFICE IF

· You or a family member has symptoms of a mouth or tongue tumor.
· The following occur after surgical treatment:
  - Fever.
  - Bleeding at the surgical site.
  - Pain.

Special notes:

_____

_____

_____

More notes on the back of this page ☐

MULTIPLE MYELOMA
(Plasma Cell Myeloma)

BASIC INFORMATION

DESCRIPTION
Cancer of the plasma cells of the bone marrow. Plasma cells normally help the body destroy germs and protect against infection. The cancer is called multiple because it usually occurs in many bones in the body. It can affect the bone marrow of all bones but is most common in the thigh, back, pelvis, or upper arms. This type of cancer occurs more often in men between ages 50 and 70.

FREQUENT SIGNS AND SYMPTOMS
• Pain in the affected bone. The pain is severe, boring, and deep. If the bone collapses, pain spreads to other parts of the body.
• Weight loss.
• Symptoms of anemia, such as weakness, paleness, tiredness, and breathlessness.

CAUSES
Unknown. The bone pain is caused by the cancerous plasma cells. The anemia is caused by damaged red blood cells and decreased platelets.

RISK INCREASES WITH
• Family history of myeloma.
• Older adults.
• Other plasma cell disease.
• Exposure to certain chemicals and high radiation doses may be risk factors.

PREVENTIVE MEASURES
No specific preventive measures.

EXPECTED OUTCOMES
Treatment can help with the symptoms and improve quality of life, but rarely produces a cure. Some patients live up to 5 years after symptoms appear. Temporary remissions may occur with treatment. Research into causes and treatment continues, so there is hope for more effective treatment and cure.

POSSIBLE COMPLICATIONS
• Recurrent infections.
• Kidney failure.
• Spontaneous bleeding.
• Bone fractures.
• Paralysis.

DIAGNOSIS & TREATMENT

GENERAL MEASURES
• Your health care provider will do a physical exam and ask questions about your symptoms and activities. Different medical tests are done to verify the diagnosis and to determine if the cancer has spread to other places in the body (called staging).

• Treatment will depend on the stage of the disease, your health, age, and preferences. Your health care provider will discuss the options and their risks and benefits. All treatments have numerous side effects.
• Watchful waiting is usually recommended if there are no symptoms. This means monitoring the cancer cells for a period of time before deciding on treatment.
• Treatment may involve radiation, chemotherapy, surgery (for complications), biologic therapy (using body's immune system), stem cell transplantation, and plasmapheresis (using patient's blood for therapy).
• Treatment may involve steps to relieve symptoms and make you comfortable, rather than treating the cancer.
• Counseling may help you cope with having cancer.
• To learn more: International Myeloma Foundation, 12650 Riverside Dr., Suite 206, North Hollywood, CA 91607; (800) 452-2873; website: www.myeloma.org or American Cancer Society, (800) ACS-2345; website: www.cancer.org.

MEDICATIONS
• Your health care provider may prescribe:
  - Anticancer and cortisone drugs (chemotherapy).
  - Pain relievers.
  - Antibiotics for infections.
  - Blood transfusions, if anemia becomes severe.
  - Drugs to treat hypercalcemia (too much calcium).

ACTIVITY
Stay as active as pain or bone complications allow.

DIET
No special diet.

NOTIFY OUR OFFICE IF

• You or a family member has symptoms of multiple myeloma.
• The following occur during treatment: fever, any sign of infection, swelling of the feet and ankles, urination problems, or unexplained bleeding.
• New, unexplained symptoms develop. Drugs used in treatment may produce side effects.

Special notes:

_____

_____

_____

More notes on the back of this page ☐

MULTIPLE SCLEROSIS

 BASIC INFORMATION

DESCRIPTION

A chronic disorder that affects the central nervous system (brain, spinal cord, and optic nerve). Multiple sclerosis (MS) more often affects adults 20 to 50, and women twice as often as men. MS types include:
- Relapsing-remitting. Most common. Patients have flare ups followed by partial or complete recovery.
- Primary-progressive. Slow and continued worsening of symptoms. May be temporary minor improvements.
- Secondary-progressive. This type follows the relapsing-remitting type. Symptoms steadily worsen.
- Progressive-relapsing. Symptoms steadily worsen from the start. Has flare ups, with or without recovery.

FREQUENT SIGNS AND SYMPTOMS
- Signs and symptoms may be mild, moderate, or severe. They vary from person to person and at times in the same person.
- Fatigue (called MS lassitude)
- Problems with walking. Lack of coordination.
- Bowel and bladder problems.
- Vision problems or hearing problems (less often).
- Vague loss of sensation or numbness and tingling.
- Mood swings and depression.
- Sexual problems.
- Difficulty with memory, concentration, attention, and problem solving.
- Speech or swallowing problems (sometimes).

CAUSES
Unknown. It is believed to be an autoimmune disorder. In these disorders, the immune system attacks the body itself by mistake and in different ways. Genetic and environmental (such as a virus) factors may contribute.

RISK INCREASES WITH
- Females more than males.
- People of Northern European descent.
- Family history of MS.
- Growing up in a cold climate (compared to tropical).

PREVENTIVE MEASURES
Cannot be prevented at present.

EXPECTED OUTCOMES
Multiple sclerosis is incurable. The course of the disorder will be different for each person. Some will be favorable and others unfavorable. Symptoms can often be relieved or controlled.

POSSIBLE COMPLICATIONS
Numerous complications can occur. They often result from problems such as immobility, chronic urinary-tract infections, difficulty with swallowing and breathing, and mental and emotional disorders.

 DIAGNOSIS & TREATMENT

GENERAL MEASURES
- Your health care provider will do a physical exam and ask questions about your symptoms, activities, and medical history. No specific test is available to diagnose MS. Medical tests may include blood, urine, and spinal fluid studies. An MRI scan of the brain and spinal cord will usually show typical changes that indicate MS. Often, a specialist called a neurologist is needed to make the diagnosis.
- Treatment may include one or more drugs to treat symptoms, prevent complications, or slow progression of the disorder. Physical therapy may be recommended. Plasma exchange (a blood treatment) may be of help.
- Multiple sclerosis will affect every aspect of your life. You will need to educate yourself about your specific symptoms and what to expect and how to adjust to the disease. The more you can learn, the better able you will be to cope with the changes in your life.
- Counseling may be helpful for you and your family.
- Joining a support group is a way to share feelings.
- To learn more: National Multiple Sclerosis Society, 733 Third Ave., New York, NY 10017, (800) 344-4867; website: www.nationalmssociety.org.

MEDICATIONS
- Drugs called disease-modifying agents are often prescribed. The options will be discussed with you.
- Cortisone drugs may be prescribed for inflammation.
- Drugs for symptoms will be prescribed as needed.

ACTIVITY
Get enough rest. Exercise to the extent possible. It helps physical and emotional well-being. It keeps muscles limber and strong, and helps balance and coordination.

DIET
Eat a healthy diet that is high in fiber to prevent constipation.

 NOTIFY OUR OFFICE IF

- You or a family member has symptoms of multiple sclerosis.
- After diagnosis, any symptoms cause you concern.

Special notes:

_____

_____

_____

More notes on the back of this page ☐

MUMPS

BASIC INFORMATION

DESCRIPTION

A mild, contagious viral disease that causes painful swelling of the glands located between the ear and jaw. These are the parotid salivary glands. Mumps can affect all ages, but is more common in children (2 to 12 years). Mumps infections are now rare because of the routine vaccines given to infants. About 10% of adults are susceptible to mumps.

FREQUENT SIGNS AND SYMPTOMS

Mumps without complications:
· Inflammation, swelling, tenderness, or pain of the glands. The glands feel firm, and discomfort increases with chewing or swallowing.
· Fever.
· Headache.
· Sore throat.

Mumps symptoms with complications:
· Painful, swollen testicles.
· Abdominal pain.
· Severe headache, if the brain or meninges (lining of the brain) are involved.

CAUSES

Person-to-person transmission of the mumps virus (*paramyxovirus*). The virus can be passed anytime from 48 hours before symptoms begin to 6 days after symptoms appear. Virus incubation is 14 to 24 days after contact; the average is 18 days.

RISK INCREASES WITH

· Epidemics in nonvaccinated area.
· Lack of immunization.

PREVENTIVE MEASURES

· Obtain routine mumps vaccines for infants.
· If you have not had mumps or been vaccinated, and a close family member has mumps, seek advice from your health care provider.

EXPECTED OUTCOMES

Recovery in about 10-12 days. After having it once, a person almost always has lifetime immunity to mumps.

POSSIBLE COMPLICATIONS

· Complications are rare, and if they occur are usually in persons over age 19. Complications can involve the testicles, thyroid, brain, spinal cord, prostate, pancreas, and the breasts. Testicle involvement may rarely lead to infertility in males.
· Mumps in the first trimester of pregnancy may lead to miscarriage.
· Hearing loss in children.

DIAGNOSIS & TREATMENT

GENERAL MEASURES

· Your health care provider can usually diagnose mumps by the signs and symptoms. Blood studies may be done to confirm the diagnosis.
· You do not need to keep the infected person away from the family. By the time symptoms appear, the disease has usually already spread.
· Apply heat or ice, whichever feels better, to the swollen, painful glands. Use a hot-water bottle, hot towel, or ice-pack.
· Stay out of school, daycare, or work until no longer contagious (about 9 days after symptoms begin).

MEDICATIONS

· Once the infection begins, it must run its natural course. There is no safe or effective drug that can treat mumps.
· For minor pain, you may use nonprescription drugs such as acetaminophen or ibuprofen.
· If testicles are involved, stronger pain relievers and other drugs may be prescribed.

ACTIVITY

Allow as much activity as strength and feeling of well-being allow. Patients are no longer contagious when swelling disappears.

DIET

Soft food diet is helpful if chewing causes pain. Increase daily fluid intake to at least 6 to 8 glasses of liquid a day.

NOTIFY OUR OFFICE IF

· You or a family member has symptoms of mumps.
· Fever rises above 101°F (38.3°C).
· The following occur during the illness:
  - Vomiting or abdominal pain.
  - Severe headache.
  - Drowsiness or inability to stay awake.
  - Swelling or pain in the testicles.
  - Twitching of the face muscles.
  - Convulsion.
  - Discomfort or redness in the eyes.

Special notes:

_____

_____

_____

More notes on the back of this page ☐

MUSCULAR DYSTROPHY

 BASIC INFORMATION

DESCRIPTION

A group of inherited disorders that cause muscle weakness and wasting (decrease in size). There are nine major types of muscular dystrophy (and some subtypes within those types). Duchenne is one of the most common types. The disorders are usually diagnosed in children (most often boys), and less often in teens or adults.

FREQUENT SIGNS AND SYMPTOMS

Early symptoms:
- Weakness.
- Duck-like gait. Lack of coordination.
- Falling, with difficulty getting up.
- Muscles appear larger and stronger but are weaker than normal.

Later symptoms:
- Muscle loss severe enough to require use of a wheelchair by age 9 to 12.
- Severe distortion of the body.
- Recurrent respiratory infections.

CAUSES

Inherited. Muscular dystrophy is a genetic abnormality. It can be carried by a female who does not have symptoms, but passes it on to male children. In other cases, it may be passed on by one or both parents. In still other cases, there is no family history.

RISK INCREASES WITH

Family history of muscular dystrophy.

PREVENTIVE MEASURES

- If you have a family history of muscular dystrophy:
  - Obtain genetic counseling before starting a family.
  - If pregnant, consider testing to determine whether the fetus is male and the disorder is present.
  - Carriers can be detected with medical tests because their blood contains high levels of a certain enzyme.

EXPECTED OUTCOMES

Outcome varies depending on the type of muscular dystrophy. Some types are more mild, progress slowly, and patients may have a normal lifespan. Other types progress more rapidly, lead to disability and a shortened lifespan. Research is ongoing for causes, prevention, effective treatments, and possible cures.

POSSIBLE COMPLICATIONS

- Muscle weakness that leads to wheelchair use.
- Fractures or injuries from falls.
- Spinal curvature caused by weak spine muscles.
- Pneumonia.
- Heart problems.
- Muscle shortening and tightening (contractures).

 DIAGNOSIS & TREATMENT

GENERAL MEASURES

- Your child's health care provider will do a physical exam and ask questions about the symptoms. Medical tests may include blood studies and muscle biopsy. A biopsy involves removal of a small amount of tissue for viewing under a microscope. A electromyogram (measures electrical impulses in muscles) and nerve conduction study may be done.
- There is no cure for muscular dystrophy. Treatment can help improve the symptoms and help prevent complications. A child will need to be assisted in many ways to make the most of his abilities and keep his independence to the extent possible.
- Your child will need a health care team. This may include physical, occupational, speech, and respiratory therapists as well as routine medical care. Illnesses are more common and need to be watched for and treated.
- Surgery may be needed to release tight, painful muscles. If heart problems develop, a pacemaker may be surgically implanted to help the heart beat normally.
- Counseling can help parents cope with the diagnosis. It can help children if emotional problems develop.
- Support groups are a good place to share problems.
- To learn more: Muscular Dystrophy Association, 3300 E. Sunrise Drive, Tucson, AZ 85718; (800) 572-1717; website: www.mdausa.org.

MEDICATIONS

Drugs may be prescribed to slow muscle loss, improve lung function, treat heart problems, for constipation, to treat infections, or for other complications.

ACTIVITY

The patient should be as physically and mentally active as possible. Many devices can help overcome handicaps caused by weakness. Braces may help.

DIET

Eat a well-balanced diet. Being overweight should be avoided (it adds more burden to already weak muscles).

 NOTIFY OUR OFFICE IF

- Your child develops symptoms of muscular dystrophy.
- After diagnosis, symptoms develop that cause concern.

Special notes:

_____

_____

_____

More notes on the back of this page ☐

MYASTHENIA GRAVIS

 BASIC INFORMATION

DESCRIPTION

A disorder of the muscles that causes muscle weakness of varying degrees. It often involves the muscles around the eyes, mouth, and throat, and the arms and legs. It can affect the breathing muscles also. Myasthenia gravis more often affects young adults and is more common in females.

FREQUENT SIGNS AND SYMPTOMS

- Drooping eyelids.
- Double vision.
- Loss of normal facial expression.
- Swallowing difficulty.
- Weakness of the arms and legs.
- Difficulty speaking clearly.
- Breathing difficulty.
- Most flare-ups appear after a brief period of normal muscle function and worsen as the muscle is used.

CAUSES

- One of a group of autoimmune disorders. In these disorders, the immune system attacks the body itself by mistake. With myasthenia gravis, there is a miscommunication between the nerves and the muscles.
- Tumor of the thymus (newborns only).

RISK INCREASES WITH

- Family history of myasthenia gravis.
- Newborns and infants of mothers with myasthenia gravis. They show symptoms in 2 to 3 weeks.

PREVENTIVE MEASURES

Cannot be prevented at present.

EXPECTED OUTCOMES

Symptoms may get worse and then improve for a period of time. Symptoms can be helped with treatment. Patients usually live many years with the disease. Research into causes and treatment continues, so there is hope for effective treatment and cure.

POSSIBLE COMPLICATIONS

- Choking from swallowing difficulty.
- Increased breathing difficulties.
- Pneumonia.

 DIAGNOSIS & TREATMENT

GENERAL MEASURES

- Your health care provider will do a physical exam and ask questions about your symptoms and activities. Medical tests may include studies of blood antibodies, electrical tests on muscle, and x-rays of the chest.
- Treatment will help control symptoms. It may involve extra rest, drug therapy, surgery, or plasmapheresis.
- Surgical removal (thymectomy) of the thymus gland may be recommended. It can improve symptoms in some patients, and even cure the disease in others.
- Plasmapheresis involves removal of blood from the patient, treating the blood, and reinjecting it.
- Acute flare-ups (myasthenia crises) may require emergency hospital care for breathing problems.
- Avoid exposure to infections and try to avoid stress.
- To learn more: Myasthenia Gravis Foundation, 1821 University Ave., W., Suite S256, St. Paul, MN 55104; (800) 541-5454; website: www.myasthenia.org.

MEDICATIONS

- Anticholinesterase drugs to help improve muscle function are usually prescribed.
- Immunosuppressive drugs may be prescribed at times when symptoms worsen.
- Intravenous immune globulin (IVIG) may be used for some patients to suppress the immune system.

ACTIVITY

- Plan activities to make the most of energy peaks. Frequent rest periods are important. Day-to-day changes in symptoms are common.
- Avoid strenuous activities and too much exposure to the sun or to cold weather.

DIET

Eat foods high in potassium. These include oranges, tomatoes, bananas, broccoli, and apricots. Soft diet may be helpful if chewing and swallowing are difficult.

 NOTIFY OUR OFFICE IF

- You or a family member has symptoms of myasthenia gravis.
- You develop swallowing or breathing difficulty.

Special notes:

_____

_____

_____

More notes on the back of this page ☐

MYOCARDITIS

 BASIC INFORMATION

DESCRIPTION

Inflammation of the heart muscle (myocardium). It can lead to poor heart function. Myocarditis usually occurs as a complication of another illness. It can affect any age, but often affects middle-aged men.

FREQUENT SIGNS AND SYMPTOMS

· No symptoms or symptoms may be mild and vague.
· Fatigue.
· Shortness of breath with physical activity.
· Irregular heartbeat.
· Fever.
· Chest pain or discomfort.
· Muscle aches.
· If myocarditis causes congestive heart failure, the following symptoms may also occur:
  - Swollen feet and ankles.
  - Distended (sticking out) neck veins.
  - Rapid heartbeat, even when at rest.
  - Breathing difficulty while resting or lying down.

CAUSES

The inflammation can result from numerous medical conditions. A viral infection is the most common cause.

RISK INCREASES WITH

· Viral infection, such as Coxsackie, adenovirus, measles, influenza, herpes simplex, hepatitis, varicella, HIV, or others.
· Bacterial infections, such as tetanus, gonorrhea, typhoid fever, tuberculosis, or diphtheria.
· Immune system disorders (lupus, arthritis, others).
· Parasitic infections.
· Radiation therapy.
· Certain drugs.
· Pregnancy.
· Rheumatic fever.
· Exposure to certain toxins or chemicals.

PREVENTIVE MEASURES

No specific preventive measures. Avoid risk factors where possible.

EXPECTED OUTCOMES

Mild cases caused by a virus usually clear up on their own in about 2 weeks. Mild cases from other causes are usually treated successfully. In more severe cases, the outcome will depend on the underlying cause, patient's health status, and treatment.

POSSIBLE COMPLICATIONS

· Congestive heart failure.
· Pulmonary edema (fluid in the lungs).
· Heart rhythm problems.
· Inflammation of muscles (myositis).
· Sudden death due to abnormal heart rhythm.

 DIAGNOSIS & TREATMENT

GENERAL MEASURES

· Your health care provider will do a physical exam. Medical tests may include blood studies, chest x-ray, and heart function tests. A biopsy may be done. This involves removal of a small amount of tissue for viewing under a microscope.
· There is no specific treatment for myocarditis. Treatment usually involves rest, treating symptoms, and drugs for a diagnosed infection. Hospital care may be needed for more severe symptoms.

MEDICATIONS

· Your health care provider may prescribe:
  - Antibiotics for a bacterial infection.
  - Steroid drugs to reduce inflammation.
  - Diuretics to reduce fluid build up.
  - Digitalis to stimulate a stronger heartbeat.
  - Anticoagulants to prevent clot formation.
  - Pain remedies.
  - Drugs to reduce the heart's workload.

ACTIVITY

· Rest in bed until symptoms improve. Recovery time varies, depending on the underlying cause.
· After recovery, resume normal activities gradually.

DIET

A low-salt diet may be recommended.

 NOTIFY OUR OFFICE IF

· You or a family member has symptoms of myocarditis.
· Symptoms get worse or don't improve with time or treatment.
· New, unexplained symptoms develop. Drugs used in treatment may produce side effects.

Special notes:

_____

_____

_____

More notes on the back of this page ☐

NARCOLEPSY

 BASIC INFORMATION

DESCRIPTION

A disorder of sleep that affects the control of sleep and wakefulness. Types of symptoms and their severity vary among different people who have the disorder. It usually begins in the teen years or young adulthood. Both young children and the elderly can also be affected. Often, it goes undiagnosed for years.

FREQUENT SIGNS AND SYMPTOMS

- Excessive daytime sleepiness (hypersomnia).
- Uncontrollable sleep attacks that may occur up to 10 times a day. They may last from 30 seconds up to 30 minutes or more. An attack leaves the person feeling refreshed, but another may occur again quickly. Attacks occur while driving, talking, working, or at social events.
- Hallucinations (seeing things that aren't there) when first going to sleep or waking up. This is called hypnagogic or hypnopompic.
- A short period of paralysis (sudden loss of muscle strength) when falling asleep or just before awakening.
- A few seconds of paralysis not related to sleep when feeling sudden emotion, such as anger, fear, or joy. This is called cataplexy.
- Nighttime sleep is disturbed by leg jerks, tossing and turning, nightmares, and frequent awakenings.

CAUSES

It is a neurologic (nervous system) disorder. The exact cause is being researched. A problem with certain brain chemicals that tell the body when to sleep and wake up appears to be a cause. There is also a genetic link.

RISK INCREASES WITH

- A family history of narcolepsy.
- Genetic factors.

PREVENTIVE MEASURES

No known preventive measures.

EXPECTED OUTCOMES

The disorder appears to be life-long. There is no cure. Drugs and lifestyle changes can help improve the symptoms. Most people with the disorder can lead a near-normal lifestyle.

POSSIBLE COMPLICATIONS

- Accidental injury during a sudden sleep attack.
- The disorder may affect all aspects of one's life. This includes work, social life, personal relationships, and emotional health.

 DIAGNOSIS & TREATMENT

GENERAL MEASURES

- Your health care provider will do a physical exam and ask about your symptoms and activities. You may be asked to keep a 2-week diary about your sleep patterns. An overnight study in a sleep clinic may be done.
- Treatment usually involves lifestyle changes along with drugs to help control the drowsiness. It may take several weeks or months to achieve the best results.
- Schedule a regular time for going to bed and getting up. Stick to the schedule. Get at least 8 hours of sleep.
- Take regular naps 2 to 3 times during the day. One 15-minute nap after lunch and another at around 5:30 PM may help symptoms.
- Don't do shift work.
- Avoid over-stimulating activities, if possible.
- Wear a medical alert type bracelet or pendant to indicate you suffer from this disorder.
- To learn more: Narcolepsy Network, 10921 Reed Hartman Hwy., Ste. 119, Cincinnati, OH 45242; (513) 891-3522 not toll-free; website: www.narcolepsynetwork.org.

MEDICATIONS

- Stimulants that increase levels of daytime alertness may be prescribed.
- Modafinil (Provigil) for narcolepsy symptoms may be prescribed.
- Antidepressants or sodium oxybate (Xyrem) for cataplexy or other symptoms may be prescribed.
- New drugs for this disorder are being studied.

ACTIVITY

- Don't engage in any activity that carries the risk of injury from a sudden sleep attack. These include activities such as driving long distances, climbing ladders, or working around dangerous machinery.
- Exercise regularly, but not within 3 hours of bedtime.

DIET

No special diet. Avoid alcohol and caffeine.

 NOTIFY OUR OFFICE IF

- You or a family member has symptoms of narcolepsy.
- New, unexplained symptoms develop. Drugs used in treatment may produce side effects.

Special notes:

_____

_____

_____

More notes on the back of this page ☐

NASAL POLYPS

Information From Your Health Care Provider

 BASIC INFORMATION

DESCRIPTION
A nasal polyp is a benign (noncancerous), soft tissue growth that develops inside the nose. Polyps look like small grapes and can grow alone, but usually occur in clusters. They often affect both sides of the nose. Nasal polyps are more common in adults than in children.

FREQUENT SIGNS AND SYMPTOMS
- Obstruction of air through the nose (chronic "stuffy-nose" feeling).
- Sense of smell is reduced.
- Nasal discharge.
- Sneezing.
- Facial pain or headaches.
- Feeling of fullness in the face.
- Itchy eyes.
- Large polyps may cause the nose to be deformed.

CAUSES
Chronic inflammation of the lining of the nose and sinuses. Inflammation is normally a reaction to injury, infection, or irritation. Why it occurs in the nose and sinuses and causes polyps is not clearly understood.

RISK INCREASES WITH
- Chronic sinus, nasal, or lung disorders. This can include asthma, allergic rhinitis, cystic fibrosis, sinusitis, fungal infections, and others.
- Aspirin sensitivity. This is not a true allergy, but it may cause allergy-like reactions (such as hives, swelling, and asthma). People with this sensitivity need to avoid aspirin and other nonsteroidal anti-inflammatory drugs.

PREVENTIVE MEASURES
No specific preventive measures. Getting treatment for allergies, infections, or other nose and sinus problems may help reduce the risk factors.

EXPECTED OUTCOMES
Treatment with drugs or surgery can help improve the symptoms.

POSSIBLE COMPLICATIONS
- Polyps may recur after surgery.
- Recurrent or chronic sinusitis.

 DIAGNOSIS & TREATMENT

GENERAL MEASURES
- Your health care provider will do an exam of the nasal passages. Medical tests may include a CT or endoscopy (small, lighted telescopic instrument) to see inside the nose. Allergy testing may be done in some cases.
- Treatment may involve drugs to temporarily shrink the polyps and help relieve the symptoms.
- Try to avoid any substances that you know you are allergic to, such as dust mites, pollen, mold, etc.
- Surgery is often done to remove polyps. The type of surgery will depend on the location, size, and the number of polyps involved. Your health care provider will discuss the options, the risks, and benefits with you.

MEDICATIONS
- For minor pain, you may use acetaminophen.
- Nonprescription antihistamines may help relieve symptoms, but they do not treat the polyps.
- Corticosteroid drugs in oral form may be prescribed for a short period to attempt to shrink the polyps.
- Corticosteroid drugs in nasal spray may be prescribed for treatment of smaller polyps. They are also prescribed following surgery to help prevent recurrence of polyps.
- Antibiotics or antifungal drugs may be prescribed for treatment of infection.

ACTIVITY
No limits.

DIET
If you have food allergies, be sure to avoid those foods.

 NOTIFY OUR OFFICE IF

- You or a family member has symptoms of nasal polyps.
- Any new symptoms develop or other symptoms get worse after treatment is started.

Special notes:

_____

_____

_____

More notes on the back of this page ☐

Copyright © 2005 by Elsevier.
All rights reserved.

NASAL SEPTUM, DEVIATED

 BASIC INFORMATION

DESCRIPTION

The septum is the structure that divides the nose into two parts. In some people it is significantly off-center, or deviated. This can result in the obstruction of normal airflow through the nasal passages. The septum is made up of cartilage (toward the tip) and bone (closer to the forehead). Ideally, the septum should divide the right and left side of the nose into two equal parts. It is estimated that 80% of all nasal septa are slightly off-center. These are usually not noticed and do not normally cause any problems.

FREQUENT SIGNS AND SYMPTOMS
- An apparently crooked nose.
- Obstruction of air through one or both nostrils.
- Nasal congestion or discharge.
- Nosebleeds, headaches, or facial pain may occur.
- Sinus infections.
- Often, there are no symptoms.

CAUSES
Trauma to the nose, or it may be congenital (being born with a deviated septum).

RISK INCREASES WITH
None known.

PREVENTIVE MEASURES
Protect yourself from nose injury. Wear protective headgear for contact sports or cycling. Buckle your auto seat belt.

EXPECTED OUTCOMES
Usually treatable with surgery. If symptoms are not troublesome, surgery is usually not needed.

POSSIBLE COMPLICATIONS
- Recurrent nosebleeds.
- Recurrent nasal or sinus infections.

 DIAGNOSIS & TREATMENT

GENERAL MEASURES
- Your health care provider can usually diagnose the problem by an exam of the nose. The exam involves the use of a bright light and nasal speculum (an instrument that spreads the nostril open). Medical tests may be done to confirm the diagnosis.
- No treatment may be needed if there are no symptoms or if symptoms are mild.
- Surgery to correct the deviation may be recommended if the deviated septum is causing symptoms such as sinus infections or nosebleeds. Your health care provider will discuss the options with you. Surgery may involve:
  - Submucosal removal, which relieves obstruction.
  - Rhinoplasty, which corrects anatomical deformity.
  - Septoplasty, which relieves nasal obstruction and improves appearance.

MEDICATIONS
- For minor discomfort, you may use nonprescription drugs, such as decongestants, to decrease nasal secretions.
- Antibiotics to fight infection may be prescribed.
- Caution: Avoid over-the-counter nasal sprays.

ACTIVITY
No limits, unless surgery is needed. If so, resume your normal activities gradually.

DIET
No special diet.

 NOTIFY OUR OFFICE IF

- You or a family member has symptoms of a deviated nasal septum, especially recurrent nosebleeds, or nasal and sinus infections.
- New symptoms develop after surgery.

Special notes:

_____

_____

_____

More notes on the back of this page ☐

NAUSEA & VOMITING IN PREGNANCY
(Morning Sickness During Pregnancy)

 ## BASIC INFORMATION

DESCRIPTION
50% to 80% of pregnant women suffer from nausea and vomiting in pregnancy. The symptoms often occur in the morning (from 6 to 9 a.m.), but they may occur at any time during the day.

FREQUENT SIGNS AND SYMPTOMS
· Mild to severe nausea with or without vomiting.
· It usually occurs during the first 12 to 14 weeks of pregnancy.
· It may continue longer, and for some women, last throughout pregnancy.
· By the end of the third month, most women stop having most of the symptoms.

CAUSES
Exact causes of nausea and vomiting during pregnancy are unknown. Nausea may result from changes in the body or hormonal changes that take place for normal growth of the baby.

RISK INCREASES WITH
Being pregnant with more than one baby.

PREVENTIVE MEASURES
Do not let your stomach get empty; eat something every 2 hours if needed.

EXPECTED OUTCOME
Morning sickness usually stops after the first 3 to 4 months of pregnancy. Your baby's well-being is not affected as long as you're able to keep food down, eat a well-balanced diet, and drink plenty of fluids.

POSSIBLE COMPLICATIONS
Hyperemesis gravidarum. This is a rare condition of pregnancy that involves severe nausea, vomiting, and weight loss.

 ## DIAGNOSIS & TREATMENT

GENERAL MEASURES
· Usually self diagnosis and self-care are all that are needed. Talk to your obstetric provider if the symptoms are a concern.
· Try to identify any odors or foods that are most upsetting, and avoid them. Many pregnant women figure out what they can and cannot eat, and how many times they need to eat during the day.
· Keep rooms well aired out to rid your home of cooking smells or other odors.
· Don't smoke. Ask your family and friends not to smoke while you are suffering from morning sickness.
· Try to keep a positive attitude. If you have problems that you cannot resolve, ask for help from family, friends, or counselors.

· Keep a daily record of your weight.
· Try acupressure bands. You can find these soft cotton wristbands at drugstores.
· Consider getting a device that regularly stimulates the underside of your wrist with a mild electric current. The devices are safe and they seem to work well for some women. One or more of these devices allow you to adjust the amount of stimulation (e.g., ReliefBand Device).
· Acupuncture may be a helpful option for some women.

MEDICATION
· Drugs are not usually prescribed for this disorder. If the symptoms are severe, your obstetric provider may prescribe certain drugs for the nausea.
· Nonprescription remedies (oral drugs or rectal suppositories) may ease the problem. Don't take or use any of these products without medical advice.
· A trial of vitamin B6 may be recommended, which appears safe at the present.
· If taking your pregnancy vitamin pill causes nausea, ask your obstetric provider about stopping it for a period of time.

ACTIVITY
No limits. Resting in a dark and quiet room provides some relief for most patients.

DIET
· The following may help lessen the nausea:
 - At night, place a small, quick-energy snack, such as soda crackers, at your bedside. Eat it before getting up.
 - Eat a small snack at bedtime and when you get up to go to the bathroom during the night.
 - Eat a snack every hour or two during the day. Avoid large meals.
 - Drink ginger ale or ginger tea.

 ## NOTIFY OUR OFFICE IF

· You have morning sickness that does not improve, despite the self-help measures.
· You vomit blood or material that resembles coffee grounds.
· Abdominal pain, cramping, or fever occurs.
· You lose more than 1 or 2 pounds.

Special notes:

_____

_____

_____

More notes on the back of this page ☐

NEPHROTIC SYNDROME

(Nephrosis)

 BASIC INFORMATION

DESCRIPTION

A condition that results from damage to tiny blood vessels in the kidneys called glomeruli. Normally, the glomeruli filter the waste and excess water from blood and into urine. When they are damaged, they do not filter properly. This causes substances (proteins) in the blood and urine to become imbalanced. Fluid then builds up in the body, instead of being passed into the urine and out of the body. Nephrotic syndrome affects all age groups, and males more than females. In children, it is more common from ages 2 to 6.

FREQUENT SIGNS AND SYMPTOMS

- Fluid retention (edema). At first, it causes puffy eyes and ankles, which followed by general puffiness of the skin, and then, a swollen abdomen.
- Weight gain due to fluid retention.
- Reduced urine output (as low as 20% of normal).
- Appetite loss, weakness, and general ill feeling.
- Frothy (foamy) urine.

CAUSES

The cause of the kidney damage is often unknown. It may be due to numerous underlying disorders. In children, it is usually due to minimal change disease.

RISK INCREASES WITH

- Disorders that affect kidney function. These include diabetes, lupus erythematosus, cancers, glomerulonephritis, autoimmune disorders, serum sickness and other severe allergic disorders, blood clot in the kidney, numerous types of infections, sickle cell anemia, congenital heart disease, severe high blood pressure, other disorders, and drugs that are toxic to the kidneys.
- Weak immune system due to illness or drugs.
- Family history of renal failure.
- Exposure to some chemical toxins.

PREVENTIVE MEASURES

- Obtain medical treatment for any risk factors listed.
- Drugs may be prescribed to help prevent nephrotic disorder in persons at risk.

EXPECTED OUTCOMES

The outcome will depend on the underlying cause diagnosed. If it is treatable, such as an infection, the outcome is often good. In children with minimal disease, almost all patients respond to treatment. In other cases, the outcome may be less favorable and kidney failure and other complications may occur.

POSSIBLE COMPLICATIONS

- Infections, kidney failure, heart or lung disorders.
- Nutrients the body needs may be lost in urine and cause bone problems, brittle hair and nails, hair loss, and stunted growth in children.

 DIAGNOSIS & TREATMENT

GENERAL MEASURES

- Your health care provider will do a physical exam and ask about your symptoms and activities. Medical tests may include urine and blood studies. A kidney biopsy may be done to diagnose any kidney disorder. A biopsy involves removal of a small amount of kidney tissue or fluid for viewing under a microscope.
- Treatment will be prescribed for any underlying disorder diagnosed. This may improve the symptoms of nephrotic syndrome. Treatment is usually with drugs and sometimes, diet changes (if needed).
- To learn more: National Kidney Foundation, 30 E. 33rd St., Suite 1100, New York, NY 10016; (800) 622-9010; website: www.kidney.org.

MEDICATIONS

- Your health care provider may prescribe:
  - Cortisone or immunosuppressive drugs.
  - Diuretics to reduce fluid retention.
  - Drugs to treat infections.
  - Angiotensin-converting enzyme (ACE) inhibitors to reduce protein loss.
  - Drugs for high blood pressure or high cholesterol.
  - Anticoagulants for blood clots.
  - Stopping the use of any drug that is the cause.

ACTIVITY

After the swelling decreases, be as active as your strength and health condition allows.

DIET

You will be advised about any limits on fat, salt, protein, and fluid intake, depending on your individual case.

 NOTIFY OUR OFFICE IF

- You or a family member has symptoms of nephrotic syndrome.
- After diagnosis, any of the following occur:
  - Signs of infection, such as fever, headache, sores on the skin, cough, or burning during urination.
  - Failure to pass at least 1 quart of urine in a 24-hour period.
  - Fluid retention, vomiting, diarrhea, or nausea.

Special notes:

_____

_____

_____

More notes on the back of this page ☐

NEVI, DYSPLASTIC

BASIC INFORMATION

DESCRIPTION

Nevi is another word for moles. Dysplastic nevi are moles that are atypical. This means they do not have the appearance of common moles, and that they are a risk for melanoma. Melanoma is a serious type of skin cancer. A large number of dysplastic nevi increase the melanoma risk. The melanoma risk is even higher for a person with dysplastic nevi along with a family history of melanoma. This is called familial atypical mole/melanoma (FAMM). It is also known as dysplastic nevus syndrome.

FREQUENT SIGNS AND SYMPTOMS

Dysplastic nevi may have the following appearance:
- Borders are irregular and ill defined.
- Have both flat and elevated areas.
- Are larger than common moles.
- Color may range from tan to dark brown or have other various shades of color within them.
- They can appear anywhere on the body, but most often are found on the back, chest, buttocks, breast, and scalp. They are found in sun-exposed as well as sun-protected areas.
- A person may have one (nevus), or a few, or more than 100 dysplastic nevi. (An average person with common moles has 15 to 20.)

CAUSES

Dysplastic nevi are acquired. A person is not born with them. The exact cause is unknown. Sunlight damage may play a part, but is not always a factor. Dysplastic nevi can appear on the buttocks and female breasts, which are generally covered. The tendency to develop dysplastic nevi does run in families.

RISK INCREASES WITH

Family history of dysplastic nevi or melanoma.

PREVENTIVE MEASURES

- There are no specific preventive measures.
- Routine use of sunscreens may help reduce risks. Use one with an SPF of 15 or higher and that protects against both ultraviolet A and ultraviolet B radiation.
- If you have a family history of dysplastic nevi or skin cancer, get regular medical skin exams to detect any new moles or changes in existing ones. Exams may be as often as every 3 months for high-risk persons.
- Perform routine skin self-exams to check for any changes in skin appearance. Have a family member help check the areas of your body that you cannot see.

EXPECTED OUTCOMES

Prompt diagnosis and treatment, if needed, can help reduce the risk of melanoma.

POSSIBLE COMPLICATIONS

Melanoma.

DIAGNOSIS & TREATMENT

GENERAL MEASURES

- Your health care provider will do a physical exam of the skin. A biopsy may be done of a nevus (single mole) if skin cancer is suspected. Biopsy involves removing all or a portion of a nevus for viewing under a microscope. If the biopsy shows cancer, the whole nevus is removed.
- Other dysplastic nevi may be removed or watched over time to see if they change. Most dysplastic nevi will not develop into melanoma; removing all of them is unnecessary. If the nevi look like melanoma, have changed over time, or are new and look abnormal, then removal may be the recommended treatment.
- In some cases, nevi may be removed because of bleeding, irritation, or they are a cosmetic concern.
- Removal usually involves excision (cutting out) of the nevi. The procedure is done in a medical office while the patients is under a local anesthetic. Sometimes stitches are required. A small scar may remain. If there are numerous nevi to be removed, it may be done over several office visits. Plastic surgery may be needed if the skin area involved is extensive.
- Color photographs may be taken of your body, so that on future office visits any changes can be verified.

MEDICATIONS

No drugs are needed for this disorder.

ACTIVITY

Be sure to use sunscreens and protective clothing for any exposure to the sun. Avoid sun exposure between 10 a.m. and 3 p.m., if possible.

DIET

No special diet.

NOTIFY OUR OFFICE IF

- You or a family member has nevi (moles) that have changed in appearance or new ones developed and cause concern.
- New nevi appear after treatment.

Special notes:

_____

_____

_____

More notes on the back of this page ☐

NOSE FRACTURE

 BASIC INFORMATION

DESCRIPTION
Fracture or damage to the bones and cartilage of the nose. This often happens when other facial bones are also fractured. The injury may be to the front or the side of the nose. Males are more often affected than females.

FREQUENT SIGNS AND SYMPTOMS
- Pain in the nose.
- Nosebleed.
- Swollen, discolored nose.
- Bruising around the eyes.
- Difficulty in breathing through the nose.
- Crooked or misshapen nose (sometimes).

CAUSES
Injury or trauma to the nose. This is usually from a motor vehicle accident, being hit on the nose, running into a hard object, or from a fall.

RISK INCREASES WITH
Previous nose injury.

PREVENTIVE MEASURES
- Wear protective headgear for contact sports or when riding motorcycles or bicycles.
- Use seat belts in motor vehicles.

EXPECTED OUTCOMES
Minor fractures with no deformity usually heal on their own. Major fractures can be repaired with treatment. Most of the swelling will be gone in 10 to 20 days, but some swelling may last for months. The nose may feel tender for about a month.

POSSIBLE COMPLICATIONS
- Infection of the nose and sinuses.
- Persistent breathing difficulty.
- Permanent change in appearance.
- Deviated nasal septum. This occurs when the structure that divides the nose in half is off-center.
- Septal hematoma. Blood becomes trapped in the septum. This can lead to complications if it is not drained.

 DIAGNOSIS & TREATMENT

GENERAL MEASURES
- First aid steps: Have the person sit down and lean forward to keep blood from going down the back of the throat. Have them breathe through the mouth. Apply cold compresses or an ice pack to the nose to reduce swelling. Do not try to move displaced bones in an attempt to straighten the nose. If a nosebleed is heavy or cannot be stopped, seek emergency medical care to get it under control.
- Your health care provider will do a physical exam of the face and nose. X-rays may or may not be needed depending on the type of injury.
- A minor nose fracture with no displacement may not require further medical treatment. It will heal on its own. Rest at home. Apply ice several times a day until the swelling is gone. Use two pillows when lying down to keep the head above the heart. This helps with pain.
- Treatment may involve reduction (correction) of the fracture. This can be done right after the injury, before any swelling occurs. It can also be done days later, when the swelling is gone. A local or general anesthetic is used.
- The reduction may be done by manipulating the nose into place with finger pressure. It may require the use of two probes inserted into the nose to move the bones back into place. More severe fractures may require surgery. An incision (cut) is made on the front of the nose. The bones are put back together with special tools. Wires, plates, or screws may be used to hold the bones in place. A splint may be needed.
- Plastic surgery can be done at a later date if there is a problem with the cosmetic appearance of the nose.

MEDICATIONS
- For minor discomfort, you may use nonprescription drugs such as acetaminophen.
- Stronger pain relievers may be prescribed.
- Antibiotics may be prescribed to prevent or treat an infection.
- Decongestants may be prescribed, to reduce swelling.

ACTIVITY
- Rest until any bleeding stops.
- Most activities can be resumed right away.
- You can usually return to non-contact sports in two weeks, and contact sports in three weeks. Protective gear may need to be worn. Follow any medical advice.

DIET
No special diet.

 NOTIFY OUR OFFICE IF

- You or a family member has symptoms of a fractured nose.
- New symptoms develop after treatment.

Special notes:

_____

_____

_____

More notes on the back of this page ☐

NOSEBLEED

(Epistaxis)

 BASIC INFORMATION

DESCRIPTION

Sudden bleeding from one or both nostrils. The bleeding involves blood vessels (arteries and veins) in the nose. Nosebleeds may occur close to the nose opening or deeper in the nose. They can affect all ages, but are twice as common in children as in adults.

FREQUENT SIGNS AND SYMPTOMS

- Blood oozing from the nostril. If the broken vessel is close to the nostril, the blood is bright red. If the broken vessel is deeper in the nose, the blood may be bright or dark red.
- Lightheadedness from a large amount of blood loss (rare).
- Rapid heartbeat, shortness of breath, and pallor (with significant blood loss only).
- Black stool from swallowed blood.

CAUSES

Injury to the nose, breathing dry air, allergies, illnesses, or for no apparent reason.

RISK INCREASES WITH

- Injury to the nose.
- Nasal or sinus infection.
- A foreign body in the nose.
- Dry mucous membranes in the nose from any cause, such as low humidity.
- Bleeding tendencies associated with some illnesses.
- Allergic rhinitis (hay fever) or nonallergic rhinitis.
- Use of certain drugs, such as anticoagulants, aspirin, or prolonged use of nose drops.
- Exposure to irritating chemicals.
- Excess alcohol use.
- High altitude or dry climate.

PREVENTIVE MEASURES

- Avoid injury if possible.
- Get medical treatment for sinus or allergy problems.
- Humidify the air if you live in a dry climate or at high altitude.
- Avoid picking at nose or vigorous nose blowing.
- Avoid aspirin if you have frequent nosebleeds.

EXPECTED OUTCOMES

Most nosebleeds are harmless, even though it seems like a lot of blood is lost. They are usually controlled with self-care by applying pressure to the nose.

POSSIBLE COMPLICATIONS

Bleeding may rarely be severe and require medical care.

 DIAGNOSIS & TREATMENT

GENERAL MEASURES

Self-care:
- Sit up with your head bent forward.
- Clamp your nose closed with your fingers for 5 uninterrupted minutes. During this time, breathe through your mouth.
- If bleeding stops and recurs, repeat, but pinch your nose firmly on both sides for 8 to 10 minutes. Holding your nose tightly closed allows the blood to clot and seal the damaged blood vessels.
- You may apply cold compresses or an ice pack at the same time you are applying pressure.
- Don't blow your nose for 12 hours after bleeding stops to avoid dislodging the blood clot.
- Don't swallow blood. It may upset your stomach or make you "gag," causing you to inhale blood.
- Don't talk (also to avoid gagging).

Medical care:
- Seek emergency treatment if self-care is not successful. Gauze packing may be inserted to absorb blood, stop the dripping, and exert pressure on the ruptured blood vessels. Continued or recurrent bleeding may require cauterization (use of heat to seal off blood vessels).
- Surgery (for severe bleeding only) to tie off the artery feeding the bleeding area.

MEDICATIONS

Drugs are not needed for a nosebleed. They may be prescribed to treat an underlying disorder.

ACTIVITY

Resume your normal activities as soon as symptoms improve.

DIET

No special diet.

 NOTIFY OUR OFFICE IF

- You or a family member has a nosebleed that won't stop with self-care steps.
- After the nosebleed, you become nauseous or vomit, or your temperature rises to 101°F (38.3°C) or higher.

Special notes:

_____

_____

_____

More notes on the back of this page ☐

OBESITY & OVERWEIGHT

BASIC INFORMATION

DESCRIPTION

Obesity is defined as having an unhealthy amount of body fat. *Overweight* is defined as an excess amount of body weight as compared to an acceptable weight. The common tool to measure obesity and overweight is the body mass index (BMI). It measures body weight in relation to height. Note: A BMI may indicate a person is overweight, but it could be due to lean muscle and not excess body fat (such as with an athlete).

FREQUENT SIGNS AND SYMPTOMS

- Low energy levels.
- Breathing/snoring problems, sleep apnea.
- Appearance of large body size.
- Fatigue and joint pain from supporting excess weight.

CAUSES

Obesity and overweight occur when a person consumes more calories then he or she burns. Other risk factors can affect this imbalance in different people.

RISK INCREASES WITH

- Genetic factors. Obesity runs in families.
- Emotional feelings. Some people eat when they are depressed, upset, angry, sad, or bored.
- Eating disorder, such as binge eating.
- Metabolic and endocrine disorders.
- Drugs (steroids, some antidepressants, and others).
- Rarely, neurologic disorders.

PREVENTIVE MEASURES

- Proper diet and nutrition. Regular exercise.
- Behavior and lifestyle changes, as needed.

EXPECTED OUTCOME

Obesity and overweight can be controlled if motivation is maintained for life.

POSSIBLE COMPLICATIONS

- High risk for many major physical health problems that can lead to disability and death.
- Emotional problems. These can include depression, and feeling unattractive, rejected and shameful.
- Prejudice or discrimination at work, school, social occasions, and travel.

DIAGNOSIS & TREATMENT

GENERAL MEASURES

- The body mass index (BMI) formula uses height and weight to measure weight status.
    - Adult BMI of 25 to 29.9 = overweight.
    - Adult BMI of 30 or more = obese.
    - BMI formula: *(weight, in pounds, times 703) divided by (height in inches squared)*. Website to calculate BMI: www.cdc.gov/nccdphp/dnpa/bmi/bmi-adult.htm.

- Waist size (circumference) measures abdominal fat. Over 40 inches (102 cm) in men and over 35 inches (88 cm) in women indicates health and obesity risk factors.
- Treatment steps depend on health status, age, degree of obesity or overweight, and motivation. Steps can include a combination of diet, exercise, behavior modification, and drugs. Gastrointestinal surgery may be recommended with severe obesity.
- You and your health care provider can develop a weight-loss plan based on your individual needs. Keep a food and activity diary to keep track of your progress.
- Books, websites, and weight-loss programs are available to help with weight-loss. Diet plans should provide proper nutrition, information on exercise and behavior changes, and maintaining the weight-loss long-term.
- Behavior changes start with identifying the behaviors that lead a person to overeat and be inactive. Then learn how to change and maintain the new behaviors. Support groups or a weight-loss counselor can help.
- Gastric surgery to reduce weight may be recommended after other weight loss methods fail.
- To learn more: Weight Control Information Network, 1 Win Way, Bethesda, MD 20892-3665; (877) 946-4627; website: www.niddk.nih.gov/health/nutrit/nutrit.htm.

MEDICATION

Drug therapy as an aid to weight loss is usually not helpful. Drugs for obesity may be prescribed on a trial basis to see if they help. Amphetamine compounds are not recommended for treating obesity.

ACTIVITY

Increase physical activity. Start with a daily 10 minute walk. Aim for 20 to 30 minutes of activity 3 to 5 times a week, plus muscle strengthening 2 times a week.

DIET

- Choose an eating plan that will work for you. Diets need to be healthy, help you lose weight, and maintain the new weight. A dietitian can help you choose a plan.
- A realistic weight-loss rate is 1 pound per week. It is normal to have periods when no weight is lost on your plan. Don't stop; weight loss will begin again.

NOTIFY OUR OFFICE IF

You or a family member wants help with weight loss.

Special notes:

_____

_____

_____

More notes on the back of this page ☐

OBSESSIVE-COMPULSIVE DISORDER

 BASIC INFORMATION

DESCRIPTION

A disorder that involves recurrent, intrusive, and unwanted thoughts (obsessions), and repetitive, ritualistic behaviors (compulsions). People with obsessive-compulsive disorder (OCD) realize that their behavior is excessive, disruptive, and unreasonable, but are unable to change it or explain it. It causes significant distress or impairment and can consume most of a person's time. It may begin gradually in childhood or early adult life.

FREQUENT SIGNS AND SYMPTOMS

- Obsessions that recur. Trying to ignore or resist them is unsuccessful. Obsessions can include:
  - Fears of infection (from germs, dirt, etc.) and fear of serious illness.
  - Doubts (Is the door shut/locked? Is the iron on?).
  - Excessive orderliness or symmetry.
  - Fear that one's actions hurt other people or cause bad thing to happen.
  - Inappropriate sexual and aggressive thoughts.
- Compulsions are repetitive, purposeful behaviors to try to suppress the anxiety caused by obsessions. Compulsions include:
  - Asking for assurances.
  - Avoiding places or actions.
  - Doubts and checking (ovens, locks, doors, lights).
  - Excessive washing (hands or bathing).
  - Hoarding possessions.
  - Repeating behaviors such as dressing rituals.
  - Counting/cleaning/ordering/arranging.

CAUSES

The cause is unknown. It may be due to a low level of serotonin (a brain chemical). Serotonin is involved in sending impulses from one nerve cell to the next, and in regulating repetitive behavior.

RISK INCREASES WITH

- Problems with work, school, relationships, living situation, abuse, or illness.
- Family history of the disorder.

PREVENTIVE MEASURES

No specific prevention methods known.

EXPECTED OUTCOME

OCD continues for life. Symptoms may ease up for a while, or become more severe. Effective and specific therapy is now available. It may not lead to a cure, but can reduce symptoms.

POSSIBLE COMPLICATIONS

- Unable to develop and maintain normal work and personal relationships.
- Depression, anxiety, and panic episodes.
- Housebound and limited lifestyle due to symptoms.

 DIAGNOSIS & TREATMENT

GENERAL MEASURES

- Your health care provider may do a physical exam and ask questions about the symptoms. No medical tests can diagnose the disorder. A patient's description of the behavior offers the best clues to diagnosis.
- Treatment is aimed at reducing anxiety, resolving inner conflicts, relieving depression, learning ways of dealing with stress, building self-esteem, and gaining an understanding of the compulsive behavior.
- Behavioral therapy (usually a process known as "exposure and response prevention") is used in treatment. It is often combined with drugs to achieve satisfactory results.
- Family education about the disorder is important.
- Group therapy may be helpful for some patients.
- A patient who is severely affected (and who does not respond to drug therapy) may benefit from precise, localized brain surgery (rare).
- To learn more: Obsessive-Compulsive Foundation, 676 State St., New Haven, CT 06511; (203) 401-2070 (not toll free); website: www.ocfoundation.org.

MEDICATIONS

- Antidepressants are often effective and may be prescribed. Complete benefits may not be seen for 3 weeks. About 10% of patients are unable to tolerate the side effects of the drugs, but an adverse response to one does not mean there will be problems with another.
- Antianxiety or tranquilizer drugs may also be prescribed.

ACTIVITY

No limits.

DIET

No special diet.

 NOTIFY OUR OFFICE IF

- You or a family member has symptoms of obsessive-compulsive disorder.
- Symptoms continue or worsen after during treatment.
- Drugs used in treatment produce side effects.

Special notes:

_____

_____

_____

More notes on the back of this page ☐

ORAL CANCER

BASIC INFORMATION

DESCRIPTION

Growth of malignant cells in the mouth or tongue. These are rare, but dangerous. Oral cancer can involve the lips, gums, palate, tongue, membranes inside the lip or cheek, floor of the mouth, or tonsillar area. It is more common in adults over 40. It is increasing in young people who chew smokeless tobacco.

FREQUENT SIGNS AND SYMPTOMS

· A pale lump, usually painless, with a hard rim that appears in any part of the mouth or tongue.
· Lump grows larger, becomes an open sore, and bleeds easily.
· Dentures may not fit properly.
· Lump may make the tongue stiff and difficult to control, causing speaking and swallowing difficulty.

CAUSES

Unknown.

RISK INCREASES WITH

· Use of tobacco in any form (including smokeless).
· Family history of oral cancer.
· Past history of oral cancer.
· Excess alcohol use.
· Sun exposure (cancer on the lower lip).
· Serious periodontal (gum) disease.

PREVENTIVE MEASURES

· Don't use tobacco in any form; and drink alcohol in moderate amounts, if at all.
· To help diagnose a cancer at an early stage, see your dental care provider or health care provider if you have any sore patches or lumps on the lips or in the mouth that do not heal in two weeks.
· Practice good oral hygiene and get regular dental checkups.

EXPECTED OUTCOMES

Recovery depends on where the cancer is located, if it has spread, and patient's general health. The outcome is more favorable with early diagnosis, as compared to diagnosis of advanced disease. Early diagnosis improves the success rate of treatment.

POSSIBLE COMPLICATIONS

· Slow healing after surgery.
· Spread to lymph nodes in the neck, requiring head and neck surgery.
· Speech and swallowing problems.
· Cancer may recur.
· The five-year survival rate is about 50% for those diagnosed with oral cancer.

DIAGNOSIS & TREATMENT

GENERAL MEASURES

· Your health care provider will do an exam of the mouth and neck area. Medical tests may include blood studies, x-rays of the head, a biopsy, and other tests. Biopsy involves removal of a small amount of tissue for viewing under a microscope. The larger the lump at the time of diagnosis, the greater the chance that it has metastasized (spread) to other places in the body.
· Treatment will vary depending on location of the cancer (lips, tongue, palate, etc.), if the cancer has spread, and the patient's age and health.
· Surgery is a common treatment for oral cancer. If needed, a person's normal facial appearance can often be restored by plastic surgery.
· Radiation therapy and/or anticancer drugs may be recommended.
· Newer treatments such as hyperthermia (using heat on cancer cells) and gene therapy are being studied.
· Follow-up therapy may be needed to help adjust to new ways of eating and talking.
· To learn more: American Cancer Society, (800) ACS-2345; website: www.cancer.org or National Cancer Institute, (800) 4-CANCER; website: www.nci.nih.gov.

MEDICATIONS

· Your health care provider may prescribe:
  - Anticancer drugs (chemotherapy).
  - Pain relievers after surgery.
  - Antibiotics, if infection occurs.

ACTIVITY

Resume your normal activities gradually after surgery.

DIET

· Depends on the extent of the disease and your ability to chew or swallow. A soft diet may be required.
· A liquid diet may be needed for a few days after surgery.

NOTIFY OUR OFFICE IF

· You or a family member has any signs of oral cancer.
· The following occur after treatment: increasing pain, fever, new lumps or sores, or excessive bleeding.

Special notes:

_____

_____

_____

More notes on the back of this page ☐

OSGOOD-SCHLATTER DISEASE
(Osteochondrosis)

 BASIC INFORMATION

DESCRIPTION

A common, temporary condition involving the knee and tibia (shin bone). It occurs often in young athletes (boys more than girls) during the pre-teen or teenage growing years. Usually, only one knee is affected. Osgood-Schlatter disease (OSD) is named for the two doctors who first described it.

FREQUENT SIGNS AND SYMPTOMS

• Swelling, pain, and tenderness below the knee joint and over the shin bone. The symptoms may be mild to severe.
• Pain worsens with activity and gets better with rest. Pain may occur with jumping, kneeling, running, climbing stairs, or anytime the knee is bent and extended.
• Bony bump may be felt just below the kneecap. It may feel tender, warm, and hurt when pressed.

CAUSES

A combination of rapid growth and stress on the knee joint due to overuse. The tendon in the kneecap that connects it to the tibia becomes inflamed due to constant pulling by the quadriceps muscles. The tendon may stretch and tear away (called avulsion) from the tibia and take a piece of bone with it.

RISK INCREASES WITH

• Sports and activities that involve running, jumping, cutting, or jogging.
• Boys between 11 and 18. As more girls participate in sports, their risk of OSD increases.
• Rapid skeletal growth.

PREVENTIVE MEASURES

No specific preventive measures. Encourage a child to exercise moderately, avoiding extremes.

EXPECTED OUTCOMES

Usually resolves on its own within 1 to 2 years. Some discomfort may persist for 2 to 3 years or until growth is completed. A permanent, painless bump may remain below the knee.

POSSIBLE COMPLICATIONS

• In a few cases, chronic pain may occur.
• About 60% of adults who have had OSD have some pain when kneeling.

 DIAGNOSIS & TREATMENT

GENERAL MEASURES

• Your health care provider will do a physical exam of the leg and ask questions about your symptoms and activities. Medical tests may include an x-ray or bone scan of the knee to confirm the diagnosis.
• Treatment may involve ice or heat, drugs (if needed for pain), rest, and limits on sports activities.
• Apply ice to the affected area several times a day for the first 2 to 3 days to reduce swelling and pain.
• After a few days, heat may help discomfort. Use warm compresses, a heating pad, or take warm baths.
• Stretching exercises may be prescribed.
• Occasionally, other treatments may be recommended depending on symptoms. These may include using crutches, having a leg cast or splint, or wearing an elastic knee brace.
• Surgery (rarely needed) if other treatment fails.

MEDICATIONS

For minor discomfort, you may use nonprescription drugs such as ibuprofen.

ACTIVITY

• Your health care provider will advise you of the limits on sports and activities. Each individual case is different. The usual recommendation is to stop any sports or activities that cause pain. Participation may be permitted when it does not cause pain. Resuming some activities too quickly could make the symptoms worse.
• When you return to normal sports activities, recommendations may include wearing a knee brace, special insoles in your shoes, using heat before and ice on your knee after your activity, and stretching and strengthening exercises.

DIET

No special diet.

 NOTIFY OUR OFFICE IF

• Your child has symptoms of Osgood-Schlatter disease.
• The following occur during treatment:
 - Pain increases.
 - Fever.

Special notes:

_____

_____

_____

More notes on the back of this page ☐

344

OSTEOARTHRITIS

(Degenerative Joint Disease)

BASIC INFORMATION

DESCRIPTION

Gradual deterioration (degeneration) of cartilage in a joint. Osteoarthritis is most common in weight-bearing joints (feet, ankles, knees, hips). It also affects fingers, wrists, shoulders, and spine. It can occur at any age, but is more likely in adults over age 45.

FREQUENT SIGNS AND SYMPTOMS

- Joint stiffness and pain, including backache. Weather changes, such as cold and damp, may increase aching.
- Joints have limited movement and less flexibility.
- No redness, heat, or fever in affected joints (usually).
- May have swelling of affected joints, such as fingers.
- May have cracking or grating sounds in joints.

CAUSES

The cartilage normally forms a soft protective layer between the bones of a joint. When the cartilage deteriorates, it allows the bones to rub together. This causes the pain and limited movement.

RISK INCREASES WITH

- Age. 50% of people over age 60 have some signs of osteoarthritis.
- Obesity.
- Activities that stress joints (e.g., dancers, football players, instrumental musicians, carpet layers, and others).
- Injury to the joint.
- Family history of osteoarthritis.

PREVENTIVE MEASURES

- Maintain normal weight for height and body structure.
- Be physically active, but avoid activities that lead to joint injury, especially after age 40. Try regular stretching or yoga exercises.

EXPECTED OUTCOMES

Symptoms can usually be relieved, but joint changes are permanent. Pain may begin as a minor irritant, but it can become severe enough to interfere with daily activities and sleep. The disorder worsens over time.

POSSIBLE COMPLICATIONS

- Crippling (sometimes).
- Symptoms can lead to limits in daily activities, affect the ability to work, bring on stress and depression, and restrict social and recreational activities.

DIAGNOSIS & TREATMENT

GENERAL MEASURES

- Your health care provider will do a physical exam and ask questions about your symptoms and activities. Medical tests may include studies of joint fluid (to rule out inflammatory forms of arthritis) and x-rays of joints.

- Treatment goals are to control pain, slow progression of the disorder, and improve mobility and function.
- Treatment may include lifestyle changes, drugs, self-care steps, and surgery.
- Lifestyle changes may involve diet (to maintain healthy weight), exercises, and using mechanical aids.
- Mechanical aids can include: shock-absorbing or orthopedic shoes, canes, crutches, or walkers. They may include splints, braces, or elastic supports to help joints; neck brace, collar, or corset to help back pain.
- Heat can ease discomfort or pain. Use heating pads or warm soaks several times a day for 10 minutes at a time.
- Cold can help reduce swelling and inflammation. Use an ice pack several times a day for 20 to 30 minutes.
- Sleep on your back on a firm mattress or place 3/4-inch thick plywood between your box spring and mattress.
- Avoid outdoor activity in cold weather, if possible.
- Acupuncture may help some people.
- Surgery for osteoarthritis may be recommended for some patients. There are different options. Your health care provider will discuss the risks and benefits.
- To learn more: Arthritis Foundation, local chapter, or contact them at P.O. Box 7669, Atlanta, GA 30357-0669; (800) 283-7800; website: www.arthritis.org.

MEDICATIONS

- Nonsteroidal anti-inflammatory drugs. These drugs may be nonprescription or prescribed. All have some side effects. You may need to try more than one to see what works best for you and has the least side effects.
- Glucosamine and chondroitin supplements may help. They should be taken at least 6 weeks as a trial.
- Cortisone injections into joints may be prescribed.
- Other drugs may be prescribed as needed.

ACTIVITY

Exercise is beneficial. Your health care provider can advise you about an exercise program. Swimming or water aerobics are good. They don't stress the joints.

DIET

If you are overweight, any weight loss will help joints.

NOTIFY OUR OFFICE IF

- You or a family member has joint pain or stiffness.
- Symptoms worsen after treatment starts.

Special notes:

_____

_____

_____

More notes on the back of this page ☐

OSTEOMYELITIS

 BASIC INFORMATION

DESCRIPTION
Infection of the bone and bone marrow. Osteomyelitis can involve any bone in the body. In a child, it usually affects the femur (upper leg bone), tibia (lower leg bone), the humerus or radius (bones in the arm). In an adult, it usually affects the pelvis or spine. It occurs in both sexes and all ages (often children and the elderly).

FREQUENT SIGNS AND SYMPTOMS
- High fever.
- Pain, swelling, redness, warmth, and tenderness in the area over the infected bone, especially when moving a nearby joint. Nearby joints, such as the knee, may also be red, warm, and swollen.
- May have limited use or not be able to use an infected extremity (arm or leg).
- Child may guard or protect area from being touched.
- General ill feeling.
- Excessive sweating, chills, back pain (sometimes).

CAUSES
Bacterial infection is the most common cause. Fungal or other infections are more rare. Bones can be infected by: bacteria in the bloodstream from infection in another body part; bacteria in soft body tissue located next to the bone; and bacteria that directly infects the bone.

RISK INCREASES WITH
- Recent injury or surgery.
- Diabetes or sickle cell anemia.
- Infection that occurs in another part of the body.
- People on dialysis (hemodialysis).
- Weak immune system due to illness or drugs.
- Intravenous (IV) drug abuse.

PREVENTIVE MEASURES
Obtain prompt medical treatment of any bacterial infection to prevent its spread to bone or other body parts.

EXPECTED OUTCOMES
Outcome will depend on severity of infection, effectiveness of drug treatment, results of surgical procedures, and general health of patient. Treatment success rates have increased and new therapies are being studied.

POSSIBLE COMPLICATIONS
- Chronic osteomyelitis. It may last for months or years and be difficult to treat. It can cause periodic bone pain, tenderness, and abscess (area of pus) that may drain through the skin. Treatment may require more surgery and drugs for an extended period of time.
- Reduced function of the affected limb and joint.
- Recurrence of the infection.
- Rarely, treatment is unsuccessful and infection continues. Surgery may be done to fuse the joint or amputate the limb.

 DIAGNOSIS & TREATMENT

GENERAL MEASURES
- Your health care provider will do a physical exam of the affected area. Medical tests include blood studies and cultures to identify the bacteria. Samples of pus, joint fluid, and infected bone may be removed and used for tests to confirm the diagnosis. Imaging studies such as bone scans or x-rays may be done.
- Treatment usually involves hospital care, drug therapy, rest, and other supportive measures.
- The affected bone and joint may be immobilized (not allowed to move). Bracing may be used for the spine.
- Surgery may be done to drain an abscess, remove dead bone tissue or infected bone, and to stabilize the spine. Bone or skin grafts may be required.
- An artificial joint that is infected may need to be removed and replaced.
- A patient may be placed in a sealed chamber where high-pressure oxygen is used for treatment.

MEDICATIONS
- Antibiotics will be prescribed to treat the infection. They are sometimes given through a vein (IV) while in the hospital. The drugs usually need to be continued at home after the hospital stay. This may be done by continuing the IV drugs or with drugs that are taken by mouth.
- Pain relievers may be prescribed.

ACTIVITY
- Rest in bed until symptoms get better. Resume your normal activities gradually.
- Physical therapy may be recommended to help affected limbs and joints regain function and flexibility.

DIET
No special diet.

 NOTIFY OUR OFFICE IF

- You or a family member has symptoms of osteomyelitis.
- Symptoms persist or recur despite treatment.
- New, unexplained symptoms develop. Drugs used in treatment may produce side effects.

Special notes:

_____

_____

_____

More notes on the back of this page ☐

OSTEOPOROSIS

 BASIC INFORMATION

DESCRIPTION

Loss of normal bone density, bone mass, and bone strength. Osteoporosis (porous bones) is a progressive disease that leads to increased thinning of bones and risk of fractures (broken bones). It occurs in both sexes, but is most common in women after menopause due to a decrease in the hormone estrogen. Estrogen protects against bone loss.

FREQUENT SIGNS AND SYMPTOMS

· Osteoporosis does not cause pain, and there are usually no obvious symptoms. It is called a "silent" disease.
· People don't realize they have osteoporosis until they fall and suffer a fracture, or a spontaneous fracture occurs in a back-bone. Pain from fractures may be mild to severe. The pain may stop when the fracture heals or it may be chronic due to permanent bone damage.

CAUSES

Loss of bone mass and density occurs due to a decrease of calcium (a mineral) and other substances that are needed for maintaining bone strength. A number of risk factors can contribute to the decrease.

RISK INCREASES WITH

· Females; advanced age; Asian or white persons.
· Early menopause (either naturally or due to surgery).
· Lack of exercise (sedentary lifestyle).
· A broad range of diseases and drugs.
· Poor nutrition. Lack of calcium, protein, and vitamins.
· Women with a small body frame or are quite thin.
· Eating disorders (bulimia or anorexia).
· Family history of osteoporosis.
· Smoking.
· Excess alcohol use.
· Men with low testosterone levels.

PREVENTIVE MEASURES

· Preventive measures need to start at a young age.
· Adequate calcium intake (1200 to 1500 mg a day) with milk and dairy products or calcium supplements.
· Regular exercise, such as walking (which is weight-bearing, and is better for preventing osteoporosis).
· Avoid risk factors such as alcohol and smoking.
· Preventive drugs may be prescribed in high-risk cases.

EXPECTED OUTCOME

There is no cure for osteoporosis. Treatment (no matter what age) can help halt and may reverse some bone loss. Pain symptoms can usually be helped with drugs.

POSSIBLE COMPLICATIONS

· Falls and bone fractures, such as hip, spine and wrist.
· Severe, disabling pain.
· Deformed spinal column and bent back (sometimes called Dowager hump). Loss of height.

 DIAGNOSIS & TREATMENT

GENERAL MEASURES

· Medical tests may include bone x-rays, ultrasound, and bone density studies. If bone density studies show bone loss is 10% or more, the diagnosis is osteoporosis.
· Treatment is aimed at stopping further bone loss, preventing fractures, relieving pain (if needed), and bone rebuilding. Treatment steps include drugs, lifestyle changes, and medical care for any underlying disorder. A treatment plan will be based on your individual case.
· Lifestyle changes may include diet changes, exercise, modifying behaviors, and home safety to prevent falls.
· Stop smoking. Find a way to quit that works for you.
· Stop excess alcohol use.
· If a drug you take is a risk factor for osteoporosis, the medical advice may be to stop the drug, reduce the dosage, or use an alternative drug.
· To learn more: National Osteoporosis Foundation, 1150 17th St., Suite 500 NW, Washington, DC 20036, (800) 223-9994; website: www.nof.org.

MEDICATION

· Different prescription drugs are used to prevent and treat bone loss. If one drug causes problems or is not effective, another drug can be prescribed.
· For minor pain, use nonprescription drugs such as acetaminophen or ibuprofen. Stronger pain drugs may be prescribed.
· Calcium and vitamin D supplements may be needed.

ACTIVITY

Exercise strengthens muscles and bones and improves balance. Aerobic and weight-bearing exercises should be part of a daily 30-minute program.

DIET

Eat a healthy, well-balanced diet.

 NOTIFY OUR OFFICE IF

· You or a family member has symptoms of osteoporosis.
· Pain develops, especially after an injury.

Special notes:

_____

_____

_____

More notes on the back of this page ☐

OTOSCLEROSIS

BASIC INFORMATION

DESCRIPTION
Slow formation of abnormal, spongy bone growth in the middle ear. The growth prevents one of the small bones in the middle ear from transmitting sound waves. This can lead to hearing loss. Otosclerosis usually affects both ears. It occurs in all ages and both sexes, but is more common in females from ages 15 to 30.

FREQUENT SIGNS AND SYMPTOMS
- Slow, continuing hearing loss. Early on, the disease is called otospongiosis.
- Ringing or other types of noises in the ears (tinnitus).
- Dizziness or imbalance if the vestibular portion of the ear is affected.

CAUSES
Appears to be an inherited disease. Sixty percent of those affected have a positive family history of the disorder. In other cases, the cause is unknown. A viral infection may be a factor.

RISK INCREASES WITH
- Family history of hearing loss.
- Genetics. Otosclerosis affects to some degree about 10% of all white persons.
- Pregnancy, which may trigger the onset.
- Osteogenesis imperfecta (a bone disease of the ear).

PREVENTIVE MEASURES
Cannot be prevented at present. Obtain genetic counseling before starting a family if you or your spouse has otosclerosis.

EXPECTED OUTCOMES
Surgical treatment can help restore or improve hearing in most patients. In patients not needing or unable to have surgery, hearing aids can be of benefit.

POSSIBLE COMPLICATIONS
- Without surgery, some degree of hearing loss may continue for years. Total deafness is a rare complication.
- Hearing loss can cause problems with work, social events, and family relationships. Emotional distress may occur.

DIAGNOSIS & TREATMENT

GENERAL MEASURES
- Your health care provider will do a physical exam of the ears and ask questions about your symptoms and family history of hearing problems. Diagnosis is based on hearing tests such as an audiogram and Rinne test (study of bone conduction). A CT (an imaging study) of the head may be done to rule out other disorders.
- Treatment will depend on the degree of hearing loss. It may involve surgery and/or hearing aids, and sometimes fluoride supplements.
- If the hearing loss is minor, no treatment is usually needed. Hearing tests will be given periodically to see if hearing loss is progressing.
- Treatment usually involves surgery (stapedectomy) to remove a part or all of the stapes (a bone in the middle ear) and replace it with prosthesis (artificial substitute). The hearing is improved in almost all cases.
- Hearing aids will benefit many patients. Different types are available. A hearing specialist can help you choose what will work best for your individual needs.
- A bone anchored hearing aid (BAHA) may be recommended. It is an implantable hearing aid that takes minor surgery to put in place.
- To learn more: American Speech-Language-Hearing Association, 10801 Rockville Pike Rd., Rockville, MD 20852; (800) 638-8255; website: www.asha.org.

MEDICATIONS
- Antibiotics may be prescribed after surgery.
- Sodium fluoride may be prescribed to prevent further hearing loss by hardening the spongy bone. It won't, however, improve hearing.

ACTIVITY
After surgery, resume your normal activities gradually.

DIET
No special diet.

NOTIFY OUR OFFICE IF

- You or a family member has symptoms of otosclerosis.
- Sudden hearing loss or dizziness occurs.
- New symptoms occur after surgery.

Special notes:

_____

_____

_____

More notes on the back of this page ☐

OVARIAN CANCER

 BASIC INFORMATION

DESCRIPTION
A malignant growth in the ovary that is likely to spread to other body parts and threaten life. It affects females of all ages, but is most common after age 50. There are many different types of ovarian cancer. Epithelial tumors account for the majority, and they grow more rapidly. Other ovarian cancers are slow growing, or they have spread from other cancer in the body.

FREQUENT SIGNS AND SYMPTOMS
- Often no symptoms occur until late in the disease.
- Discomfort in the lower abdomen, gas, and indigestion.
- Pelvic pain, or swelling in the abdomen with no pain.
- Feeling of being constipated or unable to have a bowel movement.
- Irregular menstrual periods; bleeding from the vagina.
- Pain with intercourse.
- A need to urinate often.
- Excess hair growth.
- Nausea, loss of appetite, not being able to eat, and weight loss. Sometimes a weight gain occurs.

CAUSES
The exact cause is unknown.

RISK INCREASES WITH
- Personal history of breast cancer. A family history of breast and/or ovarian cancer, colon, lung, prostate, and uterine cancers.
- Women who carry mutated genes such as BRCA1 and BRCA2.
- Advancing age.
- Women who began to menstruate before age 12 and/or start menopause after age 50.
- Women who have used ovulation-stimulating fertility drugs have a slightly increased risk of ovarian cancer.
- Late pregnancies (over age 30).
- Never having had children.

PREVENTIVE MEASURES
- No specific preventive measures. Having yearly pelvic exams may aid in earlier diagnosis and treatment.
- For women with a family history of ovarian cancer, screening tests and genetic counseling may be recommended. In some cases, ovary removal may be discussed if a woman has a strong family history of breast or ovarian cancer and pregnancy is not desired.
- Birth control pills may help with prevention.

EXPECTED OUTCOME
The outcome depends on the stage of the disease when it is first diagnosed. Other factors that affect the outcome are a woman's age and her general health.

POSSIBLE COMPLICATIONS
- Pleural effusion (excess of fluid in the lining of the lungs) or ascites (excess fluid in the peritoneal cavity).
- Spread of cancer to other places in the body. This can lead to excess pain, other complications, and death.
- Infertility if both ovaries are removed.
- Recurrence of cancer.

 DIAGNOSIS & TREATMENT

GENERAL MEASURES
- Your health care provider will do a physical exam and ask questions about your symptoms. A number of medical tests will be done. The tests help diagnose the cancer and also determine if it has spread (staging).
- Treatment varies and depends on the location and size of a tumor, any spread of the cancer, health, age and preferences of the patient. Treatment may include chemotherapy (anticancer drugs) and/or radiation therapy, surgery, and biologic therapy.
- Chemotherapy uses drugs and radiation therapy uses radiation to attack the cancer cells. Biologic therapy uses the body's immune system to fight cancer.
- The goal of surgery is to remove as many of the cancer cells as possible so that chemotherapy will be more effective. In patients who desire pregnancy, surgery may remove only the ovary and the fallopian tube.
- Treatment may involve steps to relieve symptoms and make you comfortable, rather than treating the cancer.
- Counseling may help you cope with having cancer.
- To learn more: American Cancer Society, (800) ACS-2345; website: www.cancer.org or National Cancer Institute, (800) 4-CANCER; website: www.nci.nih.gov.

MEDICATIONS
Anticancer drugs (chemotherapy) and pain relievers, as needed, may be prescribed.

ACTIVITY
No limits after recovery from surgery.

DIET
Eat a normal, well-balanced diet.

 NOTIFY OUR OFFICE IF

You or a family member has symptoms of ovarian cancer.

Special notes:

_____

_____

_____

More notes on the back of this page ☐

OVARIAN TUMOR, BENIGN

 ## BASIC INFORMATION

DESCRIPTION
• The ovaries are the female reproductive organs that hold and release eggs and produce female hormones. An abnormal growth in the ovary that is solid is called a tumor. It is different from a cyst. An ovarian cyst contains fluid. However, in the ovary, some tumors may have fluid areas within them and are called cystic tumors. Ovarian tumors are usually small, but in some cases, may grow large enough to make a woman appear pregnant.
• In some cases, the tumor may have features that suggest it will behave as a cancer, but over a long period of time (10 to 20 years). These are called low malignant-potential (LMP) ovarian tumors or borderline ovarian tumors.

FREQUENT SIGNS AND SYMPTOMS
May not cause symptoms. If symptoms occur, they may include:
• Mild pelvic pain.
• Pain in the lower back.
• Discomfort with sexual intercourse.
• Changes in menstrual flow, the length of periods, and time between periods.
• Excess hair growth, deep voice, and weight gain (sometimes).
• If a large ovarian tumor twists or ruptures, it can cause severe pain, rigid muscles, and swelling.

CAUSES
• Usually, unknown. It is likely to be related to problems of female hormone production and secretion.
• Endometriosis.

RISK INCREASES WITH
Unknown.

PREVENTIVE MEASURES
No specific preventive measures. Use of oral contraceptives may decrease risk.

EXPECTED OUTCOME
Most ovarian tumors require no treatment and disappear on their own within a few months. In other cases, treatment usually provides a complete cure. Benign or noncancerous tumors do not invade nearby tissue the way cancerous tumors do.

POSSIBLE COMPLICATIONS
• Complications from surgery may occur.
• Tumor may recur after treatment.

 ## DIAGNOSIS & TREATMENT

GENERAL MEASURES
• Your health care provider will do a physical and pelvic exam. Medical tests can include blood studies, ultrasound, and laparoscopy (a telescope-like tool is used to look inside the abdomen).
• Treatment may not be needed, except to have regular pelvic exams. The tumor's growth can be monitored.
• Some tumors require surgery to diagnose accurately, rule out cancer, or for treatment purposes. If one ovary must be removed, normal conception and childbirth is possible as long as a normal ovary remains on the other side.
• To learn more: try the library or perform a web search. A good site to start with is www.4women.gov.

MEDICATION
Female hormones may be prescribed. These help shrink or destroy some tumors. Oral contraceptives are often used as the first step in treatment.

ACTIVITY
No limits unless surgery is necessary.

DIET
No special diet.

NOTIFY OUR OFFICE IF

• You or a family member has symptoms of an ovarian tumor
• Severe pain and abdominal distention occurs.
• New, unexplained symptoms develop. Drugs used in treatment may produce side effects.

Special notes:

_____

_____

_____

More notes on the back of this page ☐

PAGET'S DISEASE OF BONE
(Osteitis Deformans)

BASIC INFORMATION

DESCRIPTION
A gradual, progressive bone disease. It usually involves the bones of the skull, spine, legs, collar bone, and pelvis. It can affect both sexes and is most common in middle-aged people. It is named for an English doctor who first described the disease. Paget's disease of the breast is a different disorder.

FREQUENT SIGNS AND SYMPTOMS
· Most often, there are no early symptoms.
· Bone pain (especially at night).
· Skin over the bones is warm.
· Joint pain or stiffness.
· Headaches.
· Hearing loss and tinnitus (noises in the ear).
· Fractures (may occur from minor trauma).
· Bowing (deformity) of extremities, such as of the legs.
· Nerve problems, from pressure on the nerves.

CAUSES
Unknown. It may involve genetics and/or a virus. The affected bone breaks down and then abnormal bone growth occurs. The new bone is weak, fragile, enlarged, and deformed.

RISK INCREASES WITH
Family history of Paget's disease.

PREVENTIVE MEASURES
· No specific preventive measures.
· Those with family history should have a blood-screening test periodically to help with early diagnosis.

EXPECTED OUTCOMES
· There is no cure, but treatment can control or reduce symptoms. With early treatment (before major bone changes occur), the outlook is generally good.
· Research into causes and treatment continues, so there is hope for better treatment and, perhaps a cure.

POSSIBLE COMPLICATIONS
Many complications can occur that affect different organs and body parts. Complications include arthritis, heart disease, hearing loss, kidney stones, bone cancer, vision changes, spinal disease, enlarged head, loose teeth, and others.

DIAGNOSIS & TREATMENT

GENERAL MEASURES
· Your health care provider will do a physical exam. Medical tests may include blood and urine studies, x-rays of affected bones, and a bone scan. Hearing and vision testing may be done if the skull is involved.

· Treatment may include physical therapy, use of assistive devices, drugs, exercise, home care, and surgery.
· If there are no symptoms, treatment may not be needed. Follow-up exams will monitor the disease status.
· Physical therapy helps maintain and improve muscle strength, range of motion, flexibility, and endurance.
· Walkers, canes, crutches, special shoes, or shoe inserts may help if walking is a problem.
· Use heat to relieve pain (warm compresses, or soaks).
· Transcutaneous electrical nerve stimulation (TENS) or massage may help muscle pain and tightness.
· Accident-proof your home. Avoid throw rugs and slippery floors. Install hand rails next to the tub. Other changes may be needed depending on patient's needs.
· Hearing aid may be useful if hearing loss occurs.
· Rarely, splinting may be needed for severely affected areas to prevent fractures.
· Bone surgery may be needed to treat fractures, correct deformities, or treat arthritis.
· To learn more: Paget Foundation, 120 Wall St., Suite 1602, New York, NY 10005-4001; (800) 237-2438; website: www.paget.org.

MEDICATIONS
· Drugs will usually be prescribed that help slow the rate of bone turnover. Several options are available and their risks and benefits will be discussed with you.
· Nonprescription drugs for pain can be used. Stronger ones may be prescribed (if needed).
· Calcium and vitamin D are often recommended.

ACTIVITY
Home exercises will help maintain mobility. Avoid stress on affected bones. Follow instructions provided by your physical therapist or health care provider.

DIET
Eat a healthy diet. Avoid weight gain.

NOTIFY OUR OFFICE IF

· You or family member has symptoms of Paget's disease of bone.
· The following occur during treatment: fever, severe pain, or unexpected weight loss.
· New, unexplained symptoms develop. Drugs used in treatment may produce side effects.

Special notes:

_____

_____

_____

More notes on the back of this page ☐

PANCREATIC CANCER

 BASIC INFORMATION

DESCRIPTION

Growth of cancer cells in the pancreas. The pancreas is an organ in the upper-middle part of the abdomen. It produces intestinal enzymes (juices) to help digest food, and insulin to control blood sugar. This cancer usually affects adults ages 35 to 70, and men more than women.

FREQUENT SIGNS AND SYMPTOMS

- Usually no symptoms occur in early stages of cancer.
- Weight loss. Loss of appetite.
- Pain in the back or upper abdomen.
- Fatigue.
- Jaundice (yellow skin and eyes). Intense itching may occur with jaundice.
- Nausea, vomiting, and problems with digestion.
- Depression, though not caused by cancer, may occur.

CAUSES

Unknown. It may be to be a combination of hereditary factors and environmental factors.

RISK INCREASES WITH

- Chronic pancreatitis (inflammation of the pancreas).
- Diabetes.
- Genetic factors. It is more common in African-Americans than in whites, Asians, or American Hispanics.
- Smoking.
- Excess alcohol use.
- Diet high in fat and low in fruits and vegetables.
- Obesity and lack of physical activity.
- Exposure to industrial chemicals, such as urea, naphthalene, or benzidine.
- Certain hereditary disorders.

PREVENTIVE MEASURES

No specific preventive measures. To reduce cancer risks: get recommended screening tests, maintain healthy weight, eat a healthy diet, exercise regularly, and don't smoke.

EXPECTED OUTCOMES

- The diagnosis often comes too late for effective treatment. Survival for more than 1 or 2 years is unlikely. However, symptoms can be relieved or controlled.
- Research into causes and treatment continues. There is hope for improved treatment and a cure.

POSSIBLE COMPLICATIONS

- Spread (metastasis) of cancer to other places in the body. This has often already occurred by the time of diagnosis.
- Surgical complications.
- Malnutrition (lack of nutrients needed by the body).
- Increased pain.

 DIAGNOSIS & TREATMENT

GENERAL MEASURES

- Your health care provider will do a physical exam and ask questions about any symptoms. A number of medical tests will be done. The tests help to diagnose the cancer, and then determine if it has spread (staging).
- Treatment varies and depends on location and size of tumor, any spread of the cancer, your health, age, and preferences. Treatment may include chemotherapy (anticancer drugs) and/or radiation therapy, surgery, and biologic therapy.
- Chemotherapy uses drugs and radiation therapy uses radiation to attack the cancer cells. Biologic therapy uses the body's immune system to fight cancer.
- Surgery may be performed to remove the tumor if the cancer has not spread to other places in the body.
- Treatment may involve steps to relieve symptoms and make you comfortable, rather than treating the cancer.
- Counseling may help you cope with having cancer.
- To learn more: American Cancer Society, (800) ACS-2345; website: www.cancer.org, or National Cancer Institute, (800) 4-CANCER; website: www.nci.nih.gov.

MEDICATIONS

- Your health care provider may prescribe:
    - Pain relievers.
    - Chemotherapy (anticancer drugs).
    - Pancreatic enzymes to replace those that the pancreas cannot manufacture.
    - Sedatives for sleep if needed.
    - Vitamin supplements.

ACTIVITY

Remain as active as you can. It helps your quality of life.

DIET

- Low-fat diet may be recommended.
- Loss of appetite may make eating difficult. Try eating several small meals each day. Choose foods easy to digest and have healthy snacks available.

 NOTIFY OUR OFFICE IF

- You have symptoms of pancreatic cancer.
- After diagnosis, new symptoms occur.

Special notes:

_____

_____

_____

More notes on the back of this page ☐

PANCREATITIS

BASIC INFORMATION

DESCRIPTION
Inflammation of the pancreas. The pancreas supplies digestive juices and hormones for the body. Acute pancreatitis occurs suddenly and lasts for a short period. If injury to the pancreas occurs, chronic pancreatitis develops.

FREQUENT SIGNS AND SYMPTOMS
Acute pancreatitis:
- Extreme abdominal pain.
- Vomiting.
- Abdominal swelling and gas.
- Fever.
- Muscle aches.
- Drop in blood pressure.

Chronic pancreatitis:
- Persistent mild or severe pain, often after meals, in the upper abdomen. Pain sometimes spreads to the back or over the entire body. Pain is aching, burning, gnawing, or stabbing. Pain episodes may last days or weeks, but rarely less than 1 day.
- Mild jaundice (yellow skin and eyes), sometimes.
- Rapid weight loss.

CAUSES
The inflammation is a reaction to injury, infection, or irritation of the pancreas. It can be brought on by a number of different factors. Sometimes the cause is unknown.

RISK INCREASES WITH
- Alcoholism.
- Disease of the gallbladder or bile ducts.
- Obstruction of the pancreatic duct by stones, scarring, or slow-growing cancer (rare).
- Abdominal injury.
- Viral, bacterial, or parasitic infection.
- Hyperlipidemia (high fat levels in the blood).
- Tumor.
- Trauma or surgery or certain medical procedures.
- Peptic ulcer disease.
- Use of drugs, such as sulfa drugs, azathioprine, chlorothiazide, or cortisone drugs.

PREVENTIVE MEASURES
Avoid risk factors where possible.

EXPECTED OUTCOMES
Acute pancreatitis is often curable with treatment. Chronic pancreatitis may have recurrent attacks for years. Drugs and diet changes can help symptoms.

POSSIBLE COMPLICATIONS
Complications may occur from acute and chronic pancreatitis. They can affect the heart, lungs, kidneys, and other body organs, and could be fatal in a few cases.

DIAGNOSIS & TREATMENT

GENERAL MEASURES
- Your health care provider will do a physical exam and ask questions about your symptoms and activities. Medical tests may include blood, stool, and urine studies; x-rays of the abdomen; CT scan or ultrasound of the pancreas; and others.
- Acute pancreatitis normally requires hospital care for intravenous (IV) fluids and control of pain and vomiting. Oxygen or breathing support with a machine may be needed for breathing problems. Surgery may be required for gallstones, perforated peptic ulcer, or to drain a source of infection.
- Chronic pancreatitis may be treated as an outpatient with drugs, diet controls, and avoidance of alcohol. In some cases, surgery may be needed to control pain.
- To learn more: National Digestive Diseases Information Clearinghouse, 2 Information Way, Bethesda, MD 20892, (800) 891-5389; website: www.digestive.niddk.nih.gov.

MEDICATIONS
- Your health care provider may prescribe:
  - Pain relievers.
  - Digestive enzymes that the damaged pancreas cannot manufacture.
  - Antibiotics, if bacterial infection develops.
  - Drugs to reduce stomach acid.
  - Insulin, if diabetes is present.

ACTIVITY
For acute pancreatitis, bed rest or rest sitting in a chair, if that is more comfortable. Increase activities gradually as symptoms resolve. No limits for chronic pancreatitis.

DIET
Small, frequent, and low-fat meals. Abstain completely from drinking alcohol.

NOTIFY OUR OFFICE IF

- You or a family member has symptoms of acute pancreatitis.
- Jaundice (yellow skin and eyes), fever of 101°F (38.3°C) or higher, continued weight loss, muscle cramps, or seizures occur.

Special notes:

_____

_____

_____

More notes on the back of this page ☐

PANIC DISORDER

 BASIC INFORMATION

DESCRIPTION

Repeated and unexpected episodes of irrational fear and panic. Panic disorder is a type of anxiety. It occurs with attack-like symptoms (often during sleep). Most attacks last 2 to 10 minutes, but some may extend as long as an hour or two. Many people may have one panic attack and never have another.

FREQUENT SIGNS AND SYMPTOMS

Physical symptoms:

• Pounding, racing or skipping heartbeat, chest pains, and shortness of breath.

• Choking feeling, lump in the throat feeling, weakness, faintness, dizziness, lightheaded, and sweating.

• Trembling, numbness, tingling, flushes, or chills.

• Muscle spasms or contractions in the hands and feet.

• Feeling of "butterflies" in the stomach. Nausea.

Emotional symptoms:

• Intense fear of losing one's mind (fear of going crazy), an urge to flee, fear of dying.

• Sense of terror, doom, or dread.

• Sense of unreality, loss of contact with people and objects, and fear of losing control.

• Fear of having another panic attack.

CAUSES

The brain's "alarm system" appears to be affected by a combination of biologic/genetic factors, illnesses, drugs, and one's personal history of traumatic events.

RISK INCREASES WITH

• Stress (emotional or physical); feelings of guilt, fatigue, or overwork; illness; alcohol or drug abuse.

• Personal history of other emotional problems and family history of panic disorder.

PREVENTIVE MEASURES

No specific measures to prevent a first panic attack. Treatment helps prevent repeated attacks.

EXPECTED OUTCOME

For many, this disorder gets better at times and worse at other times. Treatment can help reduce or completely prevent the attacks. Sometimes it recurs after treatment, but repeated treatment can be successful.

POSSIBLE COMPLICATIONS

• Without treatment, it can negatively affect all aspects of life (work, family, friends, social, and recreational).

• Chronic anxiety or depression; phobias, including agoraphobia (fear of being alone or in public places).

• People with this disorder often feel that there is a physical problem causing their symptoms. They will go from doctor to doctor to get a diagnosis. Despite being assured that they are in good health, they continue to believe otherwise.

 DIAGNOSIS & TREATMENT

GENERAL MEASURES

• Your health care provider will do a physical exam and ask questions about your symptoms and activities. Medical tests may be done to rule out other disorders. A variety of physical disorders can mimic panic attacks.

• Treatment may involve psychotherapy (treatment of emotional and mental problems), self-care, and drugs.

• Cognitive-behavioral therapy may help. Cognitive therapy teaches how to change thoughts, behaviors or attitudes. Behavioral therapy teaches ways to reduce anxiety with deep breathing and muscle relaxation.

• Self-care steps may include:

- Talking to a friend or family member about your feelings. This may sometimes defuse your anxiety.

- Keep a journal about your anxious thoughts or emotions. Consider the causes and possible solutions.

- Join a self-help group.

- Learn relaxation techniques. For some people, meditation is effective.

- Reduce stress in your life, where possible.

• To learn more: National Institute of Mental Health; 6001 Executive Blvd, Bethesda, MD 20892-9663; (800) 647-2642; website: www.nimh.nih.gov.

MEDICATION

Your health care provider may prescribe an antidepressant, benzodiazepine, or beta-blocking agent. The drug may be slowly reduced or stopped, after 6 months to a year, to determine if the panic attacks will return. If they do not return, the drug can be discontinued.

ACTIVITY

Get regular physical exercise and adequate sleep.

DIET

• Consider giving up caffeine (coffee, tea, soft drinks). You may have withdrawal symptoms of headache or tiredness, but they will stop in a few days.

• Don't use alcohol as a way to numb your feelings.

 NOTIFY OUR OFFICE IF

• You or a family member has panic attacks.

• Symptoms return after treatment.

Special notes:

_____

_____

_____

More notes on the back of this page ☐

PARKINSON'S DISEASE

 BASIC INFORMATION

DESCRIPTION

A chronic disease of the central nervous system that affects the movements of the body. Parkinson's usually starts after age 50, but can occur in younger adults. It is named for the doctor who first described it.

FREQUENT SIGNS AND SYMPTOMS

- Tremors (worse with rest and better with moving).
- General muscle stiffness (rigidity) and slowness.
- Shuffling, wide-based walk, and balance problems.
- Stooped posture.
- Loss of facial expression.
- Voice changes. It becomes weak and high pitched.
- Swallowing difficulty, drooling.
- Mental functioning can slowly decease.
- Depression and nervousness.

CAUSES

- Dopamine is a brain chemical that helps control normal muscle movement. With primary (or idiopathic) Parkinson's disease, less dopamine is produced due to a loss of nerve cell function. It is unknown why this loss of nerve cell function occurs.
- Secondary Parkinson's disease can be due to drugs, brain injury, tumors, encephalitis, slow-virus infection, some toxins, and carbon-monoxide poisoning.

RISK INCREASES WITH

- Unknown for the primary type.
- For secondary type, risk factors are listed in Causes.

PREVENTIVE MEASURES

No preventive measures for primary type. For secondary type, avoid risk factors, where possible.

EXPECTED OUTCOMES

- There is no cure for primary type. It is progressive, but unpredictable. There may be good days and bad days. It is not a fatal disease in itself. Symptoms can generally be relieved or controlled with treatment.
- Outcome for secondary type depends on the cause.

POSSIBLE COMPLICATIONS

- Dementia.
- "Freezing" (sudden, but temporary inability to move).
- Falls and fractures.
- Debilitation (weakness and loss of strength).

 DIAGNOSIS & TREATMENT

GENERAL MEASURES

- Your health care provider will do a physical exam and ask questions about your symptoms and activities. There is not a special test to diagnose the disorder. Medical tests may be done to rule out other disorders. If symptoms get better with the drug levodopa, it usually

means a person has Parkinson's disease.
- Treatment options may involve various types of therapy, exercise, self-care, drug therapy, and surgery. Individual treatment will vary depending on a person's age, stage of the disease, and symptoms.
- Counseling can help treat emotional symptoms such as depression, anxiety, stress, anger, and frustration.
- Physical therapy, occupational therapy (help with daily activities), and speech therapy may be helpful.
- Surgery may be an option for severe symptoms or when drugs are not helping. It is not a cure, but it may relieve symptoms.
- Accident-proof your home to help prevent falls and injuries. Install handrails, remove area rugs, keep cords out of the way, and carry a cordless phone with you.
- Getting dressed can be a problem. Choose clothes that are easy to slip on. Wear clothes and shoes that have Velcro fasteners. Allow plenty of time to dress.
- To learn more: American Parkinson Disease Association, 1250 Hylan Blvd., Suite 4B, Staten Island, NY 10305; (800) 223-2732; website: www.apdaparkinson.org or National Parkinson Foundation, 1501 NW 9th Ave., Miami, FL 33136; (800) 327-4545; website: www.parkinson.org.

MEDICATIONS

- One or more of a variety of drugs can be prescribed to treat the symptoms. Your health care provider will discuss the options and the risks and benefits. If one does not help or stops being effective, others can be tried.
- Vitamins or other supplements may be prescribed.

ACTIVITY

Exercises will help maintain mobility, balance, range of motion, and well-being. Follow instructions provided by your physical therapist or health care provider.

DIET

Eat a healthy diet. Add fiber to the diet and increase fluid intake to prevent constipation. If chewing is a problem, take small bites, eat slowly, and chop up food.

 NOTIFY OUR OFFICE IF

- You or a family member has symptoms of Parkinson's disease or symptoms worsen during treatment.
- New, unexplained symptoms develop.

Special notes:

_____

_____

_____

More notes on the back of this page ☐

PARONYCHIA

BASIC INFORMATION

DESCRIPTION
Inflammation of tissue folds that surround a nail. The inflammation can be from bacterial or fungal infection, and is not contagious. It usually occurs on the hands and less often on the feet.

FREQUENT SIGNS AND SYMPTOMS
Bacterial paronychia:
- Pain or tenderness, redness, warmth, and swelling of tissue adjacent to the fingernail.
- Central whitish area produced by pus.

Fungal paronychia:
- Redness and swelling around the fingernail.
- No pain, warmth, itching, or pus.

CAUSES
- Bacterial paronychia is preceded by injury, such as a torn hangnail. The infecting bacteria are usually *Staphylococcus.*
- Fungal paronychia is caused by a fungus or yeast infection.

RISK INCREASES WITH
- Injury around the fingernail.
- Work exposure to constant wetness (dishwashers, bartenders, housewives).
- Diabetes.
- Nail biting or finger sucking.
- Artificial nails.
- Shoes that bind or pinch the toes.

PREVENTIVE MEASURES
- Protect hands from wetness.
- Leave hangnails alone.
- Avoid fingertip injury.
- Avoid tight shoes.

EXPECTED OUTCOMES
- Bacterial paronychia is curable with treatment in 2 weeks.
- Fungal paronychia is chronic and may require 6 months to heal.
- Recurrence is common with both forms.

POSSIBLE COMPLICATIONS
If untreated, may permanently damage the fingernail and nail bed. Rarely, the infection may enter bone or bloodstream.

DIAGNOSIS & TREATMENT

GENERAL MEASURES
- Your health care provider will do an exam of the affected nail. Medical studies, such as a culture of the discharge, may be done to identify the germ.
- Treatment involves avoiding factors that may be the cause, self-care, and drug therapy.
- Sometimes part, or all, of a toenail may need to be removed.
- Use warm-water soaks several times a day.
- If an abscess (pus-filled area) occurs, it may require incision (cutting) and drainage.
- Wear heavy-duty vinyl gloves to prevent contact with irritating substances, such as water, soap, detergent, metal scrubbing pads, scouring pads, scouring powder, and other chemicals.
- Dry the insides of gloves after use. Discard gloves if they develop a hole. A glove with a hole harms the hand more than not wearing a glove.
- Wear vinyl gloves when you peel or squeeze lemons, oranges, grapefruit, tomatoes, or potatoes.
- Wear leather or heavy-duty fabric gloves for housework or gardening.
- Avoid contact with irritating chemicals, such as paint, paint thinner, turpentine, and polish for cars, floors, shoes, furniture, or metal.
- Use lukewarm water and very little mild soap to shower or bathe. All soaps are irritating. Expensive soaps offer no more protection against irritation than less-expensive ones.

MEDICATIONS
- For minor pain, you may use nonprescription drugs, such as ibuprofen or acetaminophen.
- Antibiotics may be prescribed for bacterial infection.
- Topical antifungals and topical steroids may be prescribed for fungal infection.

ACTIVITY
No limits.

DIET
No special diet.

NOTIFY OUR OFFICE IF

- You or a family member has symptoms of paronychia.
- Pain is not helped by treatment.

Special notes:

_____

_____

_____

More notes on the back of this page ☐

PELVIC INFLAMMATORY DISEASE

(PID; Salpingitis)

BASIC INFORMATION

DESCRIPTION

Pelvic inflammatory disease (PID) is an infection of the upper genital area (fallopian tubes, ovaries, and uterus). Any sexually active female may be affected. It mostly occurs in the late teens and early 20's. PID is one of the most common and serious complications of sexually transmitted diseases (STDs) in women. Up to 40% of untreated genital infections progress to PID. Salpingitis (fallopian tube inflammation) is another term for PID.

FREQUENT SIGNS AND SYMPTOMS

- Some women have no symptoms.
- Pain or cramps in the lower abdomen.
- Vaginal discharge (may have a foul odor).
- Painful intercourse or pain when urinating.
- Irregular menstrual bleeding.
- Fever, nausea, and vomiting.

CAUSES

Bacterial infection (usually chlamydial or gonorrheal). The bacteria infection starts in the vagina and cervix and then spreads to the upper genital area. PID usually develops from 2 days to 3 weeks after exposure to the bacteria, but can take months to develop. The infection may be transmitted by an infected sexual partner.

RISK INCREASES WITH

- Women who have a sexually transmitted disease.
- Teenagers (more at risk than older women).
- Multiple sexual partners, or exposure to a single partner who is infected.
- Use of an intrauterine contraceptive device (IUD).
- Prior episode of PID.
- Abortion.
- Pelvic surgery.
- Women who douche once or twice a month. This may push bacteria into the upper genital area.

PREVENTIVE MEASURES

- Use latex (rubber) condoms to help prevent sexually transmitted infections.
- Oral contraceptives may help to decrease the risk.
- Get routine medical check-ups for sexually transmitted diseases if you have multiple sexual partners.
- Get medical care for abnormal vaginal discharge, unusual odor, fever, and bleeding between periods.
- Have your sexual partner tested and treated if needed. Don't resume sexual activity with your partner until tests show no infection, or it has been treated.

EXPECTED OUTCOME

With early diagnosis and treatment, most women recover with no complications. Late treatment or incomplete treatment can lead to serious complications.

POSSIBLE COMPLICATIONS

- Chronic pelvic pain.
- Infertility or ectopic pregnancy.
- Recurrent PID.
- Abscess (pus-filled area). It can be life threatening.

DIAGNOSIS & TREATMENT

GENERAL MEASURES

- Your health care provider will do a physical and a pelvic exam. Medical tests may include blood studies, culture of the vaginal discharge, and a pregnancy test. Other tests may be done to confirm the diagnosis, and rule out other disorders.
- Treatment is with drugs and hospital care (if needed).
- Treatment may be done on an outpatient basis if infection is mild. It is important to follow your treatment schedule. Close medical follow-up care is needed.
- If you have a sexually transmitted disease (STD), your partner needs treatment (even if he has no symptoms).
- Use sanitary pads to absorb the discharge or menstrual flow. Don't douche during treatment.
- Hospital care may be needed for severe illness, more diagnostic tests, an abscess, pregnancy, HIV infection, or if drugs are to be given in a vein (IV).
- Surgery to drain a pelvic abscess may be needed.
- Surgery may help chronic PID or pelvic pain.
- Counseling can be helpful if infertility occurs.
- To learn more: National STD Hotline (800) 227-8922; website: www.ashastd.org/NSTD/index.html.

MEDICATION

Antibiotics (by injection or taken by mouth) for bacterial infection will be prescribed. Finish taking all the entire drug prescribed for a complete cure.

ACTIVITY

Avoid sexual intercourse until treatment is completed for you and your sexual partner.

DIET

No special diet.

NOTIFY OUR OFFICE IF

You or a family member has symptoms of pelvic inflammatory disease or symptoms recur after treatment.

Special notes:

_____

_____

_____

More notes on the back of this page ☐

PENIS CANCER

BASIC INFORMATION

DESCRIPTION

Malignant tumor of the penis including the glans (tip), corona (rounded border of the glans), or prepuce (foreskin covering the glans). Penis cancer is uncommon. It most often affects men over age 50.

FREQUENT SIGNS AND SYMPTOMS

· A small, circular lesion (resembles a pimple) or persistent, painless sore on the penis. The lesion is easily visible in a circumcised male, but it may go unnoticed in an uncircumcised male.
· Pain, bleeding, or discharge.
· Discomfort with urination.
· Enlarged lymph nodes in the groin.

CAUSES

Unknown. A human papillomavirus (HPV) may play a role in the cause. The virus can be sexually transmitted.

RISK INCREASES WITH

· Cigarette smoking.
· Having unprotected sexual relations with multiple partners. This increases the risk of HPV infection.
· AIDS (acquired immunodeficiency syndrome).
· Psoriasis (skin disorder) treatment that uses drugs along with ultraviolet light.

PREVENTIVE MEASURES

· No specific preventive measures. Avoid risk factors where possible. Practice good genital hygiene to reduce risks of infection or irritation. If uncircumcised, retract the foreskin and clean the entire penis when bathing.
· Do a self-exam of the penis and testicles monthly. This can help detect cancers early, when treatment is most successful. See your health care provider for any sign of infection or sores on the penis.

EXPECTED OUTCOMES

Will depend on the extent of the cancer at diagnosis. Early diagnosis and treatment has a more favorable outcome. Recurrence is possible after treatment.

POSSIBLE COMPLICATIONS

Men may delay treatment due to denial, fear of surgery, and loss of sexual function. Treatment delay increases the risk of the cancer spreading.

DIAGNOSIS & TREATMENT

GENERAL MEASURES

· Your health care provider will do a physical exam of the penis and ask questions about any symptoms. A number of medical tests will be done. The tests help to diagnose the cancer and then determine if it has spread (staging).

· Treatment varies and depends on the location and size of tumor, any spread of the cancer, health, age, and preferences. Treatment may include chemotherapy (anticancer drugs) and/or radiation therapy, surgery, and biologic therapy.
· Chemotherapy uses drugs and radiotherapy uses radiation to attack the cancer cells. Biologic therapy uses the body's immune system to treat cancer.
· Surgery to remove the tumor. Local tumors of the foreskin may require circumcision only. Invasive tumors require part or total removal of the penis and some lymph nodes. Urine will still be able to exit the body.
· Treatment may involve steps to relieve symptoms and make you comfortable, rather than treating the cancer.
· Counseling may help you cope with having cancer.
· To learn more: American Cancer Society, (800) ACS-2345; website: www.cancer.org or National Cancer Institute, (800) 4-CANCER; website: www.nci.nih.gov.

MEDICATIONS

Anticancer drugs may be prescribed. They may be used on the skin, taken by mouth, or given by injection.

ACTIVITY

Resume normal activities as soon as possible after treatment. Sexual relations are possible if enough penile tissue remains after surgery. If the total penis is removed, sexual pleasure is still possible using special techniques.

DIET

No special diet.

NOTIFY OUR OFFICE IF

· You or a family member has any lump or sore on the penis.
· Excessive bleeding occurs at the surgical site.
· New, unexplained symptoms develop. Drugs used in treatment may produce side effects.

Special notes:

_____

_____

_____

More notes on the back of this page ☐

PERICARDITIS

 ## BASIC INFORMATION

DESCRIPTION

Inflammation of the pericardium. The pericardium is a sac (thin membrane) around the heart. It has two layers, with a small amount of "lubricating" fluid between them. The fluid lets the heart move around within the sac. With inflammation, the heart can become squeezed inside the sac. The disorder occurs more often in men ages 20 to 50.

FREQUENT SIGNS AND SYMPTOMS

· Dull or sharp pain in the front of the chest. The pain moves to the neck, arm, and shoulder. The pain worsens with movement and eases when sitting up or leaning forward.
· Rapid breathing.
· Cough.
· Fever, sweating, and chills.
· Weakness.
· Anxiety.

CAUSES

The inflammation is a reaction to injury, infection, or irritation of the heart lining. It can be caused by a number of different factors. In many cases, the cause is unknown.

RISK INCREASES WITH

· Rheumatic fever and other diseases of connective tissue, such as lupus erythematosus.
· Complication of a heart attack.
· Complication following heart surgery.
· Complication of a chest injury.
· Viral, bacterial, tuberculous, amebic, toxoplasmotic, or fungal infection.
· Chronic kidney failure.
· Spread of cancer to the pericardium.
· Radiation therapy.

PREVENTIVE MEASURES

No specific preventive measures. To avoid risk factors, get treatment for disorders that may lead to pericarditis.

EXPECTED OUTCOMES

Usually curable with treatment. Allow 2 to 3 weeks for healing. It may recur one or more times in the next 6 to 12 months.

POSSIBLE COMPLICATIONS

· Pericarditis becomes chronic if it lasts for 6 to 12 months following the initial (acute) episode.
· Excess fluid in the pericardial sac impairs heart function.
· Pericardium becomes thick and scarred.
· Blood circulation problems.

 ## DIAGNOSIS & TREATMENT

GENERAL MEASURES

· Your health care provider will do a physical exam and ask questions about your symptoms and activities. Medical tests may include blood studies, chest x-ray, heart tests (electrocardiogram and echocardiogram), and others.
· Treatment is aimed at relieving symptoms and treating the underlying disorder. Treatment may include drugs and, sometimes, hospital care.
· Home care is usually sufficient.
· Hospital care may be needed if there are complications. A needle may be used to draw off excess fluid if it is causing problems for heart function. Rarely, surgery may be needed on the pericardium.
· Apply a heating pad or warm compresses to the chest to relieve pain.
· To learn more: American Heart Association, 7272 Greenville Ave., Dallas, TX 75231; (800) 242-8721; website: www.americanheart.org.

MEDICATIONS

· Nonsteroidal anti-inflammatory drugs to reduce pain and inflammation are usually prescribed.
· Steroid drugs for severe forms of pericarditis may be prescribed.
· Stronger pain drugs may be prescribed.
· Drugs to treat any infection (bacterial, fungal, etc.) will be prescribed.

ACTIVITY

· Rest in bed until fever and pain subside.
· Resume your normal activities gradually.
· Resume sexual relations once fever and pain are gone.

DIET

No special diet.

 ## NOTIFY OUR OFFICE IF

· You or a family member has symptoms of pericarditis.
· The following occur during treatment: Fever, shortness of breath and rapid heartbeat, cough (with blood), unexplained weight loss, or increased pain.

Special notes:

_____

_____

_____

More notes on the back of this page ☐

PERIODONTITIS
(Gum Inflammation)

 BASIC INFORMATION

DESCRIPTION

Inflammation and infection of the gums, causing loss of bone around the teeth. Periodontitis is responsible for more tooth loss than tooth decay. It can occur at any age, but is most common in adults.

FREQUENT SIGNS AND SYMPTOMS

- There may be no symptoms.
- Unpleasant taste in the mouth and bad breath.
- Bleeding of the gums.
- Loosening of teeth in the sockets.
- Aching teeth and gums when eating hot, cold, or sweet food.

CAUSES

Plaque (a sticky deposit of food, bacteria, and mucus) builds up on the teeth. It turns hard and becomes tartar (calculus). Bacteria in the plaque and tartar can cause a gum infection called gingivitis. If untreated, gingivitis infection spreads to the bones that support the teeth causing periodontitis. Pockets of infection occur around the roots of the teeth.

RISK INCREASES WITH

- Poor dental hygiene.
- Clenching or grinding teeth.
- Weak immune system due to illness or drugs.
- Smoking.
- Certain drugs.
- Pregnancy.
- Diabetes.
- Poor nutrition (not eating a healthy diet).
- Family history of gum disease.
- Tongue or lip piercing.

PREVENTIVE MEASURES

- Practice good oral hygiene daily. Visit your dental care provider on a regular basis for dental exams and cleaning of teeth to remove plaque and tartar.
- To brush teeth: Scrub the clear, sticky plaque off teeth daily with a soft toothbrush. A soft brush is less likely to damage teeth and gums than a hard brush. Place the brush at the gum line and gently rotate it, pointing the bristles toward the gum. Brush one section of teeth at a time.
- To floss teeth: Wind waxed or unwaxed dental floss around one finger on each hand. Force the dental floss between teeth. Gently clean the tooth surfaces with a back-and-forth, sawing motion at the gum line. Floss between all lower teeth, using your fingers as guides. Next, loosen the floss and place it on the tops of your thumbs. Floss between all upper teeth, using your thumbs as guides.

EXPECTED OUTCOMES

Usually curable with a combination of dental treatment and maintaining a good oral hygiene program.

POSSIBLE COMPLICATIONS

- Without treatment, teeth loosen so much that they may fall out or need to be removed.
- Recurrence of periodontitis.
- Tooth abscess (pus-filled area).
- Mouth infections.

 DIAGNOSIS & TREATMENT

GENERAL MEASURES

- Your dental care provider will do an exam of the teeth, gums, and supporting bones. X-rays may be done to check for any bone loss.
- Treatment may involve correcting dental problems, scaling, planing, and surgery. Your dental care provider will discuss a treatment plan with you.
- Dental work may be done for rough or jagged teeth.
- Dental appliances may need to be repaired.
- Scaling and root planing involves cleaning of deep pockets and smoothing the roots of the teeth.
- Gum surgery may be needed. Pockets of infection may need to be cut open and cleaned. Loose teeth may need to be removed. Bone and tissue grafts may be needed to help support the teeth.
- Dental implants may be recommended for lost teeth.
- To learn more: American Dental Association, 211 E. Chicago Ave., Chicago, IL 60611-2678; (800) 947-4746; website: www.ada.org.

MEDICATIONS

- For minor pain, you may use nonprescription drugs such as acetaminophen.
- Antibiotics may be prescribed for infection.

ACTIVITY

No limits.

DIET

No special diet.

 CALL YOUR DENTIST IF

You or a family member has symptoms of periodontitis.

Special notes:

_____

_____

_____

More notes on the back of this page ☐

PERIPHERAL NEUROPATHY

(Peripheral Neuritis)

BASIC INFORMATION

DESCRIPTION

A group of symptoms caused by damage to sensory nerves or motor nerves in the peripheral nervous system. This system is made up of nerves that branch out of the spinal cord and go to all parts of the body. Peripheral neuropathy usually affects the fingers, toes, hands, feet, lower arms, and legs. It may affect bladder or bowel control.

- Sensory nerve damage affects sensations (such as heat, cold, and pain). The sensations may be abnormal, decreased, or lacking.
- Motor nerve damage affects muscle movement or function. It results in muscle weakness, decreased movement, or loss of control of movement.

FREQUENT SIGNS AND SYMPTOMS

- Burning, tingling, and numbness in a localized area, frequently in the hands and feet.
- Shooting pain that is often worse at night. Pain is made worse by touch or temperature changes.
- Muscle weakness throughout the body on one or both sides. It is often in the same place on both sides.
- Painless ulcers on the toes or fingers.
- Pale, dry skin that becomes sensitive to touch.
- Severe back pain or loss of bladder or bowel control, if caused by back disk disease.

CAUSES

Damage may be from nerve destruction, pressure, or degeneration. The damage may be to one nerve or nerve group. Nerves become damaged due to a number of causes. Sometimes, no cause is found.

RISK INCREASES WITH

- Adults over 60.
- Exposure to certain chemicals or toxic substances.
- Certain drugs.
- Poor nutrition (not eating a healthy diet).
- Poor control of diabetes.
- Alcoholism.
- Family history of neuropathies.
- Nerve disorders, nerve injury, or pressure on nerves.
- Autoimmune disorder, or connective tissue disease.
- Infections, kidney or liver failure, and some cancers.
- Bone fractures or ruptured disk.
- Some hereditary disorders.

PREVENTIVE MEASURES

No specific preventive measures.

EXPECTED OUTCOMES

Mild cases may be cured if nerve damage is limited and the underlying cause is diagnosed and treated. More severe cases may be incurable, but treatment can often help symptoms improve.

POSSIBLE COMPLICATIONS

Complications can cause chronic pain, disability, and may sometimes be life-threatening.

DIAGNOSIS & TREATMENT

GENERAL MEASURES

- Your health care provider will do a physical exam and ask questions about your symptoms and activities. Medical tests may be done to discover any underlying medical disorder.
- The most important aspect of treatment is to identify any underlying cause and, if possible, treat it.
- Other treatments may include drugs, physical and occupational therapy, diet and exercise, assistive devices, relaxation techniques (such as biofeedback training), surgery to relieve pressure, and others.
- Your health care provider will discuss your diagnosis and a specific treatment plan with you. No one plan works for everyone.
- For self-care: Inspect hands and feet daily for unnoticed wounds. Keep feet clean and toenails trimmed properly. Wear shoes that fit well. Take measures to make your home a safe place for you.
- Surgery is helpful in some cases.

MEDICATIONS

- For minor pain, use nonprescription ibuprofen or acetaminophen. Other pain drugs may be prescribed.
- A variety of drugs can be used to treat the symptoms. Your health care provider will discuss the options and the risks and benefits.
- Drugs to treat underlying disorder may be prescribed.

ACTIVITY

Physical therapy and exercises to do at home may be recommended. If you have difficulty maintaining balance, walk with a cane or other support.

DIET

If poor nutrition is a cause, eat a healthy diet.

NOTIFY OUR OFFICE IF

- You or a family member has symptoms of peripheral neuropathy.
- Symptoms persist or worsen despite treatment.

Special notes:

_____

_____

_____

More notes on the back of this page ☐

PERITONITIS

 BASIC INFORMATION

DESCRIPTION
A serious inflammation of part or all of the lining of the abdominal cavity (peritoneum). The abdominal cavity contains such organs as the stomach, intestines, spleen, gallbladder, liver, appendix, kidneys, and pancreas.

FREQUENT SIGNS AND SYMPTOMS
- Pain in one area of, or all through, the abdomen. Pain usually starts suddenly and becomes more severe with time. Pain may be cramp-like at first and then steady. The patient often prefers to lie quietly on the back because movement or pressure on the abdomen increases pain.
- Shoulder pain (sometimes).
- Chills and fever (often high).
- Dizziness and weakness.
- Rapid heartbeat and rapid breathing.
- Low blood pressure.
- Nausea and vomiting.

CAUSES
The inflammation is a reaction to infection (most often), injury, or irritation of the abdominal lining. It can be caused by a number of different factors involving any of the organs in the abdomen.

RISK INCREASES WITH
- Infection inside the abdomen (e.g., appendicitis or bowel infection).
- Inflammation of the stomach, gallbladder, or pancreas.
- Penetrating injury to the abdominal wall, such as from a knife or bullet wound.
- Peptic ulcer.
- Pelvic inflammatory disease.
- Rupture of an ectopic pregnancy.
- Recent abdominal surgery.
- Bowel obstruction.
- Advanced liver disease.
- Hernia.
- Tuberculosis.
- Ovarian cyst or abscess.

PREVENTIVE MEASURES
No specific preventive measures. Get medical treatment for any disorder that could lead to peritonitis.

EXPECTED OUTCOMES
Usually curable with early diagnosis and treatment. Treatment delay and complications can be fatal. Outcome depends on age, length of illness, cause, and any pre-existing condition(s).

POSSIBLE COMPLICATIONS
- Shock.
- Blood poisoning (septicemia).
- Intestinal obstruction caused by adhesions (bands of scar tissue).
- Kidney or liver failure.

 DIAGNOSIS & TREATMENT

GENERAL MEASURES
- Your health care provider will do a physical exam and ask questions about your symptoms. Blood tests, x-rays, and other medical tests are usually done to help diagnose the underlying disorder.
- Hospital care is needed to treat this condition and any underlying disorder. You may require treatment for dehydration, breathing support, drugs injected into a vein (IV), blood transfusions, and surgery.
- Surgery may be needed to help diagnose the cause of the inflammation, and repair organ damage or injury.

MEDICATIONS
- Antibiotics to fight infection are usually prescribed.
- Pain relievers (sometimes) after diagnosis or surgery.

ACTIVITY
Rest in bed, after treatment, until symptoms disappear. If surgery is needed, resume your activities gradually after surgery.

DIET
While in the hospital, fluids and nutrients may be given through a vein. Oral feedings will resume when your system can tolerate them.

 NOTIFY OUR OFFICE IF

- You or a family member has symptoms of peritonitis. This is an emergency! Early diagnosis and treatment of the underlying disorder are essential.
- Any new symptoms occur after treatment.

Special notes:

_____

_____

_____

More notes on the back of this page ☐

PERSONALITY DISORDERS

 BASIC INFORMATION

DESCRIPTION

A group of conditions that are not illnesses, but ways of behaving. Each condition is defined by its main symptoms. Persons with these conditions have patterns of abnormal behavior, thought, and emotion. These patterns interfere with daily activity, personal relationships, and social and work functioning. The person feels their behavior patterns are "normal" and "right." The behaviors may lead to trouble with the law.

FREQUENT SIGNS AND SYMPTOMS

• Paranoid—Shows unwarranted suspiciousness and distrust of others; is defensive, oversensitive.
• Schizoid and schizotypal—Cold (emotionally); has difficulty forming relationships; is withdrawn, shy, superstitious, or socially isolated.
• Compulsive—Perfectionist, rigid in habits, indecisive; needs control.
• Histrionic—Dependent, immature, excitable, vain; constantly craves stimulation and attention; communicates by appearances or behavior (not verbally).
• Narcissistic—Has an exaggerated sense of one's own importance; is preoccupied with power; lacks interest in others; demands attention; feels entitled to special consideration.
• Avoidant—Fears and overreacts to rejection; has low self-esteem; is socially withdrawn; dependent.
• Dependent—Passive, overaccepting, unable to make decisions; lacks confidence.
• Passive-aggressive—Stubborn, sulking; fears authority; procrastinates; is chronically late, argumentative, helpless, clinging.
• Antisocial—Selfish, callous, promiscuous, impulsive, reckless; unable to learn from experience; fails at school and work.
• Borderline—Impulsive; has unstable and intense interpersonal relationships; displays inappropriate anger, fear, and guilt; lacks self-control; has identity problems; may self-mutilate (cut or burn oneself to relieve tension); is suicidal (sometimes).

CAUSES

Unknown. May be multiple factors, including genetics, type of parenting in childhood, one's own personality traits, and early social experiences (such as abuse).

RISK INCREASES WITH

• History of abuse as a child.
• Family history of mood disorders.

PREVENTIVE MEASURES

There are no specific preventive measures.

EXPECTED OUTCOME

Treatment can be effective for some patients, bringing about a gradual change in behavior. For others, prognosis is guarded; and for some, the outcome is poor.

POSSIBLE COMPLICATIONS

• Difficulty maintaining personal relationships and jobs; anxiety and depression.
• Drug and alcohol abuse.
• Noncompliance with treatment.
• Suicide.

 DIAGNOSIS & TREATMENT

GENERAL MEASURES

• Diagnostic measures may include observation of symptoms by other people. Diagnosis may include medical history, behavioral history, physical exam, and psychological evaluation by your health care provider.
• Treatment requires a trusting relationship between the therapist and patient. This can be difficult, as motivation for treatment often comes from someone other than the person with the disorder.
• Psychotherapy provides help with thoughts, feelings, and behavior. It may include:
  - Family and group therapy, group living situations, and self-help groups.
  - Behavior-changing techniques involve the learning of social skills, reinforcement of appropriate behavior, setting limits on inappropriate behavior, learning to express feelings, self-analysis of behavior, and accepting accountability for actions.

MEDICATIONS

• No drugs will cure a personality disorder. Drugs may be prescribed for treatment of specific symptoms:
  - Antidepressants or antianxiety drugs.
  - Antipsychotic drugs for psychoses.

ACTIVITY

No limits.

DIET

No special diet.

 NOTIFY OUR OFFICE IF

• You or a family member has symptoms of a personality disorder.
• Symptoms continue or worsen during treatment.

Special notes:

_____

_____

_____

More notes on the back of this page ☐

PHARYNGITIS

 BASIC INFORMATION

DESCRIPTION
Inflammation or infection of the pharynx. The pharynx is the hollow passage at the back of the throat. It is made up of the nasopharynx, which leads to the nose and oropharynx which leads to the mouth. The larynx (voice box) is located below the pharynx. Pharyngitis occurs in all age groups, but most often affects children.

FREQUENT SIGNS AND SYMPTOMS
- Sore throat.
- Swallowing difficulty.
- Tickle or "lump" in the throat.
- Fever.
- Swollen glands in the neck (sometimes).
- Throat may be red or covered with a white or grayish membrane (sometimes).
- Body aches (sometimes).

CAUSES
Viral infection (most common cause) or bacterial infection (such as streptococcus). The germs are spread by person-to-person contact. Rarely, there may be other causes, such as irritation.

RISK INCREASES WITH
- Common cold, flu, or seasonal allergies.
- Weak immune system due to illness or drugs.
- Smoking or second-hand smoke.
- Chronic illness, such as diabetes.
- Close quarters, such as with military recruits, in schools, and daycare centers.

PREVENTIVE MEASURES
- Avoid close contact with anyone with a sore throat.
- Avoid germs. Wash hands often, especially children.

EXPECTED OUTCOMES
Most cases of viral infection clear up on their own in a week. Antibiotic drugs can successfully treat bacterial infections. Complications are rare.

POSSIBLE COMPLICATIONS
- Airways may become blocked.
- Abscess (pus-filled area of infection).
- Rheumatic fever, scarlet fever, or glomerulonephritis, if pharyngitis is caused by streptococcal bacteria and does not receive adequate antibiotic treatment.

 DIAGNOSIS & TREATMENT

GENERAL MEASURES
- Your health care provider will do an exam of the throat, ears, nose, neck, and lungs. Medical tests may include blood study and throat culture (from a swab of the throat), or rapid strep test find the type of infection.
- Treatment will include self-care measures and antibiotic drugs for bacterial infections. Antibiotics will not help viral infections.
- To relieve the sore throat, gargle frequently with warm or cold double-strength tea or warm salt water (mix one-half teaspoon of salt in one cup of water).
- Wash hands often to help prevent the spread of germs to other family members. Avoid kissing or sharing cups or other utensils.

MEDICATIONS
- For minor discomfort, you may use nonprescription drugs such as ibuprofen. Don't give aspirin to a child.
- Nonprescription throat lozenges (for patients over age 3) may help ease discomfort.
- Antibiotic drugs are usually prescribed for bacterial infection. Finish entire course of drugs even if symptoms improve.

ACTIVITY
Return to normal activities as symptoms improve. A person can no longer spread the germs if they have taken the antibiotic drug for at least 24 hours.

DIET
Drink plenty of fluids. If swallowing solid food is painful, try a liquid or soft diet for a few days.

 NOTIFY OUR OFFICE IF

- You or a family member has symptoms of pharyngitis.
- The following occur during treatment:
  - Breathing/swallowing difficulty or chest pain.
  - Fever worsens or severe headache develops.
  - Thick mucus drainage from the nose.
  - Cough that produces colored or bloody sputum.
  - Skin rash.
  - Dark urine.

Special notes:

_____

_____

_____

More notes on the back of this page ☐

PHEOCHROMOCYTOMA

 ## BASIC INFORMATION

DESCRIPTION

A rare type of tumor of the adrenal glands. There are two adrenal glands, each located above a kidney. They produce hormones for important body functions. The tumor usually affects one adrenal gland. In some cases, it may develop outside the glands. This type of tumor is most often benign (90%), but can be cancerous. It affects adults of both sexes, usually ages 30 to 50.

FREQUENT SIGNS AND SYMPTOMS

• Episodes of at least some of these symptoms may occur several times a day or may occur less often (up to 2 months apart). Symptoms increase as tumor grows.
• High blood pressure episodes.
• Severe headaches.
• Rapid heartbeat following exercise, emotional upset, or exposure to cold.
• Tremors and nervousness.
• Feelings of doom.
• Feelings of hunger.
• Episodes of flushing.
• Sweating, paleness.
• Weakness and fatigue.
• Unexplained weight loss.
• Nausea and vomiting.

CAUSES

Hormones produced by adrenal glands work with the central nervous system to control heart rate, blood pressure, and other vital body functions. When a tumor (the pheochromocytoma) exists, even though it is benign, excess hormones are produced. The excess hormones cause symptoms. Cause of the tumor is unknown.

RISK INCREASES WITH

• Unknown for most cases.
• A disorder called multiple endocrine neoplasia (MEN) syndrome.

PREVENTIVE MEASURES

No specific preventive measures.

EXPECTED OUTCOMES

The outlook is generally good for those with benign tumors removed by surgery. For those tumors that are cancerous, the outlook is more guarded.

POSSIBLE COMPLICATIONS

• Tumor may recur.
• Stroke, caused by very high blood pressure.
• High blood pressure may continue after surgery. It can be treated with drugs.
• Kidney, brain, heart damage, and death caused by unrecognized and untreated pheochromocytoma.

 ## DIAGNOSIS & TREATMENT

GENERAL MEASURES

• Your health care provider will do a physical exam. Medical tests may include studies of urine and blood to measure hormone production, x-ray, CT, MRI, and other tests. These help diagnose the tumor and also determine if it is benign or cancer and any spread of the cancer.
• Treatment will depend on the diagnosis. It may include surgery, chemotherapy (anticancer drugs), and radiation.
• Surgery is usually done to remove the tumor.

MEDICATIONS

• Drugs are sometimes prescribed before surgery to suppress the effect of hormones.
• Drugs to treat high blood pressure may be needed.
• Anticancer drugs may be prescribed.

ACTIVITY

No limits after recovery from surgery.

DIET

Prior to surgery, a high-salt diet may be recommended to increase blood volume.

 ## NOTIFY OUR OFFICE IF

• You or a family member has symptoms of pheochromocytoma.
• Symptoms recur after treatment.

Special notes:

_____

_____

_____

More notes on the back of this page ☐

PHOBIAS

BASIC INFORMATION

DESCRIPTION

• A type of anxiety disorder involving intense and/or unrealistic fears. The fears may involve an object, situation, activity, event, or even a bodily function.

• When fears are real (due to danger or a threat to life), the body's alarm system switches on and is ready to help protect us. With phobias, this alarm system switches on when there is no real threat or danger. Phobias can cause minor or major problems in a person's life. Most people with phobias recognize that the fear is not appropriate to the situation. Phobias are classified as:

- Social–fear of embarrassment in social situations, such as public speaking or using a public bathroom.
- Agoraphobia–fear of being in crowds or fear of public places.
- Specific (simple)–fear of a specific object or situation, such as animals, insects, heights, flying, or closed places.

FREQUENT SIGNS AND SYMPTOMS

• The following anxiety symptoms occur when exposed to, or thinking of the phobic stimulus:
- Palpitations (irregular and rapid heartbeat).
- Desire to flee.
- Sweating, tremors.
- Flushing.
- Nausea.
- Negative thoughts and scary images.

CAUSES

Exact cause is unknown. It may involve genetics, family influence, traumatic events, medical conditions, or imbalance of certain brain chemicals.

RISK INCREASES WITH

• Family history of anxiety.
• Persons with other anxiety disorders.
• Women more than men.

PREVENTIVE MEASURES

No specific preventive measures to prevent the phobia. After diagnosis, treatment can help prevent or control the reaction.

EXPECTED OUTCOME

• Specific phobias–some stop on their own as the person ages. Others do not cause any problems if the object can be avoided (such as snakes). Some get better as people go through their fearful situations (such as flying). Others can be cured or helped with treatment.

• Social phobias–usually can be resolved with treatment. Drugs are often helpful.

• Agoraphobia–it is more difficult to treat because the person has so many fears, but treatment can help.

POSSIBLE COMPLICATIONS

• Limits in lifestyle due to avoiding the phobic stimulus. Agoraphobia, especially, restricts an person's activities and is severely disabling.

• Overuse of drugs or alcohol to relieve anxiety.

DIAGNOSIS & TREATMENT

GENERAL MEASURES

• Your health care provider will usually do a physical exam and ask about your symptoms and activities. Medical tests may be done to rule out other disorders.

• Treatment may involve psychotherapy, drug therapy, and self-help methods. No treatment may be needed if the phobia is not interfering with daily life.

• Cognitive-behavioral therapy may help. Cognitive therapy teaches how to change thoughts, behaviors or attitudes. Behavioral therapy teaches ways to reduce anxiety with deep breathing and muscle relaxation.

• Self-help suggestions if you feel your fear taking hold:
- Shift your thought from the negative ("The dog will bite") to one that is real and positive ("The dog is on a leash").
- Do something you can control–count backward from 1000, read a book, talk aloud, or take deep, measured breaths.
- Shift your thoughts to pleasant ones.
- Practice relaxation techniques.

• Joining a support group is helpful for some patients.

• To learn more: Anxiety Disorders Association of America, 8730 Georgia Ave., Suite 600, Silver Spring, MD 20910; (240) 485-1001 (not toll free); website: www.adaa.org.

MEDICATION

Drugs are sometimes helpful. Your health care provider will discuss the options, the risks, and benefits.

ACTIVITY

No limits.

DIET

No special diet. Avoid caffeine and alcohol.

NOTIFY OUR OFFICE IF

• You or a family member has symptoms of a phobia.
• Symptoms of the phobia return after treatment.

Special notes:

_____

_____

_____

More notes on the back of this page ☐

PHOTOSENSITIVITY
(Sun Poisoning)

BASIC INFORMATION

DESCRIPTION
Skin that reacts abnormally to light. A reaction may occur after only a few minutes of exposure. This is likely to be a problem for those taking part in hot-season sports such as swimming, surfing, sailing, tennis, or water skiing. The most common form is called polymorphous light eruption (PMLE), or sun poisoning.

FREQUENT SIGNS AND SYMPTOMS
· Red or pink skin rash, sometimes with small blisters, in areas exposed to sunlight.
· Rash may itch or burn.

CAUSES
Symptoms are triggered by exposure to sun (ultraviolet light). It is not known why the body develops this reaction. The sunlight exposure may come through glass (such as in an automobile) or thin clothing. Some people react to winter daylight as well. Tanning booths are a source of ultraviolet light.

RISK INCREASES WITH
· Use of drugs, herbs, or products that cause increased sensitivity to ultraviolet light. The most common drugs include tetracycline antibiotics, thiazide diuretics, antihistamines, sulfa drugs, nonsteroidal anti-inflammatory drugs, and birth control pills. The herb St. John's Wort can also cause the problem.
· Some sunscreens and some cosmetics, including lipstick, perfume, and soaps.
· Skin disorders such as porphyria.
· Previous episodes of photosensitivity.
· Systemic lupus erythematosus (an immune disorder).
· Weak immune system due to drugs or illness.

PREVENTIVE MEASURES
· Stay out of the sun when possible if you have a history of photosensitivity. Avoid tanning booths.
· Wear dark colored clothing that is tightly woven when in sunlight. Wear a hat with a wide brim.
· Sunscreen may help. Use with care. Some sunscreens cause a reaction in photosensitive persons.
· Avoid the drugs or products known to cause photosensitivity. Not all individuals who use these drugs will have a photosensitive reaction. Also, a reaction will be different in different people. A person may have a one time reaction and not experience it again.

EXPECTED OUTCOMES
In most cases, it takes up to 1 week for recovery if further sun exposure is avoided. If a drug or other product is the problem, symptoms usually stop after it is discontinued. In other photosensitivity cases, symptoms may come and go depending on sun exposure.

POSSIBLE COMPLICATIONS
Chronic rash and other symptoms when exposed to the sun—even for short periods—especially in spring and summer.

DIAGNOSIS & TREATMENT

GENERAL MEASURES
· Many people with mild symptoms may self-treat.
· See your health care provider if you have concerns about the symptoms or they are severe. A physical exam of the affected skin area will be done. Questions will be asked about your sun exposure, products you use, and drugs that you take. A medical test may be done to check your skin's reaction to ultraviolet light.
· Switching temporarily to different drugs or skin care products may be recommended. This will help determine a cause for the reaction.
· Apply cool, moist compresses to the affected area.
· Stay out of the sun during the hours of strongest ultraviolet light (10 a.m. to 2 p.m.).
· In some cases, phototherapy may be prescribed. This treatment (done in a medical office) gradually exposes your skin to ultraviolet light. This is done over several weeks and helps to lessen the skin's sensitivity.
· PUVA therapy may be recommended. This treatment involves use of a drug, along with ultraviolet light.

MEDICATIONS
· You may use aspirin (if over age 18), acetaminophen, or an antihistamine to relieve mild pain or itching.
· Beta-carotene taken orally helps some people.
· Your health care provider may prescribe steroid drugs for severe cases, or other drugs which can reduce the photosensitivity.

ACTIVITY
No limits, except to avoid prolonged sun exposure.

DIET
No special diet. Drink extra fluids.

NOTIFY OUR OFFICE IF

· You or a family member has symptoms of photosensitivity.
· Symptoms don't improve even with treatment.

Special notes:

_____

_____

_____

More notes on the back of this page ☐

PICA

 ## BASIC INFORMATION

DESCRIPTION

Craving, eating, or mouthing items that are not food. Pica can occur in adults, but usually affects children between ages 2 and 6, and persons with developmental disorders. Pica does not apply to infants 18 months to 2 years old who "put everything" in the mouth. That is normal.

FREQUENT SIGNS AND SYMPTOMS

- Eating non-food substances, such as starch, clay, ice, plaster, paint, cigarette ashes, hair, gravel, chalk, needles, string, pencil erasers, and others.
- Stomach pain (sometimes).

CAUSES

The exact cause is unknown. Factors that may contribute to the cause include physical, emotional, nutritional, family, social, economic, and cultural factors.

RISK INCREASES WITH

- Family history of pica.
- Poor nutrition or a vitamin deficiency.
- Poverty.
- Developmental disorders.
- Anemia.
- Pregnancy.
- Cultures where clay eating is a common practice.
- People on diets who try to ease hunger with nonfood items.

PREVENTIVE MEASURES

There are no specific preventive measures. To reduce risks, provide a well-balanced diet for yourself and your children.

EXPECTED OUTCOMES

- It may go on for years with no harmful effects.
- It may stop on its own in a few months.
- In some cases, it can be helped with treatment.
- For others, it may continue (even with treatment) into the teenage years. This occurs more often with developmental disorders.
- Pica during pregnancy usually ends with childbirth.

POSSIBLE COMPLICATIONS

- Lead poisoning from paint or plaster.
- Intestinal infections from parasites in soil.
- Anemia.
- Malnutrition (not getting enough nutrients).
- Intestinal obstruction.

 ## DIAGNOSIS & TREATMENT

GENERAL MEASURES

- Your health care provider will usually do a physical exam. Medical tests may include blood studies, x-rays, and other tests to rule out medical disorders. There is no diagnostic test for pica.
- Treatment usually includes behavior and diet changes, if needed. Several different types of behavioral training are used to treat pica. Your health care provider will discuss the options with you depending on your individual situation.
- Childproof your home by removing nonfood substances the child is eating. Repaint homes in which lead-base paints have been used. Don't use older baby cribs painted with lead-base paint.

MEDICATIONS

Drugs are usually not needed for this disorder.

ACTIVITY

No limits.

DIET

A well-balanced diet will be prescribed. A dietitian may help plan meals if any nutritional deficiency is diagnosed.

 ## NOTIFY OUR OFFICE IF

- You or a family member has symptoms of pica.
- You are pregnant and have symptoms of pica.
- Pica does not improve in 2 weeks, despite treatment.

Special notes:

_____

_____

_____

More notes on the back of this page ☐

PILONIDAL DISEASE

 ## BASIC INFORMATION

DESCRIPTION

An infection in the skin, just above the crease of the buttocks. It starts with a pilonidal cyst (a sac) under the skin. The cyst can becomes infected and form an abscess (pus-filled area). An opening (sinus) may also develop that goes from the abscess to the outside skin. The disease affects both sexes, but is more common in males, from teenagers to age 40.

FREQUENT SIGNS AND SYMPTOMS

· Symptoms may go unnoticed in mild cases.
· Pain, redness, tenderness, and swelling in the area.
· Fever and chills.
· Discharge of pus.
· Sitting or walking may be difficult.

CAUSES

It was thought for many years that people were born with the cysts. Now the theory is that they are acquired. There is still much unknown about them. In some cases, hairs growing inside the cyst may lead to infection. In other cases, no hair is found in the cyst and the cause is unknown.

RISK INCREASES WITH

· Obesity.
· Men more than women.
· Family history of pilonidal disease.
· Sedentary lifestyle (lack of exercise).
· Repeated trauma (injury) to the tailbone area.
· Work that requires a lot of sitting.
· Activities such as biking or motorcycle riding that can cause sweating and friction to the tailbone area.
· Heavy growth of body hair.

PREVENTIVE MEASURES

· Bathe or shower daily to keep the area clean. Warm tub baths seem more effective in preventing infection of the cyst than showers.
· Avoid risk factors where possible.

EXPECTED OUTCOMES

Mild cases may need no treatment. In cases of abscess or recurrence of the disease, treatment can help. Healing time may take weeks to months, depending on treatment procedure.

POSSIBLE COMPLICATIONS

The disease recurs in about 40% of the patients after the initial treatment. It may clear up on its own after age 40.

 ## DIAGNOSIS & TREATMENT

GENERAL MEASURES

· Your health care provider will do a physical exam of the cyst. Medical tests may include blood studies and a culture of the discharge from the cyst.
· Treatment may involve self-care, incision and drainage of the cyst, drugs, and surgery. Your health care provider will discuss the options with you.
· Treatment may not be needed for mild disease. Use extra care in keeping that area of the body clean. You may be advised to shave or use a hair remover product to keep the area free of hair. Soaking in a tub of warm water may help if there is discomfort or pain.
· Incision and drainage may be recommended. This involves opening the cyst so that any hair or pus can be removed. The opening is then packed with gauze. Healing may take several weeks.
· Surgical removal (excision) of the cyst or sinus may be recommended. Several different surgical methods can be used. Healing time will depend on the procedure. You will be advised about follow-up home care.

MEDICATIONS

Antibiotics may be prescribed for infection.

ACTIVITY

No limits, unless the cyst becomes infected. Then, limit activities until the infection is cured. Use a special doughnut cushion if sitting is uncomfortable.

DIET

No special diet.

 ## NOTIFY OUR OFFICE IF

· You or a family member has symptoms of a pilonidal disease.
· Symptoms recur after treatment.

Special notes:

_____

_____

_____

More notes on the back of this page ☐

PINWORMS

(Enterobiasis; Seatworm; Threadworm; Oxyuriasis)

 ## BASIC INFORMATION

DESCRIPTION
Infestation with intestinal parasites, a common occurrence in children. Pinworms are more a nuisance than a major health problem. The body parts involved are the cecum and other portions of the large and small intestine, the anus, and the skin around the anus.

FREQUENT SIGNS AND SYMPTOMS
- Some people may be infected and have no symptoms.
- Skin irritation and painful itching around the anus, especially during sleep.
- Restless sleep.
- Vaginal discharge, itching and discomfort if pinworms migrate into the vaginal opening.

CAUSES
- Infestation of the intestine by a very small worm about 1/4 to 1/2 inch long. Pinworms travel from the intestine to the rectum to lay eggs around the anus and buttocks. If a person scratches the area, the eggs can get under the fingernails and be passed to anything or anyone that person touches.
- Pinworms are easy to catch from someone who is infected. Eggs are passed to others on toilet seats or by hand-to-hand or hand-to-mouth contact. They may drift in the air, where they are inhaled or swallowed. Eggs hatch and the larvae travel to the large intestine, where they mature, mate, and repeat the cycle.

RISK INCREASES WITH
Groups of children, as in daycare, school, or at camps.

PREVENTIVE MEASURES
- Wash hands carefully before meals and after using the toilet.
- Keep the nails short and clean.
- Bathe daily, right after waking up. This helps rid the body of any eggs before they can be spread.
- Have children wear clean underwear and pajamas daily.
- Don't scratch the anus or put fingers near the nose or mouth.
- Vacuum children's play area frequently.
- Wash bedding and pajamas on a regular basis.

EXPECTED OUTCOMES
The infection is curable in two weeks with treatment. If worms reappear soon after treatment, it usually means a new infection, not treatment failure. A second treatment can be effective.

POSSIBLE COMPLICATIONS
No serious complications expected.

 ## DIAGNOSIS & TREATMENT

GENERAL MEASURES
- You may help diagnose the pinworms yourself.
- They look like small pieces of white or yellow thread.
- They may sometimes be seen on a child's stool.
- Since they are active at night, check your child a few hours after bedtime. Shine a flashlight on the rectal area and you may see the worms in action.
- Perform a tape test for the eggs:
  - Your health care provider may give you a tongue depressor with clear tape on it and a glass slide. If you do not have this, use your own clear (scotch) tape.
  - Place tape against your child's anal skin first thing in the morning (before washing or activity) to collect eggs.
  - Then place the sticky side of the tongue depressor tape on the glass slide. If your own tape was used, place it in a plastic bag and seal it.
  - Take slide or bag to the medical office for viewing under a microscope to check for pinworm eggs.
- Once the pinworm diagnosis is confirmed, the infection is usually treated with a drug to kill the worms. All family members should be treated even if they have no symptoms.
- On the day of treatment, wash sheets, towels, and clothing, especially bedclothes, in hot water. Cut and clean fingernails.

MEDICATIONS
- A two-dose course of an antiworm drug is usually prescribed. The second dose is taken 2 weeks after the first dose.
- Nonprescription creams or lotions to relieve itching may be helpful.

ACTIVITY
No limits.

DIET
No special diet.

 ## NOTIFY OUR OFFICE IF

- Anyone in your family has symptoms of pinworms.
- Pinworms reappear after treatment.

Special notes:

_____

_____

_____

More notes on the back of this page ☐

PITUITARY GLAND, UNDERACTIVE
(Hypopituitarism)

 BASIC INFORMATION

DESCRIPTION
The pituitary is a small, dime-sized gland located just below the brain. It works with the hypothalamus in the brain to regulate body functions. Hormones released by the pituitary are used in many of these functions. An underactive pituitary fails to release enough of one or more of these hormones. If all hormones are absent, it is called panhypopituitarism. Hormones include:
- Growth hormone—for growth of tissue and bones.
- Prolactin hormone—for female breast development and milk production.
- Thyroid-stimulating hormone—used by the thyroid gland for metabolism functions.
- Adrenocorticotropic hormone—used by the adrenal gland to control blood pressure.
- Luteinizing hormone and follicle-stimulating hormones—control sexual function in males and females.
- Antidiuretic hormone—affects the kidneys in the production of urine.
- Oxytocin—for contractions of the uterus during childbirth and the release of milk during breast-feeding.

FREQUENT SIGNS AND SYMPTOMS
- Decrease in appetite and weight loss.
- Abdominal pain; nausea.
- More sensitive to cold or heat.
- Persistent headaches.
- Mental changes.
- Changes in vision.
- Women may have menstrual period changes, failure to produce milk, hot flashes, and infertility.
- Men may have decreased sexual interest.
- Severe thirst and lack of urination.
- Failure of growth (seen after age 6 months).
- Lack of secondary sexual features that develop in puberty. These include voice changes, breast development, and growth of pubic hair.

CAUSES
Usually caused by disorders that affect the pituitary, the hypothalamus, or surrounding structures. Sometimes the cause is unknown.

RISK INCREASES WITH
- Tumors.
- Head injury.
- Infection (tuberculosis, syphilis, or meningitis).
- Blocked blood supply to the pituitary.
- Immune system problem.
- Pregnancy and delivery.
- Radiation or surgery.
- Congenital defect (a problem present since birth).

PREVENTIVE MEASURES
None specific. Obtain medical care for any risk factors.

EXPECTED OUTCOMES
It is usually a lifelong disorder. Outcome is generally favorable if an underlying disorder is successfully treated and hormone-replacement therapy is continued.

POSSIBLE COMPLICATIONS
Hormonal failure and possible death without treatment. Other complications depend on the underlying cause.

 DIAGNOSIS & TREATMENT

GENERAL MEASURES
- Your health care provider will do a physical exam and ask about your symptoms and activities. Medical tests may include blood studies of hormone levels and hormone function. CT or MRI scans may be done.
- Treatment is aimed at treating the cause of the pituitary failure (which may include drugs or surgery) and hormone replacement as needed.
- Surgery to remove underlying tumors or blood clots, if needed.
- Wear a medical alert-type bracelet or neck pendant indicating your hormone deficiencies and their proper treatment.

MEDICATIONS
- Hormones are usually prescribed to replace those the pituitary is not producing.
- Drugs may be prescribed for treatment of an underlying disorder.

ACTIVITY
Stay as active as your condition allows.

DIET
No special diet.

 NOTIFY OUR OFFICE IF

- You or a family member has symptoms of an underactive pituitary gland.
- After surgery, signs of infection develop, such as fever, lethargy, and muscle aches.
- New, unexplained symptoms develop. Drugs used in treatment may produce side effects.

Special notes:

_____

_____

_____

More notes on the back of this page ☐

PITUITARY TUMOR

 ## BASIC INFORMATION

DESCRIPTION
• The pituitary is a small, dime-sized gland located just below the brain. It works with the hypothalamus to regulate body functions from within the brain. Hormones released by the pituitary are used in many of these functions. Pituitary tumors are usually benign (noncancerous) tumors called adenomas. Other, less-common types may be cancerous. Tumors are also classed as functioning (producing hormones) or nonfunctioning (not producing hormones). Pituitary tumors can affect both sexes and all ages, but are more common in ages 30 to 50. Hormones released by the pituitary include:
• Growth hormone–for growth of tissue and bones.
• Prolactin hormone–for female breast development and milk production.
• Thyroid-stimulating hormone–used by the thyroid gland for metabolism functions.
• Adrenocorticotropic hormone–used by the adrenal gland to control blood pressure.
• Luteinizing hormone and follicle stimulating hormones–control sexual function in males and females.
• Antidiuretic hormone–affects the kidneys in the production of urine.
• Oxytocin–for contractions of the uterus during childbirth and the release of milk during breast-feeding.

FREQUENT SIGNS AND SYMPTOMS
• Symptoms may occur due to tumor growth. It can put pressure on eye nerves causing vision problems, headaches, and other symptoms.
• Numerous symptoms may occur due to an over-production or under-production of any of the hormones listed above. No symptoms are specific for diagnosing a tumor. Often, symptoms may go unnoticed, fail to cause alarm, or be attributed to another illness.

CAUSES
Unknown. Some types are part of a hereditary disorder.

RISK INCREASES WITH
Unknown.

PREVENTIVE MEASURES
No specific preventive measures.

EXPECTED OUTCOMES
Outcome will depend on the type of tumor, and the patient's age and general health status. Early diagnosis and treatment offer the most favorable outcome.

POSSIBLE COMPLICATIONS
• Spread of the tumor to other parts of the brain.
• Blindness due to pressure from tumor.
• Recurrence of tumor after treatment.

 ## DIAGNOSIS & TREATMENT

GENERAL MEASURES
• Your health care provider will do a physical exam and ask about your symptoms. Medical tests may include cerebrospinal fluid and blood studies, x-rays of the skull, CT scan or MRI of the brain, and vision tests.
• Treatment may involve a combination of surgery to remove the tumor, radiation treatment, hormone therapy, or other drugs.
• Different types of surgery are used to treat the tumors. The procedure depends on the type of tumor, its location and its size. Your health care provider will explain the options with you.
• Radiation therapy may be used in combination with surgery. It may also be used for people who, for medical reasons, are not able to have surgery.
• Wear a medical alert-type bracelet or neck pendant indicating your hormone deficiencies and their proper treatment.

MEDICATIONS
• Pain relievers may be prescribed.
• Hormone-replacement drugs may be prescribed. They may require frequent dosage adjustments.
• Drugs may be prescribed that reduce hormone production.
• Anticancer drugs may be prescribed.

ACTIVITY
Resume your normal activities gradually after surgery.

DIET
No special diet.

 ## NOTIFY OUR OFFICE IF

• You or a family member has symptoms of a pituitary tumor.
• The following occur after surgery:
  - Bleeding at the surgical site.
  - Signs of general infection, such as fever, chills, headache, and muscle aches.
  - Clear discharge from the nose.
  - There is a recurrence of any symptoms.

Special notes:

_____

_____

_____

More notes on the back of this page ☐

PITYRIASIS ALBA

 BASIC INFORMATION

DESCRIPTION
A common disorder of the skin. It causes a temporary loss of pigmentation (coloring) in patches found usually on the cheeks and sometimes, the neck and shoulders. *Pityriasis* means "scaly" and *alba* means "white" in Latin. It occurs mostly in children, but may appear in adults up to ages 20 to 30.

FREQUENT SIGNS AND SYMPTOMS
· Small white or light-pink patches with vague borders. They sometimes have pinpoint-sized white papules (small, raised bumps). Patches feel smooth.
· Patches are most apparent in summer because the areas do not tan. Tanning increases the contrast between the areas.
· There may be 1 to 20 patches at a time.
· Patches may itch occasionally, but they are not painful.

CAUSES
Unknown. The tendency may be inherited.

RISK INCREASES WITH
· Family history of allergies of any kind.
· Skin that us extra dry and sun exposure may be risk factors.

PREVENTIVE MEASURES
No specific preventive measures.

EXPECTED OUTCOMES
Patches may come and go for years. Between ages 20 and 30, they disappear completely.

POSSIBLE COMPLICATIONS
None expected.

 DIAGNOSIS & TREATMENT

GENERAL MEASURES
· Your health care provider can usually diagnose the disorder by an exam of the affected skin. Medical tests are generally not needed.
· No truly effective therapy is available. Some skin-care products may help the dry skin.
· Use sunscreen and protective clothing to prevent sunburn in affected areas.

MEDICATIONS
· Moisturizers may improve roughness or dryness, but do not improve the color.
· Prescription or nonprescription topical steroid drug(s) to control itching may be recommended.

ACTIVITY
No limits.

DIET
No special diet.

NOTIFY OUR OFFICE IF

You or a family member has symptoms of pityriasis alba.

Special notes:

_____

_____

_____

More notes on the back of this page ☐

PITYRIASIS ROSEA

 BASIC INFORMATION

DESCRIPTION

A common skin disorder with a faint rash that lasts weeks to months. *Pityriasis* means "scaly" and *rosea* means "pink" in Latin. It affects all ages, but is most common in adolescents and young adults. Women are affected more often than men are.

FREQUENT SIGNS AND SYMPTOMS

· A faint rash (often found in skin creases) of oval or round, pale-pink or light-brown areas. One larger patch (the "herald patch") may appear first. They may evolve into a "Christmas tree" pattern on the chest or back.
· Mild fatigue.
· Itching, usually mild.
· Occasional slight fever and headache.

CAUSES

Unknown, but may be caused by a virus or autoimmune disorder. It does not appear to be highly contagious (easily spread from one person to another).

RISK INCREASES WITH

· Fall and spring seasons.
· Weak immune system due to illness or drugs.

PREVENTIVE MEASURES

Cannot be prevented at present.

EXPECTED OUTCOMES

Pityriasis rosea usually runs its natural course in 5 weeks to 4 months. No drug or treatment is available to shorten its course, but itching and discomfort can be relieved. New rash areas continue to break out for several weeks. Once over, it is unlikely to recur.

POSSIBLE COMPLICATIONS

· Affected skin areas may have color changes in darker-skinned persons.
· Rarely, bacterial infection may occur in affected skin.

 DIAGNOSIS & TREATMENT

GENERAL MEASURES

· Your health care provider can usually diagnose the disorder by an exam of the affected skin. Medical tests may include blood studies. A scraping of the skin or a sample of the skin may be removed for viewing under a microscope.
· No specific treatment will cure the disorder.
· Treatment can help relieve the itching. In more severe cases, treatment with ultraviolet light or moderate exposure to sunlight may be recommended.
· Bathe as usual with a mild soap. Use warm water, as hot water may increase the itching. Oatmeal baths may help.

MEDICATIONS

· For minor discomfort, you may use nonprescription drugs, such as:
   - Calamine lotion, to decrease itching.
   - Steroid cream, to control more severe itching.
   - Acetaminophen, to reduce fever.
· Other topical or oral steroids and antihistamines may be prescribed.

ACTIVITY

Avoid activities that cause excess sweating. This can make the rash worse.

DIET

No special diet.

 NOTIFY OUR OFFICE IF

You or a family member has symptoms of pityriasis rosea.

Special notes:

_____

_____

_____

More notes on the back of this page ☐

374

PLACENTA PREVIA

 ## BASIC INFORMATION

DESCRIPTION

The placenta normally attaches high on the uterus wall, away from the cervix. In placenta previa, the placenta is covering or near the cervical opening (os). It can block the cervical opening to the vagina (birth canal). Placenta previa carries a risk of excessive bleeding, which can threaten the well-being of the mother and the baby. A low-lying placenta diagnosed in early pregnancy usually self-corrects as the uterus enlarges. Types of placenta previa include:

- Total placenta previa: The placenta completely covers the opening of the cervix. This type presents the most serious risk to the mother.
- Partial placenta previa: The placenta partially covers the opening of the cervix.
- Marginal placenta previa: The placenta just reaches the cervix.

FREQUENT SIGNS AND SYMPTOMS

- Sudden, painless bleeding during the second or third trimester of pregnancy. Bleeding may be mild at the start and become severe. Bleeding may not occur until after labor begins in some cases.
- Cramping may occur in some patients.

CAUSES

The exact cause of placenta previa is unknown. There may be a number of factors involved.

RISK INCREASES IN/WITH

- Previous uterine surgery involving the lining of the uterus. This includes dilation and curettage (D & C) and cesarean section.
- Smoking.
- Prior induced abortion.
- Multiple previous pregnancies and births.
- Pregnancy with twins or other multiples.
- Mothers over age 35.
- Previous placenta previa.

PREVENTIVE MEASURES

Placenta previa cannot be prevented. Good prenatal care during pregnancy can help identify it early.

EXPECTED OUTCOME

With prompt care, the outcome for mothers and term infants is good. Outcome for premature baby will depend on number of weeks of gestation and the baby's condition at birth.

POSSIBLE COMPLICATIONS

- Poor fetal growth, due to an abnormal placenta providing a decrease in blood flow and oxygen delivery.
- Premature delivery, or (possibly) fetal death.
- Rarely, blood loss could lead to maternal shock and death.

 ## DIAGNOSIS & TREATMENT

GENERAL MEASURES

- If bleeding occurs, medical tests may include blood studies and ultrasound to determine the exact location of the placenta. Rarely, a vaginal exam may be done.
- Treatment will depend on the type of previa, amount of bleeding, fetal age, condition and presentation, and the presence or absence of labor.
- Hospital care that includes blood transfusions, intravenous (IV) fluids, and oxygen may be needed with severe bleeding.
- If the bleeding is heavy or the pregnancy is at term, delivery is usually done. There may be a trial of labor for vaginal delivery or a cesarean delivery.
- If the pregnancy is between 34 and 37 weeks and the mother and fetus are stable, amniocentesis may be done to check fetal lung maturity. With mature lungs, the newborn will not need breathing support.
- If the baby's lungs are immature or the pregnancy is less than 34 weeks, the treatment may involve medical observation for a period. You may be placed on bed rest at home. Follow your obstetric provider's instructions carefully.

MEDICATION

- Steroids may be prescribed to help fetal lungs mature.
- Drugs to delay labor may be used in some cases.

ACTIVITY

Rest in bed until bleeding stops or you deliver your child. Avoid sexual intercourse or douching.

DIET

No special diet.

 ## NOTIFY OUR OFFICE IF

You or a family member has symptoms of placenta previa. Report any bleeding immediately. This is an emergency!

Special notes:

_____

_____

_____

More notes on the back of this page ☐

PLANTAR FASCIITIS

 ## BASIC INFORMATION

DESCRIPTION

Plantar fasciitis is an inflammation (red, sore, swollen) of the plantar fascia. The plantar fascia is a thick band of tissue on the bottom of the foot. It extends from the heel bone to the base of the toes. Plantar refers to the sole of the foot. Fascia describes thin, fibrous, supportive tissue. Plantar fasciitis can affect anyone, of any age, no matter their fitness level. It is a common foot problem, and is different from heel spurs. But, a person may have both of these foot problems at the same time.

FREQUENT SIGNS AND SYMPTOMS

· Pain and tenderness in the heel and sole of the foot under the heel bone.
· Pain often occurs after resting or after rising in the morning. There may be no pain when sitting.
· One or both feet can be affected.
· It hurts worse when running faster or when weight is on the ball of the foot.

CAUSES

Overuse or stress to the foot causes the plantar fascia to become stretched, irritated, and inflamed.

RISK INCREASES WITH

· People over age 40. Women more often than men.
· Athletes who overtrain, wear improper shoes, or fail to warm up).
· Running, jumping, or walking on hard surfaces.
· Having flat feet or high arches.
· Previous foot or ankle injury.
· Wearing high heeled, poorly fitting, or worn-out shoes.
· Being on the feet for many hours a day.
· Overweight.

PREVENTIVE MEASURES

· Wear proper footwear for sports, exercise, and work.
· Do stretching exercises for the Achilles tendon (tendon from the heel to the calf).
· With any new exercise or sport, build up your pace gradually. Warm up before exercise.
· Maintain a healthy weight for your height.

EXPECTED OUTCOMES

Usually curable for most people. Different types of treatment work for different people. Complete healing may take from weeks to months. Other methods of treatment are being studied and may be available in the future.

POSSIBLE COMPLICATIONS

Pain continues which may cause limping and other walking problems. This can limit everyday activities as well as sports and fitness activities.

 ## DIAGNOSIS & TREATMENT

GENERAL MEASURES

· Your health care provider will examine your foot and ankle and ask about your symptoms. The bottom of your foot will be touched and pressed to identify the cause of the pain. X-rays and other tests may be done to check for other disorders.
· There are a variety of treatment options. Follow your health care provider's advice. Basic ideas are listed here.
· Massage an ice pack over the painful area. Do this for 15 minutes, 3 or 4 times a day, and after activities.
· Before getting out of bed, use a towel to pull toes back toward the ankle. Count to 10, and do it 10 times.
· While sitting, grab a towel with your toes or roll your foot back and forth over a can of frozen juice. Stand on the ball of your foot on the edge of a step and raise and lower leg.
· Try heel cushions or arch supports. Use them in both shoes so other problems don't develop. Custom orthotics (special shoe inserts) may be prescribed.
· Taping helps some people. Apply athletic tape as directed on the product's instructions.
· Night splints are products that keep the muscles stretched while sleeping. They may help.
· Buy shoes that fit well. Sandals help some people.
· If other treatments fail after 6 months, shock wave therapy (nonsurgical) or surgery may be options.

MEDICATIONS

· For minor pain and inflammation, use nonprescription drugs, such as ibuprofen or aspirin (if over age 18).
· Steroids may be injected into the foot.

ACTIVITY

Stay off your feet as much as possible until symptoms are better. Try swimming or cycling for exercising.

DIET

If your weight is a problem, begin a weight-loss diet.

 ## NOTIFY OUR OFFICE IF

· You or a family member has symptoms of plantar fasciitis.
· Symptoms don't improve despite treatment.

Special notes:

_____

_____

_____

More notes on the back of this page ☐

PLEURISY

(Pleuritis; Pleurodynia)

 ## BASIC INFORMATION

DESCRIPTION

Inflammation and irritation of the pleura. The pleura is a thin, two-layered membrane that lines the lung and chest cavity. Pleurisy is not a disease, but may be a symptom of many different disorders. Fluid (pleural effusion) may develop at the site of inflammation, between the two membrane layers. This is called wet pleurisy. If there is no fluid build up, it is dry pleurisy.

FREQUENT SIGNS AND SYMPTOMS

• Sudden chest pain that worsens with breathing and coughing. The pain varies from vague discomfort that occurs only with deep breathing or coughing to intense, stabbing pain. Pain is usually over the area of pleural inflammation, but it may also occur in the lower chest or abdomen.
• Fever (sometimes).
• Discomfort on moving the affected side.
• Rapid, shallow breathing.
• Breathing difficulty if pleural effusion develops.

CAUSES

Pleurisy can be caused by infection (e.g., bacterial, fungal, or viral), injury, irritation, blood clot, or disease. Sometimes, no cause is found.

RISK INCREASES WITH

• Lung or chest infection (e.g., pneumonia, bronchitis, tuberculosis).
• Blood clot in the lung.
• Injury to the chest or rib fracture.
• Cancer in other parts of the body.
• Collagen vascular disease, such as systemic lupus erythematosus or rheumatoid arthritis.
• Collapse of a part of the lung.
• Kidney, liver, or pancreas disorders.
• Weak immune system due to illness or drugs.
• Smoking.

PREVENTIVE MEASURES

No specific preventive measures. Obtain medical treatment for any causes listed above to reduce the risk of pleurisy.

EXPECTED OUTCOMES

Outcome depends on successful treatment of the disorder causing it. Sometimes, pleurisy symptoms clear completely on their own in 1 to 2 weeks.

POSSIBLE COMPLICATIONS

• Fluid build up (pleural effusion).
• Pneumonia.
• Scar tissue (adhesions) may form that cause pain and shortness of breath.

 ## DIAGNOSIS & TREATMENT

GENERAL MEASURES

• Your health care provider will do a physical exam and ask about your symptoms and activities. Medical tests may include blood and pleural fluid studies, x-rays of the chest, and others to diagnose the cause.
• The main treatment is aimed at the underlying cause. Other treatment may help the symptoms of pleurisy.
• For chest pain, wrap the entire chest with two or three nonadhesive, 6-inch-wide elastic bandages.
• Lie with the sore side down, on a firm surface. This will help ease the pain.
• Quit smoking. Find a way to stop that works for you.
• Holding a pillow firmly against the chest wall helps ease the pain when coughing.
• Excess fluid in the pleura may need to be removed. This is done with a needle inserted into the pleura to draw out the fluid.

MEDICATIONS

• You may take nonsteroidal anti-inflammatory drugs, such as aspirin (if over age 18) or ibuprofen, to relieve pain and inflammation.
• Antibiotics, bronchodilators, or stronger pain relievers may be prescribed.

ACTIVITY

Reduce activity until pain and cough get better. Then resume normal activities gradually.

DIET

No special diet.

 ## NOTIFY OUR OFFICE IF

• You or a family member has symptoms of pleurisy.
• The following occur during treatment:
  - Fever.
  - Increased pain.
  - Increased breathlessness.
  - Cough that is dry and non-productive.
  - Blue or dark fingernails, toenails, or lips.
  - Blood in the sputum.

Special notes:

_____

_____

_____

More notes on the back of this page ☐

PNEUMOCONIOSIS

 BASIC INFORMATION

DESCRIPTION

Lung inflammation caused by breathing industrial dusts. Inhaling such particles for many years may cause little patches of irritation to form in one or both lungs. The scar tissue formed by the irritation may make the lungs less flexible and porous. Pneumoconiosis is not contagious. It usually takes at least 10 years of exposure and sometimes up to 25 years for it to develop. Only a few persons exposed to the dusts actually become ill. It usually affects men over age 40.

FREQUENT SIGNS AND SYMPTOMS

Early symptoms:
- Shortness of breath.
- Cough that produces little or no sputum.
- General ill feeling.

Late symptoms:
- Restless sleep.
- Appetite and weight loss.
- Chest pain.
- Hoarseness; coughing up blood.
- Bluish nails.

CAUSES

- Exposure to small particles of industrial dusts cause the following forms of pneumoconiosis:
  - Coal dust causes black-lung disease (coal miner's pneumoconiosis, anthracosis).
  - Beryllium and its compounds (once used in manufacturing fluorescent lamp bulbs, ceramics, and chemicals) cause berylliosis.
  - Talc, iron, cotton, synthetic fiber, and aluminum dusts cause a rare form of pneumoconiosis.
  - Asbestos and silica cause asbestosis and silicosis.

RISK INCREASES WITH

- Smoking.
- Greater amounts of dust inhaled over the years.

PREVENTIVE MEASURES

- Practice safety during exposure to industrial dusts. Wear a protective mask or external-air-supplied hood. Get an x-ray once a year.
- Don't smoke. Avoid second hand smoke.

EXPECTED OUTCOMES

This condition is currently considered incurable. Symptoms can be relieved or controlled. It reduces life span, but many patients live into their 60s and 70s.

POSSIBLE COMPLICATIONS

- Congestive heart failure.
- Lung collapse, pleurisy, or other lung disease.
- Tuberculosis (in the late stages).
- Lung cancer.

 DIAGNOSIS & TREATMENT

GENERAL MEASURES

- Your health care provider will do a physical exam and ask questions about your symptoms and activities. Be sure to tell your provider about your work history and any exposure to industrial dusts. Medical tests may include a chest x-ray, pulmonary function tests, and others to confirm diagnosis and check for complications.
- Drugs and lung therapy may help the symptoms and treat complications.
- Avoid any further exposure to industrial dusts.
- Quit smoking. Find a way to stop that works for you.
- Get medical care for any respiratory infection (such as a cold). Get influenza and pneumococcal vaccines.
- Chest physical therapy (such as controlled coughing) and bronchial drainage help clear secretions. Get medical training about these procedures.
- To learn more: American Lung Association, 61 Broadway, 6th Floor, New York, NY 10006, (800) 586-4872; website: www.lungusa.org.

MEDICATIONS

- Antibiotics may be prescribed for infections.
- Bronchodilators (inhaled or oral) with inhalation therapy may be prescribed. This is supervised at first by an inhalation therapist.
- For minor discomfort, you may use nonprescription drugs, such as acetaminophen or aspirin (for adults).

ACTIVITY

No limits, except those caused by symptoms.

DIET

No special diet. Maintain high fluid intake.

 NOTIFY OUR OFFICE IF

- You or a family member has symptoms of pneumoconiosis.
- The following occur during treatment:
  - Temperature of 101°F (38.3°C) or more.
  - Increased chest pain or shortness of breath.
  - Blood in sputum.
  - Continuing weight loss.
  - Unexplained symptoms develop.

Special notes:

_____

_____

_____

More notes on the back of this page ☐

PNEUMONIA, BACTERIAL

 ## BASIC INFORMATION

DESCRIPTION

Infection and inflammation of the lungs with bacterial germs. It causes fluid to collect in the air sacs (alveoli), making it difficult to breathe. Bacterial pneumonia is not usually contagious. It can affect all ages but is most severe in young children and adults over age 60.

FREQUENT SIGNS AND SYMPTOMS

- High fever (over 102°F or 38.9°C) and chills.
- Shortness of breath.
- Cough with sputum that may contain blood or blood streaks.
- Rapid breathing.
- Chest pain that worsens with inhalations.
- Abdominal pain.
- Fatigue.
- Bluish lips and nails (rare).
- Loss of appetite and weight loss.

CAUSES

Infection with bacteria, such as *Pneumococci, Haemophilus, Streptococci* or *Staphylococci*. The germs are usually breathed in, but may be spread in other ways.

RISK INCREASES WITH

- Age (newborns, infants, and adults over 60).
- Use of anticancer drugs.
- Smoking.
- Chronic diseases.
- Recent surgery.
- Poor general health from any cause.
- Weak immune system due to illness or drugs.
- Hospital care, for any reason.

PREVENTIVE MEASURES

- Obtain prompt medical care for respiratory infections.
- Arrange for pneumococcal and influenza vaccines.
- Avoid risk factors where possible.

EXPECTED OUTCOMES

Usually curable, in otherwise healthy persons, in 1 to 2 weeks with treatment. It may take longer for the very young, elderly, or those with other disorders.

POSSIBLE COMPLICATIONS

- Pleurisy and pleural effusion (problems of the membrane layers that cover the lung).
- Bronchiectasis (damaged airways in the lungs).
- Spread of infection.
- Pulmonary abscess (pus-filled area).
- Complications, including death, are more likely in older persons who have other respiratory disorders or serious diseases.

 ## DIAGNOSIS & TREATMENT

GENERAL MEASURES

- Your health care provider will do a physical exam and ask questions about your symptoms. Medical tests may include sputum culture, a blood study, x-rays of lungs, and lung scan.
- Hospital care is often needed for more severe cases. Treatment may include breathing support, fluids and/or drugs injected into a vein (IV), and removing excess fluids from the lung. Some cases may be treated at home.
- Don't suppress the cough with a drug if the cough produces sputum or mucus. It is useful in ridding the body of lung secretions.
- Use a heating pad on low heat or warm compresses to relieve chest pain.
- Quit smoking. Find a way to stop that works for you.
- To learn more: American Lung Association, 61 Broadway, 6th Floor, New York, NY 10006, (800) 586-4872; website: www.lungusa.org.

MEDICATIONS

- Antibiotics for infection will be prescribed.
- You may use nonprescription drugs, such as acetaminophen, to relieve minor discomfort.

ACTIVITY

Rest in bed, until fever declines and pain and shortness of breath disappear. Then resume normal activities gradually.

DIET

No special diet. Increase fluid intake. Extra fluid helps thin the lung secretions so they are easier to cough up.

 ## NOTIFY OUR OFFICE IF

- You or a family member has symptoms of pneumonia.
- The following occur during treatment:
  - Fever, pain or shortness of breath increases.
  - Dark or bluish fingernails, toenails, or skin.
  - Blood in the sputum.
  - Nausea, vomiting, or diarrhea.

Special notes:

_____

_____

_____

More notes on the back of this page ☐

PNEUMONIA, MYCOPLASMA

(Atypical Pneumonia; Walking Pneumonia)

 BASIC INFORMATION

DESCRIPTION

A lung inflammation caused by infection with *Mycoplasma pneumoniae,* an organism (germ) that is similar to bacteria. The disorder is also called walking pneumonia, because a patient is usually not confined to bed or in need of hospital care. Some people may not even realize they have pneumonia, as the symptoms are often mild. It can affect all ages, but is more common in ages 5 to 20 and males more than females.

FREQUENT SIGNS AND SYMPTOMS

- Cough that is dry at first and then produces sputum.
- Fever.
- Sore throat.
- Stuffy nose.
- Chest or ear pain may occur.
- Headache.
- Wheezing.
- Muscle aches and fatigue.

CAUSES

Mycoplasma pneumonia is infectious and is spread through close contact with an infected person. Germs are spread into the air when the infected person coughs or sneezes. Symptoms may begin 15 to 25 days after being exposed to the germs.

RISK INCREASES WITH

- Close living conditions (military barracks, college dorms, and families).
- Weak immune system due to illness or drugs.

PREVENTIVE MEASURES

No specific preventive measures. Avoid exposure to persons who are ill with respiratory infections. Wash hands often to prevent spread of any type of germs.

EXPECTED OUTCOMES

Symptoms usually clear up in about two weeks. Some symptoms, such as cough or fatigue, may persist for 4 to 6 weeks. The disorder will heal on its own, but treatment with antibiotics can help speed recovery. Once a person has had the infection, there is some immunity, but it is not life-long.

POSSIBLE COMPLICATIONS

- Skin rash.
- Ear infection or sinus inflammation.
- Asthma.
- Hemolytic anemia (lack of red blood cells).
- Severe pneumonia.
- Other, less common complications may occur.

 DIAGNOSIS & TREATMENT

GENERAL MEASURES

- Your health care provider will do a physical exam and ask questions about your symptoms. Medical tests may include blood studies, sputum culture, and chest x-rays.
- Treatment may include extra rest, treatment of symptoms, and antibiotics. For most patients, treatment can be done at home. Hospital care may be needed for someone with severe symptoms or complications.
- Use a heating pad on low heat or warm compresses to relieve chest pain.
- To learn more: American Lung Association, 61 Broadway, 6th Floor, New York, NY 10006, (800) 586-4872; website: www.lungusa.org.

MEDICATIONS

- Antibiotics, such as erythromycin, clarithromycin, azithromycin, or tetracycline (for ages over 8), may be prescribed. They will shorten the duration of fever and other symptoms, but you can carry the germs for weeks in spite of treatment.
- Cough medicine, nose drops, sprays or oral decongestants may be recommended.
- You may use acetaminophen or ibuprofen for fever or minor pain.

ACTIVITY

Get extra rest until symptoms improve. Normal activities should be resumed gradually. Children may return to school once symptoms improve.

DIET

No special diet. Extra fluid helps thin lung secretions so they can be coughed up more easily.

 NOTIFY OUR OFFICE IF

- You or a family member has symptoms of mycoplasma pneumonia.
- The following occur during treatment:
  - High fever, increased pain, or shortness of breath.
  - Dark or bluish fingernails, toenails, or skin.
  - Blood in the sputum, nausea, vomiting or diarrhea.
  - Rash or earache.
  - Severe headache.

Special notes:

_____

_____

_____

More notes on the back of this page ☐

PNEUMONIA, PNEUMOCYSTIS CARINII

BASIC INFORMATION

DESCRIPTION

Inflammation of the lungs caused by infection with *Pneumocystis carinii* germs. It occurs in children (including infants) and adults with a weakened immune system. They are usually AIDS patients. Most people have been exposed to these germs by age four, but their immune systems are able to fight off any infection.

FREQUENT SIGNS AND SYMPTOMS

- Dry, nonproductive cough.
- Fever.
- Difficulty in breathing.
- Fatigue.
- Weight loss.
- Night sweats.
- Tightness in the chest.
- Lips, fingernails, or skin may turn blue or gray.

CAUSES

Pneumocystis carinii (believed to be a fungus). It is most likely transmitted through the air. It is unknown if it lives in soil or other places. It is also unknown how long it takes symptoms to start after exposure. Person to person spread is a possibility, but is not yet proven.

RISK INCREASES WITH

- HIV (human immunodeficiency virus) and AIDS (acquired immunodeficiency syndrome).
- People with weak immune systems due to illness or drugs.
- Cancer chemotherapy (anticancer drugs).
- Long-term steroid drug use.
- Severe malnutrition (any disorder of nutrition).
- History of *Pneumocystis carinii* pneumonia.

PREVENTIVE MEASURES

It is almost entirely preventable with drugs. Preventive drugs can be prescribed for those at risk.

EXPECTED OUTCOMES

With prompt diagnosis and treatment, the outlook is generally good for mild cases. With more severe cases, the risk of complications is higher.

POSSIBLE COMPLICATIONS

- Prolonged illness, sometimes fatal.
- Side effects of drugs, especially skin rash and low white blood cell count.

DIAGNOSIS & TREATMENT

GENERAL MEASURES

- Your health care provider will do a physical exam and ask questions about the symptoms. Medical tests may include x-rays, a study of a specimen of sputum, and high resolution CT scan. A bronchoscopy may be done. This involves inserting a tube down the throat to view the lungs and to get a sample of tissue for diagnosis.
- Treatment is with drugs given by mouth or given through a vein (IV).
- Treatment may be done at home for mild cases. For more severe infection, hospital care may be needed.
- To learn more: American Lung Association, 61 Broadway, 6th Floor, New York, NY 10006, (800) 586-4872; website: www.lungusa.org.

MEDICATIONS

- Antibiotics, such as trimethoprim/sulfamethoxazole or pentamidine (oral or aerosol) will be prescribed.
- Corticosteroids may be prescribed.
- Cough medicine may be recommended.

ACTIVITY

Bed rest is recommended until fever subsides. Normal activities should be resumed gradually.

DIET

No special diet. Extra fluid helps to thin lung secretions so they can be coughed up more easily.

NOTIFY OUR OFFICE IF

- You or a family member has symptoms of *Pneumocystis carinii* pneumonia.
- The following occur during treatment:
  - Higher fever.
  - Pain becomes worse.
  - Increased shortness of breath.
  - Dark or bluish fingernails, toenails, or skin.
  - Blood in the sputum.
  - Nausea, vomiting, or diarrhea.
- New, unexplained symptoms develop. Drugs used in treatment may produce side effects.

Special notes:

_____

_____

_____

More notes on the back of this page ☐

PNEUMONIA, VIRAL

 BASIC INFORMATION

DESCRIPTION

Lung inflammation caused by a virus infection. It causes fluid to collect in the air sacs (alveoli) making it difficult to breathe. It can affect all ages, but can be more severe in young children and adults over age 60.

FREQUENT SIGNS AND SYMPTOMS

- Fever, chills, and sweating.
- Muscle aches and fatigue.
- Cough, with or without sputum, or "croup."
- Rapid, difficult (sometimes) breathing.
- Sore throat.
- Loss of appetite.
- Enlarged lymph glands in the neck.

CAUSES

Viral infection. These include influenza, chickenpox, and respiratory syncytial virus (especially in adults); respiratory viruses, measles, and cytomegalovirus (especially in infants).

RISK INCREASES WITH

- Newborns and infants.
- Adults over 60.
- Weak immune system due to illness or drugs.
- Persons with chronic diseases.
- Smoking.
- Crowded living conditions.
- Recent upper respiratory infection.

PREVENTIVE MEASURES

- No specific preventive measures.
- Measles vaccines for children, chickenpox vaccine, and annual flu vaccines can help prevent infections that can lead to pneumonia.
- Wash hands often to prevent spread of any germs.

EXPECTED OUTCOMES

Usually clears up on its own in 1 to 3 weeks. In more severe cases, recovery may take longer. Some people are fatigued and weak for up to 6 weeks after recovery.

POSSIBLE COMPLICATIONS

- Bacterial infection of the lungs.
- Other lung disorders such as bronchitis.

 DIAGNOSIS & TREATMENT

GENERAL MEASURES

- Your health care provider will do a physical exam and ask questions about your symptoms. Medical tests may include a sputum culture, blood studies, and x-rays.

- Most patients can be treated at home. Hospital care may be needed for more severe cases.
- Coughing and deep breathing is recommended to help clear secretions. Dispose of tissues carefully.
- Use a heating pad on low heat or warm compresses to relieve chest pain.
- Use a cool-mist ultrasonic humidifier (if advised) to increase air moisture and loosen lung secretions. Use pure water; don't put drugs in the humidifier. Clean the humidifier daily.
- Quit smoking. Find a way to stop that works for you.
- To learn more: American Lung Association, 61 Broadway, 6th Floor, New York, NY 10006, (800) 586-4872; website: www.lungusa.org.

MEDICATIONS

- Antiviral drugs may be prescribed depending on the virus and how long it's been since symptoms started.
- For minor pain, fever, and congestion, you may use nonprescription drugs, such as acetaminophen or decongestant nose drops, nasal sprays, or tablets.
- Antibiotics do not cure viral infections. They may be prescribed to prevent or treat a complicating bacterial infection.

ACTIVITY

Bed rest is helpful until fever, pain, and shortness of breath have been gone at least 48 hours. Then normal activity may be resumed slowly.

DIET

No special diet. Drink plenty of fluids. This helps to thin lung secretions so they are easier to cough up.

 NOTIFY OUR OFFICE IF

- You or a family member has symptoms of viral pneumonia.
- The following occur during treatment:
  - Temperature rises over 102°F (38.9°C).
  - Pain gets worse.
  - Nausea, vomiting, or diarrhea.
  - Increasing shortness of breath.
  - Blood in the sputum.
  - Increasingly bluish nails and skin.

Special notes:

_____

_____

_____

More notes on the back of this page ☐

PNEUMOTHORAX

BASIC INFORMATION

DESCRIPTION

Air in the chest between the two layers of the pleura (thin membranes that cover the lung). When air gets into the pleural space, the pressure becomes greater than the pressure in the lung. This causes a partial or a complete collapse of the lung. Pneumothorax types:
· Spontaneous—it occurs without a cause. It is common in young men age 20 to 40.
· Secondary spontaneous—complication of lung disease.
· Traumatic—caused by an injury to the chest.
· Tension—excessive pressure builds up around lung. Air gets in, but cannot get out. It can be life-threatening.

FREQUENT SIGNS AND SYMPTOMS

· The symptoms vary according to the degree of lung collapse and extent of other lung disease. Symptoms may be less acute if the pneumothorax develops slowly.
· Sharp chest pain. Pain may extend to a shoulder or across the chest or abdomen.
· Shortness of breath and rapid breathing.
· Anxiety.
· Dry, hacking cough (sometimes).
· Bluish nails.
· Coughing bloody sputum (sometimes).
· Rapid pulse.
· Fainting and shock (in tension pneumothorax).

CAUSES

Air may get into the pleural space due to a rupture of the small air or fluid sacs in the lungs. Air may also enter the chest from the outside, such as with a chest wound. The air may result from medical procedures performed on the chest cavity. The air may result from damaged lungs due to chronic lung disease, other diseases, or injury.

RISK INCREASES WITH

· Physical exertion in a healthy person, with no obvious injury, infection, or disease. Activities most likely to produce pneumothorax include:
  - Ascent while scuba diving.
  - Diving or high-altitude flying.
  - Activities that require stretching the chest and rib cage, such as track and field events, throwing sports, and bowling.
· Asthma, emphysema, chronic bronchitis, lung abscess, empyema or other lung disease.
· A wound to the chest area, which permits outside air to rush into the pleural space.
· Removing fluid from the lung (thoracentesis).
· Smoking.
· Family history of pneumothorax.
· Use of a machine (ventilator) for breathing support.

PREVENTIVE MEASURES

No specific preventive measures. Get medical care for chronic lung disorders. Don't smoke.

EXPECTED OUTCOMES

Most patients recover fully in 2 to 4 weeks.

POSSIBLE COMPLICATIONS

· Critical illness and death with tension pneumothorax.
· Repeated pneumothorax.

DIAGNOSIS & TREATMENT

GENERAL MEASURES

· Your health care provider will do a physical exam and ask about your symptoms and activities. X-rays of the chest help to confirm the diagnosis and determine the size of the pneumothorax.
· Treatment depends on the size of the pneumothorax and the condition of the lungs.
· No treatment may be needed in some cases. Small amounts of air are reabsorbed naturally and the lung will re-expand on its own.
· Hospital care may be needed for treatment.
  - A small needle may be inserted into the chest cavity to relieve excess pressure.
  - A tube may be placed in the chest and attached to a special vacuum bottle. This allows the air to be slowly removed and the lung to re-expand.
  - Surgery may be needed if the pneumothorax has recurred or if the lung does not re-expand after 5 days.
· Don't smoke; try not to cough; avoid loud talking, laughing, or singing.
· Rest in a sitting position. It may be more comfortable.

MEDICATIONS

You may use nonprescription drugs, such as acetaminophen, for minor pain. Stronger pain relievers may be prescribed if needed.

ACTIVITY

Rest often. Allow two or more weeks for recovery.

DIET

No special diet.

NOTIFY OUR OFFICE IF

You or a family member has symptoms of pneumothorax.

Special notes:

_____

_____

_____

More notes on the back of this page ☐

POISON IVY, OAK, & SUMAC

 BASIC INFORMATION

DESCRIPTION

Poison ivy, oak, and sumac are three types of plants that cause a skin reaction (contact dermatitis). The reaction results from contact with an oily substance (resin) produced by these plants. This particular allergic reaction is the most common in the United States. About 50% of the total population has developed an allergy to these plants.

FREQUENT SIGNS AND SYMPTOMS

Skin rash with the following signs:
- Bright red spots that develop 24 to 48 hours (sometimes may take several days) after contact.
- Weeping, crusting, and swelling.
- Intense itching and burning.
- Blisters (the fluid in blisters is not contagious).
- Enough of the oily resin remains on hands or clothing so that the rash is carried to other body parts, such as the face or genitals.

CAUSES

Contact with any part of the poison ivy, poison oak, or poison sumac plants. They grow as vines or bushes and have three leaves (poison ivy and poison oak), or a row of paired leaves (poison sumac). They produce a potent resin (urushiol) that is the cause of the problem. A reaction may also occur from touching the poison substance when it is on clothing, equipment (hunting, golfing, or athletic), or animals, such as pets. It can also come from any smoke these plants give off if they are burned. This may affect the face, eyelids, throat, and lungs.

RISK INCREASES WITH

- Spring and summer (though plants are dangerous year round).
- Not wearing protective clothing.

PREVENTIVE MEASURES

- Learn to identify and avoid contact with these plants.
- When walking in areas where these plants grow, wear shoes, socks, long pants, long-sleeved shirts, and, sometimes, gloves. Wash this clothing right after you return if possible. Use a product that prevents the poison from getting on your skin.
- If you are exposed, washing the skin immediately with soap and water and sponging with rubbing alcohol may prevent the rash.

EXPECTED OUTCOMES

Itching, redness, and swelling are often improved by the second day, and complete healing occurs within 7 to 14 days.

POSSIBLE COMPLICATIONS

A skin infection may develop.

 DIAGNOSIS & TREATMENT

GENERAL MEASURES

- Sweating and heat make the itching worse, so try to stay cool.
- Apply cool compresses to the affected area.
- A soothing bath helps. Use Aveeno (a product made of oatmeal) or baking soda (about a half cup) per bath.
- Wash all clothing and shoes, and any equipment that came in contact with the plant oils, with soap and water.
- Give pets a warm, soapy bath to remove any oil from the fur.
- Consult your health care provider if rash is severe or does not improve. The diagnosis can be confirmed and if needed, drugs may be prescribed.

MEDICATIONS

- You may use calamine lotion to relieve the itching.
- Oral antihistamines may be helpful also.
- Your health care provider may prescribe topical or oral steroid drugs for severe symptoms.

ACTIVITY

No limits. Avoid activities that can cause sweating. This can worsen itching.

DIET

No special diet.

 NOTIFY OUR OFFICE IF

- You or a family member has a severe rash.
- If swelling or pain develops around the eyes, nose, or genitals.
- Rash gets worse or doesn't improve with self-care methods.

Special notes:

_____

_____

_____

More notes on the back of this page ☐

POLYARTERITIS NODOSA
(Periarteritis; Necrotizing Angiitis)

BASIC INFORMATION

DESCRIPTION
Inflammation of small and medium size arteries in the body. This decreases the blood supply to the body organs supplied by the affected arteries. Polyarteritis nodosa can affect the muscles, joints, skin, heart, brain, intestinal tract, nerves, liver, kidneys, and genitals. It is more common in adults under age 50, and it occurs in men more than women.

FREQUENT SIGNS AND SYMPTOMS
· General symptoms include weight loss, fever, fatigue, general ill feeling, muscle and joint aches, weakness, high blood pressure, and headache.
· Other symptoms may be due to the affected organ:
 - Blood in the urine (kidney involved).
 - Chest pain (heart involved).
 - Abdominal pain (intestinal tract and liver involved).
 - Numbness and tingling of the hands and feet (nerves involved).
 - Purplish rash and other skin disorders (skin involved).
 - Testicle pain (testicles involved).

CAUSES
It is considered an autoimmune disease, although the cause is unknown. Hepatitis B appears to be a factor.

RISK INCREASES WITH
· Hepatitis B and sometimes hepatitis C.
· Other autoimmune diseases.
· Methamphetamine abuse.
· Smoking.
· Use of certain drugs, including penicillin, antithyroid drugs, thiazide diuretics, and some vaccines.

PREVENTIVE MEASURES
No specific preventive measures.

EXPECTED OUTCOMES
· The disorder is chronic and progressive. Symptoms may be relieved or controlled. With treatment, about 80% of patients survive 5 years or more. Without treatment, few patients live beyond 5 years.
· Research into causes and treatment continues, so there is hope for more effective treatment and cure.

POSSIBLE COMPLICATIONS
· Kidney failure.
· Heart attack or heart failure.
· Stroke.
· Nervous system disorders.
· Intestinal perforation.
· Aneurysm rupture.
· Side effects of drugs used in treatment.

DIAGNOSIS & TREATMENT

GENERAL MEASURES
· Your health care provider will do a physical exam and ask questions about your symptoms. Medical tests may include blood and urine studies, x-ray, biopsy, and MRI. Angiography may be done–a dye is injected into the arteries to highlight the affected areas and x-rays taken.
· Treatment is with drugs to reduce the inflammation.
· Hospital care may be needed for severe cases and complications.
· Surgery may be needed if there are complications involving the intestinal tract.
· To learn more: National Institute of Arthritis & Musculoskeletal & Skin Disorders, 1 AMS Circle, Bethesda, MD, 20892-3675, (877) 226-4267; website: www.nih.gov/niams or Polyarteritis Nodosa Research & Support Network, website: www.pansupport.org.

MEDICATIONS
· Cortisone drugs and immunosuppressive drugs are usually prescribed. They need to be continued even after symptoms improve. The dosage may be reduced once the symptoms are controlled. Some patients want to stop the drugs because of side effects. Without drugs, however, the disorder will progress and cause complications.
· Drugs to treat other disorders such as hepatitis B, heart drugs, or drugs for high blood pressure may be prescribed.

ACTIVITY
Resume your normal activities gradually as symptoms improve.

DIET
No special diet unless advised by your health care provider.

NOTIFY OUR OFFICE IF

· You or a family member has symptoms of polyarteritis nodosa.
· New, unexplained symptoms develop. Drugs used in treatment may produce side effects.

Special notes:

_____

_____

_____

More notes on the back of this page ☐

POLYCYSTIC OVARIAN SYNDROME

(PCOS; Stein-Leventhal Syndrome)

BASIC INFORMATION

DESCRIPTION

Polycystic ovarian syndrome (PCOS) is an endocrine (hormone) condition. It is not a disease itself. It is a set of signs and symptoms, that when combined, make up the condition. PCOS affects 5% to 10% of all women of childbearing age. It may begin during puberty and become more severe with time.

FREQUENT SIGNS AND SYMPTOMS

· Irregular menstrual bleeding. This results in periods of light flow along with heavy flow. There is increased time between periods, often up to several months.
· Hirsutism—increased hair growth on the face, arms, legs, and from pubic area to navel.
· Thinning of the scalp hair (alopecia).
· Overweight or obesity.
· Trouble getting pregnant; miscarriages.
· Acne.
· Dark patches of skin or skin tags (small skin growths).
· Polycystic ovaries. These are fairly common and involve enlarged ovaries from many small cysts.
· Anovulation (absence of ovulation). The monthly release of the egg from the ovary fails to take place.

CAUSES

The cause of PCOS is unclear. Hormone imbalances, insulin production, and hereditary factors all seem to play a role.

RISK INCREASES WITH

· Lifestyle problems such as obesity, poor diet, and physical inactivity.
· Family history of PCOS or diabetes.

PREVENTIVE MEASURES

Cannot be prevented at present.

EXPECTED OUTCOME

Treatment, along with weight control and exercise, can relieve or eliminate symptoms. Pregnancy (if desired) can be achieved in many patients.

POSSIBLE COMPLICATIONS

· Infertility (unable to get pregnant) or miscarriages.
· Depression and anxiety.
· High cholesterol and triglyceride levels.
· Heart and blood vessel disease; high blood pressure.
· Diabetes.
· Cancer of the breast or uterus.

DIAGNOSIS & TREATMENT

GENERAL MEASURES

· Your health care provider will usually do a physical exam and a pelvic exam. Questions will be asked about your symptoms, menstrual cycle, and pregnancies. Medical tests may include studies of blood for levels of hormones, glucose, insulin, and fats (cholesterol and triglyceride). Other tests such as an ultrasound may be done to rule out other disorders. There is no specific test to diagnose PCOS.
· Treatment goals: regulate menstrual cycle, reduce hair growth and acne problems, help with fertility (if pregnancy desired), and prevent long-term problems.
· A diet and exercise program for overweight or obese women will help improve physical and mental health.
· Infertility is usually treated successfully through diet and exercise, weight loss, and drug therapy. If these steps are not successful, other options are available.
· Quit smoking. Find a way to stop that works for you.
· Counseling may help you cope with emotional stress.
· Options for removing excess hair from your face, arms, and legs include drugs, bleaching, electrolysis, laser therapy, plucking, waxing, and depilation.
· More information is available from a variety sites on the Internet dedicated to PCOS.

MEDICATION

· Diabetic drugs (such as metformin), birth-control pills, or other drugs may be prescribed.
· Drugs to help with fertility may be prescribed.
· Vaniqa (eflornithine cream) for excess facial hair) or spironolactone for excess body hair may be prescribed.

ACTIVITY

No limits on activity, including sexual intercourse. Physical activity is important. Exercise daily.

DIET

Low-carbohydrate diet may be recommended. Begin a weight-loss diet if you are overweight.

NOTIFY OUR OFFICE IF

· You or a family member has symptoms of polycystic ovarian syndrome.
· New symptoms occur after treatment.

Special notes:

_____

_____

_____

More notes on the back of this page ☐

386

POLYCYTHEMIA

 BASIC INFORMATION

DESCRIPTION

An increase of red blood cells in the body. It more often affects adults over age 50 (but has a range of ages from 15 to 90), and it is more common in men. The disease has 3 forms:

• Polycythemia vera, which involves overproduction of red blood cells, white blood cells, and platelets.

• Secondary polycythemia (reactive polycythemia), which is a complication of diseases or factors other than blood-cell disorders.

• Stress polycythemia (pseudopolycythemia), which involves decreased blood plasma.

FREQUENT SIGNS AND SYMPTOMS

• Some patients have no symptoms. Others may have any of the following:

- Fatigue, headache, drowsiness, or dizziness.
- Itching or flushed skin.
- Enlarged spleen.
- Unexplained bleeding.

CAUSES

• Polycythemia vera: unknown.

• Secondary polycythemia: congenital heart disease, chronic lung disease, cigarette or cigar smoking, living at high altitude.

• Stress polycythemia: use of diuretic drugs, smoking, or dehydration.

RISK INCREASES WITH

• Some anticancer drugs used to treat cancer.
• Jewish ancestry.
• Exposure to radiation.
• Family history of polycythemia.

PREVENTIVE MEASURES

Polycythemia cannot be prevented at present.

EXPECTED OUTCOMES

• Polycythemia vera is incurable, but symptoms can be controlled. With treatment, average survival ranges from 7 to 15 years, with some patients living 20 or more years.

• Other forms of polycythemia can usually be cured if the causes can be eliminated.

POSSIBLE COMPLICATIONS

• Blood clots in veins or arteries.
• Gout.
• Stroke.
• Heart attack.
• Peptic ulcer.
• Kidney stones.
• Leukemia.

 DIAGNOSIS & TREATMENT

GENERAL MEASURES

• Your health care provider will do a physical exam and ask questions about your symptoms. Medical tests may include studies of bone marrow and blood (red-blood cell count, hematocrit), x-ray of the kidneys, and others to confirm the diagnosis.

• Treatment steps will depend on the age of patient, disease duration, type of polycythemia, complications, disease activity, and response to treatment.

• Treatment steps to keep the red blood cell range near normal and prevent clotting or hemorrhage include phlebotomy (withdrawal of excess blood) and drug therapy.

• For secondary or stress polycythemia, proper treatment of the underlying cause is important. Drug therapy or surgery may be recommended.

• Quit smoking. Find a way to stop that works for you.

MEDICATIONS

• Your health care provider may prescribe:

- Drugs to suppress production of red blood cells and platelets.
- Allopurinol if uric acid levels are high.
- Low-dose aspirin for ages over 18 (sometimes).
- Anti-itching drugs, such as antihistamines.
- Drugs for stomach acidity.

ACTIVITY

Resume normal activity when symptoms improve.

DIET

No special diet. Drink 6 to 8 oz. of fluid every 2 hours to maintain adequate body fluid.

 NOTIFY OUR OFFICE IF

• You or a family member has symptoms of polycythemia.

• Symptoms recur after treatment.

• New, unexplained symptoms develop. Drugs used in treatment may produce side effects.

Special notes:

_____

_____

_____

More notes on the back of this page ☐

POLYMYALGIA RHEUMATICA & GIANT CELL ARTERITIS

 BASIC INFORMATION

DESCRIPTION
Polymyalgia rheumatica (PMR) and giant cell arteritis (GCA) seem to be related inflammatory disorders. They often occur together. In PMR, inflammation affects the whole body. In GCA, certain arteries, such as those in the head and neck, are inflamed. It usually affects white adults over 50, and it affects women more than men.

FREQUENT SIGNS AND SYMPTOMS
- The symptoms may resemble those of an infection such as influenza. Symptoms can come on suddenly.
- Low fever and weakness.
- Muscle stiffness or aches and pains, especially in the morning. The muscles involved are usually those of the trunk, upper arms, and legs.
- Headache (usually in one temple).
- Pain in the temples or scalp, and sometimes, the jaw and tongue.
- Blurred or double vision; loss of vision in one eye.
- Appetite loss and weight loss.

CAUSES
Exact cause of the inflammation is unknown. It may involve the immune system, or be due to viral, genetic, or environmental factors.

RISK INCREASES WITH
White adults over age 50, especially women.

PREVENTIVE MEASURES
No specific preventive measures.

EXPECTED OUTCOMES
With treatment, the symptoms can clear up quickly and complications are unlikely. Treatment with drugs needs to continue for months to years depending on each individual patient. An active lifestyle is expected.

POSSIBLE COMPLICATIONS
- PMR may recur. It can be successfully treated again with drugs. GCA rarely recurs after treatment.
- Without treatment for GCA, there is a risk for loss of vision, stroke, heart failure, chest pain, and aneurysm.
- Adverse effects of steroid treatment (osteoporosis, high blood pressure, cataracts, and others).

 DIAGNOSIS & TREATMENT

GENERAL MEASURES
- Your health care provider will do a physical exam and ask questions about your symptoms. There is no specific diagnostic test for either disorder. Medical tests may include blood studies, tests for anemia, CT or MRI, and a biopsy. Biopsy involves the removal of a small amount of tissue or fluid for viewing under a microscope.

- Treatment involves drug therapy and exercise.
- For headache relief, apply heat to the painful side of the head. For muscle stiffness, apply heat directly to the affected area or take warm baths.
- To learn more: Arthritis Foundation, P.O. Box 7669, Atlanta, GA 30357-0669, (800) 283-7800; website: www.arthritis.org.

MEDICATIONS
- Cortisone drugs in high doses until the acute phase ends. These relieve symptoms by reducing inflammation. Adverse effects may occur. For ongoing treatment with cortisone, the dosage will be reduced as low as possible to keep symptoms under control.
- Methotrexate may be prescribed.
- Nonsteroidal anti-inflammatory drugs may be prescribed for polymyalgia rheumatica. They may not completely control symptoms.

ACTIVITY
Exercise regularly. Swimming, walking, biking, and stretching exercises will help keep muscles strong, flexible, and functional. Avoid straining the muscles (such as doing heavy lifting). Adequate rest is also important. Don't overdo physical activities.

DIET
No special diet.

 NOTIFY OUR OFFICE IF

- You or a family member has symptoms of polymyalgia rheumatica or giant cell arteritis.
- The following occur during or after treatment:
  - Any changes in vision. Call immediately!
  - Temperature of 101°F (38.3°C).
  - Blood in the urine.
  - Shortness of breath.
  - Chest pain.
  - Bloody bowel movements.
  - Severe abdominal pain.
  - Any illness with fever.
- New, unexplained symptoms develop. Drugs used in treatment may produce side effects.

Special notes:

_____

_____

_____

More notes on the back of this page ☐

388

POLYMYOSITIS & DERMATOMYOSITIS

 ## BASIC INFORMATION

DESCRIPTION

Polymyositis is muscle inflammation that leads to a gradual weakening of the muscles. When the disorder involves the skin, it is called dermatomyositis. Women are affected more often than men. It usually begins between ages 30 and 60. It may also occur in children.

FREQUENT SIGNS AND SYMPTOMS

- Symptoms vary from person to person and may be mild to severe. Their onset may be sudden or slow.
- Muscle weakness that often begins in the hip, thighs, and shoulder muscles. Other muscles may be affected.
- Frequent falls and difficulty in getting up.
- Muscle pain.
- Skin rash that may itch on the face, shoulders, arms, and over joints. The rash may be red or violet.
- Cold hands and feet.
- Speaking or swallowing difficulty.

CAUSES

Exact cause is unknown. They may be autoimmune disorders. In these disorders, the immune system by mistake attacks the body. Other factors may be involved such as viral, genetic, or environmental causes.

RISK INCREASES WITH

- Females over age 30.
- Family history of autoimmune disorders.

PREVENTIVE MEASURES

No known preventive measures.

EXPECTED OUTCOMES

The outcome varies. Symptoms can improve at times and get worse at other times. Earlier diagnosis and treatment improves the outcome. Some patients recover completely. Others have persistent symptoms, such as weakness. Others may have complications that can lead to disability and be life threatening.

POSSIBLE COMPLICATIONS

- Progressive muscle weakness.
- Heart, gastrointestinal, and lung problems.
- Adverse effects of drugs.
- Skin ulcers (open sores), infections, and scarring.
- Cancer.

 ## DIAGNOSIS & TREATMENT

GENERAL MEASURES

- Your health care provider will do a physical exam and an exam of any affected skin. Medical tests may include blood studies, heart tests, x-ray, and MRI. A biopsy may be done, which involves removal of a small amount of muscle tissue for viewing under a microscope. An electromyogram may be done. This test studies the electrical activity of muscles.
- Treatment usually involves drugs, physical therapy, or other therapy to help with activities of daily living.
- To learn more: Myositis Society of America. 1233 20th St. NW, Suite 402, Washington, DC 20036; (202) 887-0088 (not toll free); website: www.myositis.org.

MEDICATIONS

- Your health care provider may prescribe:
  - Cortisone drugs, in high doses until acute symptoms diminish, then in lower doses.
  - Drugs to suppress the immune system.
  - Drugs to help control itching.
  - Drugs for pain.
  - Drugs for bone building.

ACTIVITY

Physical therapy may be prescribed. It helps keep muscles flexible, strong, and functional. Follow instructions for exercises to do at home. Swimming is a good exercise. Don't overdo any activity. Rest as needed.

DIET

No special diet. Avoid weight gain.

 ## NOTIFY OUR OFFICE IF

- You or a family member has symptoms of polymyositis or dermatomyositis.
- Symptoms don't improve or recur despite treatment.
- New, unexplained symptoms develop. Drugs used in treatment may produce side effects.

Special notes:

_____

_____

_____

More notes on the back of this page ☐

PORPHYRIA

BASIC INFORMATION

DESCRIPTION

Any of a group of disorders in which the body has too much porphyrin. Porphyrin is a chemical that works with enzymes in the body to make heme. Heme is the part of blood that makes it red and carries the oxygen. Poryphia can affect both sexes. Types include:
- Acute intermittent porphyria (AIP).
- Variegate porphyria (VP).
- Hereditary coproporphyria (HCP).
- ALAD dehydratase porphyria (ADP).
- Porphyria cutanea tarda (PCT).
- Erythropoietic porphyria (EPP).
- Congenital erythropoietic porphyria (CEP).
- Hepatoerythropoietic porphyria (HEP).

FREQUENT SIGNS AND SYMPTOMS

- Symptoms vary and can appear over hours or days. A variety of factors can trigger an attack. Symptoms usually affect the nervous system or the skin.
- Chest, abdominal, or leg pain.
- Muscle cramps and weakness.
- Numbness and tingling in the feet and hands.
- Emotional and mental changes including depression, mania, anxiety, agitation, confusion, and others.
- Skin changes, including itching, blistering, and sensitivity to the sun.
- Excessive hair growth.
- Urine turns color (dark-red, purplish, or brown).

CAUSES

Porphyrin builds up in the body due to enzyme deficiencies. Enzymes are required to complete the porphyrin-heme process. There are several different types of enzyme deficiencies. Most types are inherited. Others develop during a person's life.

RISK INCREASES WITH

Family history of porphyria.

PREVENTIVE MEASURES

- Cannot be prevented at present.
- Porphyria attacks may result from drugs, alcohol, smoking, infection, reduced calorie intake, stress (physical and emotional), excess iron, hepatitis C, pregnancy, and before a menstrual period. Talk to your health care provider about avoiding these factors where possible.

EXPECTED OUTCOMES

There is no cure. Some people with porphyria never have symptoms. In others, the symptoms may be mild to severe. Symptoms can usually be relieved with treatment. A few patients may have complications.

POSSIBLE COMPLICATIONS

A variety of complications may occur that cause physical problems as well as psychological problems.

DIAGNOSIS & TREATMENT

GENERAL MEASURES

- Your health care provider will do a physical exam and ask questions about your symptoms and activities. Medical tests are done to measure porphyrins in the urine, blood, and stool.
- Treatment involves medical care during attacks, preventing attacks, and counseling if needed. Specific treatment will depend on the type of porphyria.
- Don't take any drugs, herbs, or supplements without medical advice.
- Avoid bright sunlight. If you must be in bright sun, use a hat and protective clothing.
- Phlebotomy may be done. A unit of blood is removed on a regular basis to get rid of excess iron in the body.
- Hospital care may be required for severe symptoms.
- Wear a medical alert type bracelet or pendant identifying your medical problem.
- Genetic counseling before starting a family is advised.
- To learn more: American Porphyria Foundation, P.O. Box 22712, Houston, TX 77227, (713) 266-9617 (not toll free); website: www.porphyriafoundation.com.

MEDICATIONS

- Your health care provider may prescribe:
  - Intravenous (IV) glucose or heme to help prevent or treat acute attacks.
  - Drugs for depression or anxiety.
  - Drugs to reduce nausea and vomiting.
  - Drugs to reduce the excess porphyrin in the body.
  - Drugs to help reduce premenstrual attacks.
  - Drugs for anemia (if needed).
  - Beta carotene for skin symptoms.

ACTIVITY

No limits except for the sunlight restrictions.

DIET

Eat a normal or high carbohydrate diet. If weight loss is desired, ask your health care provider for diet advice.

NOTIFY OUR OFFICE IF

- You or a family member has symptoms of porphyria.
- Any symptoms of an attack occur.
- New, unexplained symptoms develop.

Special notes:

_____

_____

_____

More notes on the back of this page ☐

POSTMENOPAUSAL BLEEDING

 ## BASIC INFORMATION

DESCRIPTION

Unexpected bleeding that begins 6 to 12 or more months after menopause. This is not a normal condition and can be a symptom of a serious medical problem.

FREQUENT SIGNS AND SYMPTOMS

· Vaginal bleeding. It may be a light-brown discharge or heavy, red bleeding (with or without clots).
· Mucus may be a part of the bleeding.
· Bleeding episodes vary in length.
· Pelvic pain (sometimes).

CAUSES

· Atrophy of the lining of the uterus (endometrium) or the vagina. Atrophy means shrinking or wasting away of tissue.
· Hormone therapy. Using estrogens (female hormones).
· Cancer.
· Endometrial hyperplasia (the uterine lining becomes overgrown).
· Endometrial or cervical polyps (benign growths).
· Myoma (benign fibroid tumor in the uterus).
· Trauma (injury) to the vagina.

RISK INCREASES IN/WITH

· Women over 60, due to fragile blood vessels and thin vaginal or uterine lining.
· Obesity.
· Hormone therapy. Women are likely to have some bleeding the first year.

PREVENTIVE MEASURES

No specific preventive measures.

EXPECTED OUTCOME

The outcome will depend on the cause of the bleeding. In the majority of cases, the cause is not cancer. Benign conditions can usually be treated and bleeding symptoms should clear up.

POSSIBLE COMPLICATIONS

If cancer is the cause, the outcome will depend on the type of cancer and the stage at which it is diagnosed. Many of these cancers are caught early, when treatment is more effective.

 ## DIAGNOSIS & TREATMENT

GENERAL MEASURES

· Your health care provider will usually do a physical exam, including a pelvic exam. (Be sure to tell your health care provider about nonprescribed substances that you take, such as soy protein.) Unexplained postmenopausal bleeding requires further medical testing. Tests start with blood studies and a Pap smear. Additional tests may include:
   - Biopsy of a small amount of tissue removed from the uterine lining. This is done with a thin suction device.
   - Ultrasound of the pelvic area.
   - Sonohystogram, an ultrasound with a saline (salt-water solution) injected into the uterus.
   - A hysteroscopy. A telescopic instrument with a special light is used to look inside the uterus.
   - A dilatation and curettage, referred to as D & C (dilatation of the cervix and a scraping out of the uterus with a curette). It may be both diagnostic and a treatment to relieve the bleeding.
· Specific therapy, usually drugs or surgery, is dependent on the cause. Sometimes, even after testing, no clear-cut reason for the bleeding is found.
· Surgery (hysterectomy) to remove the uterus may be needed.

MEDICATION

· If hormone drugs are currently being taken, the dose may need to be adjusted. In other cases, hormones may be prescribed.
· Drugs may be prescribed to treat any underlying disorder diagnosed.

ACTIVITY

· No limits unless advised by your health care provider.
· Sexual relations may be resumed as soon as desired after diagnosis and treatment.

DIET

No special diet.

 ## NOTIFY OUR OFFICE IF

You or a family member has unexplained bleeding after menopause or bleeding persists, despite treatment.

Special notes:

_____

_____

_____

More notes on the back of this page ☐

POSTPARTUM MOOD DISTURBANCES
(Postpartum Blues, Depression, & Psychosis)

BASIC INFORMATION

DESCRIPTION
Mood disturbances following the birth of a baby affect nearly half of all new mothers. The symptoms are most common 3 to 10 days following delivery, but can occur anytime in the first 6 months. Types include:
- Postpartum blues (baby blues), which involves mild symptoms that last a short time.
- Postpartum depression symptoms are sometimes described as baby blues that deepen and last longer.
- Postpartum psychosis is a rare and severe depression.

FREQUENT SIGNS AND SYMPTOMS
The symptoms vary, but can include:
- Mild sadness, crying spells, and mood swings.
- Appetite loss and weight loss, or weight gain.
- Sleep problems; unable to sleep when baby is sleeping, or waking up and having trouble returning to sleep.
- Loss of energy; fatigue.
- Irritability; anxiety, or feelings of tension or anger.
- Slow speech and thought, unable to make decisions.
- Frequent headaches, and other physical discomfort.
- Confusion about one's ability to improve life.
- Feelings of hopelessness, worthlessness, or gloom.
- Fears about personal health and infant's health.
- Poor personal hygiene.

CAUSES
Exact cause is unknown. It may involve physical, emotional, social, genetic, and hormone factors.

RISK INCREASES WITH
- Personal or family history of depression.
- Postpartum depression with a prior pregnancy.
- Physical and emotional stress, lack of sleep; poor nutrition, or problems with the baby's health.
- Severe pregnancy complications (e.g., preterm birth).
- Lack of support from one's partner, family, or friends.

PREVENTIVE MEASURES
- There is no specific way to prevent depression. Screening tests may help identify women at risk for it.
- If you have had depression before, ask your obstetric provider about ways to help guard against a recurrence.

EXPECTED OUTCOME
- It's common for mothers to have some degree of baby blues. It clears up on its own within about 10 days.
- For most women, postpartum depression is temporary and treatable. It may last a few weeks to months.

POSSIBLE COMPLICATIONS
- Lack of bonding between mother and baby.
- Children of depressed mothers are more at risk for developmental problems.
- Relationship problems with partner.
- Depression may become chronic or recurrent.
- Postpartum psychosis. A mother may harm herself or her baby.

DIAGNOSIS & TREATMENT

GENERAL MEASURES
- Your health care provider will ask questions about your symptoms and history to help with diagnosis. A depression-screening test may be given. Blood tests may be done to check for any physical problems.
- Treatment may involve counseling (psychotherapy), drugs, self-help, and education. Individual treatment will depend on the type and degree of the symptoms. Rarely, hospital care is needed.
- Counseling and/or group therapy may be prescribed.
- Don't feel guilty if you have mixed feelings about motherhood. Adjustment and bonding take time.
- Schedule frequent outings, such as walks and short visits with friends or family so that you don't feel alone.
- Ask for daytime help from family or friends who will shop for you or care for the baby while you rest.
- Find time for you and your partner to be alone.
- Sharing your feelings with your partner, friends, other mothers, or a support groups can help.
- To learn more: Depression After Delivery; (800) 944-4773; website: www.depressionafterdelivery.com.

MEDICATION
Antidepressant drugs may be prescribed. These are effective when used for 3 to 4 weeks. Breast-feeding mothers should get medical advice before using drugs.

ACTIVITY
Try to get some exercise each day. It will help physical and emotional well-being,

DIET
Eat a well-balanced diet. Avoid alcohol and caffeine.

NOTIFY OUR OFFICE IF

- You or a family member has symptoms of a postpartum mood disturbance.
- You have thoughts of hurting yourself or the baby, hear voices, see things, or feel unable to cope, or if a new mother talks of these feelings. Seek help promptly!

Special notes:

_____

_____

_____

More notes on the back of this page ☐

POST-TRAUMATIC STRESS DISORDER (PTSD)

BASIC INFORMATION

DESCRIPTION

A type of anxiety sometimes seen in people who have experienced an event that is extremely distressing. Such events (e.g., natural disasters, murder, rape, war, imprisonment, torture, accidents) produce psychological (emotional) stress in everyone. PTSD involves a persistent re-experiencing of the trauma and other symptoms. The symptoms may begin right after the event or develop months or years later. PTSD can affect all ages. It is more common in women than men.

FREQUENT SIGNS AND SYMPTOMS

· Recurrent, intrusive, and distressing memories of the event. A sense of reliving the event (flashbacks).
· Recurrent dreams or nightmares relating to the event.
· Chronic anxiety.
· Insomnia.
· Difficulty in concentrating and memory problems.
· A sense of personal isolation (feeling alone).
· Lack of interest in activities previously enjoyed.
· Phobic (fearful) reactions to situations or avoiding activities that recall memories of the event.
· Emotional effects (irritability, restlessness, tearfulness, explosive outbursts of behavior including violence, a numbness of feelings, or painful guilt feelings).

CAUSES

Exact cause is unknown. Exposure to an overwhelming, distressing event is a main factor. Other factors may involve a person's personality type, chemical imbalance in the brain, environmental stresses, and genetics.

RISK INCREASES WITH

Event:
· The type, severity, and duration of the event.
· Proximity of event (direct involvement or witness).
Personal:
· Emotional problems (such as low self-esteem).
· Lack of support from family, friends, or community.
· Childhood history of alcoholic parents, neglect, abuse, separation of parents, poverty, or violence.
· Previous experience with trauma.
· Personal or family history of mental disorders.
· Alcohol or drug abuse.

PREVENTIVE MEASURES

· Counseling and crisis intervention right after a traumatic event may prevent the development of PTSD.
· Debriefing soon after an event. Persons involved discuss the event, their emotions and their reactions.

EXPECTED OUTCOME

For some patients, the symptoms go away on their own after 6 months. Most patients can be helped with treatment. In others, the disorder may become chronic.

POSSIBLE COMPLICATIONS

· Marriage and family conflicts, difficulty in parenting children effectively, loss of friends, and unemployment.
· Depression, anxiety, phobias, drug or alcohol abuse.
· Self-inflicted violence and suicide.

DIAGNOSIS & TREATMENT

GENERAL MEASURES

· Your health care provider will do a physical exam and ask questions about your symptoms and exposure to a traumatic event. Medical tests may be done to rule out physical disorders. Mental health tests may be done.
· Treatment may include medical care (if needed for injuries or substance abuse), counseling (psychotherapy), drugs, education, self-help, and support groups. Individual treatment depends on your situation (safety from harm), your symptoms, and your health status.
· Cognitive-behavioral therapy is often recommended. Cognitive therapy teaches how to change thoughts, behaviors or attitudes. Behavioral therapy teaches ways to reduce anxiety with deep breathing and muscle relaxation. Other types of therapies can be effective.
· Learn relaxation techniques.
· Talking about the event may help you cope. Talk to family, friends, clergy, or join a support group.
· To learn more: National Institute of Mental Health; 6001 Executive Blvd, Bethesda, MD 20892-9663; (800) 647-2642; website: www.nimh.nih.gov.

MEDICATION

Antidepressant, antianxiety drugs, or drugs to treat insomnia may be prescribed (for a short time).

ACTIVITY

· A routine exercise program is helpful for physical and mental well-being. 30 minutes each day is a good goal.
· Go to bed and wake up at the same time every day.

DIET

No special diet.

NOTIFY OUR OFFICE IF

· You or a family member has symptoms of post-traumatic stress disorder.
· Symptoms don't improve or worsen with treatment.

Special notes:

_____

_____

_____

More notes on the back of this page ☐

POTASSIUM IMBALANCE

 BASIC INFORMATION

DESCRIPTION
Higher or lower than normal levels of potassium in the blood, body fluids, and body cells. Important electrolytes, including potassium, sodium, and calcium, maintain normal heart rhythm and regulate the body's water balance. They also help control muscle contractions and nerve impulses.

FREQUENT SIGNS AND SYMPTOMS
For above-normal levels (hyperkalemia):
- Tingling in hands and feet. Weakness and numbness.
- Extreme weakness and paralysis.
- Dangerously rapid, irregular heartbeat or heart attack.

For below-normal levels (hypokalemia):
- Mild weakness and muscle cramps, often following or during exercise.
- Discomfort in the legs while sitting.
- Confusion and disorientation.
- Extreme weakness and paralysis.
- Life-threatening rapid, irregular heartbeat.

CAUSES
Electrolytes need to be in a certain balance to maintain the health and proper functioning of the body. A high or low potassium level results in an electrolyte imbalance and can cause the heart and muscle symptoms.

RISK INCREASES WITH
Hyperkalemia:
- Kidney or renal disease.
- Severe burns, infections, or crushing muscle injuries.
- Acidosis (high acid concentration in the blood).
- Rhabdomyolysis (involves muscle and kidney injury).
- Chemotherapy (anticancer drugs).
- Adrenal gland disorders.
- Certain drugs that decrease potassium excretion.
- Rarely, strenuous exercise.

Hypokalemia:
- Use of diuretic drugs for medical or other purposes. Athletes may use diuretics to meet certain weight limits before competing (e.g., jockeys, boxers, wrestlers).
- Excessive, sweating vomiting, or diarrhea.
- Eating disorders; laxative abuse.
- Prolonged fasting or starvation.
- Alcoholism (poor diet may cause low potassium).
- Hyperaldosteronism, Cushing's syndrome, inherited kidney defects, and eating too much black licorice.

PREVENTIVE MEASURES
If you take diuretics or have renal or kidney disease, have frequent blood studies to check potassium levels.

EXPECTED OUTCOMES
Some potassium imbalances are temporary and correct themselves. Treatment can help other imbalances.

POSSIBLE COMPLICATIONS
- Treatment of hypokalemia may result in hyperkalemia and vice versa.
- Cardiac arrest and death.

 DIAGNOSIS & TREATMENT

GENERAL MEASURES
- Your health care provider may do a physical exam. Medical tests may include blood and urine studies of potassium and other electrolytes. An ECG (electrocardiogram) may be done. It measures the electrical activity of the heart.
- Treatment usually involves drugs to correct the potassium imbalance.
- Most cases are treatable at home. Hospital care and intravenous (IV) therapy may be needed for severe cases of hypokalemia or hyperkalemia. Dialysis (a way to clean the blood) may be required if kidneys fail.
- If you take diuretics and digitalis, your family members should learn cardiopulmonary resuscitation (CPR). Learn to count your own pulse at the wrist or neck.

MEDICATIONS
- Your health care provider may prescribe:
  - Oral or intravenous (IV) potassium supplements to raise low levels.
  - Diuretics to increase urination and decrease high potassium levels.
  - Intravenous (IV) fluids (electrolytes) to correct a serious imbalance.
  - Drugs to treat an underlying disorder.
  - Changes in your current drugs if they are causing the potassium imbalance.

ACTIVITY
Resume normal activities once symptoms improve.

DIET
Depends on the condition. You may be advised to eat more or less high-potassium foods, such as orange juice, bananas, melons, carrots, tomato juice, and papaya.

 NOTIFY OUR OFFICE IF

You or a family member has symptoms of a potassium imbalance.

Special notes:

_____

_____

_____

More notes on the back of this page ☐

PREECLAMPSIA & ECLAMPSIA
(Pregnancy-Induced Hypertension; Toxemia)

BASIC INFORMATION

DESCRIPTION
A serious problem of pregnancy. It involves blood pressure, kidney function, and the central nervous system. Preeclampsia (pregnancy-induced hypertension) may occur from the 20th week of pregnancy until 7 days after delivery. Eclampsia is severe preeclampsia.

FREQUENT SIGNS AND SYMPTOMS
Mild preeclampsia:
- Significant blood pressure rise, even if still in the normal range.
- Puffiness in the face, hands, and feet that is worse in the morning.
- Excessive weight gain (more than a pound a week during the last trimester).

Preeclampsia that is more severe:
- Continued blood pressure rise.
- Continued swelling and puffiness.
- Blurred vision.
- Headache.
- Irritability.
- Abdominal pain.

Eclampsia:
- Worsening of above symptoms.
- Muscle twitching.
- Seizures or coma.

CAUSES
Unknown. A dysfunction of the placenta may start the process that leads to other problems.

RISK INCREASES WITH
- Diabetes prior to pregnancy or diabetes gestational.
- High blood pressure before becoming pregnant.
- Kidney or renal disease or blood vessel disease.
- First pregnancy or first pregnancy with a new partner.
- Preeclampsia in a previous pregnancy.
- Family history of preeclampsia or eclampsia, heart disease, or high blood pressure.
- Obesity.
- Multiple gestation (twins, triplets, etc.).
- Mother's age over 40 or less than 20.
- African American women.

PREVENTIVE MEASURES
None specific. Low-dose aspirin may help. Regular prenatal care will help find abnormal blood pressure early.

EXPECTED OUTCOME
The cure is to deliver the baby. Complications for mother and baby can often be prevented with prompt diagnosis and treatment. The symptoms usually resolve days to weeks after delivery. If premature labor occurs, the newborn's survival chances depend on its maturity.

POSSIBLE COMPLICATIONS
- Mother—Stroke, kidney failure, seizures, high blood pressure, hemorrhage, pulmonary edema, heart failure, and death.
- Baby—Premature birth, low birth weight, intrauterine growth restriction, and stillbirth.

DIAGNOSIS & TREATMENT

GENERAL MEASURES
- Diagnostic tests may include blood pressure tests, blood studies, 24-hour urine study (to check the protein levels), and ultrasound (to assess fetal development).
- Treatment will depend on the severity of the symptoms and the maturity of the fetus. Mild symptoms may be treated at home. Hospital care is needed if the condition worsens or for early delivery. Eclampsia, because of seizure activity, usually requires hospital care and rapid delivery. A cesarean section may be required.
- If you are at home, weigh yourself daily and keep a record. Use a home test to check for protein in the urine (instructions will be provided).
- To learn more: Preeclampsia Foundation, 12727 NE 20th St., Suite 16, Bellevue, WA 98005; (800) 665-9341; website: www.preeclampsia.org.

MEDICATION
- Antihypertensive (blood pressure) drugs may be prescribed.
- Anticonvulsants to prevent seizures. Magnesium sulfate may be prescribed or given by vein (IV) if labor has started.

ACTIVITY
Rest often. This is important to control preeclampsia. Rest on your left side to help blood circulation.

DIET
You will be advised if a special diet is needed.

NOTIFY OUR OFFICE IF
- You or a family member has symptoms of preeclampsia at any stage of pregnancy.
- The following occur during treatment: Severe headache or vision changes, weight gain of 3 or more pounds in 24 hours, nausea, vomiting, diarrhea, cramping abdominal pains, or excessive irritability.

Special notes:

_____

_____

_____

More notes on the back of this page ☐

PREMATURE EJACULATION

 BASIC INFORMATION

DESCRIPTION

Male orgasm and ejaculation prior to the wishes of both sexual partners. There is no precise duration (or time) for sexual relations and reaching a climax. There are many variables that affect individual couples. Premature ejaculation (PE) is a common problem affecting all age groups. It is called primary if a male has always had the problem. It is called secondary if a male was previously able to have ejaculatory control and is now not able.

FREQUENT SIGNS AND SYMPTOMS

· Repeated episodes of premature ejaculation.
· Feelings of self-doubt, inadequacy, and guilt.

CAUSES

The exact cause is unknown. It may involve psychological (mental or emotional) factors (most likely) or physical factors (less likely).

RISK INCREASES WITH

· Poor relationship with sexual partner or poor communication (not able to talk things over).
· Fear of pregnancy of sexual partner.
· Fear of contracting a sexually transmitted disease.
· Anxiety about sexual performance.
· Cultural or religious conflicts.
· Belief that sex is sinful or dirty.
· May be due to underlying physical disorder (such as prostatitis).

PREVENTIVE MEASURES

No specific preventive measures.

EXPECTED OUTCOMES

The couple, and not just the man, needs to work on the problem together. It is usually curable in most people within 6 months with treatment.

POSSIBLE COMPLICATIONS

· Low self-esteem.
· The problem can recur after successful treatment.
· Stress with the marriage or other personal relationship.

 DIAGNOSIS & TREATMENT

GENERAL MEASURES

· Your health care provider may do a physical exam and ask questions about your symptoms and sexual history. Medical test results are usually normal, as most males with this problem are healthy individuals.
· Treatment may involve counseling for the patient and his partner, and drugs.
· Your health care provider may have you try the following methods. They are recommended by sex researchers and therapists Masters and Johnson. These measures often lead to ejaculatory control for 5 to 10 minutes or longer.

- Sensate-focus exercises, in which each partner caresses the other's body without intercourse to learn relaxed, pleasurable aspects of touching.
- Mutual physical exam of each other's bodies to acquaint both partners thoroughly with anatomy. This helps reduce shameful feelings about sex.
- Stop-and-start technique, in which the man is stimulated through controlled intercourse or masturbation until he feels an impending ejaculation. Stimulation is stopped and then resumed in 20 to 30 seconds.
- Squeeze technique, in which the woman squeezes her partner's penis with her thumb and forefinger when he feels an impending ejaculation. When ejaculatory feelings pass, intercourse is resumed. This is repeated as often as needed until the man can control ejaculation to the satisfaction of both partners.
· Work on ways to improve communication with your partner and try to reduce your performance anxiety.
· Counseling from a qualified sex therapist may be recommended if other methods are not successful.

MEDICATIONS

· There is no specific drug to treat the problem. A class of antidepressants called selective serotonin reuptake inhibitors (SSRIs) helps some men delay sexual climax. Your health care provider may prescribe one of these drugs for you. It may be used as a single dose prior to sexual intercourse or taken on a daily basis.
· A topical anesthetic agent may be recommended. It may help to reduce penile sensitivity and delay ejaculation. An example is lidocaine. It can be applied to the penis under a condom about 30 minutes before intercourse. Follow instructions provided with the product.

ACTIVITY

No limits.

DIET

No special diet.

 NOTIFY OUR OFFICE IF

· You or a family member has repeated episodes of premature ejaculation.
· Problem continues despite treatment.

Special notes:

_____

_____

_____

More notes on the back of this page ☐

PREMATURE LABOR & PREMATURE BIRTH

BASIC INFORMATION

DESCRIPTION
Premature labor is labor that begins before the 37th week of pregnancy. Premature birth may follow premature labor.

FREQUENT SIGNS AND SYMPTOMS
· Uterine contractions at regular intervals that begin before the 37th week of gestation (3 weeks prior to due date) and premature opening (dilation) of the cervix.
· Passage of mucus (may be bloody).
· A feeling of pelvic pressure; low back pain; cramping.
· Flow of fluid (amniotic fluid) from the uterus (sometimes). This may occur with a gush or may be only a steady watery discharge.
· Some degree of vaginal bleeding or spotting.

CAUSES
In most cases, the exact problems that cause premature labor are not well-known. Many obstetric, medical, and anatomic disorders are factors for premature labor.

RISK INCREASES WITH
· Premature rupture of the membranes ("water breaks").
· Abnormally small fetus relative to gestational age.
· Large fetus or more than one fetus.
· Illness of the mother, including preeclampsia, high blood pressure or diabetes.
· Abnormal shape or size of the uterus; weak cervix.
· Hormone imbalance.
· Vaginal infection that spreads to the uterus.
· Problems of the placenta, such as placenta previa.
· Excessive amniotic fluid (polyhydramnios).
· Poor nutrition (more so if it occurs with weight loss).
· Previous premature labor.
· Smoking, excess alcohol use, or drug abuse.
· Injury to the uterus.
· Urinary-tract infection, such as kidney infection (pyelonephritis).
· Mother-to-be is under age 18, older than 40, or was considered seriously underweight before pregnancy.

PREVENTIVE MEASURES
· Obtain good prenatal care throughout pregnancy.
· Don't smoke, abuse drugs, or drink alcohol.
· Eat a normal, well-balanced diet during pregnancy. Take prescribed prenatal vitamins.
· Don't use drugs of any kind, including nonprescription drugs, without medical advice.
· If you have a weak cervix, which is sometimes evident before pregnancy, get medical advice about a minor operation to strengthen the cervix.
· Rest more and decrease activity in the 3rd trimester, especially if you have blood spotting or irregular contractions.

EXPECTED OUTCOME
· In about 50% of cases, the premature labor ceases, either on its own or with treatment.
· Labor can often be stopped with treatment to allow more time for the fetus to mature.
· In some cases delivery must proceed; sometimes by cesarean section. Outcome depends on fetal maturity.

POSSIBLE COMPLICATIONS
· Premature infant.
· Uterine infection after delivery.
· Fetal death.

DIAGNOSIS & TREATMENT

GENERAL MEASURES
· Diagnostic tests may include amniocentesis to determine fetal maturity and to check for infection inside the uterus that could be causing the symptoms. Ultrasound is used to determine fetal weight, age, growth, and position. Blood and urine studies are done to check for infection.
· Hospital care may be necessary for any underlying risk factors (such as infections or dehydration).
· Immediate cesarean delivery may be needed.
· Treatment may continue until the 36th or 37th week of pregnancy when there is less risk for the baby.

MEDICATIONS
· Drugs to stop labor may be prescribed.
· Antibiotics if an infection develops. Antibiotics may also be used to help protect the fetus from infection.
· Corticosteroid therapy may be considered to help fetal lung maturity.

ACTIVITY
Complete bed rest is needed once signs of premature labor begin. Discontinue work or other physical activities. Avoid any sexual activity.

DIET
If labor starts, drink only clear liquids until you deliver.

NOTIFY OUR OFFICE IF

· You or a family member has symptoms of premature labor. Call immediately. This is an emergency!
· Any symptoms develop that cause concern.

Special notes:

_____

_____

_____

More notes on the back of this page ☐

PREMENSTRUAL DYSPHORIC DISORDER (PMDD)

 ## BASIC INFORMATION

DESCRIPTION

Premenstrual dysphoric disorder (PMDD) is a severe form of premenstrual syndrome (PMS). Symptoms of PMDD interfere with daily activities, and can cause problems with personal relationships. PMDD is also called late-luteal dysphoric disorder.

FREQUENT SIGNS AND SYMPTOMS

• The symptoms occur 5 to 14 days before, and go away a few days after, the start of menstruation.
• Symptoms vary for every woman, and vary at times in the same woman. Most of the symptoms involve emotional or behavioral factors. Symptoms may include:
- Being irritable or angry.
- Feeling depressed, sad, and hopeless.
- Feelings of tension or anxiety.
- Mood swings marked by periods of crying.
- Lack of interest in daily activities and relationships.
- Trouble paying attention and unable to concentrate.
- Fatigue or lack of energy.
- Food cravings or overeating.
- Trouble sleeping.
- Feeling out of control.
- Physical symptoms, such as bloating, breast tenderness, headaches, and joint or muscle pain.

CAUSES

No single cause has been found. It may be a response to hormone changes related to the menstrual cycle or low levels of serotonin, a chemical in the brain. Research into the cause is ongoing.

RISK INCREASES WITH

• Women with a personal or family history of mood disorders, such as depression or postpartum depression.
• Stressful life events.

PREVENTIVE MEASURES

None known.

EXPECTED OUTCOME

Treatment can help reduce some PMDD symptoms. Treatment may be needed for at least a year. There are a variety of treatment options. It is important to find what works for you.

POSSIBLE COMPLICATIONS

The symptoms may get worse over time and last until menopause (when menses ceases).

 ## DIAGNOSIS & TREATMENT

GENERAL MEASURES

• Your health care provider will do a physical exam (including a pelvic exam). Questions will be asked about your symptoms and lifestyle. To aid in the diagnosis, you may be asked to keep a symptom diary for two or more months. List the dates of your period and which symptoms you have (and their severity) on the days before and after your period.
• Treatment options for PMDD include lifestyle changes, counseling, drugs, and use of alternative therapies. No single treatment works for every woman.
• Lifestyle changes include diet changes, stopping smoking, aerobic exercise, and steps to reduce stress.
• Counseling may help a woman find ways to cope with the PMDD symptoms.
• Biofeedback, acupuncture, and massage may help some women. Relaxation techniques may be used as treatment for stress. Phototherapy (treatment with light) may help in some cases.
• Join a support group. Talking about your PMDD symptoms with others can help.
• To learn more, do an Internet search or visit a library.

MEDICATION

• Antidepressant drugs may be prescribed. These help the symptoms of PMDD.
• Other drugs may be prescribed for specific symptoms such as headaches, anxiety, pain, and bloating.
• Vitamins and supplements may be recommended.

ACTIVITY

Do aerobic exercise (20 to 30 minutes) daily, or at least three times per week.

DIET

• Eat a healthy diet. Try eating frequent, small meals.
• Reduce or eliminate salt, caffeine, sugar, and alcohol.

 ## NOTIFY OUR OFFICE IF

• You or a family member has symptoms of PMDD.
• Symptoms get worse or new ones develop despite treatment.

Special notes:

_____

_____

_____

More notes on the back of this page ☐

PREMENSTRUAL SYNDROME
(Premenstrual Tension; PMS)

BASIC INFORMATION

DESCRIPTION
Premenstrual syndrome (PMS) involves symptoms that begin 7 to 14 days prior to a menstrual period and usually stop when menstruation begins. About half of all women experience PMS at some time, some very frequently. It most often affects women ages 25 to 40.

FREQUENT SIGNS AND SYMPTOMS
- Depressed mood.
- Nervousness and irritability.
- Dizziness or fainting.
- Fatigue.
- Emotional instability; mood swings.
- Increased or decreased sex drive.
- Headaches.
- Tender, swollen breasts.
- Bloating, constipation, or diarrhea.
- Other digestive disturbances.
- Fluid retention (edema) in ankles, hands, and face.
- Higher incidence of minor infections such as colds.
- Acne outbreaks.
- Decreased urination.
- Many other symptoms (over 150) have been attributed to PMS.

CAUSES
Unknown, but may be due to changes in the level of hormones (especially estrogen and progesterone). These changes cause retention of sodium in the bloodstream, resulting in edema in body tissues including the brain. Increased levels of prostaglandin (a chemical) in the bloodstream may be a factor. More theories about the basis of PMS include emotional, diet, changes in brain chemicals, and other factors.

RISK INCREASES WITH
- Increased levels of emotional stress.
- Caffeine and high fluid intake may worsen symptoms.
- Smoking may also intensify or increase symptoms.
- PMS risk increases with age.
- May occur with other disorders such as depression.

PREVENTIVE MEASURES
No specific preventive measures. Try to avoid stressful situations at the expected time of PMS. Also share your feelings and needs with a close friend or spouse.

EXPECTED OUTCOME
Treatment may be effective. Drugs can sometimes help control some symptoms. PMS stops with menopause.

POSSIBLE COMPLICATIONS
- Severe emotional stress that disrupts a woman's life.
- Premenstrual dysphoric disorder (symptoms are more severe than with PMS).

DIAGNOSIS & TREATMENT

GENERAL MEASURES
- Your health care provider may do a physical exam to rule out other disorders. Diagnosis usually depends on a history of symptoms. Keep a menstrual diary. Write down your symptoms and when they occur, your physical and emotional changes, and the pain involved.
- Treatment steps involve education about PMS, diet, exercise, lifestyle changes, and drugs.
- Reduce stress where possible. Learn relaxation techniques. Reduce activities on days you have symptoms.
- Quit smoking. Find a way to stop that works for you.
- Individual or couple counseling helps some patients.
- Join a support group. Talking about your PMS symptoms with others can help.
- To learn more, do an Internet search or visit a library.

MEDICATION
- These are used with varying degrees of success:
  - Nonsteroidal anti-inflammatory drugs (NSAIDs) to decrease prostaglandin levels.
  - Antidepressants or antianxiety drugs.
  - Diuretics to reduce fluid retention.
  - Pain drugs such as acetaminophen or ibuprofen.
  - Vitamin B6, vitamin E, magnesium, or calcium.
  - Hormones to suppress ovarian function.
  - Certain herbal products, such as evening primrose oil.
  - Oral contraceptives.

ACTIVITY
- Begin a regular, aerobic exercise program (such as walking or biking). Exercise can help relieve or reduce PMS symptoms.
- Go to sleep and wake up at the same times each day.

DIET
Eat a low-fat, low-salt, high complex carbohydrate diet with frequent small meals. Limit use of caffeine.

NOTIFY OUR OFFICE IF

- You or a family member has symptoms of PMS that interfere with normal activities or relationships.
- Symptoms don't improve, despite treatment.
- New, unexplained symptoms develop.

Special notes:

_____

_____

_____

More notes on the back of this page ☐

PRIAPISM

 BASIC INFORMATION

DESCRIPTION

A persistent erection of the penis without sexual arousal or desire. It is a serious condition that requires medical care to prevent complications. It can affect all ages, including children.

FREQUENT SIGNS AND SYMPTOMS

A prolonged, usually painful erection. The erection may last hours to days.

CAUSES

It may be associated with certain diseases or use of drugs. Sometimes, no cause is found. Two types occur:
- Low-flow: blood becomes trapped in the penis causing its engorgement.
- High-flow (rarer): occurs when the blood in the penis does not circulate properly. It is usually due to an injury.

RISK INCREASES WITH

- Drugs that are used to treat impotence.
- Blood disease (sickle-cell disease or thalassemia).
- Cancer (leukemia or multiple myeloma).
- Certain drugs used to treat other disorders (such as chlorpromazine, prazosin, trazodone, some corticosteroids, anticoagulants, and antihypertensives).
- Spinal tumor, injury, or anesthesia.
- Carbon monoxide poisoning,
- Black widow spider bite.
- Malaria.
- Cocaine, marijuana, ecstasy, and alcohol abuse.
- Use of anabolic steroids.
- Prolonged sexual activity.

PREVENTIVE MEASURES

No specific preventive measures. Avoid risk factors where possible.

EXPECTED OUTCOMES

With prompt, effective medical care, the outcome is generally good. Delayed treatment can lead to increased risk of erectile dysfunction.

POSSIBLE COMPLICATIONS

- Impotence.
- Recurrence of priapism.
- Infection.
- Complications from surgical procedures may occur.

 DIAGNOSIS & TREATMENT

GENERAL MEASURES

- Emergency treatment is necessary because of the risk of permanent damage to the penis. Your health care provider will do a physical exam and an exam of the penis. Questions will be asked about your symptoms, activities, and drug use. Medical tests may include a small amount of blood taken from the penis for study. Ultrasound or angiogram (special type of x-ray) tests may be done.
- Treatment may include drug therapy, aspiration of the blood, or surgery. Any underlying cause will also need treatment. Patients with sickle-cell disease may need a blood transfusion. Spinal anesthesia is sometimes helpful.
- As a temporary measure, ice packs may be applied to the penis and perineum to help reduce swelling. Walking up a flight of stairs may help divert blood flow.
- Aspiration involves using a needle to remove blood from the penis. This will reduce pressure and swelling.
- Surgery may be needed if other treatment measures are not effective. A shunt (passageway) may be inserted to divert the blood flow. In high-flow priapism, surgery may be done to tie off an injured artery to restore normal blood flow.

MEDICATIONS

- Decongestant drugs may be prescribed. They are injected into the penis or taken by mouth. They narrow the veins in the penis and cause the swelling to subside.
- If a drug you take is the cause of priapism, it may be discontinued. An alternative drug may be prescribed.

ACTIVITY

Rest until erection is relieved.

DIET

No special diet.

 NOTIFY OUR OFFICE IF

You or a family member has an erection that persists for no apparent reason. Do not waste time trying to get it down with cold compresses. Go immediately to an emergency room.

Special notes:

_____

_____

_____

More notes on the back of this page ☐

PRICKLY HEAT
(Miliaria Rubra)

 BASIC INFORMATION

DESCRIPTION
A skin disorder caused by obstructed sweat-gland ducts. It affects all ages, but it is most common in infants.

FREQUENT SIGNS AND SYMPTOMS
Clusters of vesicles (small, fluid-filled skin blisters that may come and go within a matter of hours) or red rash without vesicles in areas of heavy sweating.

CAUSES
Obstruction of sweat-gland ducts for unknown reasons.

RISK INCREASES WITH
- Obesity.
- Hot, humid weather.
- Genetic factors, such as fair, sensitive skin.
- Plastic bedsheets.
- High fever.

PREVENTIVE MEASURES
Avoid risk factors where possible.

EXPECTED OUTCOMES
Usually curable with treatment. Recurrence is common.

POSSIBLE COMPLICATIONS
A bacterial skin infection may develop.

 DIAGNOSIS & TREATMENT

GENERAL MEASURES
- Take frequent cool showers or tub baths.
- Apply lubricating ointment or cream to skin 6 or 7 times a day.
- Use cool-water soaks to relieve itching and hasten healing. Pat skin dry, and dust with cornstarch after and between soaks.
- Wear cotton socks and leather-soled footwear rather than shoes made of synthetic materials.
- Expose the affected skin to air as much as possible.
- Don't use binding materials, such as adhesive tape, or wear tight clothing.
- Change diapers on infants as soon as they are wet.
- Avoid sunburn once you have had prickly heat. The body's inflammatory reaction to sunburn may trigger a new outbreak of prickly heat.
- Provide a cool, dry environment.
- See your health care provider if skin symptoms cause concern.

MEDICATIONS
- Nonprescription steroid cream applied 2 or 3 times a day (only upon recommendation of your physician).
- Oral antibiotics may be prescribed if there is a secondary bacterial infection.

ACTIVITY
Decrease activity during hot, humid weather or until skin heals.

DIET
No special diet.

 NOTIFY OUR OFFICE IF

Prickly heat doesn't improve in 10 days, despite home care.

Special notes:

_____

_____

_____

More notes on the back of this page ☐

PROCTITIS

BASIC INFORMATION

DESCRIPTION
Inflammation of the rectum and tissues around the anus. It affects adolescents and adults of both sexes, but it is more common in males around age 30.

FREQUENT SIGNS AND SYMPTOMS
· Rectal pain.
· Constant urge to have a bowel movement, often when little or no stool is present.
· Blood or mucus discharge from the rectum.
· Cramping pain in the left lower abdomen.
· Fever.

CAUSES
· Gonorrhea.
· Syphilis (usually secondary).
· Herpes simplex virus.
· Candidiasis.
· Chlamydia.
· Papilloma virus.
· Amebiasis.
· Nonspecific sexually transmitted infection.
· Radiation therapy.

RISK INCREASES WITH
· Anal intercourse.
· Use of laxatives.
· Rectal injury, rectal drugs.
· Radiation therapy.
· Endocrine disorders.
· Ulcerative colitis (early stages).
· Chronic constipation.
· Cancer of the rectum.
· Food allergy.

PREVENTIVE MEASURES
· Avoid anal intercourse.
· Practice safe sex methods. Unsafe sexual activity may increase the risk of an HIV infection.
· To prevent constipation, establish a regular pattern for bowel movements. Eat a high-fiber and diet drink plenty of fluids each day.
· Don't use laxatives regularly.
· Don't eat foods to which you are sensitive.
· Sexually transmitted diseases, such as gonorrhea and syphilis, must be reported to the local health department to prevent their spread. Information is kept confidential.

EXPECTED OUTCOMES
The outcome of proctitis depends on the treatment of the underlying cause. Infections can usually be cured with antibiotics. Symptoms of other disorders can be relieved or controlled with treatment.

POSSIBLE COMPLICATIONS
· Anal scarring and stricture (permanent narrowing of the anus).
· Chronic ulcerative colitis.

DIAGNOSIS & TREATMENT

GENERAL MEASURES
· Your health care provider will do a physical exam. Medical tests may include blood studies, stool cultures, tests for gonorrhea, syphilis, and other sexually transmitted diseases and stool cultures. Diagnostic tests such as proctoscopy or sigmoidoscopy may be done to rule out other disorders. These procedures use a telescope-like instrument to look inside the rectum, colon, and bowels.
· Treatment will usually be with drug therapy for the underlying cause.
· Keep the anal area clean with frequent bathing.
· Take sitz baths often to relieve pain. Sit in a tub of warm water for 10 to 15 minutes as often as needed.

MEDICATIONS
· Your health care provider may prescribe:
 - Antibiotics for sexually transmitted infections. If the cause is a gonorrheal infection, drugs may need to be injected into a muscle.
 - Acyclovir for herpes simplex infection.
 - Steroid suppositories or rectal foam to reduce inflammation from other causes.
· You may use nonprescription topical anesthetics to relieve discomfort.

ACTIVITY
No limits.

DIET
· Eat a high-fiber diet.
· Drink at least 8 glasses of water a day.
· Don't eat foods to which you are sensitive.

NOTIFY OUR OFFICE IF

· You or a family member has symptoms of proctitis, or symptoms recur after treatment.
· New, unexplained symptoms develop. Drugs used in treatment may produce side effects.

Special notes:

_____

_____

_____

More notes on the back of this page ☐

PROSTATE CANCER

BASIC INFORMATION

DESCRIPTION

Growth of malignant (cancerous) cells in the prostate gland. The prostate is about the size of a walnut and is located just below the urinary bladder in men. It helps form semen. This cancer often grows very slowly and may never cause symptoms. In some cases, it grows more rapidly, such as in younger men. Prostate cancer usually affects men over age 50.

FREQUENT SIGNS AND SYMPTOMS

• No symptoms (usually). Most prostate cancers are discovered during a routine rectal exam.
• Difficult, frequent, weak, or painful urination.
• Pain in the low back or pelvis from spread of cancer.
• Painful ejaculation.

CAUSES

Unknown.

RISK INCREASES WITH

• Age over 50.
• Family history of prostate cancer.
• High-fat diet.
• African American more than whites or others.

PREVENTIVE MEASURES

No specific preventive measures. A yearly rectal exam after age 40 and PSA testing may help detect early prostate cancer. A healthy diet may have some preventive benefit, but it has not yet been proven.

EXPECTED OUTCOMES

Often curable with surgery if treated before cancer spreads. If the cancer has spread, treatment can relieve symptoms and prolong life.

POSSIBLE COMPLICATIONS

• Fatal spread to bone, bladder, and other organs.
• Cancer may recur after treatment.
• Urinary incontinence.
• Sexual impotence after surgery (sometimes).

DIAGNOSIS & TREATMENT

GENERAL MEASURES

• Your health care provider will do a digital rectal exam (DRE). During a DRE, a gloved, lubricated finger is inserted into the rectum to check the prostate gland for lumps. Blood levels of prostate-specific antigen (PSA) will be checked. PSA, a protein produced by the prostate, is higher than normal in prostate diseases. Ultrasound, biopsy, CT, and other tests may be done to confirm the cancer diagnosis and to see if it has spread to other places in the body (staging).

• Treatment depends on the cancer stage, age, the health status and personal preferences of the patient.
• Treatment may include surgery, radiation, hormone therapy, chemotherapy (sometimes), and watchful waiting. It helps to discuss your options with family and friends and/or support groups.
• Watchful waiting. This means monitoring the disorder for a time before deciding on treatment. Some prostate cancers grow quite slowly.
• Surgery to remove the prostate gland and surrounding tissues, if the cancer has not spread. Other surgery may just remove the cancerous area and not the entire prostate. Your health care provider will explain the options, the risks and benefits.
• Cryosurgery may be recommended. It treats cancer that has not spread by freezing the cancer cells.
• Radiation or hormone treatment if the cancer has spread or for patients unable to undergo surgery.
• Tiny "seeds" may be inserted in the prostate. They deliver a dose of radiation over 3 to 6 months.
• Counseling, if sexual difficulties occur after treatment.
• To learn more: American Cancer Society, (800) ACS-2345; website: www.cancer.org or National Cancer Institute, (800) 4-CANCER; website: www.nci.nih.gov.

MEDICATIONS

• Hormones (usually estrogens or leutinizing hormone releasing hormone) to slow cancer growth.
• Chemotherapy (anticancer drugs) may be prescribed if the cancer has spread.
• Drugs for pain may be prescribed.

ACTIVITY

Resume your normal activities gradually after surgery. Follow medical advice about resuming sexual relations.

DIET

A low-fat diet may be recommended.

NOTIFY OUR OFFICE IF

• You or a family member has symptoms of prostate cancer.
• During treatment, any sign of urinary-tract infection occurs, such as frequent, difficult, or painful urination, fever and chills, aching around the genitals or rectum, or backache.
• Drugs used in treatment cause side effects.

Special notes:

_____

_____

_____

More notes on the back of this page ☐

PROSTATIC HYPERPLASIA, BENIGN

(BPH; Prostate Hypertrophy)

 ## BASIC INFORMATION

DESCRIPTION

Enlargement of the prostate gland. The prostate is about the size of a walnut and is located just below the urinary bladder in men. An enlarged prostate presses against the urethra (tube that carries urine outside) making it narrower. The bladder muscle becomes thicker and more sensitive, causing a need to urinate more often. BPH occurs more often in men over age 50.

FREQUENT SIGNS AND SYMPTOMS

- Increased urinary urgency and frequency, especially at night.
- Weak urinary stream.
- Stopping and starting again while urinating.
- Straining and dribbling during urination.
- Feeling that the bladder cannot be emptied completely.
- Leaking of urine and sometimes blood in the urine.

CAUSES

Exact cause unknown. It is common for the prostate to enlarge as a man ages.

RISK INCREASES WITH

Aging.

PREVENTIVE MEASURES

No specific prevention measures are known.

EXPECTED OUTCOMES

Symptoms may improve, worsen, or stay the same. A variety of treatments are available that can help to relieve the symptoms.

POSSIBLE COMPLICATIONS

- Urinary retention.
- Urinary stones.
- Urinary-tract infections.
- Reduced kidney function.

 ## DIAGNOSIS & TREATMENT

GENERAL MEASURES

- Your health care provider will do a digital rectal exam (DRE). During a DRE, a gloved, lubricated finger is inserted into the rectum to feel the prostate gland's size and check for lumps. Blood levels of prostate-specific antigen (PSA) will be checked. Other medical tests may include urine flow rate study, urinalysis, urine culture, x-ray of the urinary tract, and ultrasound.
- A question and answer interview is done about your symptoms. This can help in making treatment decisions. After treatment, it provides a good idea of how much the symptoms have improved.

- Treatment may include watchful waiting, nonsurgical treatment, surgery, or drug therapy. Emergency treatment may be needed if all urine output is blocked.
- Watchful waiting is an option. This means monitoring the symptoms for a time before deciding on treatment.
- Several types of nonsurgical procedures are available. They include balloon dilation, prostatic stents, microwave therapy, needle ablation using radiofrequency, electrovaporization, and laser therapy. Your health care provider will explain and discuss these options.
- Surgery may be recommended if there are more severe symptoms, complications occur, or there is a health risk. Several surgical options are available. The choice usually depends upon the size of the enlarged prostate. Surgery removes the enlarged part of the prostate. The rest is left intact.

MEDICATIONS

- Finasteride or dutasteride may be prescribed. They cause the prostate to shrink.
- Alpha-adrenergic blockers may be prescribed. They help relax the muscles in the prostate.
- Antibiotics if you develop a urinary-tract infection.
- Read labels on all nonprescription drugs. Avoid those that state "not recommended if you have prostatic hypertrophy." Examples are antidiarrheals and antihistamines.

ACTIVITY

No limits on activities.

DIET

No special diet. Avoid spicy foods and pepper, which irritate the urethra.

 ## NOTIFY OUR OFFICE IF

- You or a family member has symptoms of BPH.
- During treatment, any sign of urinary-tract infection occurs. This includes frequent, difficult, or painful urination, fever and chills, aching around the genitals or rectum, or backache.
- New, unexplained symptoms develop. Drugs used in treatment may produce side effects.
- Any new symptoms develop following surgery.

Special notes:

_____

_____

_____

More notes on the back of this page ☐

PROSTATITIS

BASIC INFORMATION

DESCRIPTION

Inflammation of the prostate. The prostate is about the size of a walnut and is located just below the urinary bladder in men. Inflammation causes swelling of the prostate. The swelling can occur gradually or come on suddenly. Symptoms occur when the swollen prostate presses against the urethra. This is the tube that carries urine from the bladder outside. Prostatitis is a common disorder in adult males. Types include:
- Acute bacterial prostatitis.
- Chronic bacterial prostatitis.
- Chronic nonbacterial prostatitis/chronic pelvic pain syndrome.
- Asymptomatic prostatitis.

FREQUENT SIGNS AND SYMPTOMS
- Urgency to urinate. Burning or pain with urination.
- Frequent urination. Waking at night to urinate.
- Difficulty starting urination and emptying the bladder completely.
- Fever, chills, tiredness, and muscle and joint aches.
- Pain between the scrotum and anus.
- Blood in the urine (sometimes) or in the semen.
- Low back pain.
- Not enjoying sex; unable to get and keep an erection.

CAUSES
- Acute and chronic bacterial types are caused by bacteria infection. In some cases, it is sexually transmitted.
- In nonbacterial types, the causes are unclear. It is not contagious, nor infectious, and does not cause cancer.

RISK INCREASES WITH
- Urinary-tract infection or sexually transmitted disease.
- Diabetes.
- Weak immune system due to illness or drugs.
- Use of a catheter (tube to remove urine) after surgery.

PREVENTIVE MEASURES
None specific. Avoid infections and sexually transmitted diseases.

EXPECTED OUTCOMES
Outcome is generally good for bacterial prostatitis. Treatment may take weeks or longer and different drugs may be tried. Other types can be more difficult to treat, and the outcomes will vary.

POSSIBLE COMPLICATIONS
- Prostatitis often recurs.
- Chronic prostatitis.
- Abscess (pus-filled infection).
- Bladder obstruction and urinary retention.
- Urinary-tract infection.
- Infertility.
- Blood poisoning.

DIAGNOSIS & TREATMENT

GENERAL MEASURES
- Your health care provider will do a digital rectal exam (DRE). During DRE, a gloved, lubricated finger is inserted into the rectum to feel the prostate gland's size and to check for lumps. Medical tests may include urinalysis and culture of secretions obtained during the DRE.
- Treatment may include drugs, lifestyle changes, hospital care, counseling and rarely, surgery.
- To relieve discomfort, sit in a tub with 6 to 8 inches of warm water for 15 minutes at least 3 times a day.
- Use an inflatable donut cushion for sitting.
- Counseling may help with stress or sexual dysfunction problems. Support groups may help some patients.
- Hospital care may be needed for severe symptoms.
- Ejaculating every 3 days or prostatic massage may help drain excess prostate fluid. Ask your health care provider about these options.
- Rarely, surgery to drain an abscess of the prostate or to remove the prostate if other treatment fails.

MEDICATIONS
- Your health care provider may prescribe:
  - Antibiotics for bacterial infection. In severe cases, they may be given through a vein (IV). Take the full course of antibiotics to help prevent recurrence.
  - Nonsteroidal anti-inflammatory drugs for pain.
  - Steroids for inflammation.
  - Drugs to help improve bladder or prostate function.
  - Tranquilizers, if stress is a concern.
  - Stool softeners to avoid constipation.

ACTIVITY
Stay active. Walking is a good exercise if it doesn't cause pain. You will be advised about sexual activity limits.

DIET
Avoid alcohol, coffee, and spicy foods. These irritate the urethra. Drink plenty of fluids.

NOTIFY OUR OFFICE IF

- You or a family member has symptoms of prostatitis.
- Symptoms don't improve after 3 days of treatment.

Special notes:

_____

_____

_____

More notes on the back of this page ☐

PRURITUS ANI

 BASIC INFORMATION

DESCRIPTION
Itching or burning around the anus and genitals. It is much more common in men than in women.

FREQUENT SIGNS AND SYMPTOMS
- Itching, often intense and worse at night.
- There may be some seepage from the anus.

CAUSES
- Unknown (often).
- Yeast infection.
- Pinworms, scabies, or lice.
- Contact dermatitis caused by soaps, contraceptive foam or jelly, perfumed toilet paper, deodorant sprays, douches, or underwear made of synthetic fabric.
- Various skin disorders, including psoriasis or seborrheic dermatitis.
- Fissures, fistulas, proctitis, prolapsing hemorrhoids, skin tags, and dysfunction of the sphincter muscle.
- Vaginal discharge or skin atrophy in women caused by low estrogen levels.
- Chronic diarrhea.
- Excessive coffee intake.

RISK INCREASES WITH
- Diabetes.
- Excessive sweating.
- Antibiotic drug use.
- Food allergy.
- Overweight.

PREVENTIVE MEASURES
- Avoid causes and risk factors where possible.
- Follow steps listed in Diagnosis & Treatment section.

EXPECTED OUTCOMES
Symptoms can be controlled with treatment, even if the cause cannot be found. It may take weeks to months for the itching to stop.

POSSIBLE COMPLICATIONS
- Skin damage, allowing a secondary bacterial infection to develop.
- Skin-thickening and chronic inflammation.
- Recurrence is common.

 DIAGNOSIS & TREATMENT

GENERAL MEASURES
- Your health care provider will do an exam of the affected area. Medical tests may include studies, such as cultures for fungi, or a microscopic exam for pinworm eggs or scabies in skin burrows.
- Treatment will be provided for any specific infection or problem that is diagnosed and for the itching.
- Keep showers or baths brief to reduce dryness and soap irritation. Don't overclean the anal area by rubbing or using too much soap. Use plain, unscented soap, or avoid soap entirely.
- Keep the rectal area clean, dry, and cool. Clean carefully after bowel movements. Use moist wipes or moistened toilet paper. Dry toilet paper can be irritating.
- Avoid contact with substances to which you are sensitive.
- Wear loose clothing and underclothing. Wear underwear with a cotton crotch or underwear made of cotton, rather than nylon or other synthetics.
- Women may be more comfortable using tampons for menstrual periods rather than sanitary napkins.
- Wear soft mittens on your hands at night, if you are scratching while asleep.

MEDICATIONS
- You may use nonprescription cortisone ointment or cream. Apply 3 times a day, and rub in gently until it disappears. Discontinue use once itching stops.
- Stronger topical cortisone drugs may be prescribed.
- Drugs to treat an infection or other medical problem may be prescribed.

ACTIVITY
Avoid activities that cause excess sweating.

DIET
Avoid spicy or highly-seasoned foods and coffee. These irritate mucous membranes of the anus. Eat plenty of high-fiber foods to help avoid constipation.

 NOTIFY OUR OFFICE IF

- You or a family member has symptoms of pruritus ani that persist, despite self-care.
- The skin area seems infected.

Special notes:

_____

_____

_____

More notes on the back of this page ☐

PRURITUS VULVAE

BASIC INFORMATION

DESCRIPTION
Pruritus vulvae is an acute or chronic itching of the skin around the vulva (the vaginal lips) and anus. It is not contagious. It often affects female adolescents and adults, especially after menopause.

FREQUENT SIGNS AND SYMPTOMS
· Itching that may be severe and burning. The itching may be continuous or come and go.
· Sensitivity and irritation in the genital area.
· The skin may be dry.
· Thin, white vaginal discharge (sometimes).
· Discomfort during sexual intercourse.

CAUSES
It may be a symptom of an infection or other health problem. It may develop without any known cause.

RISK INCREASES WITH
· Skin disease, such as psoriasis or lichen planus.
· Systemic disease, such as diabetes.
· Atrophy and dryness caused by lack of estrogen.
· Skin reaction to irritants such as toilet tissue, sanitary pads, soap, douches, deodorants, powders, perfume, and fabric.
· Systemic allergies, including food allergies.
· Disorder of the vagina or rectum, such as vaginitis or hemorrhoids.
· Genital warts.
· Vulvar cancer (rare).
· Days prior to menstruation.
· Hot, humid weather.
· Obesity.
· Lack of urinary control (incontinence).

PREVENTIVE MEASURES
No specific preventive measures. Obtain medical care for any underlying disorders to reduce risk factors.

EXPECTED OUTCOME
Treatment can help symptoms, but it may be long term.

POSSIBLE COMPLICATIONS
· Secondary bacterial infection of the inflamed skin.
· Pruritus may be chronic (persisting for a long time).

DIAGNOSIS & TREATMENT

GENERAL MEASURES
· Your health care provider will do an exam of the affected area and ask questions about your symptoms and activities. Medical tests may include study of vaginal discharge and, if needed, a biopsy of the vulva (removal of a small amount of tissue for viewing under a microscope). In some cases, the exact cause is not found.

· Treatment for the underlying cause and topical skin-care products are usually recommended.
· Avoid the irritants listed among the risk factors.
· Wear cotton underpants rather than nylon or other synthetic material.
· Keep the area as dry and cool as possible. Wear loose clothing. Don't douche.
· Don't scratch the itchy area. Scratching will aggravate soreness and cause more irritation.
· Wash the genital area with water and unscented soap only once a day.
· Use a lubricant, such as K-Y Lubricating Jelly or petroleum jelly, during intercourse. Avoid intercourse if it is painful.
· After urinating or having a bowel movement, clean the genital area gently with moist cotton or antiseptic wipes. Wipe from front to back (vagina to anus).
· During menstruation, insert tampons carefully. Change sanitary napkins frequently.
· Sit in bathtub of warm (tepid, not hot) water several times a day to help relieve itching.

MEDICATION
· Drugs may be prescribed for any infection.
· Use nonprescription steroid creams or ointments. Follow instructions on the label.
· Stronger steroid creams or lotions, or hormone ointment may be prescribed.
· Hormone therapy or topical application of estrogen is sometimes recommended for postmenopausal women.
· Sedating antihistamines may be recommended to help in sleeping at night.

ACTIVITY
Avoid excess sweating.

DIET
Avoid foods that produce allergic reactions. Avoid caffeine beverages. Also avoid tomatoes and peanuts.

NOTIFY OUR OFFICE IF

· You or a family member has symptoms of pruritus vulvae.
· Symptoms don't improve in 2 weeks, despite treatment or if scratching leads to skin infection.

Special notes:

_____

_____

_____

More notes on the back of this page ☐

PSEUDOGOUT

 BASIC INFORMATION

DESCRIPTION

An acute, inflammatory form of arthritis that usually involves the large joints of the body. It often affects the elderly and is more common in men than in women. It usually occurs in acute attacks, but often the disease may progress without the attacks.

FREQUENT SIGNS AND SYMPTOMS

- Acute attacks of swelling, pain, and warmth in one or more of the joints.
- Joints involved most often are the knee (50% of the time), ankle, wrist, and shoulder.
- Attacks may last for 2 or more days.
- Freedom from pain or less severe pain between attacks.
- Limited range of motion of the joints.
- Fever.

CAUSES

Pseudogout, like gout, involves deposits of calcium crystals in and around the joints. The medical term is calcium pyrophosphate dihydrate (CPPD). Why the crystals form is unknown. The joint becomes inflamed leading to problems with cartilage, tendons, ligaments, and muscles that all connect to the joint.

RISK INCREASES WITH

- Stroke, heart attack, or surgery.
- Aging.
- Metabolic diseases (e.g., hypothyroidism, hyperthyroidism, gout, and amyloidosis).
- Family history of pseudogout.
- Eating too much calcium is not a risk factor.

PREVENTIVE MEASURES

None known.

EXPECTED OUTCOMES

There is no cure. Treatment can usually help relieve the symptoms.

POSSIBLE COMPLICATIONS

- Recurrences of the attacks.
- Permanent joint damage.
- Depression or other emotional problems may occur.

 DIAGNOSIS & TREATMENT

GENERAL MEASURES

- Your health care provider will do a physical exam of the affected area and ask questions about your symptoms and activities. Medical tests may include blood studies, a microscopic exam of a sample of joint fluid, and x-rays.
- Treatment may include drugs, physical therapy, exercise, and self-care.
- Apply ice to the affected area several times a day for the first 2 to 3 days to reduce swelling and pain.
- After a few days, heat may help discomfort. Use warm, moist compresses, heating pad, or take warm baths.
- Drainage of fluid from the inflamed joint if needed.
- Rarely, joint surgery may be recommended.
- To learn more, do an Internet search or visit a library.

MEDICATIONS

- Nonsteroidal anti-inflammatory drugs (NSAIDs) may be prescribed for pain and inflammation.
- Stronger pain medicine may be prescribed.
- A corticosteroid injection into the joint may help relieve symptoms.
- A colchicine injection may be prescribed to reduce inflammation.

ACTIVITY

- Rest as needed during an acute attack.
- If an affected joint cause pain when walking, use a cane, crutches, or a walker temporarily.
- Physical therapy may be prescribed to help maintain range of motion. You may be taught exercises to do at home. These will help keep joints and muscles flexible, strong, and functioning as well as possible.
- Swimming, water aerobics, or riding an exercise bike are good forms of exercise.
- Avoid heavy lifting or other tasks that put too much stress on your joints.

DIET

Avoid gaining weight. If your weight is a problem, a weight-loss diet may be recommended.

 NOTIFY OUR OFFICE IF

- If you or a family member has symptoms of pseudogout.
- Symptoms worsen after treatment begins.
- New or unexplained symptoms develop. Drugs used in treatment may cause side effects.

Special notes:

_____

_____

_____

More notes on the back of this page ☐

PSEUDOMEMBRANOUS ENTEROCOLITIS

BASIC INFORMATION

DESCRIPTION
A rare, severe illness that involves the bowels. It affects the lining and deeper layers of the intestines. It is normally caused by an overuse of antibiotics.

FREQUENT SIGNS AND SYMPTOMS
- Symptoms may be mild to severe.
- Watery diarrhea (sometimes bloody) with stomach cramps.
- Fever.
- Drop in blood pressure, sometimes to shock levels, with weak pulse and rapid heartbeat.
- Nausea and vomiting.
- Disorientation.
- Symptoms usually begin 3 to 9 days after starting antibiotic treatment. In some cases, they may appear days to weeks after treatment has stopped.

CAUSES
Most often the bacterial germ, *Clostridium difficile*. This germ is found in about 5% of healthy persons and normally causes no problems. It lives in a delicate balance in the bowels with other bacteria. When antibiotics are used for treating bacterial infections, they can upset this bacterial balance of the intestinal tract. This allows *Clostridium difficile* to grow rapidly and produce a toxin that damages the intestinal wall.

RISK INCREASES WITH
- Adults over age 60.
- Recent surgery.
- A stay in a hospital.
- Cancer treatment.
- Poor general health.
- Use of antibiotics, especially lincomycin, clindamycin, ampicillin, chloramphenicol, cephalosporins, penicillin, or sulfa drugs.

PREVENTIVE MEASURES
No specific preventive measures. Maintaining good health can help prevent the need for treatment with antibiotics.

EXPECTED OUTCOMES
Almost all patients recover. Symptoms will usually disappear in 1 to 2 weeks with treatment. Some may have a relapse, which can be treated successfully.

POSSIBLE COMPLICATIONS
- Shock and severe dehydration.
- Peritonitis caused by perforation of the intestine.
- In people who are elderly and have a serious illness, it can sometimes be fatal.

DIAGNOSIS & TREATMENT

GENERAL MEASURES
- Your health care provider will do a physical exam. Medical tests may include blood studies, stool cultures, and x-rays. An endoscopy with biopsy may be done. This involves using a lighted, tube-like instrument to see inside the intestines. It is also used to remove a small bit of tissue for viewing under a microscope.
- Treatment usually involves drug therapy, supportive care, hospital care if needed, and discontinuing or changing the antibiotic causing the problem.
- Mild cases can be treated at home.
- Hospital care for moderate to severe cases. Fluids given through a vein (IV) may be required to prevent dehydration.
- In rare cases, surgery may be needed due to complications of the bowels and to prevent or treat a perforation (a tear in the wall of the intestine).

MEDICATIONS
- Vancomycin, metronidazole, or other drugs may be prescribed to treat the *Clostridium difficile* infection. They may be taken by mouth or given by injection. Sometimes, repeat treatments may be needed.
- Don't take drugs for the diarrhea unless prescribed. They can prolong the infection.
- Supplements (such as lactobacilli capsules) that help healthy bacteria grow in the intestines may be recommended.

ACTIVITY
Rest in bed until symptoms of the illness get better. Move legs often while in bed to reduce the risk of deep-vein blood clots. Resume normal activities gradually.

DIET
- Patients in the hospital may need nutrition given through a vein (IV) for a few days. Then a soft diet may be prescribed until intestinal tract is back to normal.
- Patients at home need to drink plenty of fluids.

NOTIFY OUR OFFICE IF

- You or a family member has symptoms of pseudomembranous enterocolitis.
- Symptoms return after treatment.

Special notes:

_____

_____

_____

More notes on the back of this page ☐

PSITTACOSIS
(Parrot Fever; Ornithosis)

 ## BASIC INFORMATION

DESCRIPTION
An infection transmitted by birds. The infection may be mild to severe. It is primarily a lung disease, but it may affect other organs. It can occur in all age groups, including children.

FREQUENT SIGNS AND SYMPTOMS
- Fever and chills.
- General ill feeling.
- Appetite loss.
- Cough without sputum that progresses to a cough with occasional discolored sputum.
- Shortness of breath.

CAUSES
Infection by the germ, *Chlamydia psittaci*, a special type of bacteria. Psittacosis is found in psittacine birds (parrots, parakeets, and lovebirds), poultry, pigeons, canaries, and some sea birds. Birds may not appear to be sick. Germs enter the human body by breathing in air that contains the germ or by a bite from an infected bird. Symptoms start 5 to 14 days after exposure. Human to human transmission is rare but possible.

RISK INCREASES WITH
- Bird owners.
- Pet shop employees.
- Veterinary clinic employees.
- Poultry farmers or ranchers.
- Zoo workers.
- Working in poultry processing plants.

PREVENTIVE MEASURES
- Avoid dust from bird feathers and cage contents.
- Don't handle any sick bird. Imported psittacine birds must be treated for 45 days with feed that contains chlortetracycline. This eliminates the germs from the birds' blood and feces.

EXPECTED OUTCOMES
Usually curable in 7 to 14 days with treatment.

POSSIBLE COMPLICATIONS
- Hepatitis.
- Heart inflammation.
- Nervous system complications.
- Infection may recur.
- Kidney failure.
- Severe or fatal pneumonia (rare).

 ## DIAGNOSIS & TREATMENT

GENERAL MEASURES
- Your health care provider will usually do a physical exam and ask questions about your exposure to birds. Medical tests may include blood studies or a sputum culture. X-rays of the lungs may be done.
- Treatment usually involves drugs and supportive care for symptoms.
- Hospital care may be needed in severe cases. Breathing support may be required and fluids may be given through a vein (IV).
- Use a heating pad or warm, moist compresses on the chest to relieve pain.
- Don't smoke.
- Public health agencies will be notified about cases of psittacosis.

MEDICATIONS
- Doxycycline, tetracycline, or other antibiotic drug will be prescribed. They may be taken by mouth or given through a vein (IV). Take the full course of drugs prescribed, even if symptoms improve in a day or two.
- For minor pain, take nonprescription drugs such as acetaminophen or ibuprofen.

ACTIVITY
Usually no limits unless hospital care is needed. Fatigue and weakness may persist for several weeks for some patients.

DIET
No special diet. Increase fluid intake to at least one glass of fluid every hour. This helps to thin lung secretions so they can be coughed up more easily.

 ## NOTIFY OUR OFFICE IF

- You or a family member has symptoms of psittacosis.
- Symptoms get worse or do not improve despite treatment.

Special notes:

_____

_____

_____

More notes on the back of this page ☐

PSORIASIS

BASIC INFORMATION

DESCRIPTION
A chronic, scaly skin disorder. It affects the skin of the scalp, elbows, knees, chest, back, arms, legs, toenails, fingernails, and the fold between the buttocks. Psoriasis begins in late childhood or young adulthood and continues throughout life. There are several types. The most common is plaque (discoid) psoriasis.

FREQUENT SIGNS AND SYMPTOMS
· Skin areas that are slightly raised, have red borders, and are covered with large white or silver-white scales. The areas crack and become painful.
· Itching (sometimes).
· Joint pain.

CAUSES
Unknown. It is thought to be one of a group of autoimmune disorders. In these disorders, the immune system by mistake attacks the body itself.

RISK INCREASES WITH
· Family history of psoriasis.
· Rheumatoid arthritis.
· Injury to the skin.
· Infections (viral and bacterial) elsewhere in the body.
· Smoking or alcohol use.
· Genetic factors. People with psoriasis have HLA antigens, and the incidence is highest among white people.

PREVENTIVE MEASURES
· Cannot be prevented at present.
· After diagnosis, avoid trigger factors (such as smoking, stress, or too much sun) to help prevent a flare-up.

EXPECTED OUTCOMES
Symptoms can be controlled, but not cured. There may be long periods of inactivity.

POSSIBLE COMPLICATIONS
· It can cause embarrassment and self-consciousness about one's appearance.
· Drugs used in treatment can cause adverse effects.
· Pustular psoriasis (skin has pus-filled blisters).
· Psoriatic arthritis (inflammation in the joints).

DIAGNOSIS & TREATMENT

GENERAL MEASURES
· Your health care provider can diagnose the disorder with an exam of the affected skin. A biopsy may sometimes be done. It involves removing a small amount of skin tissue for viewing under a microscope.
· No permanent cure exists. Steps in treatment depend on the type of psoriasis, extent of the disease, your response to it, and the effect on your lifestyle.

· Treatment steps include drugs to be used on the skin or taken by mouth, phototherapy, and self-care.
· Maintain good skin hygiene with daily baths or showers. Avoid skin injury, including harsh scrubbing, which can trigger new outbreaks.
· Avoid skin dryness to decrease the risk of recurrences. To reduce scaling, use nonprescription, waterless cleansers and hair products that contain coal tar or cortisone. Use a moisturizer after bathing.
· Oatmeal baths may loosen scales. Use one cup of oatmeal to a tub of warm water.
· Phototherapy may be prescribed. It involves use of sunlight or artificial light. Expose skin to moderate amounts of sunlight as often as possible. Artificial light may be used. This can be done at a medical office, or, in some cases, patients may have a unit they use at home.
· Get counseling if needed for emotional problems.
· To learn more: National Psoriasis Foundation, 6600 SW 92nd Ave., Suite 300, Portland, OR 97223, (800) 723-9166; website: www.psoriasis.org.

MEDICATIONS
· No one drug therapy works for everyone. You may be prescribed one or more of the following:
  - Topical drugs including corticosteroids, forms of vitamin D-3, coal tar, anthralin, retinoids, or salicylic acid. Some of these may be combined into one product.
  - Drugs to suppress the immune system (more severe cases). They may be taken by mouth or by injection.
  - PUVA (combines use of a psoralen drug and exposure to ultraviolet light–wavelength A).
  - Combination of tar baths with UVB (ultraviolet therapy wavelength B).
  - Antihistamines to relieve itching.

ACTIVITY
No limits.

DIET
No special diet.

NOTIFY OUR OFFICE IF

· You or a family member has symptoms of psoriasis.
· Symptoms do not improve with treatment.
· New, unexplained symptoms develop. Drugs used in treatment may produce side effects.

Special notes:

_____

_____

_____

More notes on the back of this page ☐

PSORIATIC ARTHRITIS

 BASIC INFORMATION

DESCRIPTION
Joint inflammation that occurs along with psoriasis (a skin disorder). Psoriatic arthritis can affect joints in any part of the body. It usually affects finger joints, low-back, and neck joints in the spine. The disorder is usually mild and tends to begin between ages 30 to 35. It continues off and on throughout life.

FREQUENT SIGNS AND SYMPTOMS
· Pain, swelling, limited movement, tenderness, and warmth in the affected joints.
· Psoriasis. Skin areas that are slightly raised, have red borders, and are covered with large white or silver-white scales. The areas crack and become painful. (Rarely, a person may have psoriatic arthritis without obvious signs of psoriasis.)
· Tiredness and fever (sometimes).

CAUSES
Unknown. It is thought to be one of a group of autoimmune disorders. In these disorders, the immune system by mistake attacks the body itself. Genetic (family) factors may be involved. In some cases, it may be linked to an infection.

RISK INCREASES WITH
· Psoriasis.
· Family history of psoriasis.

PREVENTIVE MEASURES
No specific preventive measures.

EXPECTED OUTCOMES
There is no cure for this disorder. The symptoms often go away and then return. Symptoms can be relieved or controlled with treatment.

POSSIBLE COMPLICATIONS
· May progress to chronic arthritis and severe crippling may occur (rare).
· Drugs used in treatment may have adverse effects.

 DIAGNOSIS & TREATMENT

GENERAL MEASURES
· Your health care provider will do a physical exam and ask about your symptoms. There is no one test that will diagnose the disorder. Medical tests may include blood studies, joint fluid studies, x-rays, CT, or MRI.
· Treatment may include drugs, physical therapy, exercise, and self-care. Psoriasis therapy will continue also.
· Use heat to relieve joint pain. Warm soaks, heating pads, or warm compresses may help. If heat does not help, try cold compresses. Ultrasound or diathermy (heat therapy) may be prescribed.
· Splints for the affected joints may be recommended.
· Physical therapy can help with joint range of motion, flexibility, stretching, and muscle strength.
· In some cases, surgery may be recommended for severe joint problems or for joint replacement.
· To learn more: National Psoriasis Foundation, 6600 SW 92nd Ave., Suite 300, Portland, OR 97223, (800) 723-9166; website: www.psoriasis.org.

MEDICATIONS
· For minor discomfort, you may use nonprescription drugs such as aspirin (if over age 18).
· Nonsteroidal anti-inflammatory drugs, cortisone injections into inflamed joints, and drugs to suppress the immune system may be prescribed to reduce joint inflammation.
· Drugs will be prescribed for psoriasis at the same time as treatment for the arthritis symptoms.

ACTIVITY
Rest during flare-ups, then resume your normal activities gradually. Exercise regularly to help keep your strength and flexibility. Swimming is a good exercise.

DIET
No special diet.

 NOTIFY OUR OFFICE IF

· You or a family member has symptoms of psoriatic arthritis.
· Symptoms do not improve with treatment.
· Drugs used in treatment produce side effects.

Special notes:

_____

_____

_____

More notes on the back of this page ☐

412

PUERPERAL INFECTION

(Puerperal Fever; Postpartum Infection)

 BASIC INFORMATION

DESCRIPTION

Bacterial infection following delivery of a baby. Infection most often occurs in the uterus and causes inflammation (endometritis). It can also affect the vagina, vulva, perineum (area between the vagina and rectum), cervix, or peritoneum (membrane that covers abdominal organs).

FREQUENT SIGNS AND SYMPTOMS

· Fever and chills for two or more days after the first postpartum day (first day after delivery).
· Headache and muscle aches.
· Appetite loss.
· Vaginal discharge with a foul odor.
· Stomach (abdominal) pain.
· General ill feeling.

CAUSES

Infection by bacteria normally found in a healthy vagina. These bacteria can infect the uterus, vagina, adjacent tissues, and kidney.

RISK INCREASES WITH

· Cesarean delivery.
· Genital or urinary tract infection prior to delivery.
· Use of a fetal scalp electrode during labor.
· Anemia, either before pregnancy, or from loss of blood during delivery.
· Poor nutrition during pregnancy.
· Long delay between water break (rupture of the placental membranes) and delivery (more than 24 hours).
· A small part of the placenta is left in the uterus.
· Extra-long labor.
· Multiple vaginal exams.
· Obesity.
· Diabetes.

PREVENTIVE MEASURES

· No specific preventive steps. To reduce risk factors:
  - Avoid anyone with an active infection for the last 2 weeks of pregnancy.
  - Notify your obstetric provider as soon your water breaks. Don't have sexual intercourse after this occurs.
  - Wash the genital area often during the first week after delivery.

EXPECTED OUTCOMES

Usually curable in 7 to 10 days with treatment.

POSSIBLE COMPLICATIONS

· Deep-vein blood clot in the pelvis or pelvic abscess.
· Shock.
· Scarring
· Infertility.
· Blood poisoning (although rare, could be fatal).

 DIAGNOSIS & TREATMENT

GENERAL MEASURES

· Your health care provider will do a physical exam including a pelvic exam. Medical tests may include blood and urine studies and studies of the vaginal discharge. Other tests may be done if drug treatment fails.
· Treatment usually involves antibiotics for the infection. Hospital care may be needed for severe infection.
· To relieve pain, place a heating pad or hot-water bottle on the abdomen or back. Take frequent, warm baths to relax muscles and help relieve pain.
· Use sanitary pads, rather than tampons, for the vaginal discharge.
· Surgery may be done to remove fragments of placenta or to treat an abscess or blood clot. An infected episiotomy (incision made during delivery) may need to be opened and drained.
· If you breast-feed, ask your health care provider about continuing to do so during treatment.

MEDICATIONS

· One or more antibiotics for infection will be prescribed. They may be taken by mouth or given through a vein (IV).
· Drugs to reduce fever and relieve pain may be prescribed.
· Anticoagulants may be prescribed to prevent blood-clots from forming.

ACTIVITY

· Rest in bed, except to use the bathroom, until fever and other signs of infection clear up. You will probably be more comfortable if you lie on your left side.
· Abstain from sexual relations until signs of infection have been gone for 7 days.

DIET

Drink lots of fluids to prevent dehydration.

 NOTIFY OUR OFFICE IF

· You or a family member has symptoms of a puerperal infection, even several hours after delivery.
· Symptoms of infection recur after treatment.

Special notes:

_____

_____

_____

More notes on the back of this page ☐

PULMONARY EDEMA

 ## BASIC INFORMATION

DESCRIPTION
A condition of excess fluid (edema) in the lungs. It more often affects middle-aged and elderly adults.

FREQUENT SIGNS AND SYMPTOMS
· Sometimes, the symptoms begin suddenly in the middle of the night and worsen rapidly.
· Extreme shortness of breath, sometimes with wheezing.
· Rapid breathing.
· Restlessness and anxiety.
· Paleness and sweating.
· Bluish nails and lips.
· Weakness and fatigue.
· Swollen feet and ankles.
· Cough. This may be unproductive at first, but later it can produce frothy, blood-stained sputum.
· Fever (sometimes).

CAUSES
Lungs are normally air-filled. They take in oxygen and pass it on to the blood for transport to all cells in the body. When fluid builds up in the lungs, it interferes with oxygen intake. This can affect all body functions. Pulmonary edema can be caused by a number of different disorders, but heart disorders are the most likely.

RISK INCREASES WITH
· Heart disorders (such as heart failure or heart attack) can cause fluid to build up in veins in the lungs. Pressure causes the veins to leak excess fluid into the lungs.
· Pneumonia (lung infection).
· Pulmonary embolism (blood clot).
· Drug overdose (such as from heroin or narcotics).
· Shock.
· High altitude illness.
· Drowning.
· Pancreatitis (inflammation of the pancreas).
· Kidney problems, liver problems, or thyroid disease.
· Inhaled toxins.

PREVENTIVE MEASURES
Get treatment for any illness or disease that could be a risk factor for pulmonary edema.

EXPECTED OUTCOMES
In most cases, symptoms can be controlled with treatment. The underlying disease causing pulmonary edema may require lifelong treatment.

POSSIBLE COMPLICATIONS
Heart attack, heart rhythm problems, shock, adverse effect of drugs, or death (if treatment is delayed or unsuccessful).

 ## DIAGNOSIS & TREATMENT

GENERAL MEASURES
· Your health care provider will do a physical exam and ask questions about your symptoms. Medical tests may include blood studies, blood-oxygen levels, chest x-ray, pulmonary function studies, and heart function studies.
· Treatment is designed to reduce the excess fluid, improve lung and heart function, and treat any underlying disorder.
· Hospital care is almost always needed. Emergency treatment is often required.
· Hospital treatment may include supplemental oxygen, breathing support with a ventilator (breathing machine), fluids given through a vein (IV), drugs, and special diet. Patients are sometimes more comfortable sitting with legs dangling over the side of the bed.

MEDICATIONS
· Your health care provider may prescribe:
 - Narcotics to relieve anxiety, decrease blood flow to the lung, and reduce oxygen demand of the body.
 - Diuretics to help remove excess fluid from the bloodstream and the lungs.
 - Drugs such as beta-blockers, ACE inhibitors, nitrates, calcium-channel blockers, digoxin, and others to reduce workload on the heart.
 - Drugs to treat any underlying disorder.

ACTIVITY
Rest in bed until your symptoms get better. After treatment, resume your normal activities gradually. Walking is a good activity to help increase strength. Resume sexual relations when you have medical approval.

DIET
In the hospital, sodium and fluids are usually restricted. After recovery, a low-salt, low-fat diet and reduced fluid intake may be recommended.

 ## NOTIFY OUR OFFICE IF

You or a family member has symptoms of pulmonary edema that appear suddenly. This is an emergency! Call 911 first.

Special notes:

_____

_____

_____

More notes on the back of this page ☐

PULMONARY EMBOLISM

 ## BASIC INFORMATION

DESCRIPTION

A blood clot in one of the arteries carrying blood to the lungs. The blood clot usually begins in a deep vein of the leg, or less often, another place in the body. The clot moves through the bloodstream, passing through the heart and into an artery in the lungs. The blockage reduces breathing ability and can destroy lung tissue. Rarely, other types of clots form that are made up of fat, air bubbles, tissue from a tumor, or bacteria. Pulmonary embolism is more common in adults.

FREQUENT SIGNS AND SYMPTOMS

- Sudden shortness of breath.
- Faintness or fainting.
- Pain in the chest.
- Cough (sometimes with bloody sputum).
- Rapid heartbeat.
- Low fever.
- These symptoms are often preceded by swelling and pain in the leg.

CAUSES

Deep-vein thrombosis, which can occur anytime blood pools in a vein.

RISK INCREASES WITH

- Previous embolism or deep-vein thrombosis.
- Any injury or illness that requires prolonged bed rest.
- Sitting for long periods, as on car or plane trips.
- Recent surgery.
- Heart disease, high blood pressure, or lung disorders.
- Bone fractures, such as hip fracture.
- Overweight.
- Pregnancy.
- Use of birth-control pills; risk increases with smokers.
- Cancer.
- Smoking.
- Family history of tendency to form blood clots.

PREVENTIVE MEASURES

- Avoid prolonged bed rest during illnesses. Wear compressive stockings during recovery (in or out of bed).
- Start moving legs and walking as soon as possible after surgery.
- Don't smoke, especially if you are a woman age 35 or older who takes birth-control pills.
- When traveling, stand and walk every 1 to 2 hours.

EXPECTED OUTCOMES

Usually curable with treatment. Embolism may recur.

POSSIBLE COMPLICATIONS

- High blood pressure in the lungs (pulmonary hypertension).
- Heart damage (a condition called cor pulmonale).
- Death (from a large clot that blocks the artery).

 ## DIAGNOSIS & TREATMENT

GENERAL MEASURES

- Your health care provider will do a physical exam and ask questions about your symptoms and activities. Medical tests may include chest x-ray, lung scan, pulmonary angiogram (a special x-ray study of blood flow), CT, blood studies, and other tests as needed.
- Treatment is aimed at maintaining heart, blood vessel, and lung functions as well as preventing clot recurrence.
- Hospital care is necessary. Supplemental oxygen will be provided, and drugs will be given through a vein (IV).
- Surgery may be necessary to tie off the big vein leading to the heart and lungs (vena cava) or to insert a filter to trap recurrent clots.
- Self-care steps (if advised by your health care provider). Wear elastic or compressive stockings or leg wraps with elastic bandages. Don't sit with your legs or ankles crossed. Elevate your feet higher than your hips if sitting for long periods. Raise the foot of your bed.

MEDICATIONS

- Anticoagulant drugs to treat the clots will be prescribed. You may need indefinite treatment with these drugs to prevent a recurrence. Your health care provider will explain their risks and benefits.
- Clot-dissolving (clot buster) drugs may be prescribed. They break down the blood clots.
- Drugs to treat other disorders may be prescribed.

ACTIVITY

Rest in bed until all symptoms of the clot improve. While in bed, move your legs often.

DIET

No special diet. Drink plenty of fluids.

 ## NOTIFY OUR OFFICE IF

- You or a family member has symptoms of pulmonary embolism. This is an emergency! Call 911.
- The following occur during treatment: Chest pain or coughing up blood, shortness of breath, or increased swelling and pain in the leg.

Special notes:

_____

_____

_____

More notes on the back of this page ☐

PURPURA, ALLERGIC

(Anaphylactoid Purpura; Henoch-Schönlein Purpura)

 BASIC INFORMATION

DESCRIPTION

An allergic disorder involving sudden bleeding into the skin or intestines. It can involve the joints (usually knees, ankles, hips, wrists, and elbows); the gastrointestinal tract; kidneys; and the skin of the legs, thighs, and abdomen. It usually affects children ages 2 to 11, most often boys. Adults are rarely affected.

FREQUENT SIGNS AND SYMPTOMS

· Headache, fever, and loss of appetite may occur first.
· Itching, red skin rash that seems to be just beneath the skin surface. The rash usually consists of large hives with small bruises or blood spots in the centers. The rash is most often on the legs, thighs, and lower abdomen, but it may be scattered over the body. The rash turns a bruised, purple color. (That is why the name purpura is given to the disorder.)
· Joint pain and swelling at the knees, ankles, hips, wrists, or elbows.
· Cramping stomach (abdominal) pain and vomiting.
· Blood in urine or stools.

CAUSES

Purpura is probably an autoimmune reaction in the inflamed small blood vessels in the body. The allergic trigger is not known. Attacks often follow an upper respiratory infection or the use of some drugs.

RISK INCREASES WITH

· Recent illness such as cold or flu. Both viral and bacterial infections have preceded allergic purpura.
· Use of certain drugs. These include antibiotics such as penicillin and ampicillin, and some vaccines, such as typhoid, measles, yellow fever, and cholera.
· Bee stings, some chemical toxins, cold exposure, and food allergies have also preceded allergic purpura.

PREVENTIVE MEASURES

No specific preventive measures. Avoid any of the risk factors where possible.

EXPECTED OUTCOMES

Most children recover completely. Mild cases may last a few days. Usually, recovery takes 1 to 4 weeks. In about 50% of cases, the disorder will recur.

POSSIBLE COMPLICATIONS

· Kidney damage. It may occur years later.
· The disorder can cause complications in almost every organ system. These include gastrointestinal, cardiovascular (heart and blood vessels), and the lungs.

 DIAGNOSIS & TREATMENT

GENERAL MEASURES

· Your health care provider will do a physical exam and ask questions about the symptoms. Medical tests may include blood and urine studies. X-rays or CT testing may be done to assess complications.
· Most patients require hospital care. This is important to help watch for, and prevent, complications.
· Treatment involves discontinuing any drugs or trigger factors that could be the cause, along with supportive therapy to relieve symptoms.
· At home, use warm soaks to relieve joint pain.

MEDICATIONS

· There is no specific drug to treat the disorder. Drugs to reduce inflammation (such as ibuprofen or naproxen), or to treat an infection may be prescribed.
· In some cases, corticosteroids may be prescribed.

ACTIVITY

When fever and pain are gone, the child may gradually resume normal activities as strength and well-being will allow.

DIET

Eat a normal, well-balanced diet.

 NOTIFY OUR OFFICE IF

· Your child has symptoms of allergic purpura.
· The following symptoms occur after treatment:
  - Increased abdominal pain.
  - Blood in the stool or black, tarry stools.
  - New bleeding under the skin.
  - Blood in the urine.

Special notes:

_____

_____

_____

More notes on the back of this page ☐

RABIES
(Hydrophobia)

BASIC INFORMATION

DESCRIPTION
A serious viral infection of the central nervous system, transmitted by the bite of infected animals. In two-thirds of patients, symptoms may appear 1 to 3 months after the bite. Sometimes they may appear in as short as 5 days or as long as 5 years.

FREQUENT SIGNS AND SYMPTOMS
Early symptoms are:
- Restlessness and irritability.
- Fatigue.
- Slight fever.
- Cough.
- Sore throat.
- Increased saliva and tears.

2 to 10 days later:
- Violent spasms of throat muscles that make swallowing impossible.
- Hyperactivity and violent behavior.
- Confusion.
- High fever.
- Irregular heartbeat.
- Irregular breathing.

CAUSES
- A virus in the saliva of infected animals passes to humans through broken skin or a mucous membrane. The virus travels slowly from the bite area to the brain.
- Animals that are commonly infected include dogs (especially wild dogs), bats, skunks, foxes, coyotes, and raccoons. Other animals can also be infected, so consult your local health department after any animal bite.

RISK INCREASES WITH
Professions or activities that may involve exposure to wild animals (cave exploration, hunting, farm or ranch workers, forest rangers, some laboratory workers, and veterinarians).

PREVENTIVE MEASURES
- Vaccinate your dog or cat against rabies.
- Report stray animals in the neighborhood, and teach children to avoid them.
- Have a rabies immunization if your work involves animals.
- Keep tetanus immunizations current.
- Avoid wild animals. In the United States, bats, skunks, and raccoons are the most likely to be infected, but any carnivore can carry the disease.

EXPECTED OUTCOMES
Rabies can be prevented with early treatment following exposure to animal bites.

POSSIBLE COMPLICATIONS
Once symptoms begin, survival is unlikely.

DIAGNOSIS & TREATMENT

GENERAL MEASURES
- For animal bites or scratches:
  - Wash the bite area for 10 minutes with soap and water to remove all saliva.
  - Cover the wound with a clean bandage.
  - Immediately call your health care provider's office or emergency room for advice.
  - Call your local animal-control center to catch the animal, if possible.
  - Seek medical help if you have been exposed to a bat (such as waking up and finding one in the room) even if you have no bite or scratch marks.
  - Don't panic. The incubation period allows time for diagnosis and treatment.
- Your health care provider will examine the wound. Medical tests may include blood tests and fluid and electrolyte studies. An exam of the animal's tissue (if available) will be done. Your own observation of the animal's behavior is important. Determine if the animal was provoked. Animals that attack without reason are more likely to be infected.
- Treatment will be determined by type of exposure (bite or nonbite), the risk of rabies in the type of animal, circumstances of the biting incident, and vaccination status of animal.
- Hospital care is needed for serious wounds. Surgery may be done to clean and repair the bite wound.

MEDICATIONS
- Injections of rabies-immune globulin. (Painful injections in the abdomen are no longer used.)
- Injections of human-diploid-cell-strain vaccine, if the animal is proven rabid.
- Tetanus booster will be prescribed if needed.

ACTIVITY
No limits.

DIET
No special diet.

NOTIFY OUR OFFICE IF

Anyone is bitten by an animal or has other exposure to an animal that may have rabies.

Special notes:

_____

_____

_____

More notes on the back of this page ☐

RADIATION SICKNESS

 BASIC INFORMATION

DESCRIPTION
Side effects that develop from radiation treatment for cancer or after accidental exposure to radiation. Symptoms vary widely and are often temporary, depending on the radiation dosage and area radiated.

FREQUENT SIGNS AND SYMPTOMS
Symptoms may include:
- Nausea, vomiting and diarrhea.
- Headache.
- Fatigue and shortness of breath.
- Rapid heartbeat.
- Yeast infection in the mouth.
- Dry mouth and loss of taste.
- Swallowing difficulty.
- Worsening of tooth or gum disease.
- Hair loss; dry cough.
- Heart inflammation with chest pain.
- Burning, inflammation, or scarring of the skin.
- Permanent skin darkening.
- Bleeding spots anywhere under the skin.
- Anemia; sexual impotence.

CAUSES
Radiation damage to the immune system and to healthy tissues.

RISK INCREASES WITH
- Dose and rate of radiation treatment exposure.
- Amount of body area exposed to radiation treatment.

PREVENTIVE MEASURES
- If you work around radiation, learn and observe all safety regulations for yourself and for patients.
- Avoid unnecessary radiation exposure.

EXPECTED OUTCOMES
- With radiation treatment, most side effects or complications disappear gradually afterward.
- With radiation accidents not severe enough to cause immediate death, side effects may not appear for years.

POSSIBLE COMPLICATIONS
- Increased risk of infections due to poor immune system function.
- Sterility or birth defects may occur.
- Increased risk of cancer especially bone-marrow cancer or leukemia.
- With radiation treatment, other complications depend upon the area involved. Modern radiation equipment makes serious complications unlikely.

 DIAGNOSIS & TREATMENT

GENERAL MEASURES
- Your health care provider may do a physical exam. Medical tests may include blood studies of hemoglobin, platelet counts and white-blood-cell counts, x-rays of treated areas, and dosimetry (a test to detect and measure exposure to radiation).
- Hospital care is usually needed. Treatment is aimed at controlling symptoms and preventing infections. Treatment may include drugs, fluids given through a vein (IV), blood transfusions, and surgery.
- Surgery to treat wounds or bone-marrow transplant may be needed for severe exposure.
- Use effective birth-control measures to prevent pregnancy until it is determined that it is safe to have children. Genetic counseling may be recommended.

MEDICATIONS
- Your health care provider may prescribe:
  - Antinausea drugs.
  - Pain relievers.
  - Blood transfusions for anemia.
  - Antibiotics to fight infections.
  - Antidiarrheal drugs.
  - Sedatives if sleeping is a problem.

ACTIVITY
Be as active as your strength allows. Rest often.

DIET
Eat a balanced diet. You may need a liquid diet for a short time or you may want to prepare food in a blender if you have trouble swallowing. Intravenous (IV) feeding or use of a small stomach tube is also possible until you can resume normal eating.

 NOTIFY OUR OFFICE IF

- You or a family member is accidentally exposed to radiation.
- Feelings of illness occur during radiation treatment, especially if there are unexpected symptoms.
- Signs of infection develop, such as fever and chills, muscle aches, headache, and dizziness, during or after exposure or treatment.

Special notes:

_____

_____

_____

More notes on the back of this page ☐

RAPE TRAUMA SYNDROME

BASIC INFORMATION

DESCRIPTION

The physical and emotional effects of rape. The term rape refers to forcible sexual intercourse with an unwilling partner. Rape involves varying degrees of physical and emotional trauma. In most cases, the rapist is a man and the victim is a woman.

FREQUENT SIGNS AND SYMPTOMS

Right after the rape:
- Physical injuries such as cuts, bruises, or other injuries, including vaginal and rectal tears.
- Fear, anger, crying, or unusual behavior such as laughter.
- No outward emotional signs (sometimes).

Later effects (may be weeks to months):
- Feelings of self-blame and guilt.
- Depression and withdrawal, even from family and friends.
- Mood swings; feelings of grief, shame, and revenge.
- Loss of appetite.
- Fear of intercourse; fear of men.
- Nightmares and sleep disorders.
- Fear of being alone.
- Anxiety.

CAUSES

Rape is extremely traumatizing. All rape victims will suffer physical and emotional effects.

RISK INCREASES WITH

Any victim of rape or attempted rape.

PREVENTIVE MEASURES

- There is no prevention for rape trauma syndrome.
- The scope of rape prevention is complex. It involves individuals, society, and the government.

EXPECTED OUTCOME

- It takes most rape victims a long time to feel like they've returned to a normal existence. Some never do, and some say that they are completely changed people.
- Length of recovery time varies depending on the individual and previous life experiences. Recovery may involve two stages:
  - *Acute.* This involves dealing with the immediate physical and emotional effects.
  - *Reorganization.* This involves reorganizing life after the rape and learning to cope again. The personality of the individual, support system, existing life-problems, and prior sexual assaults, are all factors in recovering.

POSSIBLE COMPLICATIONS

- Sexually transmitted diseases.
- Emotional trauma that may last years.
- Pelvic injury.
- Pregnancy.

DIAGNOSIS & TREATMENT

GENERAL MEASURES

Immediate care:
- Emergency medical care will be provided for your physical injuries. A general physical exam and pelvic exam will be done according to specific medical guidelines. A report is normally made to local law agencies.
- Ask for help from a rape crisis center (or similar agency). They provide support and help you through the medical, emotional, and legal necessities.
- Medical personnel will discuss:
  - Risks of pregnancy, sexually transmitted diseases, HIV/AIDS, hepatitis B, and other infections.
  - What measures are available to prevent the risks and what follow-up tests may be required.

After the medical care:
- Get counseling help. This is important for your emotional recovery. Don't just try to put the matter out of your mind, and don't try to "go it alone." Suppressing your feelings can increase distress.
- Keeping a journal or diary about your feelings, thoughts, and reactions may be helpful. Talk over your feelings with trusted friends and family.
- Prepare yourself as much as possible for legal proceedings that force you to relive the trauma.
- To learn more: National Sexual Assault Hotline (800) 656-HOPE (4673) which connects callers to a nearby rape crisis center; website: www.rainn.org.

MEDICATION

Your health care provider may prescribe:
- Antibiotics, if infection is suspected or diagnosed.
- Emergency contraception.
- Sedatives or tranquilizers to reduce anxiety.
- Tetanus prevention.

ACTIVITY

No limits.

DIET

No special diet.

NOTIFY OUR OFFICE IF

- You or someone you know has been raped.
- Emotional and/or physical problems become worse.

Special notes:

_____

_____

_____

More notes on the back of this page ☐

RAYNAUD DISEASE & PHENOMENON

 ## BASIC INFORMATION

DESCRIPTION
• Primary Raynaud or Raynaud disease is a disorder of the circulatory system. It is more common in females ages 20 to 40.
• Secondary Raynaud or Raynaud phenomenon is a circulatory system disorder that occurs as a complication of other diseases. It can affect anyone who has the underlying disease.
• Both types involve small blood vessels in the body. They usually affect blood circulation to the fingers, but they may affect the toes, and rarely, nose, lips, nipples, knees, and ears. Symptoms may develop over a period of years. In secondary Raynaud, symptoms may begin suddenly.

FREQUENT SIGNS AND SYMPTOMS
• When exposed to cold or after emotional stress, fingers turn pale followed by a bluish tinge, then redness.
• Numbness and tingling occur along with the color changes. Pain is not common, but can occur.
• Warmth helps relieves these symptoms. Hands may become swollen and painful when warmed.

CAUSES
The exact cause is unknown. The blood vessels may constrict (narrow) due to cold or emotional stress, or there may be increased thickness to the blood.

RISK INCREASES WITH
• Smoking, which impairs circulation to hands and feet.
• Autoimmune disorders, such as scleroderma, lupus erythematosus, rheumatoid arthritis, or others.
• Environmental factors, such as use of vibrating tools or exposure to certain chemicals or toxins.
• Infections, such as hepatitis B and C.
• Cancers, such as leukemia and lymphoma.
• Metabolic disorders, such as diabetes.
• Heart, blood vessel, or nerve disorders.
• Certain drugs.

PREVENTIVE MEASURES
• Don't smoke. It triggers the disorder. Raynaud is rare among nonsmokers. Avoid secondhand smoke.
• Obtain medical care for disorders listed as risk factors.

EXPECTED OUTCOMES
• Most persons cope well with Raynaud disorder and live a normal life span. In about half of the patients, the disease may improve or disappear after several years.
• Secondary Raynaud may be curable if the underlying cause can be cured.

POSSIBLE COMPLICATIONS
• Fingertip or toe ulcers (open sores).
• Smooth skin on fingertips or toes.
• Gangrene and amputation (most severe cases only).

 ## DIAGNOSIS & TREATMENT

GENERAL MEASURES
• Your health care provider will do a physical exam of the affected areas and ask questions about your symptoms and activities. Medical tests may include blood studies and a cold challenge test (putting hands in cold water). A nailfold capillary test may be done to check tiny blood vessels in the skin at the base of a fingernail.
• Treatment involves treating any underlying cause, lifestyle changes, and drugs.
• Stop smoking. Symptoms will improve if you do.
• Avoid trigger factors, such as use of vibrating tools.
• Avoid exposure to cold if possible. Wear mittens or gloves outdoors and when handling ice or frozen foods. Wear comfortable, roomy shoes and wool socks.
• Avoid drugs which can worsen symptoms (such as beta-blockers, ergot drugs, and clonidine)
• Use caution in handling iced drinks or being in air-conditioned rooms.
• Avoid stressful situations. Learn relaxation techniques.
• Biofeedback training to teach you how to raise skin temperature may be helpful.
• Surgery to sever (cut) sympathetic nerves to the involved hands or feet (rare).
• To learn more: Raynaud's Association, 94 Mercier Ave., Hartsdale, NY 10530; (800) 280-8055; website: www.raynauds.org.

MEDICATIONS
• Vasodilator drugs may be prescribed. They help dilate (widen) blood vessels to improve blood circulation.
• Topical drugs to be applied to the fingertips may be prescribed to protect them from skin ulcers.

ACTIVITY
No limits, except to keep warm. A regular exercise program is recommended. Exercise improves circulation.

DIET
No special diet.

 ## NOTIFY OUR OFFICE IF

• You or a family member has symptoms of Raynaud.
• Discomfort worsens, despite treatment.
• Ulcers that do not heal appear on fingers or toes.

Special notes:

_____

_____

_____

More notes on the back of this page ☐

420

RECTAL PROLAPSE

 ## BASIC INFORMATION

DESCRIPTION

Protrusion (bulging) of rectal tissues outside the anus. Partial prolapse is protrusion of the mucosa alone. Complete prolapse (procidentia) is protrusion of the entire thickness of the rectum. It can affect adults usually over age 60, and children ages 1 to 3. Rectal prolapse in infants can be a sign of cystic fibrosis.

FREQUENT SIGNS AND SYMPTOMS

· A vague sense of fullness in the lower abdomen or rectal area.
· A mucus discharge sometimes tinged with blood from the rectum.
· A firm mass of tissue that can be felt at the anus after a bowel movement.
· Pain when having bowel movements.

CAUSES

Exact cause is unknown. There are known risk factors.

RISK INCREASES WITH

· Cystic fibrosis (children).
· Aging.
· Weak pelvic or rectal muscles.
· Weak anal sphincter.
· Previous surgery on the rectum or vagina.
· Constipation and straining to have bowel movements.
· Multiple sclerosis.
· Stroke, paralysis, or spinal tumor.
· Lower back or pelvic injury; lumbar disc disease.
· Chronic obstructive pulmonary disease.
· Pelvic floor dysfunction.
· Multiple pregnancies.
· Benign prostatic hypertrophy.
· Parasitic infections.
· Congenital (born with) rectal structure problems.

PREVENTIVE MEASURES

· Women can practice pelvic-strengthening exercises (Kegel exercises) to prevent recurrences.
· Do not strain when having bowel movements. Avoid constipation and diarrhea.

EXPECTED OUTCOMES

Good prognosis with treatment. In children, there is usually complete recovery.

POSSIBLE COMPLICATIONS

· Ulceration (sores) and bleeding in tissue that protrudes.
· Bowel incontinence.
· Rectal prolapse may occur with another prolapse, such as the uterus or the bladder.
· Rectal prolapse may recur.

 ## DIAGNOSIS & TREATMENT

GENERAL MEASURES

· Your health care provider will do an exam of the rectal area. Medical tests may include barium enema (special x-ray) and exam of the rectal area by colonoscopy or proctosigmoidoscopy. These two are visual exams of the anus and colon with the lighted tip of an optical instrument. Cystic fibrosis tests may be done in children.
· Treatment varies according to underlying cause. Causes of straining need to be corrected.
· In children, prolapse is usually temporary.
· Occasionally, minor prolapse can be reversed by gently pushing the protruding tissue back into the rectum.
· For most patients, surgery is usually needed to repair the prolapse. There are several different options available. Your health care provider will explain them to you and discuss the risks and benefits. Surgery is usually done under a general anesthetic.
· Use sanitary napkins or absorbent pads for mucus discharge.

MEDICATIONS

To prevent constipation, bulk-formers or stool softeners may be prescribed.

ACTIVITY

· Recovery from surgery may take 4 to 6 weeks. Then resume normal activities gradually.
· Practice pelvic-strengthening exercises to prevent a recurrence.

DIET

Drink at least 8 glasses of water a day. Eat a diet high in fiber to prevent constipation.

 ## NOTIFY OUR OFFICE IF

· You or a family member has symptoms of rectal prolapse.
· Rectal pain or bleeding occur.
· Fever or chills develop, indicating infection.
· Symptoms return after treatment.

Special notes:

_____

_____

_____

More notes on the back of this page ☐

REFLEX SYMPATHETIC DYSTROPHY SYNDROME

 BASIC INFORMATION

DESCRIPTION

A chronic disorder that often affects the arms or legs, and rarely, other parts of the body. It involves the nerves, skin, muscles, blood vessels, and bones. Symptoms vary in severity and how long they last. Reflex sympathetic dystrophy can occur at any age, but is more common in ages 40 to 60. The number of cases among teens and young adults is increasing.

FREQUENT SIGNS AND SYMPTOMS

- Pain (may be burning or aching) and swelling. These symptoms may increase over time.
- Changes in skin. It may be sweaty or cold. Color may change from pale to purple/blue or gray. Affected area may be tender, thin, and shiny.
- Hair and nail growth is increased. These symptoms may decrease with time.
- Stiff joints and muscle spasms.

CAUSES

The exact cause is unknown. It usually occurs after major or minor injuries to an arm or leg. It can occur following an illness, such as a heart attack. The pain that occurs is more severe than would be expected from the injury. The sympathetic nervous system that controls blood flow and sweat glands appears to play a role in the cause.

RISK INCREASES WITH

- Genetic factors may increase the risk.
- A tendency towards increased sympathetic activity. This includes cold hands, excessive sweating, or a history of fainting.
- Major or minor injury to an arm or leg.
- Heart attack, stroke, pancreatic cancer, herpes zoster, arthritis, or nerve compression disorder.
- Chest, neck, or shoulder injury.
- The period following surgery.
- Prolonged time in a cast or splint.

PREVENTIVE MEASURES

No specific preventive measures.

EXPECTED OUTCOMES

Outcome will vary in different people. Some may be helped with treatment, some cases clear up on their own, and others have ongoing pain despite treatment.

POSSIBLE COMPLICATIONS

- Disabling pain that may affect an entire arm or leg.
- Muscle wasting (atrophy) and severe joint damage.
- Skin damage that cannot be reversed.
- Tightening of the muscles as they lose their tone. Hand and fingers or foot and toes may contract into a fixed position.
- Depression and anxiety due to chronic pain.

 DIAGNOSIS & TREATMENT

GENERAL MEASURES

- Your health care provider will do a physical exam and ask questions about your symptoms and activities. This is often enough for diagnosis. An anesthetic injection may be given and if relief of symptoms occurs within 30 minutes, it helps to confirm the diagnosis. Other tests may be done to check for complications.
- There is no cure, but there is a variety of treatment options. These include drugs, counseling, physical therapy, splinting, surgery, spinal cord stimulation, implanted drug pumps, and others. Your health care provider will devise a treatment plan based on your symptoms.
- TENS (transcutaneous electrical stimulation) may be recommended. It uses brief pulses of electricity applied to nerve endings under the skin to relieve pain.
- Applying cold may relieve swelling and sweating. If the affected area is cool, applying heat may offer relief.
- Massage therapy will often help with symptoms.
- Biofeedback may help. It is a technique that involves learning to become more aware of your body to help you relax and to relieve painful symptoms.
- Counseling may help you learn ways to cope with the chronic pain. Joining a support group may also help.
- To learn more: Reflex Sympathetic Dystrophy Syndrome Association website: www.rsds.org.

MEDICATIONS

- You may take nonprescription drugs for pain and inflammation such as ibuprofen or naproxen.
- Steroids to reduce swelling and inflammation, drugs that widen blood vessels, injections of local anesthetic, or stronger pain drugs may be prescribed.

ACTIVITY

- Maintain normal daily activities as best you can.
- Physical therapy may be prescribed to help keep muscles flexible, strong, and mobile.

DIET

Eat a healthy diet to help maintain physical well-being.

 NOTIFY OUR OFFICE IF

You or a family member has symptoms of reflex sympathetic dystrophy or pain continues despite treatment.

Special notes:

_____

_____

_____

More notes on the back of this page ☐

REITER'S SYNDROME

BASIC INFORMATION

DESCRIPTION
A disorder that can include inflammation of the joints (arthritis), the urinary tract (urethritis), the eye (conjunctivitis), and may also involve the skin. Two forms are recognized:
• A sexually transmitted form (most often *Chlamydia* infection). It usually affects male adolescents and young adults (12 to 40 years).
• A form that follows an gastrointestinal bacterial infection (such as *Salmonella*, *Shigella*, *Yersinia* and *Campylobacter*). It affects men and women equally and can occur in children.

FREQUENT SIGNS AND SYMPTOMS
• Symptoms may or may not appear at the same time.
• Inflammation of the urethra (tube that takes urine from the bladder to the outside).
• Discharge from the penis or vagina. It often occurs 1 to 2 weeks after sexual contact.
• Pain or discomfort when urinating.
• Painful, swollen joints, especially in the knees, ankles, feet, and wrists.
• Stiffness and pain in the back and neck due to inflammation of the spine.
• Small ulcers (sores) inside the mouth, tongue, and on the penis tip.
• Red, itchy, burning and tearing of the eyes.
• Skin rash similar to psoriasis on the soles, palms, and around fingernails and toenails.
• Diarrhea may occur before other symptoms.
• General ill feeling.

CAUSES
Unknown. It appears to be a combination of genetic factors and various disease agents. A genetic marker (the HLA-B27 gene) is found in numerous patients.

RISK INCREASES WITH
• Recent gastrointestinal illness with diarrhea.
• Previous sexually transmitted infections.
• Family history of Reiter's syndrome.
• Weak immune system due to illness or drugs.
• Genetic factors.

PREVENTIVE MEASURES
Men can use rubber (latex) condoms during sexual intercourse or abstain from sex.

EXPECTED OUTCOMES
Symptoms may range from mild to severe. Arthritis symptoms may continue up to 4 months, others may clear up sooner. Most patients recover in 2 to 16 weeks. Many patients have recurrences over the years.

POSSIBLE COMPLICATIONS
• Chronic or recurrent symptoms that lead to disability.

• Heart, lung, or nervous system problems (rare).
• Severe eye disease that could lead to blindness.
• Ankylosing spondylitis (arthritis of the spine).
• Deformities of the feet.

DIAGNOSIS & TREATMENT

GENERAL MEASURES
• Your health care provider will do a physical exam and ask questions about your symptoms and activities. Medical tests may include blood studies (to look for the genetic marker) and a culture of the urethral discharge. X-rays may be done in some cases.
• There is no treatment to cure Reiter's. Symptoms are managed with drug therapy and physical therapy.
• Physical therapy is often recommended to help maintain range of motion of the joints.
• Usually, no treatment is needed for eye symptoms, unless they are severe or chronic.

MEDICATIONS
Your health care provider may prescribe:
• Nonsteroidal anti-inflammatory drugs for arthritis symptoms.
• Antibiotics, such as tetracyclines, for urethritis.
• Corticosteroid injections for painful joints.
• Corticosteroid eye drops if eye symptoms are severe.
• Topical corticosteroid drugs for skin symptoms.
• Drugs that suppress the immune system.
• Drugs called tumor-necrosis factor inhibitors that are used for other forms of arthritis.

ACTIVITY
• After inflammation improves, exercise the affected joints daily with stretching and strengthening routines. Follow medical instructions. Maintain good posture.
• To relieve foot pain, wear cushion pads and arch supports in your shoes.

DIET
No special diet.

NOTIFY OUR OFFICE IF

• You or a family member has symptoms of Reiter's syndrome.
• Symptoms recur or new symptoms develop.

Special notes:

_____

_____

_____

More notes on the back of this page ☐

RENAL FAILURE, ACUTE
(Kidney Failure, Acute)

BASIC INFORMATION

DESCRIPTION
Sudden failure of the kidneys to function. Kidneys have several important functions. They produce certain hormones and help rid the body of waste products. When kidneys fail, the waste products build up and cause symptoms that vary in severity. This disorder usually has a short, sometimes severe course.

FREQUENT SIGNS AND SYMPTOMS
Early stages:
- Reduced urine output and increased thirst.
- Fatigue and listlessness.

Later stages:
- Little or no urine output.
- Nausea, vomiting, diarrhea, and appetite loss.
- Mental changes, including irritability, stupor, or coma.
- Convulsions.
- Severe itching.
- High or low blood pressure.
- Unexplained bruising, bleeding spots under the skin or unexpected bleeding.
- The symptoms of the underlying cause (see below) will also be present.

CAUSES
Conditions in the kidney, or in other areas of the body, that cause the kidneys to stop functioning. This leads to a buildup of waste products in the blood and tissues. Underlying conditions include:
- Shock with very low blood pressure.
- Blood poisoning (septicemia).
- Congestive heart failure.
- Fluid and electrolyte imbalance.
- Blood-transfusion reaction.
- Severe accident with severe muscle injury.
- Acute glomerulonephritis (kidney inflammation).
- Multiple myeloma (bone cancer).
- Obstruction of blood vessels that supply the kidney.
- Kidney stones that obstruct the ureters or the urethra.
- Prostate enlargement.
- Use of certain drugs.
- Overdose of poisons or drugs, such as drugs of abuse.

RISK INCREASES WITH
- People with one kidney.
- Recent surgery.
- Accidents with severe injuries.
- Medical history of conditions that affect the kidney, such as diabetes or gout.

PREVENTIVE MEASURES
No specific preventive measures. Seek medical care for causes and risk factors when possible.

EXPECTED OUTCOME
If the underlying condition can be controlled and the kidney failure can be treated promptly, complete recovery is likely. Recovery time may take days to weeks.

POSSIBLE COMPLICATIONS
Shock, infections, uremia, seizures, coma, heart or lung problems, chronic kidney failure, or death.

DIAGNOSIS & TREATMENT

GENERAL MEASURES
- Your health care provider will do a physical exam and ask questions about your symptoms and activities. Medical tests may include blood and urine studies that measure kidney function, and fluid and electrolyte balance. Ultrasound, x-ray, heart studies, and other tests may be done to diagnose any complications.
- Emergency hospital care may be needed to provide fluid and electrolyte therapy and dialysis.
- Treatment will be determined by cause of the failure.
- Surgery, if the cause can be corrected by surgery.
- Dialysis (artificial method of removing waste products from the blood) may be required until the kidneys recover their function.
- To learn more: National Kidney Foundation, 30 E. 33rd St., New York, NY 10016; (800) 622-9010; website: www.kidney.org.

MEDICATION
Diuretics (to remove excess fluid) and drugs to treat the underlying condition may be prescribed.

ACTIVITY
Rest in bed until the condition is cured. Then resume your normal activities as soon as symptoms improve.

DIET
Food and water intake is controlled to stop fluid and electrolyte imbalance and to reduce buildup of body wastes. A diet high in carbohydrates and low in protein (main source of waste products), to reduce kidneys' work load, may be a part of the treatment.

NOTIFY OUR OFFICE IF

- You or a family member has renal failure symptoms.
- Symptoms recur after treatment.

Special notes:

_____

_____

_____

More notes on the back of this page ☐

RENAL FAILURE, CHRONIC
(Kidney Failure, Chronic)

 BASIC INFORMATION

DESCRIPTION
Gradual failure (over months to years) of the kidneys to function. Kidneys have several important functions. They produce certain hormones and help rid the body of waste products. When kidneys fail, the waste products build up and cause symptoms that vary in severity. Kidney failure can affect all ages (often the elderly).

FREQUENT SIGNS AND SYMPTOMS
· None or few symptoms until 60% to 75% of the kidney function fails. The symptoms listed may then occur.
· Listlessness, mental confusion, and drowsiness.
· Mild shortness of breath.
· Sudden weight loss
· Nausea and vomiting.
· Itching, dry skin, and easy bruising.
· Headaches.
· Frequent hiccups.
· Changes in urine flow.
· Muscle cramps, twitches, or pain. Bone or joint pain.
· Numbness or tingling in hands or feet.
· Anemia with paleness and fatigue.
· Unusual bleeding.
· High blood pressure.

CAUSES
Many conditions (in the kidney, or in other areas of the body) can cause the kidneys to slowly lose their ability to function normally.

RISK INCREASES WITH
· High blood pressure.
· Diabetes or gout.
· Disorders that cause kidney inflammation such as systemic lupus erythematosus.
· Glomerulonephritis (kidney inflammation).
· Polycystic kidney disease; other hereditary disorders.
· Chronic kidney stones and infections.
· Use of certain drugs that are toxic to the kidneys.
· Blood-vessel diseases and various cancers.
· Previous kidney surgery.
· HIV, sickle-cell disease, and amyloidosis.
· Heroin abuse.

PREVENTIVE MEASURES
None specific. Avoid risk factors where possible or get medical care for diseases that can lead to kidney failure.

EXPECTED OUTCOME
Kidney failure is a condition that worsens gradually. Treatment can help slow the progress. Kidney dialysis or kidney transplant will eventually be needed.

POSSIBLE COMPLICATIONS
· Kidney failure can affect almost any body function.
· End stage renal disease (ESRD).

 DIAGNOSIS & TREATMENT

GENERAL MEASURES
· Your health care provider will do a physical exam and ask questions about your symptoms and activities. Medical tests may include blood and urine tests that measure kidney function and fluid and electrolytes. Ultrasound, x-ray, heart studies, and other tests may be done to diagnose underlying disorder or complications.
· Treatment is aimed at slowing the progress of the disease, treating the underlying disorder, treating complications, and replacing kidney function.
· Treatment steps may include hospital care, drugs, diet changes, dialysis, and kidney transplant.
· Hospital care may be needed for severe symptoms.
· Dialysis to filter and remove waste products from the blood may be needed for advanced kidney failure. Hemodialysis uses a machine. Peritoneal dialysis uses the body's abdominal lining as a filter.
· A kidney transplant may be recommended.
· To learn more: National Kidney & Urologic Diseases Information Clearinghouse, 3 Information Way, Bethesda, MD 20892, (800) 891-5290; website: www.kidney.niddk.nih.gov.

MEDICATION
· Your health care provider may prescribe:
  - Diuretics to reduce fluid build up in the body.
  - Drugs to lower high blood pressure, treat anemia, treat an underlying disorder, prevent bone loss, treat symptoms (such as itchy skin), or treat complications.
  - Changes in drugs you now take that may be toxic to the kidneys.

ACTIVITY
Reduce activity as needed. Get adequate sleep.

DIET
Limits on protein, salt, and fluids are usually needed. A dietitian can be helpful in providing instructions.

 NOTIFY OUR OFFICE IF

· You or a family member has symptoms of chronic renal failure.
· Chest pain, fainting, difficulty breathing, severe vomiting, bleeding, weakness, or a change in alertness occur.

Special notes:

_____

_____

_____

More notes on the back of this page ☐

RESPIRATORY SYNCYTIAL VIRUS (RSV)

 BASIC INFORMATION

DESCRIPTION

A viral infection of the nose, throat, and lungs that is easily spread from one person to another. It occurs mainly in the winter and spring months. RSV is common and most children have had an infection by age three. Symptoms are usually mild, but can be quite serious, especially in infants. A person can get it more than once, but the symptoms tend to be milder.

FREQUENT SIGNS AND SYMPTOMS

Early symptoms (are like a common cold):
- Runny nose and low-grade fever.
- Feeling tired and loss of appetite.
- Cough, sometimes with wheezing.

Later symptoms:
- Infant or child refuses to eat.
- There is an increase in coughing and wheezing.
- Ear-ache.
- Much less active and sleeping more than usual.
- Serious breathing problems. Skin color may be bluish.
- Spells of apnea (breathing stops for 10 to 15 seconds).

CAUSES

The virus is spread by close contact with an infected person, such as holding hands. It is also spread by touching a surface or object, such as a toy, that an infected person has handled. The germs can live on an object, a hard surface, or on used facial tissues for several hours and on hands for 30 minutes or longer.

RISK INCREASES WITH
- Infants and young children.
- Daycare centers. Both children and teachers.
- Living, working, or being in crowded places.

PREVENTIVE MEASURES
- Fight germs by washing your hands often.
- Take care to throw away used facial tissues.
- Cover your mouth when coughing or sneezing.
- Avoid crowds and tobacco smokers during seasonal outbreaks.
- Avoid close contact with people with cold symptoms.
- Preventive injections may be prescribed for young children at risk of a severe RSV illness.

EXPECTED OUTCOMES

Most cases are mild, need no special treatment, and last about 7 to 10 days.

POSSIBLE COMPLICATIONS
- Ear infection.
- Pneumonia or bronchiolitis, which are serious lung disorders. They are more likely to occur in premature infants, or children and adults who have heart or lung problems. Most everyone recovers, but they can be life threatening.

 DIAGNOSIS & TREATMENT

GENERAL MEASURES
- Most people who have mild symptoms, or who have a child with the symptoms, treat the illness as a cold. If there are any concerns, call your health care provider.
- Your health care provider may confirm an RSV diagnosis with a physical exam. Generally they know when there is an outbreak of RSV in the area. Medical tests are normally not required for healthy patients. They may be done for people who have a risk of complications.
- Treatment of mild symptoms in otherwise healthy people is the same as for a cold. Get extra rest and drink plenty of fluids until the symptoms are better. Be alert for any serious problems that might develop.
- Avoid being around cigarette smoke.
- Use salt (saline) nose drops for a stuffy nose.
- Hospital care may be needed for those with more severe symptoms. Oxygen, special drugs, and fluids to prevent dehydration are usually required.

MEDICATIONS
- Children may be given acetaminophen. Other drugs should be approved by their health care provider.
- A child in a hospital may be given virazole (brand name Ribavirin) for severe symptoms of the virus.
- Adults may take nonprescription drugs for pain or cold remedies.
- Antibiotics don't help a virus infection. They may be prescribed if a bacterial infection does develop.

ACTIVITY

Reduce daily activity until you feel better.

DIET

No special diet is needed. Drink plenty of fluids.

 NOTIFY OUR OFFICE IF

- You or your child has symptoms of respiratory syncytial virus, and you are worried about the illness.
- Any of the following occur during the illness: Fever rises, cough or wheezing gets worse, difficulty breathing, feeling very tired or weak, infant refuses any foods or liquids, not sleeping, or periods of sleep apnea.

Special notes:

_____

_____

_____

More notes on the back of this page ☐

RESTLESS LEGS SYNDROME

BASIC INFORMATION

DESCRIPTION
· Restless legs syndrome (RLS) is a disorder that causes unpleasant sensations in the legs. RLS occurs more often in women than in men. It may begin at any age, even as early as infancy. Patients with severe symptoms are usually middle-aged or older.
· More than 80% of people with RLS also have a more common condition known as periodic limb movement disorder (PLMD). PLMD involves involuntary leg twitching or jerking movements during sleep. They typically occur every 10 to 60 seconds, sometimes throughout the night. People have no control over them.

FREQUENT SIGNS AND SYMPTOMS
· The main symptom of RLS involves sensations in the legs. They are often described as burning, creeping, tugging, or like insects crawling inside the legs.
· They usually occur deep inside the leg, between the knee and ankle. More rarely, they occur in the feet, thighs, arms, and hands. The sensations usually affect both sides of the body.
· The sensations range in severity from uncomfortable, to irritating, to painful. They may come and go.
· Lying down and trying to relax causes the symptoms.
· Symptoms may be less apparent during the day and more severe in the evening or at night. They cause difficulty in falling, and staying, asleep.
· Long car trips, sitting in a movie theater, long airplane trips, or relaxation exercises can trigger the symptoms.

CAUSES
In most cases, the cause of RLS is unknown. In others, there are certain factors or conditions that may be related to RLS, but it is unknown if they actually cause it.

RISK INCREASES WITH
· Family history of RLS.
· Low iron levels or anemia.
· Chronic diseases such as kidney failure, diabetes, Parkinson's disease, and peripheral neuropathy.
· Pregnancy.
· Certain drugs.
· Caffeine, alcohol, and tobacco may aggravate or trigger symptoms in some patients.

PREVENTIVE MEASURES
None known.

EXPECTED OUTCOMES
· There is no cure. Symptoms may disappear for weeks or months, but usually return. Treatment can reduce the symptoms and increase periods of restful sleep.
· With pregnancy, RLS usually stops by 4 weeks after delivery.

POSSIBLE COMPLICATIONS
· Left untreated, the condition causes exhaustion and daytime fatigue.
· Symptoms may gradually worsen with age.

DIAGNOSIS & TREATMENT

GENERAL MEASURES
· Your health care provider will do a physical exam and ask questions about your symptoms and activities. Medical tests may be done to identify any medical disorder that may be a factor in the symptoms.
· Treatment will be given for any disorder diagnosed.
· Treatment options for RLS may include lifestyle changes and drugs or supplements.
· Don't smoke. Find a plan that will help you to quit.
· A regular sleep pattern can help reduce symptoms. Try to go to bed and get up at the same times each day.
· Taking a hot bath, massaging the legs, or using a heating pad or ice pack may help relieve symptoms.
· To learn more: Restless Legs Syndrome Foundation, 819 Second Street, SW, Rochester, MN 55902-2985; (507) 287-6465 (not toll free); website: www.rls.org.

MEDICATIONS
· No one drug works for everyone with RLS. There are several options and your health care provider will discuss their benefits and side effects with you. If one type doesn't help, another can be tried.
· Diet supplements may be recommended.
· If a drug you take could be a cause of RLS, you may be advised to change the dose or take a different drug.

ACTIVITY
A program of regular, moderate exercise may help you sleep better. Excessive exercise may worsen symptoms.

DIET
Avoid caffeine and alcohol. They may trigger symptoms.

NOTIFY OUR OFFICE IF

· You or a family member has symptoms of restless legs syndrome.
· Symptoms continue despite treatment.

Special notes:

_____

_____

_____

More notes on the back of this page ☐

RETINAL DETACHMENT

 BASIC INFORMATION

DESCRIPTION
A separation or tear of the retina (the light-receptive tissue at the back of the eye) from the remainder of the eye. It can affect all ages (most often ages 40 to 70) and both sexes. Retinal detachment is a medical emergency.

FREQUENT SIGNS AND SYMPTOMS
The following symptoms usually affect one eye, but sometimes both are affected:
- Light flashes in the field of vision.
- Floating spots in the field of vision.
- Blurred vision.
- Wavy visual images (sometimes).
- Gradual loss of vision. This may not be noticed because it is so gradual.
- No pain.

CAUSES
Retinal detachments may develop in eyes with retinas weakened by a hole or a tear. This allows fluid to seep underneath and weaken the attachment, so that the retina then becomes detached.

RISK INCREASES WITH
- Aging.
- Eye injury.
- Diabetes (which can lead to diabetic retinopathy).
- Vascular disease.
- Previous retinal detachment.
- Family history of retinal detachment.
- Extreme nearsightedness (myopia).
- Complications of eye surgery.
- Tumors or inflammation.
- Glaucoma.

PREVENTIVE MEASURES
- No specific preventive measures.
- Patients at risk should have regular eye exams.
- If you have diabetes or vascular disease, obtain medical care to control the disorder.

EXPECTED OUTCOMES
Usually curable with prompt treatment.

POSSIBLE COMPLICATIONS
- Without treatment, partial or complete blindness in the affected eye may occur.
- With delayed treatment, detachment may extend to the macula (the area of most detailed vision). This can cause permanent loss of detailed (central) vision.
- Detachment may recur. This can occur within a few months of surgery. Treatment will need to be repeated.

 DIAGNOSIS & TREATMENT

GENERAL MEASURES
- Your eye doctor (ophthalmologist) will diagnose the detachment by an exam of the eye. An ultrasound may be done in some cases.
- Treatment will depend on location and severity of the detachment. There are several procedures available. Sometimes, a combination of one or more procedures is used. The procedures are most often done as an outpatient, but hospital care may be needed for surgery. A local or general anesthetic may be used. Your eye doctor will explain the procedures to you.
- The retina may be reattached using special lasers or cryotherapy (using below-freezing temperatures).
- A gas bubble may be injected into the eye. It holds the retina in place while, over a period of days, the fluid that seeped in is resolved. The gas bubble is eventually absorbed by the body. This procedure may require the head to remain in a certain position for days to weeks.
- More advanced detachments may require surgery. Scleral buckle or vitrectomy are two types of surgery that may be recommended.
- Recovery of vision may take weeks to months. If vision was good before the detachment, good vision should return. If vision was poor prior to the detachment, the return may be slow and remain poor.

MEDICATIONS
Drugs are usually not needed for this disorder.

ACTIVITY
You will be advised about limits on activity depending on the type of procedure used. Follow all instructions carefully.

DIET
No special diet.

 NOTIFY OUR OFFICE IF

- You or a family member has flashes or floating spots in your field of vision. Do not delay in getting medical help. This can be an emergency.
- Any sign of infection occurs (bleeding, redness, pain, swelling, or fever) or vision worsens after surgery.

Special notes:

_____

_____

_____

More notes on the back of this page ☐

REYE'S SYNDROME

 ## BASIC INFORMATION

DESCRIPTION

A rare disease that involves the brain, liver, and other major organs. It can occur at any age, but it most often affects children and young teenagers.

FREQUENT SIGNS AND SYMPTOMS

- Vomiting.
- Lethargy.
- Drowsiness.
- Confusion.
- Delirium.
- Personality changes (such as irritability).
- Seizures.
- Arm or leg weakness, or unable to move them.
- Double vision.
- Speech problems.
- Coma.

CAUSES

Unknown. Reye's syndrome usually occurs following a virus infection. Studies link most cases to the use of salicylate drugs, such as aspirin, during a viral illness, especially chickenpox and influenza.

RISK INCREASES WITH

- Recent illness, such as chickenpox, influenza, or other respiratory illness.
- Use of aspirin with the viral illness.

PREVENTIVE MEASURES

Don't give a child under the age of 18 aspirin for fever until it has been diagnosed. If the illness is diagnosed as viral, never use aspirin.

EXPECTED OUTCOMES

Some patients will have a mild illness with complete recovery. Others may have more severe symptoms and develop varying degrees of brain damage. Early diagnosis is important to help prevent complications.

POSSIBLE COMPLICATIONS

- Pneumonia.
- Respiratory failure.
- Heart rhythm problems or heart attack.
- Seizures.
- Permanent brain damage, coma, or death caused by pressure on the brain.

 ## DIAGNOSIS & TREATMENT

GENERAL MEASURES

- Your health care provider will do a physical exam. Medical tests may include blood studies of liver function and a study of cerebrospinal fluid (CSF). An EEG (electroencephalogram, which measures electrical activity of the brain) may be done.
- There is no specific treatment that will cure the disorder. Hospital intensive care is needed. Treatment steps are aimed at preventing complications such as swelling of the brain. This may involve inserting a feeding tube, intravenous (IV) fluids, urinary catheter, mechanical breathing support, kidney dialysis, blood transfusion, cardiovascular (heart and blood vessel) monitoring, and therapies to reduce pressure on the brain.
- To learn more: National Reye's Syndrome Foundation, 426 N. Lewis, P.O. Box 829, Bryan, OH 43506, (800) 233-7393; website: www.reyessyndrome.org.

MEDICATIONS

- Your health care provider may prescribe:
  - Steroids or other drugs to reduce pressure and swelling of the brain.
  - Diuretics to help remove excess fluid from the body.
  - Glucose solutions to maintain normal levels of glucose.

ACTIVITY

Bed rest is needed until the symptoms improve. Normal activities may then be resumed gradually.

DIET

Nothing by mouth at first. After recovery, no special diet is required.

 ## NOTIFY OUR OFFICE IF

- Your child has symptoms of Reye's syndrome. Call at the first sign of confusion, lethargy, or other mental changes!
- After hospital care, any symptoms of Reye's syndrome recur or the child develops a fever.
- New, unexplained symptoms develop. Drugs used in treatment may produce side effects.

Special notes:

_____

_____

_____

More notes on the back of this page ☐

RH ISOIMMUNIZATION
(Erythroblastosis Fetalis)

BASIC INFORMATION

DESCRIPTION
Incompatibility between an infant's blood type and that of its mother. This results in the destruction of the infant's red blood cells during pregnancy and after birth by antibodies from its mother's blood.

FREQUENT SIGNS AND SYMPTOMS
Signs during pregnancy:
· Decreased fetal growth.
· Decreased fetal movement.
Signs in a newborn:
· Paleness.
· Jaundice (yellow skin and eyes) that begins within 24 hours after delivery.
· Unexplained bruising or blood spots under the skin.
· Tissue swelling (edema).
· Breathing difficulty.
· Seizures.
· Lack of normal movement.
· Poor reflex response.

CAUSES
The baby of an Rh-negative (blood type) mother and an Rh-positive father may be Rh-positive. If the father is known to be Rh negative, there is no concern. During pregnancy, but more commonly during delivery, a small amount of the infant's blood is absorbed by the mother through the placenta, stimulating her body to produce antibodies against Rh-positive blood. The antibodies are produced after delivery, so the first infant is not affected. With each subsequent pregnancy, anti-Rh antibodies cross the placenta and may destroy fetal blood cells. The resulting anemia can be severe enough to cause fetal death. If the fetus survives, antibodies can cross to the baby during birth, causing jaundice and other symptoms shortly after birth.

RISK INCREASES WITH
Each pregnancy after the first one that involved different blood types.

PREVENTIVE MEASURES
Medical care early in pregnancy is important to determine the risk of Rh incompatibility and provide treatment if needed.

EXPECTED OUTCOME
With prompt diagnosis, monitoring, and treatment, the outcome is generally good.

POSSIBLE COMPLICATIONS
· Complications may develop from procedures such as amniocentesis or cordocentesis.
· Emergency delivery of the baby may be required.
· Hydrops fetalis in the newborn. This involves severe edema (swelling), heart, lung, and liver problems.

DIAGNOSIS & TREATMENT

GENERAL MEASURES
· Blood tests are done to type the mother's, father's, and infant's blood, measure the mother's Rh-positive antibodies, and to detect anemia in the infant's blood.
· Amniocentesis may be done. A small amount of amniotic fluid is withdrawn from the amniotic sac that surrounds the unborn child in the uterus for a diagnostic procedure. It can be used sometimes to determine the fetal blood type.
· Cordocentesis (percutaneous umbilical blood sampling [PUBS]) may be recommended. It is done to determine fetal blood type and the degree of anemia.
· Intrauterine blood transfusions (sometimes).
· Transfusion to completely exchange the infant's blood after birth.
· Hospital care. The newborn child will remain in the hospital up to 2 weeks after an exchange transfusion.
· If you have an Rh-negative blood type, tell any health care provider who treats you. Be sure this information is in your medical records. Wear a medical alert type bracelet or pendant to identify your medical problem.

MEDICATION
If you are pregnant and have Rh-negative blood type, you will be prescribed an anti-Rh gamma globulin injection (RhoGAM) at 28 weeks and again within 72 hours after delivery or at the end of a pregnancy for any reason. You may have antibody titer drawn during pregnancy to see if you are producing anti-Rh antibodies. You do not need RhoGAM if your fetus is Rh-negative.

ACTIVITY
No limits after treatment.

DIET
No special diet.

NOTIFY OUR OFFICE IF

You have further questions about RH isoimmunization.

Special notes:

_____

_____

_____

More notes on the back of this page ☐

RHEUMATIC FEVER

 ## BASIC INFORMATION

DESCRIPTION

An inflammatory disorder that affects many parts of the body, especially the joints and heart. It occurs following group A streptococcal pharyngitis (strep throat). Strep infections are contagious, but rheumatic fever is not. It can affect all ages, but it is more common in children.

FREQUENT SIGNS AND SYMPTOMS

- Joint inflammation that causes pain, redness, swelling, and warmth. Wrists, elbows, knees, or ankles are most often affected. The symptoms may move from one joint to another.
- Fever; fatigue; paleness.
- Appetite loss; general ill feeling.
- Stomach (abdominal) pain; chest pain.
- Mild skin rash on the chest, back, and abdomen.
- Small, painless bumps just under the skin in bony areas such as the elbows or knees.
- Uncontrolled arm and leg movement (chorea).
- If the heart is involved:
  - Shortness of breath.
  - Fluid build up that causes swelling of legs and back.
  - Rapid heartbeat, especially when lying down.

CAUSES

Rheumatic fever is caused by a preceding strep infection in the throat that occurs 1 to 6 weeks prior to the start of symptoms. It is probably an autoimmune disorder in which antibodies produced by the body to attack the strep bacteria also attack tissues of the joints or heart.

RISK INCREASES WITH

- Family history of rheumatic fever.
- Crowded or unclean living conditions.
- Poor nutrition.

PREVENTIVE MEASURES

Obtain prompt antibiotic treatment of any strep infection, including those of the skin. Strep infections must be treated with antibiotics.

EXPECTED OUTCOMES

Strep infections are usually curable with treatment. Rheumatic fever is treatable, but not curable. It usually resolves in 2 to 12 weeks. Some cases may take 15 weeks.

POSSIBLE COMPLICATIONS

- Rheumatic heart disease. In some cases, rheumatic fever may damage the heart valves. It may take 10 to 30 years for symptoms of valve damage to appear. A damaged valve can usually be replaced with surgery.
- Chronic heart disease that may lead to disability.
- Rheumatic fever may recur following reinfection with strep.

 ## DIAGNOSIS & TREATMENT

GENERAL MEASURES

- Your health care provider will do a physical exam and ask questions about your symptoms and previous illnesses. Medical tests may include blood studies, a throat culture, and x-rays of the chest and heart. An ECG (electrocardiogram) may be done. This test measures electrical activity of the heart. No test is specific to diagnose rheumatic fever.
- Treatment includes rest and drugs to treat the symptoms and to prevent rheumatic fever from recurring. Home care is recommended for most cases. Hospital care may be required for more severe cases.
- To learn more: American Heart Association, 7272 Greenville Ave., Dallas, TX 75231; (800) 242-8721 website: www.americanheart.org.

MEDICATIONS

- Your health care provider may prescribe:
  - Drugs to reduce inflammation.
  - Diuretics to reduce fluid build-up in the body.
  - Drugs for congestive heart failure if it occurs.
  - Antibiotics for strep bacteria. Once rheumatic fever reaches the inactive stage, low-dose antibiotics may be continued indefinitely to prevent recurrence. They may be taken by mouth or given as an injection.

ACTIVITY

Bed rest normally (or very limited activity) until studies show the disease has subsided. Then return to normal activities gradually. Your health care provider will advise when to return to school.

DIET

- A liquid or soft diet in the early stages. Then provide a normal diet high in protein, calories, and vitamins.
- A low-salt diet may be recommended if patient has carditis (inflammation of the heart).

 ## NOTIFY OUR OFFICE IF

- You or your child has symptoms of rheumatic fever.
- The following symptoms occur during treatment:
  - Swelling of the legs or back.
  - Shortness of breath, cough, or fever.
  - Vomiting, diarrhea, or severe abdominal pain.

Special notes:

_____

_____

_____

More notes on the back of this page ☐

RINGWORM
(Tinea)

 BASIC INFORMATION

DESCRIPTION

Fungal (tinea) infection of the skin. Ringworm can involve the scalp (tinea capitis), skin (tinea corporis), groin skin (tinea cruris), nails (tinea unguium), feet (tinea pedis), and skin with beard (tinea barbae). It affects children and adults and is more common in males than females.

FREQUENT SIGNS AND SYMPTOMS

- Lesions (sores) that itch (sometimes).
- On the scalp—lesions cause patchy hair loss and scaling scalp.
- On body skin—lesions are red, circular, flat, scaling, and have well-defined borders.
- On the bearded area of the face—lesions cause an itchy, scaling rash under the beard.
- On the feet—in the skin between the toes, a soft scaling (may be blistered), itchy rash.
- Of the nails—thickened, yellow, dull nails with crusting at the free edge.

CAUSES

Fungal infection with one or more of 5 different fungi. They are found almost everywhere. Transmission is by person-to-person contact or by contact with infected surfaces, such as towels, shoes, or shower stalls. Worms have nothing to do with the infection.

RISK INCREASES WITH

- Crowded living conditions.
- Contact with infected persons or animals.
- Daycare centers or schools.
- Weak immune system due to illness or drugs.
- Chronic moisture and irritation of the skin.
- Warm, humid climates.

PREVENTIVE MEASURES

- The fungi are so prevalent that total prevention is impossible. To reduce risk:
  - Get treatment for pets that have skin problems.
  - Carefully dry feet after bathing in a tub or shower or after swimming. Apply antiperspirant to your feet if they perspire excessively.
  - Good personal hygiene.
  - Don't share headgear (hats, combs, brushes).
  - Avoid tight shoes or underwear that may rub or irritate the skin.

EXPECTED OUTCOMES

Usually curable with treatment. It may take weeks to months depending on the location. Recurrence is common and ringworm becomes chronic in 20% of cases.

POSSIBLE COMPLICATIONS

Bacterial infection of ringworm lesions.

 DIAGNOSIS & TREATMENT

GENERAL MEASURES

- In most cases, self-treatment is all that is needed. See your health care provider if self-care does not help.
- Your health care provider can usually diagnose the disorder by an exam of the affected skin. Medical tests may include microscopic exam of skin scrapings and exam with ultraviolet light (Wood's lamp) for ringworm on the scalp.
- Treatment is usually with topical drugs. Other specific care depends on location of infection.
- For infection on the body: Carefully launder all clothing, towels, or bed linens that have touched the lesions.
- Keep the skin dry. If the area is red, swollen, and weeping, use compresses made of 1 teaspoon salt to 1 pint water. Apply 4 times a day for 2 to 3 days before starting the local antifungal medication.
- For infection of the scalp, shampoo the hair daily.
- For infected feet, expose feet to air whenever possible. Wear sandals or leather shoes, wear cotton socks. Wash and dry your feet at least twice a day.
- For an infected beard, let the beard grow. If necessary to shave, use an electric shaver and not a blade.
- For nail infection, keep nails short.

MEDICATIONS

- Use topical antifungal drugs in the form of creams, lotions, or ointments. Treatment may continue after symptoms clear up to help prevent a recurrence.
- In widespread infections or nail infections, an oral antifungal may be prescribed.
- Topical steroids may be prescribed for itching or inflammation.
- Antibiotics may be prescribed for a bacteria infection.

ACTIVITY

No limits.

DIET

No special diet.

 NOTIFY OUR OFFICE IF

- You or a family member has symptoms of ringworm.
- Lesions become redder, painful, and ooze pus.
- Symptoms don't improve in 3 or 4 weeks.

Special notes:

_____

_____

_____

More notes on the back of this page ☐

ROCKY MOUNTAIN SPOTTED FEVER

(Tick Typhus)

BASIC INFORMATION

DESCRIPTION

An acute illness with fever caused by a germ transmitted by infected ticks. This is not contagious from person to person. It can involve the skin, central nervous system, gastrointestinal tract, and muscles. It can affect all ages but is more likely to occur in children and young adults. The disease gets its name from the area where it was first identified.

FREQUENT SIGNS AND SYMPTOMS

The following occur 3 to 12 days after a tick bite:
- Fever, often high, with chills.
- Red skin rash that begins on hands and feet and spreads to ankles, wrists, legs, trunk, and abdomen.
- Headache that may be severe.
- Muscle aches and weakness; stiff back.
- Nausea and vomiting.
- Mental confusion; coma.

CAUSES

Rickettsia germs that live inside ticks. People are infected through tick bites, usually in the spring or summer. *Rickettsia* also infect rodents, squirrels, and chipmunks. The disease occurs in all states of the United States, especially on the East coast from Georgia to Maryland, and in heavy brush areas, such as Long Island.

RISK INCREASES WITH

- Outdoor activities in tick-infested areas.
- Contact with dogs.

PREVENTIVE MEASURES

- Wear protective clothing in tick-infested areas, and use insect repellent.
- During outdoor activity, carefully inspect the body frequently to remove ticks. If ticks are removed within 4 hours, it will reduce the risk of infection. Remove the tick with tweezers by grabbing as close to the skin as possible. Disinfect the bite site and wash hands with soap and water. Do not remove ticks by squeezing, using petroleum jelly (Vaseline), or burning them with a match. Save the tick in a plastic bag in a freezer. If illness occurs, it may be used to help with diagnosis.

EXPECTED OUTCOMES

Curable, if treatment is begun in the early stages. Those with severe illness are more likely to develop complications.

POSSIBLE COMPLICATIONS

- Brain infection.
- Seizures.
- Kidney failure.
- Hepatitis.
- Rocky Mountain spotted fever can be fatal if untreated (due to pneumonia or heart failure).

DIAGNOSIS & TREATMENT

GENERAL MEASURES

- Your health care provider will do a physical exam and ask questions about your symptoms and activities. Medical tests may include blood studies and skin biopsy (small piece of skin is removed to view under a microscope). The history of a tick bite or travel to a tick-infested area helps confirm diagnosis.
- Treatment is with drugs and supportive care.
- Patients with mild disease may be treated at home. Moderate to severe infections require hospital care. Treatment may include mechanical breathing support, blood transfusions, and close watch for complications such as kidney failure.
- Good mouth care is important.
- To learn more: Centers for Disease Control & Prevention, 1600 Clifton Rd, Atlanta, GA 30333; (800) 311-3435; website: www.cdc.gov/ncidod/dvrd/rmsf/.

MEDICATIONS

Antibiotics, such as doxycycline, tetracycline, or chloramphenicol will be prescribed.

ACTIVITY

Rest in bed until fever and other symptoms clear up.

DIET

No special diet. Very ill patients may require intravenous (IV) feedings. For others, small frequent meals may be needed.

NOTIFY OUR OFFICE IF

- You or a family member has symptoms of Rocky Mountain spotted fever.
- New, unexplained symptoms develop. Drugs used in treatment may produce side effects.

Special notes:

_____

_____

_____

More notes on the back of this page ☐

ROSEOLA INFANTUM
(Exanthem Subitum)

 BASIC INFORMATION

DESCRIPTION
A common, contagious childhood disease. It usually affects infants and young children (ages 1 to 3 years). 90% of cases occur before age two.

FREQUENT SIGNS AND SYMPTOMS
· Fever, often high, for several days. It may be the only symptoms until the rash appears.
· Flat, reddish skin rash after 3 to 5 days of high fever. When the rash appears, fever disappears. Some children may never develop the rash.
· Irritability.
· Drowsiness.
· Loss of appetite.

CAUSES
It is caused by a type of herpes virus. (It is not the same herpes virus that causes cold sores.) The fever begins 5 to 15 days (usually 9 days) after exposure. A child is infectious during the fever phase of the illness. It is not known exactly how the infection is spread from one person to another.

RISK INCREASES WITH
· Daycare center.
· Exposure to others in public places.

PREVENTIVE MEASURES
There is no specific way to prevent the infection.

EXPECTED OUTCOMES
The illness heals on its own in about 1 week.

POSSIBLE COMPLICATIONS
· Rarely, convulsions caused by high fever. They will not cause brain damage and will stop after the fever subsides.
· Infection of the brain or hepatitis (both rare).

 DIAGNOSIS & TREATMENT

GENERAL MEASURES
· Parents can usually treat the disorder without medical care. Call your child's health care provider if you have any concern about the symptoms. The disorder can usually be diagnosed without any medical tests, but a blood or urine study may be done.
· There is no specific treatment for roseola. Rest at home, drink extra fluids, and drug therapy to reduce the fever if needed.
· Lukewarm water bath or sponge bath may be used to reduce the fever if it reaches 102°F (38.9°C) or higher.

MEDICATIONS
· For relief from minor discomfort and to reduce fever, you may use nonprescription drugs such as acetaminophen or ibuprofen. Don't give aspirin to children under age 18.
· Antibiotics will not help a virus infection.
· Anticonvulsant drugs (if child has seizure) may be prescribed.

ACTIVITY
The child should rest in bed until the fever disappears.

DIET
The child should eat a normal, well-balanced diet. Encourage extra fluid intake. Continue baby-vitamin supplements if the child is accustomed to taking them.

 NOTIFY OUR OFFICE IF

· Your child has symptoms of roseola.
· High fever occurs.
· Twitching or other signs of a convulsion begin.
· The child refuses liquids.
· The child cries loudly and persistently, and does not stop when picked up.
· The child is listless and has a stiff neck.

Special notes:

_____

_____

_____

More notes on the back of this page ☐

ROUNDWORMS
(Ascariasis & Other Roundworms)

 ## BASIC INFORMATION

DESCRIPTION
Roundworms thrive in the gastrointestinal tract (and sometimes in the lungs). They are contagious and affect all ages, but are most common in children.

FREQUENT SIGNS AND SYMPTOMS
- Often, there may be no symptoms.
- Irritability.
- Restlessness at night.
- Erratic or poor appetite.
- Frequent fatigue.
- Weight loss or lack of weight gain.
- Stomach (abdominal) discomfort.
- Diarrhea (sometimes).
- Cough and wheezing (rare).
- Worms may sometimes be seen in bowel movements or in the child's bed. Rarely, one may be vomited.
- Fever.

CAUSES
There are several types of roundworms (or nematodes). Some can be seen by the human eye, and others can only be seen with a microscope. Their eggs can enter the human body through contaminated water, food, or soil-contaminated hands. In some types, the larvae (young worms) enter through the skin.

RISK INCREASES WITH
- Crowded or unclean living conditions.
- Using human feces as a fertilizer.

PREVENTIVE MEASURES
- Wash hands often, and always before eating and after using the bathroom.
- Keep fingers away from the mouth.
- Have pets treated for worms. Avoid strange animals.

EXPECTED OUTCOMES
Usually curable in one week with treatment.

POSSIBLE COMPLICATIONS
- If untreated:
  - Worms migrate to other body parts.
  - Intestinal obstruction (rare).

 ## DIAGNOSIS & TREATMENT

GENERAL MEASURES
- Your health care provider may do a physical exam. Medical tests may include studies of the stool or a study of an adult worm, if passed, to identify the worm. X-ray of the lungs or an ultrasound may be done in some cases.
- Treatment can be given at home and involves anti-worm drugs.
- Wash hands carefully after using the toilet or before meals. Keep fingers away from the mouth. Keep nails short and clean.
- In rare cases, surgery may be needed for complications, such as a bowel perforation (tear).

MEDICATIONS
Drugs called anthelmintics that kill roundworms will be prescribed. Follow the instructions provided for taking the drug.

ACTIVITY
No limits.

DIET
No special diet.

 ## NOTIFY OUR OFFICE IF

- You or your child has symptoms of roundworms.
- Roundworms reappear after treatment.
- New, unexplained symptoms develop. Drugs used in treatment may produce side effects.

Special notes:

_____

_____

_____

More notes on the back of this page ☐

RUBELLA
(German Measles)

 BASIC INFORMATION

DESCRIPTION

A mild, contagious, viral illness. It can affect all ages, but has been most common in children. Use of the rubella vaccine has reduced the number of cases in the United States by 99%. Rubella is likely to cause serious birth defects in the unborn baby of a pregnant woman who develops the disease in the first 3 or 4 months of pregnancy.

FREQUENT SIGNS AND SYMPTOMS

- Fever.
- Muscle aches and stiffness, especially in the neck.
- Fatigue and headache.
- Reddish rash on the head and body after the 2nd or 3rd day. The rash lasts 1 or 2 days.
- Swollen lymph glands, especially behind the ears and at the back and sides of the neck.
- Joint pain (adults).

CAUSES

The rubella virus is spread by person-to-person contact. It takes 14 to 23 days after exposure before symptoms appear. Patients are contagious from one week before the rash appears until one week after it started.

RISK INCREASES WITH

- Young, unimmunized adults.
- Crowded living conditions.
- School or daycare.
- Weak immune system due to illness or drugs.

PREVENTIVE MEASURES

- Vaccination:
  - For children, rubella vaccine is usually given with the measles and mumps vaccine (MMR).
  - Nonpregnant women of childbearing age should be vaccinated if they have not had rubella or have not been vaccinated before. Pregnancy should be prevented for one month after vaccination. A blood test can be done if a woman is unsure about her rubella immunity.
  - Health care workers and daycare workers should get vaccinated if they have not been, or if their vaccination history is unknown. Young adults, such as college students should get two doses of MMR if not previously vaccinated.
- A person should not be vaccinated if he or she has a weak immune system, as occurs with cancer patients, currently takes cortisone or anticancer drugs, is receiving radiation therapy, or has a serious illness.
- A person, especially a pregnant woman, who is exposed to rubella and has not had it, or been vaccinated against it, should consult their health care provider right away.

EXPECTED OUTCOMES

No specific treatment is needed. The illness will heal on its own in one week in children, sometimes longer in adults. Complications are rare.

POSSIBLE COMPLICATIONS

- Encephalitis (brain inflammation).
- Thrombocytopenia (a blood disorder).
- Agranulocytosis (reduction in white blood cells).
- Rubella infection in a pregnant woman may cause miscarriage or birth defects. The baby may have growth restriction; mental retardation; deafness; or liver, spleen, and bone marrow problems.

 DIAGNOSIS & TREATMENT

GENERAL MEASURES

- Your health care provider can usually diagnose the disorder with a physical exam. Medical tests are normally not done for rubella. If needed, cultures of the throat, blood, urine, or cerebrospinal fluid can confirm the presence of the virus.
- Usually no specific treatment is required. Get extra rest and drink plenty of fluids.
- Be sure to contact any pregnant woman who has been exposed to the patient. Exposure includes contact with the infected person 1 week prior to, during, or 1 week after the start of symptoms. This woman should consult her obstetric care provider right away.

MEDICATIONS

For minor discomfort, you may use nonprescription drugs such as acetaminophen or ibuprofen.

ACTIVITY

Get extra rest until the symptoms get better.

DIET

No special diet.

 NOTIFY OUR OFFICE IF

- You or a family member has symptoms of rubella.
- The following occur during treatment: high fever, red eyes, cough, shortness of breath, severe headache, drowsiness, lethargy, or convulsion.
- Unusual bleeding occurs 1 to 4 weeks after the illness (from gums, nose, uterus, or blood specks on the skin).

Special notes:

_____

_____

_____

More notes on the back of this page ☐

SALIVARY GLAND INFECTION

 BASIC INFORMATION

DESCRIPTION

An infection of a salivary gland. The salivary glands are located around the mouth and they produce saliva. Saliva is the moisture in the mouth that helps with chewing and swallowing. There are three pairs of salivary glands and the largest is called the parotids.

FREQUENT SIGNS AND SYMPTOMS

- Pain and swelling of parotid gland (behind ear) or sublingual (under tongue) salivary gland.
- Dry mouth.
- May be hard to open mouth wide.
- Food may taste strange.
- There may be a bitter tasting pus, which is a creamy fluid, in the mouth caused by the infection.
- Fever.

CAUSES

- Usually a bacterial infection, which results from poor mouth care.
- The gland could become blocked by tiny, stone-like substances.
- Mumps is a virus that can infect the glands. Mumps is much less common now because of the childhood vaccine against it.

RISK INCREASES WITH

- Poor oral hygiene.
- Adults over age 60.
- Smoking.
- Dehydration.
- Poor eating habits, especially a lack of vitamins.
- Recent or chronic illness, such as a mouth infection, that lowers the body's germ-fighting ability.
- Diabetes.
- Use of certain drugs that cause a dry mouth.

PREVENTIVE MEASURES

- Brush and floss teeth often and use germ-killing mouthwash, especially when ill.
- Visit your dentist regularly for checkups.

EXPECTED OUTCOMES

Usually can be cured in two weeks with treatment.

POSSIBLE COMPLICATIONS

If the gland becomes blocked with a stone or scar tissue, surgery may be needed before the infection can clear. This is rare.

 DIAGNOSIS & TREATMENT

GENERAL MEASURES

- Your health care provider will do a physical exam of the head, neck, mouth, and throat. Tests may be done on a sample of the fluid from the infected gland.
- For pain control, apply warm soaks or a heating pad on low setting.
- Rinse the mouth with warm salt water a few times a day. Use one-half teaspoon of salt in one cup of warm water. This may help ease the pain.
- Suck on hard candy, such as lemon drops to increase moisture in the mouth.

MEDICATIONS

- Antibiotics will be prescribed to fight any bacterial infection.
- For minor pain, you may use nonprescription drugs such as acetaminophen.

ACTIVITY

No limits. Resume normal activities when fever disappears.

DIET

No special diet. Try to drink at least six to eight glasses of fluid a day.

 NOTIFY OUR OFFICE IF

- You or a family member has symptoms of a salivary gland infection.
- The infection does not improve in four days or symptoms get worse despite treatment.
- Fever persists or recurs after treatment.
- There is pain or swelling in the mouth.

Special notes:

_____

_____

_____

More notes on the back of this page ☐

SALIVARY GLAND TUMOR

 BASIC INFORMATION

DESCRIPTION

A type of growth in the salivary glands. The salivary glands are located around the mouth and they make saliva, the moisture in the mouth that helps you chew and swallow. Most salivary-gland tumors are benign (do not have cancer cells) and take several years to grow. Even cancer cell tumors rarely spread to other places in the body. The tumors can involve the parotid glands, which are the salivary glands in the jaw or other salivary glands in the floor of the mouth.

FREQUENT SIGNS AND SYMPTOMS

· A soft or firm mass in the jaw or in the floor of the mouth.
· There may be pain or swelling.

CAUSES

Unknown.

RISK INCREASES WITH

· Dehydration.
· Poor oral hygiene.
· Smoking.
· Salivary duct stone.
· False teeth.

PREVENTIVE MEASURES

Most can't be prevented, but the risk may be reduced by:
· Not smoking.
· Keeping the mouth healthy with careful brushing and flossing of the teeth. Drink water each day and suck on hard candy to stop dry mouth.

EXPECTED OUTCOMES

· Tumors with cancer cells are usually cured with surgery, radiation treatment, or anticancer drugs.
· Tumors that are not cancerous are usually cured with surgery alone.

POSSIBLE COMPLICATIONS

· Infection at the surgical site.
· Cancer cells spread to other places in the body (rare).

 DIAGNOSIS & TREATMENT

GENERAL MEASURES

· Your health care provider will do a physical exam of the head, neck, mouth, and throat. Medical tests may include x-rays to check whether the tumor has cancer cells in it.
· Surgery may be done to remove the tumor and remove lymph glands in the neck, if cancer cells have spread there.
· After surgery, keep the mouth clean with salt water mouthwashes. At least three or four times a day, rinse the mouth with a solution of one-half teaspoon salt in one cup of warm water.

MEDICATIONS

Your health care provider may prescribe:
· Pain medicine if needed.
· Drugs for any infection.
· Anticancer drugs to help destroy cancer cells.

ACTIVITY

Resume your normal activities as soon as possible after surgery.

DIET

After surgery, a liquid diet may be needed for a short time until your mouth heals.

NOTIFY OUR OFFICE IF

· You or a family member has symptoms of a salivary gland tumor.
· After surgery, signs of infection occur in your mouth, such as feeling warmer or tender, redness, pain, and swelling.
· New or unusual symptoms occur. Drugs used in treatment may produce side effects.

Special notes:

_____

_____

_____

More notes on the back of this page ☐

438

SALMONELLA INFECTIONS

 ## BASIC INFORMATION

DESCRIPTION

An illness caused by a bacteria named *Salmonella*. This is a type of germ sometimes found in food or drinks. The illness can cause symptoms that affect the stomach and the intestines (digestive tract). A group of people may get sick at the same time if they all eat the same infected food at a picnic, a party, or at a restaurant. A mild *Salmonella* illness may feel like a simple upset stomach for some people.

FREQUENT SIGNS AND SYMPTOMS

· Diarrhea, often with stomach cramps. Diarrhea is an abnormal increase in the number and looseness of stools or bowel movements a day.
· Nausea, vomiting, and fever.
· Blood in the stool (sometimes).
· Headache.
· Some people may have a rash.

CAUSES

· Symptoms start 6 to 72 hours after eating food such as meat, chicken, eggs, or drinking raw (unpasteurized) milk, or water that contains the *Salmonella* germs. This germ can stay alive even in frozen foods, but careful cooking will kill it.
· The illness can also be passed from person to person.
· Pet turtles, lizards, and other pets or animals can carry the germ and cause illness in humans.

RISK INCREASES WITH

· Living in a place with many other people such as a school dorm, or living in a place that is not kept very clean.
· People older than age 60, young children, and infants.
· An illness or the use of certain drugs that can stop your body from fighting off germs.

PREVENTIVE MEASURES

· Keep the kitchen area where you prepare meals very clean. Kill germs on knives and other items you use for cooking by washing them with hot water and soap.
· Stay away from pets or animals that might be sick.
· Drink only milk that is pasteurized.
· Always wash your hands after you go to the bathroom, before you handle any food, and if you have touched an animal or pet.
· Avoid being around someone who has this illness.

EXPECTED OUTCOMES

In most cases, the illness is mild and over in 2 to 7 days.

POSSIBLE COMPLICATIONS

· Dehydration from diarrhea and vomiting. This can be serious for infants and older persons.
· People who have a severe case of this illness or have complications may need treatment in a hospital.

 ## DIAGNOSIS & TREATMENT

GENERAL MEASURES

· Your health care provider may do a physical exam and may want to have a medical test done on a sample of the stool (bowel movement).
· Most patients recover by getting some extra rest and replacing the fluids one's body loses due to the diarrhea.
· Keep the ill person away from other people in the house, if possible.

MEDICATIONS

· Medicine is not needed for mild cases, but may be prescribed for severe cases and for patients who have other health problems.
· Do not use any drugs for the diarrhea unless your health care provider tells you to do so. The diarrhea is the way your body gets rid of the germs.

ACTIVITY

Rest in bed, except for trips to the bathroom, until the symptoms get better. Then begin your normal routine slowly, day by day.

DIET

Replace the fluids lost from the body due to diarrhea with sports drinks such as Gatorade or a special children's product such as Pedialyte. Begin to eat regular food within 12 to 24 hours or when you feel better.

 ## NOTIFY OUR OFFICE IF

· You or a family member has symptoms of a *Salmonella* illness.
· An infant has signs of dehydration, such as dry, wrinkled skin, less urine output, or dark urine.
· A patient has a fever 102°F (38.9°C) or higher, yellow skin or eyes, cough with blood, or diarrhea gets worse.

Special notes:

_____

_____

_____

More notes on the back of this page ☐

SCABIES

 BASIC INFORMATION

DESCRIPTION

A skin disorder caused by little bugs called mites (the "itch" mite). Scabies is very contagious and can be spread from person-to-person or by sharing clothing, towels, or bedding. It may take as long as four to six weeks after you have been exposed for the rash to first appear.

FREQUENT SIGNS AND SYMPTOMS

• A rash with small, very itchy, red bumps or blisters. They may look like pimples. Scabies usually infects the skin of the finger webs, and folds under the arms, breasts, elbows, genitals, and buttocks.
• Sores can form on the skin where it has been scratched.

CAUSES

A mite that burrows into deep skin layers, where the female mite lays her eggs. Eggs grow into adult mites in three weeks. Mites are so tiny that they can only be seen under a microscope. If you scratch the skin area, the mites and eggs get under the fingernails and then get spread to other places in the body.

RISK INCREASES WITH

• Living in a place with many other people such as a school dorm, or living in a place that is not kept very clean.
• Children in child care centers.
• Standing close to or touching the skin of a person who has scabies. It can be spread by sexual contact.

PREVENTIVE MEASURES

• Avoid being close to persons or linen and clothing that you suspect may be infected with scabies.
• Keep yourself as clean as possible:
  - Bathe daily, or at least two to three times a week.
  - Wash hands before eating.
  - Wash clothes often.

EXPECTED OUTCOMES

The skin will usually heal in about two weeks with treatment. The itching can last for up to four weeks even after treatment.

POSSIBLE COMPLICATIONS

• Sores from scratching the itchy skin may become infected with bacteria.
• You can be reinfected with scabies.

 DIAGNOSIS & TREATMENT

GENERAL MEASURES

• Your health care provider can diagnose scabies by looking at the affected skin area. Sometimes the skin may be scraped to gather the mites so they can be viewed under a microscope.
• Treatment is with a drug to be used on the skin.
• Use hot water to wash all clothes, towels, bedding and washable toys used two days before and during treatment. You don't need to clean furniture or floors with special care. Put items you can't wash in plastic bags for two weeks to kill the mites.

MEDICATIONS

• Several different lotions or creams can be used for treatment. Infants and pregnant women may need a milder lotion than that used for other family members. These are general directions (follow your health care provider's instructions or read the directions that come with the product):
  - Take a bath or shower before applying the lotion.
  - Apply from the neck down, and cover the entire body. Wait 15 minutes before dressing.
  - Leave lotion on the skin for 8 to 12 hours, then take a bath or shower to remove it.
  - Your family or other close contacts should be treated at the same time.
  - You may need to repeat the lotion treatment if the rash does not go away in a few weeks or if it gets worse after being treated.
• In some cases, an anti-itching drug may be prescribed.

ACTIVITY

No limits.

DIET

No special diet.

 NOTIFY OUR OFFICE IF

• You or a family member has symptoms of scabies.
• After treatment, the skin shows signs of infection (redness, pus, swelling, or pain).

Special notes:

_____

_____

_____

More notes on the back of this page ☐

SCARLET FEVER

 ## BASIC INFORMATION

DESCRIPTION
Scarlet fever is a childhood (usually ages 2 to 10) skin rash disorder caused by a streptococcal (strep) bacteria infection. It is very contagious.

FREQUENT SIGNS AND SYMPTOMS
Symptoms may vary in different children. The following is the usual course of the disease:
· Day 1
  - Fever as high as 104°F (40°C); a red sore throat, swollen tonsils (tonsils may have a whitish coating), enlarged lymph glands in the neck, cough, vomiting.
· Day 2
  - Bright red rash on the face, except around the mouth.
· Day 3
  - Reddened tongue ("strawberry tongue") and rash in body creases, which spreads to the neck, chest, back, and then the entire body. The rash looks like a sunburn with bumps.
· Day 6
  - The rash fades and skin may begin peeling, which can go on for 10 to 14 days.

CAUSES
· Streptococcal or strep infection caused by a type of germ that produces a scarlet fever toxin (poison). Germs are spread by contact with an infected person, breathing in germs in the air, or touching an object with germs on it.
· Very few strep infections lead to scarlet fever. Not everyone is susceptible to the toxin that produces the rash. In a family, one child may get scarlet fever, a second may have only a strep throat, and a third may carry the germ and spread it to others, but not be sick.

RISK INCREASES WITH
· Strep infections that recur often.
· Living in a place with many other people such as a school dorm.
· Exposure to others in public places.
· Children ages 2 to 10.

PREVENTIVE MEASURES
· Cannot be prevented completely, because some healthy persons will carry the strep germ without being ill. However, some ways to help prevent it include:
  - Antibiotic drug for 10 days for strep infection.
  - Avoid persons with sore throats.

EXPECTED OUTCOMES
With treatment, it is usually cured in about 10 days.

POSSIBLE COMPLICATIONS
Without treatment, infections that are more serious can occur.

 ## DIAGNOSIS & TREATMENT

GENERAL MEASURES
· Your health care provider will do a physical exam. Tests may include throat culture or blood test for strep bacteria. Testing may done on other family members if they have symptoms.
· Treatment is with drugs. Care may be given at home.
· Keep the ill person away from other people, including family members. After the patient has taken the antibiotic drug for 24 hours, they are no longer contagious and can return to school or child-care. The rash is not contagious.
· Use a cool-mist, ultrasonic humidifier (if advised) to relieve the sore throat. Clean the humidifier daily.

MEDICATIONS
· Antibiotics will be prescribed. Be sure to take all the doses even if the symptoms improve.
· Use acetaminophen for pain relief and fever. Do not give aspirin to children under age 18.

ACTIVITY
Extra rest is a good idea until symptoms improve.

DIET
No special diet. Drink plenty of fluids.

 ## NOTIFY OUR OFFICE IF

· You or your child has symptoms of strep throat or scarlet fever.
· The following occur during treatment:
  - Fever goes away and then returns.
  - New symptoms begin, such as nausea; vomiting; earache; cough; headache; thick, colored, nasal drainage; chest pain; or difficulty breathing.

Special notes:

_____

_____

_____

More notes on the back of this page ☐

SCHIZOPHRENIC DISORDERS

 BASIC INFORMATION

DESCRIPTION

A group of disabling mental disorders. Schizo means "split", and phrenia refers to the mind. The person can't tell fact from fantasy, and therefore does not behave rationally. Symptoms may begin in the early teen years or early adulthood. Symptoms may take months or years to become apparent.

FREQUENT SIGNS AND SYMPTOMS

- Delusions (fixed false, unreal beliefs).
- Hallucinations (hearing voices or seeing things that are not there).
- Becomes more withdrawn and wants to be alone.
- Lack of energy and desire to do things.
- Showing few emotions, or showing emotions that are not appropriate.
- Disordered thoughts that are shown in disorganized or disjointed speech.
- A belief that other people hear and "steal" one's thoughts or that one is being controlled by others.
- Suspicious and paranoid behavior (in paranoid schizophrenia).

CAUSES

Exact cause is unknown. It may involve abnormal amounts of some chemicals in the brain. Research is ongoing to find the cause and a possible cure.

RISK INCREASES WITH

Family history of schizophrenia.

PREVENTIVE MEASURES

No specific preventive measures are known.

EXPECTED OUTCOME

Treatment is effective for many patients and helps them to return to varying degrees of independence. About 30% return to normal lives and work. Sometimes the condition completely disappears. The majority of people with the disorder are not prone to violence.

POSSIBLE COMPLICATIONS

- Life-long disability.
- Drugs may not be effective in treatment.
- Patients stop taking the drugs because of side effects, impaired thinking, or they because they feel they don't need them.
- Self-inflicted injuries; suicide.
- Hostile behavior toward others.
- Relapse, neglect, homeless, or ending up in prison.

 DIAGNOSIS & TREATMENT

GENERAL MEASURES

- Your health care provider will do a physical exam and ask questions about the symptoms and activities. Some information about behavior may be supplied by family members. There is no specific test to diagnose schizophrenia. At times, it is difficult to tell one mental disorder from another. Medical tests will be done to rule out other medical problems.
- The goal of therapy is to help the person get back in touch with reality. Treatment often begins with drugs to reduce the symptoms.
- Once symptoms are improved, treatment continues to help the person learn to cope with daily aspects of life. Treatment depends on the patient's needs and the severity of their symptoms. It may include social and work skills training, self-help groups, and counseling.
- The family or other important persons in the patient's life should also be involved in the therapy. This will help them understand the problem and what they can do to help the patient. Schizophrenia patients are sometimes difficult to live with.
- To learn more: National Alliance for the Mentally Ill, (800) 950-6264; website: www.nami.org or National Institute of Mental Health, (301) 443-4513 (not toll free); website: www.nimh.nih.gov.

MEDICATIONS

Antipsychotic drugs are usually prescribed. Some are taken by mouth. Others may be injected. If side effects are too severe with one drug or the symptoms are not controlled, a different drug is prescribed. The dose is reduced as symptoms improve. For most patients, the drugs may need to be taken for life.

ACTIVITY

Normally no limits. unless directed by your health care provider.

DIET

Eat a regular healthy diet. Drink plenty of fluids.

 NOTIFY OUR OFFICE IF

- You or a family member has symptoms of schizophrenia.
- Symptoms continue or worsen after treatment is started.
- New, unexplained symptoms develop. Drugs used in treatment may produce side effects.

Special notes:

_____

_____

_____

More notes on the back of this page ☐

SCLERODERMA
(Progressive Systemic Sclerosis)

BASIC INFORMATION

DESCRIPTION
A disease in which the skin and other body parts change gradually, becoming thick, stiff, and hard. Scleroderma has two main classes, localized and systemic. Localized affects only certain parts of the body such as the skin and its tissues. Systemic affects the whole body, including blood vessels and major organs. These are subgroups defined within these two classes. Scleroderma affects adults of both sexes, but is more common in women between ages 30 and 50.

FREQUENT SIGNS AND SYMPTOMS
- Patches on the skin that start in one place and spread.
- Fingers, toes, cheeks, nose, and ears may have numbness, pain, and color changes. Symptoms may be brought on by cold weather or emotional upset. This is called Raynaud's phenomenon.
- Skin—hardening and thickening, especially in the face, which becomes tight, losing its elasticity.
- Digestive system problems—swallowing difficulty, poor food absorption, bloating after eating, weight loss, heartburn, and a feeling that food sticks in the chest.
- Feet and hands may be swollen.
- Feeling weak and tired.
- Joint pain, stiffness, and swelling.

CAUSES
The exact cause is unknown. It appears that the body's immune system, which normally protects the body against germs, becomes faulty and causes problems. With scleroderma, it produces too much collagen, a fibrous type of protein found in connective tissues.

RISK INCREASES WITH
Unknown.

PREVENTIVE MEASURES
Cannot be prevented at present.

EXPECTED OUTCOMES
The course of the disorder is variable and unpredictable.

POSSIBLE COMPLICATIONS
It is often slowly progressive and affects the gastrointestinal system, heart, lungs, and kidneys.

DIAGNOSIS & TREATMENT

GENERAL MEASURES
- Your health care provider will do a physical exam and check the affected skin. Questions will be asked about your symptoms. Medical tests may include blood studies and a biopsy. With a biopsy, a small amount of tissue is removed and viewed under a microscope.

Other tests may be done to confirm the diagnosis or to check for any complications.
- There is no cure for the disorder. The goals of treatment are to help with the symptoms and stop the progression of the disease. Follow the prescribed treatment plan (this list is general).
- Physical therapy and occupational therapy (to help with day-to-day living activities) may be prescribed.
- Wear warm clothing, such as heavy socks, and gloves if going out in the cold. Cover your head and face.
- Sleep on 2 or 3 pillows, or raise the head of your bed 5 to 8 inches to prevent digestion problems.
- Stop smoking. Find a way to quit that works for you.
- Use heat to relieve joint stiffness.
- Seek counseling to help adjust to living with the disease. Joining a support group may help.
- To learn more: Scleroderma Foundation, 12 Kent Way, Suite 101, Byfield, MA 01922; (800) 722-4673; website: www.scleroderma.org.

MEDICATIONS
- Different drugs may be prescribed, depending on your symptoms. Drugs can improve circulation, help with joint stiffness and pain, improve the immune system, aid digestive problems, and lower high blood pressure.
- Use skin lotions, lubricants, and bath oils to soften skin.

ACTIVITY
- Be as active as your strength permits; avoid fatigue.
- Regular exercise (or movement) helps keep skin flexible, helps blood circulation, and prevents fixed joints.

DIET
Eat frequent, small meals to minimize bloating, heartburn, and stomach discomfort. A soft diet is sometimes helpful. Drink extra fluids to help with swallowing. A dietitian can help plan a nutritious diet.

NOTIFY OUR OFFICE IF

- You or a family member has symptoms of scleroderma.
- Any sign of infection occurs.
- Symptoms get worse or new ones develop.

Special notes:

_____

_____

_____

More notes on the back of this page ☐

SCOLIOSIS
(Curvature of the Spine)

 BASIC INFORMATION

DESCRIPTION

A sideways curve (or twisting) of the spinal column. It can involve the thoracic (middle) spine, the lumbar (lower) spine, or the thoracolumbar (between the two areas). It most often affects children after age 10, and is more common in girls than in boys.

FREQUENT SIGNS AND SYMPTOMS

Early stages:

· No obvious symptoms or signs. It comes on gradually. Scoliosis can be detected by a health care provider with a simple screening test. Schools sometimes have scoliosis screening programs.

Later stages:

· Visible curving of the upper body. The spine becomes S-shaped or C-shaped.
· Shoulders become uneven and rounded.
· Sunken chest.
· Swayback.
· One side of the pelvis thrusts forward.
· Back pain.

CAUSES

· Most often the cause is unknown. Scoliosis is sometimes a result of:
   - A disease of the central nervous system, such as cerebral palsy or muscular dystrophy.
   - Congenital (being born with) defects of the spine.
   - Uneven leg length.

RISK INCREASES WITH

Family history of scoliosis.

PREVENTIVE MEASURES

Cannot be prevented at present.

EXPECTED OUTCOMES

Mild curves may not require treatment. If treatment is done, the outcome is usually successful.

POSSIBLE COMPLICATIONS

· Severe curving of the spine and ribs.
· Social embarrassment, due to wearing a brace.
· Complications such as lung and heart damage, loss of bone strength, and back pain may occur. These are more likely when scoliosis is more severe and goes untreated.

 DIAGNOSIS & TREATMENT

GENERAL MEASURES

· Your child's health care provider can diagnose scoliosis with a physical exam. An x-ray may be done to confirm the diagnosis. The amount of curve in the spine is measured by degrees.
· Treatment will depend on the age of the child, how severe the curve is, and how much it is progressing.
· Many cases of scoliosis are minor (less than 20 degrees) and require no treatment. Follow up medical exams will be done to see if the problem is progressing.
· For children with more of a curve (usually 25 to 40 degrees), treatment often involves wearing an orthopedic back brace. Sometimes this is needed for several years. Some braces are less visible and permit the person to wear regular clothes.
· Surgery to correct scoliosis is usually advised if the curve is more than 40 to 50 degrees or bracing is not helping. Surgery helps improve posture and back function.
· For adults with scoliosis, physical therapy or exercises to strengthen back muscles are sometimes helpful. Talk to your health care provider.
· To learn more: National Scoliosis Foundation, 5 Cabot Place, Stoughton, MA 02072; (800) 673-6922; website: www.scoliosis.org.

MEDICATIONS

Drugs will not correct this disorder.

ACTIVITY

Special exercises may be part of therapy. If a brace is necessary, sports participation will be restricted. Some activities, such as swimming, may help since they tone and strengthen the back.

DIET

No special diet.

 NOTIFY OUR OFFICE IF

You suspect your child is developing scoliosis.

Special notes:

_____

_____

_____

More notes on the back of this page ☐

SEASONAL AFFECTIVE DISORDER (SAD)

 BASIC INFORMATION

DESCRIPTION

A mood disorder that occurs during the winter months and stops when spring begins. Light plays a major part in its origin and in its treatment. It can affect both adults and children, and is more common in women. In rarer instances, the seasonal disorder symptoms occur in the summer months and may be caused by intolerance to heat.

FREQUENT SIGNS AND SYMPTOMS

• Symptoms usually begin in September when days begin to shorten, and last through the winter into March when the days begin to get longer again.
• Depression.
• Feeling tired, sluggish, and needing more sleep.
• Increased appetite (especially for carbohydrates).
• Weight gain.
• Irritability and feeling less cheerful.
• Being less social.
• Decreased interest in sex and physical contact.
• Joint aches, stomach problems, and more infections.

CAUSES

It is thought that the lack of bright light in winter months causes changes in the brain chemistry. Melatonin, a substance produced at night by the pineal gland, normally helps with sleep. When too much melatonin is produced due to longer nights, it can cause symptoms of depression.

RISK INCREASES WITH

• The area of the country where a person lives. People in northern latitudes are more susceptible to SAD.
• Other depressive illness.

PREVENTIVE MEASURES

No measures are known to prevent the disorder.

EXPECTED OUTCOME

With correct diagnosis and treatment, symptoms can be helped.

POSSIBLE COMPLICATIONS

Problems in coping with life as a result of the symptoms.

 DIAGNOSIS & TREATMENT

GENERAL MEASURES

• Your health care provider will do a physical exam and ask questions about your symptoms and activities. Diagnosing SAD can be difficult.

The same symptoms can arise from other types of depression. Blood tests may be done to rule out other medical disorders. Diagnosis usually requires a three-year pattern of mood changes that begin in the autumn and stop in the spring.
• Mild symptoms may be helped with simple measures. Keep drapes and blinds open in your house and sit near windows and gaze outside often. Turn on bright lights on cloudy days. Keep a diary or journal of your mood changes so that any changes or patterns can be tracked. Stay social, visit friends, and stay busy with activities.
• Treatment may involve light therapy (phototherapy). Duration and intensities of this therapy will vary for each person. It is recommended that light therapy not be used without medical advice. Examples include:
  - Sitting in a very bright light (equal to 10 or more 100-watt bulbs) for a period in the morning and, sometimes, in the evening. The term lux (Latin for light) is the unit of measure for the light therapy.
  - Installing a computerized system of lighting in a patient's bedroom that creates an artificial dawn. The light goes from very dim to bright like a sunrise.
• Other forms of treatment include drugs or counseling to help the person cope with the symptoms.
• To learn more: National Organization for Seasonal Affective Disorder, P.O. Box 40133, Washington, DC 20016; website: www.nosad.org.

MEDICATION

Antidepressants may be prescribed.

ACTIVITY

• Stay as active as your energy permits. Physical activity is almost always good for mood disorders.
• Get outside as much as possible, especially in the early morning light.
• Take vacations in the winter months.

DIET

Eat a normal well-balanced diet to maintain good health.

 NOTIFY OUR OFFICE IF

• You or a family member has symptoms of seasonal affective disorder.
• Symptoms continue or worsen, despite treatment.

Special notes:

_____

_____

_____

More notes on the back of this page ☐

SEBACEOUS CYST
(Epidermoid Cyst; Wens)

 ## BASIC INFORMATION

DESCRIPTION
A cyst is a closed sac beneath the skin. A sebaceous cyst is filled with a soft substance made up of oil and dead cells. The cysts usually involve the skin of the trunk, face, neck, and scalp. They can affect all ages, but are most common in teens and adults. They may occur with acne.

FREQUENT SIGNS AND SYMPTOMS
A cyst with the following features:
· The cyst has sloped sides or is dome-shaped, is firm, and has a smooth surface. It normally does not hurt.
· The cyst is whitish or skin-colored.
· If the cyst becomes injured or infected, it may become bright red and painful.

CAUSES
Sebaceous cysts are caused by clogged hair follicles. They may enlarge from hormone changes or injury.

RISK INCREASES WITH
No specific risk factors.

PREVENTIVE MEASURES
Cannot be prevented at present.

EXPECTED OUTCOMES
· Most cysts do not cause symptoms and do not require any medical treatment. Some may disappear on their own.
· Sometimes cysts can be irritated by clothes rubbing against them or by shaving. Cysts that are causing problems, are infected, or are injured can be treated.

POSSIBLE COMPLICATIONS
· Infection of a cyst can turn into an abscess (be filled with pus).
· Cysts can recur after treatment.

 ## DIAGNOSIS & TREATMENT

GENERAL MEASURES
· Your health care provider will diagnose the cyst based on its appearance.
· If needed, cysts can be removed through a simple incision in the skin lying over the cyst. The sac is removed and the incision closed with stitches. If the entire cyst wall is removed, it should not recur.
· For infected cysts, an incision may be needed to drain the pus.

MEDICATIONS
· Drugs are usually not necessary for this disorder.
· If a cyst becomes infected, antibiotics may be prescribed.
· For some, small infected cysts, treatment may include an injection of a steroid drug.

ACTIVITY
No limits.

DIET
No special diet.

 ## NOTIFY OUR OFFICE IF

· You or a family member has new skin growths or there is a change in any existing skin growth.
· After treatment, the treated skin becomes hot, red, and painful.
· The treated area does not appear to be healing well within one week.

Special notes:

_____

_____

_____

More notes on the back of this page ☐

SEVERE ACUTE RESPIRATORY SYNDROME (SARS)

 ## BASIC INFORMATION

DESCRIPTION

Severe acute respiratory syndrome (SARS) is a type of respiratory illness. Respiratory refers to the lungs and breathing. In 2003, SARS was first diagnosed in Asia and then spread to other countries, including the United States.

FREQUENT SIGNS AND SYMPTOMS

• Fever higher than 100.4°F (38.0°C). The fever starts 2 to 7 days after being infected.
• May include headache, an overall feeling of discomfort, and body aches.
• Some people also have mild breathing problems.
• After 2 to 7 days, patients may develop a dry cough and have more trouble breathing.

CAUSES

• The cause is a new form of the coronavirus. It is one of a family of viruses that in humans usually cause mild infections like common colds. How the new type came into being is unknown.
• SARS germs spread by close, person-to-person contact. A cough or sneeze can spread the germs into the nearby air and be breathed in by someone. They are also spread if you touch the skin of an infected person or objects that have the germs on them, and then touch your eyes, nose, or mouth. SARS may spread more broadly in the air or by other ways that are not now known. Also unknown is the time period that an infected person can spread germs to others.

RISK INCREASES WITH

• Travel to an area where the infection is present.
• Close contact with an infected person.

PREVENTIVE MEASURES

• Check for any travel precautions for the area you plan to visit. The Centers for Disease Control & Prevention has updated information about travelers health; website: www.cdc.gov or toll free hotline (877) 394-8747.
• If you are in an area where this infection is present, wash your hands often or use alcohol-based hand wipes. Avoid crowds if possible.
• Wearing a facemask or other protective device may be helpful.

EXPECTED OUTCOMES

Outcome varies depending on the severity of the symptoms. Most people will recover from the infection.

POSSIBLE COMPLICATIONS

• Severe breathing problems that may lead to death.
• It is unknown if people who recover from SARS suffer permanent lung damage.

 ## DIAGNOSIS & TREATMENT

GENERAL MEASURES

• The symptoms for SARS are like those for other viral illnesses, such as cold and flu. If you have been exposed to SARS or have recently been traveling, and symptoms occur, seek medical help right away. Advise any health care provider in advance of your visit about the SARS exposure. Arrangements can be made, as needed, to prevent the spread of germs to others.
• Your health care provider will do a physical exam and have blood and urine studies done. An x-ray and other medical tests may be needed. Specific tests to diagnose SARS are still being developed.
• Once a SARS infection is diagnosed, hospital treatment is needed. This may be in an intensive care unit.
• Treatment is aimed at assistance with the breathing problems. Oxygen is provided through a facemask. Some patients require breathing support with a ventilator (a device to help the lungs).
• Research is ongoing to develop a rapid diagnostic test, effective drug therapies, and a vaccine for the disease.

MEDICATIONS

Drugs are not available to cure the infection. Drugs to treat the symptoms will be given while in the hospital.

ACTIVITY

Resume normal activities slowly once symptoms improve.

DIET

May require feeding through a vein (IV) while in the hospital. Then return to a regular diet with recovery.

 ## NOTIFY OUR OFFICE IF

You or a family member has symptoms of SARS. You should seek emergency care. Be sure to advise any health care providers in advance of your visit about the SARS exposure.

Special notes:

_____

_____

_____

More notes on the back of this page ☐

SEXUAL DYSFUNCTION, FEMALE

 BASIC INFORMATION

DESCRIPTION
Female sexual dysfunction is not a disease. It is a term used to describe problems with sexual desire, arousal, orgasm, and sexual pain in women. It can affect women of any age. Over 40% of women have sexual problems at some time in their lives.

FREQUENT SIGNS AND SYMPTOMS
- Lack of sexual desire or no interest in sex.
- Not able to feel aroused. There may be no sexual response in the body, or it may start, and then stop.
- Failure to achieve orgasm (climax), even when sexually aroused.
- Pain with sexual intercourse.

CAUSES
Sexual dysfunction is usually due to a variety of factors involving a woman's mind, body, and sexual partner.

RISK INCREASES WITH
- Depression, stress, or anxiety. Worries about family problems, finances, career, childcare, marital problems.
- Previous sexual abuse or trauma.
- Feelings of shame or guilt about sex.
- Pregnancy (during and after), or a fear of pregnancy.
- Lack of experience or knowledge about sex on the part of either partner.
- Male sexual partner is having sexual problems.
- Not enough or ineffective foreplay. Feeling boredom with the same sexual routine.
- Couples differ in what they expect from sex, and their attitude toward sex.
- Other people close by in the home (children, mother-in-law).
- Fatigue (e.g., working and caring for small children).
- Medical conditions such as cancer, diabetes, heart disease, thyroid disorders, arthritis, and others.
- Drug abuse, including alcohol.
- Heavy smoking.
- Gynecology factors (infection or other disorders).
- Side effects of some drugs.
- Intercourse causes pain.
- Hysterectomy with removal of ovaries.
- Menopause (reduced estrogen levels affect sexual function).

PREVENTIVE MEASURES
- Avoid the risk factors where possible.
- Get counseling for any anxieties or fears about sex.
- Maintain good communication with sexual partner.

EXPECTED OUTCOME
Some sexual problems go away on their own. Others are helped with treatment and the support of a caring partner. Some problems are more difficult to resolve.

POSSIBLE COMPLICATIONS
- Ongoing inability to enjoy sex.
- Relationship problems with partner.

 DIAGNOSIS & TREATMENT

GENERAL MEASURES
- Your health care provider will do a physical exam and ask questions about your symptoms and sexual history. It may be difficult to discuss your sexual concerns, but it is important to be open and honest. Medical tests may be done to check for any health problems.
- Treatment will depend on the type(s) of dysfunction and the causes. Your health care provider will discuss the options regarding treatment steps.
- Treatment will be provided for any medical disorder. This includes vaginal dryness or other physical problems that may be causing painful intercourse.
- Counseling may be suggested for emotional problems such as stress, anxiety, depression, or sexual fears.
- Sex education may be needed for the woman and her partner. Learning about the female anatomy, sexual response, and arousal can help both partners.
- Treatment with a sex therapist may be helpful. Partners can learn techniques to help stimulate each other, perform self-stimulation, use sexual aids, new sexual routines, and communicate about sexual desires.
- A small vacuum device to improve blood flow to the clitoris may be prescribed. It may help sexual arousal.

MEDICATION
Nonprescription vaginal lubricants may help. Hormone therapy may be prescribed. Other drugs are currently being tested for female sexual problems.

ACTIVITY
Exercise daily. It can reduce stress, improve your physical well-being, and may lead to better sexual health.

DIET
Eat a well-balanced diet.

 NOTIFY OUR OFFICE IF

You or a family member has sexual dysfunction problems and wants help in resolving them.

Special notes:

_____

_____

_____

More notes on the back of this page ☐

SEXUALLY TRANSMITTED DISEASES (STDs)

BASIC INFORMATION

STD FACTS:

· Sexually transmitted diseases (STDs) affect more than 12 million men and women in the United States each year. Many are teenagers or young adults.

· Using drugs or alcohol increases your chances of getting STDs. These substances can interfere with your judgment and your ability to use a condom correctly.

· Intravenous (IV) drug use puts a person at higher risk for human immunodeficiency virus (HIV) and hepatitis B, because IV drug users usually share needles.

· The more sexual partners you have, the higher your chance of being exposed to HIV or other STDs. This is because it is difficult to know if a person is infected, or has had sex with people who are more likely to be infected due to IV drug use or other risk factors.

· Sometimes, early in an infection, there may be no symptoms. Also, symptoms may be easily confused with other illnesses.

· You can not tell by looking at someone whether he or she is infected with HIV or another STD.

· Sexually transmitted diseases include HIV, chancroid, chlamydial infections, trichomoniasis, genital herpes, pubic lice, genital warts, gonorrhea, lymphogranuloma venereum, syphilis, viral hepatitis, scabies, candidiasis, molluscum contagiosum, and others.

STDs CAN CAUSE:

· Pelvic inflammatory disease (PID). It can damage a woman's fallopian tubes and result in pelvic pain and being unable to have children.

· Tubal pregnancies (where pregnancy grows in the fallopian tube instead of the womb). It is sometimes fatal to the mother and always fatal to the fetus.

· Sterility—the inability to have children—in both men and women.

· Cancer of the cervix in women.

· Damage to major organs, such as the heart, kidney, and brain, if STDs go untreated.

· Death (e.g., with HIV infection).

RISKS:

High-risk behaviors include having sex—vaginal, anal, or oral—with:

· A person who has an STD. This is the most risky behavior. If you know your partner is infected, avoid intercourse (including oral sex). If you do decide to have sex with an infected person, always be sure to use a new condom from start to finish, every time.

· Someone who has shared needles to inject drugs with an infected person.

· Someone with a past partner(s) who was/were infected. If your partner had sexual contact with a person infected with HIV, he or she could pass it on to you. This can happen even if the prior sexual contact was a long time ago—as long as 10 years. Your partner may seem perfectly healthy. HIV can be in the body a long time before a person feels sick.

PREVENTION:

· Reduce the chance of being infected with HIV or other STDs. People who take part in risky sexual behavior should always use a condom.

· Use of a condom is also important for an uninfected pregnant woman. It can help protect her and her unborn child from STDs.

SEE A HEALTH CARE PROVIDER IF YOU HAVE ANY OF THESE STD SYMPTOMS:

· Discharge from the vagina, penis, or rectum.

· Pain or burning during urination or intercourse.

· Pain in the abdomen (women), testicles (men), and buttocks and legs (both men and women).

· Blisters, open sores, warts, rash, or swelling in the genital or anal area, or the mouth.

· Persistent, flu-like symptoms. These include fever, headache, aching muscles, or swollen glands. These symptoms may precede STD symptoms.

ADDITIONAL RESOURCES FOR INFORMATION:

· National AIDS Hotline (800) 342-2437; website: www.cdc.gov/hiv/dhap.htm.

· Sexually Transmitted Diseases Hotline (800) 227-8922.

NOTIFY OUR OFFICE IF

You or a family member has questions or concerns about STDs.

Special notes:

_____

_____

_____

More notes on the back of this page ☐

SHIN SPLINTS
(Medial Tibia Stress Syndrome)

 BASIC INFORMATION

DESCRIPTION
Pain in the lower leg brought on by exercise or athletic activity. *Shin splints* is a common term that has been used to describe a variety of different leg injuries and it is generally being replaced by more specific diagnostic terms. The most common shin pain is caused by medial tibia stress syndrome (MTSS). The tibia (shin bone) is the larger of the two bones between the knee and the ankle. Medial refers to the inside part of the tibia (the most common injury site).

FREQUENT SIGNS AND SYMPTOMS
• Pain, dull ache, or tenderness, and some-times swelling, redness, and warmth, in the inner side (medial), back side (posterior), or outer side (anterior) of the lower leg.
• Pain may come and go as activity continues.

CAUSES
It is an overuse condition that can be caused by several factors. This shin problem usually develops gradually over weeks to months or could occur after a single excessive or intense training session. The problem is exercise-induced, but the specific cause of the pain is difficult to pinpoint. It may be periostitis (inflammation of the outer layer of the bone), myositis (muscle inflammation), tendinitis (inflammation of the muscle-tendon complex) or a combination of two of these. Faulty foot mechanics contribute to the injury.

RISK INCREASES WITH
• Sports involving running (e.g., runners and sprinters, football, basketball, soccer, and rugby players); jumping activities such as gymnastics or figure skating.
• Training too quickly, too hard, and for too long.
• Training that involves switching from one type of sport to another (e.g., a triathlon).
• High impact aerobics or aerobic dancing.
• Poorly fitting or worn-out running shoes.
• Foot arches that are flat (pronated) or high (supinated), or muscle imbalance in leg muscles.

PREVENTIVE MEASURES
• Stretch and strengthen the muscles in the lower leg.
• Stretch before and after running.
• Avoid hard and uneven surfaces. Use soft surfaces such as dirt or grass for jogging, running, and walking.
• Warm up before the activity and avoid overtraining.
• Wear shoes that fit well, with good arch support.
• Try sports activities, such as swimming or biking that have less impact on the shins.

EXPECTED OUTCOMES
Healing time may range from a few days to two weeks to two months.

POSSIBLE COMPLICATIONS
• May progress to stress fracture.
• Shin splints may recur.

 DIAGNOSIS & TREATMENT

GENERAL MEASURES
• Use ice massage over the painful area (in a circle about the size of a softball). Do this for 15 minutes at a time three or four times a day.
• After a few days, apply heat if you want. Use hot soaks, hot showers, or heating pads.
• Massage area gently and often to provide comfort and decrease swelling.
• See your health care provider if self-care does not help. A physical exam and x-ray or bone scan may be done to rule out a stress fracture.

MEDICATIONS
• For minor discomfort, use nonprescription anti-inflammatory drugs such as aspirin (not for children) or ibuprofen.
• Other nonsteroidal anti-inflammatory drugs may be prescribed.

ACTIVITY
• Discontinue sports or exercise until the pain is gone. Return to pre-injury activity level slowly.
• In some cases, severe pain may require the use of crutches for a short period of time.
• If foot mechanics are a problem, such as excessive pronation, special shoes, heel lifts, or orthotics (inserts for the shoes) may be prescribed. Orthotics can be non-prescription products. In some cases, custom-made orthotics are recommended.
• Try different exercises (cross-training) such as swimming or walking in water, bicycle riding, or regular walking.

DIET
No special diet.

 NOTIFY OUR OFFICE IF

• You or a family member has painful shin splints.
• Mild symptoms don't improve within 2 to 3 weeks.

Special notes:

_____

_____

_____

More notes on the back of this page ☐

450

SHOCK

 BASIC INFORMATION

DESCRIPTION
The heart and blood vessels are unable to supply enough blood and oxygen to meet the demands of the body. Shock can be caused by several different conditions and is a medical emergency.

FREQUENT SIGNS AND SYMPTOMS
- Cold hands and feet.
- Fast, weak pulse.
- Not knowing where you are or confusion.
- Anxiety with feelings of impending doom.
- Skin that is pale, moist and sweaty.
- Shortness of breath and rapid breathing.
- Lack of urination.
- Low blood pressure.

CAUSES
- Hypovolemic shock is a sudden loss of blood or body fluids. The bleeding may be visible, or bleeding that occurs inside the body. Sudden fluid loss occurs with severe burns, severe vomiting, and/or diarrhea.
- Cardiogenic shock is due to damaged heart function. This includes heart attack or heart failure.
- Anaphylactic shock is an adverse reaction to a substance to which the body is sensitive. These can include drugs such as penicillin, insect bites, or food allergies.
- Septic shock is caused by blood poisoning or major infections in the body.
- Neurogenic shock is caused by damage to the nervous system, such as a spinal cord injury.
- Shock can be caused by exposure to extreme heat or cold for too long.

RISK INCREASES WITH
- Serious injury, illness, or surgery.
- Heart disorders.
- Contact with a substance you are allergic to.
- Overdose of mind-altering drugs.
- Excess alcohol consumption.

PREVENTIVE MEASURES
- You can't prevent shock. You can avoid the risk factors where possible.
- You may be able to help someone in shock, or prevent shock, until emergency medical help is available if you are prepared. To prepare yourself:
  - Take a first aid course.
  - If you or a family member has a severe allergy, be sure there is an emergency kit available and that you know how to give the injection.
  - Carry emergency supplies, such as a first aid kit, in your car or truck.
- Wear a medical alert tag if you have a serious medical or allergy problem.

EXPECTED OUTCOMES
The outcome will depend on how severe the symptoms are and receiving prompt treatment.

POSSIBLE COMPLICATIONS
- Heart or lungs are unable to function.
- Permanent brain damage.
- Death.

 DIAGNOSIS & TREATMENT

GENERAL MEASURES
- Get emergency help right away. Shock requires immediate medical care.
- Emergency care in the hospital will include fluids given through a vein, oxygen for breathing support and drugs. A careful physical exam will be done. Treatment will be provided for the injuries or other causes of the shock. The patient will be watched closely for any complications until the risk is over.

MEDICATIONS
- If shock is from blood or fluid loss, treatment includes blood transfusion or fluids given through a vein.
- If blood pressure is at a dangerous low level, drugs to raise blood pressure may be given.
- If infection is present, antibiotics will be used.

ACTIVITY
Rest in bed until completely recovered. Move legs actively while in bed to decrease the likelihood of blood clots.

DIET
Diet will depend on your medical condition.

 NOTIFY OUR OFFICE IF

You or a family member has symptoms of shock or observe them in someone else. Call 911 immediately. This is a life-threatening emergency!

Special notes:

_____

_____

_____

More notes on the back of this page ☐

SHOULDER, FROZEN
(Adhesive Capsulitis)

 ## BASIC INFORMATION

DESCRIPTION

A general term used to describe pain and stiffness in the shoulder joint that leads to loss of shoulder movement. Adhesive capsulitis is the medical term. It affects the shoulder capsule (tissues surrounding the ball and socket joint) and the ligaments that attach the shoulder bones to each other. Sometimes both shoulders are affected. Frozen shoulder occurs more often in people over age 40, and in women more than men. It can last a few months to a year or longer.

FREQUENT SIGNS AND SYMPTOMS

• Stage 1 (painful)–Ache or pain in the shoulder, often mild. It progresses to severe pain that interferes with sleep and normal activities. Pain gets worse with shoulder movement. This stage may last for 2 to 9 months.
• Stage 2 (adhesive)–Less pain occurs, but stiffness increases in the shoulder. This prevents normal range of motion movement. Reduced movement increases stiffness. This stage may last 4 to 12 months.
• Stage 3 (recovery)–Healing starts. For most patients, the range of motion begins to increase. This stage may last for 12 months or up to several years.

CAUSES

The cause is unknown. It may be due to an inflammatory process. In some cases, it may result from an injury that leads to lack of use due to pain. Adhesions (a type of scar tissue) grow between the joint surfaces, causing restricted motion. There is less synovial fluid. It normally lubricates the shoulder joint to help it move.

RISK INCREASES WITH

• A shoulder injury, fracture, or trauma (could be very minor).
• Diabetes.
• Heart disease, stroke or lung conditions, thyroid problems, Parkinson's disease, and depression.
• Being immobile (prolonged inactivity) due to trauma, overuse injuries, or surgery.

PREVENTIVE MEASURES

• Obtain early medical treatment for any shoulder injury, pain, or stiffness.
• Do regular stretching exercises.

EXPECTED OUTCOMES

Most patients can expect increased shoulder mobility and function with time and treatment. It may take many months to see the improvement. You may need help in performing daily activities that require lifting your arms.

POSSIBLE COMPLICATIONS

Some permanent shoulder disability and pain may occur despite treatment.

 ## DIAGNOSIS & TREATMENT

GENERAL MEASURES

• Your health care provider will do an exam of the affected shoulder and ask questions about your symptoms and activities. X-rays or other tests may be done to confirm the diagnosis.
• Exercises, and sometimes, drugs are used in treatment to restore joint movement and reduce the pain.
• Apply heat (warm compresses or heating pad) to the affected area or apply ice packs if it feels better.
• Physical therapy and stretching exercises will help improve joint movement. They may be uncomfortable to do, but should not cause excess pain. You will be instructed about exercises to do at home.
• Other treatments sometimes used include acupuncture, ultrasound therapy, and electrical stimulation.
• Manipulation may help some patients. This procedure can be done under a local or general anesthesia. The shoulder joint capsule is stretched to break up scar tissue. It helps right away, but exercise is still needed.
• If other treatment does not help the symptoms after several months, your health care provider may recommend shoulder surgery. This is usually done with an arthroscope (small instrument) through tiny incisions.

MEDICATIONS

• Nonsteroidal anti-inflammatory drugs or muscle relaxers may be prescribed. Injections of cortisone or local anesthesia into joints may help to reduce severe pain.
• For minor pain, you may use nonprescription drugs such as ibuprofen or aspirin (not for children).

ACTIVITY

• Be sure to follow instructions for home exercises.
• Resume athletic or fitness activities as your symptoms ease and you have medical approval.

DIET

No special diet.

 ## NOTIFY OUR OFFICE IF

• You or a family member has symptoms of a frozen shoulder.
• Shoulder symptoms get worse after treatment starts.

Special notes:

_____

_____

_____

More notes on the back of this page ☐

SICKLE CELL ANEMIA & SICKLE CELL TRAIT

BASIC INFORMATION

DESCRIPTION

Sickle cell anemia is an inherited blood disorder. It causes chronic anemia, periods of severe pain, high risk of infections, and general poor health. It usually begins at about 6 months of age and is a lifelong disorder. People with the sickle cell trait usually have no symptoms of the disorder, but may pass it onto their children.

FREQUENT SIGNS AND SYMPTOMS

- Swollen hands or feet, fever, and paleness.
- Shortness of breath; rapid heartbeat; fatigue.
- Episodes of pain in any organ or joint.
- Frequent infections, especially pneumonia.
- Eye problems.
- Delayed growth and development in children.
- Jaundice (yellow skin and/or eyes).

CAUSES

A gene that causes defective hemoglobin (blood cells). The gene occurs mostly in African Americans (about 8% are carriers) and some Hispanics. Defective hemoglobin changes blood cells from smooth and round to a stiff, sickle shape. These abnormal cells cause blood flow in blood vessels to become blocked. This leads to the symptoms and sickle crisis (severe pain episode). A chronic short supply of red blood cells causes anemia.

RISK INCREASES WITH

Family history of sickle cell anemia. If both parents have the gene, their child may have sickle cell anemia. If one parent has the gene, the child will not get the disorder, but may carry the sickle cell trait.

PREVENTIVE MEASURES

- If you have a family history of sickle cell anemia, ask for testing. If the condition is present, obtain genetic counseling before starting a family.
- Early pregnancy test to see if the baby has inherited the double-dose gene (both parents are carriers).

EXPECTED OUTCOMES

There is no cure for sickle cell anemia. Life span is reduced, but has gradually increased to over 40 years. More effective treatments are helping.

POSSIBLE COMPLICATIONS

Infections, other medical problems, stroke, and death.

DIAGNOSIS & TREATMENT

GENERAL MEASURES

- Blood tests can diagnose sickle cell anemia. Screening tests are done on newborns in most states. If the screening test shows sickle hemoglobin, a second test is done to confirm diagnosis.

- A health care provider with special knowledge of this disorder may be recommended for ongoing health care.
- Home treatment involves good nutrition and hygiene, rest as needed, and steps to avoid infection and stress. Encourage a child to lead as normal a life as possible.
- Some things may worsen symptoms. These include an injury or infection, pregnancy, surgery, traveling to high altitudes (as in driving up a mountain, or an airplane trip).
- See your health care and dental care providers on a regular basis. Keep all vaccines and flu shots up to date.
- Wear a medical alert type bracelet or pendant to identify the medical disorder.
- Counseling may be helpful in adapting to this condition, especially for children. Support groups may help.
- Hospital care may be required at times of severe attacks for intravenous (IV) therapy and oxygen therapy and, sometimes, blood transfusions.
- Bone marrow transplants may be an option for some.
- To learn more: Sickle Cell Disease Association of America, 200 Corporate Pointe, Ste 495, Culver City, CA 90230; (800) 421-8453; website: www.sicklecelldisease.org.

MEDICATIONS

- No drugs are effective for the disease. Drugs are prescribed to treat symptoms and prevent complications.
- Use nonsteroidal anti-inflammatory drugs or acetaminophen for pain.
- Penicillin started in infancy helps prevent infection.
- Adults should be treated promptly for infections.
- Hydroxyurea helps to reduce the frequency of painful crisis. It may be prescribed for certain patients.
- Daily vitamin supplements are often recommended.

ACTIVITY

- Avoid strenuous exercise. Avoid being out in very hot or cold temperatures. Rest in bed during acute attacks.
- Activity may be somewhat limited due to chronic anemia and poor muscular development.

DIET

Eat a healthy diet. Drink plenty of fluids.

NOTIFY OUR OFFICE IF

- After diagnosis, any signs of infection occur, pain increases, or symptoms develop that cause concern.
- You want to know if you have the sickle cell gene.

Special notes:

_____

_____

_____

More notes on the back of this page ☐

SILICOSIS

 BASIC INFORMATION

DESCRIPTION

A chronic lung condition due to breathing silica (quartz) dust. Silicosis is the most common form of pneumoconiosis. This is a group of lung diseases caused by inhaling certain mineral dusts.

FREQUENT SIGNS AND SYMPTOMS

Early symptoms:
- Shortness of breath.
- Cough that produces little or no sputum.
- General ill feeling.

Later symptoms:
- Fitful sleep.
- Appetite loss.
- Chest pain.
- Hoarseness.
- Coughing blood.
- Symptoms of heart failure.
- Bluish nails.

CAUSES

Chronic breathing in of small particles of free crystalline silica dust. The dust may be invisible to the naked eye. It is so light that it can remain in the air for a long time. The disorder causes lung inflammation and then scarring of lung tissues. It usually takes 20 to 30 years of exposure to develop silicosis. If exposure is extremely high, it may take less than 10 years.

RISK INCREASES WITH

- Work such as mining, granite-cutting, concrete mixing and drilling, manufacturing pottery, metal-grinding, tunneling, sand-blasting, and others.
- Smoking adds to possible lung damage.

PREVENTIVE MEASURES

- Be aware of the risks and follow all training and preventive instructions provided for your work. Get health screenings on a regular basis.
- Employers are required to take certain preventive measures to reduce exposure for workers.
- Don't smoke.

EXPECTED OUTCOMES

There is no cure and silicosis causes increasing lung problems. Outcome will vary for each individual depending on amount of lung damage. Symptoms can sometimes be relieved or controlled.

POSSIBLE COMPLICATIONS

- Pulmonary tuberculosis (late stages of silicosis).
- Chronic obstructive pulmonary disease (COPD).
- Lung fibrosis (scar tissue).
- Heart failure.

 DIAGNOSIS & TREATMENT

GENERAL MEASURES

- Your health care provider will do a physical exam and ask questions about your symptoms and activities. Be sure to tell your provider about your work history and any exposure to silica. Medical tests may include x-ray of the chest, pulmonary function tests, and others to confirm the diagnosis and check for complications.
- No specific treatment is known for silicosis. Drugs and lung therapy may help the symptoms and treat complications.
- Avoid any further exposure to silica dust.
- Quit smoking. Find a way to stop that works for you.
- Obtain medical treatment for any respiratory infection, including the common cold.
- Get influenza and pneumococcal vaccines.
- Consider moving to a warm, dry climate if you have advanced disease.
- Chest physical therapy (such as controlled coughing) and bronchial drainage help clear secretions. Get medical training about these procedures.
- To learn more: American Lung Association, 61 Broadway, 6th Floor, New York, NY 10006, (800) 586-4872; website: www.lungusa.org.

MEDICATIONS

- Antibiotics may be prescribed for infections.
- Bronchodilators (inhaled or oral) with inhalation therapy may be prescribed. This is supervised at first by an inhalation therapist.
- For minor discomfort, you may use nonprescription drugs, such as acetaminophen or aspirin.

ACTIVITY

No limits, except those caused by symptoms.

DIET

No special diet. Maintain high fluid intake.

 NOTIFY OUR OFFICE IF

- You or a family member has symptoms of silicosis.
- Fever, increased chest pain or breathing problems, blood in the sputum, or other new symptoms develop.

Special notes:

_____

_____

_____

More notes on the back of this page ☐

454

SINUSITIS
(Sinus Infection or Inflammation)

 BASIC INFORMATION

DESCRIPTION
Infection or inflammation (redness and soreness) of the sinuses. Sinuses are air-filled spaces that make mucus to help clean the air we breathe. They are located behind the eyebrows, inside each cheekbone, and between the eyes. Sinuses open into the nose for mucus and air exchange. Sinusitis can be acute (short illness), or chronic if it continues for several weeks or recurs often.

FREQUENT SIGNS AND SYMPTOMS
- Nasal congestion with white or greenish-yellow (sometimes blood-tinged) discharge.
- Feeling of pressure inside the head.
- Eye pain.
- Headache that is worse in the morning or when bending forward.
- Cheek pain that may resemble a toothache.
- Post-nasal drip.
- Cough (sometimes) that is usually non-productive.
- Disturbed sleep (sometimes).
- Fever (sometimes).
- Swelling of the sinus openings, blocking the discharge, and increasing pain.

CAUSES
- Bacterial infection. A common cold or allergic reaction can cause the sinuses to swell and increase the amount of mucus they produce. Bacteria begin to grow in the excess mucus in the swollen sinuses and causes the symptoms.
- Fungal infection, such as aspergillosis, may occur in people who have a weakened immune system.
- Allergies that cause swelling of sinuses.

RISK INCREASES WITH
- Common cold or other viral illness.
- A weakened immune system due to illness or drugs.
- Swimming or diving.
- Using nasal decongestant sprays too often.
- Growths (polyps) in the nose or a deviated septum.
- People with asthma or an allergic disease.
- Smoking.
- People with cystic fibrosis.
- Dental problems.

PREVENTIVE MEASURES
Prompt treatment of any cold or other viral infection.

EXPECTED OUTCOMES
Will often clear up on its own, but may be treated with drugs, or surgery if needed.

POSSIBLE COMPLICATIONS
- Sinusitis may become chronic.
- Rarely, infection may spread into bones, eyes, or brain.

 DIAGNOSIS & TREATMENT

GENERAL MEASURES
- Your health care provider will do a physical exam and ask questions about your symptoms and recent illnesses, such as a cold. Diagnosis can usually be made based on this information. Medical tests may be done in certain cases, such as repeated infections.
- Drug treatment is aimed at improving symptoms and curing the infection.
- Apply moist heat to relieve pain in the sinuses and nose. Take a warm shower once or twice a day.
- Sinusitis not responding to drug treatment may require surgery to drain blocked sinuses.
- Surgery may be done for polyps or a deviated septum.
- Sinusitis caused by a fungus may require surgery.

MEDICATIONS
- For stuffy nose, use nonprescription nasal decongestants. Limit use to 3 days in a row. Saline nasal sprays may be used several times a day. Nonprescription antihistamines are sometimes helpful.
- For minor pain, you may use drugs such as acetaminophen.
- Drugs to reduce congestion may be prescribed.
- Antibiotics for the infection may be prescribed.

ACTIVITY
Resume your normal activities gradually. Exercise can help to clear your head.

DIET
Drink extra fluids to help thin secretions.

 NOTIFY OUR OFFICE IF

- You or a family member has symptoms of sinusitis.
- The following occur during treatment:
  - Fever; bleeding from the nose; severe headache.
  - Swelling of the face (forehead, eyes, side of the nose, or cheek).

Special notes:

_____

_____

_____

More notes on the back of this page ☐

SJÖGREN'S SYNDROME

 BASIC INFORMATION

DESCRIPTION

One of a group of autoimmune disorders. In these disorders, the immune system by mistake attacks the body itself. Sjögren's syndrome mainly affects the glands that produce moisture, but it can affect the body as a whole. Symptoms may be mild or severe. It occurs mostly in women (about 90% of cases) with an average age of 50.

FREQUENT SIGNS AND SYMPTOMS

• Dry eyes. It may cause foreign body sensation, gritty feeling, redness, burning, sensitivity to light, itching, feeling that there is a "film" across the field of vision, and eye discharge.

• Dry mouth, nose, and throat. This can cause problems in swallowing and talking, changes in taste, thirst, ulcers (sores), or dental cavities. Nosebleeds, hoarseness, chronic nonproductive cough, ear infection, other infections may occur.

• Vaginal dryness can cause painful intercourse.

• Dry skin.

• Severe fatigue.

• Parotid glands become enlarged (sometimes referred to as "chipmunk face" or "chipmunk cheeks").

• Joint pain and stiffness.

• Other symptoms include hair loss, low-grade fever, itching skin, and muscle aches or pain.

CAUSES

Unknown. Genetic, immunologic, hormonal and environmental factors may contribute to its cause. Viral infection may trigger the disorder in some people. It may occur alone or along with other autoimmune disorders such as rheumatoid arthritis, scleroderma, systemic lupus erythematosus, or polymyositis.

RISK INCREASES WITH

• Family history of autoimmune disorders.

• Having other autoimmune disorders.

PREVENTIVE MEASURES

No specific preventive measures known.

EXPECTED OUTCOME

Sjögren's syndrome is a chronic disorder. Symptoms sometimes stay the same, worsen, or sometimes disappear for a period. Treatment can relieve symptoms and help prevent complications.

POSSIBLE COMPLICATIONS

• Damage to the kidneys, blood vessels, lungs, liver, eyes, pancreas, and brain may occur.

• Children born to some younger women with the disorder may be at risk for heart defects.

 DIAGNOSIS & TREATMENT

GENERAL MEASURES

• Your health care provider will do a physical exam and ask questions about your symptoms. Medical tests of blood, tear production, saliva production, an eye exam, and others may be done to confirm the diagnosis.

• Treatment is directed to relieving the dryness symptoms and preventing complications.

• Brush and floss teeth daily. Use a fluoride mouthwash. See the dentist for frequent checkups.

• Wear sunglasses when outside to help protect eyes from dust, wind, and strong light. See your eye care provider for regular exams.

• Warm compresses or heating pad may help ease joint pain or swollen gland discomfort.

• To learn more: Sjögren's Syndrome Foundation, 8120 Woodmont Ave., Suite 530, Bethesda, MD 20814; (800) 475-6473 (voice mail); website: www.sjogrens.org.

MEDICATION

• Use artificial tears for dry eyes. Use an eye ointment at night. Other drugs for dry eyes may be prescribed.

• Use nonprescription saliva substitutes and mouth-coating products for dry mouth.

• Vaginal lubricant (not petroleum jelly) will help vaginal dryness.

• Use aspirin or other nonsteroidal anti-inflammatory drugs for joint pain and muscle aches.

• Avoid decongestants and antihistamines. They can cause dry mouth or eyes.

• Steroids and other drugs may be prescribed.

ACTIVITY

Mild exercise daily helps keep joints flexible.

DIET

• Chew sugarless gum or suck on sugarless candies.

• Drink or sip fluids all during the day.

• If mouth soreness prevents eating regular foods, drink high-calorie, high-protein liquid supplements.

 NOTIFY OUR OFFICE IF

• You or a family member has symptoms of Sjögren's syndrome.

• Symptoms worsen or don't improve with treatment.

Special notes:

_____

_____

_____

More notes on the back of this page ☐

SKIN CANCER, BASAL CELL

BASIC INFORMATION

DESCRIPTION

Skin cancer in the skin's basal layer. The basal layer is at the bottom of the skin's outer layer (epidermis). The cancer usually involves the skin of face, ears, backs of hands, shoulders, and arms. Adults over age 40 are most often affected, and men are more often affected than women. It is the most common type of skin cancer.

FREQUENT SIGNS AND SYMPTOMS

· A sore that does not heal within 3 weeks. It may bleed, ooze, or have a crust.
· An area or patch of skin that is reddish or irritated. It might have a crust.
· A shiny, pearly looking bump on the skin. The color is usually pink, red, or white. On some people, the color may be tan, black or brown, and look like a mole.
· A skin growth that is pink with a slightly raised, rolled border. The center is crusted and is lower than the border. Tiny blood vessels may be seen, as it grows larger.
· An area that looks like a white or yellow scar. The skin is shiny and looks tight. This type is more rare.

CAUSES

Chronic sun exposure. The ultraviolet light in sunlight damages the skin, and causes the cells to change and grow into skin cancers.

RISK INCREASES WITH

· Exposure to excess sunlight from work or play.
· People with fair skin and blue eyes.
· Living in an area where there is lots of sunlight.

PREVENTIVE MEASURES

· Limit exposure to sunlight. Protect skin with a hat, clothing, and sunscreen with SPF of 15 or more. Reapply sunscreen every 2 hours during sun exposure.
· Perform a skin self-exam once a month. Check for new growths or changes in growths already present.

EXPECTED OUTCOMES

The cancer seldom spreads beyond the skin and is almost always harmless. It is curable in just about all cases. People who have had skin cancer are at higher risk for new skin cancers elsewhere on the skin.

POSSIBLE COMPLICATIONS

· Skin cancer may recur in the same place after surgery.
· Scarring from the surgery.

DIAGNOSIS & TREATMENT

GENERAL MEASURES

· Your health care provider will examine the affected skin area. All or part of the affected skin tissue may be removed for biopsy. The tissue is viewed under a microscope to see if it is cancerous.

· Treatment varies with appearance, extent, and location of the skin cancer. The treatment method chosen will often be decided by you and your health care provider together. Options include:
  - Curettage and electrodesiccation–local anesthetic applied, then cutting out or shaving of the cancer, followed by high-frequency electrical current to destroy tissue with heat.
  - Surgical excision–local anesthetic is applied, then skin is marked for surgery, and a scalpel is used for the excision.
  - Moh's surgery–a special type of surgery is used to treat high-risk cancers, especially on the head and face.
  - Cryosurgery–use of liquid nitrogen to freeze and kill the cells. A local anesthetic is sometimes used.
  - Laser treatment–is sometimes used.
  - Radiation treatment–used if cancer location requires it, such as locations near lips and eyelids.
  - Photodynamic therapy uses drugs and special light.
· Healthy skin from elsewhere on the body may be used to replace skin removed in surgery (skin graft).
· Your health care provider will advise you of any follow-up care needed after the procedure.
· To learn more: American Cancer Society, (800) ACS-2345; website: www.cancer.org or National Cancer Institute, (800) 4-CANCER; website: www.nci.nih.gov.

MEDICATIONS

· Use nonprescription pain-relief drugs for minor pain.
· Skin cancer drugs (chemotherapy) applied to the skin may be prescribed.
· Antibiotic for the skin to prevent infection may be prescribed.

ACTIVITY

No limits.

DIET

No special diet.

 ## NOTIFY OUR OFFICE IF

· You or a family member has signs of skin cancer.
· After treatment, the treated skin becomes hot, red, and painful.

Special notes:

_____

_____

_____

More notes on the back of this page ☐

SKIN CANCER, SQUAMOUS CELL

BASIC INFORMATION

DESCRIPTION

A skin cancer in the squamous cells that make up the skin's outer layer (epithelium). The cancer usually involves the skin of the face, ears, backs of hands, shoulders, and arms. Adults over age 40 are most often affected, and men moreso than women. It is the second most common type of skin cancer.

FREQUENT SIGNS AND SYMPTOMS

• A sore that does not heal within 3 weeks. It may bleed or ooze or have a crust.
• An area or patch of skin that is reddish or irritated. It might have a crust.
• A shiny, pearly looking skin bump. The color is usually pink, red, or white. On some people, the color may be tan, black, or brown and look like a mole.
• A skin growth that is pink with a slightly raised, rolled border. The center is crusted and is lower than the border. Tiny blood vessels may be seen as it grows larger.
• An area that looks like a white or yellow scar. The skin is shiny and looks tight. This type is more rare.

CAUSES

Chronic sun exposure. The ultraviolet light in sunlight damages the skin and causes the cells to change and grow into skin cancers.

RISK INCREASES WITH

• Exposure to excess sunlight from work or play.
• People with fair skin and blue eyes.
• Living in an area where there is lots of sunlight.

PREVENTIVE MEASURES

• Limit exposure to sunlight. Protect skin with a hat, clothing and sunscreen with SPF of 15 or more. Reapply sunscreen every 2 hours during sun exposure.
• Perform a skin self-exam once a month. Check for new growths or changes in growths already present.

EXPECTED OUTCOMES

It is curable in just about all cases. People who have had skin cancer are at higher risk for new skin cancers elsewhere on the skin.

POSSIBLE COMPLICATIONS

• Skin cancer may recur in the same place after surgery.
• Scarring from the surgery.
• Cancer may spread to nearby lymph nodes.

DIAGNOSIS & TREATMENT

GENERAL MEASURES

• Your health care provider will examine the skin growth for any abnormal appearance. All, or part, of the skin tissue may be removed for biopsy. The tissue is viewed under a microscope to see if it is cancerous.

• Treatment varies with appearance, extent, and location of the skin cancer. The treatment method chosen will often be decided by you and your health care provider together. Options include:
 - Curettage and electrodesiccation–local anesthetic applied, then cutting out, or shaving, of the cancer, followed by high-frequency electrical current to destroy tissue with heat.
 - Surgical excision–local anesthetic is applied, then skin is marked for surgery, and a scalpel is used for the excision.
 - Moh's surgery–a special type of surgery is used to treat high-risk cancers, especially on the head and face.
 - Cryosurgery–use of liquid nitrogen to freeze and kill the cells. A local anesthetic is sometimes used.
 - Laser treatment–is sometimes used.
 - Radiation treatment–used if cancer location requires it, such as locations near the lips and eyelids.
 - Photodynamic therapy uses drugs and special light.
• Healthy skin from elsewhere on the body may be used to replace skin removed in surgery (skin graft).
• Your health care provider will advice you of any follow up care needed after the procedure.
• To learn more: American Cancer Society, (800) ACS-2345; website: www.cancer.org or National Cancer Institute, (800) 4-CANCER; website: www.nci.nih.gov.

MEDICATIONS

• Use nonprescription pain-relief drugs for minor pain.
• Skin cancer drugs (chemotherapy) applied to the skin may be prescribed.
• Antibiotic for the skin to prevent infection may be prescribed.

ACTIVITY

No limits.

DIET

No special diet.

NOTIFY OUR OFFICE IF

• You or a family member has signs of skin cancer.
• After treatment, the treated skin becomes hot, red, and painful.

Special notes:

_____

_____

_____

More notes on the back of this page ☐

SLEEP APNEA

 BASIC INFORMATION

DESCRIPTION

Episodes during sleep in which breathing stops for 10 seconds, or longer. In most cases, the person is unaware of the condition. It can affect all ages, but is more common in adults over 60.

FREQUENT SIGNS AND SYMPTOMS

· Periods of not breathing while asleep. This can happen hundreds of time each night. This causes less oxygen to get to the lungs and eventually triggers the lungs to suck in air. The person may make a gasping or snorting sound, but is usually not fully awake.
· Snoring and restless sleep.
· Daytime sleepiness and fatigue.
· Sexual dysfunction.
· Morning headaches.
· Mental or emotional problems such as memory loss, feeling irritable, poor judgment, or depression.

CAUSES

· Obstructive apnea. Breathing stops because the airway collapses and prevents air from getting into the lungs. Airway collapse may be due to several factors. There may be excess tissue at the back of the throat (large tonsils). The tongue may fall back and close off the airway. The muscles controlling the airway have become weakened.
· Central sleep apnea. Is less common and caused by a problem in the central nervous system.
· Mixed apnea. The two types occur together.

RISK INCREASES WITH

· Overweight.
· Family history of sleep apnea.
· Persons having a large neck, recessed chin, or abnormal structure of the upper airway.
· Smoking.
· Use of alcohol or sedative drugs.
· African Americans, Pacific Islanders, and Mexicans.
· Acid reflux may contribute to sleep apnea.

PREVENTIVE MEASURES

No specific preventive measures. Avoid risk factors such as smoking and alcohol.

EXPECTED OUTCOMES

Outcome depends on the individual and how severe the symptoms are. Treatment can help improve apnea.

POSSIBLE COMPLICATIONS

· Heart failure, high blood pressure, and stroke. Other health effects may occur. It is unclear if apnea is the cause.
· Emotional problems and reduced quality of life.
· Sleep quality of bed partner is affected. This can cause sleepiness and fatigue for that person.

 DIAGNOSIS & TREATMENT

GENERAL MEASURES

· A bed partner may be the first to notice the symptoms. Your health care provider may do a physical exam and ask questions about your symptoms and lifestyle. Tests to check your airways may be done. An overnight study at a sleep center may be prescribed. Diagnostic devices to be used at home may be used.
· Treatment will depend on severity of apnea, other health problems, and daytime sleepiness.
· Steps should be taken to treat any underlying medical problems, such as heart or lung disorders.
· Sleep on your side, not your back. Pillows may help. Or sew a pocket on the back of your pajama top. Place a ping-pong ball or tennis ball in it.
· Weight loss program for an overweight patient.
· Quit smoking. Find a way to stop that works for you.
· A special dental device may be prescribed.
· Devices to keep the airway open may help. Continuous positive airway pressure (CPAP) is often prescribed. A mask is worn over the nose and mouth during sleep. A small air-compressor forces air into the nasal passages to keep airway open.
· For severe apnea, surgery may be an option. Your health care provider will discuss the risks and benefits.
· To learn more: American Sleep Apnea Association, 1424 K St. NW. Ste. 302, Washington, DC 20005; (202) 293-3650 (not toll free); website: www.sleepapnea.org.

MEDICATIONS

· Specific drugs are not available for this disorder. Drugs may be prescribed for depression, acid reflux, or other medical problems.
· Avoid drugs like sedatives, hypnotics, barbiturates, narcotics, and alcohol. Nasal strips do not treat apnea.

ACTIVITY

Get regular exercise, but not right before bedtime.

DIET

Lose weight, if you are overweight.

 NOTIFY OUR OFFICE IF

You suspect you have sleep apnea or observe signs of sleep apnea in another family member.

Special notes:

_____

_____

_____

More notes on the back of this page ☐

SLEEP DISORDERS

 BASIC INFORMATION

DESCRIPTION

Difficulty falling asleep or remaining asleep, being awake off and on, early-morning awakening, or a combination of these. Sleep disorders affect all age groups, but are more common in the elderly. Over 70 sleep disorders have been identified. The main one is insomnia.

FREQUENT SIGNS AND SYMPTOMS

- Feeling restless when trying to fall asleep.
- Brief sleep followed by wakefulness.
- Normal sleep until very early in the morning (such as 3AM to 4AM), then being wide awake (often with frightening thoughts).
- Periods of no sleep that alternate with periods of excess sleep.
- Feeling sleepy and tired during the day.

CAUSES

Sleep is a normal and natural function of the human body. Nerve cells in the brain control whether you are asleep or awake. When something affects the balance or normal rhythm of these nerve cells, changes in sleep patterns can occur.

RISK INCREASES WITH

Emotional problems:
- Depression.
- Anxiety.
- Stress.

Physical problems:
- Sleep apnea (a breathing problem), restless leg syndrome, or narcolepsy (daytime sleepiness).
- Allergies and early-morning wheezing. Other health problems that cause shortness of breath.
- Heartburn or gastroesophageal reflux disease (GERD).
- Painful disorders, such as fibromyalgia or arthritis.
- Medical problems that require urination or bowel movements during the night.
- Alcoholism.
- Use of certain drugs, such as decongestants.
- Drug abuse, including overuse of sleep-inducers.
- Use of stimulants, such as coffee, tea, or cola drinks.
- Withdrawal from addictive substances.
- Obesity.

Lifestyle problems:
- Erratic work hours.
- New environment or location.
- Jet lag after travel.
- Noisy environment (including a snoring partner).
- Lack of physical exercise.

PREVENTIVE MEASURES

Maintain a healthy lifestyle that includes good sleep habits. Avoid risk factors of sleep disorders.

EXPECTED OUTCOME

Most persons can establish good sleep patterns if the underlying cause of the problem is treated or stopped.

POSSIBLE COMPLICATIONS

- Short-term sleep disorders may become chronic.
- Excess daytime sleepiness can affect all aspects of life.

 DIAGNOSIS & TREATMENT

GENERAL MEASURES

- Sometimes, self-care steps are all that is needed.
- Set a routine schedule of going to bed and waking up.
- Try to find ways to reduce stress in your life.
- Relax in a warm bath before bedtime.
- Create a comfortable sleep setting. It should be dark, cool, and quiet. Don't turn your bedroom into an office.
- Turn off your mind. Focus on peaceful and relaxing thoughts. Play soft music or relaxation tapes.
- Use ear plugs, eye shades, or an electric blanket.
- If self-help fails, see your health care provider. A physical exam and medical tests may be done to help find the cause. An overnight sleep study may be prescribed.
- Your treatment plan will depend on the cause. It may include lifestyle changes, drugs, medical devices, or counseling.
- To learn more, do an Internet search or visit a library.

MEDICATION

- Your health care provider may prescribe sleep-inducing drugs for a short period of time.
- Melatonin, a nonprescription product, may help some people. Ask your health care provider.
- Drugs may be prescribed if a disorder is diagnosed.

ACTIVITY

Exercise regularly, but not within 2 hours of bedtime.

DIET

Don't eat within 3 hours of bedtime if indigestion is a problem. A glass of warm milk before bedtime may help. Avoid caffeine.

 NOTIFY OUR OFFICE IF

- You or a family member has symptoms of any type of sleep disorder.
- Sleep problems don't improve, despite treatment.

Special notes:

_____

_____

_____

More notes on the back of this page ☐

SMOKING CESSATION

 BASIC INFORMATION

DESCRIPTION
Cigarette smoking is an addiction disorder and the cause of many serious health problems.

FREQUENT SIGNS AND SYMPTOMS
· An average smoker smokes 15 to 20 cigarettes a day. The more one smokes, the greater the health risks. Someone who smokes even 1 to 4 cigarettes a day has more risks for health problems than nonsmokers.
· Certain activities also become linked with smoking. These include smoking after a meal, when drinking coffee, while on the phone, relaxing, or if stressed.

CAUSES
There are many chemicals in cigarette smoke. Among them are tar, nicotine and carbon monoxide (a poisonous gas). These three substances are a health risk to the person smoking and to those who breathe in the second-hand smoke. Tar condenses into a sticky substance in the lungs. Nicotine is the addictive component of tobacco smoke. Carbon monoxide decreases the oxygen carried by the red blood cells in the body.

RISK INCREASES WITH
· Teenagers. Smoking often begins as a social behavior and an adventure. Teens feel pressure from friends; they want to be socially accepted in certain groups, and to appear more mature.
· People who are under stress or feel nervous.
· Less education (high school dropouts are more likely to smoke than college graduates).
· Lower economic group.
· Ages 25 to 44. They have highest smoking rates.
· Blue-collar occupations.
· Risk taking and outgoing personality types.
· Family history of smoking.
· Alcoholics.

PREVENTIVE MEASURES
· Education about health risks.
· Prohibiting smoking in public places.

EXPECTED OUTCOME
It is never too late to quit. Anyone who smokes should make every attempt to quit. If you do, it can reverse most of the health risks and bring about a better quality of life.

POSSIBLE COMPLICATIONS
· Cancer, heart, blood vessel, and lung diseases.
· Problems with infertility.
· Problems in pregnancy, and risks to the baby's health.
· Earlier menopause and possible osteoporosis.
· Skin becomes rougher, thicker, and more wrinkled.
· Second-hand smoke is harmful to others.
· Home fire deaths (most all are caused by smoking).

 DIAGNOSIS & TREATMENT

GENERAL MEASURES
· Smokers can quit on their own or be helped by a variety of methods. No one method works for everyone.
· See your health care provider for help and advice.
· Self-help steps in quitting: 1) Think about your smoking habits and when and why you smoke. 2) Make up your mind to quit. 3) Choose the day and quit on that day. 4) Use any kind of substitute (gum, hard candy). Give up those activities, for now, that you link with smoking. 5) Reward yourself for not smoking (buy yourself something special). 6) During the first few weeks, eat plenty of low-calorie snacks; drink lots of water.
· Call the local office of the American Cancer Society or the American Lung Association for help in quitting.
· Join a support group or a smoking cessation program.
· Try out other ideas, such as hypnosis or acupuncture.
· Concerns about quitting: 1) *Weight gain.* Average amount is 5-8 pounds over 5 years (for some, there is no weight gain). 2) *Stress.* It may occur. Get counseling or help with managing stress. 3) *Withdrawal.* Physical symptoms stop in about 10 to 14 days. Psychologic symptoms may go on for months or longer. 4) *Fear of failure.* Relapse is common. Many people have had to try more than once, and by more than one method.

MEDICATION
· Stop smoking aids include nicotine gum, skin patches, nasal sprays, or inhalers. They can help reduce withdrawal symptoms. Discuss the risks and benefits with your health care provider. These aids are to be used along with counseling or a smoking-cessation program.
· Antidepressants may be prescribed for a short time.

ACTIVITY
Exercise daily. It helps to control weight, reduces stress, and lessens the craving for cigarettes.

DIET
No special diet. Eat healthy, low-fat, high-fiber foods.

 NOTIFY OUR OFFICE IF

You or a family member is a cigarette smoker and wants help in quitting.

Special notes:

_____

_____

_____

More notes on the back of this page ☐

SNAKEBITE

 BASIC INFORMATION

DESCRIPTION

Bite from a venomous snake, such as a rattlesnake, copperhead, water moccasin, or coral snake. Bites on the legs and feet are more common. Bites on the head and trunk are more dangerous. Snakes are more likely to bite runners, joggers, walkers, hikers, backpackers, fishers, boaters, and campers or anyone playing or working where snakes live.

FREQUENT SIGNS AND SYMPTOMS

· If the bite is from a coral snake, it will have multiple fang marks and small cuts; symptoms may not appear for 3 to 4 hours. If the bite is from another snake, it will have deep single or double fang marks, and symptoms will begin quickly.
· Severe pain and swelling around the bite.
· Skin color around the bite looks bruised.
· Bleeding spots under the skin, all over the body.
· Numbness and tingling around the mouth and in the hands and feet.
· Excessive sweating; fever.
· Low blood pressure and life-threatening shock.
· Breathing difficulty.
· Blurred vision; headache.
· Seizures; coma.

CAUSES

Snakes use their fangs to bite a person. Venomous snakes inject a venom through the fangs.

RISK INCREASES WITH

Bites from venomous snakes occur during outdoor activities in warm months in areas where snakes are known to live. People handling snakes or trying to capture snakes put themselves at risk.

PREVENTIVE MEASURES

· Wear protective shoes, boots and clothing for hiking, camping, fishing, and hunting. Consider taking a snakebite kit with instructions with you.
· Don't try to pick up or handle snakes.

EXPECTED OUTCOMES

Usually curable with rapid medical care. Skin tissue affected by the bite may take weeks to months to heal.

POSSIBLE COMPLICATIONS

· Wound infection and skin loss.
· Heart, lung, blood, or kidney complications.
· Compartment syndrome (loss of blood circulation to muscles in a closed body space).
· Reaction to the antivenin includes anaphylaxis (severe allergic) and delayed serum sickness.
· Death from snakebite is rare.

 DIAGNOSIS & TREATMENT

GENERAL MEASURES

· If possible, identify the snake, but don't waste time looking for it.
· Don't panic! Venom will spread more quickly through the body if the victim runs or gets excited.
· Call 911 for emergency help. If help cannot get there right away, go to the nearest emergency center.
· Follow snakebite kit instructions if one is handy.
· Some basic first aid steps include: Remain calm. Keep bitten area below or at heart level, if possible. Remove jewelry and tight clothing. Do not cut or suction the bite. Cover area with a clean, dry pad. Do not use a tourniquet. If elastic bandage is available, wrap firmly around the area. Don't use ice on the area (cool compresses may be used). Cover victim with a blanket. Don't give victim food or drink, especially alcohol.
· In the hospital, the treatment may include:
  - Breathing support with a machine if needed.
  - Treatment to prevent any complications.
  - Surgical debridement (removal of dead or infected tissue) after 3 or 4 days. Skin grafts may be needed.

MEDICATIONS

· Your health care provider may prescribe:
  - Antivenin to counter the snake poison.
  - Tetanus booster injection.
  - Antibiotics to prevent infection.
  - Pain relievers. Narcotics cannot be used for coral snake bites. They may cause shock.

ACTIVITY

Resume normal activities as soon as symptoms improve.

DIET

No special diet.

 NOTIFY OUR OFFICE IF

New, unexplained symptoms develop after snakebite treatment.

Special notes:

_____

_____

_____

More notes on the back of this page ☐

SODIUM IMBALANCE

BASIC INFORMATION

DESCRIPTION
Above-normal sodium level (hypernatremia) or below-normal sodium level (hyponatremia) in the blood. Sodium helps regulate the body's water balance and maintains normal heart rhythm. It is responsible for the conduction of nerve impulses, and the contraction of muscles.

FREQUENT SIGNS AND SYMPTOMS
- Confusion.
- Restlessness and anxiety.
- Weakness.
- Muscle cramps (usually in the legs).
- Changes in pulse rate and blood pressure.
- Tissue swelling (edema).
- Stupor or coma (if severe imbalance).
- Sodium imbalance may be part of a disease with other symptoms, such as fever, vomiting, diarrhea, or excessive sweating.

CAUSES
Hyponatremia (below-normal sodium):
- Prolonged loss of body fluids from vomiting or diarrhea.
- Addison's disease.
- Congestive heart failure.
- Prolonged, excessive drinking of water. This is usually a psychiatric condition.
- Some cancers of the adrenal glands.
- Infections with high fever.

Hypernatremia (above-normal sodium):
- Inability to drink water, as with stroke or gastrointestinal diseases.
- Use of cortisone drugs.
- Excess intake of salty food or liquid, as in near drowning in salt water.
- Inappropriate secretion of anti-diuretic hormone.

RISK INCREASES WITH
- Diabetes.
- Congestive heart failure.
- Use of diuretics (drugs to remove excess fluid).
- Kidney diseases. Healthy kidneys can usually control sodium levels.

PREVENTIVE MEASURES
- Sodium imbalance is the result of an underlying disease. Medical treatment for that disorder will help prevent sodium imbalance.
- If you have a disorder or take drugs that affect sodium balance, learn as much as possible about your drugs and your condition. Learn how to prevent a sodium imbalance.

EXPECTED OUTCOMES
Usually, the imbalance can be corrected and the underlying disorder treated to prevent a recurrence.

POSSIBLE COMPLICATIONS
Shock, which can be life threatening.

DIAGNOSIS & TREATMENT

GENERAL MEASURES
- Your health care provider may do a physical exam. Medical tests may include blood and urine studies of sodium and other electrolytes.
- Treatment will depend on the underlying cause.
- If a drug is the cause for sodium imbalance (above or below normal), it may be stopped or the dose lowered.
- For below-normal sodium levels, water restriction is usually the therapy. This will increase the sodium levels in the body. It is important that the treatment not over-correct the sodium levels, as that can be dangerous.
- For above-normal levels of sodium, providing fluids (such as dextrose in water) to return sodium levels to normal is the usual therapy.

MEDICATIONS
- Your health care provider may prescribe:
  - Intravenous (IV) sodium, if sodium levels are low.
  - Diuretics to decrease high sodium levels.
  - Drugs to correct underlying disorders.

ACTIVITY
Bed rest until stable, or underlying condition resolved or controlled. Resume normal activities after recovery.

DIET
No special diet for low sodium levels. Most persons with high sodium levels benefit from a low-salt diet. Low-salt diets contain enough sodium to prevent hyponatremia. However, sodium levels are not influenced by diet alone.

NOTIFY OUR OFFICE IF

- You or a family member has symptoms of a sodium imbalance.
- You are having problems with a disorder that affects sodium levels.

Special notes:

_____

_____

_____

More notes on the back of this page ☐

SORES, PRESSURE

(Bed Sores; Decubitus Ulcers)

 BASIC INFORMATION

DESCRIPTION
Sores that affect the skin over pressure points in the lower back, buttocks, elbows, knees, shoulders, heels, and ankles. They can affect all ages, but occur most often in the elderly.

FREQUENT SIGNS AND SYMPTOMS
Spots of the skin that are red and shiny. Spots progress to blisters, then ulcers (deep sores), leading to a breakdown of tissue under the ulcer.

CAUSES
Constant pressure on the skin, especially over bony areas. Pressure reduces the blood supply, causing death in the tissue layers. Pressure sores usually develop in persons who cannot move because of chronic illness or disability that confines them to bed.

RISK INCREASES WITH
- Elderly people who are frail, disabled, ill, or immobile.
- Being confined to bed or a chair for long, or even short periods of time. Sores can start within 24 hours.
- Poor nutrition and low body weight.
- Impaired mental status.
- Skin that is too dry or too moist.
- Illness that reduces blood flow in the body.

PREVENTIVE MEASURES
- Provide good nursing care for the disabled.
- Daily skin inspection in good light.
- Frequent changes of position in bed or wheelchair (hourly may be needed).
- Keep skin clean. Clean the skin of any urine or fecal matter as soon as possible. Apply moisturizers.

EXPECTED OUTCOMES
Usually curable with treatment. Sores heal in 2 to 4 weeks, or sometimes longer. Healing time varies with the site and size of the ulcer and the patient's general health.

POSSIBLE COMPLICATIONS
- Infection develops in the pressure sores.
- Infection of bone (osteomyelitis) next to the ulcer.

 DIAGNOSIS & TREATMENT

GENERAL MEASURES
- Your health care provider can diagnose pressure sores by an exam of the affected area.
- Treatment involves relieving the pressure, treating the sores, and improving nutrition, or other conditions. Your health care provider will discuss the steps to take.

- Relieve pressure by not lying on the sores. Other options include protective, soft padding, such as gel flotation pads or sheepskin, over the affected area.
- A water mattress, egg-crate rubber mattress, alternating-pressure mattress, or special airbed may be recommended.
- Clean the area with mild soap and warm water and pat dry. Avoid harsh soaps, tincture of benzoin, or hexachlorophene. Cover the sore with bandage or dressing.
- Apply a skin product if prescribed. Apply a thin layer of the cream, ointment, or lotion 3 or 4 times daily. Rub in gently for several minutes, until it disappears.
- Special dressings for pressure sores, such as Gelfoam or Duoderm, may be prescribed.
- Dead skin and tissue may need to be removed. This can be done in different ways and can be painful to the patient.

MEDICATIONS
- Antibiotics will be prescribed if infection develops.
- Ointments, dressings, and drying agents may be recommended.
- Drugs for pain may be needed when dead skin tissue is removed.
- Vitamin and mineral supplements may be needed.

ACTIVITY
- Change the position of an immobilized patient every 1 to 2 hours. A wheelchair patient should change position every hour.
- Passive or active exercises (if the patient is able). Instructions will be provided by your health care provider or physical therapist.

DIET
Normal, well-balanced diet that includes extra protein. Good nutrition is important in prevention and healing.

 NOTIFY OUR OFFICE IF

- You or a family member has symptoms of pressure sores or observe them in someone else.
- The following occur during treatment:
  - Skin sores become worse or don't improve.
  - Signs of infection, such as pain, redness, tenderness, swelling, or increased warmth of the affected area.
  - Fever.

Special notes:

_____

_____

_____

More notes on the back of this page ☐

SPINAL CORD TUMOR

BASIC INFORMATION

DESCRIPTION
An abnormal growth that presses on the spinal cord or its nerve roots. The growth may be benign (noncancerous) or malignant (cancerous). A benign tumor may be as damaging as a malignant tumor if it is not treated.

FREQUENT SIGNS AND SYMPTOMS
• Symptoms may come on gradually and then suddenly be more severe.
• Dull, burning, or aching pain due to tumor putting pressure on the spinal cord. Pain may be constant and, sometimes, severe. It may feel like it's coming from various parts of the body.
• Pain may be located near the level of the tumor on the spinal cord. Midway affects the chest, higher affects arms and neck, and lower affects the back and legs.
• A loss of sensation that may include a feeling of numbness and skin being less sensitive to heat and cold.
• Muscle weakness or stiffness.
• Urination problems or incontinence (unable to control urination or bowel movements).
• If not treated, muscle wasting (loss of tissue) and paralysis may occur.

CAUSES
• A spinal cord tumor usually comes from cancer that has spread from another part of the body. The cancer may have started in the lung, breast, intestinal tract, prostate, kidney, thyroid, or lymphatic system.
• Tumors that start first (primary tumors) in the spinal cord are more rare, especially in childhood or old age. Their cause is often unknown. A few may result from a genetic disease or radiation exposure.

RISK INCREASES WITH
Cancer in any of the body places listed above.

PREVENTIVE MEASURES
• No specific preventive measures. Steps to help reduce your cancer risk or diagnose the cancer early include:
   - Not smoking.
   - Eating a healthy diet. Maintaining a healthy weight.
   - Get the recommended cancer screening exams.
   - Learn the warning signs and symptoms of cancer.

EXPECTED OUTCOMES
Early diagnosis and early treatment offer the most favorable outcome for cancerous tumors. Many benign tumors are cured with surgery.

POSSIBLE COMPLICATIONS
Paralysis, spread of cancer to other body organs, surgery complications, infections, and other medical problems.

DIAGNOSIS & TREATMENT

GENERAL MEASURES
• Your health care provider will do a physical exam and ask questions about your symptoms. This exam may include checking: your eye movement, reflexes, hearing, sense of touch and balance. Medical tests may include x-ray, CT, MRI, and others to help confirm the diagnosis.
• Treatments include monitoring (no treatment right away), surgery, radiation and/or chemotherapy (anticancer drugs). It depends on the tumor type, your health, other cancer treatment, and your preferences.
• A slow-growing, benign tumor may be monitored for a period of time. It may have been found on a routine exam and not be causing symptoms, or the symptoms are mild.
• Surgery is often the first option if the tumor can be removed without damage to the spinal cord or nerves. Several different types of surgery are available. If the tumor is benign, surgery can provide a cure.
• Radiation therapy is usually done after surgery for a cancerous tumor. Radiation may also be done if the tumor cannot be removed with surgery.
• Research is ongoing for improved treatment options.
• To learn more: American Cancer Society, (800) ACS-2345; website: www.cancer.org or National Cancer Institute, (800) 4-CANCER; website: www.nci.nih.gov.

MEDICATIONS
• Pain relievers may be prescribed.
• Cortisone drugs to decrease swelling around the tumor and reduce pressure on the spinal cord.
• Anticancer drugs, if the tumor is malignant.

ACTIVITY
Activity levels will depend on your physical well-being. Be as active as your energy permits.

DIET
Eat a normal, well-balanced diet.

NOTIFY OUR OFFICE IF

You or a family member has any symptoms of a spinal cord tumor.

Special notes: _____

_____

_____

_____

More notes on the back of this page ☐

SPONDYLITIS, ANKYLOSING
(Marie-Strumpell Disease; AS)

 BASIC INFORMATION

DESCRIPTION
A chronic, progressive, rheumatic disease of the joints. Ankylosing means "fusing together." Spondylitis means "inflammation of the vertebrae" (bones in the spine). Males are affected more often than females. The onset is usually in the late teens or early twenties.

FREQUENT SIGNS AND SYMPTOMS
Early stages:
- Recurrent episodes of low backache. Pain can also occur along the sciatic nerve (along the leg).
- Stiffness in the spine. It may be worse in the morning.
- The symptoms can be mild and a person may think it is just a common backache.

Later stages:
- Symptoms gradually become worse. Pain often spreads from the lower back to the middle back, or higher in the neck. Joints in the arms, legs, feet, and hands may be affected.
- It can bring about a "bent forward" posture caused by stiffening of the spine and support structures.
- Muscle stiffness.
- Fatigue; weight loss.
- Iritis (eye redness and soreness).

CAUSES
Unknown. It may be genetic or an autoimmune disorder (immune system goes wrong). The disorder causes some or all the bones of the spine to fuse together.

RISK INCREASES WITH
- Family history of ankylosing spondylitis.
- Having a certain gene called HLA-B27.

PREVENTIVE MEASURES
No specific preventive measures. Consult your health care provider if you have a family history of the disorder and have ongoing back or joint pain.

EXPECTED OUTCOME
There is no cure for this disorder. Symptoms change with mild or moderate flare-ups and they may stop for periods of time. With treatment, symptoms can be relieved or controlled. Most patients can lead normal, productive lives. For some, the disease is severe and incapacitating due to deformities.

POSSIBLE COMPLICATIONS
- Heart and lung problems.
- Eye inflammation.
- Difficulty walking and standing.
- Osteoporosis and fractures of the spine.
- Anemia.
- Permanent disability.

 DIAGNOSIS & TREATMENT

GENERAL MEASURES
- Your health care provider will do a physical exam and ask questions about your symptoms. Medical tests may include blood studies and x-rays of the spine.
- Physical therapy, exercise, and drugs can help delay or prevent deformity, ease pain, and maintain function.
- Physical therapy includes exercises for breathing techniques, to maintain proper posture, and to build up muscle groups (to oppose the direction of possible deformities).
- Sleep on your back on a firm mattress. Use a small pillow or none at all.
- Take hot baths or use heat compresses before exercising or to relieve pain. Get regular massages, if possible.
- Quit smoking. Find a way to stop that works for you.
- See your eye care provider for regular exams.
- Surgery to replace a damaged hip or to insert bone grafts in the spine (advanced stages only).
- To learn more: Spondylitis Association of America, PO Box 5872, Sherman Oaks, CA 91413; (800) 777-8189; website: www.spondylitis.org.

MEDICATION
- Use nonprescription, nonsteroidal anti-inflammatory drugs to help ease discomfort.
- Drugs to treat arthritis symptoms, stronger pain drugs, and muscle relaxants may be prescribed.

ACTIVITY
- Exercise to maintain good posture and retain as much upright carriage as possible.
- Swim regularly, if possible. Your buoyancy in water will allow you to move stiff, painful areas more easily.
- Avoid activity that puts stress on the back. Avoid contact sports (too much risk of spinal injury).

DIET
No special diet.

 NOTIFY OUR OFFICE IF

- You or a family member has symptoms of ankylosing spondylitis.
- Increasing back pain or stiffness, or eye pain occur.

Special notes:

_____

_____

_____

More notes on the back of this page ☐

SPOROTRICHOSIS

 ## BASIC INFORMATION

DESCRIPTION
A fungal infection that affects the skin. Sporotrichosis is not contagious from person to person. It can affect all ages, and occurs in equal numbers of men and women.

FREQUENT SIGNS AND SYMPTOMS
· A small, movable, non-tender bump (nodule) usually on the fingers, hands, or arms. It starts at the place where the fungus entered the skin. The color may be pink, red, or purple.
· More bumps occur around the same area.
· The bumps may ulcerate (become open sores).
· The skin infection can spread in a line-like formation up the fingers, hands or arms. They spread along what is called lymphatic channels.

CAUSES
· Infection by a fungus, *Sporotrichum schenckii*, that lives in soil, sphagnum moss, weeds, baled hay, and decaying organic vegetation. It enters the skin through small cuts or punctures, such as from thorns. The infection may appear on the skin 1 to 12 weeks after exposure.
· Research has shown that a pet cat may have the infection and pass it to a human through a bite or scratch.

RISK INCREASES WITH
· Farm laborers, plant nursery workers, gardeners, and others who handle rosebushes, sphagnum moss, hay bales, or barberry bushes.
· Kids playing among hay bales.
· Those with weak immune system due to illness or drugs are more at risk for complications.

PREVENTIVE MEASURES
· Wear gloves and long sleeves when working with plants with thorns, hay bales, pine seedlings, or other materials that could cause minor skin breaks.
· Avoid skin contact with sphagnum moss. It has been the cause of some outbreaks.

EXPECTED OUTCOMES
Curable with treatment, but it can take several months to heal completely.

POSSIBLE COMPLICATIONS
Spread of the fungal infection to joints, lungs, and central nervous system. This is rare, but may occur in those who have diabetes or weak immune systems.

 ## DIAGNOSIS & TREATMENT

GENERAL MEASURES
· Your health care provider will do a physical exam of the affected skin. Medical tests may include a culture of fluid from the sores or a small bit of tissue is removed for viewing under a microscope.
· The disorder is treated with antifungal drugs.
· You may be advised to apply warm compresses or a heating pad to the affected skin for 40 to 60 minutes a day. This can help control the skin symptoms.
· Cover lesions with loose-fitting bandages to prevent secondary infection with bacteria.
· Rarely, hospital care may be needed if complications occur.

MEDICATIONS
Oral (taken by mouth) antifungal drugs are usually prescribed. Drugs may be continued for 1 to 2 months or more after the skin symptoms have cleared up.

ACTIVITY
No limits.

DIET
No special diet.

 ## NOTIFY OUR OFFICE IF

· You or a family member has symptoms of sporotrichosis.
· Any new sores occur after treatment starts.
· New, unexplained symptoms develop. Antifungal drugs used in treatment may produce side effects.

Special notes:

_____

_____

_____

More notes on the back of this page ☐

SPRAINS & STRAINS

 BASIC INFORMATION

DESCRIPTION

A sprain is a stretched or torn ligament. A strain is a stretched or torn muscle or tendon. Sprains occur most often in ankles, knees, or fingers, although any joint can be sprained. Strains often occur in the back or hamstring muscles (at the back of the thigh). It is sometimes difficult to know if the injury is a sprain and strain.

FREQUENT SIGNS AND SYMPTOMS

• Pain or tenderness in the area of injury; severity varies with the extent of injury.
• Swelling of the affected joint.
• Redness or bruising in the area of injury, either right away, or several hours after injury.
• Loss of normal mobility in the injured joint.

CAUSES

• Strains are often caused by twisting, pulling, or overuse injuries. Pulled muscle is another term used.
• Sprains usually occur as a result of trauma (fall, twisting injury, or automobile accident). The ankle is injured most often because of its normal weakness, its exposed position and the stress it sustains in sports and other activities.

RISK INCREASES WITH

• Sports requiring running, jumping, and change of direction.
• High-risk activities such as skateboarding, contact sports, ice and roller skating, mountain biking, skiing and, rock climbing.
• Overweight.
• Trauma.
• Excessive exercise.
• Poor conditioning.
• Poor fitting shoes and high-heeled shoes.

PREVENTIVE MEASURES

• Maintain good level of physical fitness.
• Maintain a healthy weight.
• To avoid injury:
  - Wear proper shoes and other protective gear for the sport or activity.
  - Stretch muscles before and after exercise.
  - Strengthen weak muscles with special exercises.
  - Accident-proof your home.

EXPECTED OUTCOMES

With treatment and rest, it takes 6 to 8 weeks for recovery. It may take longer if the injury is severe.

POSSIBLE COMPLICATIONS

• Joint may remain unstable.
• Arthritis may develop later on in the joint.

 DIAGNOSIS & TREATMENT

GENERAL MEASURES

• Your health care provider will do an exam of the injured area. Questions will be asked about your symptoms and activities that lead to the injury. Tests may include x-rays or other special scans of the injured area.
• Treatment for a sprain or strain will depend on how mild or severe the injury is. It may range from simple self-care, to wearing a cast or brace, to having surgery.
• Use RICE therapy—Rest, Ice, Compression, Elevation.
  - Rest and reduce activities as needed. Crutches or a cane may be required to get around.
  - Apply ice. Place ice in a plastic bag and separate it from the skin with a thin towel. Continue the ice treatment for 20 minutes at a time at 2-hour intervals. After 24 hours, continue ice treatment or switch to heat.
  - Compression may be done with elastic wrap. Also, special boots, casts, or splints may be prescribed.
  - Elevate the injured area on a pillow, above the heart level if possible, to help reduce swelling.
• Rehabilitation for a sprain or strain starts after the pain and swelling improve. The goals are to restore complete joint function and a return to full activity levels. You and your health care provider will work out a recovery and exercise plan for your individual needs.

MEDICATIONS

You may take pain relievers such as acetaminophen. If the sprain is severe, a stronger pain reliever may be prescribed. Avoid aspirin, as it may increase the tendency to bleed.

ACTIVITY

You will be taught exercises to do several times a day at home. Physical therapy may be needed. Don't return to previous activity level until advised to do so. You risk a re-injury and chronic joint problems.

DIET

No special diet.

 NOTIFY OUR OFFICE IF

• You or a family member has a joint injury.
• Pain, swelling or bruising, increases.

Special notes:

_____

_____

_____

More notes on the back of this page ☐

STOMACH CANCER
(Gastric Carcinoma)

BASIC INFORMATION

DESCRIPTION
Growth of cancer cells in the stomach. Stomach cancer most often affects adults over age 50 and is more common in men than in women. Most people do not have symptoms until the disease is advanced.

FREQUENT SIGNS AND SYMPTOMS
Early stages:
- Vague symptoms of indigestion, such as fullness, burping, nausea, and poor appetite.

Later stages:
- Unexplained weight loss.
- Loss of appetite.
- Vomiting blood.
- Black stools.
- Fullness after eating small amounts.
- Pain in the stomach.
- Mass in the stomach that can be felt (sometimes).

CAUSES
Exact cause is unknown. *Helicobacter pylori* infection, a bacteria infection of the stomach, appears to be a factor. Dietary factors are believed to play a role.

RISK INCREASES WITH
- Age over 50. Men are more at risk than women.
- Excess alcohol or tobacco use.
- Previous stomach surgery.
- Diet that includes high amounts of smoked, pickled, and salted foods; and low amounts of protein, fresh fruits, and green, leafy vegetables.
- Pernicious anemia (unable to absorb vitamin B12).
- Family history of stomach cancer.
- Being overweight.
- People with type A blood.

PREVENTIVE MEASURES
- There are no specific preventive measures. Changing some lifestyle behaviors can help lower the risks.
- Eat a nutritious, well-balanced diet with plenty of fresh fruits and vegetables. Lose weight if overweight.
- Decrease alcohol use if you drink more than 1 or 2 drinks a day. Don't smoke. If you do smoke, try to quit.
- To help find stomach cancer early, don't ignore symptoms of indigestion that last more than a few days. Do a yearly home test for blood in the stool.
- Treatment for ongoing *Helicobacter pylori* infection as a cancer-preventive step is being researched.

EXPECTED OUTCOMES
Often, the cancer is diagnosed too late for effective treatment. New developments in treatment may offer hope in some cases. If the cancer is found early, and surgery removes the entire tumor, recovery may be complete.

POSSIBLE COMPLICATIONS
- Excess fluid in the abdomen (ascites).
- Spread of cancer to lymph nodes, liver, pancreas, and colon.
- The 5-year survival rate is poor, even with treatment.

DIAGNOSIS & TREATMENT

GENERAL MEASURES
- Your health care provider will do a physical exam and ask questions about your symptoms. Medical tests may include blood studies, CT, and x-rays of the stomach, esophagus, and small intestine. The stomach may be examined with a endoscope (a viewing tube passed down the esophagus to the stomach). A small amount of tissue may be removed for a biopsy.
- Your health care provider will discuss treatment options with you. They depend on the location of the cancer, how advanced it is, your overall health, and your own preferences.
- Surgery to remove part or all of the stomach may be recommended, if the cancer has not spread.
- Drugs to treat the cancer or radiation therapy may achieve a temporary response.
- Treatment may involve steps to relieve symptoms and make you comfortable, rather than treating the cancer.
- To learn more: American Cancer Society, (800) ACS-2345; website: www.cancer.org or National Cancer Institute, (800) 4-CANCER; website: www.nci.nih.gov.

MEDICATIONS
- Anticancer (chemotherapy) drugs may be prescribed.
- Pain relievers may be prescribed.

ACTIVITY
As tolerated by your energy level.

DIET
Eat frequent, small meals of soft foods. Try to maintain a high calorie intake.

NOTIFY OUR OFFICE IF

- You or a family member has symptoms of stomach cancer.
- Indigestion or other symptoms occur after surgery.

Special notes:

_____

_____

_____

More notes on the back of this page ☐

STOMATITIS

 ## BASIC INFORMATION

DESCRIPTION

A common, and painful condition that affects the lining of the mouth. It may involve the cheeks, gums, lips, tongue, roof, and floor. The two main types are acute herpetic stomatitis and aphthous stomatitis (canker sore), which is the most common. Stomatitis may be a sign of a more serious, underlying disorder.

FREQUENT SIGNS AND SYMPTOMS

- Inflammation (redness, swelling, and soreness) of the mouth.
- Mouth sores that are shallow, usually red, and may have a white coating over them.
- Mild to severe pain.
- Bleeding (sometimes).
- Bad breath.

CAUSES

The condition can be caused by a variety of factors. For canker sores, the exact cause is unknown.

RISK INCREASES WITH

- Infection.
- Trauma (injury) and burns, such as from hot food or drink.
- Dryness of the mouth and nasal passages.
- Irritants.
- Toxic agents.
- Autoimmune conditions.
- Vitamin deficiency.
- Anemia.
- Allergies to food or drugs.
- Smoking.
- Dentures, jagged or sharp teeth.
- Emotional stress, anxiety.
- Poor nutrition.
- Radiation or chemotherapy (anticancer drugs).
- Excess alcohol.
- Excess eating of hot foods or spices.
- Sensitivity to mouthwashes, candy dyes, or lipstick.
- Side effect of certain drugs.
- Diseases such as HIV, Behçet's, Crohn's, and others.
- Family history of canker sores.

PREVENTIVE MEASURES

No specific preventive measures. Avoid risk factors where possible.

EXPECTED OUTCOMES

- Usually heals in 1 or 2 weeks, or longer. Some may require treatment, and others heal on their own.
- Some outcomes will depend on underlying disorders.

POSSIBLE COMPLICATIONS

- May recur after treatment.
- Underlying disorder may have complications.

 ## DIAGNOSIS & TREATMENT

GENERAL MEASURES

- Most people will let the sores heal on their own or use self-treatment methods.
- See your health care provider if sores persist or cause pain so that you you can't eat. An exam of the mouth will be done. Medical tests such as smears or cultures of the sores may be done to check for infection or other cause.
- Treatment will vary depending on the cause.
- Infections may be treated with drugs.
- Careful oral hygiene is important. Use a soft-bristled toothbrush. Brush teeth and gums gently.
- Avoid mouthwash or toothpaste that may be a cause.
- Quit smoking. Find a way to stop that works for you.
- Have your dental care provider correct problems with jagged or sharp teeth, or ill-fitting dentures.

MEDICATIONS

- Drugs may be prescribed for the underlying cause, where it can be determined.
- Mouth rinses or oral lozenges may be prescribed.
- Nonprescription drugs for canker sores that are applied to the sores may help some people.
- Vitamins, iron, or folate will be prescribed if needed.
- Use ibuprofen or acetaminophen for minor pain.

ACTIVITY

No limits.

DIET

- Avoid spicy foods or foods that are hard, sharp, or dry (such as potato chips, tacos, or peanuts).
- Avoid any foods that cause an allergic reaction.
- Drink plenty of fluids.

 ## NOTIFY OUR OFFICE IF

- You or a family member has signs or symptoms of stomatitis.
- Symptoms don't improve with treatment.

Special notes:

_____

_____

_____

More notes on the back of this page ☐

STRABISMUS

(Cross-Eyes)

BASIC INFORMATION

DESCRIPTION

The eyes are not aligned together, and eyes point in different directions. One or both eyes may turn inward (crossed eyes), outward ("walleye"), upward, or downward. The ability of the eyes to focus is not fully mature at birth. A true eye problem shows up from 3 or 4 months of age. It also may occur in childhood or later. Strabismus may be constant (occurs all the time) or intermittent (occurs some of the time).

FREQUENT SIGNS AND SYMPTOMS

· Eye movement that is not coordinated.
· Child may look at you with one eye closed, squint, or with the head turned to one side.
· Adults may have double vision, eyestrain, headaches, and/or an abnormal head position (from trying to see properly).

CAUSES

· Eye movement is controlled by brain signals to six muscles around each eye. Loss of coordinated movement may result from:
  - Muscle imbalance between the eyes.
  - Lack of equal focusing ability in the eyes. The brain gets a different picture from each eye, so it blocks the one from the weaker eye. The weaker eye becomes more useless from disuse, and a "lazy," or wandering eye results.
  - Brain damage or head injury (rare).

RISK INCREASES WITH

· Family history of strabismus.
· Down syndrome
· Cerebral palsy.
· Eye tumor.
· Damage to fetal central nervous system.
· Birth trauma (injury).
· In adults, thyroid disease, stroke, myasthenia gravis, diabetes, brain tumor, other neurological disease.

PREVENTIVE MEASURES

No specific preventive measures.

EXPECTED OUTCOMES

· With early diagnosis and treatment, strabismus can be corrected. It can take many months or even years. Without prompt treatment, vision loss in one eye may become permanent.
· Many persons adapt well to single-eye vision and learn to drive a car as well as other activities. If vision is lost in one eye, take extra care against injury in the other eye. Wear goggles for sports and other activities, such as carpentry, or welding, which carry the risk of injury.

POSSIBLE COMPLICATIONS

Loss of normal vision in one eye.

DIAGNOSIS & TREATMENT

GENERAL MEASURES

· Your health care provider will do an exam of the eyes. Medical tests may include a visual acuity test, a retina exam, and others.
· Treatment has three goals: to obtain the best possible vision, gain the best eye alignment, and provide the best chance for binocular (both eyes) vision.
· Glasses or an eye patch may be used over the stronger eye to correct focusing imbalance. These force the weak eye to work. This treatment may be done for only a few hours a day or all waking hours (full-time).
· Eye-muscle exercises (called orthoptics) will improve the eye muscles to help straighten the eyes.
· Vision therapy involves exercises that help the eye and brain learn to work together better.
· Surgery to correct the condition of the eye muscles may be recommended. Sometimes a second operation is required. Your eye care provider will explain the risks and benefits of the surgery.
· A therapy for adults involves the use of eyeglasses overlaid with thin plastic prisms. These are used by a patient prior to surgery. They help determine the amount of adjustment needed on the eye muscles.
· To learn more: American Academy of Ophthalmology, PO Box 7424, San Francisco, CA 94120; website: www.aao.org/aao/public.

MEDICATIONS

Botulinum toxin injections may sometimes be recommended for adults. They are injected into an eye-turning muscle, outside the eye, by using a special needle.

ACTIVITY

No limits. Protect your child against falls or injury while he or she adjusts to an eye patch.

DIET

No special diet.

NOTIFY OUR OFFICE IF

· You or a family member has symptoms of strabismus.
· Signs of infection develop after eye surgery (redness, pain, fever).

Special notes: _____

_____

_____

More notes on the back of this page ☐

STREP THROAT
(Streptococcal Sore Throat)

 ## BASIC INFORMATION

DESCRIPTION

Infection of the throat (the pharynx) by group A streptococcus (GAS) bacteria. Strep throat can spread from person to person and is most common in children. Infection can be present in someone with no symptoms, but who can still spread the germs (carrier state).

FREQUENT SIGNS AND SYMPTOMS

· Rapid onset of throat pain.
· Throat pain that is worse when you swallow.
· Headache, fever, general ill feeling.
· Children may have nausea and vomiting.
· Tender, swollen glands in the neck.
· Bright-red tonsils that may have specks of pus.

CAUSES

Streptococcal bacteria. Germs are spread by contact with an infected person, breathing in germs in the air, or touching an object with germs on it. A person usually has symptoms in 2 to 5 days of exposure. Strep throat is one of the most common types of infection caused by group A streptococcus. It can also cause skin infections and other health problems.

RISK INCREASES WITH

· Recent strep infection in a family member.
· Crowded living conditions such as a dorm.
· Being in daycare center or attending school.

PREVENTIVE MEASURES

· Avoid close contact with anyone with strep throat.
· Avoid germs. Wash hands often, especially children.

EXPECTED OUTCOMES

Curable with treatment. Symptoms are usually better within the first few days of treatment. Any complications are rare.

POSSIBLE COMPLICATIONS

· Ear infection.
· Sinusitis.
· Rheumatic fever or scarlet fever.
· Glomerulonephritis (a kidney disorder).

 ## DIAGNOSIS & TREATMENT

GENERAL MEASURES

· Your health care provider will examine the throat. A sore throat (pharyngitis) can also be caused by virus infection, allergies, or other problems. Further tests are usually needed. A throat culture or rapid strep test can confirm a strep infection.
· Treatment for strep infection is with antibiotic drugs.
· To relieve the sore throat, gargle frequently with warm or cold double-strength tea or warm salt water (mix one-half teaspoon of salt in one cup of water).

MEDICATIONS

· Penicillin or another antibiotic will be prescribed. Complete the course prescribed, even if symptoms get better. This helps prevent any complications or having the infection recur.
· Use nonprescription pain medicine, such as ibuprofen if needed. Don't give aspirin to children under age 18.
· Throat lozenges for sore throats are available from drugstores and may help with pain relief.

ACTIVITY

Return to normal activities as symptoms improve. A person can no longer spread the germs if they have taken the antibiotic drug for at least 24 hours.

DIET

A liquid diet may be helpful while the throat is sore. Drink plenty of fluids, including milk shakes, soups, tea, carbonated drinks, or iced coffee. Any type and amount of solid food is fine as long as you can swallow it without too much pain.

 ## NOTIFY OUR OFFICE IF

· You or a family member has symptoms of strep throat.
· The following occur during treatment:
  - Fever recurs after being normal for a few days.
  - New symptoms appear, such as nausea, vomiting, earache, cough, swollen glands, skin rash, severe headache, nasal drainage, or shortness of breath.
  - Joints become red or painful.

Special notes:

_____

_____

_____

More notes on the back of this page ☐

STRESS

 BASIC INFORMATION

DESCRIPTION

Stress is the physical, mental, and emotional reactions you experience due to changes and demands in your life. The changes and demands can be large or small and each person will respond to them differently. Some people are more prone than others to stressful situations. Positive stress can be a motivator. Negative stress occurs when these changes and demands are overwhelming to you.

FREQUENT SIGNS AND SYMPTOMS

• Physical symptoms include muscle tension, headache, chest pain, upset stomach, diarrhea or constipation, racing heartbeat, cold clammy hands, fatigue, profuse sweating, rashes, rapid breathing, shaking, tics, jumpiness, changes in appetite, weakness, tiredness, and dizziness.

• Emotional reactions include anger, low self-esteem, depression, lack of interest, irritability, fear and phobic responses, difficulty concentrating, guilt, worry, agitation, anxiety, and panic.

• Behavioral reactions may lead to alcohol or drug abuse, an increase in smoking, sleep disorders, overeating, memory loss, or confusion.

CAUSES

In stressful times, the body increases the production of certain hormones. These cause changes in the heart rate, blood pressure, metabolism, and physical activity.

RISK INCREASES WITH

Common causes of stress include:
• Recent loss of a loved one (spouse, child, friend).
• Holidays, such as Christmas.
• Injuries or severe illnesses.
• Problems with work or school.
• Recent move to a new city or state.
• Sexual difficulties between you and your partner.
• Business or financial problems; buying a new home.
• Regular conflict between you and a spouse or family member, close friend, or business associate.
• Constant fatigue.
• Demands on your time and energy levels by other family members leaving little time for self-care.
• World or national events such as war or disasters.

PREVENTIVE MEASURES

• To help prevent negative stress, try to take charge of those aspects of your life that you can manage.
• Since stress cannot always be prevented, learn coping techniques to protect your mental and physical health.

EXPECTED OUTCOME

Usually resolved with time, self-treatment, or medical care.

POSSIBLE COMPLICATIONS

Chronic stress can cause problems with your work and family relationships. Stress can also lead to high blood pressure, and risk of stroke and heart attack.

 DIAGNOSIS & TREATMENT

GENERAL MEASURES

• Diagnosis is often by your own or others' observation of symptoms. Sometimes medical tests may be needed to rule out medical problems that could cause the symptoms. A person may not realize they are stressed.

• Counseling may be recommended. Talking about your problems is one way of relieving stress.

• Here are some tips to help reduce stress:
  - Learn a meditation or relaxation technique and practice it regularly, daily if possible.
  - Share your feelings with a friend. You are not alone.
  - Arrange daily schedules to make them less stressful.
  - Decide what is important and has to get done and what can be put off, left undone or passed on to others.
  - Take a short time away from any stressful situation you encounter during a day. A short walk can help.
  - Learn and practice a muscle-tensing and muscle-relaxing technique. Take warm, relaxing baths.
  - Make lists of what needs to be done each day, and then cross the items off as they are completed.
  - Take time for some form of enjoyable recreation.
  - Avoid taking problems home or to bed with you. At the end of the day, take a few minutes and review the day. Let go of negative emotions. Decide about undone activities. Release mental or muscular tension.

• To learn more: National Mental Health Association, (800) 969-6642; website: www.nmha.org.

MEDICATION

If symptoms are severe, drugs may be recommended.

ACTIVITY

Exercise 20 to 30 minutes daily. It helps relieve stress.

DIET

Eat a normal, well-balanced diet. Don't skip meals.

 NOTIFY OUR OFFICE IF

You or a family member has symptoms of stress.

Special notes:

_____

_____

_____

More notes on the back of this page ☐

STROKE
(Cerebrovascular Accident; CVA)

 BASIC INFORMATION

DESCRIPTION
A sudden decrease in the blood supply to part of the brain. This causes damage to the brain so it cannot function normally. Adults over 55 are most often affected.

FREQUENT SIGNS AND SYMPTOMS
The symptoms may vary in different people:
- Inability to speak.
- Inability to move part of the body.
- Loss of consciousness.
- Sudden heavy feeling in an arm or leg, or feeling numb and unable to control muscles.
- Headache.
- Vision changes.
- Confusion.
- Dizziness.
- Loss of bowel and bladder control.

CAUSES
- Blood flow to the brain is blocked. It may be from a blood clot that forms in the brain itself due to narrowed arteries. It may be from a blood clot that forms elsewhere in the bloodstream and travels to the brain.
- Hemorrhage (bleeding) due to ruptured blood vessel. The bleeding may occur in the brain or in the space between the brain and the skull.

RISK INCREASES WITH
- Age over 55. Males have more strokes than females.
- Diabetes.
- Prior stroke.
- Family history of stroke.
- Cigarette smoking.
- High blood pressure.
- Heart disease.
- Previous transient ischemic attacks (mini strokes).
- Excess alcohol use and certain types of drug abuse.

PREVENTIVE MEASURES
- Exercise regularly.
- Eat a healthy diet.
- Don't smoke.
- Get treatment for diabetes, heart disease, or other chronic disorders.
- Have your blood pressure checked regularly. If it is high, see your health care provider.
- Get medical advice about taking aspirin daily.

EXPECTED OUTCOMES
Stroke causes death, permanent damage, or disability in two-thirds of all cases. The long-term outlook depends on the extent of brain damage. In some cases, complete recovery without long-term disability is possible.

POSSIBLE COMPLICATIONS
Serious physical and mental health problems. Major lifestyle changes that affect work, family, and social life.

 DIAGNOSIS & TREATMENT

GENERAL MEASURES
- Call 911 if you think you might be having a stroke or have someone take you to an emergency center. The first few hours are critical for effective treatment.
- Emergency care will include a physical exam and medical tests to check heart, brain, and other body functions. Treatment may include drugs, oxygen to help with breathing, and sometimes, surgery. You will stay in the hospital until symptoms improve. Long-term care may be needed for some patients.
- Early rehabilitation after a stroke will help improve physical abilities. Outcome will depend on the extent of the brain injury. Physical therapy, occupational therapy, and speech therapy may be needed. Patient attitude and family support are important in the success.
- To learn more: American Stroke Association, 7272 Greenville Ave., Dallas, TX 75231; (888) 478-7653; website: www.strokeassociation.org.

MEDICATIONS
- Drugs to break up clots, control brain swelling, and prevent complications may be given in the hospital.
- Drugs for high blood pressure, clot prevention, and other preventive drugs may be prescribed.

ACTIVITY
If you have lost muscle control, therapy will help you learn to use affected limbs. You can often regain basic skills, such as eating, dressing, and toilet functions.

DIET
At first, you may require feeding tube, then progress to a pureed, soft, and to a regular diet.

 NOTIFY OUR OFFICE IF

- You or a family member has symptoms of a stroke or observe them in someone else. This is an emergency!
- New symptoms develop after treatment.

Special notes:

_____

_____

_____

More notes on the back of this page ☐

STYE
(Hordeolum)

BASIC INFORMATION

DESCRIPTION
A stye is an infection or inflammation (red, sore, swollen) of the upper or lower eyelid. It is typically harmless. The medical term for stye is hordeolum.

FREQUENT SIGNS AND SYMPTOMS
· A bump on the edge of the eyelid.
· The eyelid area is red, swollen, painful, or tender. The head of the stye is usually on the outside, but it may be on the underside of the lid.
· Eye may be sensitive to bright light.
· A gritty feeling in the eye.
· Eye may water.

CAUSES
Bacterial infection (most often, staphylococcal) in a hair follicle or a gland in the corner of the eye. The infection may be limited to the eyelid or may have spread from somewhere else in the body.

RISK INCREASES WITH
· Having diabetes or other health problem.
· Blepharitis (infection of eyelid margin).
· High cholesterol.
· History of styes.
· Certain chronic skin problems.

PREVENTIVE MEASURES
· Use a mild shampoo on eyelashes when bathing or washing face.
· Don't share eye makeup with anyone.

EXPECTED OUTCOMES
The infection usually heals on its own. It will drain in about two days. Styes often recur, even with treatment.

POSSIBLE COMPLICATIONS
· Spread of infection to other glands in the eyelid.
· Ongoing infection that may not respond to treatment.

DIAGNOSIS & TREATMENT

GENERAL MEASURES
· Use warm-water soaks to relieve pain and inflammation and hasten healing. Apply soaks for 10 minutes, then rest at least 1 hour. Repeat as often as needed.
· Don't squeeze the stye. It will soon open and release the pus, bringing relief from the pain.
· Do not wear contact lenses until the infection is resolved.
· Consult your health care provider if the stye does not drain or is spreading. Your eye will be examined to make sure there is not another eye problem. Sometimes minor surgery to drain the stye or drugs may be needed to help heal the infection.

MEDICATIONS
Antibiotic ointments or creams may be prescribed. Apply according to package instructions.

ACTIVITY
No limits.

DIET
No special diet.

NOTIFY OUR OFFICE IF

· You or a family member has a stye does not drain on its own.
· Pain occurs in the eye.
· Vision changes.

Special notes:

_____

_____

_____

More notes on the back of this page ☐

SUBCONJUNCTIVAL HEMORRHAGE

 ## BASIC INFORMATION

DESCRIPTION
Sudden appearance of blood in the white area of the eye. Although the bleeding may seem alarming, it is not serious. The bleeding is from the thin, clear membrane (conjunctiva) that covers the white of the eye (the sclera). Often, a person discovers the problem after waking up in the morning.

FREQUENT SIGNS AND SYMPTOMS
· A small, usually painless spot of bright red blood in the white of the eye. It may first appear as a patch, but may spread to cover the entire white area of the eye.
· Swelling may occur in that part of the eye.
· There are no vision problems.

CAUSES
When one of the tiny, unseen blood vessels in the conjunctiva breaks, it can bleed and cause the problem. There is often no obvious reason why the vessel breaks. It may follow coughing, sneezing, vomiting, heavy lifting, diving under water, or rubbing of the eyes.

RISK INCREASES WITH
Certain disorders such as high blood pressure, diabetes, or use of blood thinner drugs can be risk factors.

PREVENTIVE MEASURES
No specific preventive measures.

EXPECTED OUTCOMES
The blood will go away by itself. It should be absorbed in 1 to 3 weeks. The blood may change color from red to yellow before disappearing.

POSSIBLE COMPLICATIONS
None expected.

 ## DIAGNOSIS & TREATMENT

GENERAL MEASURES
· No treatment is necessary, except time.
· Cool compresses may be applied at first. After 24 hours, you may use warm compresses applied to the eye to help hasten the removal of the blood.

MEDICATIONS
· Drugs are usually not needed for this disorder.
· Nonprescription artificial tears may help if there is any irritation.

ACTIVITY
No rest is needed and you may continue with your regular activities.

DIET
No special diet.

 ## NOTIFY OUR OFFICE IF

· You or a family member has symptoms of subconjunctival hemorrhage with eye pain, your vision changes, or both eyes are affected.
· Your subconjunctival hemorrhage does not get better within 3 weeks, or it recurs often.

Special notes:

_____

_____

_____

More notes on the back of this page ☐

476

SUBSTANCE ABUSE

BASIC INFORMATION

DESCRIPTION

The continuing misuse of any mind altering substances or chemicals. There is a loss of self-control and a compulsion to continue despite adverse personal, physical, mental, and social outcomes that may result.

FREQUENT SIGNS AND SYMPTOMS

Depends on the substance of abuse. Most produce:
- A temporary pleasant mood.
- Relief from anxiety.
- False feelings of self-confidence and being in control.
- Increased sensitivity to sights and sounds (including hallucinations).
- Altered activity levels—either lethargy and sleeplike states, or frenzied states (being very active).
- Unpleasant or painful symptoms when the abused substance is no longer used (withdrawal).
- Tolerance (need more of the substance to get "high").
- People may observe new and odd behavior changes.

CAUSES

- Substances of abuse may produce addiction or dependence. Common substances of abuse include:
  - Nicotine and alcohol.
  - Marijuana.
  - Amphetamines; barbiturates; cocaine.
  - Opiates. These include codeine, heroin, opium, morphine, methadone, hydrocodone, and oxycodone.
  - Psychedelic or hallucinogenic drugs (club drugs), including PCP ("angel dust"), mescaline, GHB, and LSD.
  - Volatile substances, such as glue, solvents, and paints that are inhaled.
  - Misuse of the cough remedy dextromethorphan.

RISK INCREASES WITH

- Family history of drug or alcohol abuse.
- Family problems (conflict, stress, lack of closeness, poor parenting, loss of job, physical or sexual abuse).
- Genetic factors (may be more prone to addiction).
- Peer pressure, especially in teenagers.
- Fatigue or overwork; problems at work or school.
- Ease of obtaining the substances of abuse.
- Emotional problems, including depression, dependency, poor self-esteem, anxiety, and stress.

PREVENTIVE MEASURES

- Don't socialize with persons who abuse drugs.
- Get medical help for emotional or mental problems.
- Caring parents need to help kids stay drug free.
- Drug education and prevention programs.

EXPECTED OUTCOME

Successful recovery from substance abuse can improve all aspects of one's life. It is not easy, but it can be done.

POSSIBLE COMPLICATIONS

- Accidents, infections and other health problems.
- Loss of job or family. Legal problems.
- Relapse to using substance of abuse.
- Death caused by overdose.

DIAGNOSIS & TREATMENT

GENERAL MEASURES

- Treatment can be voluntary or involuntary. Family, legal, or job factors may lead a person into treatment.
- Your health care provider may do a physical exam. Medical tests may include blood studies and substance abuse screening studies.
- No single treatment works for everyone. A plan needs to address the person's type of abuse, their physical and emotional health, and job, social, and legal aspects. A person is rarely able to quit without some help.
- The plan may require a combination of counseling, drug therapy, other medical services, family therapy, parenting instruction, job training, social and legal services. Treatment may take 3 months, or up to a year.
- Counseling (group or alone) is important in recovery.
- Physical symptoms of withdrawal will be treated.
- You may be monitored for use of the substance of abuse during treatment.
- Join local support group (e.g., Narcotics Anonymous).
- Learn more: National Clearinghouse for Alcohol & Drug Information, (800) 729-6686; website: www.health.org.

MEDICATION

Your health care provider may prescribe drugs to help you through withdrawal symptoms. Other drugs may be prescribed to treat emotional or mental problems.

ACTIVITY

No limits. Try to exercise 20 to 30 minutes every day.

DIET

Eat a normal, well-balanced diet. Take vitamins.

NOTIFY OUR OFFICE IF

- You or a family member has a problem with, or has symptoms of, substance abuse.
- New, unexplained symptoms develop. Drugs used in treatment may produce side effects.

Special notes:

_____

_____

_____

More notes on the back of this page ☐

SUNBURN

 ## BASIC INFORMATION

DESCRIPTION
Redness and soreness of the skin that follows excess exposure to the sun or tanning devices.

FREQUENT SIGNS AND SYMPTOMS
- Sunburn symptoms develop 2 to 4 hours after exposure.
- Red, swollen, and (sometimes) blistered skin. Pain occurs and is worse in the first 6 to 48 hours.
- Fever, nausea, and feeling faint (sometimes).

CAUSES
Melanin, a pigment, in the skin helps to protect the skin from exposure to the ultraviolet light from the sun. When there is overexposure, the melanin is unable to keep up the protection, and sunburn occurs.

RISK INCREASES WITH
- Being of fair skin, blue eyes, and red or blonde hair.
- Exposure to the sun from 10:00 a.m. to 3:00 p.m.
- Certain drugs, soaps, or cosmetics may cause a photosensitive reaction. This causes the skin to be even more sensitive to the sun.

PREVENTIVE MEASURES
- Avoid the sun from noon to 3 p.m. Sunburn can occur even on cloudy days. Ultraviolet light is not blocked by thin clouds on overcast days. It is partially screened by smoke and smog. A great deal of ultraviolet light can reflect from snow, water, sand, and sidewalks.
- Use sunscreen daily. Use products with a sun-protective factor (SPF) of 15 or more. Some of these resist water and perspiration. Reapply them every 2 hours or after swimming. Baby oil, mineral oil, or cocoa butter offer no protection from the sun.
- For the best protection, use a physical barrier agent such as zinc-oxide ointment. Reapply after swimming and at frequent intervals during exposure. Barrier agents are helpful on skin areas that are more likely to burn. These include the nose, ears, backs of the legs, and back of the neck.
- Wear clothing that covers your whole body. Protect your face with a wide-brimmed hat. Wear sunglasses.
- If you feel you must get a tan, do it very gradually.

EXPECTED OUTCOMES
Recovery in 3 days to 3 weeks. Tanning or peeling of the skin usually occurs, depending on how severe the burn was.

POSSIBLE COMPLICATIONS
- Blisters may become infected.
- Years of over-exposure to the sun can lead to wrinkled, saggy and leathery skin. The risk of skin cancer is greatly increased.

 ## DIAGNOSIS & TREATMENT

GENERAL MEASURES
- To reduce heat and pain, dip gauze or towels in cool water and lay these on the burned areas. Take cool showers.
- Soak in a tub of cool water to which an oatmeal product (Aveeno) or baking soda has been added. Pat skin dry, do not rub. Use a moisturizer to keep the skin from feeling dry.
- See your health care provider for severe sunburn or if you have other symptoms such as nausea, vomiting, or swelling. An exam of the affected area will be done and treatment prescribed for any complications.

MEDICATIONS
- Use nonprescription drugs, such as antihistamines, aspirin (not for children), or acetaminophen to help relieve discomfort.
- Ask your health care provider about using nonprescription burn remedies that contain local anesthetics such as benzocaine or lidocaine. They can produce allergic reactions in some persons.
- Drugs for pain or cortisone drugs to use briefly may be prescribed.

ACTIVITY
Rest in any comfortable position until symptoms get better. Cover yourself with an upside-down "cradle" or tent of cardboard or other material. This will keep bed linens off the burned skin.

DIET
No special diet. Increase fluid intake.

 ## NOTIFY OUR OFFICE IF

You or a family member has sunburn that seems severe or there are other symptoms from sun exposure.

Special notes:

_____

_____

_____

More notes on the back of this page ☐

478

SURGICAL WOUND INFECTION

 ## BASIC INFORMATION

DESCRIPTION
Infection that develops after a surgical procedure. Infections after surgery occur in 1.5% to 30% of cases, depending on the type of procedure. The medical term is surgical site infections (SSIs).

FREQUENT SIGNS AND SYMPTOMS
• Symptoms usually begin within 5 to 10 days after surgery, but in some cases, they begin weeks later.
• Pain, redness, and heat around the surgical wound.
• Pus and other collections of fluid around the incision.
• Red streaks in the skin around the wound.
• Fever, chills (sometimes).

CAUSES
Infection with bacteria, including *streptococci*, *staphylococci*, or other germs. These sometimes cause infection, in spite of careful preventive measures.

RISK INCREASES WITH
• Very young and very old persons.
• Poor nutrition (weakness from not being able to eat).
• A pre-existing illness, such as diabetes.
• Weak immune system due to illness or drugs.
• Obese patients.
• Smoking.
• Other infection at the time of surgery.
• Type of surgery being performed.
• Type of surgery wound. It may range from clean to contaminated, depending on several medical factors.
• Increased length of time for the surgery.
• Emergency surgery.

PREVENTIVE MEASURES
• Surgery team members need to follow all medical guidelines for preventing wound infections.
• In some cases, antibiotic drugs may be given to help prevent infections.

EXPECTED OUTCOMES
In most patients, surgical wounds heal in about 2 weeks.

POSSIBLE COMPLICATIONS
• Delayed healing.
• Sepsis (also called blood poisoning) is a bloodstream infection.
• Chronic infection in some patients.

 ## DIAGNOSIS & TREATMENT

GENERAL MEASURES
• Your health care provider will do a physical exam of the surgical wound area. Medical tests may include a culture of pus or blood from the infection site.
• Treatment may include antibiotic drugs and wound-cleaning procedures.
• Surgery to open the wound and remove infected or damage tissue or treat an abscess may be required.
• After treatment, relieve pain with heat. Use a heating pad or warm compress 3 or 4 times a day for 30 to 40 minutes.
• Change wound dressings as directed.

MEDICATIONS
• Antibiotics may be prescribed for an infection. They may be taken by mouth or given intravenously (into a vein).
• Vitamin and mineral supplements to hasten healing.
• Pain relievers. You may use nonprescription drugs, such as acetaminophen, to relieve minor pain.

ACTIVITY
Rest in bed until signs of infection disappear.

DIET
Usually, no special diet required.

 ## NOTIFY OUR OFFICE IF

• You or a family member has symptoms of a surgical-wound infection.
• High fever occurs and a general ill feeling, or infection seems to worsen after treatment.
• New, unexplained symptoms develop. Drugs used in treatment may produce side effects.

Special notes:

_____

_____

_____

More notes on the back of this page ☐

SYPHILIS

 BASIC INFORMATION

DESCRIPTION

A sexually transmitted disease. Syphilis is known as the "great mimic," because its symptoms are like those of many other diseases. There are two types. Congenital form occurs in babies (age 0 to 2 weeks) born to mothers with syphilis. Contagious form is the type that affects persons of all ages and both sexes who get it by sexual contact. There may be no symptoms or very mild ones. A person may not know they are infected.

FREQUENT SIGNS AND SYMPTOMS

• *Primary stage* (contagious; begins 9 to 90 days after exposure; usually at about 3 weeks):
- A painless, red sore (chancre) on the genitals, mouth, or rectum. The sore usually affects the penis in males and vagina or cervix in females.
• *Secondary stage* (occurs if not treated; contagious; begins 2 to 8 weeks after the chancre appears):
- Enlarged lymph glands in the neck, armpit, or groin.
- Headache, sore throat, and feeling tired.
- Rash on skin and mucous membranes of the penis, vagina, or mouth. The rash has small, red, scaly bumps.
- Fever (sometimes).
• *Latent stage or hidden stage* (can be 2 to 30 years after second stage; may be contagious):
- There are no signs or symptoms.
• *Tertiary stage* (rare; not contagious; may appear 2 to 30 years after other stages):
- The infection can seriously damage the heart, brain, nervous system, eyes, skin, bones, and joints.

CAUSES

• A germ (bacteria) called *Treponema pallidum*.
• Contagious form is spread by sexual contact (vaginal, anal, or oral sex) with someone who has the sores or rash. Germs cannot be spread from toilet seats, towels, or other objects.
• Congenital form passes to a baby by infected mother.

RISK INCREASES WITH

Unsafe sex.

PREVENTIVE MEASURES

• Latex male condoms used during sexual contact help stop the risk, but do not provide 100% protection.
• Avoid sexual contact with an infected person or a person whose health history you don't know.
• Obtain blood test for syphilis early in pregnancy. If infected, get treatment right away.

EXPECTED OUTCOMES

Curable with antibiotic treatment.

POSSIBLE COMPLICATIONS

• After penicillin treatment, a Jarisch-Herxheimer reaction may occur. Previous symptoms get worse, but only for about 24 hours.
• Treatment in a few patients may need to be repeated.
• Syphilis sores makes it easier to get an HIV infection.
• Without treatment, the disease may progress to the next stage. A number of medical problems and death may occur with tertiary syphilis.

 DIAGNOSIS & TREATMENT

GENERAL MEASURES

• Your health care provider will do a physical exam. Blood tests and microscope studies of material from a sore are usually done to confirm the diagnosis. Tests for other sexually transmitted diseases are often done.
• Syphilis is treated with drugs.
• Be sure that all your sexual partners obtain treatment. The public health department will help you if needed.
• After drug treatment, blood tests will be done at regular intervals to verify that you are no longer infectious.
• The tertiary stage of syphilis generally requires treatment in a hospital.
• To learn more: Sexually Transmitted Diseases Hotline (800) 227-8922 or the Centers for Disease Control and Prevention (CDC) website: www.cdc.gov.

MEDICATIONS

Penicillin will be given by injection for all stages. If someone is allergic to penicillin, other antibiotics can be equally effective.

ACTIVITY

Avoid sexual intercourse until cured.

DIET

No special diet.

 NOTIFY OUR OFFICE IF

• You or a family member has symptoms of syphilis.
• The following occur during or after treatment: fever, skin rash, sore throat, or swelling in any joint, such as the ankle or knee.
• You have had sexual contact with someone who has syphilis.

Special notes:

_____

_____

_____

More notes on the back of this page ☐

480

TAPEWORM

BASIC INFORMATION

DESCRIPTION

A parasitic infection of the digestive tract or other organs. Tapeworms are typically acquired from eating undercooked meat or fish.

FREQUENT SIGNS AND SYMPTOMS

- Most people with this problem have no symptoms.
- Pain in the upper abdomen.
- Diarrhea.
- Unexplained weight loss.
- Symptoms of anemia (weakness, fatigue, and shortness of breath).
- Bowel movements containing worm eggs and worm body parts.

CAUSES

- Parasites: *Taenia saginata* from beef, *Taenia solium* from pork, and *Diphyllobothrium* from fish. People become infected by eating improperly cooked or raw food infected with the parasite.
- *Echinococcus* tapeworm is found in dogs and some livestock (often in sheep). Humans can get an infection (echinococcosis) from this tapeworm. Infected dogs leave feces in soil or water. Humans are infected by eating food grown in the soil or drinking the water. It can also be spread by handling an infected dog or livestock. The infection causes cysts (sores), usually in the liver. Symptoms may not develop for 10 to 20 years after exposure.

RISK INCREASES WITH

Travel to places such as Asia, Africa, or Latin America. This disorder is uncommon in the United States.

PREVENTIVE MEASURES

- Cook beef, pork, and fish thoroughly. Additional information available from the National Center for Nutrition (800) 366-1655 or the Department of Agriculture Meat and Poultry Hotline (800) 535-4555.
- Buy only meat that has been inspected.
- Wash your hands after handling any raw meat or fish.
- Keep pet dogs clean and dewormed. Wash hands after handling pets or livestock.

EXPECTED OUTCOMES

Usually curable with appropriate treatment.

POSSIBLE COMPLICATIONS

- Cysticercosis, a more widespread infection from tapeworm larvae (rare).
- Obstruction of intestine (rare).
- Echinococcosis can cause severe health problems including death.

DIAGNOSIS & TREATMENT

GENERAL MEASURES

- Your health care provider may do a physical exam. Medical tests usually include a study of a stool sample to check for eggs or worms. If echinococcosis is suspected, an x-ray or blood study may be done.
- The usual treatment is with drugs.
- Cysts from echinococcosis infection may need to be removed surgically.
- Have all family members examined for possible infection.

MEDICATIONS

Anthelmintic drug to kill the parasite. The drug can cure with a single dose. Medical tests should be repeated in 3 to 6 weeks to make sure the disorder is cured.

ACTIVITY

No limits.

DIET

No special diet.

NOTIFY OUR OFFICE IF

- You or a family member has symptoms of a tapeworm.
- New, unexplained symptoms develop. Drugs used in treatment may produce side effects.

Special notes:

_____

_____

_____

More notes on the back of this page ☐

TAY-SACHS DISEASE

 BASIC INFORMATION

DESCRIPTION

An inherited, rare disorder of the central nervous system in infants and young children. The classic form causes progressive impairment and early death. Less than 100 children are born with the disease each year in the United States.

FREQUENT SIGNS AND SYMPTOMS

• The child seems normal at birth. Symptoms begin to appear before 6 months.
• Loss of alertness and retarded mental development.
• Loss of muscle strength, such as difficulty sitting up or turning over.
• Deafness.
• Blindness.
• Severe constipation caused by an impaired nerve supply to the colon.
• Seizures.

CAUSES

• An inherited disease resulting from a recessive gene that causes enzyme deficiency. If both parents have the gene, they have a 25% chance of having a child with Tay-Sachs disease. If only one parent is a carrier, the children will not have the disease. The gene occurs in 1 out of 60 people of Ashkenazi Jewish or French Canadian ancestry.
• Other forms of Tay-Sachs include:
  - Juvenile form which appears about ages 2 to 5. Symptoms are like the classic form and death occurs by age 15.
  - Chronic form may appear at age 5. Symptoms are like the classic form but are milder.
  - Adult form, which appears between teens and 30s. Symptoms are like chronic the form.

RISK INCREASES WITH

Genetic factors. Many parents who carry the recessive gene are of Eastern European Jewish (Ashkenazi) or French Canadian origin.

PREVENTIVE MEASURES

• A simple blood test can identify Tay-Sachs carriers. It can not be used in pregnant women. For pregnant women, an amniocentesis or chorionic villus testing can be done.
• Obtain genetic counseling if you or your spouse have a family history of Tay-Sachs or are of Ashkenazi or French Canadian background.
• Assisted reproductive technologies can be used to help at-risk couples have a non-affected baby.

EXPECTED OUTCOMES

There is no cure or treatment. Death usually occurs before age 5 with the classic form. Research is ongoing.

POSSIBLE COMPLICATIONS

Symptoms progress to loss of all voluntary movement, which eventually causes death.

 DIAGNOSIS & TREATMENT

GENERAL MEASURES

• To make the diagnosis, your baby's health care provider will do a physical exam and an eye exam. A cherry-red spot at the back of the eye occurs in a baby with Tay-Sachs disease. A blood test will be done to confirm the diagnosis.
• Treatment consists of providing comfort and support for the baby.
• Counseling may help parents and siblings to learn to cope with the distress produced by this condition.
• Seek out support groups for families of Tay-Sachs victims.
• To learn more: National Tay-Sachs and Allied Disease Association, 2001 Beacon St., Suite 204, Brookline, MA 02146; (800) 906-8723; website: www.ntsad.org.

MEDICATIONS

• Anticonvulsants to control seizures.
• Stool softeners and laxatives to relieve constipation.
• Other drugs to help with complications as they arise.

ACTIVITY

In the early stages, encourage the child to be as active as possible. Increasing loss of mental, nervous, and muscular functions will eventually confine the child to bed much of the time.

DIET

Provide plenty of fluids and a normal, high-fiber diet to reduce constipation. Feeding by tube usually becomes necessary as the disease progresses.

 NOTIFY OUR OFFICE IF

• You are concerned about your infant's mental and physical development.
• You think you or any member of your family carries the abnormal gene. A genetic counselor can advise you on how to prevent having children with this disease.

Special notes:

_____

_____

_____

More notes on the back of this page ☐

TEAR DUCT INFECTION OR
BLOCKAGE (Dacryocystitis or Dacryostenosis)

 ## BASIC INFORMATION

DESCRIPTION

An infected or blocked tear duct causes tears to gather or pool in the eyes and then run down the cheeks even though the person is not crying. Infection of the tear duct is called dacryocystitis. It occurs in all ages, but it is most common in children. A blocked tear duct is called dacryostenosis. It may occur in infants at 3 to 12 weeks of age or in older children and adults.

FREQUENT SIGNS AND SYMPTOMS

- Increased tearing of one or both eyes.
- Mucus and pus drains out of the tear duct. It may drain on its own or come out when pressure is put on the area.
- Pain, redness, or swelling of the eye area.
- Fever (sometimes).

CAUSES

Tears are stored in a sac (lacrimal sac) and are released into the eyes to help keep them clean, for protection, and to provide lubrication. The tears drain out of the eyes through small pinpoint openings in the corner of the eyes. They then flow through a duct or tube into the nose. The duct is called the nasolacrimal duct. When infection or blockage occurs in the duct, the tears can not drain normally and they back up.

RISK INCREASES WITH

- Tear duct is not fully developed or formed properly in a newborn.
- Bacterial infection of the duct.
- Sinus or nasal infection, or abnormal growths or tumors.
- Surgery on the face, nose, or sinuses.
- Eye injury.
- Conjunctivitis (pink eye).
- Fracture of the nose or facial bones.
- Thickening of the tear duct lining as a person ages.

PREVENTIVE MEASURES

No specific preventive measures. Always get prompt medical treatment for eye, nose, or sinus infections. For contact sports, wear helmets and facemasks to protect the face from injury.

EXPECTED OUTCOMES

Infected or blocked tear ducts are usually cured with treatment. Blocked tear ducts in an infant are usually outgrown when they are 9 to 12 months of age.

POSSIBLE COMPLICATIONS

A blocked tear duct may cause chronic infection. Minor surgery is sometimes needed.

 ## DIAGNOSIS & TREATMENT

GENERAL MEASURES

- Your health care provider will do a physical exam of the eye area. A sample of the discharge may be tested to check for the germs causing the infection. To confirm the diagnosis, a harmless dye may be placed in the eye. This helps determine if tears are flowing normally. Other tests may be needed in adults.
- Treatment may involve drugs for infection, massaging the area, and, for some, surgery to open the duct. In some cases, no treatment is needed.
- Clean any drainage from the eye with a cotton ball or washcloth moistened with warm water. Gently wipe away any pus or crusted areas.
- For a child with a blocked duct, massage can help. Do it several times a day for 2 months, or as directed. Wash your hands carefully. Place your index finger along side the nose and firmly massage down toward the corner of the nose. Use a warm compress on the eye area to provide comfort and promote drainage.
- If there is excessive tearing, surgery may be recommended to probe the tear duct. A thin wire is passed through the duct to open any obstruction.
- Other surgery options involve placing tubes in the tear duct that stay in for about 6 months or inserting a balloon to stretches the tear duct and then is removed.
- In adults, tear ducts damaged by chronic infection may need to be surgically replaced by creating a new passage or inserting an artificial duct. Tumors or nasal polyps may need to be removed with surgery.

MEDICATIONS

Antibiotics for infection may be prescribed. These may be eyedrops, eye ointment, or drugs taken by mouth.

ACTIVITY

No limits unless advised by your health care provider.

DIET

No special diet.

 ## NOTIFY OUR OFFICE IF

- You or a family member has symptoms of a tear duct infection or blockage.
- Symptoms don't improve or vision changes.

Special notes:

_____

_____

_____

More notes on the back of this page ☐

TEETHING
(Cutting Teeth; Tooth Eruption)

 BASIC INFORMATION

DESCRIPTION
The process of the appearance of baby teeth and adult teeth. New teeth erupt continually from around age 6 months to 3 years. Between ages 6 and 12, children lose baby teeth, which are replaced with adult teeth. On average, the first set of teeth is complete soon after the second birthday.

FREQUENT SIGNS AND SYMPTOMS
- Excess saliva production, drooling, and chewing on anything the baby can hold.
- Pain. (This symptom cannot be proven, but probably does occur.)
- Gums may become red or swollen.
- Irritability.
- Fretful and clinging.
- Difficulty in sleeping.
- Crying more than usual.
- Teething should never be considered the cause of fever, vomiting, diarrhea, prolonged loss of appetite, earache, convulsions, cough, or diaper rash. These are symptoms of an illness.

CAUSES
Teething is normal. There are 20 baby (or primary) teeth and 32 permanent teeth.

RISK INCREASES WITH
Teething problems are not related to any known risk factor.

PREVENTIVE MEASURES
- Teething problems cannot be prevented, but the symptoms can be relieved.
- The timing of teeth eruption is highly variable. However, the sequence of normal tooth eruption in children is:
   - First teeth (lower front teeth) at about 6 months, sooner in girls than boys. Teething may start as early as one month or as late as one year. Rarely, a baby is born with one or more teeth.
   - Complete set of baby teeth by about age two and a half.
   - First adult teeth at about age 6.
   - Bicuspids (side teeth) between ages 10 and 12.
   - Permanent molars at about age 12.

EXPECTED OUTCOMES
Teething discomfort can be partially relieved.

POSSIBLE COMPLICATIONS
None expected.

 DIAGNOSIS & TREATMENT

GENERAL MEASURES
- Your baby's health care provider will examine the baby's mouth and gums and any new teeth at well-baby check ups. Follow any special instructions.
- Rub the child's gums with a clean finger; this is very comforting.
- Freeze a wet washcloth for the baby to chew on.
- Offer the child a safe, one-piece teething ring. It can be cooled in the refrigerator (don't freeze the ring).
- Don't put anything into the baby's mouth that might cause choking. Don't tie anything around the neck.
- Sucking a thumb, finger, or pacifier will not harm the baby's teeth. If sucking continues after age four, talk to your child's dentist to see if there are any concerns.
- Clean new teeth and gums with your finger using a soft washcloth. When the teeth are bigger, start brushing them with a baby's toothbrush.
- Begin regular dental visits at about age one.
- At age five, explain to the child that losing baby teeth is normal. This prevents the child from becoming concerned when tooth loss begins.

MEDICATIONS
- Medicine is not usually needed for teething.
- Your baby's health care provider may suggest:
   - Acetaminophen for the pain.
   - A cream or ointment rubbed on the gums to ease discomfort.

ACTIVITY
No limits.

DIET
- Don't let your baby go to bed or walk around with a bottle with milk in it. Milk that stays in contact with the teeth for a long time can cause decay.
- Start your baby or toddler off to a healthy diet that will promote healthy teeth. Avoid too many sweets, sticky foods, or constant snacks during the day.

 NOTIFY OUR OFFICE IF

- Your child's temperature rises above normal.
- Signs of infection such as pain, pus, a lot of swelling, or very red gums occur.

Special notes:

_____

_____

_____

More notes on the back of this page ☐

TEMPOROMANDIBULAR JOINT (TMJ) DISORDER

BASIC INFORMATION

DESCRIPTION

Pain in the temporomandibular joint. This is the joint on either side of the lower jaw that opens and closes the mouth. The disorder affects adults of both sexes, but it is more common in women.

FREQUENT SIGNS AND SYMPTOMS

· Symptoms may come on slowly; they may begin suddenly if there is an injury to the area.
· Dull, aching pain on one side of the jaw. It occurs below or in front of the ear, in the temples, in back of the head, and along the jaw line.
· It may hurt to chew.
· "Clicking" or "popping" joint sounds.
· Unable to open the jaw all the way or rarely, jaw may "lock" in open position.
· Headache, dizziness, and toothache.
· Ears feel pressured, clogged, aching, or you may hear ringing.
· Tired facial muscles from yawning, speaking, or when waking up. Head, shoulder, and neck muscles may ache.

CAUSES

Normally the jaw, the skull, the muscles that attach to and move the jaw, and the involved nerves work together in a smooth relationship. For a variety of reasons, an imbalance occurs in the way one or more of these parts function. This brings about the symptoms.

RISK INCREASES WITH

· Physical and emotional stress.
· Joint is affected by jaw, head, or neck injuries.
· Grinding or clenching teeth (sometimes during sleep).
· Chewing gum or biting nails.
· Tension of the masticatory (chewing) muscles.
· Faulty alignment ("bite") between the upper and lower jaws (disk derangement).
· Osteoarthritis, rheumatoid arthritis, or gout.
· Work habits such as holding a phone between shoulder and ear.

PREVENTIVE MEASURES

No specific preventive measures. Avoid risk factors where possible.

EXPECTED OUTCOMES

The symptoms often clear up on their own in about 2 weeks. In most other cases, simple treatment measures can relieve symptoms.

POSSIBLE COMPLICATIONS

· Arthritis of the joint.
· Chronic pain of the face.

DIAGNOSIS & TREATMENT

GENERAL MEASURES

· Your health care provider will do a physical exam of the jaw area and ask questions about your symptoms and habits. Medical tests may include jaw range-of-motion studies, x-rays, and others.
· Treatment plans may include lifestyle changes, drugs for pain, diet changes, and simple jaw exercises. For tooth or denture problems, see a dental care provider.
· Try to limit jaw movements and learn to relax the jaw. Don't open it wide. Block a yawn by putting your fist under your chin. Don't chew gum.
· Ice and/or heat may be of benefit in relieving discomfort. Try one and then the other to see what works best for you. Massage the TMJ muscle area.
· Counseling may be helpful for stress problems.
· Simple jaw exercises may help. You will be instructed on how to do stretching and relaxing exercises.
· You may be fitted with a special splint or biteplate that will help reduce clenching or teeth grinding.
· A procedure to wash out the joint or inject pain drugs may be done in a medical office with local anesthesia.
· Severe cases that do not respond to simpler measures may need surgery to reconstruct the joint (rare).
· To learn more: TMJ Association, PO Box 26770, Milwaukee, WI 53226; (414) 259-3223 (not toll free); website: www.tmj.org.

MEDICATIONS

· For pain and inflammation, use nonprescription drugs such as aspirin (not for children) or ibuprofen.
· Muscle relaxants, drugs for pain, or steroids may be prescribed for a short time.

ACTIVITY

No limits.

DIET

Eat a soft diet until symptoms improve. Avoid hard, chewy foods such as bagels.

NOTIFY OUR OFFICE IF

· You or a family member has symptoms of temporomandibular joint disorder.
· Symptoms do not improve with treatment.

Special notes:

_____

_____

_____

More notes on the back of this page ☐

TENDINITIS & TENOSYNOVITIS

 BASIC INFORMATION

DESCRIPTION
Inflammation of a tendon (tendinitis) and the lining of the tendon sheath (tenosynovitis). They often occur at the same time. Tendons are made up of tough, fibrous, cord-like tissue. A typical skeletal muscle has a tendon on each end that attaches to the bone.

FREQUENT SIGNS AND SYMPTOMS
· Limited movement, tenderness, pain, and swelling around the inflamed tendon. Common sites are the shoulder, elbow, Achilles' tendon (heel), or hamstring.
· Weakness in the tendon caused by calcium deposits that often accompany tendinitis.

CAUSES
Inflammation or a small tear in a tendon. The tendons become inflamed for a variety of reasons. Inflammation is a reaction of the body's tissues to injury, infection, or irritation. The four signs of inflammation are redness, swelling, heat, and pain.

RISK INCREASES WITH
· Injury or overuse, usually from an athletic activity, exercising, or during work.
· Incorrect movement and strain during activity. For example, repeatedly holding and swinging a tennis racket incorrectly may cause tendinitis at the elbow (tennis elbow).
· Certain joint diseases (rheumatoid arthritis, scleroderma, gout, and Reiter's disease).
· Aging (tendons are more prone to injury).

PREVENTIVE MEASURES
· Gradually build up the intensity and frequency of an activity.
· Avoid overuse of muscles and tendons. Maintain strength and flexibility. Warm up before each workout and stretch afterwards.
· Learn the proper techniques for any exercise or sport you intend to do regularly.
· Wear proper gear for any sport or exercise activity including well-fitting shoes.

EXPECTED OUTCOMES
Usually curable with treatment and rest of the affected tendon area. Pain and swelling usually decrease in a few days. Allow 6 weeks for complete healing.

POSSIBLE COMPLICATIONS
· Chronic disability.
· Tendon rupture.
· Frozen shoulder.

 DIAGNOSIS & TREATMENT

GENERAL MEASURES
· Many cases of tendinitis are self-treated.
· See your health care provider if symptoms persist or are more severe. A physical exam of the affected area will be done and questions asked about your symptoms and activities. X-rays do not show tendon problems, but they may be done if an injury occurred.
· Treatment may involve rest, ice or heat, drugs, range-of-motion exercises, and steps to prevent recurrence.
· When resting, sleeping, or sitting, place the injured area on a pillow—at or above heart level.
· Wrap the area in a compressive (Ace) bandage to reduce swelling.
· Apply ice packs to the affected area. Do this several times a day for the first 24 to 48 hours. Then, apply them twice a day until pain is gone. You can apply heat if it feels good. Take hot showers, soak in a warm bath, apply warm compresses, or use a heating pad.
· You may want to use a sling or splint for an arm or shoulder to limit movement. Use crutches, a cane or a brace, for affected leg, knee, or heel if needed.
· Surgery may be recommended in chronic tendinitis. Physical therapy helps to regain strength and flexibility.

MEDICATIONS
· Use nonprescription nonsteroidal anti-inflammatory drugs and pain relievers such as ibuprofen.
· Steroid injection for painful tendons may be prescribed. This reduces pain and inflammation and allows movement. Injections are done just a few times because steroids can weaken the tendon.

ACTIVITY
· Resume normal activities as symptoms improve.
· After a few days, begin range-of-motion exercises to prevent stiffness in the area. Do them 3 to 4 times a day.

DIET
No special diet.

 NOTIFY OUR OFFICE IF

· You or a family member has symptoms of tendinitis.
· Pain and swelling increase despite treatment.

Special notes:

_____

_____

_____

More notes on the back of this page ☐

TENNIS ELBOW
(Epicondylitis, Lateral)

BASIC INFORMATION

DESCRIPTION

Inflammation of the tendons on the outside of the elbow at the epicondyle. The epicondyle is the bony area on the outside of the elbow. This is where muscles of the forearm attach to the bone of the upper arm. When the muscles and bones of the elbow are involved as well as the tendons, it is called epicondylitis.

FREQUENT SIGNS AND SYMPTOMS

- Pain and tenderness over the bony part of the elbow.
- Unable to straighten the arm completely.
- Stiffness in elbow in the morning.
- Pain when bending or twisting the hand and arm.
- Weak grip (even when grabbing a light object such as a coffee cup).

CAUSES

The tendon becomes inflamed due to a variety of reasons. Small tears in the tendon may lead to the problem. Inflammation is a reaction of the body's tissues to injury, infection, or irritation. The four signs of inflammation are redness, swelling, heat, and pain.

RISK INCREASES WITH

- Work or activity that requires repetitive forearm movement such as hedge clipping or tennis.
- Work or activity that requires excessive, constant gripping or squeezing.
- Poor physical condition.
- Sudden strain on the forearm.

PREVENTIVE MEASURES

- Don't play sports, such as tennis, for long periods until you are in good condition. Learn proper playing techniques. Tennis racquets can aggravate tennis elbow. Choosing a different size or type (larger, more flexible, larger grip) may help.
- For work or sports activity requiring elbow movement, warm up the arm for 5 to 10 minutes. Take frequent breaks. Use ice pack on elbow if pain develops.
- Do flexibility and strength exercises for the arm and elbow.

EXPECTED OUTCOMES

Usually curable, but it takes time. Healing may require 3 to 6 months or longer.

POSSIBLE COMPLICATIONS

- Recurrence of tennis elbow.
- Rarely, surgery may be needed for some patients.

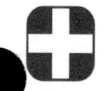

DIAGNOSIS & TREATMENT

GENERAL MEASURES

- Mild cases may be self-treated if desired.

- See your health care provider if symptoms persist or are more severe. A physical exam of the affected area will be done and questions asked about your symptoms and activities. X-rays do not show tendon problems, but they may be done if an injury occurred.
- Treatment may involve rest, ice or heat, massage, drugs, exercises, and steps to prevent recurrence.
- When resting, sleeping, or sitting, place the injured area on a pillow—at or above heart level.
- Wrap the thickest portion of the forearm in a compressive (Ace) bandage to reduce swelling. Massage the area several times a day.
- Apply ice packs to the affected area (several times a day) for the first 24 to 48 hours. Then, apply heat if it feels good. Take hot showers, soak in a bath, apply hot compresses, or a heating pad.
- You may need to wear a forearm splint to immobilize the elbow. Do the following exercise 3 or 4 times a day while wearing the splint. Stretch your arm, flex your wrist, and then press the back of your hand against a wall. Hold for 1 minute.
- Surgery possibly (if other methods of treatment fail).

MEDICATIONS

- Use nonprescription nonsteroidal anti-inflammatory drugs and pain relievers such as ibuprofen or aspirin (not for children).
- Steroid injection for painful tendons may be prescribed. This reduces pain and inflammation and allows movement. Injections are done just a few times as steroids can weaken the tendon.

ACTIVITY

Don't repeat the activity that caused tennis elbow until symptoms clear up. Stretching and strength exercises are often prescribed to do at home. Do them daily or as directed.

DIET

No special diet.

NOTIFY OUR OFFICE IF

- You or a family member has symptoms of tennis elbow.
- Symptoms don't improve in 2 weeks with treatment.

Special notes:

_____

_____

_____

More notes on the back of this page ☐

TESTICLE TORSION

 BASIC INFORMATION

DESCRIPTION

Twisting of the spermatic cord of the testicle. This may damage the testicle. Testicle torsion usually occurs on one side only. Prompt treatment is necessary to save the affected testicle. It affects males of all ages, but it is most common in ages 12 to 20.

FREQUENT SIGNS AND SYMPTOMS

· Sudden pain in one testicle. it often starts in the night. Some prior pain may have been felt off and on, but it went away on its own.
· Swelling, redness, and tenderness of the scrotum.
· Nausea and vomiting.
· Sweating.
· Fever (sometimes).

CAUSES

Usually unknown. It may be a problem of weak connective tissue whereby the testicle is not attached firmly within the scrotum. The testicle is more movable and more likely to become twisted.

RISK INCREASES WITH

· Undescended testicles.
· Trauma to the scrotum.
· Strenuous exercise.

PREVENTIVE MEASURES

No specific preventive measures. Wear an athletic supporter or cup when participating in contact sports to prevent genital injury.

EXPECTED OUTCOMES

Curable with prompt diagnosis and treatment.

POSSIBLE COMPLICATIONS

· The testicle is usually injured beyond repair unless surgery is done within about 6 hours after symptoms begin. If one testicle must be removed, the remaining healthy testicle should provide enough hormones for normal male growth, sex life, and fertility.
· Infection in the scrotum and testicle.

 DIAGNOSIS & TREATMENT

GENERAL MEASURES

· Your health care provider will do a physical exam of the scrotum area and ask questions about your symptoms and activities. Medical tests may be done to confirm the diagnosis.
· Immediate surgery is the usual treatment.
· In some cases, gentle manipulation by hand may undo the twisting. This is a temporary measure and is usually followed up with surgery to stop recurrence.
· Surgery is done to untangle the twisted spermatic cord. The affected testicle is attached to the inside scrotal wall, which prevents recurrence. The surgery will probably also include treatment on the unaffected testicle to prevent torsion.
· After surgery, use ice packs to relieve pain and swelling. Wrap the ice in plastic. Apply it to the affected side, separating the ice from the skin with a cloth towel. Apply ice 5 to 10 minutes at a time. Repeat as often as necessary.

MEDICATIONS

After surgery, pain relievers may be prescribed.

ACTIVITY

Resume your normal activities gradually after surgery.

DIET

No special diet.

 NOTIFY OUR OFFICE IF

· You or a family member has symptoms of testicular torsion. This is an emergency!
· Signs of infection begin after surgery. These include fever, chills, muscle aches, headache, dizziness, and a general ill feeling.
· Excessive bleeding occurs at the surgical site.

Special notes:

_____

_____

_____

More notes on the back of this page ☐

TESTICLE, UNDESCENDED
(Cryptorchidism)

BASIC INFORMATION

DESCRIPTION
While in the uterus, a baby boy's testicles grow in his abdomen and then move down (descend) into his scrotum. Sometimes at birth, one or both testicles have not descended into the scrotum. Over 3% of full-term newborn males, and 30% of premature newborn males have undescended testes. The medical term for the condition is cryptorchidism.

FREQUENT SIGNS AND SYMPTOMS
One or both testicles can't be felt in the normal position in the scrotum. "Testes" is another name for testicles.

CAUSES
Unknown. It may be related to a hormone deficiency in the mother or fetus.

RISK INCREASES WITH
· Family history of undescended testicle.
· Premature birth.
· Low birth weight.

PREVENTIVE MEASURES
No specific preventive measures.

EXPECTED OUTCOMES
Most testicles will descend without treatment by 3 to 6 months of age. If they remain undescended, treatment can usually correct the problem.

POSSIBLE COMPLICATIONS
· Inguinal hernia (weak area in wall of abdomen where intestines may protrude).
· Increased risk of testicular cancer as an adult.
· Sterility or reduced fertility rate.
· Emotional problems, about the physical appearance of an empty scrotum, may develop as a boy gets older.
· Testicular torsion (twisting).

DIAGNOSIS & TREATMENT

GENERAL MEASURES
· Your child's health care provider will do a physical exam. One or both testicles will not be in the scrotum, but they can often be felt above it. If they cannot be located, medical testing may be needed. Follow-up exams are done to check if they have descended.
· If the testicle lies in the scrotum at times and then occasionally retracts, the problem normally resolves itself by puberty. No treatment is needed.
· Surgery (called orchiopexy) to move the testicles into the scrotum is usually recommended. Surgery is normally performed between 6 and 24 months of age and is successful in most cases. Your child may have the surgery, which takes about one hour, and go home the same day. Follow-up care instructions will be provided.
· In cases where a testicle is missing or cannot be moved surgically, artificial ones (implants) are available.
· Adult men with undescended testicles may have them removed or left in place. Your health care provider will discuss options with you.

MEDICATIONS
· Hormone therapy may be prescribed in some cases. It helps increase male hormones, which may cause the testicles to descend.
· Pain relief drugs may be prescribed following surgery.

ACTIVITY
No limits, except those following surgery.

DIET
No special diet.

 NOTIFY OUR OFFICE IF

Your child has undescended testicle. Call as soon as you find symptoms of this problem.

Special notes:

_____

_____

_____

More notes on the back of this page ☐

TESTICULAR CANCER

 ## BASIC INFORMATION

DESCRIPTION
Growth of malignant cells in the testicle. Testicles are the male sex glands and are located in the scrotum. This cancer can affect all ages, but it is found more often in ages 18 to 32. It is the most common form of cancer in young men.

FREQUENT SIGNS AND SYMPTOMS
- A firm swelling in one testicle discovered by accident or by self-examination.
- No pain (90% of cases).
- Sense of fullness in the scrotum.
- A rarer type of the cancer may cause breast tenderness or swelling and loss of sexual desire.
- If cancer has spread, there may be back or chest pain, cough, and shortness of breath.

CAUSES
Unknown. There are several types of testicular cancer depending on the cells where it develops. The most common type is called germ cell. It develops in cells that produce sperm. Rarely are both testicles affected.

RISK INCREASES WITH
- Undescended testicles in infancy even if the testicle was surgically moved into the scrotum.
- Caucasian race.
- Being a younger male. Men over age 40 are less likely to get this form of cancer.
- Personal or family history of testicular cancer.
- Klinefelter's syndrome (a congenital disorder).
- Testicles that did not develop normally.

PREVENTIVE MEASURES
Males should examine testicles routinely at least once a month. This will not prevent the cancer, but the self-exam may detect a tumor early enough for effective treatment. Your health care provider can give you instructions on how to do a self-exam.

EXPECTED OUTCOMES
Most types of testicular tumors are curable with early diagnosis and treatment. Removal of one testicle does not interfere with normal sexual function or the ability to have children.

POSSIBLE COMPLICATIONS
- Without treatment, cancer may spread to other places in the body.
- Cancer recurs or develops in the other testicle.
- Patient is more at risk for other forms of cancer.

 ## DIAGNOSIS & TREATMENT

GENERAL MEASURES
- Your health care provider will do a physical exam of the genital area. Different medical tests are usually done to verify the diagnosis and to determine if cancer has spread (called staging).
- Treatment often involves surgery (called orchidectomy) to remove the cancerous testicle. Radiation therapy and/or chemotherapy (anticancer drugs) may be prescribed depending on the type and stage of the cancer. Bone marrow transplantation is a newer form of treatment.
- Some patients may want to arrange to have their sperm frozen in a sperm bank before treatment. This will allow them to produce children (if fertility is lost).
- Testicular prosthesis (implants) may be a choice of some patients after surgery. They are made of saline and are implanted in the scrotum to look and feel natural.
- To learn more: American Cancer Society, (800) ACS-2345; website: www.cancer.org or National Cancer Institute, (800) 4-CANCER; website: www.nci.nih.gov.

MEDICATIONS
- Chemotherapy may be prescribed.
- Pain medicine if needed.

ACTIVITY
- Resume your normal activities as soon as possible. Radiation and chemotherapy may cause temporary fatigue requiring extra rest.
- Resume sexual relations when you are able.

DIET
No special diet.

 ## NOTIFY OUR OFFICE IF

- You have a firm swelling or mass in the scrotum.
- New, unexplained symptoms develop due to a treatment procedure.

Special notes:

_____

_____

_____

More notes on the back of this page ☐

TETANUS
(Lockjaw)

 ## BASIC INFORMATION

DESCRIPTION
An infection in a wound that causes severe muscle spasms and can lead to death. Tetanus cannot be spread from person to person. It is now rare, due to tetanus immunization.

FREQUENT SIGNS AND SYMPTOMS
- Stiffness of the jaw.
- Muscle pain and frequent, severe spasms.
- Headache.
- Sore throat and difficulty in swallowing.
- Difficulty using chest muscles to breathe.
- Fast pulse.
- Profuse sweating.
- Stiff neck, arms, and legs.

CAUSES
Bacteria (*Clostridium tetani*) that are present almost everywhere, especially in soil, manure, or dust. Bacteria may enter through any break in the skin, including burns or puncture wounds. The wound can be tiny such as with a splinter. Toxins produced by the bacteria travel to nerves that control muscle contraction, producing muscle spasms and seizures.

RISK INCREASES WITH
- Lack of up-to-date tetanus immunization.
- Newborn infants born to non-immunized mothers.
- Use of street drugs with unclean needles and syringes.
- Burns, surgical wounds, and skin ulcers.
- Outdoor work or outdoor sports activity.

PREVENTIVE MEASURES
- Obtain tetanus vaccination. It is given in a series of shots in combination with a diphtheria and pertussis vaccine in children. Booster shots are recommended every 10 years thereafter.
- An additional booster shot may be needed at the time of an injury.

EXPECTED OUTCOMES
With early diagnosis and treatment, full recovery is likely in mild or moderate tetanus. Allow 4 weeks for recovery. The death rate from severe tetanus is about 50%.

POSSIBLE COMPLICATIONS
- Pneumonia.
- High blood pressure.
- Severe pain with muscle spasms.
- Irregular heartbeat.
- Bone fractures.
- Coma.
- Infection.
- Brain damage.
- Respiratory paralysis and death.

 ## DIAGNOSIS & TREATMENT

GENERAL MEASURES
- Your health care provider will do a physical exam and ask questions about your symptoms and activities. Medical tests may include blood and culture studies.
- Hospital care is required. A quiet, dark room may be recommended. Treatment may include the use of breathing tubes, a respirator (machine to help breathing), intravenous (IV) fluid support, and drugs.
- Surgery to remove infected tissue may be needed.

MEDICATIONS
You may be given:
- Antitoxins to neutralize the nerve toxin.
- Muscle relaxants to control spasms.
- Sedatives to relieve anxiety.
- Anticonvulsants.
- Antibiotics.
- Tetanus combination vaccine.

ACTIVITY
During hospital time, bed rest is needed with as little disturbance as possible. During recovery, activities should be resumed gradually.

DIET
Intravenous (IV) fluids will be needed because of difficulty in swallowing.

 ## NOTIFY OUR OFFICE IF

- You or a family member has symptoms of tetanus or observes them in someone else. Call immediately. This is an emergency!
- You or someone in your family needs basic or booster tetanus immunizations.
- You have a puncture wound or injury that breaks the skin, and you have not had an immunization or booster in 5 years.

Special notes:

_____

_____

_____

More notes on the back of this page ☐

THORACIC OUTLET SYNDROME (TOS)

 BASIC INFORMATION

DESCRIPTION
Thoracic outlet syndrome (TOS) is a general term used to describe symptoms that occur due to pressure on nerves and blood vessels in the neck area. The thoracic outlet is a space between the rib cage and the collarbone.

FREQUENT SIGNS AND SYMPTOMS
· Numbness, tingling, or prickling feelings in the neck, shoulders, arms, and hands.
· There may be no pain or mild to more severe pain.
· Weakness and tiredness in the arms and hands.
· Poor blood flow that causes coldness, swelling, and blueness in the hands and fingers (rare).
· Sense of touch may be lost.

CAUSES
Nerves and blood vessels that supply the shoulder, arms, and hands begin in the neck. They then pass as a bundle near the cervical ribs and collarbone. Pressure on this nerve and blood vessel bundle creates symptoms. There are multiple problems that can lead to the pressure.

RISK INCREASES WITH
· An extra rib in the body. It may have fiber-like bands attached to it.
· Overextending arm or shoulder or repeated overhead arm movements. This may be due to work activities or exercise.
· Carrying heavy loads.
· Fracture of clavicle (collarbone) or first rib.
· Muscle weakness and drooping shoulders or head.
· Tumor or blood clots.
· Other health or emotional disorders may make a person more at risk for TOS.

PREVENTIVE MEASURES
No specific preventive measures. Try to avoid repetitive arm and shoulder activities and overhead arm tasks. Exercise daily to maintain good physical fitness.

EXPECTED OUTCOMES
Symptoms can be relieved in most patients with treatment.

POSSIBLE COMPLICATIONS
· Problem can recur.
· If surgery is performed, it may have complications.
· Chronic pain syndrome, disability, and depression may occur in some patients.
· Some loss of function in arm and shoulders.

 DIAGNOSIS & TREATMENT

GENERAL MEASURES
· Your health care provider will do a physical exam and ask questions about your symptoms and activities. You may be asked to make certain movements with the head, arm, and shoulders to help find the cause of the symptoms. Other medical tests may be done to rule out problems that could cause similar symptoms.
· Treatment may involve physical therapy, stretching and strengthening exercises, drugs, ultrasound therapy, electrical stimulation, manipulation, or (rarely) surgery. Your health care provider will discuss an individual plan for you depending on your symptoms.
· Use heat to help relieve pain. Use a heating pad, warm showers, or warm, moist compresses.
· Surgery may be a final option when other treatments are not helpful. It may relieve pressure on the nerves and blood vessels.

MEDICATIONS
· You may use nonprescription drugs, such as acetaminophen or aspirin (not for children), to relieve pain. Drugs cannot correct the underlying condition.
· Other drugs or injections for specific symptoms may be prescribed.

ACTIVITY
· Physical therapy and exercise will be prescribed to promote shoulder muscle function and improve any posture faults. These are usually recommended for 2 to 3 months.
· Avoid straining or heavy activity for 3 months.

DIET
No special diet. If weight is a problem, a weight-loss diet is recommended.

 NOTIFY OUR OFFICE IF

· You or a family member has symptoms of thoracic outlet syndrome.
· Symptoms don't improve in 2 weeks, despite treatment.

Special notes:

_____

_____

_____

More notes on the back of this page ☐

492

THROMBOCYTOPENIA

BASIC INFORMATION

DESCRIPTION
A decrease in the number of platelet cells in the blood. Platelets (thrombocytes) play a vital role in the control of bleeding at the site of an injury. With thrombocytopenia, there is a tendency to bleed, mainly from the smaller blood vessels. This causes abnormal bleeding into the skin and other body places. There are several forms of the disorder, including idiopathic thrombocytopenic purpura (ITP) and thrombotic thrombocytopenic purpura (TTP).

FREQUENT SIGNS AND SYMPTOMS
· Petechiae. These are small round, nonraised, purple-red spots on the skin.
· Bruising easily.
· Bleeding in the mouth and nosebleeds.
· Heavy or prolonged menstrual periods.
· Blood in the urine or stool.

CAUSES
Platelets are normally produced in the bone marrow and are removed or destroyed by the spleen when not needed. A number of underlying conditions may interfere with the production, function, and destruction of the platelets. If no underlying condition is found, it is called idiopathic.

RISK INCREASES WITH
· Infection.
· HIV infection.
· Taking aspirin or other nonsteroidal anti-inflammatory drugs.
· Taking drugs such as quinidine, sulfa preparations, oral antidiabetic agents, gold salts, rifampin, etc.
· Hypersplenism (a disorder of the spleen).
· Hypothermia (exposure to cold temperatures).
· Blood transfusion or blood poisoning.
· Excess alcohol use.
· Preeclampsia (a disorder of pregnancy).
· Disorders such as systemic lupus erythematosus, anemia, leukemia, cirrhosis, certain cancers, and others.
· Exposure to x-ray or radiation.
· Children ages 2 to 4 for idiopathic thrombocytopenic purpura.

PREVENTIVE MEASURES
· Avoid drugs, when possible, that are risk factors.
· For patients with thrombocytopenia, avoid trauma, and get medical care if trauma occurs.

EXPECTED OUTCOMES
· Will depend on the underlying condition. Recovery occurs within two months for most cases of idiopathic thrombocytopenic purpura.
· For chronic cases, symptoms may come and go.

POSSIBLE COMPLICATIONS
· Severe blood loss.
· Anemia due to blood loss.
· Adverse effects of drug therapy.

DIAGNOSIS & TREATMENT

GENERAL MEASURES
· Your health care provider will usually do a physical exam and ask questions about your symptoms and activities. Medical tests may include blood studies and other tests to check for an underlying disorder.
· Treatment will be provided for any specific disorder that is diagnosed.
· Watchful waiting is an option. This means monitoring the symptoms for a time before deciding on treatment.
· Stop using any drug that could be the cause. An alternative drug may be prescribed. Avoid aspirin products.
· Surgery to remove the spleen (splenectomy) may be recommended for persistent cases.
· Pregnant women may require special treatment.
· Platelet transfusions may be prescribed. This may be for patients with serious bleeding, those planning major surgery, and those with chronic thrombocytopenia.
· To learn more: Platelet Disorder Association, PO Box 61533, Potomac, MD; (877) 528-3538; website: www.itppeople.com.

MEDICATIONS
A number of drugs are used for treatment. Your health care provider will discuss the options, risks, and benefits before prescribing them.

ACTIVITY
If platelet counts are very low, bed rest and reduced activity to avoid injury may be recommended.

DIET
No special diet.

NOTIFY OUR OFFICE IF

· You or a family member has symptoms of thrombocytopenia.
· Symptoms worsen during treatment. Severe blood loss is an emergency situation.
· New or unexplained symptoms develop.

Special notes:

_____

_____

_____

More notes on the back of this page ☐

THROMBOPHLEBITIS, SUPERFICIAL
(Phlebitis; Phlebothrombosis)

 BASIC INFORMATION

DESCRIPTION
Inflammation (redness and swelling) and blood clots in a superficial vein. Superficial means the vein is near the surface of the skin. Superficial thrombophlebitis occurs most often in the veins in the legs, and it sometimes occurs in the arms.

FREQUENT SIGNS AND SYMPTOMS
- Tenderness, redness, and pain in the affected area. The symptoms usually come on slowly.
- Vein may feel like a tender hard cord under the skin.
- Fever (sometimes).
- In some cases, there are no symptoms.

CAUSES
When a vein is damaged due to injury, surgery, or infection, the normal flow of blood is slowed down or blocked. Blood clots can then form.

RISK INCREASES WITH
- Illness or surgery with a lot of time spent in bed.
- Long car rides or airplane trips where you are sitting for long periods.
- Smoking.
- Elderly.
- Use of birth control pills.
- Overweight.
- Varicose veins.
- Injuries, burns, or infections.
- Pregnancy.
- Chronic illnesses, heart problems, and some cancers.
- Intravenous (IV) drug abusers.

PREVENTIVE MEASURES
- Avoid risk factors where possible.
- On long trips, walk when you can, move legs often, and wear support stockings to prevent swollen legs. Ask your health care provider about taking aspirin before a long trip.

EXPECTED OUTCOMES
Usually curable in several days to 3 weeks.

POSSIBLE COMPLICATIONS
Serious complications are rare. The main concern is about blood clots forming in deep veins (deep venous thrombosis). They can have serious complications.

 DIAGNOSIS & TREATMENT

GENERAL MEASURES
- Your health care provider will examine the affected area of the leg and ask questions about your symptoms.

Medical tests may be done to make sure there are no other medical problems. These include blood tests and ultrasound (using sound waves to check the blood flow).
- Treatment usually involves rest and elevation of the affected leg or arm and, sometimes, drugs (depending on the cause).
- Apply heat with warm compresses. Wet a towel in hot water, wring it out, and place it on the affected area.
- Wearing support stockings may help. Some types can be purchased at a drugstore. Your health care provider may prescribe prescription-type support stockings.
- If you smoke, this is a good time to stop. Talk to your health care provider about programs to help you quit.
- If varicose veins are a problem, they may need treatment.

MEDICATIONS
- Use nonsteroidal anti-inflammatory drugs, such as aspirin (not for children)or ibuprofen, to decrease swelling, redness, and pain.
- Anticoagulants (drugs to prevent blood clots) may be prescribed.
- Antibiotics may be prescribed if there is an infection.

ACTIVITY
Rest with the affected leg or arm elevated as much as possible for 1 or 2 days. Move the feet, ankles, and legs often. When the symptoms begin to get better, resume normal activity slowly. Rest often. Don't sit or stand for prolonged periods, and don't cross your legs.

DIET
No special diet.

 NOTIFY OUR OFFICE IF

- You or a family member has symptoms of superficial thrombophlebitis.
- The following occur during treatment: Fever of 102°F (38.9°C) or higher, pain gets worse, coughing blood, shortness of breath, chest pain, or swelling of leg or foot.
- New, unexplained symptoms develop. Drugs used in treatment may produce side effects.

Special notes:

_____

_____

_____

More notes on the back of this page ☐

THROMBOSIS, DEEP VEIN

 BASIC INFORMATION

DESCRIPTION
A blood clot (thrombus) that forms inside a deep vein. It may partially or completely block blood flow, or it could break off and travel to the lung. Deep vein thrombosis often occurs in the lower legs (calves). Less often it occurs in the arm or pelvis.

FREQUENT SIGNS AND SYMPTOMS
· Sometimes no symptoms occur.
· Swelling, tenderness, or pain in the leg, especially the calf muscle.
· Warmth or redness of the leg.
· Soreness or pain when walking. The soreness does not disappear with rest.
· Pain when raising the leg and flexing the foot.
· Fever (sometimes).

CAUSES
Pooling of blood in the vein, which triggers blood-clotting mechanisms. The pooling may occur after prolonged bed rest, following surgery, or from long-lasting illness, such as heart attack, stroke, or bone fracture.

RISK INCREASES WITH
· Persons over 60.
· Obesity.
· Smoking.
· Estrogen use in birth control pills or for replacement after menopause. More of a risk with smokers.
· Surgery and surgery recovery.
· Long (usually over 4 hours) auto or airplane trips.
· During pregnancy and right after childbirth.
· Cancer, heart failure, stroke, and polycythemia.
· Bed rest for an extended time, burns, or injuries.
· Intravenous (IV) drug abuse.
· Blood disorders that increase the risk of blood clots.

PREVENTIVE MEASURES
· Avoid prolonged bed rest if possible. Move legs as often as possible after surgery or during a long illness.
· On long auto or airplane trips, exercise your legs at least once every hour. Elevate legs when possible. Drink plenty of fluids. Avoid alcohol.
· Stop smoking, especially if you take estrogen.
· Wear special compression stockings.

EXPECTED OUTCOMES
Usually curable with treatment.

POSSIBLE COMPLICATIONS
· Pulmonary embolism (blood clot travels to the lung).
· Embolism to another part of the body.
· Post-thrombotic syndrome due to vein damage. Blood pools in lower leg, causing swelling and pain in leg.
· Excessive bleeding from blood-thinner drugs.

 DIAGNOSIS & TREATMENT

GENERAL MEASURES
· Your health care provider will do a physical exam of the affected area. Questions will be asked be about your symptoms and activities. Medical tests, such as ultrasound, may be done to confirm the diagnosis.
· Small clots located in the calf may not need treatment right away. These clots often clear up on their own.
· In many cases, hospital care is required for drug injections and to watch for complications.
· A surgical procedure may be done to insert a filtering device ("umbrella") into the vena cava (main vein to the lungs). It will trap clots before they reach the lungs.
· Special compression stockings may be recommended. They help prevent pain, swelling, and complications.

MEDICATIONS
· Usually, an intravenous (IV) anticoagulant (blood thinner) drug is prescribed. This stops a clot from growing and prevents new clots. Blood tests will be ongoing to check the anticoagulant level. Oral anticoagulants may be prescribed for 6 months or longer.
· Thrombolytic drugs, which dissolve the clots, may be prescribed in more severe cases.

ACTIVITY
· Rest at home as advised by your health care provider. While resting, make it a habit to move leg muscles, bend ankles, and wiggle toes.
· Elevate the feet higher than the hips when sitting or when in bed. Place a cushion under the feet or raise the foot of bed higher.

DIET
No special diet.

 NOTIFY OUR OFFICE IF

· You or a family member has symptoms of deep vein thrombosis.
· The following occur during treatment: Unexpected bleeding anywhere, chest pain, coughing up blood, shortness of breath, continued or increased swelling, and pain.

Special notes:

_____

_____

_____

More notes on the back of this page ☐

THROMBOSIS & EMBOLUS, ARTERIAL

BASIC INFORMATION

DESCRIPTION
Thrombosis is a blood clot that forms in an artery. If all or part of the clot breaks away and travels to another part of the artery, it is an embolus. Clots may occur in the large or medium arteries anywhere in the body. The arteries in the neck or the arteries that go to the brain, intestine, legs, arms, or kidney are more often affected.

FREQUENT SIGNS AND SYMPTOMS
Symptoms depend on where the embolus lodges:
· Brain: Temporary blindness, speaking difficulty, partial paralysis, hearing-loss, headache, and dizziness.
· Arms or legs: Pain in the arm or calf after exercise; weakness, numbness, burning and tingling sensations; or weak or absent pulse beyond the blocked blood flow. Symptoms ease up with rest.
· Intestine: Abdominal pain, nausea, vomiting, and shock.

CAUSES
Clots may form with any condition that damages the smooth lining of the heart or a blood vessel. As the clot grows—small or large portions break away and are carried by the bloodstream to the brain, abdomen, arms, legs, or other areas. Conditions that damage the blood-vessel lining include:
· Atherosclerosis (hardening of the arteries).
· Injury to a blood vessel from an accident or from surgery.
· Heart valve disease.
· Heart attack.
· Atrial fibrillation.

RISK INCREASES WITH
· Adults over 60.
· Smoking.
· High blood pressure.
· Diabetes.
· Previous transient ischemic attacks.

PREVENTIVE MEASURES
· If you have high blood pressure or diabetes, adhere to your treatment plan to control the disease.
· Take anticoagulant (blood thinner) drugs for a short time after injury or surgery to prevent blood clots.
· Exercise regularly to help keep blood vessels healthy.

EXPECTED OUTCOMES
Depends on the organs affected, size of the affected blood vessel, and size of the clot. Clots in the arms or legs can be removed with surgery, to relieve symptoms. Clots to the brain, kidney, and intestines may cause death or permanent disability before they can be removed.

POSSIBLE COMPLICATIONS
When blood flow is blocked in an artery, it can cause damage and death to the body tissues involved.

DIAGNOSIS & TREATMENT

GENERAL MEASURES
· Your health care provider will usually do a physical exam. Medical tests may include x-rays of the blood vessels after injection of a special substance.
· Early treatment is needed and usually requires drugs or surgery (embolectomy).
· Surgery to repair or replace damaged blood vessels or to remove an embolus by suction or bypass.

MEDICATIONS
· Drugs to break up the clot may be given through a catheter (tube) directly into the artery involved.
· Anticoagulants to thin the blood and reduce the chance of clots forming may be prescribed.
· Vasodilators (drugs to widen blood vessels) may be prescribed.

ACTIVITY
Complete rest is necessary until blood flow is re-established by surgery or other treatment.

DIET
No special diet during recovery.

NOTIFY OUR OFFICE IF

· You or a family member has symptoms of arterial thrombosis or embolus. This is an emergency! Get medical help immediately.
· Symptoms return after surgery.
· New, unexplained symptoms develop. Drugs used in treatment may produce side effects.

Special notes:

_____

_____

_____

More notes on the back of this page ☐

THRUSH
(Oral Candidiasis)

 BASIC INFORMATION

DESCRIPTION
A fungal infection of the mouth. It is common in newborns and infants. In adults, it is usually a result of an underlying condition.

FREQUENT SIGNS AND SYMPTOMS
· Patches (plaques) appear in the mouth.
· Patches are white to creamy-yellow, and slightly raised. They are similar to milk curds, but they don't wipe off.
· Usually no pain, but may have mild discomfort.
· If patches are rubbed off, they can leave small, painful ulcers (sores).
· The mouth is dry.
· Infant may have trouble feeding.

CAUSES
A fungus called *Candida albicans*. It is usually present in small numbers in the mouth. Certain factors may cause it to multiply out of control:
· Treatment with antibiotics. This may upset the natural balance of germs in the mouth and allow thrush to develop.
· Birth. Newborns may acquire the infection during passage through the birth canal, especially if the mother has a vaginal yeast infection. Thrush can appear within hours or up to 7 days after birth.
· Aging. Older persons develop thrush because of their lower natural resistance.

RISK INCREASES WITH
· Infants.
· People with poor nutrition.
· AIDS. Thrush in adults is part of the criteria used to diagnose AIDS.
· Diabetes.
· Dentures.
· Weak immune system due to illness or drugs.
· Chronic steroid drug use (oral or inhaled).

PREVENTIVE MEASURES
· Good oral hygiene.
· Avoid antibiotics, unless prescribed for you.
· People at risk for thrush may be prescribed a preventive drug.

EXPECTED OUTCOMES
Usually clears up in a few days, but it has a tendency to recur.

POSSIBLE COMPLICATIONS
Complications are rare. They are more likely to occur in those with underlying conditions.

 DIAGNOSIS & TREATMENT

GENERAL MEASURES
· Your health care provider will do a physical exam of the mouth and ask questions about your symptoms and recent use of antibiotics or other drugs. Medical tests may include a scraping of the patch for viewing under a microscope.
· Treatment is aimed at improving an underlying condition and relieving the symptoms of thrush.
· Brush teeth with a soft toothbrush.
· If an infant has the infection, sterilize any objects that may be placed in the baby's mouth.

MEDICATIONS
· Nystatin oral suspension may be prescribed. Follow instructions that are provided with the product. Mothers who are nursing an infant with thrush should use the prescribed drug on her nipples. This prevents the infection from being spread back to the infant.
· Other antifungal drugs are effective and may be prescribed for adults.

ACTIVITY
No limits.

DIET
No changes in infants. Older children and adults should maintain a good fluid intake with milk, liquid gelatin, ice cream, custard, water, tea, or other beverages and foods that are easy to swallow. Use a straw for drinking if the patches are painful.

 NOTIFY OUR OFFICE IF

· You or a family member has symptoms of thrush.
· Signs of dehydration (sunken eyes, poor elasticity of the skin, and lethargy) appear in a child.
· Fever develops.

Special notes:

_____

_____

_____

More notes on the back of this page ☐

THUMB SUCKING

 BASIC INFORMATION

DESCRIPTION
Placing the finger or thumb on the roof of the mouth behind the teeth and sucking with lips and teeth closed. Thumb sucking is common in infants and young children and is a behavior, not a disorder.

FREQUENT SIGNS AND SYMPTOMS
Sucking of the thumb. It is most likely to occur before going to sleep, watching TV, or when hungry, ill, or tired.

CAUSES
Thumb sucking is one of the first acts that an infant can do that brings pleasure. The need to suck is present in all babies. They will suck on almost anything that they can bring into contact with their mouths.

RISK INCREASES WITH
None known.

PREVENTIVE MEASURES
• Thumb sucking is normal and does not need to be prevented. The behavior is calming and soothing to a baby.
• Provide pacifiers early in infancy if you desire. They cause no health problems. Once your child no longer needs a pacifier for their sucking need, you can start to wean them from pacifier use.

EXPECTED OUTCOMES
Some babies stop thumb sucking by age one. In most cases, the habit is given up by the time a child is 3 or 4 years old.

POSSIBLE COMPLICATIONS
Thumb sucking that continues past age 6. It could cause problems with your child's mouth or teeth. Also, the child may get teased by others about the baby-like behavior. Parents should work with the child to change the habit for the sake of appearance and dental health.

 DIAGNOSIS & TREATMENT

GENERAL MEASURES
• No treatment or action is usually necessary. Talk to your child's health care provider if you have any questions or concerns about thumb sucking.
• For a child over age 6 or 7 who sucks the thumb or fingers, follow the advice of your child's health care provider, or try those listed here:
  - Give the child extra attention.
  - Watch the child's behavior to see if conflicts or anxiety seems to provoke sucking. Help the child explore other ways to cope with stress.
  - If the child decides to try to stop sucking, help the child set goals. Give rewards for any progress toward the goal. Reward is not a bribe, but something earned through effort.
  - Methods such as scolding, shaming, and nagging are usually of no avail. Other methods do not always work either. These include mittens, bad-tasting substances on the thumb, elbow splints, and others.
  - Consult your child's dentist for help as well. The dentist may fit a training device in the child's mouth to prevent the thumb from touching the roof of the mouth.

MEDICATIONS
Drugs are usually not necessary for this disorder.

ACTIVITY
No limits.

DIET
No special diet.

 NOTIFY OUR OFFICE IF

Your child wishes to stop thumb sucking and self-help methods are not working.

Special notes:

_____

_____

_____

More notes on the back of this page ☐

THYROID NODULE

BASIC INFORMATION

DESCRIPTION
Nodules (lumps) involving the thyroid gland located in the front of the neck. Most often, the nodules are benign. Less than 10% are malignant (cancerous). Nodules are common and can affect both sexes (women more than men) and all age groups.

FREQUENT SIGNS AND SYMPTOMS
- Most nodules have no symptoms. They are sometimes found during routine physical exams.
- Swelling or lump in the throat.
- Pain and tenderness in the thyroid gland.
- Difficulty swallowing if a large nodule is pressing on the windpipe or esophagus.
- Hyperthyroidism (overactive thyroid) symptoms if the nodule produces too much thyroid hormone. Symptoms can include weight loss, sleep problems, and being irritable.
- Hoarseness (rare).

CAUSES
The thyroid gland produces hormones that help regulate different body functions. For unknown reasons, the tissue in the thyroid develops into the nodules. There are several different types of nodules that develop. They may be cystic (fluid filled) or solid. There may be one nodule or many. Thyroid nodules can cause a goiter (an enlarged thyroid).

RISK INCREASES WITH
- Radiation treatment during childhood, even in small doses, to the head, neck, and upper chest.
- Exposure to nuclear radiation.
- Family history of thyroid tumors.

PREVENTIVE MEASURES
No specific preventive measures.

EXPECTED OUTCOMES
- Benign nodules can be treated successfully.
- Most thyroid cancers are curable.

POSSIBLE COMPLICATIONS
- Side effects of treatment can lead to hypothyroidism or hyperthyroidism.
- Rarely, spread of a malignant tumor to other places in the body.
- Injury to the vocal cords during surgery.
- Permanent hoarseness or loss of voice following surgery.

DIAGNOSIS & TREATMENT

GENERAL MEASURES
- Your health care provider will do a physical exam and ask about your symptoms and history of radiation exposure. Medical tests are usually done to rule out cancer.
- Treatment will depend on the type of nodules.
- Watchful waiting is an option if the nodule is benign. This means monitoring the thyroid with testing for a time before deciding if treatment is needed.
- Drug treatment may be prescribed to help shrink benign nodules.
- Surgery (thyroidectomy) is usually performed for malignant nodules. It is usually done also for larger benign nodules or nodules where the diagnosis is unclear if they are or are not cancerous. Thyroid hormone replacement therapy will be required for life after the thyroid is removed.
- To learn more: American Thyroid Association, 6066 Leesburg Pike, Suite 650, Falls Church, VA 22041; (800) 849-7643; website: www.thyroid.org or Thyroid Foundation of America, 410 Stuart St., Boston, MA. 02116; (800) 832-8321; website: www.tsh.org.

MEDICATIONS
- Radioactive iodine or drugs to suppress (stop) the thyroid from producing hormones may be prescribed.
- Injections may be recommended for benign nodules to shrink them. It may require one or more injections over a few months.
- Antithyroid drugs or replacement thyroid hormone may be prescribed.

ACTIVITY
No limits, unless surgery is performed.

DIET
No special diet.

NOTIFY OUR OFFICE IF

- You or a family member has symptoms of thyroid nodules or thyroid enlargement.
- New, unexplained symptoms develop. Drugs used in treatment may produce side effects.

Special notes:

_____

_____

_____

More notes on the back of this page ☐

THYROIDITIS

 BASIC INFORMATION

DESCRIPTION

Thyroiditis is a group of inflammatory thyroid disorders. The thyroid gland is a hormone-producing organ at the base of the neck, next to the trachea (windpipe). The disorders often affect women between ages 30 and 50. Types include:
· Chronic lymphocytic thyroiditis (Hashimoto's thyroiditis or autoimmune thyroiditis) is the most common type.
· Subacute granulomatous thyroiditis (DeQuervain's thyroiditis). It is less common.
· Subacute lymphocytic thyroiditis (silent thyroiditis or postpartum thyroiditis). It occurs more often in women who have recently delivered a baby.
· Acute suppurative thyroiditis (rarer type).

FREQUENT SIGNS AND SYMPTOMS

· No symptoms may occur or they may be very mild.
· Enlarged thyroid gland (goiter).
· May have trouble swallowing.
· Pain or tenderness in the thyroid (sometimes).
· Fever (sometimes).
· Underactive thyroid (hypothyroidism). It may cause fatigue, weight gain, and trouble concentrating.
· Overactive thyroid (hyperthyroidism). It is less common, and may cause weight loss and sleep problems.

CAUSES

Thyroiditis can be brought on by a number of different factors. In the most common type, it is an immune system problem, but why this occurs is unknown. Other factors include viral or bacterial infections.

RISK INCREASES WITH

· Disorder of the body's immune system.
· Pregnancy.
· Family history of thyroid disease.
· Previous thyroid disorders.
· Various viruses, such as mumps or influenza.
· Bacterial infection of the thyroid gland (rare).

PREVENTIVE MEASURES

No specific preventive measures.

EXPECTED OUTCOMES

Will depend on the type. The chronic type can be treated successfully with thyroid hormone therapy. It may take several weeks of therapy for symptoms to improve. Other types of thyroiditis may clear up on their own in 4 to 6 months.

POSSIBLE COMPLICATIONS

Permanent loss of thyroid function. This requires lifelong thyroid hormone replacement.

 DIAGNOSIS & TREATMENT

GENERAL MEASURES

· Your health care provider will usually do a physical exam and ask about your symptoms. Medical tests include blood studies to check your thyroid function. Other tests may be done to confirm the diagnosis.
· Treatment, if needed, is with drugs, and will depend on the type of thyroiditis.
· If symptoms are not severe, treatment may involve watchful waiting. This means monitoring thyroid function for a few months before deciding on treatment.
· Very rarely, thyroid surgery may be an option if other treatment does not improve painful symptoms.
· With any type of thyroiditis, it is important to follow up with your health care provider for periodic exams.
· To learn more: American Thyroid Association, 6066 Leesburg Pike, Suite 650, Falls Church, VA 22041; (800) 849-7643; website: www.thyroid.org or Thyroid Foundation of America, 410 Stuart St., Boston, MA. 02116; (800) 832-8321; website: www.tsh.org.

MEDICATIONS

· Antithyroid drugs or thyroid replacement hormones, depending on the activity of your thyroid hormones.
· Beta-adrenergic blockers to suppress symptoms of an overactive thyroid may be prescribed.
· Antibiotics to fight infection, if needed.
· Cortisone drugs to decrease inflammation may rarely be prescribed.
· You may use aspirin (not for children) or ibuprofen to control mild pain.

ACTIVITY

No limits.

DIET

No special diet.

 NOTIFY OUR OFFICE IF

· You or a family member has symptoms of thyroiditis.
· New, unexplained symptoms develop. Drugs used in treatment may produce side effects.

Special notes:

_____

_____

_____

More notes on the back of this page ☐

TINEA CRURIS

(Jock Itch)

 BASIC INFORMATION

DESCRIPTION

Fungal infection of the skin in the groin. Tinea cruris is more likely to occur in men than in women.

FREQUENT SIGNS AND SYMPTOMS

· Scaling patches on the skin of the groin, thighs, and buttocks.
· Patches have well-defined edges.
· Sometimes small, pus-filled blisters appear.
· Itching of involved areas.
· Pain (if the skin also becomes infected with bacteria).

CAUSES

Infection by fungi called dermatophytes. These germs tend to grow in the darkness, warmth, and moisture of the body's groin area.

RISK INCREASES WITH

· Hot, humid weather.
· Excessive sweating.
· Tight clothing.
· Obesity, which fosters sweating.
· Friction of skin against skin from constant movement.
· Contact with infected surfaces, such as towels or benches.
· Weak immune system due to illness or drugs.
· Diabetes.
· Other fungal infection such as athlete's foot (tinea pedis).

PREVENTIVE MEASURES

· Dry completely after bathing. Use clean towel.
· Don't sit around in a wet bathing suit.
· Wear loose fitting, cotton underwear.
· Wear clean, dry athletic supporters and underwear for each workout.
· Use nonprescription tolnaftate (Tinactin) after bathing if you have had tinea cruris before. This powder can help prevent a recurrence.

EXPECTED OUTCOMES

Symptoms can be controlled in 2 to 4 weeks with treatment.

POSSIBLE COMPLICATIONS

· Recurrences are common.
· Bacterial infection in the affected area.

 DIAGNOSIS & TREATMENT

GENERAL MEASURES

· Your health care provider will do a physical exam of the affected area. Medical tests may include a microscopic exam of scraped-off scales.
· Treatment usually involves a drug applied to the skin. Use it for the length of time prescribed, even if the rash goes away.
· For home care, follow the steps listed in Preventive Measures.
· If you also have an athlete's foot infection, treat both areas with equal care.

MEDICATIONS

· You may use nonprescription, topical antifungal drugs for treatment and prevention.
· Other topical or oral (taken by mouth) antifungal drugs may be prescribed.

ACTIVITY

No limits.

DIET

No special diet.

 NOTIFY OUR OFFICE IF

· You or a family member has symptoms of tinea cruris.
· Rash worsens despite treatment.
· Infection recurs after treatment.

Special notes:

_____

_____

_____

More notes on the back of this page ☐

TINEA VERSICOLOR

 ## BASIC INFORMATION

DESCRIPTION

An infection caused by a yeast type of skin fungus that changes the color of skin that it affects. The skin of the chest, back, shoulders, upper arms, trunk, or groin (rarely, the face) is most often affected. The infection is more common in teens and young adults.

FREQUENT SIGNS AND SYMPTOMS

- Small, scaly spots (or patches) on the skin. They may appear white to pink or tan to dark. They show up differently on light skin as compared to darker skin.
- Affected skin may itch (more likely if the person gets hot).
- Spots begin small and spread. They may join together to form larger patches.
- In hot climates, a person may have the spots all year around. In other climates, they may fade during the cooler months.

CAUSES

A fungus called *Pityrosporum orbiculare*. It is present on normal skin, but it can't be seen and it normally causes no problems. Why it grows more active and causes symptoms for some people is unknown.

RISK INCREASES WITH

- Exposure to heat and high humidity.
- Excess sweating.
- Skin that is more oily.
- Weak immune system due to illness or drugs.

PREVENTIVE MEASURES

No specific preventive measures. Once you have had the infection, re-treatment can help stop a recurrence.

EXPECTED OUTCOMES

There is no permanent cure. Treatment can clear up the infection. Following treatment, the patches will remain for months after the infection has been cured.

POSSIBLE COMPLICATIONS

- Recurrence is common. The episodes of recurrence decline with age.
- The cosmetic appearance of the skin may cause some emotional distress, especially in young teens.

 ## DIAGNOSIS & TREATMENT

GENERAL MEASURES

- Your health care provider can usually diagnose the disorder by an exam of the affected skin. Medical tests may include a microscopic exam of scales scraped from the skin to confirm the diagnosis.
- Numerous topical products are effective in clearing tinea versicolor.
- Your health care provider will usually recommend a method to help prevent a recurrence. Several options are available. One method is to repeat treatment every week for 3 to 4 weeks and then once a month for 3 to 4 months.

MEDICATIONS

- Nonprescription, antifungal, topical products such as shampoos, creams, or lotions may be recommended. These are applied to the affected areas. Use product as directed on the label.
- In some cases, drugs taken by mouth may be prescribed.

ACTIVITY

No limits. Try to avoid activities that cause excess sweating. If heavy sweating occurs, shower as soon as possible.

DIET

No special diet.

 ## NOTIFY OUR OFFICE IF

- You or a family member has symptoms of tinea versicolor.
- Infection doesn't improve despite treatment.

Special notes:

_____

_____

_____

More notes on the back of this page ☐

TINNITUS

 ## BASIC INFORMATION

DESCRIPTION

A persistent sound heard in one or both ears when there is no environmental noise. Tinnitus can be a common symptom of nearly all ear disorders, as well as other medical problems.

FREQUENT SIGNS AND SYMPTOMS

A noise that may be a ringing, buzzing, roaring, whistling, or hissing sound, that is heard in one or both ears. The sound may be continuous, off and on, pulsing, or in time with the heartbeat.

CAUSES

There has probably been some sort of damage to the hearing system, but why this might cause tinnitus is unknown. Tinnitus does not cause deafness, nor does deafness cause tinnitus. They can both occur together in some patients.

RISK INCREASES WITH

- Hearing loss.
- Earache or ear infection.
- Labyrinthitis.
- Meniere disease.
- Otitis media or externa.
- Otosclerosis.
- Ototoxicity.
- Earwax blockage.
- Aneurysm or tumor in the head (rare).
- Foreign body in the ear.
- Certain drugs (antibiotics, diuretics, and others).
- High or low blood pressure.
- Head trauma.
- Anemia.
- Hypothyroidism or hyperthyroidism.
- Allergies.
- Exposure to excessively loud noise, either once or over a period of time.

PREVENTIVE MEASURES

No specific prevention known.

EXPECTED OUTCOMES

Treatment of an underlying disorder may help. Often there is no cure, and learning to cope is the only therapy. Some people tolerate the condition much better than others. Research is ongoing to find the cause and effective treatment.

POSSIBLE COMPLICATIONS

There are usually no medical complications. Emotional problems may develop due to feelings of distress for those who find the noise very difficult to live with.

 ## DIAGNOSIS & TREATMENT

GENERAL MEASURES

- Your health care provider may do a physical exam and an ear exam. Questions will be asked about your symptoms. Medical tests may be done to check for an underlying disorder.
- If tinnitus is ongoing, the treatment is basically finding methods that help to you cope with the constant noise. Try one method for a time to see if it helps. Sometimes, a combination of different methods will work.
- Try to ignore the sound by directing your attention to other things and activities. Counseling or biofeedback training may help you learn to do this technique.
- Play music in the background during the day and while falling asleep.
- Learn techniques to control stress in your life. This helps some people with tinnitus.
- Quit smoking. Find a way to stop that works for you.
- A hearing aid for any associated deafness may help mask tinnitus.
- Wear a tinnitus suppressor or masker. This is a device that fits in the ear like a hearing aid, and presents a more pleasant sound.
- Dental treatment may be recommended.
- Electrical stimulation with cochlear implant may help tinnitus, but it is usually used only for severe deafness.
- Tinnitus retraining therapy (TRT) may help. It combines counseling with sound therapy.
- To learn more: American Tinnitus Association, P.O. Box 5, Portland, OR 97207; (800) 634-8978; website: www.ata.org.

MEDICATIONS

There are no drugs for tinnitus. Drugs normally prescribed for other conditions may help some people.

ACTIVITY

No limits.

DIET

No special diet.

 ## NOTIFY OUR OFFICE IF

- You or a family member has symptoms of tinnitus.
- Feelings of distress about tinnitus worsen.

Special notes:

_____

_____

_____

More notes on the back of this page ☐

TOENAIL, INGROWN

 BASIC INFORMATION

DESCRIPTION
A common problem in which one or both edges of a nail grows into the flesh of a toe, usually the great (big) toe. This can lead to infection and inflammation.

FREQUENT SIGNS AND SYMPTOMS
Pain, tenderness, redness, swelling, and heat in the toe where the sharp nail-edge pierces the nearby fold of tissue. Once tissue around the nail becomes red and sore, infection often develops.

CAUSES
• An ingrown toenail is likely to occur with one of the following conditions:
  - The nail is more curved than normal.
  - The toenail is clipped back too far, allowing tissue to grow up over it.
  - Shoes fit poorly, forcing the toe of the shoe against the nail and surrounding tissue.
  - Injury to the nail, or infection of the nail.
  - Sports activities that requires sudden stops ("toe jamming").

RISK INCREASES WITH
Any of the causes listed.

PREVENTIVE MEASURES
• Wear roomy, well-fitting shoes and socks.
• Carefully cut toenails straight across, and not too short.
• People with diabetes or blood vessel disease have poor healing abilities. Be very careful in trimming your toenails. Foot injury is a risk with these disorders because of changes in blood flow to the feet.
• If you often handle heavy objects in your work, consider wearing work shoes with steel toe boxes.
• Keep feet clean and dry.

EXPECTED OUTCOMES
Curable with treatment.

POSSIBLE COMPLICATIONS
An ingrown toenail may become very painful, red, and swollen with pus if treatment for infection is delayed too long. Sometimes a bloody growth called proud flesh builds up on the side of the nail.

 DIAGNOSIS & TREATMENT

GENERAL MEASURES
• The following home treatment may help prevent the need for surgery:
  - Soak the toe for 20 minutes twice a day in a gallon of warm water. You may add either 2 tablespoons of Epsom salts or 2 tablespoons of a mild detergent.

  - Lift the nail corners gently, and wedge a very small piece of cotton under the ingrown nail edges. This will lift the nail slightly so it can grow past the skin tissue it is digging into. Replace the cotton daily. Do not cut a "V" in the middle of the nail. This is not helpful.
  - There are certain products you can buy that may soften the nail and the skin around it, which can help relieve the pain. Follow the directions carefully. These products should not be used if you have diabetes or a blood vessel problem.
• See your health care provider if home care does not help. Your foot and toe will be examined. If there is an infection, drugs usually relieve symptoms within 1 week. If an ingrown toenail occurs often, then surgery is often the best treatment.
• The type of surgery will depend on how severe the problem is. It may involve just removing overgrown skin tissue, removing a portion of the toenail, or complete removal of the toenail.

MEDICATIONS
• Antibiotic ointment may be prescribed to fight any infection.
• You may use ibuprofen or acetaminophen for pain.

ACTIVITY
• Resume your normal activities as soon as symptoms improve. You may need to wear sandals or a shoe with the toe cut out until the toe heals.
• If you have surgery, your health care provider will instruct you about aftercare, such as keeping the foot propped up as much as possible.

DIET
No special diet.

 NOTIFY OUR OFFICE IF

• You have symptoms of an ingrown toenail that persist despite self-treatment.
• The following occur during treatment or after surgery:
  - Fever.
  - Increased pain.
  - Signs of infection (pain, redness, heat, swelling, or tenderness) in the toe.
  - Red streaks going up the foot or ankle.

Special notes:

_____

_____

_____

_____

More notes on the back of this page ☐

TONGUE INFLAMMATION
(Glossitis)

 BASIC INFORMATION

DESCRIPTION
Acute or chronic inflammation of the tongue from a variety of causes. This is sometimes contagious, but not cancerous.

FREQUENT SIGNS AND SYMPTOMS
Any of the following:
- Bright red, swollen tongue.
- Tongue looks and feels smooth.
- Tongue may be sore and tender.
- Hairy-looking tongue, sometimes with a black surface.
- A tongue with a red tip and edges.

CAUSES
- Bacterial or viral (including herpes) infections.
- Burns.
- Injury from jagged teeth, ill-fitting dentures, mouth-breathing, or repeated biting during seizures.
- Excessive use of alcohol, tobacco, hot food or spices.
- Poor dental health.
- Allergy to toothpaste, mouthwash (especially mouthwash containing peroxide), candy, dye, or material used in dental work.
- Lack of B vitamins, resulting in B-12-deficiency anemia, pellagra, or iron-deficiency anemia.
- Adverse reaction to drugs.

RISK INCREASES WITH
- Poor nutrition, especially vitamin deficiencies.
- Smoking.
- Chemical or environmental exposure to irritating or corrosive chemicals.
- Alcoholism.
- Anxiety or depression.
- Diabetes.

PREVENTIVE MEASURES
- Practice good oral hygiene. Brush teeth and tongue at least twice a day, and floss teeth daily. Obtain regular dental checkups.
- Don't smoke.
- Prevent tongue injury by wearing protective headgear for contact sports or cycling.

EXPECTED OUTCOMES
Usually curable in 2 weeks with treatment.

POSSIBLE COMPLICATIONS
- Tongue inflammation can become chronic if not adequately treated.
- Tongue may become swollen and block the airway.

 DIAGNOSIS & TREATMENT

GENERAL MEASURES
- Your health care provider will do an exam of the mouth and tongue. Medical tests may include blood studies to check for any underlying disorder.
- Treatment will be directed at the underlying cause along with self-help measures.
- Observe if there is an association between eating specific foods and tongue symptoms. Irritating foods may include chocolate, citrus, acidic foods (vinegar, pickles), salted nuts, or potato chips.
- Rinse mouth 3 or more times a day with a salt solution (mix one-half teaspoon of salt in one cup of warm water).
- If tongue symptoms are caused by teeth or denture problems, consult your dentist. The problem won't heal until the cause is eliminated.

MEDICATIONS
- For minor pain, you may use nonprescription drugs, such as anesthetic mouthwashes or acetaminophen.
- For infection and pain, antibiotics or topical anesthetics may be prescribed.

ACTIVITY
No limits.

DIET
- No special diet, except to avoid foods that may cause the symptoms.
- Drink as many fluids and eat as well-balanced a diet as possible while healing.
- To reduce pain, sip liquids through straws. Foods or fluids that cause the least pain are milk, liquid gelatin, yogurt, ice cream, and custard.

 NOTIFY OUR OFFICE IF

- You or a family member has symptoms of tongue inflammation.
- Symptoms don't improve in 3 days despite treatment.
- Pain gets worse and isn't relieved by treatment.
- Tongue swells and interferes with swallowing.

Special notes:

_____

_____

_____

More notes on the back of this page ☐

TONSILLITIS

 ## BASIC INFORMATION

DESCRIPTION

Tonsils that are inflamed (red, sore, and swollen). The tonsils are located at the back of the throat on each side. They are small at birth, enlarge during childhood, and become smaller during the teen years. Tonsils usually help prevent infections in the nose, mouth, and throat from spreading to other places in the body. However, they themselves can become infected. Tonsillitis can be spread from person to person. It affects all ages, but is most common in children between ages 5 and 10.

FREQUENT SIGNS AND SYMPTOMS

- Sore throat and pain when you swallow.
- Tonsils are redder than normal.
- Throat may have white or yellow patches.
- Swollen glands on either side of the jaw.
- Fever.
- Headache.
- Ear pain.
- A very young child may not want to eat.

CAUSES

Usually a bacterial (often *streptococcus,* or "strep" as it is called) or a virus infection.

RISK INCREASES WITH

- Young children.
- Daycare centers (for both children and teachers).
- Living, working, or being in crowded places.
- Smoking.
- Having a chronic illness, such as diabetes.

PREVENTIVE MEASURES

Fight germs. Wash hands often.

EXPECTED OUTCOMES

Symptoms generally begin to improve in 2 to 3 days. Treatment will take longer to ensure that germs are gone. If tonsillitis is severe and occurs often, your health care provider may suggest surgery (tonsillectomy) to remove the tonsils.

POSSIBLE COMPLICATIONS

- Abscess (an infected sore on the tonsils).
- Chronic tonsillitis. It can cause ear infection and enlarged tonsils. This may lead to breathing problems and snoring.
- Rheumatic fever may occur if the cause is strep and it is not treated, or if treatment is stopped too soon.

 ## DIAGNOSIS & TREATMENT

GENERAL MEASURES

- Your health care provider will examine your head, neck, and throat. Medical tests may include a rapid strep test and a throat culture (to find which germ is the cause). Family members may also need a strep test. A person may carry the strep germ, but not have any symptoms.
- Treatment usually involves drugs and self-care.
- To relieve the sore throat, gargle frequently with warm or cold double-strength tea or warm salt water (mix one-half teaspoon of salt in one cup of water).
- Suck on hard candy such as lemon drops, to increase moisture in the mouth.
- If surgery to remove the tonsils is needed, your health care provider will discuss the details. It is usually done on an outpatient basis.

MEDICATIONS

- If the cause is strep, take prescribed antibiotic (usually penicillin) for at least 10 days, or as directed.
- To relieve pain, you may use acetaminophen. Don't give aspirin to children under age 18.

ACTIVITY

- Stay away from others until fever, pain, and other symptoms disappear.
- Bed rest if there is fever. Then return to your regular routine.

DIET

Drink plenty of fluids. While the throat is very sore, use liquids for food. This includes milk shakes, soups, and high-protein fluids (diet or instant-breakfast milk drinks).

 ## NOTIFY OUR OFFICE IF

- You or a family member has symptoms of tonsillitis. If there is any trouble with breathing, call right away.
- Symptoms worsen, or other symptoms occur during treatment.

Special notes:

_____

_____

_____

More notes on the back of this page ☐

TOOTH GRINDING

(Bruxism)

BASIC INFORMATION

DESCRIPTION

The habit of grinding or clenching the teeth. Bruxism is the medical term for the problem. Tooth grinding is often done while asleep, but grinding or tapping teeth during the day is also common. Continual tooth grinding may erode gums and supporting bones in the mouth.

FREQUENT SIGNS AND SYMPTOMS

- Pain in the jaw muscles. Earaches may occur also.
- Clenching of the jaw, or clicking noises in the jaw.
- Annoying, tooth grinding noises at night. These may be loud enough to awaken others.
- Teeth may become loose and more sensitive to cold and heat.
- Damage to teeth, supporting gums, and bone (a dentist will notice the changes in a dental exam).
- Headaches.
- Daytime sleepiness.

CAUSES

- There is no one specific cause. Anxiety, tension, and stress appear to play a role.
- Unconscious attempt to correct an abnormal "bite."
- Tooth grinding occurs in children. They may grind their teeth when they have a cold, ear ache, allergies, or other problems. The children usually outgrow the habit, and it typically causes no damage to the teeth.

RISK INCREASES WITH

- One study found that it occurs more often in people who drink alcohol at bedtime, drink more than 6 cups of coffee a day, smoked cigarettes, or suffered from depression and/or anxiety.
- Suppressed anger may be a risk factor.
- Some antidepressant or antipsychotic drugs may increase the risk.

PREVENTIVE MEASURES

Avoid stressful situations if possible.

EXPECTED OUTCOMES

Treatment can help relieve the symptoms and limit any further damage to the teeth or other complications.

POSSIBLE COMPLICATIONS

- Without treatment, teeth, bones, and gums may erode or crack from the pressure of grinding.
- Problems with the temporomandibular joint. This is the hinge-like area where your upper jaw connects to the lower jaw.
- Continued problems with disrupted sleep.

DIAGNOSIS & TREATMENT

GENERAL MEASURES

- Self-treatment options may sometimes help.
  - Cut down on alcohol and caffeine.
  - Try taking a warm bath before bedtime.
  - Use a warm washcloth to apply heat to the jaw area.
  - Decrease the stress in your life, where possible.
  - Have your spouse wake you at night when you grind your teeth. Then get up and do some simple activity for about 10 minutes before you go back to sleep.
- See your dentist if self-help measures aren't working. Your dentist will examine your teeth and the jaw areas of your face. Several treatment options may be discussed.
- Dental work can help resolve certain problems such as an abnormal bite, crooked or missing teeth.
- A night guard may be prescribed. This is a custom-made plastic device worn at night to stop upper and lower teeth from coming together.
- Your dentist may suggest a sound alarm device. It is worn at night and sounds an alarm to wake you when it senses jaw movements.
- Biofeedback training (relaxation exercises) or counseling to learn ways to cope more effectively with stress may be needed.
- Physical therapy, hypnosis therapy, or discontinuing drugs that are a risk factor may help some patients.

MEDICATIONS

Your health care provider or dentist may prescribe drugs for a short period for certain problems. These include muscle relaxants or mild sleeping aids.

ACTIVITY

No limits.

DIET

No special diet.

NOTIFY OUR OFFICE IF

- You or a family member grinds teeth at night. It is also a good idea to call your dentist.
- Once treatment begins, call your dentist if you have new symptoms or if other symptoms become worse.

Special notes:

_____

_____

_____

More notes on the back of this page ☐

TORTICOLLIS

(Wryneck)

 BASIC INFORMATION

DESCRIPTION

A problem of the neck muscles that causes a twisted head movement. Torticollis is a type of movement disorder (dystonia). It usually affects adults ages 30 to 60 (women more than men). Congenital muscle torticollis is a type that affects newborns.

FREQUENT SIGNS AND SYMPTOMS

- Symptoms may begin slowly and progress over time or develop suddenly.
- Head turns (or tilts) toward one shoulder while the chin turns toward the opposite shoulder. The head may be pulled forward or backward.
- The head may not move from the abnormal position (tonic), may have jerky head movements (clonic), or may have both types.
- Neck muscles are tense and tender.
- There may be pain in the neck, back, or shoulder.
- In a newborn, a lump may be felt in the neck muscle.

CAUSES

- In newborns, the exact cause is unknown. It may be due to a muscle injury prior to, during, or after birth. There are other possible causes. It sometimes occurs along with a hip dislocation.
- In other cases, the nerves and muscles involved are affected by various causes. Sometimes, no cause is found. This is called idiopathic spasmodic torticollis.

RISK INCREASES WITH

Newborn:
- Birth defect.
- Injury to neck muscles or vertebrae (spinal bones) at birth or later.
- Breech delivery of newborn.
- Large baby.

Others:
- Family history of torticollis.
- Cervical spine problems (injury, fractures, scar tissue, tumor, infections, ligament problems, and others).
- Inflammatory problems (such as myositis and others).
- Certain prescribed drugs.
- Some drugs of abuse.
- Infection in tissues around neck muscles.

PREVENTIVE MEASURES

No specific preventive measures.

EXPECTED OUTCOMES

- Congenital torticollis can usually be corrected with muscle-stretching exercises or surgery, if needed.
- Other forms often improve with treatment. Healing can sometimes occur, and healing time varies. Some patients may take only a few days or weeks. Other patients may have neck problems for months or years.

POSSIBLE COMPLICATIONS

Condition becomes chronic.

 DIAGNOSIS & TREATMENT

GENERAL MEASURES

- Your health care provider will do a physical exam of the affected area and ask questions about your symptoms and activities. Medical tests may include x-rays and studies of muscle movements.
- Congenital torticollis is initially treated with physical therapy, including daily passive therapy for at least a year. If therapy is not successful, then surgery to lengthen neck muscles is performed.
- For other forms of torticollis, drug therapies may help, along with physical therapy and massages.
- If a drug is causing the problem, it should be stopped.
- A neck brace or collar may be recommended.
- Relieve pain from neck spasms with heat or massage. Take hot showers or use warm, moist compresses, deep-heating ointments, or heating pad.
- Stress may worsen symptoms. Learn stress-reduction techniques, including biofeedback.
- Ultrasound therapy may be recommended.
- Rarely, a surgical procedure to denervate (cut the nerves) in the neck muscles may be recommended.
- To learn more: National Spasmodic Torticollis Association, 9920 Talbot Ave., Suite 233, Fountain Valley, CA 92708; (800) 487-8385; website: www.torticollis.org.

MEDICATIONS

- Muscle relaxants, anti-inflammatories, or other drugs may be prescribed. They may be taken by mouth or injected by your health care provider.
- Injections of botulinum toxin type A into the neck muscles may be prescribed.

ACTIVITY

Activity limits will be determined by your symptoms.

DIET

No special diet.

 NOTIFY OUR OFFICE IF

- You or a family member has symptoms of torticollis.
- You have neck pain or spasms that last over 1 week.

Special notes:

_____

_____

_____

More notes on the back of this page ☐

TOXIC SHOCK SYNDROME (TSS)

 BASIC INFORMATION

DESCRIPTION

A form of blood poisoning caused by poisons (toxins) released by bacteria. Menstrual toxic shock involves the female reproductive and respiratory systems. Nonmenstrual toxic shock can affect all ages and both sexes (up to 15% of cases occur in males).

FREQUENT SIGNS AND SYMPTOMS

- Sudden, high fever in a previously healthy person.
- Vomiting and watery diarrhea.
- Rash that resembles sunburn.
- Low blood pressure.
- Excessive thirst.
- Rapid pulse.
- Feeling of impending doom.
- Mental changes, such as confusion.
- Extreme fatigue and weakness.
- Headache.
- Sore throat.

CAUSES

Some strains of staphylococcal bacteria produce toxins that enter the bloodstream, causing sudden symptoms. Most serious cases have come from staphylococci in the vagina of women using tampons. Toxic shock syndrome can also arise from wounds or infections in the throat, skin, lungs, or bone.

RISK INCREASES IN/WITH

- Prolonged use of tampons (particularly super absorbent) during menstrual periods.
- Staphylococcal infections.
- Postpartum women.
- Postoperative patients, particularly after nasal surgery.

PREVENTIVE MEASURES

- Change tampons frequently, and alternate them at night with sanitary napkins.
- Don't use super absorbent tampons. Use those made of cotton.
- Don't use tampons if you have a skin infection, especially near the genitals.
- Wash hands thoroughly before inserting tampons. *Staphylococci* are commonly found on the hands.
- Get early medical attention for infected wounds.

EXPECTED OUTCOME

Most patients recover with early diagnosis and prompt hospital treatment, but some cases are fatal. Skin of the palms and soles often peels during recovery.

POSSIBLE COMPLICATIONS

- Severe shock.
- Kidney failure.
- Congestive heart failure.
- Respiratory distress.
- Loss of hair and nails.
- Recurrence of TSS.
- Mortality may be as high as 15% in severe cases.

 DIAGNOSIS & TREATMENT

GENERAL MEASURES

- You health care provider will do a physical exam. Medical tests may include blood studies and a culture of discharge from the vagina.
- Immediate hospital care is required to give intravenous (IV) fluids, antibiotics, and electrolytes to correct fluid and electrolyte loss and dehydration. Treatment is provided for kidney or heart problems and provide mechanical breathing support, if needed.
- Tampons, diaphragms, or other foreign bodies are removed at once.
- To learn more, perform an Internet search. A good site to start with is www.4women.gov.

MEDICATION

- Antibiotics, usually given through a vein (IV), for infection.
- Intravenous fluids and electrolytes.

ACTIVITY

Resume your normal activities as soon as symptoms improve.

DIET

No special diet after recovery.

 NOTIFY OUR OFFICE IF

- You or a family member has symptoms of toxic shock syndrome. Call immediately! Shock develops rapidly.
- New, unexplained symptoms develop. Drugs used in treatment may produce side effects.

Special notes:

_____

_____

_____

More notes on the back of this page ☐

TOXOPLASMOSIS

BASIC INFORMATION

DEFINITION

An infection in humans and animals caused by a tiny parasite, *Toxoplasma gondii*. It can live up to a year in water or moist soil. The parasite can infect most types of animals, but cats are the most often infected. Humans can get the infection in several different ways.

FREQUENT SIGNS AND SYMPTOMS

- No symptoms usually (80% to 90% of patients).
- Fever, sore throat, or fatigue.
- Swollen lymph glands.
- Muscle aches.
- Rash (sometimes).
- Inflammation (redness and soreness) of the retina (retinitis).

CAUSES

- People can get a toxoplasmosis infection by eating foods or drinking water that contain the germs. Infection can occur if you touch something, such as infected cat litter, with your hands then accidentally touch your mouth or eyes.
- Pregnant women who get the infection can transmit it to their offspring.
- Blood transfusion or organ transplantation (rare).

RISK INCREASES WITH

- Eating raw or partially-cooked meat (e.g., pork, lamb, beef, or venison). Eating raw fruits or vegetables grown in infected soil. Handling raw meats, and then touching your mouth.
- Infected cats (who usually have no symptoms). They pass germs in their stools (feces) into litter boxes, the soil in gardens, or in a child's sand box. The germs get on a person's hands when they change litter or garden. The hands then accidentally touch the mouth or eyes. Children who eat the sand or soil can become infected.
- Having a weak immune system due to illness or drugs.

PREVENTIVE MEASURES

- Cook meat thoroughly. Carefully wash any surface that raw meat has touched, including your hands. Wash raw fruits and vegetables before eating them.
- Persons with weak immune systems and pregnant women should avoid contact with cat feces. If you do change cat litter or garden, be sure to wear gloves.
- Change cat litter boxes daily. Feed indoor cats only canned, dry or cooked meat (no raw meat).
- Protect children's play areas, including sand boxes, from cat and dog feces.

EXPECTED OUTCOME

The majority of infected persons have no symptoms. Those with mild symptoms recover on their own.

POSSIBLE COMPLICATIONS

- Complications are rare. Inflammation may occur in the eyes (retinitis), the brain (encephalitis), or heart (myocarditis). People with weak immune systems are more likely to have complications.
- Pregnant women may have a miscarriage or stillbirth.
- Serious health problems or death may result for newborns who get the infection from the mother.

DIAGNOSIS & TREATMENT

GENERAL MEASURES

- Your health care provider may do a physical exam and ask questions about your symptoms and activities. A blood test is needed to confirm the diagnosis.
- Treatment is usually not needed for a healthy person with no symptoms or if their symptoms are mild.
- For an infected pregnant female, your obstetric provider will discuss the treatment available, the risks involved, and the expected outcomes.
- For a person with a weakened immune system, treatment is usually with drugs.
- Infected newborns (with or without symptoms) are usually treated with drugs to help prevent complications that may occur as they get older.
- If drugs are prescribed, your health care provider will do frequent blood tests to monitor for side effects.

MEDICATION

- Pyrimethamine and sulfadiazine are the drugs most often prescribed to treat toxoplasmosis. These or other drugs may be prescribed for a pregnant woman.
- Corticosteroids, if necessary, for inflammation.
- Other drugs are currently being tested.

ACTIVITY

Usually no limits unless symptoms are severe.

DIET

No special diet.

NOTIFY OUR OFFICE IF

- You or your child has symptoms of toxoplasmosis.
- Symptoms don't improve after diagnosis and treatment, or prescribed drugs cause any side effects.

Special notes:

_____

_____

_____

More notes on the back of this page ☐

510

TRANSIENT ISCHEMIC ATTACK (TIA)

 BASIC INFORMATION

DESCRIPTION

A type of stroke that lasts only a few minutes. They are sometimes called "mini strokes." The term transient is used to describe a condition that lasts a short time. Ischemic describes an inadequate blood flow. TIAs most often affect adults over age 40.

FREQUENT SIGNS AND SYMPTOMS

· Symptoms are brief. Most last less than 5 minutes. A few may last an hour and rarely, up to 24 hours.
· Loss of muscle function on one side of the body.
· Headache.
· Dizziness.
· Tingling in the arms and legs.
· Numbness.
· Vision disturbance or temporary blindness in one eye.
· Confusion.
· Faintness without loss of consciousness.
· Slurred speech or inability to speak.

CAUSES

TIAs happen when blood flow to a part of the brain is reduced for a short period. The reduced blood flow may be due to a small blood clot in an artery. It may be caused by a spasm of a brain artery causing it to narrow. TIAs normally do not cause lasting injury to the brain such as a stroke does.

RISK INCREASES WITH

· Aging, males or African Americans.
· Personal or family history of high blood pressure, atherosclerosis (hardening of the arteries), or stroke.
· Smoking or excess alcohol use.
· Diabetes, heart disease, or carotid artery disease.
· High cholesterol levels or high homocysteine levels.
· Obesity.
· Sedentary lifestyle (being physically inactive).

PREVENTIVE MEASURES

· Exercise daily. Maintain a healthy weight. Eat a healthy diet.
· Don't smoke or use alcohol to excess.
· Have your blood pressure checked regularly. If it is high, get medical advice for treatment to reduce it.
· Daily aspirin may help. Ask your health care provider.

EXPECTED OUTCOMES

· There are normally no lasting effects (such as weakness on one side) from a TIA. Treatment of TIAs can help reduce your risk factors for stroke.
· TIAs often recur. Symptoms of each attack may be similar or different from others.

POSSIBLE COMPLICATIONS

Stroke. Without treatment, over 30% of persons who have TIAs have strokes within 5 years.

 DIAGNOSIS & TREATMENT

GENERAL MEASURES

· Your health care provider will do a physical exam and ask questions about your symptoms and activities. Medical tests may include studies to check your heart, brain and blood vessel function.
· Emergency hospital care may be needed.
· Treatment may include drugs, taking control of risk factors (diabetes, high blood pressure, heart disease, and others), and lifestyle changes. A treatment plan will be based on your individual case.
· Stop smoking and/or alcohol use. Get counseling, join a support group, or find other methods to help you quit.
· Surgery (endarterectomy) may be needed to remove plaques (fatty deposits) from carotid arteries in the neck.
· Heart valve-replacement surgery may be needed.
· To learn more: American Stroke Association, 7272 Greenville Ave., Dallas, TX 75231; (888) 478-7653; website: www.strokeassociation.org.

MEDICATIONS

Anticoagulants (blood thinners) may be prescribed to decrease the risk of blood clots. Aspirin can help decrease the risk of future stroke. Other drugs can be prescribed for those unable to take aspirin.

ACTIVITY

· If you have frequent TIAs, you may be advised to avoid or limit certain activities that could risk injury to you or others.
· Exercise daily or as advised.

DIET

· Eat a well-balanced diet that is low in salt and fat. Include plenty of fresh fruits and vegetables, and fiber.
· A weight loss diet is recommended for obese patients.

 NOTIFY OUR OFFICE IF

· You or a family member has symptoms of a TIA. Seek emergency help.
· Other symptoms occur after treatment begins

Special notes:

_____

_____

_____

More notes on the back of this page ☐

TRANSIENT SYNOVITIS OF THE HIP

(Toxic Synovitis)

 BASIC INFORMATION

DESCRIPTION

Transient synovitis of the hip is inflammation (swelling and pain) of the tissues around the hip joint. It usually affects one hip, not both, and is a common cause of sudden hip pain in young children. It occurs more often in children ages 3 to 10, and most are boys. Transient is used to describe a condition that lasts a short time. Synovitis describes an inflamed joint in the body.

FREQUENT SIGNS AND SYMPTOMS

· Mild or more severe pain in the hip. It may start quickly or come on slowly.
· Some children may have pain in the inner thigh or knee area.
· Difficulty walking or standing.
· Walking with a limp.
· Hip is tender to the touch.
· Mild fever less than 101°F (38.3°C) may occur.

CAUSES

The exact cause is unknown. A virus, an allergic reaction, or a minor injury may be involved.

RISK INCREASES WITH

Unknown.

PREVENTIVE MEASURES

None known.

EXPECTED OUTCOMES

· The pain may start to improve within 24 to 48 hours, and is usually gone completely within 2 weeks. Some children may have minor pain for several weeks.
· A few children may get the disorder again. If it does recur, it is usually within 6 months.

POSSIBLE COMPLICATIONS

Complications are rare, but may involve other problems with hip or thigh-bones.

 DIAGNOSIS & TREATMENT

GENERAL MEASURES

· Your child's health care provider will do a physical exam with careful attention to the painful hip area. Medical tests may include blood studies, x-rays, and other tests. These are done to confirm the diagnosis and make sure that there is not another problem involved.
· The main treatment is rest at home.
· Check your child's temperature daily to see if high fever develops.

MEDICATIONS

Naproxen or ibuprofen may be prescribed for treating pain and inflammation.

ACTIVITY

Limit activities until the pain symptoms are gone.

DIET

No special diet.

 NOTIFY OUR OFFICE IF

· Your child has symptoms of transient synovitis of the hip.
· After diagnosis, your child develops a high fever, other symptoms get worse, or symptoms don't improve within 10 days.

Special notes:

_____

_____

_____

More notes on the back of this page ☐

512

TRENCH MOUTH

(Necrotizing Ulcerative Gingivitis; Vincent's Disease)

 ## BASIC INFORMATION

DESCRIPTION

Infection of tissue between the teeth. This is not contagious or cancerous. It affects both sexes and all ages, but is most common in young adults (20 to 40 years).

FREQUENT SIGNS AND SYMPTOMS

- Painful gums.
- Gums that bleed when pressed.
- Excess saliva.
- Bad breath.
- Ulcers (sores) covered with gray membrane on the gums.
- Swallowing with difficulty.
- Speaking difficulty.

CAUSES

Bacterial or other infection of the gums.

RISK INCREASES WITH

- Poor nutrition.
- Weak immune system due to illness or drugs.
- Smoking.
- Stress.
- Poor oral hygiene. Tartar, plaque, or food debris between teeth.

PREVENTIVE MEASURES

- Maintain good oral hygiene. To brush teeth: Scrub clear, sticky plaque off teeth daily with a soft toothbrush. Place the brush at the gum line and gently rotate, pointing bristles toward the gum. Brush one section of teeth at a time. Then brush tongue. A soft brush is less likely to damage teeth and gums than a hard brush.
To floss: Use waxed or unwaxed dental floss according to instructions on the package label or your dentist's instructions.
- Eat a well-balanced diet.
- Don't smoke.

EXPECTED OUTCOMES

Usually curable in two weeks with treatment. Frequent dental checkups, up to once a month, after treatment.

POSSIBLE COMPLICATIONS

- Surgery may be needed to trim rough, infected gums.
- Infection may spread to other areas of the face (cheeks, lips, and jawbone) and cause tissue damage.

 ## DIAGNOSIS & TREATMENT

GENERAL MEASURES

- Your dental care provider or health care provider will do an exam of the gums. Dental x-rays or facial x-rays may be done.
- Removal of dead tissue may be recommended as a treatment.
- Rinse your mouth with warm salt water a few times a day. Use one-half teaspoon of salt in one cup of water.
- Follow steps listed in Preventive Measures on how to brush and floss your teeth.
- Don't smoke. Find a way to quit that works for you.
- Find ways to reduce stress in your life.
- Avoid any gum irritation until gums heal completely.

MEDICATIONS

- Antibiotics may be prescribed for infection.
- You may use nonprescription drugs, such as acetaminophen, for minor pain.

ACTIVITY

Usually no limits.

DIET

- A liquid or soft diet may be necessary for two or three days because of gum tenderness. When pain subsides, eat a normal, healthy diet. Avoid spicy or hot (temperature) food.
- Drink plenty of fluids each day.

 ## NOTIFY OUR OFFICE IF

- You or a family member has symptoms of trench mouth.
- One or more of the following occur during treatment:
  - Fever.
  - Swelling of neck or face.
  - Swallowing difficulty.
  - Inability to eat.

Special notes:

_____

_____

_____

More notes on the back of this page ☐

TRICHINOSIS

 BASIC INFORMATION

DESCRIPTION

Infection caused by larvae of parasites that live in the intestines of pigs (rarely meat of bears and some marine animals). People may be infected and never have symptoms. The infection affects different places in the body:
• Gastrointestinal tract (where larvae enter).
• Lymphatic system and bloodstream (through which they are transported).
• Large muscles of the body. The diaphragm (large muscle used in breathing that separates the chest from the abdomen), arms and legs (in which the larvae become embedded).

FREQUENT SIGNS AND SYMPTOMS

Early stages (usually begin in 7 to 10 days):
• Appetite loss, nausea, vomiting, diarrhea and stomach cramps.
Later stages:
• Puffy eyelids and face.
• Muscle pain.
• Headache.
• Itching, burning skin.
• Sweating.
• High fever (102°F to 104°F or 38.9°C to 40°C).
Late stages:
• Symptoms decrease, but some muscle tissues remain permanently infected with microscopic cysts. In rare cases, these cause heart and central nervous system disorders.

CAUSES

Infection with a parasite, *Trichinella spiralis*. It is transmitted to humans when they eat infected animals. Thorough cooking kills the parasite and makes infected meat safe to eat. The parasites pass from animal to animal in contaminated food (usually raw garbage).

RISK INCREASES WITH

• Eating improperly cooked or raw pork.
• Weak immune system due to illness or drugs.

PREVENTIVE MEASURES

Don't eat raw or undercooked pork meats (including ready-to-eat pork sausage). Cook all meats thoroughly.

EXPECTED OUTCOMES

Usually curable in 5-6 weeks in most persons with rest and treatment and, in severe cases, hospital care.

POSSIBLE COMPLICATIONS

Overwhelming infection, which can lead to:
• Heart and lung complications.
• Central nervous system problems.
• Kidney damage.
• Vision or hearing disorders.
• Some deaths have been reported.

 DIAGNOSIS & TREATMENT

GENERAL MEASURES

• Your health care provider will usually do a physical exam and ask about your symptoms and diet. Medical tests including blood studies, and a muscle biopsy may be done to confirm the diagnosis. With a biopsy, a small amount of muscle tissue is removed for viewing under a microscope.
• Treatment usually includes drugs for pain and fever and rest at home. Antiworm drugs may help in some cases.
• Hospital care for severe cases. Breathing support and intravenous (IV) fluids may be needed.

MEDICATIONS

• Anthelmintic (antiworm) drugs to kill the parasites may be prescribed. They can help if larvae are in the intestinal tract. They will not help help if the muscles are infected.
• Corticosteroids for patients with severe symptoms or with central nervous system involvement.
• You may take nonprescription drugs, such as acetaminophen, to reduce fever and discomfort.

ACTIVITY

Rest in bed until symptoms improve. While confined to bed, move legs often to reduce the likelihood of deep-vein blood clots. Resume normal activities gradually.

DIET

No special diet. Drink plenty of fluids.

 NOTIFY OUR OFFICE IF

• You or a family member has symptoms of trichinosis.
• New, unexplained symptoms develop. Drugs used in treatment may produce side effects, especially nausea, vomiting, skin rash or fever.

Special notes:

_____

_____

_____

More notes on the back of this page ☐

TRICHOMONIASIS

 ## BASIC INFORMATION

DESCRIPTION

Trichomoniasis is a parasitic infection that affects both sexes, but is more common in women. Trichomoniasis is a sexually transmitted disease (STD).

FREQUENT SIGNS AND SYMPTOMS

- Women:
  - Discomfort varies greatly from woman to woman and from time to time in the same woman.
  - Foul-smelling, frothy vaginal discharge that is most apparent several days after a menstrual period.
    - Vaginal itching and pain.
    - Pain with intercourse.
    - Redness of the vaginal lips (labia) and vulva.
    - Painful and frequent urination.
- Men:
  - Infected men usually have no symptoms.
  - Rarely may have painful urination and a pale white discharge from the penis.

CAUSES

Infection from a tiny parasite, *Trichomonas vaginalis*. The infection is spread from person to person during sexual intercourse. Symptoms may start 5 to 28 days after being exposed. The parasite may also live in the body for years without producing symptoms. Since it thrives in both men and women, both sexual partners must receive treatment.

RISK INCREASES WITH

- Having multiple sexual partners.
- Having sex with someone who has, or had, multiple sexual partners.
- Engaging in unsafe sex.
- On very rare occasions, the infection can be spread by sharing moist towels, washcloths or even from Jacuzzis and hot baths.

PREVENTIVE MEASURE

- Use latex (rubber) condoms during sexual intercourse.
- Limit your sexual partners or practice abstinence. The more sex partners you have, the greater your risk of any sexual transmitted disease.

EXPECTED OUTCOME

Can be cured with treatment.

POSSIBLE COMPLICATIONS

If the infection is untreated, it can lead to other problems. Women may be more at risk for HIV infection (if exposed). If pregnant, it may cause early delivery and low birth weight baby. In men, prostate, bladder or urethra problems may occur.

 ## DIAGNOSIS & TREATMENT

GENERAL MEASURES

- Your health care provider will do a physical exam and a pelvic exam in women. Medical tests may include Pap smear, and studies of vaginal discharge and urine. Tests to check for other STDs are often done.
- Treatment is with a drug. Your sexual partner(s) must be treated at the same time. This will prevent you from getting reinfected.
- Don't douche unless prescribed for you.
- Wear cotton underpants or pantyhose with a cotton crotch.
- Take showers instead of tub baths.
- If urinating causes burning, urinate through a tubular device, such as a toilet-paper roll or plastic cup with the bottom cut out. Pour a cup of warm water over the genital area while you urinate.
- Don't sit around in wet clothing, especially in a wet bathing suit.
- To learn more: Centers for Disease Control & Prevention (CDC) National STD Hotline (800) 227-8922; website: www.cdc.gov/std.

MEDICATION

Metronidazole (Flagyl) taken for 1-14 days is usually prescribed for you and your sexual partner. Follow directions carefully. Don't drink alcohol when you take this drug. If combined, they interact and cause a reaction with nausea, vomiting, sweating, weakness and other symptoms.

ACTIVITY

Avoid too much exercise, heat, and excessive sweating. Avoid sex until treatment is complete. Allow about 10 days for recovery.

DIET

No special diet.

 ## NOTIFY OUR OFFICE IF

- You or a family member has symptoms of trichomoniasis.
- Symptoms get worse despite treatment.
- Unusual vaginal bleeding or swelling develops.

Special notes:

_____

_____

_____

More notes on the back of this page ☐

TRIGEMINAL NEURALGIA

(Tic Douloureux)

BASIC INFORMATION

DESCRIPTION
A condition involving the 5th cranial (trigeminal) nerve that causes episodes of severe facial pain. The nerve and its branches supply sensation to the face, scalp, teeth, mouth, and nose. The condition is more common in adults over age 40. Women are affected more than men.

FREQUENT SIGNS AND SYMPTOMS
• Attacks of severe facial pain, described as "jabbing" or "searing" or like an electrical shock. These attacks (or bouts) of pain usually last for seconds, or sometimes for 1 to 2 minutes. A dull ache may be felt between bouts, or there may be little or no discomfort.
• Facial spasm (or tic) often occurs at the same time as pain.
• Only one side of the face is usually affected, but it may occur at different times on both sides.
• Pain is often triggered by touching or stroking the face, brushing teeth, shaving, exposure to wind, or chewing.
• Attacks may occur several times a day. They may disappear for weeks or months.
• A less common form, called atypical trigeminal neuralgia, may cause less-intense symptoms.

CAUSES
The exact cause is unknown (often called idiopathic). It may involve a nerve or blood vessel problem such as injury, irritation, inflammation, or disease.

RISK INCREASES WITH
Multiple sclerosis.

PREVENTIVE MEASURES
No specific preventive measures.

EXPECTED OUTCOMES
Symptom relief is usually possible with treatment. Sometimes surgery may be required. A patient may experience pain-free intervals (lasting from months to years), and then the pain returns exactly as before.

POSSIBLE COMPLICATIONS
Interference with normal activities from frequent, severe pain episodes.

DIAGNOSIS & TREATMENT

GENERAL MEASURES
• Your health care provider will do a physical exam of the affected facial area and ask about your symptoms and activities. This is usually enough for diagnosis. Medical tests may be done to check for other problems.

• Most patients obtain pain relief with drugs. However, as time goes by, the drugs may become ineffective in some patients and the pain then "breaks through."
• Alternate type of treatments have been used by some, but they are not always effective. These include acupuncture, herbal remedies, chiropractic care, electrical stimulation, hypnosis, myotherapy (muscle release), and others.
• Surgery may be effective when drugs don't help. The different procedures available will be explained to you.
• Maintain good oral health with dental checkups at least twice a year.
• Learn to control stress. It may trigger or worsen pain.
• To learn more: Facial Neuralgia Resources, website: www.facial-neuralgia.org or Trigeminal Neuralgia Association, 2801 South Archer Rd., Suite C, Gainesville, GA 32608; (352) 376-9955 (not toll free); website: www.tna-support.org.

MEDICATIONS
• Anticonvulsant (antiseizure) drugs are often prescribed to help relieve the pain.
• Other drugs including antidepressants, muscle relaxants, or antispasmodics may be helpful in some cases. Ordinary pain relievers are not helpful for this disorder.
• Products applied to the skin may help some patients. These include capsaicin (Zostrix) or lidocaine. Ask your health care provider before using.
• Experimental drugs are being researched and tested.

ACTIVITY
No limits. Avoid blasts of hot or cold air.

DIET
• Try to eat foods that don't involve much chewing.
• Chew on the unaffected side.

NOTIFY OUR OFFICE IF

• You or a family member has symptoms of trigeminal neuralgia.
• New, unexplained symptoms develop. Drugs used in treatment may produce side effects.

Special notes:

_____

_____

_____

More notes on the back of this page ☐

TUBERCULOSIS (TB)

 ## BASIC INFORMATION

DESCRIPTION

A chronic bacterial infection that mainly involves the lungs. Tuberculosis (TB) is occurring more often due to AIDS, poverty, homelessness, abuse of alcohol and other drugs, and failure of infected persons to take the prescribed drugs.

FREQUENT SIGNS AND SYMPTOMS

Early stages:
- No symptoms (often).
- Flu-like symptoms.

Middle stages:
- Low fever.
- Weight loss.
- Chronic fatigue.
- Heavy sweating, especially at night.

Later stages:
- Cough, with sputum that over time becomes bloody, yellow, thick, or gray.
- Chest pain and/or shortness of breath.
- Reddish or cloudy urine (sometimes).

CAUSES

Infection by the germ, *Mycobacterium tuberculosis.* Germs are transmitted in the air from one person to another. Many persons are infected with TB that is inactive and there are no symptoms (called latent TB infection or LTBI). About 1 in 10 of these people will eventually develop active TB.

RISK INCREASES WITH

- Adults over 60. General decline in health from aging.
- Newborns and infants.
- Chronic illness that lowers resistance (e.g., AIDS).
- Use of cortisone or drugs that suppress the immune system. These may cause inactive TB to become active.
- Crowded or unclean living conditions.
- Alcohol and drug abuse.
- Homeless people.
- Living in, or coming from, third world countries.

PREVENTIVE MEASURES

- Preventive treatment for several months with isoniazid (INH) if a tuberculin skin test is positive.
- Latent TB may be treated to prevent active TB.
- A vaccine called BCG is used in countries where TB is very common. It is less often used in the United States.

EXPECTED OUTCOMES

Usually curable with treatment.

POSSIBLE COMPLICATIONS

- Lung abscess, chronic obstructive pulmonary disease, bronchiectasis, or respiratory failure.
- Spread of infection to brain, bone, spine, and kidneys.
- Without treatment, TB can be fatal.

 ## DIAGNOSIS & TREATMENT

GENERAL MEASURES

- Your health care provider will do a physical exam and ask about your symptoms. Medical tests may include TB skin test, blood studies, sputum study, and chest x-ray.
- Treatment is with drugs. It is important to take the drugs as prescribed to be sure the infection is cured. People may stop the drugs once they feel better, but the infection is still active. If this happens, the patient can spread the infection to others. In addition, this allows the TB bacteria to "outwit" the TB drugs and soon those drugs become ineffective.
- A TB infection that becomes resistant to drugs is termed multidrug-resistant TB (MDR-TB). Stronger TB drugs have to be used which have serious side effects. MDR-TB is more difficult to cure, and it can be fatal.
- If you are infectious, use tissue to cover your mouth when coughing, sleep in a separate bed, keep away from others, and don't go to work or school.
- It is sometimes necessary to isolate (separate from other persons) or have hospital care for a TB patient.
- Have regular follow-up visits with your health care provider to see if treatment is working.
- To learn more: Centers for Disease Control & Prevention (CDC), 1600 Clifton Rd., NE, Mailstop E-10, Atlanta, GA 30333; website: www.cdc.gov/nchstp/tb.

MEDICATIONS

Antitubercular drugs, usually for 6 to 12 months. Several types are given at the same time to avoid bacterial resistance to the drugs. Patients are probably not infectious after 10 days to 2 weeks of treatment. MDR-TB may need treatment for up to two years.

ACTIVITY

Rest in bed until symptoms improve. You may need to restrict activities for 6 months.

DIET

No special diet.

 ## NOTIFY OUR OFFICE IF

- You or a family member has symptoms of TB.
- Symptoms persist or worsen, despite treatment.
- New, unexplained symptoms develop.

Special notes:

_____

_____

_____

More notes on the back of this page ☐

TYPHOID FEVER

 ## BASIC INFORMATION

DESCRIPTION
A bacterial infection of the gastrointestinal tract. In the United States, people affected have usually been traveling internationally.

FREQUENT SIGNS AND SYMPTOMS
- Fever, headache, fatigue.
- Constipation and dry cough. Diarrhea is less common.
- Bloated abdomen with some discomfort.
- Confusion and feeling listless.
- Rash (rose spots) on the front of the body.
- Eye symptoms, such as vision changes (sometimes).
- Later symptoms may include foul smelling diarrhea, weight loss, weakness, slow pulse, rapid breathing, delirium, and others.

CAUSES
Infection with *Salmonella typhi*, a type of bacteria. The infection is spread by persons who are ill with the infection, or carriers who have been ill and recovered, but still carry the germs. You can become ill if you eat food or drink beverages prepared by one of these persons. Also, the germs may get into sewage and contaminate water that is used for drinking or washing foods. Shellfish from contaminated water or canned meat prepared improperly can cause outbreaks of the infection. Symptoms may appear 10 to 20 days after exposure.

RISK INCREASES WITH
- Travel to developing countries.
- Weak immune system due to illness or drugs.

PREVENTIVE MEASURES
- For travel to countries where typhoid is present, consider typhoid vaccine (injection or oral form). It is not 100% protective, so take precautions with food and water. During travel, avoid tap water, salad and raw vegetables, unpeeled fruits, and dairy products. Follow the advice—"boil it, cook it, peel it, or forget it."
- Wash your hands after using the bathroom and before handling food.

EXPECTED OUTCOMES
Usually curable in 2 to 3 weeks with treatment. Relapse may occur in 10-20% of patients. Treatment is repeated.

POSSIBLE COMPLICATIONS
- Perforation of the intestines.
- Gastrointestinal hemorrhage or abscess.
- Pneumonia.
- Bone infection.
- Congestive heart failure.
- Without treatment, it can be fatal.

 ## DIAGNOSIS & TREATMENT

GENERAL MEASURES
- Your health care provider will do a physical exam and ask about your symptoms and recent travel. Medical tests are usually done to confirm the diagnosis.
- Hospital care is needed for severe cases; others can be cared for at home. Follow any special instructions provided for preventing infection from being spread to other persons.
- Use a heating pad or warm compress to relieve abdominal cramps.
- Wash hands carefully and often.
- People in certain types of jobs, such as food handlers, health care, or child care workers, will need to be tested for the germs before they can resume their usual work. They need three negative tests.
- Surgery may be needed in severe cases if complications occur, such as bleeding or an abscess.

MEDICATIONS
- Antibiotics will be prescribed. They may be given by injection or taken by mouth.
- For severe cases, steroids will be prescribed in addition to antibiotics.
- Eye symptoms may require eye drops or ointments.

ACTIVITY
Bed rest is necessary until all symptoms have been gone at least 3 days. The legs should be moved often in bed to prevent deep-vein blood clots from forming.

DIET
Diet will be determined by the symptoms.

 ## NOTIFY OUR OFFICE IF

- You or a family member has symptoms of typhoid fever.
- New symptoms develop or other symptoms become worse, despite treatment.

Special notes:

_____

_____

_____

More notes on the back of this page ☐

518

ULCER, PEPTIC
(Duodenal Ulcer; Gastric Ulcer)

 ## BASIC INFORMATION

DESCRIPTION
An ulcer is a sore in the gastrointestinal tract. Ulcers that form in the upper part of the small intestine are duodenal ulcers. They are the most common type. Ulcers that form in the stomach are called gastric ulcers. They are less common. Ulcers can affect all ages.

FREQUENT SIGNS AND SYMPTOMS
- Pain in the upper abdomen, or sometimes, the lower chest. It may be a burning, boring, or gnawing feeling that lasts 30 minutes to 3 hours. It may be worse before or after eating. It often awakens a person during the night. The pain may come and go. Weeks of off and on pain may alternate with short, pain-free periods.
- Pain is temporarily relieved with use of antacids.
- Appetite loss and weight loss. With duodenal, it may be weight gain, as person eats more to ease discomfort.
- Vomiting (sometimes may contain blood).
- Blood in the stool.

CAUSES
- Almost all ulcers are caused by either an infection with *Helicobacter pylori* bacteria or nonsteroidal anti-inflammatory drugs. *Helicobacter pylori* bacteria is present in many healthy people. Why it causes ulcers in some is unknown.
- Ulcers are not caused by stress, or anxiety or eating spicy foods, although they may aggravate existing ulcers.

RISK INCREASES WITH
- Family history of ulcers.
- Elderly.
- Smoking.
- Excess alcohol use (possibly).
- Use of nonsteroidal anti-inflammatory drugs (e.g., aspirin).
- Type-O blood (for duodenal ulcers).

PREVENTIVE MEASURES
Avoid as many risk factors as possible.

EXPECTED OUTCOMES
Usually curable with treatment, but relapses can occur.

POSSIBLE COMPLICATIONS
- Perforation. This is an erosion of the ulcer through the intestinal wall. It can cause infection or bleeding into the abdomen.
- Bleeding into the intestine.
- Anemia from blood loss.
- Duodenal ulcers are almost always benign, while gastric ulcers may rarely become malignant.
- Intestinal obstruction.

 ## DIAGNOSIS & TREATMENT

GENERAL MEASURES
- Your health care provider will do a physical exam and ask about your symptoms and activities. Medical tests may include blood studies, gastrointestinal tract studies, and a test to check for *Helicobacter pylori*.
- Treatment is with drugs and sometimes, life-style changes.
- Discontinue the use of aspirin or nonsteroidal anti-inflammatory drugs. Use acetaminophen instead.
- Quit smoking. Find a way to stop that works for you.
- If you drink alcohol heavily, stop or cut down.
- If stress is a problem, learn ways to help you cope.
- Hospital care may be needed for complications such as bleeding ulcer or severe perforation or obstruction.
- Surgery for some patients for complications or if drug treatment is not effective.
- To learn more: National Digestive Diseases Information Clearinghouse, 2 Information Way, Bethesda, MD 20892, (800) 891-5389; website: www.digestive.niddk.nih.gov.

MEDICATIONS
- Your health care provider may prescribe:
  - Antibiotics to treat the *Helicobacter pylori* infection.
  - Antacids to help neutralize excess stomach acid.
  - H-2 blockers or proton pump inhibitors to reduce stomach acid. Long-term therapy may be required for some patients.
  - Drugs to coat and protect the lining of the stomach and the duodenum.

ACTIVITY
No limits.

DIET
- Eat small, healthy meals on a regular scheduled.
- Avoid foods that bring on pain.

 ## NOTIFY OUR OFFICE IF

- You or a family member has symptoms of an ulcer.
- Vomiting occurs that is bloody or looks like coffee grounds, or stool is bloody, black, or tarry-looking.
- You feel weak, tired, have pale skin, or back pain.

Special notes:

_____

_____

_____

More notes on the back of this page ☐

URETHRITIS

 BASIC INFORMATION

DESCRIPTION
Inflammation (redness and soreness) or infection of the urethra. The urethra is the tube that carries urine out of the bladder when you urinate. In women, it is about an inch long. In men, it is the full length of the penis. Urethritis can affect all ages and both sexes. In women, it often occurs along with a bladder infection or inflammation (cystitis).

FREQUENT SIGNS AND SYMPTOMS
· Painful or burning urination. The pain can be severe.
· Discharge that may be cloudy, yellow-green mucus, or may be watery and white.
· Genital itching.
· Frequent urge to urinate, even when there is not much urine in the bladder.
· Men may have no symptoms.

CAUSES
· An infection that is spread by a sexual transmitted disease (STD). Most common causes are gonorrhea and chlamydia. Less often, herpes virus, human papilloma virus (HPV), trichomoniasis, and other infections are the cause. Non-specific urethritis (NSU) is the term used when there is infection present, but the cause is unknown.
· Lower estrogen levels in postmenopausal women.
· Yeast infection in women.
· Other causes could be from an injury or surgery, or from a chemical such as an antiseptic. Bubble bath or bath oils have been known to cause urethritis. This type of urethritis can not be spread to anyone else.

RISK INCREASES WITH
· Bacterial infection that spreads and enters the urethra from the skin around the genitals and anal area.
· Contact with an infected sexual partner.
· Use of a urinary catheter (tube used to remove urine).
· Multiple sexual partners.
· High-risk sexual behavior.
· Current or previous sexually transmitted disease.
· Loss of estrogen in postmenopausal women.

PREVENTIVE MEASURES
· Practicing safer sexual behaviors. This includes having only one sexual partner and using rubber (latex) condoms to help protect against infections.
· Keep the genital area clean and dry. Use plain, unscented soap. Be sure sexual partner is clean.
· Avoid irritants and chemicals that cause redness, burning, or itching in the genital area.

EXPECTED OUTCOME
Proper treatment usually brings complete recovery.

POSSIBLE COMPLICATIONS
· Complications are rare, unless it is not treated, or treatment is not adequate.
· In women, urinary tract infections, pelvic inflammatory disease (PID), or infertility may occur. There is also a risk of complications in pregnancy and in a newborn.
· In men, urinary tract infections or prostatitis (prostate infection) may occur.

 DIAGNOSIS & TREATMENT

GENERAL MEASURES
· Your health care provider will usually do an exam of the genital area. Medical tests may include blood studies and a culture of urine and any discharge.
· Treatment will depend on the cause.
· Drugs may be prescribed. If infection is present, your sexual partner(s) will sometimes need treatment also.
· If the cause is trauma or chemical irritants, avoid the source of injury or irritant.
· To relieve pain, take sitz baths by sitting in a tub of warm water for 15, minutes at least twice a day.
· Keep the area around the genitals clean. Use unscented, plain soap.

MEDICATION
· Antibiotics for infection will usually be prescribed. Finish the complete dose, even if symptoms clear up.
· In cases of severe pain, phenazopyridine (Pyridium) may be prescribed. Pyridium produces bright orange (tea) colored urine.
· In menopausal women, estrogen applied to the vaginal area, or taken by mouth may be helpful.

ACTIVITY
Avoid sexual intercourse until you have been free of symptoms for 2 weeks. Otherwise, no limits.

DIET
· Drink 8 glasses of water (or other fluid) every day.
· Drink cranberry juice to acidify urine. Some drugs are more effective when urine is more acidic.

 NOTIFY OUR OFFICE IF

· You or a family member has symptoms of urethritis.
· Symptoms worsen or new symptoms occur after treatment.

Special notes:

_____

_____

_____

More notes on the back of this page ☐

UTERINE BLEEDING, DYSFUNCTIONAL
(Premenopausal Abnormal Uterine Bleeding)

BASIC INFORMATION

DESCRIPTION
Bleeding that is abnormal, irregular, and not part of a normal period. There is no tumor, infection, or pregnancy involved. It most often occurs in women over age 40 and in those under age 20.

FREQUENT SIGNS AND SYMPTOMS
• Bleeding between periods. Blood flow may be light or heavy, prolonged, and may contain clots.
• Periods last for 7 to 14 or even 18 days, and/or have spotting between periods.

CAUSES
The normal menstrual cycle depends on a balance of estrogen and progesterone. Bleeding problems occur if they get out of balance. There is too much estrogen or not enough progesterone. This happens most often due to anovulation (failure of the ovaries to produce or release eggs). Anovulation is more likely to occur in women who are close to menopause and young girls whose menstrual cycles have just started.

RISK INCREASES WITH
• Women over age 40 and under age 20.
• Polycystic ovary syndrome (cysts on the ovaries).
• Obesity.
• Athletes.
• Emotional stress.
• Eating disorders.

PREVENTIVE MEASURES
No specific preventive measures.

EXPECTED OUTCOME
Outcome will depend on the woman's medical condition, age, the severity of the problem, and treatment.

POSSIBLE COMPLICATIONS
• Anemia due to excessive bleeding.
• Cancer (rare).
• Infertility from lack of ovulation.

DIAGNOSIS & TREATMENT

GENERAL MEASURES
• Your health care provider will usually do a physical exam and a pelvic exam. Questions will be asked about your symptoms and activities. Dysfunctional uterine bleeding is diagnosed after other causes of abnormal uterine bleeding have been ruled out. These include diseases, drugs, pregnancy, eating disorders, gynecological infections, polyps or other growths, or tumors. One or more medical tests are needed to help confirm the diagnosis. These will be explained to you.

• Goals of treatment are to return periods to a normal cycle or stop the bleeding altogether. Treatment will depend on a woman's age, other medical conditions, and the severity of the bleeding.
• If bleeding is severe, a hospital stay may be needed to bring it under control.
• Treatment will be given for anemia if it exists.
• If symptoms are not severe, treatment may involve watchful waiting. This means monitoring the bleeding for a few months before treating it.
• Hormone therapy is usually the first treatment step, particularly in younger women.
• If hormones do not help the bleeding, surgery may be needed. Your health care provider will discuss options, benefits, and risks. Together, you'll choose the treatment that will work best for you:
 - Dilation and curettage (D & C) may be the recommended procedure.
 - Other surgery options include endometrial ablation (destruction or removal of the uterine lining), or hysterectomy. These procedures mean a woman can no longer become pregnant. They may be used for women who are close to menopause.
• To learn more: National Women's Health Information Center (800) 994-9662; website: www.4women.gov.

MEDICATION
• Hormone therapy may be prescribed. This includes birth control pills, hormone-replacement therapy, or progesterone.
• Iron supplements may be recommended for anemia.

ACTIVITY
No limits.

DIET
With anemia, an iron-rich diet may be recommended.

 ## NOTIFY OUR OFFICE IF

• You or a family member has abnormal uterine bleeding.
• The following occur during treatment:
 - Bleeding becomes heavy (filling a pad or tampon more often than once an hour).
 - Signs of infection develop, such as fever, a general ill feeling, headache, dizziness, or muscle aches.
• New, unexplained symptoms develop. Drugs used in treatment may produce side effects.

Special notes:

_____

_____

_____

More notes on the back of this page ☐

UTERINE MALIGNANCY
(Endometrial Carcinoma; Uterine Sarcoma)

 BASIC INFORMATION

DESCRIPTION
Endometrial carcinoma is cancer of the endometrium (lining of the uterus). It usually affects postmenopausal women ages 50 to 60 and older. It is the most common female pelvic cancer in the United States. Sarcoma is a less common type of uterine cancer. It involves the muscles and/or other supporting tissues of the uterus.

FREQUENT SIGNS AND SYMPTOMS
- Bleeding or spotting, often after sexual intercourse. This usually happens after menstrual periods have stopped for 12 months or more. A watery or blood-streaked vaginal discharge may occur before bleeding or spotting.
- Cramps (sometimes).
- Pain or mass in the pelvic area and weight loss.

CAUSES
Exact cause is unknown. Increased estrogen levels are thought to play a role.

RISK INCREASES WITH
- Diabetes.
- Obesity.
- Women who have never given birth to a child.
- High blood pressure.
- Use of estrogen without also using progesterone.
- History of breast, ovarian or colon cancer.
- Family history of endometrial cancer.
- Use of the drug tamoxifen.
- History of uterine polyps, menstrual cycles without ovulation, or other signs of hormone imbalance.
- Delayed menopause (after age 52).
- Previous pelvic radiation therapy.

PREVENTIVE MEASURES
- There are no specific measures to prevent cancer.
- Pelvic exams every 6 to 12 months may aid in early detection when treatment is more effective. Exams are very important for women with risk factors.
- Obtain medical care for any bleeding or spotting after menopause.
- Good general health measures to control diabetes, high blood pressure, and maintain ideal body weight.

EXPECTED OUTCOME
With early diagnosis and treatment, 90% of patients survive at least 5 years. Older patients and delayed diagnosis have a poorer outcome.

POSSIBLE COMPLICATIONS
- If bleeding is not treated, anemia may occur.
- Spread of cancer to other organs. This can be fatal.
- Treatment is not effective, or cancer recurs.

 DIAGNOSIS & TREATMENT

GENERAL MEASURES
- Your health care provider will do a physical exam and a pelvic exam. Medical tests are done, first to diagnose the cancer, and then to find out if it has spread to other body organs (staging). Tests will be explained to you. They may include blood tests, Pap smear, liver function tests, chest x-ray, CT scan, mammogram, barium enema, MRI, vaginal ultrasound, endometrial biopsy, and/or dilatation and curettage (D & C).
- Treatment will depend on the extent of the disease, your health and your preferences. It may involve one or more of the following: Surgery, radiation, hormone therapy, and chemotherapy (anticancer drugs).
- In some cases, other disorders, such as diabetes, high blood pressure, or anemia must be brought under control before the cancer can be treated.
- Surgery treatment may include removing the uterus and, usually, the ovaries and fallopian tubes.
- Counseling may help you cope with having cancer.
- To learn more: American Cancer Society, (800) ACS-2345; website: www.cancer.org or National Cancer Institute, (800) 4-CANCER; website: www.nci.nih.gov.

MEDICATION
- Chemotherapy or hormone therapy may be prescribed.
- Antibiotic therapy, if needed for infection.

ACTIVITY
Resume normal activities, including sexual activity, when you recover from treatment.

DIET
Eat a healthy diet, even if you lose your appetite from radiation or drug therapy.

 NOTIFY OUR OFFICE IF

- You or a family member has symptoms of cancer of the uterus.
- After surgery, you have more bleeding or signs of infection, such as fever, muscle aches, and headache.
- Drugs used in treatment produce any side effects.

Special notes:

_____

_____

_____

More notes on the back of this page ☐

522

UTERINE PROLAPSE

 ## BASIC INFORMATION

DESCRIPTION
A uterus that has fallen or dropped from its normal location. This causes it to bulge into or beyond the vagina. Other types of genital prolapse may also occur:
- Cystocele (part of bladder bulges into the vagina).
- Enterocele (small bowel bulges into the vagina).
- Rectocele (rectum bulges into the vagina).

FREQUENT SIGNS AND SYMPTOMS
- A lump in front or back of the vagina, or a lump that extends outside of the vagina.
- Vague discomfort or pressure in the pelvic region.
- Backache that gets worse with lifting.
- Frequent and painful urination.
- Stress incontinence (urine leakage when laughing, sneezing, or coughing) may occur.
- Problem in moving bowels.
- Pain with sexual intercourse.

CAUSES
Prolapse occurs when muscles and ligaments of the pelvic floor become overstretched and weak.

RISK INCREASES WITH
- Being overweight.
- Having one or more vaginal births.
- Obstetrical trauma and lacerations sustained during labor and delivery.
- Normal aging and decreased estrogen.
- Strain on the supportive muscles such as from chronic cough or chronic constipation.
- Work or other activities requiring heavy lifting.
- Tumors (rare).

PREVENTIVE MEASURES
- May not be able to prevent, but can reduce the risk.
- Maintain a healthy body weight.
- Practice pelvic floor exercises during pregnancy and after childbirth.
- Exercise on a regular basis to maintain muscle strength.
- Avoid constipation.
- Consider estrogen therapy after menopause.

EXPECTED OUTCOME
Mild prolapse usually responds to conservative treatment. A more severe prolapse can be helped with surgery.

POSSIBLE COMPLICATIONS
- The cervix may become irritated and sore.
- Higher risk of infection or injury to pelvic organs.
- Hemorrhoids from straining due to constipation.
- Problems with bladder, bowel, or sexual functions.
- Prolapse may recur.

 ## DIAGNOSIS & TREATMENT

GENERAL MEASURES
- Your health care provider can usually diagnose the prolapse with a pelvic exam. Medical tests may be done to check for other pelvic disorders or complications.
- Treatment options depend on the severity of the prolapse. Other factors to consider are the patient's age, if pregnancy is still desired, and other pelvic disorders.
- Patients with mild symptoms can usually be treated without surgery. This can includes an exercise program (e.g., Kegel), hormone therapy, or use of a pessary (supportive device).
- Avoid wearing tight girdles or clothing that increases intra-abdominal pressure.
- Get treatment for any chronic coughing problem.
- Quit smoking. Find a plan that will work for you.
- Kegel exercises. Learn to recognize, control, and develop the pelvic muscles. These are the ones you use to interrupt urination in mid-stream.
- A pessary is small device inserted into the vagina to help maintain the uterus in a normal position. They come in different shapes, and are individually fitted.
- Surgery may be needed for severe prolapse. Several methods are available and it can be performed to save the uterus if desired. Your options will be discussed.
- To learn more: National Women's Health Information Center (800) 994-9662; website: www.4women.gov.

MEDICATION
- Estrogen (cream or pills) may be prescribed. It helps improve blood flow to pelvic muscles and ligaments.
- Stool softeners may be prescribed for constipation.

ACTIVITY
- Avoid heavy lifting.
- If surgery is done, resume normal activities gradually.

DIET
- Keep your weight under control.
- Eat a diet high in fiber to help prevent constipation.

 ## NOTIFY OUR OFFICE IF

- You or a family member has symptoms of uterine prolapse.
- Symptoms don't improve, despite treatment.

Special notes:

_____

_____

_____

More notes on the back of this page ☐

VAGINAL OR VULVAR CANCER

 ## BASIC INFORMATION

DESCRIPTION
A cancer that involves the growth of malignant cells in the vagina or on the vulva. The vagina is the opening to the birth canal. The vulva is the whole area surrounding the vagina and extending to the thighs including the clitoris and vaginal lips. This type of cancer is rare and occurs mostly in women over age 50. One type (rhabdomyosarcoma) occurs in children.

FREQUENT SIGNS AND SYMPTOMS
- Vulvar itching.
- Abnormal vaginal bleeding.
- Discomfort or bleeding with intercourse.
- Small or large, firm, painless sores on the vulva that may bleed easily.
- Changes in skin color.

CAUSES
For unknown reasons, abnormal cells begin to develop and grow out of control. These abnormal cells may be benign (not cancer), precancer, or cancer cells. Certain risk factors have been identified.

RISK INCREASES WITH
- Women over age 60.
- Being born between 1938 and 1971 to a mother who took DES to control spotting or bleeding in pregnancy. DES is diethylstilbestrol, a drug prescribed up to 1971.
- Family history of cancer of reproductive organs.
- Human papillomavirus (HPV), the cause of genital warts.
- Smoking.
- Multiple sex partners.
- A history of sexually transmitted diseases.
- Other cancer.

PREVENTIVE MEASURES
- No specific preventive measures. Have a yearly pelvic exam and Pap smear to detect possible problems early.
- Become familiar with the appearance of your genitals. Use a mirror and examine once a month. Darker spots around the labia are generally not vaginal or vulvar cancer. They may be a sign of melanoma, a skin cancer. See your health care provider for any dark skin change.

EXPECTED OUTCOME
Early diagnosis and treatment offer a good chance for complete recovery. Symptoms can be relieved or controlled during treatment.

POSSIBLE COMPLICATIONS
Spread to other places in the body. Common sites of spread are lymph nodes in the groin, wall of the pelvis, bladder, rectum, bone, lungs, or liver. This could be fatal.

 ## DIAGNOSIS & TREATMENT

GENERAL MEASURES
- Your health care provider will do a physical exam and a pelvic exam and ask questions about your symptoms. Medical tests will be done to diagnose cancer and to check if it has spread to other parts of the body (called staging).
- Treatment options include surgery, radiation, and (sometimes) chemotherapy. It depends on the location and stage of the cancer, and the age and physical health of the patient. Precancer conditions may be treated.
- Surgery involves leaving normal skin while removing the cancer. Different options are used depending on the cancer stage. All or part of the vagina and vulva may be removed. Lymph node removal may be needed if cancer has spread.
- Laser therapy may be used for treatment of some vulvar cancer.
- Radiation treatment (sometimes). External radiation shrinks the primary tumor. Internal radiation (implants) affects cancer that has spread to nearby tissues.
- To learn more: American Cancer Society, (800) ACS-2345; website: www.cancer.org or National Cancer Institute, (800) 4-CANCER; website: www.nci.nih.gov.

MEDICATION
- Anticancer (chemotherapy) drugs may be given by pill, through a vein, or applied topically.
- Pain relievers (if needed) may be prescribed.
- Use stool softener (if needed) to prevent constipation.

ACTIVITY
- After surgery, resume your normal activities gradually, allowing 6 weeks for full recovery.
- Sexual relations may be resumed when healing is complete or as advised by your health care provider.

DIET
No special diet after treatment.

 ## NOTIFY OUR OFFICE IF

- You or a family member has symptoms of cancer of the vagina or vulva.
- After treatment, signs of infection, such as pain, fever, swelling, or excessive vaginal bleeding occur.

Special notes:

_____

_____

_____

More notes on the back of this page ☐

VAGINISMUS

BASIC INFORMATION

DESCRIPTION
Vaginismus involves spasms (clenching up) of the pelvic muscles. This may prevent sexual intercourse. The problem can affect females of all ages. Types:
- *Primary vaginismus:* a woman has never been able to have sexual intercourse.
- *Secondary vaginismus:* a woman has had intercourse at one time, but is no longer able to because of the spasms.

FREQUENT SIGNS AND SYMPTOMS
- Muscle spasms around the vagina and rectum. They may be quite painful.
- The vagina closes so tightly that the penis cannot penetrate for sexual intercourse. It also prevents inserting any object into the vagina, such as a tampon, diaphragm, or speculum (used for pelvic exam).

CAUSES
It may be caused by physical or mental (emotional) factors, or a combination of the two.

RISK INCREASES WITH
- An unconscious desire to prevent penile penetration. This may be due to fear of pain, anxiety, hostility, anger, or a distaste for sex.
- Being brought up to think that sex is a sin or dirty.
- Previous sexual trauma (incest, rape, sexual abuse).
- The first sexual experience for a woman.
- A sexual partner who is not sensitive; insufficient or unskillful foreplay.
- Emotional stress.
- Infections, allergic reactions, or a rigid, intact hymen.
- Surgical or postdelivery scarring.
- Endometriosis (a gynecological condition).

PREVENTIVE MEASURES
Pelvic exam by a health care provider and counseling prior to beginning of sexual activity.

EXPECTED OUTCOME
Medical treatment and counseling can help. Treating the underlying cause may clear up the condition.

POSSIBLE COMPLICATIONS
Emotional problems caused by guilt, anxiety, loss of self-esteem, and feeling inadequate. Relationship problems with your sexual partner.

DIAGNOSIS & TREATMENT

GENERAL MEASURES
- You health care provider will do a physical exam and a pelvic exam if possible. Sedation may be needed for a complete exam. A sexual history is important. This will include early childhood experiences, family attitudes toward sex, previous and current sexual responses. Contraceptive practices, reproductive goals, feelings about your sexual partner, and specifics about the pain you experience will be discussed.
- Treatment will be given for any medical problems. This is often followed by therapy to help with emotional problems, and to reduce the muscle spasms.
- One therapy involves dilating (widening) the vaginal opening gently and gradually with rubber or glass dilators. Treatments may be started at the medical office and then practiced at home.
- Prior to dilation therapy or attempted intercourse, sit in a tub of warm water for 10 to 15 minutes. Baths often relax muscles and relieve discomfort.
- Kegel exercises to control the pelvic muscles may be helpful. You will be instructed on how to do them.
- Counseling is helpful for many patients and their partners. It can help resolve any conflicts and concerns in your life, and to better communicate with your partner.
- You and your partner may try other sexual activities. This can include massage, oral sex, or masturbation.

MEDICATION
- Anti-anxiety drugs or muscle relaxants may be prescribed for short period.
- Before attempting intercourse, you and your partner should use a lubricant, such as K-Y Lubricating Jelly.

ACTIVITY
No limits.

DIET
No special diet.

NOTIFY OUR OFFICE IF

- You or a family member has symptoms of vaginismus.
- Symptoms don't improve after 3 weeks, despite treatment. Symptoms recur after treatment.

Special notes:

_____

_____

_____

More notes on the back of this page ☐

VAGINITIS
(Vulvovaginitis; Atrophic Vaginitis)

 BASIC INFORMATION

DESCRIPTION

Vaginitis is an inflammation (pain, redness, and swelling) of the vagina. Types of vaginitis include:
· *Infectious:* this is the most common type and is usually caused by a bacterial infection. It may also be due to a yeast or parasitic infection.
· *Noninfectious:* may be caused by vaginal dryness (atrophic), allergic reaction, or chemical irritation.

FREQUENT SIGNS AND SYMPTOMS

· The vagina normally has a thin, whitish or clear discharge which will change if an infection is present:
   - Texture (thick, thin, or curd-like).
   - Color (white, gray, or yellowish).
   - Odor (fishy smell).
   - Amount (heavy or light).
· Itching, burning, irritation, redness, swelling, and possibly pain in the vagina or vulva (external genitals).
· Vaginal dryness (due to atrophy).
· Pain with sexual intercourse.
· Pain and burning when urinating.
· Symptoms may vary with the menstrual cycle.

CAUSES

· Infectious vaginitis causes include: bacterial vaginosis (most common cause), vulvovaginal candidiasis (a yeast infection), or trichomoniasis (a parasitic infection).
· Noninfectious causes include a decrease of natural estrogen (at menopause), an irritant (such as clothes that rub), or an allergic reaction (such as a spermicide).

RISK INCREASES WITH

· Use of antibiotic drugs.
· Spermicide or use of an intrauterine device (IUD).
· Sexual intercourse.
· Having multiple sex partners.
· Douching.
· Changes in hormone levels (pregnancy, breast-feeding, menopause, using birth-control pills).

PREVENTIVE MEASURES

· Wear underwear and pantyhose with a cotton crotch. Avoid wearing tight jeans, pants, or panty hose.
· Keep your genital area clean and dry. Don't douche.
· Don't sit around in a wet bathing suit.
· Avoid perfumed or deodorant soap, detergents, fabric softeners, bubble baths, powder, and vaginal sprays.
· Always wipe away from the vagina–front to back–after bowel movements.
· Use a latex condom for sexual intercourse unless you and your partner are monogamous (having one mate).

EXPECTED OUTCOME

With treatment, symptoms usually clear up in 3 to 4 days.

POSSIBLE COMPLICATIONS

· Vaginitis may recur after treatment.
· Without treatment, infections can lead to more serious medical problems, be a risk factor for sexual transmitted disease, or cause pregnancy complications.

 DIAGNOSIS & TREATMENT

GENERAL MEASURES

· Don't assume you have a yeast infection and use antifungal drugs to self-treat without a diagnosis. Those drugs won't help other types of infection. In addition, a vaginal infection should not be self-treated with herbal remedies, douches, or deodorant sprays.
· Your health care provider will usually do a physical exam, a pelvic exam, and ask questions about your symptoms. Tests may be done of the vaginal discharge.
· Treatment will depend on the cause of the vaginitis. Drugs are usually prescribed for infections and sometimes for vaginal dryness or irritation. Your sexual partner needs treatment if trichomoniasis is the cause.
· If the vaginitis is due to an irritant or allergic reaction, stop using the offending product.
· To learn more: National Women's Health Information Center (800) 994-9662; website: www.4women.gov.

MEDICATION

· For infection, an antibiotic, antifungal, or antiparasitic drug may be prescribed. Take the entire drug course prescribed even if symptoms improve in a few days.
· For vaginal dryness, estrogen creams or oral tablets may be recommended.
· For vaginal irritation, steroid or hormone creams may be prescribed.

ACTIVITY

It is best to avoid sexual intercourse until treatment is complete. No other limits on activity.

DIET

No special diet.

 NOTIFY OUR OFFICE IF

· You or a family member has symptoms of vaginitis.
· Symptoms recur following treatment.

Special notes:

_____

_____

_____

More notes on the back of this page ☐

VAGINOSIS, BACTERIAL
(Gardnerella Vaginitis; Nonspecific Vaginitis)

BASIC INFORMATION

DESCRIPTION
Vaginosis is an infection of the vagina. Bacterial vaginosis (BV) means that bacteria are the cause of the infection. It affects all ages, but it most often occurs during the childbearing years. It is not thought to be a sexually transmitted disease (STD), but sexual activity has been linked to this infection. It may cause vaginitis that has symptoms of soreness, itching, and irritation.

FREQUENT SIGNS AND SYMPTOMS
· About 50% of women have no symptoms.
· Vaginal discharge that may have an unpleasant odor (referred to as a "fishy" smell). The color and amount of discharge varies from woman to woman.

CAUSES
Normally, there are a number of harmless bacteria in the vagina. They may help protect against other infections such as yeast infection. These harmless bacteria sometimes get out of balance and undesirable bacteria are able to grow. Why this occurs is unknown. Undesirable bacteria types are *Gardnerella vaginalis*, *Mycoplasma hominis*, and *Mobiluncus species*.

RISK INCREASES WITH
· Intrauterine contraceptive device (IUD).
· Smokers.
· Early age at first intercourse.
· Higher number of lifetime sexual partners.
· New sexual partner, or increase in number of sexual partners in the month before diagnosis.
· Recent use of antibiotic drugs.

PREVENTIVE MEASURES
· There are no specific preventive measures. The following general measures may help to prevent bacterial vaginosis or other vaginal disorders.
· Use condoms with new sexual partners to help protect against infections, possibly bacterial vaginosis.
· Keep the genital area clean and dry. Use plain unscented soap. Be sure sexual partner is clean. Avoid vaginal douching.
· Take showers rather than tub baths. If you take a bath, don't add oils or bubble bath to the water.
· Wear cotton underwear or pantyhose with a cotton crotch.
· Don't sit around in wet clothes, such as a bathing suit.
· After going to the bathroom, wipe from front to back (vagina to anus).
· Change tampons or sanitary pads frequently.

EXPECTED OUTCOME
Mild cases may get better without treatment. Treatment can relieve symptoms in other cases, but recurrence is common.

POSSIBLE COMPLICATIONS
· May recur, but it can be retreated.
· Infection with another vaginal disorder.
· Increased risk of infection with uterine surgery.
· May cause problems with pregnancy and delivery.

DIAGNOSIS & TREATMENT

GENERAL MEASURES
· Your health care provider will do a physical exam including a pelvic exam. because some women have no symptoms of the infection, it may be diagnosed on a routine exam. Medical tests may include studies of vaginal discharge and a Pap smear.
· Treatment is usually recommended for women who have symptoms and women who will be having surgical procedures.
· For pregnant women with the infection, your obstetric provider will discuss the diagnosis, risks, and treatment recommendations when needed.
· If you smoke, find a stop smoking plan that will work for you.
· Testing and treating male sexual partners is usually not needed.
· Douches or deodorant sprays that mask vaginal odor should not be used to treat BV. They may eliminate the odor, but they will not cure the condition.
· To learn more: National Women's Health Information Center (800) 994-9662; website: www.4women.gov.

MEDICATION
Metronidazole (Flagyl) or clindamycin (Cleocin) are often prescribed for treatment of bacterial vaginosis. They are available in both an oral and topical form.

ACTIVITY
No limits.

DIET
No special diet.

NOTIFY OUR OFFICE IF

· You or a family member has a vaginal discharge.
· Symptoms persist longer than 1 week or worsen, despite treatment.
· Unusual vaginal bleeding or swelling develops.

Special notes:

_____

_____

_____

More notes on the back of this page ☐

VALVULAR HEART DISEASE
(Heart Valve Disease)

 BASIC INFORMATION

DESCRIPTION
A complication of diseases that distort or destroy valves of the heart. The heart has four valves. The mitral and tricuspid valves (main heart valves) control blood flow into the ventricles. The aortic and pulmonic valves control blood flow out of the heart. The proper functioning of the valves is vital to the heart as a pump.

FREQUENT SIGNS AND SYMPTOMS
- No symptoms (sometimes).
- Fatigue and weakness.
- Dizziness or fainting.
- Chest pain.
- Shortness of breath, which may wake you out of a sleep.
- Lung congestion.
- Heart-rhythm problems.

CAUSES
Narrowed valves (stenosis) can obstruct blood flow. Widened or scarred valves allow blood to leak backward into the heart (insufficiency). The disorder may be inherited or caused by a variety of medical problems.

RISK INCREASES WITH
- Persons over 60.
- Family history of heart-valve disease.
- Pregnancy.
- Rheumatic fever.
- A complication of strep throat.
- Atherosclerosis.
- High blood pressure.
- Congenital (being born with) heart defects.
- Endocarditis (heart inflammation).
- Intravenous (IV) drug abuse.
- Syphilis (rare).
- Marfan's syndrome.

PREVENTIVE MEASURES
- Obtain medical care for diseases that cause heart-valve damage, such as high blood pressure, endocarditis, and syphilis.
- Take antibiotics, if prescribed, for streptococcal infections to prevent rheumatic fever.
- If you have a family history of congenital heart disease, obtain genetic counseling before starting a family.

EXPECTED OUTCOMES
Depends on the underlying condition. Many complications of valvular disease can be controlled with treatment.

POSSIBLE COMPLICATIONS
- Infection of the valves.
- Congestive heart failure.

 DIAGNOSIS & TREATMENT

GENERAL MEASURES
- Your health care provider will do a physical exam. Medical tests may include blood tests, electrocardiogram (which measures electrical activity of the heart), echocardiogram (uses sound waves to examine the heart), and x-rays of the heart, lungs, and blood flow (called angiography).
- Surgery may be recommended to repair a heart valve or to remove a diseased or damaged valve. It may be replaced by a mechanical valve, one made from human or bovine tissue, or a human valve from a donor.
- Tell any doctor, dentist, or anesthesiologist who treats you that you have heart-valve disease. Remind those involved, even if you think they know the details of your medical history.
- To learn more: American Heart Association, 7272 Greenville Ave., Dallas, TX 75231; (800) 242-8721; website: www.americanheart.org.

MEDICATIONS
- You may be prescribed:
  - Antibiotics to treat or prevent bacterial infection of abnormal heart valves.
  - Antiarrhythmic drugs or digitalis drugs for the heart.
  - Anticoagulants (blood thinners) after surgery.

ACTIVITY
You will be advised about any limits. Sometimes, no limits are needed with certain forms of the disease.

DIET
You may be advised to eat a low-fat, low-salt diet.

 NOTIFY OUR OFFICE IF

- You or a family member has symptoms of heart-valve disease.
- During treatment, signs of infection develop, such as fever, chills, muscle aches, headache, fatigue, and a general ill feeling.

Special notes:

_____

_____

_____

More notes on the back of this page ☐

VARICOCELE

 ## BASIC INFORMATION

DESCRIPTION

A varicocele is a tangled network of blood vessels, or varicose veins, in the testicles. Varicocele occurs more often in the left testicle than the right, and, less often, in both. They can take up to 20 years to grow large enough to be noticeable. This is a common condition, occurring in about 15% of men (often in their 20s or 30s).

FREQUENT SIGNS AND SYMPTOMS

· In most cases, there are no symptoms. They may be diagnosed during a routine physical exam.
· Ache in the testicle. Sometimes they cause pain.
· Feeling of heaviness or dragging in the scrotum (the pouch of skin that contains the testicles).
· Atrophy (shrinkage) of the testicle.
· Enlarged veins can be felt (like feeling a "bag of worms"), and can make the testicle look lumpy.

CAUSES

· Normally, blood in the testicles travels through a series of small veins into a large vein that goes up through the abdomen. A series of one-way valves in the veins prevents the reverse flow of blood back to the testicles. Sometimes, these one-way valves become damaged or defective. This causes the blood to flow backward. This reverse flow of blood stretches and enlarges the tiny veins around the testicle to cause a varicocele.
· Because of the varicocele, the blood does not cool as it does in a normal vein. The increased temperature of the blood raises the temperature of the testicles. This is believed to contribute to infertility, as heat can damage or destroy sperm. The raised temperature may also block production of new, healthy sperm.

RISK INCREASES WITH

Men in their 20s or 30s.

PREVENTIVE MEASURES

No known preventive measures.

EXPECTED OUTCOMES

· Successful treatment can reduce the swelling and discomfort of varicoceles that cause symptoms.
· Treatment may help with infertility. It takes about 90 days for a sufficient quantity of new sperm to be produced to permit fertilization. Semen study is usually done at 3 and 6 months after treatment.

POSSIBLE COMPLICATIONS

· Low sperm count.
· Male infertility.
· Varicocele may recur after treatment.
· Some patients develop a condition called hydrocele. This is a fluid-filled cyst that forms around the testicle. Minor surgery is used to correct the problem.

 ## DIAGNOSIS & TREATMENT

GENERAL MEASURES

· Your health care provider will do an exam of the genital area. Varicoceles may be seen with the naked eye or by palpating (feeling) the area while a patient is standing up. Small varicoceles may be diagnosed with ultrasound or other medical tests.
· No treatment may be needed if there are no symptoms or the symptoms are mild and infertility is not an issue. Wear an athletic supporter or a pair of snug-fitting underwear to provide the scrotum with support.
· Surgery or other treatment may be recommended if the varicocele causes pain, atrophy, or infertility.
· Most varicoceles can be corrected through a surgical procedure called varicocelectomy (tying off the affected spermatic veins). It is usually performed under general or local anesthesia as an outpatient.
· Laparoscopy may be an option. It involves the insertion of a thin, lighted tube (called a laparoscope) through a small incision (cut) in the abdomen to locate and tie off the varicocele.
· A nonsurgical alternative called varicocele embolization may be recommended. A small catheter (tube) is inserted into the groin. Substances that will block the flow of blood are inserted through the catheter. The affected veins are sealed off, causing the blood flow to return to its normal path.

MEDICATIONS

Drugs are normally not needed.

ACTIVITY

No limits.

DIET

No special diet.

 ## NOTIFY OUR OFFICE IF

· You or a family member has symptoms of a varicocele.
· Varicocele symptoms recur after treatment.

Special notes:

_____

_____

_____

More notes on the back of this page ☐

VARICOSE VEINS

 BASIC INFORMATION

DESCRIPTION
Veins, usually in the legs, which become permanently enlarged and often twisted. Varicose veins can involve superficial veins, deep veins, and veins that connect superficial and deep veins. The disorder is more common in adults.

FREQUENT SIGNS AND SYMPTOMS
• Enlarged, bulging, ropelike, bluish veins that are visible under the skin. They appear most often in the back of the calf or on the inside of the leg from the ankle to the groin.
• Vague discomfort and aching, or pain in the legs, especially after standing.
• Fatigue.

CAUSES
The veins of the legs contain one-way valves every few inches to help blood return against gravity to the heart. If the valves leak, blood pressure in the veins prevents blood from draining properly. Valves may fail because of previous vein disease, such as thrombophlebitis; prolonged standing; or pressure on veins in the pelvis from pregnancy, tumors, or fluid in the abdomen.

RISK INCREASES WITH
• Increasing age.
• Being overweight.
• Straining. This may be from constipation, a chronic cough, prostate problems, or urinary retention.
• Family history of varicose veins.
• Work that require, prolonged sitting or standing.
• Pregnancy or menstruation.
• Injury or prior surgery on the legs.

PREVENTIVE MEASURES
• Exercise regularly, especially by walking, swimming, or bicycling to keep circulation healthy.
• Don't sit or stand for long periods. Move around.

EXPECTED OUTCOMES
Self-care steps may help symptoms. Medical treatment has a high success rate.

POSSIBLE COMPLICATIONS
• Ulcer near the ankle (stasis dermatitis) caused by poor blood flow to the skin. This may be slow to heal.
• Deep-vein blood clot.
• Venous insufficiency. Blood does not completely return to the heart.
• Varicose veins may return after treatment.

 DIAGNOSIS & TREATMENT

GENERAL MEASURES
• Your health care provider will do a physical exam of the affected veins and ask about your symptoms. Medical tests may include ultrasound and other studies.
• Simple treatment methods may be recommended:
  - Take frequent rest periods with legs elevated.
  - Use lightweight, elastic compression hosiery. It is best to put them on before getting out of bed.
  - Don't wear girdles or other tight clothing.
  - Avoid long periods of sitting or standing. Take breaks and walk around.
  - Wear comfortable shoes and avoid high heels.
  - Cross legs at ankles and not at the knees.
• Surgery and other treatment methods may be done for pain, recurrent phlebitis (inflamed veins), skin changes, or for cosmetic reasons.
• Veins can be sealed off by using sclerotherapy (injections), laser, intense-pulsed light therapy, or radio-frequency ablation. Veins can also be removed with surgery. Your health care provider will discuss your options, the risks, and benefits of each one with you.
• Spider veins (idiopathic telangiectases) are small superficial veins. They may be treated with a laser or with injections.

MEDICATIONS
• A chemical may be injected (sclerotherapy) into small varicose veins to make them collapse and disappear over time Other veins will take over blood flow.
• Drugs for pain may be prescribed following surgery.

ACTIVITY
• Walking and being active after any treatment is important to help promote healing.
• Compression hose will usually need to be worn for a period of time after any form of treatment.

DIET
• Eat healthy. Avoid alcohol.
• Consider a weight-loss diet, if weight is a problem.

 NOTIFY OUR OFFICE IF

• You or a family member has varicose veins.
• After diagnosis, varicose veins cause any problems.

Special notes:

_____

_____

_____

More notes on the back of this page ☐

VITILIGO

 BASIC INFORMATION

DESCRIPTION

Loss of skin pigment (color) that results in white patches. This condition can affect persons of any race or ethnic group. It affects skin on the hands, face and lips, arms, armpits, legs, and sometimes, the genitals. It is more common in late childhood (9 to 12 years) to mid-adulthood.

FREQUENT SIGNS AND SYMPTOMS

· Patches of different skin color.
· They are flat, usually white, and can't be felt with the fingers. Skin texture does not change.
· They don't hurt or itch.
· They spread to form very large, irregularly shaped areas without pigment.
· The amount of skin affected differs in each person. Some may have small areas, while others may gradually lose pigment over their entire body.
· Hair color may turn gray prematurely.

CAUSES

Exact cause is unknown, but it is probably an autoimmune disorder. The immune system by mistake attacks the body itself. With vitiligo, it attacks the pigment-producing cells (melanocytes), and they become weak or die resulting in a lack of pigment production.

RISK INCREASES WITH

· Family history of vitiligo.
· Exposure to some chemicals, such as phenol. It is used in photography, and is also found in some hair color products, household stains, and other products.
· Hyperthyroidism (overactive thyroid) and hypothyroidism (underactive thyroid).
· Autoimmune disorders.

PREVENTIVE MEASURES

Cannot be prevented at present.

EXPECTED OUTCOMES

· Treatment can be prolonged and often unsatisfactory. Complete and permanent repigmentation rarely occurs. It is impossible to predict how much improvement will occur with treatment. Younger individuals (under 30) and those who obtain treatment early usually respond best. Allow 1 year to evaluate results.
· Research is ongoing to look for the causes and find new, effective forms of treatment.

POSSIBLE COMPLICATIONS

· Disorder may never disappear completely, causing permanent white skin areas.
· Emotional problems may occur.

 DIAGNOSIS & TREATMENT

GENERAL MEASURES

· Your health care provider will do a physical exam of the affected areas of the skin. Medical tests may be done to check for disorders such as a thyroid problem.
· Treatment is sometimes not needed. The disorder is benign and often more of a cosmetic concern.
· Some patients with limited disease may choose to use a make-up product. Cover the affected skin with opaque makeup, self-tanning products, or dyes to help make it less noticeable.
· Some sun exposure may help improve skin color. Ask your health care provider. If advised, use sunscreen (with SPF of 15 or higher) to avoid sunburn.
· Counseling may be helpful for patients if the disorder is causing emotional problems.
· If treatment is desired, your health care provider will discuss several options. Treatment with drugs can involve repigmenting the skin or removing the remaining pigment. Surgery involving skin grafts or tattooing the affected skin are options for some patients.
· To learn more: National Vitiligo Foundation, 611 S. Fleishel Ave., Tyler, TX 75701; (903) 531-0074 (not toll free); website: www.nvfi.org.

MEDICATIONS

· Steroid creams may help repigment small areas.
· Psoralen drugs used with exposure to ultraviolet A (UVA) may be prescribed. It is called PUVA. This stimulates pigmentation. It helps some, but not all patients. Adverse effects of these drugs are frequent.
· Monobenzyl ether of hydroquinone may be prescribed for depigmentation. It can permanently remove pigment so that skin color is uniform. It takes about 6 months to a year. Success rate is about 75%.
· Other drugs may be prescribed.

ACTIVITY

No limits.

DIET

No special diet.

 NOTIFY OUR OFFICE IF

You or a family member has symptoms of vitiligo.

Special notes:

_____

_____

_____

More notes on the back of this page ☐

VOCAL CORD NODULES
("Singer's Nodes")

BASIC INFORMATION

DESCRIPTION
Nonmalignant overgrowths of tissue on the vocal cords. The condition can be common in children and occurs in women more than men.

FREQUENT SIGNS AND SYMPTOMS
· Persistent hoarseness without pain.
· Breathy or scratchy voice.
· Singers may notice they have a voice alteration.

CAUSES
The vocal cords are located in the voice box (larynx) in the middle of the throat. They are made up of two fibrous bands that vibrate to produce sound. The bands are covered with skin-like tissue. This tissue becomes thickened when the vocal cords are used a lot. A part of the thickened tissue can grow and produce nodules. They appear as red, swollen bumps and may be the size of a pinhead up to a small pea. When nodules occur, the vocal cords cannot close completely. This causes the voice to sound hoarse.

RISK INCREASES WITH
· Continued overuse of the voice by singing, shouting, yelling, lecturing, or other forms of talking too loudly or too much.
· Excessive coughing or throat clearing.
· Using the voice incorrectly.
· People who use the voice a lot such as singers, teachers, ministers, auctioneers, cheerleaders, aerobic instructors, and others.
· Smoking or exposure to smoke.
· Chronic infection caused by allergies or irritants.
· Reflux (stomach acid backs up into throat).

PREVENTIVE MEASURES
· Take voice or speech lessons to learn proper techniques for speaking or singing.
· Don't smoke. Avoid being around smokers.
· Drink plenty of fluids.
· Try not to use the voice too long or too loudly.
· Rest your voice for a while when it appears to have been overused.

EXPECTED OUTCOMES
Almost always curable with voice therapy treatment or surgery.

POSSIBLE COMPLICATIONS
· Without treatment, permanent hoarseness or voice change may occur.
· Nodules may regrow after treatment if voice continues to be overused.

DIAGNOSIS & TREATMENT

GENERAL MEASURES
· Your health care provider will do a physical exam of the throat and vocal cords. Medical tests may include a biopsy of the nodule to rule out cancer. A biopsy involves removing a small piece of tissue for viewing under a microscope.
· Treatment usually involves voice therapy (voice behavior). This may include voice rest (using your voice less, controlling the loudness and not talking much for a few days). Therapy includes behavior training on healthy use of the voice and proper voice techniques. Therapy may take 1 to 2 sessions a week for 5 to 6 weeks.
· Surgery (rarely) to remove nodules may be needed if voice therapy is not effective. Surgery is usually not done in children under age 12.
· Quit smoking. Find a way to stop that works for you.

MEDICATIONS
Drugs are usually not needed for this disorder.

ACTIVITY
No limits except those for voice usage.

DIET
No special diet.

NOTIFY OUR OFFICE IF

You or a family member is hoarse for more than 2 weeks.

Special notes:

_____

_____

_____

More notes on the back of this page ☐

VULVOVAGINITIS BEFORE PUBERTY

BASIC INFORMATION

DESCRIPTION

Infection or inflammation (redness and soreness) of the vagina or vulva before a young girl reaches puberty. Before puberty, the skin around the vaginal area can be very sensitive, and it can easily become red and inflamed.

FREQUENT SIGNS AND SYMPTOMS

- Redness, pain, and itching around the genital area.
- Vaginal discharge. It may or may not have an odor.
- Pain with urination.
- Bleeding from the affected area (sometimes).

CAUSES

- Infections caused by bacteria, parasites (including pinworms), yeast-like fungi, or viruses.
- Allergies to synthetic fabrics, soap, or other items in contact with the genitals.
- Scratches, abrasions or genital injury from foreign body in the vagina (this could be some toilet paper).
- Genital injury from sexual abuse.
- Irritation from bubble bath or oils put in bath water.

RISK INCREASES WITH

- Poor hygiene such as infrequent bathing, not wiping, or wiping incorrectly after urinating.
- Diabetes.
- Trauma or injury to the vaginal area.
- Overweight.
- Wearing tight leotards, jeans, underwear, or bathing suits.

PREVENTIVE MEASURES

- Teach the child to wipe from the vagina toward the anus after bowel movements.
- Don't let the child sit around in wet clothing, especially a wet bathing suit. Avoid tight clothing.
- Have the child bathe or shower frequently.
- Don't use scented soap or bubble baths, dyed or perfumed toilet tissue.
- Provide the child with cotton underpants or nylon underpants with a cotton crotch.
- Teach your child to resist and report any attempted sexual contact by anyone.
- Don't wash your child's hair in the bath. Shampoo the hair over a sink instead. If you do it in the bath, wash it at the end of the bath. Be sure to rinse off any shampoo that may have gotten on the genital area.
- Use a bland ointment for protection of the skin.

EXPECTED OUTCOME

Symptoms often clear up by using preventive measures. In cases of infection, drugs will relieve symptoms.

POSSIBLE COMPLICATIONS

Symptoms may persist or other skin infections may develop. Rarely, an infection may worsen.

DIAGNOSIS & TREATMENT

GENERAL MEASURES

- Your child's health care provider will usually do a physical exam, including a gentle exam of the genital area. Medical tests may include blood studies and a culture of any vaginal discharge.
- Treatment will depend on the cause.
- It may involve removing any foreign object in the vagina.
- Stop the use of any product that may cause irritation or allergy, such as soap or bubble bath.
- Follow steps in Preventive Measures.
- Your child's health care provider will be discuss any possibility of child abuse with you.
- Prevent urine from stinging inflamed skin: The child may urinate while in the shower. Urinate through a toilet-paper roll or plastic cup with the bottom cut out. Pour a cup of warm water over the genital area while urinating.
- Taking sitz baths (warm water baths) in clear water 2 to 4 times a day may help relieve symptoms.

MEDICATION

- Nonprescription topical ointments, or 0.5% or 1% hydrocortisone cream, 3 to 4 times a day may be recommended to relieve burning and itching.
- Drugs for infection (including antibiotics, antifungal, or antiparasitic drugs) may be prescribed.

ACTIVITY

No limits.

DIET

No special diet.

NOTIFY OUR OFFICE IF

- Your child has symptoms of vulvovaginitis.
- You suspect your child has been sexually abused.
- Symptoms don't improve in 7 to 10 days or symptoms worsen, despite treatment.

Special notes:

_____

_____

_____

More notes on the back of this page ☐

VULVOVAGINITIS, CANDIDIASIS
(Vaginal Yeast Infection)

 BASIC INFORMATION

DESCRIPTION

Vulvovaginal candidiasis is an infection of the vagina and vulva (external genitals). It can affect women of all ages but occurs most often in the childbearing years. Men may have candidiasis infection with no symptoms.

FREQUENT SIGNS AND SYMPTOMS

· The symptoms vary among women and from time to time, in the same woman.
· White, "curdy" vaginal discharge (resembles lumps of cottage cheese). Odor may be unpleasant, but not foul.
· Swollen, red, tender, itching vaginal lips (labia) and surrounding skin.
· Burning during urination.
· Change in vaginal color from pale pink to red.
· Pain during sexual intercourse (dyspareunia).

CAUSES

Most often, the cause is a yeast-like fungus called *Candida albicans*. Healthy women have this yeast in their vagina (and the mouth and intestines). If the normal conditions of the vagina change, the yeast can overgrow and cause infection. Rarely, *Candida* may be passed from person to person, by sexual intercourse.

RISK INCREASES WITH

· Pregnancy.
· Diabetes.
· Drugs (antibiotics, corticosteroids, birth control pills).
· Weak immune system from drugs or disease.
· Recent illness, poor diet, or lack of sleep.

PREVENTIVE MEASURES

· There are no specific preventive measures. The following steps may help to prevent vaginal disorders.
· Use condoms with new sexual partners to help protect against some infections.
· Keep the genital area clean and dry. Use plain unscented soap. Be sure sexual partner is clean. Avoid vaginal douching.
· Take showers rather than tub baths. If you take a bath, don't add oils or bubble bath to the water.
· Wear cotton underwear or pantyhose with a cotton crotch. Avoid tight jeans, pants, or pantyhose.
· Don't sit around in wet clothes, such as bathing suits.
· After going to the bathroom, wipe from front to back (vagina to anus).
· Change tampons or sanitary pads frequently.
· Take antibiotics only when prescribed for you.

EXPECTED OUTCOME

Symptoms will normally clear up with treatment.

POSSIBLE COMPLICATIONS

· It may cause vaginitis (soreness, itching, and irritation).

· Some women may develop recurrent vulvovaginal candidiasis (RVVC). This is when four or more episodes of vulvovaginal candidiasis have occurred in one year.

 DIAGNOSIS & TREATMENT

GENERAL MEASURES

· Don't assume you have a yeast infection and use antifungal (yeast) drugs to self-treat without a diagnosis. Also, a vaginal infection should not be self-treated with douches, deodorant sprays, or herbal remedies.
· Your health care provider will usually do a physical exam and a pelvic exam and ask questions about your symptoms. Tests of the vaginal discharge may be done.
· Drug therapy is usually recommended.
· If urinating causes burning, urinate through a tubular device, such as a toilet-paper roll or plastic cup with the bottom cut out, or pour a cup of warm water over the genital area while you urinate.
· To learn more: National Women's Health Information Center (800) 994-9662; website: www.4women.gov.

MEDICATION

· Antifungal drugs, either in vaginal creams or suppositories or in oral form, may be recommended. Some nonprescription examples are miconazole nitrate (Monistat-7) and clotrimazole (Gyne-Lotrimin, Mycelex-7, and FemCare). Follow the instructions on the product. If you have tried one of these drugs and it has not worked for you, your health care provider may prescribe a prescription-only drug.
· Recurrent vulvovaginal candidiasis treatment usually involves two weeks of intensive antifungal drugs, then up to six months of a lower "maintenance" dose.

ACTIVITY

Delay sexual relations until symptoms clear up.

DIET

Some women find that eating yogurt or a low sugar diet can help in preventing or treating yeast infections.

 NOTIFY OUR OFFICE IF

· You or a family member has symptoms of vulvovaginal candidiasis.
· Symptoms get worse or recur.

Special notes:

_____

_____

_____

More notes on the back of this page ☐

WARTS
(Verruca Vulgaris)

BASIC INFORMATION

DESCRIPTION
Skin growths caused by a virus in the outer skin layer. Warts are not cancerous. They are mildly contagious from person to person and from one area to another on the same person. They can appear anywhere on the skin, but most likely on the fingers, hands, and arms. They are most common in children and young adults between ages 1 and 30, but may occur at any age. Note: this information does not discuss genital warts.

FREQUENT SIGNS AND SYMPTOMS
A small, raised bump on the skin with the following features:
- Warts begin very small and grow larger.
- Warts have a rough surface and clearly defined borders. They are usually the same color as the skin, but sometimes darker.
- Warts often appear in clusters around a "mother wart."
- If you cut into the wart surface, it contains small black dots or bleeding points.
- Warts are painless and typically don't itch.
- Plantar warts appear on the soles of the feet.

CAUSES
Infection of the outer skin layer (epidermis) by the human papillomavirus (HPV) family. The virus causes some cells to grow more rapidly than normal. Warts are very common.

RISK INCREASES WITH
- Use of public showers.
- Skin injury.
- People who have a weak immune system due to drugs or illness.

PREVENTIVE MEASURES
- To keep from spreading warts, don't scratch them. Warts spread readily to small cuts and scratches.
- Wear thong sandals in public locker rooms, swimming pools, or showers. Don't share towels.

EXPECTED OUTCOMES
There is no one specific treatment for warts that works for everybody. Some warts go away on their own, others are cured with nonprescription drugs. Some may require medical care that could include surgery. There are also many "home remedies" that may work for some people. Nonsurgical treatment for warts may take some time, so be patient.

POSSIBLE COMPLICATIONS
- Spread to other places in the body.
- Scars where warts were removed.
- Recurrence of warts after treatment.

DIAGNOSIS & TREATMENT

GENERAL MEASURES
- There are a variety of nonprescription products and home (or folk) remedies for warts. Family members or friends may recommend trying different treatments.
- Your health care provider has other options for treatment. These can be done during an office visit. Some treatments may be somewhat painful, so be sure to discuss the risks and benefits.
  - Cryotherapy (freezing) with liquid nitrogen. Freezing causes a blister to form that heals in about a week. More than one treatment may be needed for complete wart removal.
  - Electrosurgery (using heat). This treatment is often completed in one office visit. An electric needle is used to cut away the wart or destroy it.
  - Surgery with a knife (scalpel) or laser.
  - Injection of a drug into the wart.

MEDICATIONS
- There are nonprescription drugs for treatment of warts. Most are applied to skin daily for several weeks. Also available is a freezing aerosol product. Follow the instructions provided with any product that you buy.
- Your health care provider may prescribe stronger drugs or injections for removing the warts.

ACTIVITY
No limits.

DIET
No special diet.

NOTIFY OUR OFFICE IF

- You or your child has warts on the face or genital area.
- Self-treatment for warts has not worked.
- After treatment, the treated skin becomes hot, red, and painful.
- Warts don't disappear completely after treatment.
- Other warts appear after treatment.

Special notes:

_____

_____

_____

More notes on the back of this page ☐

WARTS, GENITAL
(Condylomata Acuminata; Venereal Warts)

 BASIC INFORMATION

DESCRIPTION
Warts in the genital area. The warts can affect both sexes of sexually active young people and adults. Women are affected more often than men.

FREQUENT SIGNS AND SYMPTOMS
· Warts appear on moist surfaces of the genital area. They are thin, flexible, solid raised areas of the skin, growing in stalks or clusters. They are taller than they are wide. They may be tiny or grow in larger masses. Small warts usually cause no symptoms.
· In women, they may be on the inside and outside of the vagina, on the cervix, or around the anus.
· Men may have warts on the tip or shaft of the penis or around the anus.
· They don't hurt or itch.
· Women may have a vaginal discharge.

CAUSES
· Genital warts are caused by certain types of the human papillomavirus (HPV). More than 100 types of HPV have been identified and most are harmless. About 30 types are spread through sexual contact.
· Genital warts spread very easily from one person to another. They are spread through oral, genital, or anal sex with an infected person. They have an incubation period of 1 to 6 months. Genital warts are considered a sexually transmitted disease (STD). Some types of HPV that cause genital warts can also cause, or be a risk factor for, genital cancers.

RISK INCREASES WITH
· Other venereal disease.
· Multiple sexual partners.
· Smoking.
· Early age for first sexual intercourse.
· Use of oral contraceptives.

PREVENTIVE MEASURES
· Men and women need to avoid sexual activity with a person who has visible genital warts.
· Use rubber (latex) condoms during sexual intercourse. They may reduce the risk of genital warts.
· Don't pick, squeeze, or scratch the warts. You can spread them to other places in your body.

EXPECTED OUTCOMES
Small warts often disappear on their own. Because the virus is a risk factor for genital cancer, get medical care. Treatment can get rid of the warts, but the virus stays in the body. Recurrence of warts after treatment is common. Most HPV infections do not progress to cancer.

POSSIBLE COMPLICATIONS
· Cancer.
· Problems in pregnant woman and her newborn.

 DIAGNOSIS & TREATMENT

GENERAL MEASURES
· Your health care provider will do a physical exam including a pelvic exam. Vinegar (acetic acid) may be applied to the skin area to better see any warts. A special magnifying instrument may be used to view the affected area. Medical tests may include a Pap smear. If it shows abnormal cells, further follow up will be done.
· Treatment will be determined by size and location of the warts.
· Some warts may be treated with drugs that are applied to the skin.
· Other warts may be frozen (cryotherapy), burned (electrocautery), or removed with laser treatment.
· Warts that are large and have not responded to other treatment may need to be surgically removed.
· Pregnant women with genital warts will be examined by their obstetric providers. The possible problems for mother and for the baby and options for treatment will be discussed.

MEDICATIONS
There are several types of drugs that can be used on the warts. Some are applied at a medical office and others can be used at home. Your health care provider will discuss the options, the risks, and benefits of each type. Follow instructions carefully if you decide on home treatment.

ACTIVITY
No limits, except to avoid sexual relations until warts are completely gone.

DIET
No special diet.

 NOTIFY OUR OFFICE IF

· You or a family member has symptoms of genital warts.
· The treated area becomes infected (red, swollen, painful, or tender).
· Warts return after treatment.

Special notes:

_____

_____

_____

More notes on the back of this page ☐

BASIC INFORMATION

DESCRIPTION

People who look for health and medical information have many choices on the World Wide Web. It is important to know the source and if it is reliable. Look at the web page address. The following types of addresses often have excellent websites:

· Addresses that end in *.gov* are hosted by the U.S. government.

· Addresses that end in *.org* are hosted by nonprofit organizations, such as the American Heart Association.

· Addresses ending in *.edu* are provided by universities.

Websites that advertise products (*.com*) can be good sources for medical information also, but should be read with some caution. It is often helpful to compare several different web resources on the same topic.

Information obtained from the Web is not a substitute for your health care provider's instructions and advice. Words on the computer screen can not replace the knowledge and experience that your health care provider can share with you.

SELECTED WEB SITES

This is a selected list of websites that provide medical information. There are also many others (sponsored by different types of organizations) that are useful for valid and quality medical information, patient education materials, and helpful ideas for managing your health.

· **CancerNet (National Cancer Institute)**
www.cancernet.nci.nih.gov
A source of current cancer information for patients and anyone interested in learning more about this topic.

· **Centers for Disease Control (CDC) Division of Sexually Transmitted Diseases Prevention**
www.cdc.gov/nchstp/dstd/dstdp.html
Provides information on specific diseases. An excellent starting point for finding reliable STD facts.

· **Family Doctor**
www.familydoctor.org
The American Academy of Family Physicians provides information for general educational purposes for the whole family. All of the information has been written and reviewed by physicians and patient education professionals.

· **American Dental Association**
www.ada.org/public//index.asp
The American Dental Association provides information on a variety of topics about your teeth and oral health. They include topics such as Anxiety about dental visits.

· **Healthfinder**
www.healthfinder.gov
The U.S. Department of Health & Human services along with other federal agencies designed this web site as a gateway to consumer health information. It provides access to selected online publications, clearinghouses, databases, web sites, and support and self-help groups. It also links to government agencies and not-for-profit organizations that produce reliable information for the public. Resources in Spanish are located in the section, "espanol."

· **Medem**
www.medem.com
Medem is the web site project of several organizations–including the American Medical Association, the American Academy of Pediatrics, and the American College of Obstetricians and Gynecologists. It is a comprehensive and trusted source of health care content on the Internet.

· **Medlineplus**
www.medlineplus.gov
A web site established by the National Library of Medicine, the world's largest biomedical library and creator of the Medline database. An alphabetical list of medical and health topics consists of hundreds of specific diseases, conditions and wellness issues. Health information in Spanish is also included.

· **National Women's Health Information Center (NWHIC)**
www.4woman.gov
A project of the Office on Women's Health in the U.S. Department of Health and Human Services (HHS). NWHIC is a gateway to women's health information resources that allows visitors to read and download a wide variety of materials developed by federal government agencies, and private sector resources.

· **Mayo Clinic**
www.mayoclinic.com
Sponsored by the Mayo Clinic, this site offers general information about health and medical topics. New information is added daily.

· **National Health Information center**
www.health.gov/nhic
This site is run by the U.S. Department of Health and Human Services. It provides links to many organizations that have information about specific medical topics.

Special notes:

_____

_____

_____

More notes on the back of this page ☐

WEST NILE VIRUS

 BASIC INFORMATION

DESCRIPTION

A virus that can cause a mild or, less often, a serious disease in humans. Outbreaks often occur in the summer and continue into the fall, but can happen year round. Most people who are infected will not show any symptoms. About 20% will have mild symptoms typically lasting a few days. This is called West Nile fever. A few (1 in 150 infected persons) will develop severe disease.

FREQUENT SIGNS AND SYMPTOMS

- Mild symptoms:
  - Fever.
  - Headache.
  - Body aches.
  - Nausea and vomiting.
  - Swollen lymph glands.
  - Skin rash on the chest, stomach, and back.
- Severe symptoms can include high fever, headache, neck stiffness, stupor, disorientation, coma, tremors, convulsions, muscle weakness, vision loss, numbness, and paralysis.

CAUSES

Bite of an infected mosquito. Mosquitoes are carriers that become infected when they feed on infected birds. Infected mosquitoes can then spread the infection to humans and other animals when they bite. In a very few cases, it has spread through blood transfusions, organ transplants, breastfeeding, and during pregnancy from mother to baby. It is not spread through casual contact such as touching or kissing a person with the virus. People may develop symptoms between 3 and 14 days after they are bitten by an infected mosquito.

RISK INCREASES WITH

- People who spend a lot of time outdoors.
- Presence of mosquitoes in or around the home.
- People with chronic disease, weak immune system, or the elderly are more likely to develop severe illness.

PREVENTIVE MEASURES

- When outdoors, use mosquito repellent containing DEET on the skin. Wear protective, light-colored clothing. Spray clothing with DEET or permethrin products.
- Put screens on windows and doors. Drain standing water from buckets, flower pots, and other items.
- Don't handle dead birds. Call local health department.
- Mosquito control programs in communities can help.
- Vaccines for the virus are being researched.

EXPECTED OUTCOMES

Mild symptoms clear up without treatment. In severe cases, most patients recover with hospital care, but it may be fatal.

POSSIBLE COMPLICATIONS

- Encephalitis (inflammation of the brain).
- Meningitis (inflammation of the lining of the brain).
- Meningoencephalitis (having both of the above).
- Permanent brain damage or muscle weakness, or death (rare).

 DIAGNOSIS & TREATMENT

GENERAL MEASURES

- Most people will not seek or need medical care. Mild symptoms are similar to other virus infections that people usually treat themselves.
- See your health care provider if you have any concern about the symptoms. A physical exam may be done and questions asked about your symptoms and activities. A blood test may be done if needed to confirm diagnosis.
- No treatment is available to cure the infection. Drugs may help relieve symptoms such as fever or headache.
- Severe symptoms require hospital care. Treatment can include fluids given through a vein (IV), breathing support (sometimes with a machine), and steps to prevent more complications.
- To learn more: Centers for Disease Control and Prevention, (888) 246-2675; website: www.cdc.gov, or call your local health department.

MEDICATIONS

You may use nonprescription drugs for mild symptoms such as fever, pain, or headache. Antibiotics do not help virus infections.

ACTIVITY

No limits for people with mild symptoms.

DIET

No special diet.

 NOTIFY OUR OFFICE IF

- You or a family member has symptoms of West Nile virus infection that you are concerned about.
- Symptoms are severe, get emergency care.

Special notes:

_____

_____

_____

More notes on the back of this page ☐

538

WHIPLASH
(Cervical Sprain or Strain)

BASIC INFORMATION

DESCRIPTION
Injury to the neck caused when it is whipped forcefully backward and then forward, usually in an accident. Body areas involved are the muscles, tendons, ligaments, disks, and nerves in the neck.

FREQUENT SIGNS AND SYMPTOMS
- Pain in the front and back of the neck either immediately following or up to 24 hours after injury.
- Stiffness in the neck. Difficult to move neck around.
- Pain may go into the shoulder or arm.
- Headache.

CAUSES
Injury, usually from a motor-vehicle accident or contact sports. It may also be caused by being punched or hit by a falling object, or rarely, in cases of child abuse.

RISK INCREASES WITH
- Situations that make accidents more likely, such as:
  - Driving in rainy, icy, or snowy weather.
  - "Tail-gating" or other poor driving habits.
  - Driving after excess alcohol use or use of mind-altering drugs.
- Women are more often affected than men.
- Previous neck injury.
- People who have bone or joint disease.

PREVENTIVE MEASURES
- Use seatbelts and the padded headrests in your auto. These have decreased the frequency and severity of auto whiplash injuries. Drive carefully and defensively. Don't drink alcohol and drive.
- Use proper head gear for contact sports.

EXPECTED OUTCOMES
The injury is usually not serious and permanent damage is rare. Most people recover in a few weeks to 3 months.

POSSIBLE COMPLICATIONS
- Temporary numbness and weakness in the arms, if nerve roots are injured. This may persist until recovery.
- A few may have symptoms for a year, while others may have some symptoms even after two years. It may affect quality of life for a person. Depression may occur.

DIAGNOSIS & TREATMENT

GENERAL MEASURES
- Your health care provider will do a physical exam and ask questions about your symptoms and the cause of your injury. X-rays or other tests may be done to rule out injury to the spine.
- Treatment will depend on the extent of injury. Steps may include drugs and/or injections, physical therapy, exercises, massage, chiropractor care, heat or ice, wearing a neck collar, ultrasound, or traction. You and your health care provider can discuss a treatment plan for your individual needs.
- Apply ice packs (over a towel) to the injured area for 10 to 20 minutes each hour during the first 24 hours.
- After 24 hours, use ice packs or heat to relieve pain. Heat may include warm showers twice a day, in which the water beats on your neck and shoulders for 10 to 20 minutes. Between showers, apply warm soaks to the neck several times a day for 10 to 15 minutes.
- Surgery to remove an injured spinal disk (rare).

MEDICATIONS
- Pain relievers or muscle relaxants may be prescribed.
- You may use aspirin (not for children), ibuprofen, or acetaminophen for minor pain.

ACTIVITY
People who stay active and exercise the neck muscles as directed appear to recover more quickly. Resume routine activities and work as soon as possible. Some adjustments at your job may be needed for a short time.

DIET
No special diet. Avoid alcohol.

NOTIFY OUR OFFICE IF

- You or a family member has a painful neck injury.
- Pain, numbness, tingling, or weakness develops in the arm or face.
- New, unexplained symptoms develop. Drugs used in treatment may produce side effects.

Special notes:

_____

_____

_____

More notes on the back of this page ☐

WHOOPING COUGH

(Pertussis)

 BASIC INFORMATION

DESCRIPTION

A serious, contagious infection of the nose, throat, and lungs. Pertussis is the medical name for whooping cough. It can affect all ages, but most often occurs in children. Use of a vaccine has greatly reduced the occurrence of the disease.

FREQUENT SIGNS AND SYMPTOMS

Early stages:
- Runny nose.
- Dry cough that leads to a cough with thick sputum.
- Slight fever.

Late stages:
- Severe, ongoing coughing bouts that last up to 1 minute. The face turns red or blue from lack of oxygen while coughing. At the end of each coughing effort, the person gasps for breath with a "whooping" sound.
- Vomiting and diarrhea.
- Little or no fever.

CAUSES

Bordetella pertussis bacteria. Germs are spread by contact with an infected person, breathing in germs in the air, or touching an object with germs on it. The time from being exposed to the germs to having symptoms is about 7 to 10 days, and not more than 21 days.

RISK INCREASES WITH

- Children who have not been immunized or have not completed the whole series of vaccine shots needed.
- The vaccine protection fades as children get older. Teens and adults can easily get the infection if exposed.
- A person who does not know they have the infection may spread the germs. This can happen during the first 21 days of their cough.

PREVENTIVE MEASURES

- Pertussis vaccine starting in infancy is the best way.
- Adult forms of the vaccine are being tested.
- Keep infants away from anyone with a cough illness.

EXPECTED OUTCOMES

Usually curable in about 6 weeks with treatment (may range from 3 weeks to 3 months). The usual course of illness is: 2 weeks with the cough; 2 weeks with bouts of the "whooping" cough; and 2 weeks for recovery. Some persistent coughs may continue for months.

POSSIBLE COMPLICATIONS

- Children under age one are at high risk for complications. They are less likely in older children and adults.
- Complications include severe ear infection, nosebleeds, dehydration, pneumonia, convulsions, and in rare cases, brain damage and death.

 DIAGNOSIS & TREATMENT

GENERAL MEASURES

- Your health care provider will do a physical exam. The diagnosis can be made based on the symptoms and knowing about contact with an infected person. Medical tests are usually done to confirm the diagnosis.
- Treatment depends on how severe the symptoms are.
- Severely ill infants will need hospital care.
- Children can usually be treated at home. They should get extra rest, drink plenty of fluids, take any prescribed drugs, and be watched for any complications.
- Keep an ill person at home and away from others when possible. Return to daycare, school, or work is permitted after taking antibiotics for five days. Without antibiotics, it will be 3 to 4 weeks after the start of symptoms.

MEDICATIONS

- An antibiotic, most often erythromycin, is usually prescribed. If started early in the infection, it helps improve symptoms. It also reduces the risk of spreading germs.
- Close contacts of an infected person are usually prescribed antibiotics to help prevent the infection (even if they have had the vaccine).

ACTIVITY

Resume normal activity after symptoms get better.

DIET

- Drink extra fluids, such as fruit juice, tea, carbonated drinks, and clear soups.
- No special diet. Small, frequent meals may decrease vomiting.

 NOTIFY OUR OFFICE IF

- You or a family member has symptoms of whooping cough or has been exposed to anyone with it.
- Your child's coughing is severe.
- Vomiting persists more than 1 or 2 days.
- You are concerned about any symptoms that occur.

Special notes:

_____

_____

_____

More notes on the back of this page ☐

WILMS' TUMOR

(Nephroblastoma)

 ## BASIC INFORMATION

DESCRIPTION

A malignant, mixed tumor (one that contains several cell types) of the kidneys. Only one kidney is affected in 90% of cases. The kidneys are a pair of organs that are shaped like kidney beans. They are located on either side of the backbone. Kidneys filter and clean the blood in the body and make urine. Wilms' tumor usually affects children under age 7, with a peak incidence between ages 3 and 4. Very rarely, it may not appear until teen years or adulthood.

FREQUENT SIGNS AND SYMPTOMS

- Enlarged abdomen. A large, firm, smooth tumor can usually be felt within the abdominal wall.
- Blood in the urine (urine may appear cloudy).
- Abdominal pain (sometimes).
- Repeated vomiting.
- Fever.
- Weight loss.
- High blood pressure (this may have no symptoms).

CAUSES

Exact cause is unknown. It often occurs along with other congenital (being born with) abnormalities. These include urinary-tract problems, absence of iris in the eyes (aniridia), and enlargement of one side of the body.

RISK INCREASES WITH

- Congenital abnormalities.
- African Americans are more often affected.
- Girls are more often affected than boys.

PREVENTIVE MEASURES

Cannot be prevented at present.

EXPECTED OUTCOMES

With appropriate treatment, the outlook is good. In most cases, Wilms' tumor is curable with surgery, radiation treatment, and chemotherapy (anticancer) drugs. Long-term follow-up care is needed to watch for any late effects of treatment.

POSSIBLE COMPLICATIONS

- Cancer may recur.
- Tumor may spread to lungs, bones, liver, or brain, if untreated.
- Adverse reactions, including hair loss, from radiation treatment and chemotherapy.
- Surgery procedures may have complications.
- Kidney function problems.
- Chemotherapy and radiation treatment are risk factors for developing other types of cancer.

 ## DIAGNOSIS & TREATMENT

GENERAL MEASURES

- Your child's health care provider will do a physical exam. Different medical tests are done to verify the diagnosis and to determine if the cancer has spread to other places in the body (called staging).
- The treatment plan will be determined by the stage of the cancer, the type of cancer cells, the size of the tumor, and your child's age and health status. Your child's health care provider will discuss all aspects of treatment with you.
- Surgery is usually needed for treatment. It may involve removal of the tumor and the whole affected kidney or less often, a portion of the kidney. Body tissue around the kidney and lymph nodes may need to be removed.
- Chemotherapy (anticancer drugs) may be done before and/or after surgery. Radiation may be done for certain stages of the tumor.
- To learn more: American Cancer Society, (800) ACS-2345; website: www.cancer.org or National Cancer Institute, (800) 4-CANCER; website: www.nci.nih.gov.

MEDICATIONS

Your child's health care provider may prescribe anticancer drugs, antinausea drugs, pain relievers, antibiotics (if infection occurs), and stool softeners to prevent constipation following surgery.

ACTIVITY

An active lifestyle is possible with one kidney. Sports activities that carry a risk of kidney injury (e.g., hockey or boxing) should be avoided.

DIET

No special diet.

 ## NOTIFY OUR OFFICE IF

- Your child has symptoms of Wilms' tumor.
- The following occur during treatment:
  - Vomiting, abdominal pain or constipation.
  - Shortness of breath.
  - Swelling in feet or ankles.
- New, unexplained symptoms develop. Drugs used in treatment may cause side effects.

Special notes:

_____

_____

_____

More notes on the back of this page ☐

ZINC DEFICIENCY

 BASIC INFORMATION

DESCRIPTION
Inadequate amounts of zinc in body cells. This affects the function of the testicles, liver, and muscles, and affects the structure of bones, teeth, hair, and skin. Zinc is a vital part of many enzymes that aid chemical reactions needed for normal body function. This includes immune function and skin healing. Zinc deficiency can affect all ages, but is most common in children during periods of rapid growth (10 to 18 years).

FREQUENT SIGNS AND SYMPTOMS
· Poor appetite.
· Poor growth.
· Sensations of unpleasant tastes and odors, and decreased senses of taste and smell.
· Decreased sex drive.
· Darkening of the skin all over the body.
· Sparse hair growth.
· Deformed nails.

CAUSES
· Excessive intake of substances that bind zinc and prevent its absorption from the gastrointestinal tract. These include calcium, vitamin D, high fiber-diet, and phytate enzyme (found in whole-meal bread).
· Surgical removal of any part of the gastrointestinal tract, especially the stomach.
· Parasitic infection in the gastrointestinal tract.
· Excessive milk drinking in preschool children.

RISK INCREASES WITH
· Alcoholism. Alcohol increases the excretion of zinc.
· Use of cortisone drugs increases zinc excretion.
· Pregnancy.
· Diabetes, kidney disease, or cirrhosis.
· Burns or major trauma.

PREVENTIVE MEASURES
· Adults should not drink or eat more than the recommended amounts of milk, other dairy products, or whole-meal bread. Keep calcium intake at 1500 mg or less daily.
· Don't take large doses of vitamin D supplements.
· Take zinc supplements if you have had gastrointestinal surgery.
· Obtain medical care for any parasite infections.
· Don't drink more than 1 or 2 alcoholic drinks, if any, a day.

EXPECTED OUTCOMES
Usually curable in 2 months with zinc supplements and removal or treatment of the underlying causes.

POSSIBLE COMPLICATIONS
· Iron-deficiency anemia. Zinc is necessary for iron absorption.
· Poor wound healing.
· Liver and spleen enlargement.
· Excess zinc replacement or overdose may interfere with the body's manufacture of necessary enzymes.

 DIAGNOSIS & TREATMENT

GENERAL MEASURES
· Your health care provider may do a physical exam and ask questions about your symptoms. Medical tests may include blood studies to determine zinc levels, and other tests to determine any underlying disorder.
· Treatment usually consists of correcting the cause and the use of zinc supplements.

MEDICATIONS
Zinc supplements. Take with milk or meals to prevent stomach upset.

ACTIVITY
No limits.

DIET
Eat foods high in zinc such as red meat. Avoid excessive intake of whole-meal bread.

 NOTIFY OUR OFFICE IF

You or a family member has symptoms of zinc deficiency.

Special notes:

_____

_____

_____

More notes on the back of this page ☐

DIETS

APPENDIX

ILLUSTRATIONS

PURPOSE:
This diet is designed to promote optimum health through good nutrition. It is to be used for those individuals requiring no special dietary modification or restrictions.

DESCRIPTION:
Foods from all basic food groups are included with the addition of other foods to meet energy needs and provide essential nutrients. The diet is planned to reduce the risk of chronic conditions such as heart disease, hypertension, cancer, and diabetes.

BASIC INFORMATION:
The Dietary Guidelines for Americans outline what people should eat to stay healthy. The guidelines include:

- Eat a variety of foods.
- Balance the foods you eat with physical activity—maintain or improve your weight.
- Choose a diet with plenty of grain products, vegetables, and fruits.
- Choose a diet low in fat, saturated fat, and cholesterol.
- Choose a diet moderate in sugars.
- Choose a diet moderate in salt and sodium.
- If you drink alcoholic beverages, do so in moderation.

The United States Department of Agriculture (USDA) Food Guide Pyramid is a diet plan to help individuals meet the dietary guidelines. Each of these food groups provides some, but not all, of the nutrients that people need. Foods in one group cannot replace those in another. For good health, all are needed.

The Food Guide Pyramid emphasizes foods from these food groups:

- **Bread, Cereal, Rice, and Pasta** (6 to 11 Servings Daily)
These foods are from grains and provide complex carbohydrates. Individuals need the most servings of these foods each day. Examples of a serving are 1 slice of bread, 1 ounce of ready-to-cook cereal, 1/2 cup of cooked cereal, rice, or pasta. Whenever possible, select whole grain breads and cereals.

- **Vegetables** (3 to 5 Servings daily) **& Fruits** (2 to 4 Servings Daily)
These foods are from plants. Most people need to eat more of these foods for the vitamins, minerals, and fiber they supply. Examples of a serving are 1 orange, 3/4 cup unsweetened juice, 1/2 medium cantaloupe or 1/2 cup of a vegetable or fruit. Good sources of vitamin A (beta carotene) are dark green or dark yellow vegetables. Good sources of vitamin C are citrus fruits, tomatoes, peppers, potatoes, and various greens.

- **Milk, Yogurt, Cheese** (2 to 3 Servings Daily)
These foods come from animals. They are important for protein and calcium. Examples of a serving are 1 cup of milk or yogurt, 1–1/2 ounces natural cheese or 2 ounces processed cheese. Select low-fat or fat-free dairy products when possible.

- **Meat, Poultry, Fish, Dry Beans, Peas, Eggs, Nuts** (2 to 3 Servings Daily)
These foods are important for protein, iron, and zinc. Examples of a serving are 2 to 3 ounces of cooked lean meat, poultry, or fish; 1/2 cup of cooked dry beans or 1 egg count as 1 ounce of lean meat; 2 tablespoons of peanut butter or 1/3 cup of nuts count as 1 ounce of meat.

- **Fats, Oils, & Sweets** (Use Sparingly)
These foods provide calories and little else nutritionally. Most people should use these foods sparingly.

NUTRITIONAL ADEQUACY:
This diet is designed to provide adequate amounts of calories, protein, vitamins, minerals, and other nutrients to meet the nutritional needs of healthy adults.

Suggested Meal Plan	Suggested Foods and Beverages
BREAKFAST Fruit or Citrus Juice Cereal Meat/Meat Substitute Bread - Margarine Milk Beverage	Orange Juice (1/2 cup) Oatmeal (1/2 cup) One Scrambled Egg Slice Whole Wheat Toast/Jelly/Margarine (1/2 tsp each) Skim Milk/Fat Free (1 cup) Coffee or Tea
DINNER - NOON OR EVENING MEAL Meat/Meat Substitute Potato/Potato Substitute Vegetable and/or Salad Bread - Margarine Dessert Beverage	Baked Chicken (3 oz) Sweet Potatoes (1/2 cup) Green Beans, Coleslaw (1/2 cup each) One Whole Wheat Roll, Margarine (1 tsp) Strawberries (1/2 cup) Coffee or Tea
SUPPER - EVENING OR NOON MEAL Soup or Juice Meat/Meat Substitute Potato/Potato Substitute Vegetable and/or Salad Bread - Margarine Dessert Milk/Beverage	Vegetable-Bean Soup (1 cup) Meatballs (3 oz) with Spaghetti Sauce (1/2 cup) Spaghetti (1/2 cup) Broccoli (1/2 cup) Spinach Salad (1 cup)/Dressing (1 Tbsp) Slice Garlic Bread Rice Pudding (1/2 cup) Skim Milk (1 cup) Coffee or Tea

Nutrient Analysis

Calories	1966 Kcal	Riboflavin	2.2 mg
Protein	104 gm	Thiamin	1.3 mg
Carbohydrate	263 gm	Folate	341 mcg
Fat	62 gm	Vitamin B6	2.0 mg
Saturated Fat	16 gm	Vitamin B12	4.3 mcg
Monounsaturated Fat	24 gm	Calcium	1297 mg
Polyunsaturated Fat	15 gm	Phosphorus	1541 mg
Cholesterol	379 mg	Zinc	11 mg
Dietary Fiber	33 gm	Iron	19 mg
Vitamin A	5202 IU	Sodium	2868 mg
Vitamin C	244 mg	Potassium	4109 mg
Niacin Equivalents	15 mg		

Adapted from the Southwest Diet Manual 1999

ALLERGY/FOOD SENSITIVITY DIETS

(Sheet 1 of 3)

PURPOSE:

The diet is individually tailored to omit those foods that cause an immediate or delayed allergic reaction.

DESCRIPTION:

The diet may be recommended once a recognized relationship has been established between a particular food or foods and a symptomatic reaction. Common signs and symptoms of food allergies include skin reactions (itching, erythema, hives, eczema, edema) or reactions of the gastrointestinal tract (vomiting, diarrhea, abdominal pain). Systemic anaphylactic reactions could include sneezing, wheezing, conjunctivitis, palpitations, cardiac arrhythmia, shock, or collapse. Reactions can be immediate, or take up to 72 hours to appear.

BASIC INFORMATION:

This information describes some of the more common food allergies (wheat, eggs, milk, corn). Other common food allergens include: Seafood, nuts, legumes, chocolate, cola, citrus fruit, beef, white potatoes, pork, chicken, oatmeal, rye, mustard, garlic, tomatoes, and cucumbers. The wheat-, egg-, corn-, and milk-free diets commonly use an "elimination" approach to assess potential food allergens and intolerances. Elimination diets must be planned carefully and monitored regularly.

NUTRITIONAL ADEQUACY:

If planned carefully, allergy diets are generally adequate in all nutrients. The exception would be the milk-free diet, which is inadequate in calcium and possibly vitamin D, and will likely require supplementation. The elimination diets can be deficient in calories, carbohydrates, vitamins and minerals; therefore, long-term use is not advised and monitoring of nutritional sufficiency is essential. NOTE: These diets should be utilized under the prescription and careful guidance of a health care provider and/or dietitian.

WHEAT SENSITIVITY

Avoid foods containing wheat and wheat products. These include:

- **Milk/Dairy:** Flavored milk drinks: malted milk, chocolate milk, Ovaltine.
- **Meat/Meat Substitutes:** Meat loaf, croquettes; meats, fish, and poultry breaded or prepared with wheat flour; hot dogs, sausage, luncheon meats; canned meat dishes with sauce; casseroles made with wheat-based ingredients.
- **Breads & Grains:** All dry or cooked wheat cereals, wheat germ, wheat bran; graham flour; all commercial breads, crackers, muffins, and biscuits (unless 100% rye), soy, corn, or specifically labeled "wheat free"; French toast, waffles, pancakes; flour tortillas; pasta, except those specifically labeled "wheat free."
- **Fruits & Vegetables:** Breaded, fried vegetables; scalloped tomatoes.
- **Desserts/Sweets:** All commercial cookies, cakes, pies, doughnuts, pastries; commercial pie fillings, custards, puddings thickened with wheat flour; commercial ice cream, ice cream cones; prepared cake and cookie mixes.
- **Beverages:** Coffee substitutes, Postum; flavored instant coffee mixes; instant coffee (unless 100% coffee); beer, gin, whiskey.
- **Miscellaneous:** Pretzels, seasoned potato and corn chips; cream soups; cream-cheese dips, salad dressings (thickened with wheat); commercially prepared baked beans; soy sauce; commercially prepared gravies and sauces (usually thickened with wheat flour).

EGG SENSITIVITY

Avoid foods containing eggs. These include:

- **Milk/Dairy:** Eggnog, Ovaltine, malted milk.
- **Meat/Meat Substitutes:** Meatloaf, meat balls, croquettes; breaded or batter-dipped meat, fish, poultry; egg substitutes containing eggs or egg whites; soufflé, quiche.
- **Breads & Grains:** Breads and rolls with glazed crust; muffins, sweet rolls, doughnuts; French toast, pancakes, waffles; some commercial cake, cookie, muffin mixes; egg noodles.
- **Fruits & Vegetables:** Batter dipped fruits or vegetables; fruit fritters.
- **Desserts/Sweets:** Cream pies; meringues, custards; french ice cream; commercially prepared cookies and cakes; candies made with almond paste, cream, chocolate, fondant, marshmallow; macaroons.
- **Beverages:** Some root beer; malted drinks.
- **Miscellaneous:** Salad dressings and mayonnaise unless egg-free; egg-based sauces such as hollandaise; broth, consommé, bouillon, egg-drop soup, noodle soup, stocks clarified with egg; Simplesse.

MILK SENSITIVITY

Avoid all products containing milk. These include:

· **Milk/Dairy:** Cow's milk in all forms: fresh, dry, evaporated, condensed, buttermilk; chocolate milk, cocoa, milkshakes, malted milk, eggnog; Ovaltine; flavored instant coffee mixes; yogurt; whey.

· **Meat/Meat Substitutes:** Meatloaf, cold cuts, hot dogs; creamed meats, fish, poultry; scrambled eggs, quiche, souffles; all cheeses.

· **Breads & Grains:** Commercial breads or rolls made with milk; muffins, pancakes, French toast, waffles; prepared mixes made with milk or milk products; macaroni and cheese; pasta in cream sauce.

· **Fruits & Vegetables:** Mashed, scalloped, au gratin potatoes; vegetables with cheese or cream sauce.

· **Desserts/Sweets:** Custards, puddings; cream pies; ice cream, sherbet, frozen yogurt; candies made with chocolate, caramel, or milk ingredients; cakes and cookies made with milk or milk ingredients; whipped cream.

· **Beverages:** All milk-based beverages as noted above.

· **Miscellaneous:** Butter, margarine; sour cream; milk gravy, cream sauces, cheese sauce; salad dressings made with milk or milk-based ingredients; egg substitutes made with milk-based ingredients; Simplesse.

CORN SENSITIVITY

Avoid food containing corn, corn syrup, and cornstarch. This includes:

· **Milk/Dairy:** Chocolate milk, milkshakes, milk substitutes, cheese spreads, soy milk.

· **Meat/Meat Substitutes:** Bacon, ham, cold cuts, sausage, enchiladas, tacos, tostados, tamales, commercial entrees except those specifically labeled corn-free, commercial peanut butter.

· **Breads & Grains:** Corn bread, muffins, or rolls; English muffins, corn chips, corn tortillas, graham crackers, hominy, grits, packaged mixes of all types, corn fritters, pizza crust sprinkled with cornmeal, Cheerios, Corn Chex, Toasties, presweetened ready-to-eat cereals.

· **Fruits & Vegetables:** Sweetened fruit juice and juice products; fruits canned in heavy syrup, fruit desserts thickened with cornstarch, Harvard beets, corn, mixed vegetables, succotash, potatoes fried in corn oil, polenta.

· **Desserts/Sweets:** Cakes, candied fruits, cream pie, ice cream, pastries, sherbet.

· **Beverages:** Carbonated beverages containing corn syrup, presweetened ice tea, sweetened fruit punch, ale, beer, whiskey, gin.

· **Miscellaneous:** All commercial soups, homemade soup thickened with cornstarch, cane sugar, corn syrup, imitation maple syrup, Karo syrup, confectioners sugar, jam, jelly, and preserves, corn oil, corn oil margarine, baking powder, corn starch, chewing gum, distilled vinegar, MSG (monosodium glutamate), popcorn, yeast.

WHEAT, EGGS, MILK, CORN FREE DIET - SAMPLE MENU

Suggested Meal Plan	Suggested Foods and Beverages
BREAKFAST Citrus Fruit or Juice Cereal Meat/Meat Substitute Bread - Margarine Beverage	Orange Juice (1/2 cup) Oatmeal (1 cup) Peanut Butter (no added corn syrup) (1 Tbsp) Rice Cakes (2) Coffee
DINNER - NOON OR EVENING MEAL Meat/Meat Substitute Potato/Substitute Bread Vegetable and/or Salad Dessert Beverage	Lean Beef Patty (no fillers) (3 oz) Baked Potato (1) Rye-Krisp Crackers (4) Tossed Salad (1 cup)/Cider/Vinegar/Olive Oil (2 Tbsp) Fresh Apple (1) Iced Tea
SUPPER - EVENING OR NOON MEAL Soup or Juice Meat/Meat Substitute Potato/Substitute Vegetable and/or Salad Bread - Margarine Dessert Beverage	Turkey Rice Soup (1 cup) Baked Chicken (3 oz) Rice (1/2 cup) Green Beans (1/2 cup) Slice 100% Rye Bread Gelatin Dessert (1/2 cup) Coffee
SNACK Fruit or Juice Bread	Fresh Orange (1) Rice Cakes (2)

Nutrient Analysis

Calories	1988 Kcal	Riboflavin	1.0 mg
Protein	92 gm	Thiamin	1.5 mg
Carbohydrate	264 gm	Folate	296 mcg
Fat	58 gm	Vitamin B6	1.9 mg
Saturated Fat	14 gm	Vitamin B12	2.5 mcg
Monounsaturated Fat	29 gm	Calcium	300 mg
Polyunsaturated Fat	11 gm	Phosphorus	1196 mg
Cholesterol	171 mg	Zinc	13 mg
Dietary Fiber	35 gm	Iron	16 mg
Vitamin A	395 IU	Sodium	1281 mg
Vitamin C	165 mg	Potassium	3157 mg
Niacin Equivalents	16 mg		

Adapted from the Southwest Diet Manual 1999

ATKINS DIET©

PURPOSE

The goal of this diet is to aid in weight loss by adjusting the participant's metabolism. Foods high in carbohydrates are restricted. The diet works on the principle of ketosis, a process in which the body burns its excess fat.

DESCRIPTION

This low-carbohydrate diet is divided into four phases; each phase allows more carbohydrates than the previous one.

Phase 1, the induction phase, lasts for 14 days. The goal during this phase is to change the participant's metabolism through a biological process called ketosis. During ketosis, the body thinks it is starving and begins to burn its stores of fat. To accomplish this, participants reduce their carbohydrate intake to less than 20 grams per day. The participant can expect rapid weight loss (consisting mostly of water loss) during this phase. After 2 weeks, the participant moves into the second phase (the ongoing weight-loss phase). In this phase, the participant slowly increases the intake of carbohydrates over several weeks. The goal is to determine the amount of carbohydrates the participant can eat daily and continue to lose weight. The participant remains on this phase until they are within 5 to 10 pounds of their weight loss goal. *Phase 3* of the diet is a pre-maintenance phase. The participant begins to add more carbohydrates into their diet while continuing to lose weight but at a much slower rate than in the previous phases. During this phase, the effects of ketosis will begin to diminish, and the participant will begin to feel less satiated. For this reason, participants are encouraged to indulge their cravings while continuing to eat healthy. In the fourth and final phase of the diet (the maintenance phase), participants decide how many carbohydrates they will allow themselves to eat and continue the diet under these constraints. This phase is a lifelong diet that helps maintain the participant's weight.

BASIC INFORMATION

• *Phase 1:* In this phase, the participant will limit all foods that are high in carbohydrates and sugar while eating normal-size portions of meat, certain vegetables, eggs, and cheese. Foods that are not allowed during this phase include bread, rice, potatoes, pasta, baked goods, sugar, alcohol, and caffeine. Portion sizes should be large enough to satisfy hunger.

• *Phase 2:* After 14 days on *phase 1*, the participant moves to *phase 2*, the ongoing weight loss phase. The participant begins adding five carbohydrates a week to their diet until they stop losing weight. They then stay under this carbohydrate limit to continue to lose weight. Foods that remain limited include processed carbohydrates (e.g., white bread and rice), baked goods, refined sugars, and caffeine. The participant remains on this phase until they are within 5 to 10 pounds of their weight loss goal.

• *Phase 3:* This is the premaintenance phase in which the dieter is encouraged to maintain the eating habits they have learned on this diet. In addition, foods may be introduced in this phase to learn which items trigger weight gain for them.

• *Phase 4:* This is the phase in which the participant decides how many carbohydrates they feel comfortable allowing in their diet while maintaining their weight. The participant then continues this lifelong maintenance phase using the habits learned from the previous phases to maintain their weight.

NUTRITION ADEQUACY

This diet may be too low in essential fatty acids; vitamins A, D, E; and others. Vitamin supplements are recommended. Additionally, it is recommended that a potential dieter get a medical checkup and discuss their desire to go on the diet with their health care provider.

SAMPLE MENU—INDUCTION PHASE	
BREAKFAST	
Eggs	Scrambled Eggs
Beverage	Decaffeinated Coffee
SNACKS	
	1 Slice Bacon Wrapped Around 1 Piece of Cheese
DINNER–NOON OR EVENING MEAL	
Meat	Cheeseburger, No Bun
Salad	Tossed Salad
SUPPER–EVENING OR NOON MEAL	
Shellfish	Shrimp Scampi
Meat	Steak
Vegetable	1/2 Cup Eggplant
Dessert	Sugar-Free Gelatin Dessert

Nutrient Analysis (Induction Phase Menu)

Calories	1980 Kcal	Dietary Fiber	0.12 gm	Thiamin	0.6 mg
Protein	172 gm	Vitamin A	3079 IU	Calcium	1629 mg
Carbohydrate	14 gm	Vitamin C	14 mg	Phosphorus	2047 mg
Fat	134 gm	Niacin	19 mg	Iron	13.5 mg
Cholesterol	979 mg	Riboflavin	2.15 mg	Sodium	3156 mg

SAMPLE MENU–ONGOING WEIGHT LOSS PHASE

BREAKFAST	
Juice	Tomato Juice
Vegetable	Onion Rings (No Breading)
Eggs	Omelet
Beverage	Decaffeinated Coffee or Tea
SNACKS	
	Hard-Boiled Egg
DINNER - NOON OR EVENING MEAL	
Meat	Meatloaf
Vegetable	Baked Spinach
SUPPER - EVENING OR NOON MEAL	
Salad	Caesar Salad
Fish	Smoked Trout
Vegetable	Broccoli
Dessert	1/2 Cup of Strawberries in Cream

Nutrient Analysis

Calories	3195 Kcal	Dietary Fiber	7.4 gm	Thiamin	0.79 mg
Protein	182 gm	Vitamin A	1475 IU	Calcium	728 mg
Carbohydrate	31 gm	Vitamin C	134 mg	Phosphorus	1705 mg
Fat	261 gm	Niacin	28 mg	Iron	20.4 mg
Cholesterol	1428 mg	Riboflavin	2.92 mg	Sodium	1849 mg

SAMPLE MENU–PREMAINTENANCE/MAINTENANCE PHASE

BREAKFAST	
Eggs	Fried Eggs
Fruit	1 Cup Berries
Beverage	Decaffeinated Coffee or Tea
SNACKS	
	Beef Jerky (2g Sugar or Less)
DINNER - NOON OR EVENING MEAL	
Fish/Vegetable	Tuna Salad–Stuffed Tomato
Meat	Cold Cuts
Vegetable	Sour Pickle
SUPPER - EVENING OR NOON MEAL	
Vegetable	Fried Mushrooms
Vegetable	String Beans
Fish	Poached Salmon
Dessert	Sugar-Free Frozen Fudge Bar

Nutrient Analysis

Calories	1664 Kcal	Dietary Fiber	4.1 gm	Thiamin	0.76 mg
Protein	148 gm	Vitamin A	4195 IU	Calcium	279 mg
Carbohydrate	41 gm	Vitamin C	45 mg	Phosphorus	1739 mg
Fat	100 gm	Niacin	44 mg	Iron	10.5 mg
Cholesterol	816 mg	Riboflavin	2.2 mg	Sodium	3786 mg

PURPOSE:

This diet is designed to provide adequate nutrition during treatment of inflammatory or ulcerative conditions of the esophagus, stomach, and intestines. It is intended to decrease irritation of the mucosa, aid in physical comfort, and provide increased dietary variety as individual tolerance improves.

DESCRIPTION:

The basic food groups are used for planning nutritionally adequate meals. The diet may vary due to individual food intolerances and the patient's lifestyle. Active mucosal irritants are avoided. These include caffeine, coffee, decaffeinated coffee, tea, cocoa, carbonated beverages containing caffeine, alcohol, chocolate, pepper, chili powder, and any other foods that cause individual discomfort. Some patients find acid fruits and fruit juices too irritating for regular use. Most foods stimulate gastric secretions and are therefore not useful as buffers to gastric acid. Three to five small moderate meals per day are recommended, if tolerable. Avoid bedtime snacks, which can stimulate acid production during the night.

BASIC INFORMATION:

There is no scientific evidence that foods other than those listed above will contribute to the formation or continuation of ulcerative disease.

NUTRITIONAL ADEQUACY:

The bland diet will meet the requirements for all essential nutrients. Food intolerances or habits that limit variety and quantity of food selection may cause some nutrient deficiencies. Patients on this diet will need to be individually assessed to determine if nutritional supplementation is necessary. Chronic or severe blood loss may lead to iron deficiency.

FOOD LISTS

Food Group	Foods Allowed	Foods to Avoid
Milk & Dairy	Whole, low-fat or 2%, or fat-free (skim) milk; dry or instant milk; evaporated milk; buttermilk; yogurt.	Chocolate milk or cocoa.
Meats & Meat Substitutes	Lean and tender meats with visible fat removed; beef, veal, lamb, fresh pork (cooked medium to well done). Poultry; fresh, frozen or canned fish or shellfish; organ meats—liver and sweetbreads; eggs, cottage cheese, cheese.	Fried or smoked meats. Processed ham, sausage, spiced or highly seasoned meats such as frankfurters and luncheon meats, fried eggs.
Breads & Grains	Enriched breads, cooked or ready-to-eat cereals, tortillas, rolls, English muffins, melba toast, rusks, zwieback, saltines, crackers, pasta, rice.	Fried tortillas, fry bread.
Fruits & Vegetables	All fruit, juices and vegetables as tolerated; baked (without skin), boiled, mashed, diced or creamed potatoes, yams.	Citrus fruits and gas-forming vegetables as tolerated, fried potatoes, hash brown potatoes.
Desserts & Sweets	Custard, vanilla or fruit-flavored puddings, tapioca pudding, sherbet, ice cream, frozen yogurt, or ice milk (except chocolate and peppermint), fruit ices, flavored and plain gelatin, Junket, plain or iced cakes, sponge cake, angel food or pound cake, cookies without chocolate or peppermint, sugar, jam, jelly, honey, syrup.	Any foods containing chocolate, cocoa, or other seasonings not allowed.

FOOD LISTS (continued)

Food Group	Foods Allowed	Foods to Avoid
Beverages	Decaffeinated tea; cereal beverages such as Postum and Pero, juices as tolerated, carbonated beverages as tolerated, sports beverages as tolerated.	Coffee, tea, decaffeinated coffee, chocolate drinks, carbonated beverages containing caffeine, alcoholic beverages.
Miscellaneous	Salt, lemon and lime juice, vanilla and other extracts and flavorings, sage, cinnamon, thyme, mace, allspice, paprika, vinegar, prepared mustard.	Pepper, chili powder, cocoa or chocolate; non-prescription drugs, such as aspirin, without a health care provider's advice.

SAMPLE MENU

Suggested Meal Plan	Suggested Foods and Beverages
BREAKFAST Citrus Fruit or Juice Cereal with Milk Meat/Meat Substitute Bread/Margarine Milk Beverage	Apricot Nectar (1/2 cup) Oatmeal (1/2 cup) Soft Cooked Egg (1) Slice White Toast, Margarine (1 tsp) Low-Fat (1%) Milk (1 cup) Decaffeinated Tea
DINNER - NOON OR EVENING MEAL Meat/Meat Substitute Potato/Potato Substitute Vegetable Dessert Bread/Margarine Beverage	Meat Loaf (3 oz) no Gravy Whipped Potatoes (1/2 cup) Green Beans (1/2 cup) Cooked Carrots (1/2 cup) Lemon Sponge Pudding (1/2 cup) Dinner Roll (1), Margarine (1 tsp) Low-Fat (1%) Milk (1 cup)
SUPPER - EVENING OR NOON MEAL Soup or Juice Meat/Meat Substitute Potato/Potato Substitute Vegetable and/or Salad Dessert Bread/Margarine Beverage	Vegetable Bean soup (1 cup) Baked Chicken (3 oz) Noodles (1/2 cup) Green Peas (1/2 cup) Applesauce (1/2 cup) Slice White Bread, Margarine (1 tsp) Low-Fat (1%) Milk, Decaffeinated Tea

Nutrient Analysis

Calories	1838 Kcal	Riboflavin	2.7 mg
Protein	107 gm	Thiamin	1.6 mg
Carbohydrate	238 gm	Folate	260 mcg
Fat	56 gm	Vitamin B6	1.4 mg
Saturated Fat	18 gm	Vitamin B12	5.5 mcg
Monounsaturated Fat	19 gm	Calcium	1399 mg
Polyunsaturated Fat	14 gm	Phosphorus	1809 mg
Cholesterol	432 mg	Zinc	11 mg
Dietary Fiber	28 gm	Iron	17 mg
Vitamin A	3008 IU	Sodium	2129 mg
Vitamin C	49 mg	Potassium	2884 mg
Niacin Equivalents	17 mg		

Adapted from the Southwest Diet Manual 1999

Information From Your Health Care Provider

PURPOSE:

This diet is designed to prevent or minimize the loss of bone that may occur due to aging or calcium deficiency.

DESCRIPTION:

This diet plan provides at least 1500 to 1800 mg of calcium per day. A high calcium intake is achieved by increasing servings of milk and dairy products and other foods containing appreciable amounts of calcium. Excessive amounts of fiber, protein, caffeine, alcohol, and sodium may inhibit calcium absorption or increase urinary excretion of calcium and should be limited. Weight-bearing exercises increase calcium retention and are encouraged.

BASIC INFORMATION:

A high calcium diet has been found to increase retention of calcium in the bone. Several studies clearly show that a high calcium intake can help reduce the number of fractures that may occur. To achieve a high calcium diet, the regular diet can be followed with the addition of the suggestions below to boost calcium intake to 1500–1800 mg daily.

NUTRITIONAL ADEQUACY:

This diet is designed to provide adequate amounts of calories, protein, vitamins, minerals, and other nutrients to meet the needs of healthy adults.

FOOD LISTS:

All foods are allowed on this diet, in moderation. High calcium foods are listed below and should be added liberally to the diet. In addition, the suggestions below can also help increase calcium in the diet.

• Add 1/3 cup to 1/2 cup nonfat dry milk to recipes for pancakes, breads, mashed potatoes, scrambled eggs, puddings, cookies, cakes, and other foods. The milk powder can be blended into the other dry ingredients (flour, sugar, etc.) or added along with the water or liquid milk.

• Substitute yogurt for sour cream or mayonnaise in recipes, dips, dressings, and toppings.

• Choose spinach, romaine, and other dark-colored salad greens instead of iceberg lettuce.

• Use milk or buttermilk instead of water to reconstitute canned soups, dry cereal such as Cream of Wheat, instant mashed potatoes, pancakes, or waffles from a mix, and salad dressing mixes.

• Select pudding, frozen yogurt, ice milk, custard, or milk/yogurt fruit smoothies as high calcium snacks and desserts.

• Use calcium-fortified commercial products such as calcium-fortified orange juice, pasta, and ready-to-eat cereals.

• Add milk or evaporated milk to coffee instead of cream. Or, for convenience, use nonfat dry milk powder rather than nondairy creamer.

• Select milk-based coffee drinks such as caffe latte, caffe au lait, or cappuccino; request nonfat milk or low-fat milk to reduce total fat and caloric intake.

• Top casseroles, omelets, toast, baked potatoes, and steamed vegetables with a shredded cheddar, Swiss, or mozzarella cheese for a calcium boost. Use low-fat cheese to reduce total fat intake.

Information From Your Health Care Provider

HIGH CALCIUM FOODS (Use low-fat or nonfat products, where available)

FOOD GROUPS	FOODS	Mg of CALCIUM
Dairy Products	Ice Cream or Ice Milk, 1 cup	150-250 mg
	Milk, 1 cup	280-345 mg
	Yogurt, 1 cup	415-450 mg
	Milkshake, 10–12 oz	250-350 mg
	Nonfat Dry Milk, 2 Tbsp	200 mg
Meats/Meat Substitutes/Fish	Clams, 3 1/2 oz	95 mg
	Sardines, canned w/bones, 3 1/2 oz	310 mg
	Salmon, canned w/bones, 3 1/2 oz	225 mg
	Tofu, 1/2 cup	250 mg
Legumes/Nuts	Almonds, 1 oz	150 mg
	Brazil Nuts, 1 oz	50 mg
	Hazelnuts, 1 oz	55 mg
	Kidney or Lima Beans, cooked, 1 cup	50 mg
	Navy Beans, cooked, 1 cup	125 mg
	Pinto or Refried Beans, cooked, 1 cup	80-100 mg
Cheeses	Mozzarella, 1 oz	160-180 mg
	Ricotta, 1/2 cup	250-335 mg
	Swiss Cheese, 1 oz	250 mg
	Parmesan, 1 Tbsp	70 mg
	Cottage Cheese, 1/2 cup	70 mg
	Cheddar Cheese, 1 oz	145 mg
	Hard Cheeses, miscellaneous, 1 oz	190-270 mg
Vegetables	Bok Choy, cooked 1/2 cup	80 mg
	Collard Greens, cooked, 1/2 cup	150 mg
	Kale, frozen cooked, 1/2 cup	90 mg
	Spinach, cooked, 1/2 cup	122 mg
	Broccoli, 1/2 cup	35 mg
	Okra, cooked, 1/2 cup	75 mg
	Swiss Chard, cooked 1/2 cup	50 mg
Fruits	Calcium-fortified Orange Juice, 1 cup	300 mg
	Orange, 1 medium	50 mg
	Papaya, 1 medium	70 mg
	Prunes, 10	40 mg
	Rhubarb, frozen, cooked, 1/2 cup	170 mg
Breads/Grains	Calcium-fortified Pasta, cooked, 1 cup	300 mg
	English Muffin, 1	90-100 mg
	Pancakes, 2	100-150 mg
	Tortilla, corn or flour, 1	45 mg
	Waffle, homemade, 1	90-135 mg

Adapted from the Southwest Diet Manual 1999

CHOLESTEROL- & SODIUM-RESTRICTED DIET
(Sheet 1 of 3)

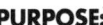

PURPOSE:
The cholesterol- and sodium-restricted diet is designed to help improve serum lipid profiles and to achieve a reduction in sodium intake necessary for the control of hypertension in salt sensitive persons or for the treatment of other disorders such as congestive heart failure.

DESCRIPTION:
This diet meets the general requirements of the National Cholesterol Education Program Step 1 Diet and the 3-gram Sodium Diet. African Americans, the elderly, and overweight adults are more likely to be salt sensitive than other patients. The level of sodium may need to be reduced further; the National High Blood Pressure Education program recommends a moderate sodium restriction (2300 mg/day), while some patients with moderate or severe congestive heart failure may require a 1 to 2 gram sodium restriction.

Foods high in total fat, saturated fat, and cholesterol are controlled. Total cholesterol intake is restricted. Limited amounts of mono- and polyunsaturated fats are used as replacements for saturated fats. Calories are to be adjusted to achieve or maintain desired body weight.

Foods high in sodium content are omitted. Depending on the degree of sodium restriction, one-half teaspoon of salt is allowed in the preparation of food or for use at the table. Spices, herbs, natural flavoring agents, and low-salt or salt-free seasonings may be used in place of table salt.

BASIC INFORMATION:
Cholesterol is found only in animal products. Saturated fats are often solid at room temperature and are usually found in animal products such as meats, poultry, butter, cheese and ice cream. Plant sources of saturated fats include palm oil, palm kernel oil, and coconut oil. Monounsaturated fats are found in products such as olives and olive oil, peanuts and peanut oil, avocado, and canola (rapeseed) oil. Polyunsaturated fats are usually liquid at room temperature and are found in safflower, sunflower, corn, soybean and cottonseed oils, seeds, and certain nuts.

Salt substitutes must be ordered by the health care provider or dietitian. Salt-free herbs and spices may be used freely. Carefully read labels as some salt-replacement seasonings contain sodium chloride. "Light" salts that are a mixture of potassium chloride and sodium chloride are also limited on sodium-controlled diets.

NUTRITIONAL ADEQUACY:
Depending on an individual's food choices, the low-cholesterol, low-sodium diet will normally be adequate in all nutrients.

FOOD LISTS:

Milk/Dairy (Limit to 2 to 3 servings a day)
· **Allowed:** Skim (nonfat) or 1% fat milk (liquid, powdered, evaporated), nonfat or low-fat yogurt, nonfat or low-fat cottage cheese, nonfat or low-fat cheese (limit to one ounce a day); nonfat cream cheese, nonfat sour cream.
· **Avoid:** Whole milk (over 3% fat) (liquid, evaporated, condensed), 2% milk, cream, half-and-half, imitation milk products, most nondairy creamers, whipped toppings; whole milk yogurt; regular cottage cheese (4% fat); natural cheeses made from whole milk (cheddar, Swiss, blue, Camembert, etc.); low-fat or regular cream cheese; low-fat or regular sour cream. NOTE: If 2% milk is used, decrease added fat by 1 teaspoon for each cup of milk.

Meat/Meat Substitute
· **Allowed:** Dried beans, split peas, lentils, pinto beans cooked without salt; poultry without the skin; fish; tuna packed in water (limit to 1.5 oz a day); lean beef (extra-lean ground beef, eye of round, sirloin, round tip, round, top round, tenderloin, top loin); lean pork (fresh not cured, tenderloin, leg, shoulder); lamb (arm, leg, loin, rib); luncheon meats (1 gram fat or less per ounce); egg whites (2 egg whites = 1 whole egg); low cholesterol egg substitutes.
· **Avoid:** Fried meats or meat substitutes; any meat, fish or poultry that is smoked, cured salted or canned (such as bacon, dried beef, corned beef, cold cuts, ham, turkey ham, hot dogs, sausages, sardines, anchovies, pickled herring); fatty cuts of beef, pork, lamb; goose, duck; liver, kidney, brains or other organ meats; sausage, bacon; regular luncheon meats; egg yolks in excess of allotments.

FOOD LISTS (continued)

Breads & Grains (6 to 11 servings a day)
- **Allowed:** Whole-grain breads (oatmeal, whole wheat, rye, bran, multigrain, etc.); English muffins, bagels, pita bread, corn and flour tortillas; rice; pasta; homemade baked goods low in fat; low-fat or fat-free unsalted crackers (rice cakes, popcorn cakes, Rye Krisp, melba toast, breadsticks); hot or cold cereals (with less than 2 grams of fat/serving), baked fat-free and salt-free chips.
- **Avoid:** High-fat baked goods (pies, cakes, doughnuts, croissants, pastries, muffins, biscuits); high-fat crackers; egg noodles; granola type cereals; cereals with more than 2 grams of fat per serving; pasta and rice prepared with cream, butter or cheese sauces; breads, rolls and crackers with salted tops; instant rice and pasta mixes; commercial stuffing; commercial casserole mixes, regular chips (corn, tortilla, potato), pretzels.

Vegetables (3 to 5 servings per day or more)
- Allowed: Any fresh, frozen, dried, or low-sodium canned; regular canned, drained vegetables—limit to 1 serving per day; low-salt vegetable juices.
- Avoid: Vegetables prepared in butter, cream or other sauces; fried vegetables; sauerkraut; pickled vegetables and others prepared in brine; regular vegetable juice; potato casserole mixes.

Fruits (2 to 4 servings per day or more)
- **Allowed:** Any that are fresh, frozen, canned, or dried.
- **Avoid:** Coconuts, avocados (except as allowed under Miscellaneous).

Desserts & Sweets (Limit to control calories if needed)
- **Allowed:** Sugar, jelly, jam, honey, molasses; low-fat or fat-free frozen desserts (sherbet, sorbet, ices, nonfat frozen yogurt, Popsicles); angel food cake; low-fat or fat-free cakes and cookies (vanilla wafers, graham crackers, ginger snaps); baking cocoa; low-fat or fat-free candy (such as jelly beans, hard candy), low-fat or fat-free puddings; gelatin desserts.
- **Avoid:** Ice cream; high-fat cakes, pies and cookies (most commercially made); puddings made from whole milk; chocolate; nut candies.

Beverages (As desired; limit high-calorie beverages if needed)
- **Allowed:** Juices, tea, coffee, decaffeinated coffee, carbonated drinks, sports beverages, and most alcoholic beverages.
- **Avoid:** Milkshakes; ice cream floats; eggnog; alcoholic beverages containing milk, cream or coconut; commercially softened water as beverage or in food preparation.

Miscellaneous
- **Allowed:** Limit fat based on total number of calories consumed (use very sparingly). Limit (1 tsp per serving): Unsaturated vegetable oils (corn, olive, canola, safflower, sesame, soybean, sunflower); margarine or shortening made from unsaturated vegetable oils; mayonnaise and salad dressings made from unsaturated oils (1 Tbsp); diet margarine (2 tsp), avocado (1/8 medium or 2 Tbsp), salt-free seeds and nuts (1 Tbsp seeds, 6 almonds, 20 small peanuts), salt-free peanut butter (1 tsp).

   No Limit: Vegetable oil sprays; fat free salad dressings; herbs, spices, pepper, salt substitute (with medical approval); mustard; vinegar; lemon and lime juice; cream sauces made with allowed ingredients, nonfat sour cream.

   Limit added salt to 1/2 teaspoon per day, may be used in cooking or at the table.
- **Avoid:** Butter; coconut oil; palm oil; palm kernel oil; lard; bacon fat; salad dressings made with egg yolk; fried snack foods (potato chips, cheese curls, tortilla chips); olives; regular cream sauces; salt, garlic salt, celery salt, onion salt, seasoned salt, sea salt, kosher salt; seasonings containing monosodium glutamate (MSG, Accent); salted nuts and seeds; salted peanut butter; canned soups.

556

Information From Your Health Care Provider

SAMPLE MENU

Suggested Meal Plan	Suggested Foods and Beverages
BREAKFAST Citrus Fruit or Juice Cereal Meat/Meat Substitute Bread - Margarine Milk Beverage	Grapefruit (half) Bran Flakes (1/2 cup) Low Cholesterol Egg Substitute (1/4 cup) 2 Slices Whole Wheat Toast Margarine/Jelly (2 tsp each) 1% Milk (1 Cup) Coffee
DINNER - NOON OR EVENING MEAL Meat/Meat Substitute Potato/Potato Substitute Vegetable and/or Salad Bread - Margarine Dessert Beverage	Salt-Free, Fat-Free Chicken Breast (3 oz) Salt-Free, Fat-Free Sweet Potato (1/2 cup) Salt-Free, Fat-Free Green Beans (1/2 cup) Whole Wheat Rolls (2), Honey (2 tsp) Strawberries (1 cup) Iced Tea
SUPPER - EVENING OR NOON MEAL Soup or Juice Meat/Meat Substitute Potato/Substitute Vegetable and/or Salad Bread - Margarine Dessert Milk Beverage	Pineapple Juice (1/2 cup) Salt-Free, Fat-Free Meatballs (3 Oz) in Salt-Free Spaghetti Sauce (1/2 cup) Spaghetti (1/2 cup) Salt-Free, Fat-Free Broccoli (1/2 cup) Raw Carrots, Red & Green Peppers (1 cup), Fat Free Dip Slice Italian Bread, Margarine (1 tsp) Fruit Sorbet (1/2 cup) 1% Milk (1 Cup) Coffee or Tea

Nutrient Analysis

Calories	1934 Kcal	Riboflavin	3.0 mg
Protein	99 gm	Thiamin	2.3 mg
Carbohydrate	310 gm	Folate	467 mcg
Fat	45 gm	Vitamin B6	3.5 mg
Saturated Fat	13 gm	Vitamin B12	5.5 mcg
Monounsaturated Fat	16 gm	Calcium	1180 mg
Polyunsaturated Fat	11 gm	Phosphorus	1898 mg
Cholesterol	162 mg	Zinc	17 mg
Dietary Fiber	50 gm	Iron	22 mg
Vitamin A	6184 IU	Sodium	2282 mg
Vitamin C	550 mg	Potassium	5300 mg
Niacin Equivalents	15 mg		

Adapted from the Southwest Diet Manual 1999

DAILY VALUES (DV) NUTRITION INFORMATION

Daily value (DV) is a dietary reference to help you plan a healthy overall diet. It will be the reference you will see used on nutrition labels for food products regulated by the Food and Drug Administration (FDA) and the U.S. Department of Agriculture (USDA). The labeling plan was devised so that the nutrition label information can be easily seen on the product, understood, and utilized in planning your daily diet.

DEFINITIONS:

· **DVs (Daily Values):** A dietary reference term that will appear on food labels. It is made up of two sets of references, DRVs and RDIs.

· **DRVs (Daily Reference Values):** A set of dietary references that applies to fat, saturated fat, cholesterol, carbohydrate, protein, fiber, sodium, and potassium.

Daily Reference Values (DRVs)*

Food Component	DRV
fat (total)	65 grams (g) (based on 30% of calories)
saturated fatty acids	20 g (based on 10% of calories)
cholesterol	300 milligrams (mg)
total carbohydrate	300 g (based on 60% of calories)
fiber	25 g
sodium	2400 mg
potassium	3500 mg
protein**	50 g (based on 10% of calories)

*Based on 2000 calories a day for adults and children over 4 only.

**DRV for protein does not apply to certain populations: Reference Daily Intake (RDI) for protein has been established for these groups: children 1 to 4 years = 16 gm; infants under 1 year = 14 gm; pregnant women = 60 gm; nursing mothers = 65 gm.

· **RDIs (Reference Daily Intakes):** A set of dietary references based on the Recommended Dietary Allowances for essential vitamins and minerals and, in selected groups, protein. The name "RDI" replaces the term "U.S. RDA" (U.S. Recommended Daily Allowance) previously used by the FDA.

Reference Daily Intakes (RDIs)*

Nutrient	Amount	Nutrient	Amount
vitamin A	5000 IU	folic acid	0.4 mg
vitamin C	60 mg	vitamin B_{12}	6 mcg
thiamin	1.5 mg	phosphorus	1.0 gm
riboflavin	1.7 mg	iodine	150 mcg
niacin	20 mg	magnesium	400 mg
calcium	1.0 gm	zinc	15 mg
iron	18 mg	copper	2 mg
vitamin D	400 IU	biotin	0.3 mg
vitamin E	30 IU	pantothenic acid	10 mg
vitamin B_6	2.0 mg		

· **RDAs (Recommended Dietary Allowances):** A set of estimated nutrient allowances established by the National Academy of Sciences. It is updated periodically to reflect current scientific knowledge.

* Based on National Academy of Sciences' 1968 Recommended Dietary Allowances.

Adapted from FDA Consumer Magazine, May 1993

FAT- & CHOLESTEROL-RESTRICTED DIET

(Sheet 1 of 3)

PURPOSE:

The low-fat/low-cholesterol diets are designed to improve serum lipid profiles for the treatment and prevention of coronary heart disease (CHD).

DESCRIPTION:

Foods high in total fat, saturated fat, and cholesterol are controlled. Total cholesterol intake is restricted. Limited amounts of monounsaturated and polyunsaturated fats are used as replacements for saturated fats. Calories need to be adjusted to achieve or maintain desired body weight. Lean meat, fish, skinless poultry, and non- or low-fat dairy products are included as well as plant sources of protein, such as legumes, dried beans, and dried peas. High-fat meats and poultry, organ meats, egg yolks, and cheese are limited. Foods high in complex carbohydrates and fiber such as fruits, vegetables, whole-grain products, and legumes are emphasized.

BASIC INFORMATION:

The National Cholesterol Education Program (NCEP) guidelines indicate that a serum total cholesterol should be measured in all adults over the age of 20 at least once every 5 years. Total cholesterol levels below 200 mg/dL are classified as "desirable blood cholesterol," those 200-239 mg/dL as "borderline high cholesterol" and those 240 mg/dL and over as "high blood cholesterol." Serum (blood-level) high density lipoprotein cholesterol (HDL-C) of at least 35 mg/dL is desirable. Elevated total serum cholesterol should be confirmed by repeat testing per your health care provider's recommendation.

Dietary treatment is the primary treatment for elevated serum cholesterol. The goals of therapy are to reduce serum cholesterol to less than 200 mg/dL and Low Density Lipoprotein (LDL) to less than 130 mg/dL for people with other heart disease risk factors and to 160 mg/dL for clients with no other risk factors. Another goal of therapy is to maintain a nutritionally adequate eating pattern.

Step I Diet Therapy of Blood Cholesterol

Nutrient	Recommended Intake
Total Fat	Less than 30% of Total Calories
Saturated Fat	8 to 10% of Total Calories
Polyunsaturated Fat	Up to 10 % of Total Calories
Monounsaturated Fat	10 to 15 % of Total Calories
Carbohydrates	At least 55% of Total Calories
Protein	Approximately 15% of Total Calories
Cholesterol	Less than 300 mg
Total Calories	To achieve and maintain desirable weight

Note: Step II Diet therapy reduces saturated fat to less than 7% of calories and cholesterol to less than 200 mg.

After starting the diet plan, patients should be checked at 4 to 6 weeks and then 3 months for cholesterol levels and diet adherence. It usually takes 6 months for results. Drug therapy may be recommended if cholesterol levels are still high.

Cholesterol is found only in animal products. Saturated fats are often solid at room temperature and are usually found in animal products such as meats, poultry, butter, cheese, and ice cream. Plant sources of saturated fats include palm oil, palm kernel oil, and coconut oil. Monounsaturated fats are found in products, such as olive oil, peanuts, flaxseed oil, and canola (rapeseed) oil. Polyunsaturated fats are usually liquid at room temperature and are found in safflower, sunflower, corn, soybean and cottonseed oils, seeds, and certain nuts.

Along with cholesterol testing, all adults should be evaluated for other CHD risk factors such as hypertension, smoking, diabetes, and obesity.

Information From Your Health Care Provider

FOOD LISTS - STEP I DIET

Milk/Dairy (Limit to 2 to 3 servings a day)
· **Allowed:** Skim (nonfat) or 1% fat milk (liquid, powdered, or evaporated), nonfat or low-fat yogurt, nonfat or low-fat cottage cheese, nonfat or low-fat cheese, nonfat sour cream; and nonfat cream cheese.
· **Avoid:** Whole milk (over 3% fat) (liquid, evaporated, or condensed); 2% milk, cream; half-and-half; imitation milk products; most nondairy creamers; whipped toppings; whole milk yogurt; regular cottage cheese (4% fat); natural cheeses made from whole milk (cheddar, Swiss, blue, Camembert, etc.); low-fat or regular cream cheese; low-fat or regular sour cream; low-fat sour cream. NOTE: If 2% milk is used, decrease added fat by 1 teaspoon for each cup of milk.

Meat/Meat Substitute (Limit to 6 oz a day from animal products; limit 4 egg yolks a week)
· **Allowed:** Cooked dried beans; split peas; lentils; pinto beans; poultry without the skin; fish; tuna packed in water; lean beef (extra lean ground beef, eye of round, sirloin, round tip, round, top round, tenderloin, top loin); lean pork (tenderloin, leg, shoulder); lamb (arm, leg, loin, rib); luncheon meats (1 gram of fat or less per ounce); egg whites (2 egg whites will equal 1 whole egg); low-cholesterol egg substitutes.
· **Avoid:** Fried meats or meat substitutes; fatty cuts of beef, pork or lamb; goose; duck; liver; kidney; brains; or other organ meats; sausages; bacon; regular luncheon meats; peanut butter (except as allowed under Miscellaneous); or egg yolks beyond allotment.

Breads & Grains (6 to 11 servings a day)
· **Allowed:** Whole-grain breads (oatmeal, whole wheat, rye, bran, multigrain, etc.); English muffins; bagels; pita bread; rice; pasta; homemade baked goods low in fat; low-fat crackers (rice cakes, popcorn cakes, Rye Krisp, Melba toast, pretzels, breadsticks); or hot or cold cereals (with 1 to 2 grams of fat or less per serving).
· **Avoid:** High-fat baked goods (pies, cakes, doughnuts, croissants, pastries, muffins, biscuits); fry bread; high-fat crackers; egg noodles; granola type cereals; cereals with more than 2 grams of fat per serving; pasta and rice prepared with cream; butter; and cheese sauces.

Vegetables (3 to 5 servings per day or more)
· **Allowed:** Any fresh, frozen, canned. or dried.
· **Avoid:** Vegetables prepared in butter, cream, and other sauces; fried vegetables.

Fruits (2 to 4 servings per day or more)
· **Allowed:** Any fresh, frozen, canned, or dried.
· **Avoid:** Coconuts, avocados, and olives except as allowed under Miscellaneous.

Desserts & Sweets (Limit to control calories)
· **Allowed:** Sugar; jelly; jam; honey; molasses; low-fat or fat-free frozen desserts (such as sherbet, sorbet, ices, nonfat frozen yogurt, and Popsicles); angel food cake; low-fat or fat-free cakes and cookies (such as vanilla wafers, graham crackers, ginger snaps [and others with less than 2 grams of fat per serving]); baking cocoa; low-fat or fat-free candy (such as jelly beans or hard candy); low-fat or fat-free puddings; gelatin desserts.
· **Avoid:** Ice cream; high-fat cakes, pies, and cookies (most commercially made); chocolate; puddings made with whole milk; and nut candies.

Beverages
· **Allowed:** Juices, tea, coffee, decaffeinated coffee, carbonated drinks, and most alcoholic beverages.
· **Avoid:** Milkshakes; ice cream floats; eggnog; and alcoholic beverages containing milk, cream, and coconut.

Miscellaneous
· **Allowed:** Limit fat based on total number of calories consumed. Generally no more than 6 to 8 servings/day of added fat such as margarine and salad dressing should be eaten; overweight, sedentary, or elderly individuals may need less.
Limit: (1 tsp per serving) Unsaturated vegetable oils (corn, olive, canola, flaxseed, safflower, sesame, soybean, or sunflower); margarine or shortening made from unsaturated vegetable oils; mayonnaise and salad dressings made from unsaturated oils (1 Tbsp); diet margarine (2 tsp); olives (10 small or 5 large); avocado (1/8 medium or 2 Tbsp); seeds and nuts (1 Tbsp seeds, 6 almonds, 20 small peanuts); peanut butter (2 tsp).

FAT- & CHOLESTEROL-RESTRICTED DIET

(Sheet 3 of 3)

No Limit: Vegetable oil sprays; fat-free mayonnaise and salad dressings, fat-free sour cream; herbs, spices, pepper, and salt substitute (with health care provider's approval); mustard; catsup; vinegar; lemon and lime juice; fat-free sauces; cream sauces made with allowed ingredients.
· **Avoid:** Butter; coconut oil; palm oil; palm kernel oil; lard; bacon fat; salad dressings made with egg yolk; fried snack foods (potato chips, cheese curls, tortilla chips); regular cream sauces.

SAMPLE MENU STEP I DIET

Suggested Meal Plan	Suggested Foods and Beverages
BREAKFAST	
Citrus Fruit or Juice	Grapefruit Half
Cereal	Bran Flakes (1/2 cup)
Meat/Meat Substitute	Low Cholesterol Egg Substitute (1/4 cup)
Bread/Margarine	2 Slices Whole Wheat Toast, Jelly (1 tsp)
Milk	1% Milk (1 cup)
Beverage	Coffee
DINNER - NOON OR EVENING MEAL	
Meat/Meat Substitute	Baked Chicken Breast (3 oz)
Potato/Potato Substitute	Sweet Potato (1/2 cup)
Vegetable and/or Salad	Fat-Free Green Beans (1/2 cup)
	Garden Salad (1 cup), Low-Fat Dressing (2 Tbsp)
Bread/Margarine	Whole Wheat Rolls (2), Honey (2 tsp)
Dessert	Strawberries (1 cup)
Beverage	Iced Tea
SUPPER - EVENING OR NOON MEAL	
Soup or Juice	Vegetable Juice (1/2 cup)
Meat/Meat Substitute	Fat-Free Meatballs (3 oz) in Spaghetti Sauce (1/2 cup)
Potato/Substitute	Spaghetti (1/2 cup)
Vegetable and/or Salad	Fat-Free Broccoli (1/2 cup)
	Spinach Salad (1 cup), Low-Fat Dressing (2 Tbsp)
Bread/Margarine	Slice Italian Bread, Margarine (1 tsp)
Dessert	Fruit Sorbet (1/2 cup)
Milk	1% Milk (1 cup)
Beverage	Coffee or Tea

Nutrient Analysis

Calories	1864 Kcal	Riboflavin	3.1 mg
Protein	99 gm	Thiamin	2.0 mg
Carbohydrate	285 gm	Folate	546 mcg
Fat	46 gm	Vitamin B6	2.7 mg
Saturated Fat	13 gm	Vitamin B12	5.7 mcg
Monounsaturated Fat	15 gm	Calcium	1227 mg
Polyunsaturated Fat	12 gm	Phosphorus	1879 mg
Cholesterol	226 mg	Zinc	16 mg
Dietary Fiber	45 gm	Iron	22 mg
Vitamin A	3781 IU	Sodium	3675 mg
Vitamin C	341 mg	Potassium	4494 mg
Niacin Equivalents	14 mg	Adapted from the Southwest Diet Manual 1999	

FIBER-ENHANCED DIET

(Sheet 1 of 2)

PURPOSE:

This diet is designed to emphasize foods rich in dietary fiber as a part of preventive and/or therapeutic nutrition. High-fiber diets may be used in the treatment of irritable bowel syndrome, uncomplicated diverticulosis, and constipation.

DESCRIPTION:

The high fiber diet is based on the Food Guide Pyramid with an emphasis on fiber-rich foods such as fruits, legumes, vegetables, whole-grain breads, and high fiber cereals. The Daily Reference Value for fiber is 25 gm (based on 2000 calorie-per-day diet). The American Diabetes Association has reported that up to 40 gm fiber daily or 25 gm per 1000 Kcal may be beneficial (National Cancer Institute recommends 25 to 30 gm a day). A maximum of 50 gm of fiber per day is suggested.

BASIC INFORMATION:

Dietary fiber is the component found in many foods that cannot be digested by the enzymes in the intestinal tract. Adequate fluid intake is important when following a high-fiber diet due to the water binding capacity of fiber. Fiber should be increased in the diet slowly to avoid unpleasant side effects (gas, abdominal bloating, cramps). Unprocessed wheat bran can increase fiber intake. Its intake should be increased slowly. It can be added to milk, cereal, yogurt, and other recipes and mixes. Dietary fiber can be divided into two separate categories: water-insoluble fiber and water-soluble fiber.

Water-Insoluble Fiber:

Water-insoluble components, such as cellulose, hemicellulose, and lignin, remain essentially unchanged during digestion. Foods containing water-insoluble fiber include the following: fruits, vegetables, cereals, and whole grain products. Research suggests that insoluble fiber may be beneficial in the prevention and/or treatment of constipation and diverticular disease and may decrease the risk of colon cancer.

Water-Soluble Fiber:

Water-soluble fiber, such as gum, pectin, and mucilages, does dissolve in water and is found in oats, beans, barley, and some fruits and vegetables. Some studies show that this type of fiber may improve blood glucose and cholesterol levels and appetite regulation.

NUTRITIONAL ADEQUACY:

The high-fiber diet is adequate in all nutrients. Some studies indicate that excessive consumption of some high-fiber foods may bind and decrease the absorption of the following minerals: calcium, copper, iron, magnesium, selenium, and zinc. However, it is believed that with a varied, well-balanced diet, mineral or nutrient imbalances are unlikely to happen in those consuming a high-fiber diet.

DIETARY FIBER CONTENT OF FOODS IN COMMONLY SERVED PORTIONS

FOOD GROUP	Less than 1 gm	1–1.9 gm	2–2.9 gm	3–3.9 gm	4–4.9 gm	5–5.9 gm	Over 6 gm
Breads 1 slice	bagel, white, French	whole-wheat, flour tortilla	bran muffin	corn tortilla			
Cereals 1 oz	Rice-Krispies, Special K, cornflakes	oatmeal, Nutri-Grain, Cheerios	Wheaties, Shredded-Wheat, Total	Cream of Wheat, Honey-Bran Malt-O-Meal	Bran Chex, 40% Bran-Flakes, Raisin-Bran	Corn Bran	All-Bran, Bran Buds, 100% Bran, Fiber 1
Pasta 1 cup		macaroni, spaghetti		whole-wheat spaghetti			
Rice 1/2 cup	white	brown					
Legumes 1/2 cup cooked				lentils	lima beans, dried peas		kidney beans, baked beans, navy beans

DIETARY FIBER CONTENT OF FOODS (continued)

FOOD GROUP	Less than 1 gm	1-1.9 gm	2-2.9 gm	3-3.9 gm	4-4.9 gm	5-5.9 gm	Over 6 gm
Vegetables (1/2 cup)	cucumber, lettuce (1 cup), green pepper, mushrooms. onions	asparagus, green beans, cabbage, cauliflower, potato (no skin), celery, sweet potato	broccoli, Brussels sprouts, carrots, corn, potato (with skin), spinach	peas			
Fruits (1 medium unless stated)	grapes (20), watermelon (1 cup), plums (5)	apricots (3), pineapple (1/2 cup), peach with skin, grape-fruit (1/2)	apple without skin, banana, orange	apple with skin, pear with skin, raspberries (1/2 cup)			

SAMPLE MENU

Suggested Meal Plan	Suggested Foods and Beverages
BREAKFAST	
Fruit Juice	Prune Juice (1/2 cup)
Cereal	All Bran Cereal (1/2 cup)
Meat/Meat Substitute	Poached Egg (1)
Bread - Margarine	Slice Whole Grain Toast & Margarine/Jam (1 tsp each)
Milk/Beverage	1% Milk (1 cup) & Coffee or Tea
DINNER - NOON OR EVENING MEAL	
Meat/Meat Substitute	Meat Loaf (3 oz)
Potato/Potato Substitute	Baked Potato (1)
Vegetable and/or Salad	Lima Beans (1/2 cup), Tossed Salad (1 cup)/Dressing (1 Tbsp)
Bread - Margarine	Slice Rye Bread & Margarine (1 tsp)
Dessert	Fig Cookies (4)
Beverage	Coffee or Tea
SUPPER - EVENING OR NOON MEAL	
Soup or Juice	Lentil Soup (1/2 cup)
Meat/Meat Substitute	Baked Chicken (3 oz)
Vegetable and/or Salad	Banana Squash (1/2 cup), Tossed Salad (1 cup)/Dressing (1 Tbsp)
Bread - Margarine	Slice Rye Bread w/Margarine (1 tsp)
Dessert	Baked Apple (1)
Milk/Beverage	1% Milk (1 cup) & Coffee or Tea

Nutrient Analysis

Calories	2039 Kcal	Riboflavin	2.6 mg
Protein	98 gm	Thiamin	1.7 mg
Carbohydrate	275 gm	Folate	394 mcg
Fat	69 gm	Vitamin B6	2.8 mg
Saturated Fat	18 gm	Vitamin B12	6.0 mcg
Monounsaturated Fat	22 gm	Calcium	1046 mg
Polyunsaturated Fat	22 gm	Phosphorus	1742 mg
Cholesterol	373 mg	Zinc	15 mg
Dietary Fiber	45 gm	Iron	23 mg
Vitamin A	1529 IU	Sodium	2820 mg
Vitamin C	100 mg	Potassium	4484 mg
Niacin Equivalents	16 mg		

Adapted from the Southwest Diet Manual 1999

PURPOSE:

This diet is designed to eliminate the protein gluten found in barley, buckwheat, bulgur, millet, oats, quinoa, rye, spelt, triticale, wheat germ, wheat, or their derivatives for individuals with gluten-sensitive enteropathy or celiac sprue and dermatitis herpetiformis. The gliadin component of gluten is believed to be the trigger for intolerance.

DESCRIPTION:

The Food-Guide Pyramid is used as the basis for meal planning. All protein sources are acceptable except those containing gluten. Products made from the flours or starches of arrowroot, corn, potato, rice, and soybean replace products made from wheat, rye, oats, and barley and those cereals and grains listed above.

Tips on Reading Labels:

The following ingredients are frequently listed on product labels. Those from wheat, rye, oat, or barley sources must be excluded from the diet. Only those from arrowroot, corn, potato, soy, or tapioca are permitted. Specific ingredient information may be obtained from manufacturers or the Celiac Sprue Association, P.O. Box 31700, Omaha. NE 68131; (877) 272-4272; website: www.csaceliacs.org. Gluten-free products are available from certain stores. Ask your pharmacist about your medications; some drugs contain gluten.

Flour or Cereal Products
Hydrolyzed Vegetable Protein (HVP) or Texturized Vegetable Protein (TVP)
Malt or Malt Flavoring
Modified Starch or Modified Food Starch
Soy Sauce or Soy Sauce Solids
Starch
Vegetable Protein
Vegetable Gum

NUTRITIONAL ADEQUACY:

This diet should be adequate in all nutrients. An added effort will need to be made to ensure adequate fiber.

FOOD LISTS

Food Groups	Foods Allowed	Foods To Avoid
Breads/Grains	Cornflakes; cornmeal; hominy; rice; puffed rice; grits; Cream of Rice; or Rice Krispies. Food items made from from rice, corn, or soybean flours, or gluten-free wheat starch, arrowroot, or tapioca. Homemade broth, vegetable, or cream soups made with allowed ingredients.	All products made from barley; buckwheat; bulgur; millet; oats; quinoa; rye; spelt; triticale wheat germ or wheat; cereals containing malt flavorings; prepared cake, cookie, bread, biscuit, muffin, pancake, or waffle mixes.
Fruits/Vegetables	All except items listed to avoid.	Any thickened or prepared (i.e., some pie fillings). Any creamed or breaded vegetables.
Milk/Dairy	All except items listed to avoid.	Commercial chocolate milk w/cereal addition; malted milk; instant milk drinks; hot cocoa mix; nondairy cream substitutes; processed cheese, cheese foods, and spreads containing a gluten source; cheese containing oat gum.
Meat/Meat Substitutes	All unprocessed meats, poultry, and fish, eggs, dried beans, and legumes, nuts, peanut butter, soybeans.	Any prepared with stabilizers or fillers, such as frankfurters, luncheon meats, sandwich spreads, sausages and canned meats; breaded fish, poultry or meats; poultry or meat prepared with hydrolyzed or texturized vegetable protein (HVP, TVP). Read labels.

FOOD LISTS (continued)

Food Groups	Foods Allowed	Foods To Avoid
Desserts/ Sweets	Ices; homemade ice-cream; custard; junket; rice pudding; tapioca; gelatin; cakes, cookies, and pastries prepared with gluten-free wheat starch; syrup; jelly; jam; hard candies; molasses; plain chocolate candies; marshmallows.	All others unless labeled gluten-free. Read labels.
Beverages	Carbonated beverages, fruit juices, tea, coffee, decaffeinated coffee to which no wheat flour was added, sports beverages.	Postum, Ovaltine, ale, beer, root beer.
Miscellaneous	Herbs; spices; pickles; vinegar; popcorn; potato chips; homemade broth; vegetable or cream soup made with allowed ingredients; jelly; jam; honey, corn syrup; butter; or margarine.	Commercial salad dressings except pure mayonnaise; chip dips; some catsup; chili sauce; soy sauce; steak sauce; mustard; horseradish; sauces and gravies with gluten sources; some dry seasoning mixes; pickles; distilled white vinegar; stabilizers; some chewing gum; malt or malt flavoring unless derived from corn; baking powder.

SAMPLE MENU

Suggested Meal Plan	Suggested Foods and Beverages
BREAKFAST Fruit Juice Cereal Meat/Meat Substitute Bread - Margarine Milk Beverage	Apricot Nectar (1/2 cup) Cream of Rice (1 cup) Poached Egg (1) Rice Cake (1)/Margarine (1 tsp) 1% Milk (1 cup) Coffee or Tea
DINNER - NOON OR EVENING MEAL Meat/Meat Substitute Potato/Potato Substitute Vegetable and/or Salad Bread - Margarine Dessert Beverage	Beef Patty (no fillers) (3 oz) Mashed Potato (1/2 cup) Frozen Peas (1/2 cup) Lettuce/Tomato Salad (1 cup)/ Salad Dressing (1 Tbsp) Slice Gluten-Free Bread/Margarine (1 tsp) Fresh Apple (1) Coffee or Tea
SUPPER - EVENING OR NOON MEAL Soup or Juice Meat/Meat Substitute Vegetable and/or Salad Bread - Margarine Dessert Milk/Beverage	Tomato Juice (1/2 cup) Baked Chicken (3 oz) Rice (1/2 cup), Spinach (1/2 cup) Corn Tortilla (1) Rice Pudding (1/2 cup) 1% Milk (1 cup), Coffee or Tea

Nutrient Analysis

Calories	1864 Kcal	Riboflavin	2.1 mg
Protein	97 gm	Thiamin	1.2 mg
Carbohydrate	244 gm	Folate	345 mcg
Fat	58 gm	Vitamin B6	2.2 mg
Saturated Fat	18 gm	Vitamin B12	5.0 mcg
Monounsaturated Fat	20 gm	Calcium	1060 mg
Polyunsaturated Fat	16 gm	Phosphorus	1507 mg
Cholesterol	397 mg	Zinc	13 mg
Dietary Fiber	19 gm	Iron	13 mg
Vitamin A	1511 IU	Sodium	1962 mg
Vitamin C	79 mg	Potassium	3868 mg
Niacin Equivalents	18 mg		

Adapted from the Southwest Diet Manual 1999

INFANT NUTRITIONAL INFORMATION
(BIRTH-12 MONTHS)

PURPOSE:
These guidelines are designed to meet the nutritional needs during the first year of life to promote optimal growth and development.

DESCRIPTION:
Exclusive breast-feeding is recommended for all normal infants from birth to 4 to 6 months of age. Breast-feeding with the appropriate introduction of other foods is recommended for the remainder of the first year, or longer if desired. Infants not receiving breast milk should receive iron-fortified formula. The American Academy of Pediatrics recommends that solids be introduced between 4 to 6 months of age.

CALORIC REQUIREMENTS

Age	Calories
0–6 months	108 calories per kilogram (kg)* (650 calories a day)
6–12 months	98 calories/kg (900 calories per day)

*One kilogram equals 2.2 pounds

BASIC INFORMATION:
Breast milk or formula fortified with iron is sufficient for healthy infants during the first six months of life. Introduction of food should begin as nutritional requirements increase with age; developmental patterns will also help to indicate this time.

Developmental signs showing the infant is ready for solids include when the baby can sit with support, poses lips to receive a spoon, closes mouth around the spoon, no longer pushes food out of mouth with tongue, maintains grasp when object is placed in hands, reaches for objects, and begins mouthing objects.

Suggested age for introduction of solids	Foods
4–6 months	add iron-enriched baby cereals (rice cereal first)
6–8 months	add one strained fruit (vitamin C-rich serving per day), vegetables; strained meats (per health care provider's advice)
8–10 months	add strained meats, fruit juices in a cup, egg yolk, plain or low sugar yogurt
10–12 months	add soft mashed table foods, crackers, cheese strips, other finger foods

There are several potential disadvantages to the early introduction of solid foods. Many health care providers and pediatric nutritionists believe the early introduction of solids increases the child's risk of developing food allergies; the solid foods may displace nutrient-rich breast milk or infant formula; inappropriate choices of solid foods may cause digestive and bowel changes; and the infant may develop a tendency to overeat.

Certain foods are not appropriate for infants; desserts and other concentrated sweets; high-sugar fruit punch, gelatin water, soda, popcorn, nuts, hot dogs, whole grapes, honey, hard candies. Plain cow's milk should not be added to an infant's diet until 12 months of age due to the increased risk of cow's milk protein allergy and gastrointestinal problems if introduced at an earlier age. If there is a family history of food allergies, some health care providers and dietitians recommend delaying the introduction of wheat, egg whites, citrus, and soy protein.

Adapted from the Southwest Diet Manual 1999

LACTOSE-CONTROLLED DIET

PURPOSE:
This diet is designed to minimize gastrointestinal (GI) disturbances such as abdominal cramps, bloating, flatulence, increased GI motility, and diarrhea associated with ingestion of the carbohydrate lactose.

DESCRIPTION:
This diet is individualized to provide the appropriate amount of lactose that a lactose-intolerant individual may tolerate. Milk and milk products including whey and milk solids are limited.

BASIC INFORMATION:
Current research indicates that most lactose-intolerant individuals can consume 15–30 grams of lactose per day (about 2 cups milk) without experiencing severe symptoms. Tolerance level is highly individualized. There are a number of commercial products that will break down lactose (milk sugar), allowing more flexibility in the diet.

NUTRITIONAL ADEQUACY:
This diet may provide adequate amounts of essential nutrients based on the use of lactose-reduced food choices. If lactose-reduced foods are not included, the diet may be deficient in calcium, vitamin D, or riboflavin.

FOOD LISTS

Food Groups	Foods Allowed	Foods to Avoid
Milk/Dairy	Milk substitutes and non-dairy products. Milk treated with lactose reducing enzymes, soy milk, as tolerated: buttermilk, acidophilus milk, yogurt.	Milk or milk products in excess of allowed amounts. Avoid or decrease intake with development of intolerance.
Meats/Meat Substitute	Any meat, fish and poultry except those listed to avoid, peanut butter, kosher hot dogs, dried beans, eggs. Cheeses as tolerated: blue, brick, Swiss, Camembert, cheddar, Colby, mozzarella, muenster, provolone.	All other cheese and cheese products, creamed meats, luncheon meats, hot dogs, other processed meats with added lactose, breaded meats, fish or poultry, casseroles and egg dishes made with milk or foods to avoid.
Breads/Grains	Breads, cereals, crackers, quick breads such as muffins, biscuits, etc., in moderation if made with milk, rice, pasta, no lactose cereals.	Excessive use of commercial products with added milk or lactose, milk or cream-based soups or pasta, cooked or dry cereal with milk, French toast, macaroni and cheese.
Fruits/Vegetables	Any fresh, canned or frozen.	Fruit juice products containing lactose and dietetic fruits with added lactose; creamed vegetables or vegetables in cheese; sauce; mashed, au gratin, scalloped potatoes.
Desserts/Sweets	Sugar, honey, jelly, jams, plain sugar candies such as gumdrops, jelly beans, marshmallows, Angel food cake, fruit ices, gelatin, commercial mixes or baked products containing milk in moderation, non-dairy frozen desserts, 1 serving milk chocolate per day.	Cream candies, tablet candies containing lactose, cream pies, products with cream fillings, cream cheese or sour cream, commercial puddings, artificial sweeteners containing lactose, toffee, caramels.
Beverages	Coffee, tea, carbonated beverages, cereal beverages, sports beverages, alcoholic beverages (if allowed by doctor), Isomil, Pregestimil, ProSobee, Ensure.	Cocoa, Ovaltine, cocoa malt, cocoa mixes, beverages containing cream, flavored instant coffee mixes.

FOOD LISTS (continued)

Food Groups	Foods Allowed	Foods to Avoid
Miscellaneous	Condiments, pure flavorings, popcorn, nuts, salt, vinegar, spices, lactate, lactic acid, lactalbumin, citric acid, MSG, margarine, butter, bacon, lard, mayonnaise, vegetable oils, vegetable shortenings, most oil-based commercial salad dressings, non-dairy whipped cream, broth type soups.	Cream sauces, milk gravies, gum, ascorbic acid tablets, spice blends with lactose added, milk or cream soups, whey, salad dressing with added milk or cheese not allowed, sour cream (alone, or in spreads and dips), cream cheese and spreads, whipped cream.

SAMPLE MENU

Suggested Meal Plan	Suggested Foods and Beverages
BREAKFAST	
Citrus Fruit or Juice	Orange Juice w/calcium (1 cup)
Cereal	Shredded Wheat (1/2 cup)
Meat/Meat Substitute	Soft-Cooked Egg (1)
Bread - Margarine	Slice Wheat Toast with Margarine (1 tsp)
Milk	Lactose Free Low-Fat Milk (1 cup)
Beverage	Coffee or Tea
DINNER - NOON OR EVENING MEAL	
Meat/Meat Substitute	Baked Chicken (3 oz)
Potato/Potato Substitute	Brown Rice (1/2 cup)
Vegetable and/or Salad	Spinach (1/2 cup), Lettuce & Tomato Salad (1 cup)/Salad Dressing (1 Tbsp)
Bread - Margarine	Slice Wheat Bread with Margarine (1 tsp)
Dessert	Angel Food Cake (1 slice), Strawberries (1/2 cup)
Beverage	Coffee or Tea
SUPPER - EVENING OR NOON MEAL	
Soup or Juice	Apple Juice (1/2 cup)
Meat/Meat Substitute	Lean Roast Beef (3 oz)
Vegetable and/or Salad	Cooked Carrots, Three Bean Salad (1/2 cup each)
Bread - Margarine	Dinner Roll (1)/ Margarine/Honey (1 tsp each)
Dessert	Raspberry Sorbet (1/2 cup)
Beverage	Coffee or Tea

Nutrient Analysis

Calories	1711 Kcal	Riboflavin	1.9 mg
Protein	92 gm	Thiamin	1.3 mg
Carbohydrate	223 gm	Folate	384 mcg
Fat	54 gm	Vitamin B6	1.9 mg
Saturated Fat	15 gm	Vitamin B12	3.9 mcg
Monounsaturated Fat	19 gm	Calcium	1002 mg
Polyunsaturated Fat	16 gm	Phosphorus	1260 mg
Cholesterol	384 mg	Zinc	15 mg
Dietary Fiber	21 gm	Iron	15 mg
Vitamin A	2987 IU	Sodium	1756 mg
Vitamin C	195 mg	Potassium	3435 mg
Niacin Equivalents	17 mg		

Adapted from the Southwest Diet Manual 1999

LIQUID DIET, CLEAR

PURPOSE:
This diet is often used to minimize digestion within the gastrointestinal tract. Fluid and energy are provided in a form that minimizes digestion.

DESCRIPTION:
The diet consists of clear liquids or foods that are fluid at body temperature. This diet is also residue-free which minimizes fecal output.

BASIC INFORMATION:
Due to the extremely restrictive nature of this diet, use should be limited to three days or less. For prolonged use, an appropriate low-residue supplement is recommended for nutritional support. Large intakes of beverages high in simple sugars, electrolytes, or amino acids may produce nausea, diarrhea, or dehydration. Liquids such as apple or grape juice, broth, and some fruit punches may need to be diluted before use with vulnerable patients.

NUTRITIONAL ADEQUACY:
This diet is extremely inadequate and is planned for brief use only. Specific items and amounts depend upon patient tolerance and should be offered frequently.

FOOD LIST

Food Groups	Foods Allowed	Foods to Omit
Milk/Dairy	None	All
Meat/Meat Substitute	None	All
Breads/Grains	None	All
Fruits/Vegetables	Clear fruit juices, such as: apple, grape, or cranberry; or strained juices such as orange, lemonade, or grapefruit; pulp-free fruit ices.	All others
Desserts/Sweets	Clear, flavored gelatin; Popsicles; clear fruit ices; sugar; honey; sugar substitutes; hard candy.	All others
Beverages	Clear coffee or tea, carbonated beverages, sports drinks.	All others including milk, nectars, cream, juices with pulp.
Miscellaneous	High-protein broth or gelatin, iodized salt, clear broth or bouillon.	

SAMPLE MENU

Breakfast	Dinner or Lunch	Supper or Lunch
Grape Juice	Apple Juice	Cranberry Juice
Clear Broth	Clear Beef Broth	Clear Chicken Broth
Flavored Gelatin	Flavored Gelatin	Flavored Gelatin
Black Coffee	Clear Tea	Clear Tea

Nutrient Analysis

Calories	512 Kcal	Riboflavin	0.3 mg
Protein	19 gm	Thiamin	0.1 mg
Carbohydrate	105 gm	Folate	18 mcg
Fat	4 gm	Calcium	56 mg
Cholesterol	0 mg	Phosphorus	203 mg
Dietary Fiber	0 gm	Zinc	1 mg
Vitamin A	1 RE	Iron	2 mg
Vitamin C	46 mg	Sodium	2346 mg
Niacin	9 mg	Potassium	888 mg

Adapted from Southwest Diet Manual 1999

PURPOSE:

This diet is intended for the patient who cannot chew or swallow solid foods or as a transition from the clear liquid to a soft or general diet.

DESCRIPTION:

This diet is a modification in the consistency or texture of the normal diet. It contains foods which are liquid or will become liquid at body temperature and are free from mechanical irritants.

BASIC INFORMATION:

Milk-based foods make up a large proportion of this diet. If milk based foods are poorly tolerated in patients, the use of low-lactose foods or a lactase product may prove beneficial. Fat tolerance will improve with use of low-fat or fat-free milk and dairy products.

NUTRITIONAL ADEQUACY:

This diet may be inadequate in niacin, folacin, and iron. If the diet is used for longer than 2 to 3 weeks, a liquid vitamin and mineral supplement is recommended. Patients with lactose intolerance should use a lactose-hydrolyzed milk or use lactose-free products.

	FULL LIQUID DIET - FOOD LIST	
Food Groups	**Foods Allowed**	**Foods to Avoid**
Milk & Dairy	All milk and milk drinks such as milk shakes and eggnogs made from commercial mix, yogurt—plain or flavored (no seeds or fruit pieces). All beverages including high-protein, high-calorie oral supplements.	Cheese, cottage cheese
Meat/Meat Substitutes	Eggnogs, custards.	All others
Breads / Grains	Thin, cooked cereal such as farina, grits, oatmeal.	All others
Fruits / Vegetables	Vitamin C sources (daily): Strained citrus and tomato juices. Vitamin A sources (alternate days): Strained carrot juice.	All others
Desserts and Sweets	Custards, puddings, plain gelatin, plain ice cream, ice milk, sherbet, sugar, hard candy, honey, Popsicle, syrup, frozen yogurt.	All others
Miscellaneous	Butter, margarine, cream, nondairy creamer.	All others

SAMPLE MENU

Suggested Meal Plan	Suggested Foods and Beverages
BREAKFAST	
Fruit Juice	Orange Juice, Strained
Cereal	Farina
Meat/Meat Substitute	Custard
Milk/Dairy	2% Milk
Beverage	Coffee
DINNER - NOON OR EVENING MEAL	
Soup	Strained Cream Soup
Juice	Tomato Juice
Salad	Lime Gelatin
Dessert	Ice Cream
Beverage	Ginger ale
SNACK	
Milk/Dairy	1 Milkshake
SUPPER - EVENING OR NOON MEAL	
Soup	Strained Cream Soup
Juice	Peach Nectar
Dessert	Popsicle
Beverage	Chocolate Milk
SNACK	
Juice	Cranberry Juice
Milk/Dairy	Vanilla Pudding, 2% Milk

Nutrient Analysis

Calories	1881 Kcal	Riboflavin	2.7 mg
Protein	60 gm	Thiamin	0.9 mg
Carbohydrate	293 gm	Folate	161 mcg
Fat	56 gm	Calcium	1822 mg
Cholesterol	311 mg	Phosphorus	1572 mg
Dietary Fiber	7 gm	Zinc	7 mg
Vitamin A	931 RE	Iron	5 mg
Vitamin C	133 mg	Sodium	3205 mg
Niacin	5 mg	Potassium	3120 mg

Adapted from the Southwest Diet Manual 1999

PURPOSE:

These diets provide adequate nutrition for the child of any developmental age and will aid in establishing good eating habits.

DESCRIPTION:

These diets are based on the basic food groups with considerations of the Recommended Dietary Allowances (RDA) for age. Food group quantities may be divided to include between-meal snacks.

BASIC INFORMATION:

The age of the child will determine consistency and amount of foods to be eaten. The toddler will take table food and finger foods in small portions. Older children will eat table foods of larger portions and additional fluids. It is at this age that positive nutritional habits can be reinforced. Adolescents will eat increased portion sizes. It is important to continue emphasizing regular meals and good nutritional habits.

Toddlers

The one-year-old begins to show a decrease in appetite and interest in food. This should not be interpreted as "poor" appetite but rather normal for this age with a decrease in growth rate. To ensure that the diet is adequate in nutrients, one must select the toddler's food carefully. The CDC (Centers for Disease Control & Prevention) recommends that children aged 1 to 5 years drink no more than 24 fl oz of milk per day to minimize risk of iron deficiency. Children should not be bribed or rewarded with food.

Adolescents

The nutritional needs during adolescence vary individually and according to gender. The period of greatest nutritional need coincides with the peak rate of growth during adolescence. The greatest need for girls is between 10 and 13-1/2 years, and for boys between 12 and 15 years. Since the growth spurt and the sequence of sexual development are related, it is useful to consider an adolescent's state of maturation to assess nutritional needs accurately.

NUTRITIONAL ADEQUACY:

If these guidelines are followed and servings are matched to age group, the RDA for children and adolescents will be met, with the exception of iron. Supplementation with iron may be recommended if food intake is inadequate, especially with adolescent girls. Fluoride supplements may be needed if amount of fluoride in the water is less than 0.7 to 1.2 parts million. Ask your health care provider about any need for supplements.

Information From Your Health Care Provider

PEDIATRIC BASIC FOOD GROUPS & SUGGESTED PORTION SIZES

Food Groups	AGE 1–3* Serving Size	AGE 4–6 Serving Size	AGE 7–11 Serving Size	AGE 12–14 Serving Size	Servings Per Day
Milk Whole, 2%, Skim, Cheese, Yogurt	4–6 oz	6 oz	8 oz	8 oz	3-4
Meat Meat, Fish, or Poultry	1–2 oz	1–2 oz	2–3 oz	3 oz	2 or more
Egg	1 medium	1 medium	1 medium	1 medium	
Cheese	1/4 cup	1–2 oz	2 oz	2 oz	
Fruit (vitamin C rich)	1/8–1/4 cup 1/2 fruit	1/2 cup 1/2 fruit	1/2 cup 1/2 fruit	1/2 cup 1 fruit	5
Vegetable**	2–4 Tbsp.	1/4–1/2 cup	1/2 cup	1/2 cup	
Bread-Cereal Whole grain, Enriched bread	1/2–1 slice	1 slice	1–2 slices	2 slices	4
Cereal, pasta, rice	1/2 cup cooked 1 oz dried	1/2 cup cooked 1 oz dried	1/2 cup cooked 1 oz dried	1/2 cup cooked 1 oz dried	
Others Fats, oils, butter, margarine, sweets, puddings, ice cream	In amounts needed to provide calories to meet growth needs.				

*Children under two years of age should be given whole milk only.

**Be sure to include a vitamin A rich vegetable every other day (dark green or dark yellow vegetables).

POTASSIUM RICH FOODS

BASIC INFORMATION:

Potassium is the predominant positively charged electrolyte in body cells. The flow of potassium and sodium in and out of the cells helps maintain the normal functioning of the heart, brain, kidney and skeletal muscles. It promotes regular heart-beat, muscle contractions and nerve transmissions. A potassium-enriched diet may be recommended for a patient with low serum (blood) potassium levels. Low levels of potassium seldom result from dietary deficiency since many foods contain potassium. Instead, the low level is usually due to illness, injury, or trauma, or from certain drugs such as some diuretics and steroids.

Foods High in Potassium	Amount of Serving	Potassium (mg)
Cereals		
Kellog's All Bran	1/2 cup	532
Nabisco 100% Bran	1/2 cup	354
Bran Flakes	1 cup	251
Shredded Wheat	1 cup	155
Fruit		
Orange juice	1 cup	479
Dried apricots	1/4 cup	454
Cantaloupe	1/4 medium	412
Prunes	1/4 cup	353
Banana	1 small	338
Grapefruit juice (canned)	1 cup	360
Tomato juice	1 cup	552
Avocado	1/2	510
Peaches, dried	4 medium halves	330
Raisins	3 tablespoons	225
Cooked Beans		
Pinto beans	1/2 cup	531
Kidney beans	1/2 cup	452
Lentils	1/2 cup	374
Black beans	1/2 cup	309
Canned beans	1/2 cup	332
Vegetables		
Baked potato	1 medium	593
Baked winter squash	1 cup	590
Baked sweet potato	3/4 cup	528
Beet greens	1/2 cup	417
Chard (large leaves)	1/2 cup	563
Peas (cooked)	1/2 cup	296
Spinach (fresh)	1/2 cup	440
Lima beans (canned or frozen)	1/2 cup	473
Other		
Canned tomato sauce	1/2 cup	459
Blackstrap molasses	2 tablespoons	1218
Sardines (canned in oil)	3 ounces	459
Chocolate (unsweetened/bitter)	1 ounce	249

According to the FDA's (Food and Drug Administration's) food labeling guidelines, the listing of the potassium content on food products is voluntary, rather than mandatory one. Therefore, even if potassium isn't shown on the label, it can still be a component.

PREGNANCY NUTRITION DIET

(Sheet 1 of 4)

PURPOSE:
This diet is designed to provide the increased nutrients during pregnancy that are essential for the health of the mother and the well being of the baby.

DESCRIPTION:
Foods from each food group in the Food Guide Pyramid are included in quantities to meet the increased nutrient needs of pregnancy. Nutrient needs that are markedly increased include protein, iron, folate, vitamin B6, and magnesium. Energy requirements increase by 300 calories a day during the second and third trimesters. Pregnant women need to emphasize foods high in nutrients. Alcohol should be avoided during pregnancy. Caffeine intake should be limited to no more than two cups of caffeine-containing beverages per day.

BASIC INFORMATION:
Weight Gain: Recommendations for the range of total weight gain and the pattern of weight gain should be based on prepregnancy weight for height. The pattern of weight gain is as important as total weight gain during pregnancy. Weight gain should be recorded on a chart that shows weight gain by gestational age.

Pregnancy Weight Gain Recommendations

Prepregnancy Weight	Total Weight Gain	Rate of Gain for 2nd and 3rd Trimesters
Normal Weight	25-35 pounds	1.0 pound/week
Underweight	28-40 pounds	more than 1.1 pound/week
Overweight	15-25 pounds	0.67 (2/3) pound/week
Twins	30-35 pounds	1 1/2 pounds/week

Nutrient Supplements
Assessment of dietary intake should be completed for every pregnant woman. The increased nutrient needs of pregnancy can generally be met with slight changes in dietary habits.

Pregnant women should receive daily supplementation of 30 mg ferrous iron in the second and third trimester. All pregnant women should consume 400 mcg folic acid from fortified foods such as folic acid-fortified grain and cereal products and/or supplements, in addition to food folate from a variety of fruits, fruit juices, and leafy green vegetables.

Prenatal vitamin and mineral supplements should be provided for women with inadequate diets and for high-risk populations. Excessive vitamin and mineral intakes should be avoided because of potential toxic effects in pregnancy. Vitamin and mineral supplements for use during pregnancy should not contain more than twice the recommended amount for adults.

Anemia
Iron deficiency is the most common cause of anemia in pregnancy. Iron needs markedly increase in pregnancy. Women taking iron supplements of more than 30 mg per day may be prescribed supplements of 2 mg copper and 15 mg zinc per day.

Eat foods high in iron such as beef, pork, lamb, and organ meats; iron fortified cereals; dried beans, peas, or lentils; dark green leafy vegetables; peanut butter and molasses. Combine foods high in vitamin C with iron-rich foods. Use cast-iron cookware, if possible.

Caffeine
Studies do not provide significant evidence that caffeine affects pregnancy outcome, however, pregnant women should eliminate or limit consumption of caffeine-containing beverages such as coffee, teas, and colas to no more than two servings a day.

Information From Your Health Care Provider

Diabetes

Pregnant women with any type of diabetes need special medical and nutritional care. Women with diabetes should achieve good blood sugar control before becoming pregnant. All other women should be screened for gestational diabetes at 24 to 28 weeks of pregnancy. Careful monitoring of blood glucose levels are critical for a healthy pregnancy outcome.

Food Safety

Foodborne illness is especially dangerous for pregnant women. To avoid exposure to *Listeria*, pregnant women should avoid unpasteurized milk and soft cheeses; carefully follow "keep refrigerated" and "use by" dates. Avoid eating raw or partially cooked meats, poultry, shellfish, and eggs. Wash hands after handling raw foods.

To avoid other foodborne diseases, proper food handling procedures should be followed including storing foods at proper temperatures; washing cutting boards and knives after contact with raw meat, poultry, and seafood; and careful handwashing before and after handling food.

Hypertension

Immediate referral for medical treatment is essential for pregnant women with increases in blood pressure. A diet to meet the nutrient needs of pregnancy with ample (but not excessive amounts) of calories and protein should be encouraged. Sodium intake should not be restricted unless specified by a health care provider.

Pica

Pica is the practice of eating substances with little or no nutritional value. Pica in pregnancy often involves consumption of ice, dirt, clay, or cornstarch. Less frequently, matches, hair, charcoal, cigarette ashes, mothballs, baking soda, and coffee grounds may be eaten.

Nutritious food may be displaced by pica substances. Items such as starch that provide calories may result in excessive weight gain. Pica substances may contain toxic elements or interfere with the absorption of minerals, such as iron.

Pica has been associated with iron deficiency. If either iron deficiency or pica is identified during pregnancy, medical tests should be initiated to see if other medical or nutritional problems exists.

Sodium

Normal sodium intake is needed during pregnancy to support the large prenatal expansion of tissues and fluids. Sodium should not be restricted unless specified by a health care provider.

Teen Pregnancy

Teens should gain weight at the upper end of the appropriate weight for height ranges. Teens are at high risk for iron deficiency and inadequate calorie intake. Eating regular meals, choosing healthy snacks, and emphasizing foods high in nutrients are especially important for pregnant teenagers.

Vegetarian Diets

Pregnant women consuming vegetarian diets need careful nutritional assessment. The type of vegetarian diet will determine the potential for nutrient deficiencies. A lacto-ova vegetarian diet that includes milk, dairy products, and eggs is more likely to meet the nutrient needs of pregnancy than the highly restrictive vegan diet, which eliminates all foods of animal origin. Vegan diets will require careful planning to consume adequate protein from complementary plant proteins. Alternate sources of Vitamin B_{12}, zinc, iron, and calcium will be needed in a vegan diet. Iron status should be carefully monitored. Low prepregnancy weight and less than optimal weight gain are common problems for vegans. High-calorie foods such as nuts, nut butter, wheat germ, avocados, dried fruit, coconut, honey, and salad dressings may be needed.

NUTRITIONAL ADEQUACY: This diet is designed to provide adequate amounts of calories, protein, vitamins, minerals, and other nutrients to meet the nutritional needs of a pregnant woman.

Information From Your Health Care Provider

Daily Food Guide for Pregnant Women

Food Group and Recommended Serving	Serving Size
Dairy Foods (3-4 Servings) Rich in calcium, protein, vitamins A & D, & phosphorus Sources: Milk, yogurt, cheese, salmon, dark leafy greens, cottage cheese; vegan calcium sources: calcium-fortified orange juice, cereal, pasta	1 cup milk or yogurt 1/3 cup dry milk powder 1 1/2 ounces cheese 2 cups cottage cheese
Protein Foods (6-7 Servings) Rich in protein, iron and B vitamins Sources: Beef, pork, lamb, chicken, fish, eggs, cheese, cottage cheese, tofu, peanut butter, dried beans or peas, nuts, seeds	1 ounce meat, chicken, or fish 1/4 cup tuna, cottage cheese or tofu 1 egg, or 1 ounce cheese 2 tablespoons peanut butter 1/2 cup dried beans or peas 1/3 cup nuts, or 1/4 cup seeds
Vitamin A Rich Fruits and Vegetables (1 Serving) Rich in vitamin A and fiber Sources: Carrots, spinach, dark leafy greens, sweet potatoes, winter squash, chili peppers, red and green peppers, tomatoes, cantaloupe, mango, papaya, apricots, vegetable juice cocktail, green onions, nectarine	1/2 cup cooked vegetables 1 cup raw dark leafy greens 2 tablespoons chili peppers 1/2 cup red pepper 2 medium tomatoes 6 ounces vegetable juice cocktail 1/2 cup raw green onions 1/4 cup dried or 3 raw apricots 1/2 medium papaya 1/4 medium cantaloupe or 1 medium mango
Vitamin C Rich Fruits and Vegetables (1 Serving) Rich in vitamin C and fiber Sources: Oranges, grapefruit, tangerines, lemons, cantaloupe, kiwi fruit, strawberries, mango, papaya, broccoli, Brussels sprouts, cabbage, cauliflower, chili peppers, red and green peppers, tomatoes	6 ounces citrus juice 1 orange or lemon 1/2 grapefruit or 2 medium tangerines 1/4 medium cantaloupe or papaya 1 medium kiwi fruit or mango 1/2 cup strawberries 1/2 cup broccoli, Brussels sprouts, or cauliflower 1 cup raw or 1/2 cup cooked cabbage 2 tablespoons raw chili pepper 1/2 cup red or green peppers 2 medium tomatoes
Other Fruits and Vegetables (3-7 Servings) Rich in other vitamins, minerals and fiber Sources: Apples, bananas, grapes, peaches, pears, pineapple, raisins, plums, watermelon, green beans, beets, corn, cucumbers, lettuce, peas, potatoes, radishes, zucchini, dried fruits	1 piece fresh fruit 1/2 cup canned or cooked fruit 1 cup raw fruit 1/4 cup dried fruit
Bread and Cereals (6-11 Servings) Rich in B vitamins, iron and fiber (if whole grain) Sources: Breads, tortillas, crackers, hot and cold cereals, rice, noodles, macaroni	1 slice bread 1 roll 1 tortilla 1/2 cup rice or pasta 3/4 cup cold cereal 1/2 cup cooked cereal 1 ounce cracker
Fats Provide vitamin E and essential fatty acids Sources: Butter, margarine, oils, lard, bacon, salad dressings, olives, avocados	As needed to meet calorie needs. Use in moderation. Fats occur normally in many foods such as meats, poultry, and dairy products.
Fluids	Drink at least 8 glasses of liquids each day. Milk, fruit juices, soups and water. **Don't drink beverages containing alcohol.**

Information From Your Health Care Provider

Suggested Meal Plan	Suggested Foods and Beverages
BREAKFAST	
Citrus Fruit or Juice	Orange Juice (1 cup)
Cereal	Oatmeal (1/2 cup)
Meat or Meat Substitute	Scrambled Egg (1)
Bread/Margarine	Slice Whole Wheat Toast/Jelly/Margarine (1 tsp each)
Milk/Beverage	Skim (Fat-free) Milk (1 cup), Decaffeinated Coffee
DINNER - NOON OR EVENING	
Meat or Meat Substitute	Baked Chicken (3 oz)
Potato/Substitute	Sweet Potato (1/2 cup)
Vegetable and/or Salad	Green Beans, Coleslaw (1/2 cup each)
Dessert	Strawberries (1/2 cup)
Bread/Margarine	Whole Wheat Roll (1)/Margarine (1 tsp)
Milk/Beverage	Skim (Fat-free) Milk (1 cup), Water
AFTERNOON SNACK	
Milk/Fruit	Fruited Yogurt (1 cup)
SUPPER - EVENING OR NOON	
Soup or Juice	Vegetable-Bean Soup (1 cup)
Meat or Meat Substitute	Meatballs (3 oz) with Spaghetti Sauce (1/2 cup)
Potato/Substitute	Spaghetti (1/2 cup)
Vegetable and/or Salad	Spinach Salad (1 cup)/Dressing (1 Tbsp), Zucchini (1/2 cup)
Dessert	Rice Pudding (1/2 cup)
Bread/Margarine	Garlic Bread (2 slices)
Milk/Beverage	Skim (Fat-free) Milk (1 cup), Decaffeinated Iced Tea
EVENING SNACK	
Meat, Bread, Fruit	Turkey Breast (1 oz), Slice Whole Wheat Toast
	Apple Juice (1/2 cup)

Nutrient Analysis

Calories	2724 Kcal	Riboflavin	2.9 mg
Protein	135 gm	Thiamin	1.4 mg
Carbohydrate	358 gm	Folate	345 mcg
Fat	64 gm	Vitamin B6	2.1 mg
Saturated Fat	22 gm	Vitamin B12	6.4 mcg
Monounsaturated Fat	21 gm	Calcium	2040 mg
Polyunsaturated Fat	16 gm	Phosphorus	2052 mg
Cholesterol	394 mg	Zinc	13 mg
Dietary Fiber	34 gm	Iron	21 mg
Vitamin A	5297 IU	Sodium	3401 mg
Vitamin C	768 mg	Potassium	6626 mg
Niacin Equivalents	17 mg		

Adapted from the Southwest Diet Manual 1999

PURPOSE:

Sodium-controlled diets are used to reduce blood pressure in salt-sensitive hypertension and to promote the loss of excess fluids in edema due to cardiovascular or renal disease and in ascites due to hepatic disease. Sodium-controlled diets may also enhance the action of some medications. Over 90% of sodium in an average diet is in the form of salt so the diet may be termed salt restriction.

DESCRIPTION: 2.0-2.5 Gram Sodium (86-109 mEq Na)

This level of sodium is used for low salt, low sodium, salt-free, and no salt diet prescriptions. Foods high in sodium content are omitted. One-fourth teaspoon of salt is allowed in the preparation of food or may be used at the table. Since sodium is widely distributed in foods, portions and number of servings are restricted according to the sodium content.

BASIC INFORMATION:

Salt substitutes should be approved by your health care provider. Salt-free herbs and spices may be used freely. Carefully reading labels is important, as some salt-replacement seasonings contain sodium chloride. "Light" salts, which are a mixture of potassium chloride and sodium chloride, are also limited on sodium-controlled diets.

Approximately 75% of the sodium Americans consume is added to foods during processing or preparation. The following list will help you interpret sodium information on food labels:
- Sodium Free - 5 mg or less of sodium per serving.
- Very Low Sodium - 35 mg or less of sodium per serving.
- Low Sodium - 140 mg or less of sodium per serving.
- Reduced Sodium - 25% less sodium per standard serving than the regular product.
- Light in sodium - 50% less sodium per standard serving than the regular product.
- No Added Salt or Unsalted - no salt is added during processing.

Water Supply

Water supplies vary in natural sodium content. Up to 25% of dietary sodium may come from drinking water. For the sodium content in your water supply, call your city's Water Department. Water softeners may add large amounts of sodium to the water. The sodium content of softened water ranges between 7 and 220 milligrams per quart. The company that installed your softener can provide sodium level information. Distilled drinking water may be used for cooking and drinking when water supplies contain more than 120 mg sodium per liter and the diet is below 2 grams.

Recommended Intake

The estimated average daily intake of sodium in the American diet ranges from 3.5 to 6.0 grams per day. The American Heart Association recommends that sodium intake should not exceed 3 grams per day. The National Heart, Lung, and Blood Institute recommends a maximum of 3.3 grams of sodium for healthy adults.

Hypertension (High Blood Pressure)

Although salt/sodium restriction is frequently used in the prevention and treatment of hypertension, not all persons respond equally to this restriction. African Americans, elderly, and hypertensive adults are more sensitive to dietary sodium than other population groups. Changing lifestyle or diet will often result in a reduction in drug requirements and thereby decrease costs and adverse reactions. Treatment for hypertension is not limited to taking medicines and the control of sodium intake. Lifestyle and dietary treatments also play a role:
- Weight reduction, even if modest.
- Increased physical activity.
- Avoidance of tobacco.
- Moderation of alcohol intake.
- Stress management.
- Maintenance of adequate potassium, magnesium, and calcium intakes.

Nutritional Adequacy

The 2.5–gram sodium controlled diet is designed to provide adequate nutrients to meet the needs of healthy adults.

FOOD LISTS - 2.5 GRAM SODIUM DIET

Milk and Dairy Products (2 to 3 servings/day)
- **Foods Allowed:** Any milk—white, low-fat, skim, chocolate and cocoa; yogurt; natural cheese (limit 1 oz per day), low sodium cheese, cottage cheese, substitute for 8 oz of milk: 4 oz evaporated milk, 4 oz condensed milk, or 1/3 cup dry milk powder.
- **Foods to Avoid:** Buttermilk, malted milk, instant cocoa or milk mixes, processed cheese.

Meats and Meat Substitutes (6 ounces/day)
- **Foods Allowed:** Fresh or fresh frozen: beef, lamb, pork, veal, and game; chicken, turkey, Cornish hen or other poultry; any fresh-water or fresh-frozen unbreaded fish and shellfish; low-sodium canned tuna or salmon; low sodium peanut butter; eggs, dried beans and peas, unsalted nuts.
- **Foods to Avoid:** Any meat, fish or poultry that is smoked, cured, salted, or canned, such as bacon, dried beef, corned beef, cold cuts, ham, turkey ham, hot dogs, sausages, sardines, anchovies, pickled items (herring, meats, or eggs), koshered meats and poultry, imitation crab, frozen/boxed entrees with more than 500 mg sodium per serving, salted nuts or peanut butter.

Breads and Grains (6 or more servings/day)
- **Foods Allowed:** Enriched white, wheat, rye, and pumpernickel bread; hard rolls, bagels, English muffins, cooked cereal without salt; dry low-sodium cereals; unsalted crackers and breadsticks; corn or flour tortillas; biscuits, muffins, cornbread, pancakes, and waffles all made with low-sodium baking powder; low-sodium or homemade bread crumbs; rice, noodles, barley, spaghetti, macaroni, and other pastas; homemade bread stuffing.
- **Foods to Avoid:** Breads and rolls with salted tops; quick breads; instant hot cereals; dry cereals with added salt; crackers with salted tops; pancakes, waffles, muffins, biscuits, and cornbread with salt, baking powder, self-rising flour or instant mixes; regular bread crumbs or cracker crumbs; commercial stuffing.

Vegetables (3 or more servings/day)
- **Foods Allowed:** Fresh, frozen, and low-sodium canned vegetables; regular canned, drained vegetables (limit to 1/2 cup serving per day); unsalted tomato sauce, low-sodium vegetable juice; sauerkraut, salt-free potato chips.
- **Foods to Avoid:** Regular canned vegetables (over 1/2 cup per day); vegetable juices; sauerkraut; pickled vegetables and others prepared in brine; instant potato products with added salt or sodium.

Fruits (3-4 or more servings a day)
- **Foods Allowed:** All fruits and juices.
- **Foods to Avoid:** None except salted prunes (saladitos).

Desserts/Sweets
- **Foods Allowed:** Any sweets like sugar, honey, jam, jelly, syrup, marmalade, hard candy; limit regular baked products (cake, pie, cookies) to 1 serving a day.
- **Foods to Avoid:** More than 1 serving a day of regular baked products.

Beverages
- **Foods Allowed:** Coffee, tea, soft drinks with less than 35 mg sodium per serving; alcoholic beverages (if your health care provider approves).
- **Foods to Avoid:** Commercially softened water as beverage or in food preparation.

Miscellaneous
- **Foods Allowed:** Limit added salt to 1/4 teaspoon per day, may be used in cooking or at the table; limit to 3 tsp salted butter or margarine per day; salt-free butter or margarine; vegetable oils, shortening, and mayonnaise; salt-free salad dressings; salt substitute (with health care provider's approval); pepper, herbs, and spices; flavorings; vinegar and lemon or lime juice; salt-free seasonings; low-sodium condiments: catsup, chili sauce, mustard, and pickles; fresh-ground horseradish; homemade or salt-free soups; low-sodium baking powder; unsalted snacks: nuts, seeds, pretzels, chips, and popcorn.
- **Foods to Avoid:** Added salt in excess of 1/4 tsp per day; light-salt; garlic salt, celery salt, onion salt, and seasoned salt; sea salt, rock salt, and kosher salt; seasonings containing salt and sodium compounds; monosodium glutamate (MSG, Accent); regular catsup, chili sauce, mustard, pickles, relishes, olives, and horseradish; Kitchen Bouquet; gravy and sauce mixes; barbecue sauce, soy and teriyaki sauce; Worcestershire and steak sauce; salted snack foods: nuts, seeds, pretzels, chips, and popcorn; commercially prepared convenience foods; regular canned or dried soups.

SODIUM-CONTROLLED DIET

(Sheet 3 of 3)

SAMPLE MENU 2.5 GRAM SODIUM DIET

Suggested Meal Plan	Menu (may use 1/4 teaspoon added salt)
BREAKFAST	
Citrus Fruit or Juice	1/2 grapefruit
Cereal	Cornflakes (1/2 cup)
Meat/Meat Substitute	Poached Egg (1)
Bread/Margarine	Whole Wheat Toast (2 slices)/Unsalted Margarine (1 tsp)
Milk/Beverage	1% Milk (1 cup)/Coffee or Tea
DINNER - NOON OR EVENING MEAL	
Meat/Meat Substitute	Salt-Free Hamburger Patty (3 oz)
Potato/Potato Substitute	Salt-Free Oven Fries (1/2 cup)
Vegetable, Salad or Soup	Garden Salad (1 cup)/Salad dressing (1 Tbsp)
	Salt-Free Vegetable Beef Soup (1 cup)
Bread/Margarine	Hamburger Bun (1)
Dessert	Oatmeal Raisin Cookies (2), Fresh Fruit (1/2 cup)
Beverage	Lemonade (1 cup); Coffee or Tea
SUPPER - EVENING OR NOON MEAL	
Soup or Juice	Salt-Free Tomato Juice (1/2 cup)
Meat/Meat Substitute	Salt-Free Herbed Baked Chicken (3 oz)
Potato/Potato Substitute	Salt-Free Brown Rice (1/2 cup)
Vegetable and/or Salad	Salt-Free Broccoli (1/2 cup)
	Salt-Free Cooked Carrots (1/2 cup)
Bread/Margarine	Whole Wheat Roll (1)/Unsalted Margarine (1 tsp)
Dessert	Strawberry Sorbet (1/2 cup)
Milk/Beverage	1% Milk (1 cup)/Coffee or Tea

Nutrient Analysis

Calories	2072 Kcal	Riboflavin	2.3 mg
Protein	94 gm	Thiamin	1.5 mg
Carbohydrate	274 gm	Folate	317 mcg
Fat	68 gm	Vitamin B6	2.4 mg
Saturated Fat	20 gm	Vitamin B12	4.6 mcg
Monounsaturated Fat	27 gm	Calcium	979 mg
Polyunsaturated Fat	17 gm	Phosphorus	1440 mg
Cholesterol	364 mg	Zinc	16 mg
Dietary Fiber	23 gm	Iron	18 mg
Vitamin A	5348 IU	Sodium	1744 mg
Vitamin C	237 mg	Potassium	3580 mg
Niacin Equivalents	19 mg		

Adapted from the Southwest Diet Manual 1999

PURPOSE:

As a progression from a full liquid diet to a general diet. The soft diet may also be used for a postoperative patient who is too ill to tolerate a general diet. The soft diet may also be needed for patients who are too weak or whose teeth are too poor to handle all foods on a general diet.

DESCRIPTION:

Food tolerances vary with individuals. Tender foods are used (not ground or pureed) unless the individual needs additional modifications to the diet. Most raw fruits and vegetables and coarse breads and cereals are eliminated.

BASIC INFORMATION:

This diet is moderately low in plant fibers. Fried foods and highly seasoned foods may cause discomfort for the immobile or postoperative patient.

NUTRITIONAL ADEQUACY:

This diet will be adequate if foods from each of the basic food groups are eaten daily.

SOFT DIET–FOOD LISTS

Food Groups	Foods Allowed	Foods to Avoid
Milk / Dairy	Milk and milk drinks, milkshakes, cottage cheese, mild cheeses.	Sharp or highly seasoned cheese.
Meat / Meat Substitute	Broiled, roasted, baked or stewed tender lean beef, mutton, lamb, veal, chicken, turkey, liver, ham, white fish, tuna, salmon, smooth peanut butter, eggs, mashed beans if tolerated.	All fried meats, fish or fowl, lunchmeats, sausages, hot dogs, meats with gristle, chunky peanut butter, beans and legumes.
Breads / Grains	Rice, noodles, spaghetti, macaroni, dry or cooked refined cereals such as farina, cream of wheat, oatmeal, grits, whole wheat cereals, plain or toasted white or wheat blend or whole grain breads, soda crackers or saltines, flour tortillas.	Wild or brown rice, coarse cereals such as bran or cereals with nuts. Bread or bread products with nuts or seeds.
Fruits / Vegetables	Fruit and vegetable juices, well cooked or canned fruits and vegetables, well ripened, easy-to-chew fruits, sweet potatoes, baked, boiled, mashed, creamed, escalloped or au gratin potatoes.	All gas-forming vegetables (corn, radishes, Brussels sprouts, onions, broccoli, cabbage, parsnips, turnips, chili peppers), fruits containing seeds and skin.
Desserts / Sweets	Simple desserts such as custard, junkets, gelatin desserts, plain ice cream, frozen yogurt, and sherbets, simple cakes and cookies, sugar, syrup, jelly, honey, plain hard candy, and molasses.	Rich pastries, any dessert containing dates, nuts, raisins or coconut, fried pastries such as doughnuts.
Beverages	Fruit and vegetable juices, lemonade, caffeine free beverages (soda drinks, coffee, tea), sports beverages.	Caffeinated beverages (soda drinks, coffee, tea).
Miscellaneous	Butter, cream, margarine, mayonnaise, oil, cream sauces, salt and mild spices.	Highly spiced salad dressings. Highly seasoned foods, Tabasco, mustard or horseradish, pepper.

SAMPLE MENU

Suggested Meal Plan	Suggested Foods and Beverages
BREAKFAST	
Citrus Fruit or Juice	Orange Juice (1/2 cup)
Cereal	Oatmeal (1/2 cup)
Meat/Meat Substitute	Soft Cooked Egg (1)
Bread - Margarine	Slice White Toast with Margarine/Jelly (1 tsp each)
Milk/Dairy/Beverage	1% Milk (1 cup)/Decaffeinated Coffee or Tea
DINNER - EVENING OR NOON MEAL	
Meat/Meat Substitute	Meat Loaf (3 oz)
Potato/Potato Substitute	Mashed Potato (1/2 cup)
Vegetable and/or Salad	Green Beans (1/2 cup)
Dessert	Lemon Pudding (1/2 cup)
Bread - Margarine	Dinner Roll (1) with Margarine (1 tsp)
Beverage	Decaffeinated Coffee or Tea
SUPPER - EVENING OR NOON MEAL	
Soup or Juice	Beef Consommé (1/2 cup)
	Apricot Nectar (1/2 cup)
Meat/Meat Substitute	Chicken Breast (3 oz)
Vegetable and/or Salad	Rice, Peas and Carrots (1/2 cup each)
Dessert	Applesauce (1/2 cup)
Bread - Margarine	Slice White Bread with Margarine (1 tsp)
Milk	1% Milk (1 cup)/Decaffeinated Coffee or Tea

Nutrient Analysis

Calories	1781 Kcal	Riboflavin	2.1 mg
Protein	89 gm	Thiamin	1.4 mg
Carbohydrate	236 gm	Folate	211 mcg
Fat	53 gm	Vitamin B6	1.6 mg
Saturated Fat	16 gm	Vitamin B12	4.4 mcg
Monounsaturated Fat	20 gm	Calcium	1041 mg
Polyunsaturated Fat	13 gm	Phosphorus	1602 mg
Cholesterol	386 mg	Zinc	10 mg
Dietary Fiber	16 gm	Iron	10 mg
Vitamin A	1455 IU	Sodium	2380 mg
Vitamin C	77 mg	Potassium	3212 mg
Niacin Equivalents	15 mg		

Adapted from the Southwest Diet Manual 1999

SOUTH BEACH DIET™

(Sheet 1 of 2)

PURPOSE

This diet is intended to assist in weight loss while teaching participants to be more aware of the nutritional value of the foods they eat. This diet is based on the theory that cravings for carbohydrates with low nutritional value create an unhealthy cycle of high-carb/sugar intake, resulting in a surge of energy that eventually declines and causes even more cravings for high-carbohydrate foods.

DESCRIPTION

The intake of high-carbohydrate foods with little nutritional value is controlled. This is done in three phases. In *phase one* the goal is to break the cycle of carbohydrate cravings. This phase involves 2 weeks of strict carbohydrate restriction, and participants experience a quick weight loss (consisting mostly of water loss). In *phase two* participants gradually add the healthier carbohydrates back into their diet while continuing to lose weight. During this phase participants learn to avoid the foods that trigger their cravings. Participants stay in *phase two* until they achieve their desired weight loss. *Phase three* is the lifetime maintenance phase. Participants are encouraged to keep eating healthily, but they are allowed to periodically indulge in high-carbohydrate/high-sugar items as long as eating such foods does not cause weight gain.

BASIC INFORMATION

• *PHASE ONE:* In this phase the participant limits all foods that are high in carbohydrates and sugar while eating normal-size portions of meat, vegetables, eggs, cheese, and nuts. Foods that are not allowed during this phase include bread, rice, potatoes, pasta, baked goods, sugar, and alcohol. Caffeine and milk are limited to 1 to 2 servings per day. Participants are encouraged to eat 3 meals, 2 snacks, and a healthy dessert each day. Portion sizes should be large enough to satisfy hunger.

• *PHASE TWO:* After 14 days on *phase one*, the participant moves to *phase two*. In this phase, some of the foods that were not allowed in *phase one* are added gradually back to the diet. Foods that remain limited include: Processed carbohydrates (e.g., white bread and rice), baked goods, refined sugars, and caffeine. Participants remain on this phase until they attain their weight loss goal.

• *PHASE THREE:* This is the lifetime maintenance phase in which participants are encouraged to maintain the eating habits they learned on this diet. Although eating anything is allowed during this phase, it is important for participants to monitor their weight for any gain.

NUTRITION ADEQUACY

This diet may be too low in calcium for some participants (especially women) during *phase one*. Calcium supplements are highly recommended

SAMPLE MENU: PHASE ONE	
BREAKFAST	
Meat Substitute	Scrambled Eggs and Mushrooms
Beverage	Decaffeinated Coffee/Tea (Nonfat Milk and Sugar Substitute)
MORNING SNACK	
Dairy	1 Mozzarella Stick
DINNER–NOON OR EVENING MEAL	
Salad	Baby Spinach Salad with Tomato and Mozzarella
Meat	Baked Chicken Breast
AFTERNOON SNACK	
Vegetable	Hummus with Celery
SUPPER–EVENING OR NOON MEAL	
Salad	Tossed Salad
Meat Substitute/Vegetable	Grilled Salmon with Vegetables
Dessert	Sugar-Free Frozen Fudge Bar

Nutrient Analysis

Calories	1540 Kcal	Niacin	59 mg
Protein	173 gm	Riboflavin	2.27 mg
Carbohydrate	51 gm	Thiamin	1.8 mg
Fat	70 gm	Calcium	935 mg
Cholesterol	619 mg	Phosphorus	2219 mg
Dietary Fiber	6 gm	Iron	10 mg
Vitamin A	1832 IU	Sodium	1252 mg
Vitamin C	126 mg		

SAMPLE MENU: PHASE TWO	
BREAKFAST	
Cereal	High-Fiber Cereal with Nonfat Milk
Fruit	Fresh Strawberries
Beverage	Decaffeinated Coffee/Tea (Nonfat Milk and Sugar Substitute)
MORNING SNACK	
Meat Substitute	Hard-Boiled Egg
DINNER–NOON OR EVENING MEAL	
Meat/Bread	Open-Faced Roast Beef Sandwich
AFTERNOON SNACK	
Dairy	Nonfat Plain Yogurt
SUPPER–EVENING OR NOON MEAL	
Salad	Caesar Salad
Meat/Vegetable	Stir-fry Chicken and Vegetables
Dessert	Sugar-Free Gelatin

Nutrient Analysis

Calories	1273 Kcal	Niacin	54 mg
Protein	105 gm	Riboflavin	5.5 mg
Carbohydrate	166 gm	Thiamin	3.7 mg
Fat	38 gm	Calcium	1042 mg
Cholesterol	408 mg	Phosphorus	2866 mg
Dietary Fiber	44 gm	Iron	24.5 mg
Vitamin A	1081 IU	Sodium	1778 mg
Vitamin C	221 mg		

SAMPLE MENU: PHASE THREE	
BREAKFAST	
Cereal	High-Fiber Cereal with Nonfat Milk
Fruit	Fresh Berries
Beverage	Decaffeinated Coffee/Tea (Nonfat Milk and Sugar Substitute)
MORNING SNACK	
Dairy/Vegetable	Cottage Cheese and Cucumbers
DINNER–NOON OR EVENING MEAL	
Meat/Bread	Chicken Salad Sandwich on Whole Wheat Bread
AFTERNOON SNACK	
Bread	Whole Wheat English Muffin
SUPPER–EVENING OR NOON MEAL	
Salad	Chef's Salad
Meat/Vegetable	Broiled Sirloin Steak with Creamed Spinach
Dessert	Vanilla Pudding

Nutrient Analysis

Calories	1775 Kcal	Niacin	58 mg
Protein	140 gm	Riboflavin	5.8 mg
Carbohydrate	252 gm	Thiamin	4.2 mg
Fat	42 gm	Calcium	1421 mg
Cholesterol	227 mg	Phosphorus	3688 mg
Dietary Fiber	51 gm	Iron	29.7 mg
Vitamin A	1846 IU	Sodium	4302 mg
Vitamin C	284 mg		

TYRAMINE-RESTRICTED DIET

(Sheet 1 of 2)

PURPOSE:
This diet is designed to promote optimum health through good nutrition. It is to be used for those individuals requiring no special dietary modification or restrictions.

DESCRIPTION:
Foods from all basic food groups are included with the addition of other foods to meet energy needs and provide essential nutrients. The diet is planned to promote the prevention of chronic diseases such as heart disease, cancer, and diabetes.

BASIC INFORMATION:
The Dietary Guidelines for Americans outline what people should eat to stay healthy. The guidelines include:

- Eat a variety of foods.
- Balance the foods you eat with physical activity—maintain or improve your weight.
- Choose a diet with plenty of grain products, vegetables, and fruits.
- Choose a diet low in fat, saturated fat, and cholesterol.
- Choose a diet moderate in sugars.
- Choose a diet moderate in salt and sodium.
- If you drink alcoholic beverages, do so in moderation.

The United States Department of Agriculture (USDA) Food Guide Pyramid is a diet plan to help individuals meet the dietary guidelines. Each of these food groups provides some, but not all, of the nutrients that people need. Foods in one group cannot replace those in another. For good health, all are needed.

The Food Guide Pyramid emphasizes foods from these food groups:

• Bread, Cereal, Rice and Pasta (6 to 11 Servings Daily)
All of these foods are from grains. Individuals need most servings of these foods each day. Examples of a serving are 1 slice of bread, 1 ounce ready-to-eat cereal, 1/2 cup of cooked cereal, rice, or pasta.

• Vegetables (3 to 5 Servings daily) & Fruits (2 to 4 Servings Daily)
All of these foods are from plants. Most people need to eat more of these foods for the vitamins, minerals, and fiber they supply. Examples of a serving are 1 orange, 1/2 cup juice, 1/2 medium cantaloupe, 1/2 cup vegetable or fruit. Good sources of vitamin A (beta carotene) are dark green or dark yellow vegetables. Good sources of vitamin C are citrus fruits, tomatoes, peppers, potatoes, and various greens.

• Milk, Yogurt, Cheese (2 to 3 Servings Daily)
All of these foods come from animals. These foods are important for protein and calcium. Examples of a serving are 1 cup of milk or yogurt, 1-1/2 ounces natural cheese, 2 ounces processed cheese.

• Meat, Poultry, Fish, Dry Beans, Eggs, Nuts (2 to 3 Servings Daily)
Most of these foods come from animals. These foods are important for protein, iron and zinc. Examples of a serving are 2 to 3 ounces of cooked lean meat, poultry, or fish; 1/2 cup of cooked dry beans or 1 egg count as 1 ounce lean meat; 2 tablespoons peanut butter or 1/3 cup of nuts count as 1 ounce of meat.

• Fats, Oils, & Sweets (Use Sparingly)
These foods provide calories and little else nutritionally. Most people should use these foods sparingly.

NUTRITIONAL ADEQUACY:
This diet is designed to provide adequate amounts of calories, protein, vitamins, minerals, and other nutrients to meet the nutritional needs of healthy adults.

Information From Your Health Care Provider

SAMPLE MENU	
Suggested Meal Plan	**Suggested Foods and Beverages**
BREAKFAST	
Fruit Juice	Orange Juice (1/2 c)
Cereal	Oatmeal (1 c)
Meat/Meat Substitute	Soft Cooked Egg (1)
Bread - Margarine	Toast - Butter or Margarine* (1 slice)
Milk/Beverage	Milk*/Decaffeinated Coffee or Tea (1 c)
DINNER - NOON OR EVENING MEAL	
Meat/Meat Substitute	Broiled Beef Patty
Potato/Potato Substitute	Mashed Potatoes
Vegetable and/or Salad	Steamed Spinach
Bread - Margarine	Whole Wheat Bread with Margarine*
Dessert	Gelatin Cubes
Beverage	Decaffeinated Coffee or Tea
SUPPER - EVENING OR NOON MEAL	
Soup or Juice	Consommé
Meat/Meat Substitute	Roast Chicken
Vegetable and/or Salad	Peas, Creamy Coleslaw
Bread - Margarine	Biscuit with Margarine*
Dessert	Fresh Apple
Milk/Beverage	Milk*/Decaffeinated Coffee or Tea

*To reduce amount of fat in your diet, omit margarine or butter and use 1% or skim milk.

Nutrient Analysis

Calories	1700 Kcal	Riboflavin	1.9 mg
Protein	102 gm	Thiamin	1.3 mg
Carbohydrate	176 gm	Folate	337 mcg
Fat	68 gm	Calcium	952 mg
Cholesterol	443 mg	Phosphorus	1493 mg
Dietary Fiber	16 gm	Zinc	12 mg
Vitamin A	1371 IU	Iron	13 mg
Vitamin C	99 mg	Sodium	2373 mg
Niacin	25 mg	Potassium	3040 mg

Adapted from the Southwest Diet Manual (revised 1999)

WEIGHT CONTROL SUGGESTIONS

Weight control diets are designed to provide a specific calorie level calculated to meet an individual's requirement to attain optimal body weight.
An exercise program is also highly recommended. Weight loss of 1-2 pounds per week is generally optimal.

The U.S. Department of Agriculture's Food Guide Pyramid diet plan can be used as a guide to healthy eating and is likely to produce desired weight loss. Weight loss diets of greater than 1,200 calories per day are generally adequate in all nutrients except iron, as long as the diet is planned to include a variety of foods from all food groups.

FOOD GUIDE PYRAMID - DAILY SERVINGS

· **Fats, Oils, & Sweets (Use Sparingly):** These foods provide calories and little else nutritionally. Most people should use these foods sparingly.
· **Milk, Yogurt, and Cheese (2 to 3 Servings) & Meat, Poultry, Fish, Dry Beans, Eggs, and Nuts (2 to 3 Servings):** Most of these foods come from animals. These foods are important for protein, calcium, iron, and zinc.
· **Vegetables (3 to 5 Servings) & Fruits (2 to 4 Servings):** All of these foods are from plants. Most people need to eat more of these foods for the vitamins, minerals, and fiber they supply.
· **Bread, Cereal, Rice and Pasta (6 to 11 Servings):** All of these foods are from grains. Individuals need the most of these foods each day.

BEHAVIORAL STRATEGIES IN MANAGEMENT OF WEIGHT CONTROL

Individuals seeking to make a lifetime commitment to improve their eating and exercise habits can succeed at long-term weight loss. Most of the successful long-term weight-loss programs include several components: behavior modification; exercise; nutrition; social support; and cognitive changes, including goal setting, assertiveness training, and coping with mistakes and motivation. Emphasis should be placed on slow, progressive weight loss.

The following is a list of behavior modification techniques that can be used to promote healthy eating, lifestyle and, in turn, weight loss.

BEHAVIOR MODIFICATION TECHNIQUES

· Evaluate what behaviors, activities, or feelings trigger eating.
· Don't use food as a reward for desired behavior.
· Drink plenty of non-caloric fluids, including water, daily.
· Change usual eating-places; avoid eating while involved in other activities.
· Make an effort to eat breakfast and small, frequent meals.
· Eat fresh fruits and raw vegetables at least four times daily.
· Exercise along with television exercise programs or during commercials when watching television.
· Eat slowly, putting your utensil down between bites.
· Weight should be checked on a weekly basis only.
· Remove high calorie, low-nutrient foods from cupboards.
· Keep busy so the focus is not on food.
· Shop from a healthy food list and not when hungry.
· Leave the table soon after eating and don't feel a need to finish everything.
· Trim fat off meat and skin off poultry.
· Place a photo of a thinner you on the mirror.
· Plan ahead, especially when attending social events.
· Keep records of intake and/or weight loss progress.
· When weight drops, give away clothes that no longer fit.
· Break the habit of nibbling while cooking or cleaning up from meals.
· Try low-fat and low-calorie food items (the taste keeps improving).

Adapted from the Southwest Diet Manual 1999

WEIGHT-REDUCTION DIET

(Sheet 1 of 2)

PURPOSE:

This is a simple "exchange list" diet for individuals who want to lose weight. The goal of diet therapy is to reduce caloric intake to a level that can be safely and comfortably tolerated. Usually diets that provide 1,200 to 1,500 calories a day are acceptable for most people. However, you and your health care provider should determine the appropriate amount of calories required for your weight, height, activity level and general health. The example shown is for a 1,400 calories per day menu. It may be modified by adding more food portions.

DESCRIPTION:

Plan your breakfast, lunch, and dinner meals by selecting items from the appropriate food list. This sample diet allows you one fruit portion, one starch, and one milk for breakfast. You may choose cereal with banana and milk. Coffee or tea is a "free" item. Amounts of each portion are indicated in each food list. Portions can be interchanged among breakfast, lunch, and dinner as long as the total for the day doesn't exceed those indicated. For example, you can eat all your fruits for breakfast if desired, but don't exceed four portions for the day.

SUGGESTED MEAL PLANS FOR APPROXIMATELY 1,400 CALORIES PER DAY DIET
DAILY PORTIONS FROM FOOD LISTS
(See lists below and following page)

BREAKFAST	LUNCH	DINNER	SNACK
1 Fruit	2 Meats	3 Meats	1 Starch
2 Starches/Bread	1 Vegetable	1 Fat	1 Fruit
1 Milk	1 Fat	2 Starches/Bread	1 Milk
	2 Starches/Bread	1 Vegetable	
	1 Fruit	1 Fruit	
	(raw vegetable	(raw vegetable	
	as desired)	as desired)	

FRUIT LIST (60 calories, 15 grams carbohydrates):

(A portion is 1 small piece or 1/2 cup unless listed)

Apples (Juice or Sauce)	Fruit Cocktail	Plums (2)
Apricots (4)	Grapefruit or Juice	Prunes (3)
Apricots, dried (7 halves)	Grapes (15)	Prune Juice (1/4 cup)
Banana (1/2)	Grape Juice	Raspberries (1 cup)
Blackberries (3/4 cup)	Lemon	Raisins (2 Tbsp)
Blueberries (3/4 cup)	Orange/Orange Juice	Rhubarb
Cantaloupe (1/3)	Peach	Strawberries (10)
Cherries (12 or 1/2 cup)	Pear	Tangerine
Dates (2)	Pineapple (3/4 cup fresh)	Watermelon (1 cup)

VEGETABLE LIST (25 calories, 5 grams carbohydrates, 2 grams protein):

(A portion is 1 cup raw or 1/2 cup cooked)

Artichoke	Celery	Peppers
Asparagus	Cucumber	Peas
Beans (green, wax or sprouts)	Eggplant	Pumpkin
Beets	Endive	Radish
Broccoli	Mixed Vegetables	Rutabaga
Brussels Sprouts	Mushrooms	Spinach
Cabbage or Sauerkraut	Okra	Squash
Cauliflower	Onions	Tomato
Carrot	Parsnips	Turnips

Note: Some vegetables are shown in the Starch List.

STARCH LIST (80 calories, 15 grams carbohydrates, 2–3 grams protein, 1–2 grams fat):

(A portion is 1/4 cup or as listed)

Angel Food Cake (1 oz)	Cornbread (2 inch cube)	Popcorn, fat-free (3 cups)
Bagel (small or 1 oz)	Cornstarch (2 Tbsp)	Potato, white (1/2 cup)
Beans, canned (1/3 cup)	English muffin (1/2)	Potato, sweet (1/3 cup)
Biscuit (2 1/2 inch size, 1)	Gelatin (1/2 cup)	Pretzels (5 small)
Bread (1 slice)	Graham crackers (2)	Rice (1/3 cup)
Bun (1/2)	Lentils, canned (1/3 cup)	Rice cakes (2)
Cereal (3/4 cup, dry;	Matzo crackers (3/4 oz)	Saltines (6)
1/2 cup hot)	Pancake (4 inch size, 1)	Taco Shell (1)
Corn (1/2 cup)	Pasta (1/2 cup)	Tortilla (one 6–inch)
Cookies (fat-free, 1 or 2 small)	Pita bread (6 inch size, 1/2)	

MEAT OR MEAT SUBSTITUTE LIST (55–70 calories, 7 grams protein, 3–5 grams fat):

(A portion is 1 ounce or 1/4 cup or as listed)

Beef (lean cuts)	Eggs (3 per week)	Pork (chops, ham, roast)
Cheese (skim milk types)	Fish (all types)	Shellfish
Cold Cuts or Frankfurters	Lamb (leg, roasted)	Soybeans, cooked (1/3 cup)
(95% fat-free)	Peanut Butter (1 Tbsp)	Veal
Cottage Cheese (1/3 cup)	Poultry (no skin)	

FAT LIST (45 calories, 5 grams fat):

(Use nonfat or low-fat products when they are available)

Bacon, crisp (1 slice)	Gravy (2 Tbsp)	Oils (1 teaspoon)
Cheese, cream* (1 Tbsp)	Margarine* (1 teaspoon)	Olives (5 large)
Coconut (2 Tbsp)	Mayonnaise* (1 teaspoon)	Salad Dressings* (1 Tbsp)
Cream, light (2 Tbsp)	Nuts (6 to 10)	Seeds (1 Tbsp)

* Portion amounts may be increased if using nonfat products (e.g., mayonnaise, 2 Tbsp)

MILK LIST (80 calories, 12 grams carbohydrates, 8 grams protein):

Skim milk (1 cup)   Yogurt (1 cup plain, nonfat, unsweetened except with sugar substitute)

FREE ITEMS: (You may have these as desired)

Beverages: Coffee, tea, sugar-free beverages
Pickles, except sweet pickles
Bouillon and consommés
All spices, herbs, flavorings, and artificial sweeteners
Catsup, mustard, soy sauce, vinegar
Worcestershire sauce
Sugar-free gelatin

Raw salad greens—lettuce, parsley, romaine,
  spinach, watercress, endive, escarole,
  cabbage, Chinese cabbage, other greens
Nonstick pan spray
Lemon or lime juice
Sugar substitutes

ADDITIONAL INFORMATION:

• Purchase fruits fresh, fresh-frozen, or canned unsweetened, or in natural juices. All juices should be unsweetened.

• Vegetable and fruit portions are for the edible amounts of the item.

• Allowed amounts of meats are after cooking; amounts shown are for edible parts only (excluding bones). Be sure to trim all extra fat away from meat before cooking. Remove skin from all poultry. Roasting or broiling of meats is preferred.

• If salt intake is limited, avoid foods high in sodium (e.g., pickles) and don't use salt at the table.

• Even though the diet should meet your nutritional needs, a vitamin and mineral supplement may be recommended by your health care provider.

• Everyone on a diet will experience an occasional setback. This doesn't mean failure. Long-term success is still possible.

• Combine your diet with eating behavior modification to help you maintain the weight loss.

BREAST SELF-EXAMINATION

FINDING BREAST CANCER EARLY

• There have been many advances made in diagnosing and treating breast cancer. More and more women are surviving the disease. In many cases, breast cancers found early and treated promptly have a better chance for a cure.

• Tools to detect breast cancer include exams by a medical professional, mammography, ultrasound, and breast self-examination (BSE). BSE has come under some debate about how effective it is. Studies have shown that there is no difference in the number of lives saved among women who did perform a BSE and those who did not. In addition, they have found that BSE may increase unneeded biopsies and anxiety.

• The American Cancer Society continues to recommend that BSE be performed monthly beginning at age 20. BSE will help a woman under age 40 learn what her breasts feel like under normal conditions. If a lump or other change is discovered, she can see her health care provider about it. There is some added benefit to women over age 40 in doing a BSE. Exams by a medical professional and mammography should have the most emphasis in early detection of breast cancer.

• Several products have been approved by the Food & Drug Administration (FDA) to help women perform monthly breast self-examinations. They may help make the exams easier for some women. Ask your health care provider about their use.

WHEN TO EXAMINE YOUR BREASTS

• Follow the same procedure once a month a few days to about a week after your period ends, when your breasts are usually not tender or swollen. Breast tissue in adult women changes throughout the month as it responds to hormone levels occurring during the menstrual cycle. Some women have normally lumpy breasts, but they can still learn the pattern of the lumps and should be able to detect new or unusual lumps.

• After menopause, check your breasts on the same day of each month. After a hysterectomy, ask your health care provider about the best time of the month.

BREAST EXAM WHILE LYING DOWN ON YOUR BACK

• To examine your right breast, put a pillow or folded towel under your right shoulder. Place your right hand under your head—this distributes breast tissue more evenly on the chest.

• Use the finger pads of the three middle fingers of your left hand. Press gently and firmly. A ridge of firm tissue in the lower curve of each breast is normal. Then move around the breast in 1) a circular pattern, 2) up and down line, or 3) in a wedge pattern. Always use the same pattern each month. Now repeat the procedure on your left breast with a pillow under your left shoulder and the left hand under your head. Notice how your breast structure feels.

• Check the area under each arm (with your elbow slightly bent). The lymph glands are in this area. They may become swollen if you are sick. If you feel a small lump that moves freely, check it daily for a few days. If it doesn't go away, call your health care provider.

• Any discharge from the nipple, clear or bloody, should be reported to your health care provider.

BREAST EXAM IN THE SHOWER

Examine your breasts during a shower (hands glide easier over wet skin). With the fingers flat, move the hand gently over every part of each breast. Use your right hand to examine the left breast, left hand for the right breast. Check for any lump, hard knot, or thickening.

BREAST EXAM IN FRONT OF A MIRROR

Inspect your breasts with arms at your sides. Next, raise your arms high overhead. Look for any changes in each breast (swelling, dimpling, or changes in the nipple).

SIGNS OF POSSIBLE PROBLEMS IN YOUR BREASTS

• Lumps, hard knots, or thickening in the breast.
• Unusual swelling, warmth, redness, or darkening that does not go away.
• Change in the size or shape of your breast.
• Dimpling or puckering of the skin.
• Itchy, scaly, sore, or rash on the nipple.
• Pulling in of the nipple or other parts of the breast.
• Nipple discharge that starts suddenly.
• Pain in one spot that does not vary or change with your monthly cycle.

WHAT TO DO

• It is important to see your health care provider as soon as possible if you find any suspicious changes in your breasts. Don't be frightened. Most breast lumps or changes are not cancer.

• Remember that a monthly breast exam is not a substitute for the other two critical parts of the guidelines for early breast cancer detection. The American Cancer Society recommends an annual mammogram after age 40, and an exam by a medical professional every three years for women ages 20–39, and annually for women over age 40. Ask your health care provider about when you should schedule a mammogram and a breast exam.

• To learn more: American Cancer Society, 1599 Clifton Rd., Atlanta, GA 30329, (800) ACS-2345; website: www.cancer.org or National Cancer Institute, (800) 4-CANCER; website: www.nci.nih.gov.

Special notes:

_____

_____

_____

More notes on back of this page ☐

CARE OF CASTS

 BASIC INFORMATION

A cast immobilizes a part of the body that has been injured. Casts are used most commonly after bone fractures. A cast is usually applied by placing a splint along the injured part and wrapping it in gauze saturated with plaster of Paris or fiberglass. Before the injury heals, it may be necessary to change the cast one or more times. The time needed for healing determines how long a cast remains in place. Some casts are needed for only two weeks. Others are worn for several months. X-rays through a cast reveal whether bone alignment is satisfactory. They are also used in later stages to check for signs of healing.

AFTER YOU LEAVE THE MEDICAL OFFICE
• Don't allow pressure on any part of the cast—no matter what type of casting material was used—until it is completely dry. Any depression that develops will create pressure on the skin underneath, making ulcer formation likely. Drying time varies depending on the type of material used, thickness of the cast, temperature and humidity. Drying can require 24 hours or longer.
• Keep the cast dry, especially at first. If a plaster cast accidentally gets wet and a soft area appears, return to your health care provider's office, emergency room, or outpatient surgical facility for repairs.
• Whenever possible, elevate the body part enclosed in the cast. This decreases the chance of tissue swelling inside the cast. Prop a leg in a cast on a pillow when in bed or on a footstool or chair when sitting. Prop an arm in a cast on a pillow placed on the chest. Elevate the foot of the bed at night for any injury requiring a cast below the abdomen.

SWELLING INSIDE A CAST
No matter how carefully the injured tissues are handled and no matter how expertly a cast is applied, swelling sometimes occurs inside a cast. Swelling should be reported immediately to your health care provider. The following are common symptoms and signs of swelling:
• Severe, persistent pain.
• Change in color of tissues beyond the cast, such as a change to blue or gray under the fingernails or toenails.
• Coldness of the tissues beyond the cast, even though the rest of the body is warm.
• Numbness or complete loss of feeling in the skin beyond the cast.
• Feeling of tightness under the cast after it dries.
• With a leg cast, inability to raise or curl the big toe.

INFECTION INSIDE A CAST
Sometimes the injured area becomes infected during healing. Detecting the infection in its early stages may be difficult if the infected area is covered by a cast. Infection should be reported immediately to the doctor. Following are common signs and symptoms of infection:
• Leakage of fluid through the cast.
• Increasing pain or soreness of the skin under the cast.
• Fever accompanied by a general ill feeling.

ITCHING INSIDE A CAST
• Itching can be a maddening problem for a person with a cast—especially during hot weather. Even if you can reach the itch, don't scratch the skin inside the cast. Because the skin is in a hot, moist environment, it is very vulnerable to damage; scratching is more likely to injure the skin than under normal circumstances. If no incision was made in the skin enclosed by the cast, you may sprinkle cornstarch into the cast to relieve itching. If an incision was made, consult your health care provider about a pain reliever. Itching is a form of mild pain.
• Although slow to relieve itching, applying an ice bag over the cast or heating it with a hair dryer may help.

BATHING WITH A CAST
• You may find bathing difficult when wearing a cast. The cast must be kept dry at all times, so do not take showers. If the cast is on a limb, such as your arm or leg, you may take baths in a tub. Position a chair or other support by the tub so you can prop the injured part out of the water while bathing. If the cast is on the trunk of the body, you should take sponge baths until the cast is removed.
• Alternately, a "rubber dam" cast cover can be used over a cast on an extremity to allow you to shower. Ask your health care provider or a pharmacist, or medical supply store for this.

 NOTIFY OUR OFFICE IF

You have questions or concern about your cast.

Special notes:

_____

_____

_____

More notes on the back of this page ☐

COMPLEMENTARY & ALTERNATIVE MEDICINE (CAM)

 ## BASIC INFORMATION

Complementary and alternative medicine (CAM) is a group of diverse medical and health care systems, practices, and products that are not presently considered part of conventional medicine. Some scientific evidence exists about certain CAM therapies. For most, there are questions about whether they are safe and whether they work for the diseases or medical conditions for which they are used.

DEFINITIONS
• Conventional:

Conventional medicine is medicine as practiced by holders of M.D. (medical doctor) or D.O. (doctor of osteopathy) degrees, and by other health professionals, such as physical therapists, psychologists, and registered nurses. Other terms for conventional medicine include allopathy; Western, mainstream, orthodox, and regular medicine; and biomedicine. Some conventional medical practitioners are also practitioners of CAM.

• Complementary:

Complementary medicine is used together with conventional medicine. An example of a complementary therapy is using aromatherapy to help lessen a patient's discomfort following surgery.

• Alternative:

Alternative medicine is used in place of conventional medicine. An example of an alternative therapy is using a special diet to treat cancer instead of undergoing surgery, radiation, or chemotherapy that has been recommended by a medical doctor.

• Integrative:

Integrative medicine combines mainstream medical therapies and CAM therapies for which there is some high-quality scientific evidence of safety and effectiveness.

CATEGORIES OF COMPLEMENTARY AND ALTERNATIVE THERAPIES
• Alternative medical systems

Alternative medical systems are built upon complete systems of theory and practice. Often, these systems have evolved apart from and earlier than the conventional medical approach used in the United States. Examples of alternative medical systems that have developed in Western cultures include homeopathic medicine and naturopathic medicine. Examples of systems that have developed in non-Western cultures include traditional Chinese medicine and Ayurveda.

• Mind-body interventions

Mind-body medicine uses a variety of techniques designed to enhance the mind's capacity to affect bodily function and symptoms. Some techniques that were considered CAM in the past have become mainstream (for example, patient support groups and cognitive-behavioral therapy). Other mind-body techniques are still considered CAM, including meditation, prayer, mental healing, and therapies that use creative outlets such as art, music, or dance.

• Biologically based therapies

Biologically based therapies in CAM use substances found in nature, such as herbs, foods, and vitamins. Some examples include dietary supplements, herbal products, and the use of other so-called "natural" yet scientifically unproven therapies (for example, using shark cartilage to treat cancer).

• Manipulative and body-based methods

Manipulative and body-based methods in CAM are based on manipulation and/or movement of one or more parts of the body. Some examples include chiropractic or osteopathic manipulation, and massage.

• Energy therapies (involve the use of energy fields). They are of two types:

- Biofield therapies are intended to affect energy fields that are thought to surround and penetrate the human body. The existence of such fields has not yet been scientifically proven. Some forms of energy therapy manipulate biofields by applying pressure and/or manipulating the body by placing the hands in, or through, these fields. Examples include qi gong, Reiki, and Therapeutic Touch.

- Bioelectromagnetic-based therapies involve the unconventional use of electromagnetic fields, such as pulsed fields, magnetic fields, or alternating current or direct current fields.

• To learn more: National Center for Complementary and Alternative Medicine Clearinghouse, P.O. Box 7923, Gaithersburg, MD 20898; (888) 644-6226; website: www.nccam.nih.gov.

 ## NOTIFY OUR OFFICE IF

You have questions about complementary or alternative medicine.

Special notes:

_____

_____

_____

More notes on the back of this page ☐

BASIC INFORMATION

WHO SHOULD USE A CONDOM?

• Condoms are used for both birth control and reducing the risk of disease. Some people think that other forms of birth control will also protect them against disease. This is not true. Even if you use another form of birth control, you need a condom to help reduce the risk of getting STDs (sexually transmitted diseases) including the human immunodeficiency virus (HIV) infection.

• Condoms do not make sex 100% safe, but, if properly used, they can reduce the chance of contracting STDs. This can mean protection not only for you and your partner, but also for any children you may have in the future.

CHOOSING A CONDOM

Read the label and look for the following:

• The condoms should be made of latex (rubber) or made of polyurethane.

• It should say that the condoms are to prevent disease, and if used properly, latex condoms help reduce risk of HIV transmission and many other STDs. If the package doesn't say anything about preventing disease, the condoms may not provide the protection you need. Novelty condoms, for example, will not be labeled for either disease- or pregnancy-prevention. Condoms that don't cover the entire penis are not labeled for disease prevention and should not be used for this purpose. For proper protection, a condom must unroll to cover the entire penis.

• Check the expiration date (EXP followed by date). The condom should not be purchased or used after that date.

• Condoms are available in many stores and from vending machines. If buying condoms from vending machines, check for proper labeling. Do not buy condoms from a vending machine located where it may be subject to extreme temperatures or direct sunlight.

• Condoms should be stored in a cool, dry place out of direct sunlight. Closets or drawers usually make good storage places. Condoms should not be kept in a pocket, wallet, or purse for more than a few hours at a time because they may be exposed to extreme temperatures.

HOW TO USE A CONDOM

• When opening a condom, handle the package gently. Don't use teeth, sharp fingernails, scissors, or other sharp instruments. These may damage the condom. Make sure you can see what you're doing!

• After you open the package, inspect the condom. If the material sticks to itself or is gummy, the condom is no good. Check the condom top for other obvious damage such as brittleness, tears, and holes. Do not unroll the condom to check it; this could damage it.

• Use a new condom at the beginning of every sexual act (vaginal or anal intercourse and oral sex).

• Put the condom on as soon as the penis is erect and before any contact is made between the penis and any part of the partner's body. Don't delay condom use. Studies have shown that while pre-ejaculatory fluid is not semen, it does contain HIV.

• If the condom does not have a reservoir tip, pinch the tip enough to leave a half-inch space for semen to collect. Make sure to squeeze out any air in the tip to help keep the condom from breaking.

• While holding the condom by the rim (and pinching the half-inch tip, if needed), place the condom on top of the penis. Then, continuing to hold it by the rim, unroll it all the way to the base of the penis. If you are using water-based lubricant, you can put more on the outside of the condom.

• If you feel the condom break, stop right away, withdraw, and put on a new condom.

• After ejaculation and before the penis gets soft, grip the rim of the condom and carefully withdraw.

• To remove the condom, gently pull it off the penis, being careful the semen doesn't spill out.

• Wrap the used condom in a tissue and throw it in the trash. Because condoms may cause problems in sewers, don't flush them down the toilet. Then wash your hands with soap and warm water.

CONDOM USAGE TO PREVENT STDs

(Sheet 2 of 2)

PRECAUTION

Condoms provide good protection for vaginal and oral sex (where the penis is in contact with the mouth). The protection they give for anal sex is questionable. The Surgeon General of the Public Health Service has said, "Condoms provide some protection, but anal intercourse is simply too dangerous a practice." Condoms may be more likely to break during anal intercourse than during other types of sex. This is due to the greater amount of friction and other stresses involved. Even if the condom doesn't break, anal intercourse is very risky because it can cause rectal tissue to tear and bleed. This allows disease germs to pass more easily from one partner to another.

SPERMICIDES

Spermicides (gels, creams, foams, or films), which kill sperm, are used for birth control, either alone or with barrier contraceptives such as the diaphragm or cervical cap. A spermicide called nonoxynol 9 has been widely used with condoms to supposedly help reduce the risk of STD transmission. Studies now show that nonoxynol 9 does not reduce the risk of transmission of the human immunodeficiency virus (HIV) or other STDs during intercourse. Some condoms come with nonoxynol-9 already added but they are not recommended for prevention of STDs. The best STD and HIV barrier is a latex condom without nonoxynol-9. Nevertheless, a condom that is lubricated with nonoxynol-9 is safer than unprotected sex with no condom at all. Condom packages are required to be labeled with the expiration date of the spermicide, and they should not be used after that date. In females, frequent use of spermicides containing nonoxynol 9 can cause vaginal irritation and lesions (sores), which may actually increase the possibility of transmitting an STD from an infected partner.

LUBRICANTS

Lubricants may help prevent condoms from breaking during use. They may prevent irritation that might increase the chance of infection. Some condoms come lubricated with dry silicone, jelly, or cream, or you can add water-based lubricants specifically made for this purpose (for example, K-Y Lubricating Jelly). If you use a separate lubricant, never use a product that contains oils, fats, or greases such as a petroleum-based jelly (for example, Vaseline), baby oil or lotion, hand or body lotion, cooking shortening, or oily cosmetics such as cold creams. These can seriously weaken latex, causing a condom to tear easily. If you use a spermicide, you do not necessarily need to use a lubricant because some spermicide acts as a lubricant.

TO LEARN MORE

Centers for Disease Control and Prevention STD Hotline (800) 227-8922; website: www.cdc.gov/std.

 NOTIFY OUR OFFICE IF

You have questions about the use of condoms.

Special notes:

_____

_____

_____

More notes on the back of this page ☐

BASIC INFORMATION

The choice to use a dietary supplement can be a wise decision that provides health benefits. Sometimes, however, these products may not be needed for good health, or they may even create unexpected risks.

DEFINITION OF DIETARY SUPPLEMENTS

· Dietary supplements are defined as products that contain one or more of the following ingredients:
  - a vitamin.
  - a mineral.
  - an herb or other botanical (plant or plant part).
  - an amino acid.
  - a dietary substance used by people to supplement the diet by increasing total dietary intake.
  - a concentrate, metabolite, constituent, and extract, or combination of any of the ingredients listed.
  - intended for ingestion in the form of a capsule, powder, softgel or gelcap, and not represented as a conventional food or as a sole item of a meal or the diet.

PURPOSE OF DIETARY SUPPLEMENTS

Dietary supplements are intended to supplement the diets of some people. They are not meant to replace the balance of the variety of foods important to a healthy diet. While you need nutrients, too much of some nutrients can cause problems.

CAUTIONS

Dietary supplements may not be risk-free in some cases. Use caution if you are pregnant, nursing a baby, or have a chronic medical condition such as, diabetes, hypertension, or heart disease. Be sure to consult your health care provider or pharmacist before buying or taking any supplement.

CHILDREN AND DIETARY SUPPLEMENTS

Vitamin and mineral supplements are widely used and generally safe for children. You may wish to check with your child's health care provider or pharmacist before giving any dietary supplements other then vitamins and minerals to your child.

TALK TO YOUR HEALTH CARE PROVIDER

If you plan to use a dietary supplement in place of drugs or at the same time as any drug, tell your health care provider first. Many supplements contain active ingredients that have strong effects in the body and their safety is not always assured in all users. If you have certain health conditions and take these products, you may be placing yourself at risk.

INTERACTIONS WITH OTHER DRUGS

· Some supplements may interact with prescription and nonprescription drugs. Taking a combination of supplements or using these products together with drugs (both prescription or nonprescription) could, under certain circumstances, produce adverse effects. Some of these interactions could be life-threatening. Ask your health care provider or pharmacist about possible interactions.

· Examples of interactions:
  - Coumadin (a prescription drug), ginkgo biloba (an herbal supplement), aspirin, and vitamin E can each thin the blood. Taking any of these products together can increase the potential for internal bleeding.
  - Combining St. John's Wort with certain HIV drugs reduces their effectiveness. St. John's Wort may also reduce the effectiveness of prescription drugs for heart disease, depression, seizures, certain cancers, or oral contraceptives.

SURGERY & DIETARY SUPPLEMENTS

Some supplements can have unwanted effects during surgery. It is important to fully inform your health care provider about the vitamins, minerals, herbals, or any other supplements you are taking, especially before elective surgery. You may be asked to stop taking these products at least two to three weeks ahead of the procedure. This will help to avoid potentially dangerous supplement/drug interactions. Interactions could cause changes in heart rate, blood pressure, and increase bleeding. Any of these could adversely affect the outcome of your surgery.

ENSURING THE SAFETY & EFFICACY OF SUPPLEMENTS

Under the law, manufacturers of dietary supplements are responsible for making sure their products are safe before they go to market. They are also responsible for making sure that the claims on their labels are accurate and truthful. Dietary supplement products are not reviewed by the government before they are marketed. The FDA (Food & Drug Administration) does have the responsibility to take action against any unsafe dietary supplement product that reaches the market. If the FDA can prove that claims on marketed dietary supplement products are false and misleading, it may take action against those products.

DIETARY SUPPLEMENTS

(Sheet 2 of 2)

DOES THE INFORMATION FOR THE DIETARY SUPPLEMENT SOUND TOO GOOD TO BE TRUE?

· Do the claims for the product seem exaggerated or unrealistic? While the Web can be a valuable source of accurate, reliable information, it also has a wealth of misinformation that may not be obvious. It is important to know what information about a product is accurate and what is misleading or false. Some advertising can be very convincing.

· Be cautious about information that comes from persons who have no formal training in nutrition or from personal reports. Information may come from store employees, friends, or online chat rooms and message boards. They may talk about incredible benefits or results obtained from using a product. Ask these people about their training and knowledge in nutrition or medicine.

· Think twice about chasing the latest headline. Sound health advice is generally based on experience and a variety of medical research (not just a single study). Be wary of results claiming a "quick fix." In addition, news stories, about the latest scientific study, especially those on TV or radio, are often too brief. They do not include important details that may apply to you or allow you to make an informed decision.

CONTACT THE MANUFACTURER FOR MORE INFORMATION

· If you cannot tell whether the product you are purchasing meets the same standards as those used in the research studies you read about, check with the manufacturer or distributor. Ask to speak to someone who can answer your questions. Questions may include:

1. What information does the firm have to substantiate the claims made for the product? Be aware that sometimes firms supply so-called "proof" of their claims by citing undocumented reports from satisfied consumers, or "internal" graphs and charts that could be mistaken for proven research.

2. Does the firm have information to share about tests it has conducted on the safety or efficacy of the ingredients in the product?

3. Does the firm have a quality control system in place to determine if the product actually contains what is stated on the label and is free of contaminants?

4. Has the firm received any adverse event reports from consumers using their products?

REPORTING ADVERSE EFFECTS

· Adverse effects from the use of dietary supplements should be reported to the FDA. You, your health care provider, or anyone may report a serious adverse event or illness directly to FDA if you believe it is related to the use of any dietary supplement product, by calling FDA at (800) FDA-1088, by fax at (800) FDA-0178 or on-line at www.fda.gov/medwatch/how.htm.

· The FDA would like to know whenever you think a product caused you a serious problem. Report it even if you are not sure that the product was the cause, and even if you do not visit a health care provider or medical clinic. In addition to contacting the FDA on-line or by phone, you may use the form available from the FDA Web site.

 ## NOTIFY OUR OFFICE IF

You have questions about using dietary supplements.

Special notes:

_____

_____

_____

More notes on the back of this page ☐

DRUGS, BUYING ONLINE

 BASIC INFORMATION

TIPS AND WARNINGS FOR CONSUMERS

With hundreds of drug-dispensing Websites in business, how can consumers tell which sites are legitimate ones, especially when it is very easy to set up a site that is very professional looking and promises deep discounts or no hassles?

IF YOU BUY MEDICAL PRODUCTS ONLINE, BE AWARE OF THE FOLLOWING DANGERS:

• Purchasing a drug from an illegal Website puts you at risk. You may receive a contaminated or counterfeit product, the wrong product, an incorrect dose, or no product at all.
• Taking an unsafe or inappropriate drug puts you at risk for possible drug interactions and other serious health problems.
• Getting a prescription drug by filling out a question and answer form without seeing a health care provider poses serious health risks. This type of form does not provide enough information for a health care provider to determine whether that drug is for you or safe to use, if another treatment is more appropriate, or if you have an underlying medical condition where using that drug may be harmful. The American Medical Association has determined that this practice is generally substandard medical care. The Food and Drug Administration (FDA) agrees.

FDA (FOOD & DRUG ADMINISTRATION) OFFERS THESE TIPS TO CONSUMERS WHO BUY HEALTH PRODUCTS ONLINE:

• Check with the National Association of Boards of Pharmacy (website: www.nabp.net, or call (847) 698-6227) to determine whether a Website is a licensed pharmacy in good standing.
• Don't buy from sites that offer to prescribe a prescription drug for the first time without a physical exam, sell a prescription drug without a prescription, or sell drugs not approved by FDA.
• Don't do business with sites that have no access to a registered pharmacist to answer questions.
• Avoid sites that do not identify with whom you are dealing and do not provide a U.S. address and phone number to contact if there's a problem.
• Don't purchase from foreign Websites at this time because generally it will be illegal to import the drugs bought from these sites, the risks are greater, and there is very little the U.S. government can do if you get ripped off.
• Beware of sites that advertise a "new cure" for a serious disorder, or a quick cure-all for a wide range of ailments.
• Be careful of sites that use impressive-sounding terminology to disguise a lack of good science or those that claim the government, the medical profession, or research scientists have conspired to suppress a product.
• Avoid sites that include undocumented case histories claiming "amazing" results.
• Talk to your health-care provider before using any drugs for the first time.

 NOTIFY OUR OFFICE IF

You have other questions about purchasing drugs online.
(Note: This information adapted in part from the Food & Drug Administration).

Special notes:

_____

_____

_____

More notes on the back of this page ☐

DRUGS, SAFE USE OF

 CHECKLIST FOR SAFER DRUG USE

INFORMATION YOU SHOULD PROVIDE

Always give the information listed in 1 and 2 below to your doctor, dentist, or other health care provider so that they can prescribe drugs properly:

1. Your medical history

Tell the important facts of your medical history dealing with drugs. Include allergic reactions, side effects, or adverse reactions you have experienced in the past. Describe the allergic problems you have such as hay fever, asthma, eye watering and itching, throat irritation, and reactions to food. People who have allergies to common substances are more likely to develop side effects or adverse reactions to drugs.

2. Drugs you are taking now

List all prescription and nonprescription drugs. Don't forget common ones such as laxatives; herbal, vitamin, or mineral supplements; skin, rectal, vaginal drugs; antacids; antihistamines; cold and cough remedies; aspirin and aspirin-containing pain pills; motion sickness remedies; weight-loss aids; salt and sugar substitutes; caffeine (in coffee, tea, cola drinks, and cocoa); oral contraceptives; sleeping pills; or "tonics."

INFORMATION TO KNOW BEFORE TAKING A DRUG

• Generic names and brand names of all the drugs you take. Write them down to help you remember. If a drug is a mixture of two or more generic ingredients, learn the names of each.

• Uses for each drug you take.

• How to take each drug—for example, with or without water, or with or without food.

• When to take it.

• What to do if you forget a dose.

• How each drug works in your body.

• Time lapse before drug works.

• Symptoms and treatment of overdose.

• Possible adverse reactions and side effects and what to do if they occur.

• Interactions with other drugs and other substances such as alcohol, food, beverages, cocaine, marijuana, and tobacco. When mixed, they can sometimes cause serious interactions.

• Know all warnings and precautions that apply to special circumstances, such as the following:

1. Reasons (called contraindications) not to take the drug in the presence of some medical conditions.

2. Special considerations for elderly patients, pregnant or breast-feeding women, infants, and children.

3. Information about long-term use, exposure to sun and sunlight, driving, piloting aircraft, hazardous work, or flying in airplanes.

4. Instructions before discontinuing the drug.

OTHER SAFETY TIPS

• Before taking any prescribed drug, discuss plans with the doctor that you may have for elective surgery, pregnancy, and breast-feeding.

• Don't hesitate to ask questions about a drug. We will be able to provide more information if we are familiar with you and your past medical history, especially regarding drugs.

• Never take a drug in the dark! It is always possible to take the wrong one. Recheck the label before each drug use.

• Notify our office about any new or unexpected symptoms you develop while taking a drug. You may need to change drugs or have a dose adjustment.

• Store all drugs out of children's reach. Keep drugs in a cool, dry place, such as a kitchen cabinet or bedroom. Avoid medicine cabinets in bathrooms—they get too moist and warm at times. Keep drugs in their original containers, tightly closed. Don't remove the labels! If directions call for refrigeration, keep the drug cool, but don't freeze it.

• Don't save leftover drugs to use later. Discard them on or before the expiration date shown on the label.

• Do not flush old drugs down the toilet or dispose in a drain. Doing so may result in traces of the drug seeping into the water supply. Throw the drugs in the trash, packaged in childproof containers and/or sealed plastic bags (out of the reach of children and pets). Another option is to check if local household hazardous-waste collection programs—where you're supposed to take motor oil and batteries—accept expired drugs.

• Don't take any drug prescribed for someone else.

• Prior to any surgery (including oral surgery or simple dental procedures), tell the doctor or dentist about all drugs you take or have taken in the past few weeks.

• If you become pregnant while taking any drug, tell your health care provider right away. Avoid all drugs when you are pregnant, if possible.

 NOTIFY OUR OFFICE IF

You have questions about taking drugs.

Special notes:

_____

_____

_____

More notes on the back of this page ☐

BASIC INFORMATION

PROTECTING YOUR CHILD AGAINST SERIOUS DISEASE
It's important that children get vaccinated (get their "shots") so they don't get childhood diseases. Your child can be vaccinated at the doctor's office or your local health department. Keep a list of the shots your child has received so that you have records for school and so you'll know if your child needs more shots.

VACCINES THAT ARE AVAILABLE
· Diphtheria.
· Whooping cough (pertussis).
· Tetanus.
· Polio.
· Measles.
· Mumps.
· German measles (rubella).
· Chickenpox (varicella).
· Hepatitis A and hepatitis B.
· HIB (*haemophilus influenzae* type B).
· *Pneumococcal* diseases.
· Influenza.
  (Some of these vaccines are being combined into single shots. Ask your health care provider.)
· In most of the United States, many of these vaccinations are required for school or day-care. The first shots for most of these illnesses should be given when the child is still a baby. This is important because most of the diseases these vaccines protect your child against can be serious or even deadly.
· Like any medicine, vaccines carry a small risk of serious harm such as a severe allergic reaction. But side effects from shots are usually mild and last only a short time. Some children have no side effects at all. None of the possible side effects should keep your child from getting shots unless your doctor says so.
· Be sure to tell your doctor if anyone in your immediate family has ever had a bad reaction to a vaccine, and ask if there are certain conditions under which vaccination is not recommended. Also talk to your doctor about whether certain reactions to vaccines can be controlled, such as by giving your child acetaminophen or ibuprofen before or after vaccination.

VACCINATIONS, THE RECOMMENDED AGE TO GET THEM AND POSSIBLE SIDE EFFECTS:

DTaP
· Protects against: Diphtheria, whooping cough (pertussis), and tetanus. The vaccines against these three diseases are combined in a single shot. The single shot may also include the polio and hepatitis B vaccine.
· Diphtheria is a serious infection of the throat, mouth, and nose, which can lead to suffocation, pneumonia, heart failure, and paralysis.

· A child who catches whooping cough develops a bad cough that sounds like a "whoop." The severe coughing can interfere with eating, drinking, and breathing. Whooping cough can be life-threatening, especially in children younger than 1 year old.
· Tetanus is caused by germs in dirt and rusty metal that get into the body through a cut. Tetanus attacks the jaw muscles first, often causing lockjaw. It can also affect the muscles used to breathe. It causes death in 3 out of 10 people who get it.
· Ages to get vaccine: Shot is given at 2 months, 4 months, 6 months, and 15-18 months, with a booster given between the ages of 4 and 6 years. After that, everyone should get a tetanus booster every 10 years throughout life.
· Possible side effects include: Fever, soreness where shot is given, and irritability. In rare cases, the shot can cause very high fever and convulsions.

POLIO
· Protects against: Polio, a virus that can cause paralysis and death. There are two kinds of polio vaccines: the inactivated polio virus (IPV), which is the shot recommended in the United States today, and a live, oral polio virus (OPV). OPV causes polio in a few people and it is believed that using OPV is no longer worth the slight risk, except in limited cases. IPV does not cause polio.
· Ages to get vaccine: Shot is usually given at 2 months, 4 months, 6-18 months, and at 4-6 years. This vaccine may be combined with other vaccines.
· Possible side effects include: The main side effect of IPV is soreness where the shot is given.

MMR
· Protects against: Measles, mumps, and German measles (rubella). The vaccines against these three diseases are combined in a single shot.
· Measles is easy to catch and causes a rash, high fever, and cough. Measles can also cause hearing loss, convulsions, brain damage, and death.
· Mumps makes the saliva glands under the jaws swell and hurt. It also usually causes fever and headache and can have serious complications. It is even more painful for teen-age boys, whose testicles may swell.
· German measles is mild in children but can damage the unborn baby if a woman gets it while pregnant.
· Ages to get vaccine: One shot is given at 12–15 months and another is usually given at 4-6 years. Women who do not know if they are immune to rubella can be tested to see if they are. If they have no immunity they should get the rubella vaccine more than three months before they plan to get pregnant.
· Possible side effects include: Pain where the shot is given and a rash. The shot can also cause swollen glands or mild joint pain, but these are rare.

Information From Your Health Care Provider

CHICKENPOX

- Protects against: Chickenpox, which is usually a mild disease that causes an itchy rash and fever. Some children experience serious complications.
- Ages to get vaccine: One shot is given between the ages of 12 months and 12 years. It is recommended that children receive the shot at 12 to 18 months of age. Adults and adolescents older than 13 who have not had chickenpox get two shots, at least 4–8 weeks apart.
- Possible side effects include: Pain where the shot is given, rash, or fever.

HEPATITIS A

- Protects against: Hepatitis A, a disease of the liver caused by the hepatitis A virus. It can be mild to severe.
- Ages to get vaccine: For children 2 years or older. Two doses are needed, the second dose given 6-18 months after the first. The vaccine is recommended for children in select areas of the United States.
- Possible side effects include: Pain or swelling where the shot is given, fatigue, or mild fever.

HEPATITIS B

- Protects against: Hepatitis B, a disease of the liver caused by the hepatitis B virus. It can cause lifelong liver problems or death.
- Ages to get vaccine: For babies, three shots are given before 18 months of age. Older children, adolescents, and adults who didn't get the shot as babies can get the first shot any time, a second shot 1–2 months later, and a third shot 4–6 months after the first shot. This vaccine may be combined with other vaccines.
- Possible side effects include: Soreness where the shot is given and fever.

HIB

- Protects against: *Haemophilus influenzae* type b, an infection that can seriously harm a child's brain, blood, bones, throat, and the area around the heart.
- Ages to get vaccine: Shot is given at 2 months, 4 months, 6 months, and 12–15 months.
- Possible side effects include: Soreness where the shot is given and fever.

PNEUMOCOCCAL CONJUGATE

- Protects against: Invasive pneumococcal diseases, which can cause brain damage and death.
- Ages to get vaccine: Shot is given at 2 months, 4 months, 6 months, and 12 to 15 months.
- Possible side effects include: Soreness where the shot is given and mild fever.

INFLUENZA VACCINE

- Protects against: Influenza ("flu"), which is a virus that spreads from infected persons to the nose or throat of others. It can be mild to severe, and may be fatal.
- Ages to get vaccine: Shot given each year to children ages 6 months and 2 years.
- Possible side effects include: Soreness, redness, or swelling where the shot is given, fever, and aches. In rare cases, an allergic reaction may occur.

RECOMMENDED IMMUNIZATION SCHEDULE

Hepatitis B

1st dose	Birth–2 months
2nd dose	1 month–4 months
3rd dose	6 months–18 months
catch-up	11–12 years

Diphtheria, Tetanus, Pertussis (DTaP)

1st dose	2 months
2nd dose	4 months
3rd dose	6 months
4th dose	15 months–18 months
5th dose	4–6 years

Tetanus, Diphtheria (Td)

11–12 years; 13–18 years

H. influenzae type b (HIB)

1st dose	2 months
2nd dose	4 months
3rd dose	6 months
4th dose	12 months–15 months

Inactivated Poliovirus (Polio)

1st dose	2 months
2nd dose	4 months
3rd dose	6 months–18 months
4th dose	4–6 years

Pneumococcal Conjugate

1st dose	2 months
2nd dose	4 months
3rd dose	6 months
4th dose	12 months–15 months

Measles, Mumps, Rubella (MMR)

1st dose	12 months–15 months
2nd dose	4–6 years
catch-up	11–12 years

Varicella (chickenpox)

1st dose	12 months–18 months
catch-up	11–12 years

Hepatitis A (in selected areas of the United States)

1 dose	24 months–14–18 years

Influenza ("flu")

1 dose (each year)	6 months–2 years

Note: Temporary shortages of some vaccines may occur. The vaccine schedule may change until the shortage is corrected. Your child's health care provider will explain how a vaccine shortage affects your child.

 NOTIFY OUR OFFICE IF

You have any questions about childhood vaccinations.

Special notes:

_____

_____

_____

More notes on the back of this page☐

KEGEL EXERCISES
(Pelvic Floor Exercises)

 BASIC INFORMATION

• Life's events can weaken pelvic muscles. Pregnancy, childbirth, and being overweight can do it. Luckily, when these muscles get weak, you can help make them strong again.

• Pelvic floor muscles are just like other muscles. Exercise can make them stronger. Women with bladder control problems can regain control through Kegel exercises (pelvic muscle exercises).

THE PELVIC MUSCLES

• Exercising your pelvic floor muscles for just 5 minutes, three times a day can make a big difference to your bladder control. Exercise strengthens muscles that hold the bladder and many other organs in place.

• The part of your body including your hip bones is the pelvic area. At the bottom of the pelvis, several layers of muscle stretch between your legs. The muscles attach to the front, back, and sides of the pelvis bone.

• Two pelvic muscles do most of the work. The biggest one stretches like a hammock. The other is shaped like a triangle. These muscles prevent leaking of urine and stool.

• You can make these pelvic floor muscles stronger with a few minutes of exercise every day.

DOING THE EXERCISES

• Find the right muscles. This is very important. Your doctor, nurse, or physical therapist will help make sure you are doing the exercises the right way.

• You should tighten the two major muscles that stretch across your pelvic floor. They are the "hammock" muscle and the "triangle" muscle. Here are three methods to check for the correct muscles.

    1. Try to stop the flow of urine when you are sitting on the toilet. If you can do it, you are using the right muscles.

    2. Imagine that you are trying to stop passing gas. Squeeze the muscles you would use. If you sense a "pulling" feeling, those are the right muscles for pelvic exercises.

    3. Lie down and put your finger inside your vagina. Squeeze as if you were trying to stop urine from coming out. If you feel tightness on your finger, you are squeezing the right pelvic muscle.

• Don't squeeze other muscles at the same time. Be careful not to tighten your stomach, legs, or other muscles. Squeezing the wrong muscles can put more pressure on your bladder control muscles. Just squeeze the pelvic muscle. Don't hold your breath.

• Repeat, but don't overdo it. At first, find a quiet spot to practice—your bathroom or bedroom—so you can concentrate. Lie on the floor. Pull in the pelvic muscles and hold for a count of 3. Then relax for a count of 3. Work up to 10 to 15 repeats each time you exercise. Healthy sphincter muscles can keep the urethra closed.

• Do your pelvic exercises at least three times a day. Every day, use three positions: lying down, sitting, and standing. You can exercise while lying on the floor, sitting at a desk, or standing in the kitchen. Using all three positions makes the muscles strongest.

• Be patient. Don't give up. It's just 5 minutes, three times a day. You may not feel your bladder control improve until after 3 to 6 weeks. Still, most women do notice an improvement after a few weeks.

• Exercise aids. You can also exercise by using special weights or biofeedback. Ask your health care provider about these exercise aids.

HOLD THE SQUEEZE UNTIL AFTER THE SNEEZE

• You can protect your pelvic muscles from more damage by bracing yourself.

• Think ahead just before sneezing, lifting, or jumping. Sudden pressure from such actions can hurt those pelvic muscles. Squeeze your pelvic muscles tightly and hold on until after you sneeze, lift, or jump.

• After you train yourself to tighten the pelvic muscles for these moments, you will have fewer accidents.

POINTS TO REMEMBER

• Weak pelvic muscles often cause bladder control problems.

• Daily exercises can strengthen pelvic muscles.

• These exercises often improve bladder control.

• Ask your health care provider or nurse if you are squeezing the right muscles.

• Tighten your pelvic muscles before sneezing, lifting, or jumping. This can prevent pelvic muscle damage.

 NOTIFY OUR OFFICE IF

You have questions about pelvic floor exercises.

Special notes:

_____

_____

_____

More notes on the back of this page ☐

LIVING LONGER & HEALTHIER

 STAYING HEALTHY

Practicing healthy behaviors can help you live a longer and healthier life. Many diseases and health problems are due, in part, to lifestyle factors that can be changed.

EAT A HEALTHY DIET
Eat a variety of foods, including fruit, vegetables, animal or vegetable protein (such as meat, fish, chicken, eggs, beans, lentils, tofu, or tempeh), and grains (such as whole wheat or brown rice). Limit the amount of saturated fat you eat. Avoid fats that say "hydrogenated."

EAT AT REGULAR TIMES
Regular meals will keep the body working at its most efficient level. Don't skip breakfast. Failing to eat because "you don't have time" or to reduce calories leads to poor health. If you get hungry between meals, don't resort to fatty, salty, or refined-sugar snacks. Instead, eat fruit, raw vegetables, or whole grain snacks.

CONTROL YOUR WEIGHT
Even small amounts of excess weight can lead to health problems. Obesity is a major factor in many diseases. If you need to reduce, do so. If your weight is ideal, work to keep it that way. Balance the number of calories you eat with the number you burn off by your activities. Remember to watch portion sizes.

BE PHYSICALLY ACTIVE
Exercise that you enjoy is most likely to be successful and continued. Walk, dance, ride a bike, rake leaves, or do any other physical activity you enjoy. Start small and work up to a total of 20 to 30 minutes most days of the week.

DRINK ALCOHOL MODERATELY OR NOT AT ALL
Alcohol abuse can cause serious diseases, and affect every aspect of your daily life. If you drink, have no more than two drinks a day. A standard drink is one 12-ounce bottle of beer or wine cooler, one 5-ounce glass of wine, or 1.5-ounces of 80-proof distilled spirits.

DON'T SMOKE
Smoking damages the human body and shortens life. It is a risk factor for many heart and lung disorders. It can cause damage to unborn children of pregnant women who smoke. If you do smoke, find a way to quit that works for you. Avoid secondhand smoke.

DON'T ABUSE DRUGS
Avoid illicit drugs completely if you want to stay mentally and physically healthy. If you have a problem with drug abuse, seek medical help.

STAY SOCIALLY INVOLVED
Talk to and visit with friends and family often. Take the initiative. Don't wait for them to call. Stay active through work, recreation, church, volunteer, and community activities.

MEDICAL HELP
Get regular medical and dental checkups. See a health care provider when you suspect a problem, either physical or emotional. Wear a medical identification bracelet or neck tag if you have any chronic disorder, have known allergies to drugs, or if you take drugs that emergency personnel would need to know about.

GET ENOUGH SLEEP
Get the right amount of sleep (average 8 hours for men, 7 for women) each night. Use the bedroom for sleep and intimacy only. Avoid taking business or private worries to bed with you. Avoid getting caught up in suspenseful reading or television while relaxing in bed. If you occasionally toss and turn and can't get to sleep, go to another room and do something productive.

SAFETY
Use seat belts when you drive or ride in any vehicle. Practice good safety measures at home to prevent fires and to avoid accidents such as falls. Avoid overexposure to sun and cold.

PRACTICE SAFE SEX
Safe sex practices are those that lower the risk of catching or giving a sexually transmitted disease (STD), or becoming pregnant. Abstinence is the only sure preventive method. If you are sexually active, use condoms to protect against STDs. Limit number of sex partners. Avoid sex with a partner who has sores, abuses IV (intravenous) drugs, or has had many sexual partners.

PREVENT INFECTIONS
• Many germs are spread by way of hand contact. Hand washing is the first line of defense against the spread of infectious diseases for adults as well as children. When you are unable to wash your hands, use alcohol-based hand rub products (wipes, lotion, or gel).
• Be sure to cover your mouth and nose when coughing or sneezing to prevent spreading infectious droplets in the air. Cough into a tissue, if available, and then throw it away.

 NOTIFY OUR OFFICE IF

You have any questions about lifestyle changes you can make to help you live longer and healthier.

Special notes:

_____

_____

_____

More notes on the back of this page ☐

PRENATAL EXERCISING

 BASIC INFORMATION

GENERAL INFORMATION

• Exercising during pregnancy can help reduce some of the discomfort that occurs with pregnancy. It can improve posture and make the body more supple. It helps blood circulation. It provides a feeling of general well being. Pregnancy is a state of health, not of illness. Properly done exercises can help maintain health and avoid problems. A well-conditioned body will perform better during the stress of advanced pregnancy, labor, and delivery. Being fit will lead to a more speedy recovery of body weight after delivery.

• Do exercises on a routine basis, rather than once in a while. Plan your exercise program with the help of your prenatal medical team. It should be based on your fitness level before pregnancy. Women who have routinely done an exercise program before pregnancy can continue it during pregnancy. Sometimes a few changes are needed. Women who were not exercising before pregnancy are advised to begin an exercise program slowly.

• Limits to your exercise program will depend on your state of health, if you have had any problems with prior pregnancies, what types of exercise activities you plan, and your dietary needs.

NORMAL CHANGES DURING PREGNANCY

• The pregnant woman's center of gravity moves forward and downward. This alters balance, stability, and alignment (standing tall and straight). Backache, a frequent complaint of pregnancy, is mainly due to poor posture.

• Hormonal changes during pregnancy soften ligaments and connective tissue. This can affect the stability and support of the spine and torso.

• The abdominal muscles are stressed by the weight of the enlarging uterus. Keeping the pelvis in proper position protects these muscles from undue stretching and possible separation.

• Proper posture and alignment will assist with better lung function, which can become limited by the enlarging uterus.

THINGS TO LOOK FOR IN AN EXERCISE PROGRAM

• A warm-up period that slowly stretches muscles to the limit of range of motion is achieved, and blood circulation to muscles and heart rate are gradually increased.

• Twenty to thirty minutes is considered a minimum time for the exercises to be effective.

• After exercising, there should be a cool-down period for muscles and heart rate to return to their pre-exercise state.

• Exercises should focus on control, rhythm, stabilization of the pelvis, and proper alignment of the pelvis.

• Swimming provides rhythm, controlled breathing, and water buoyancy. In the late second trimester and in the third trimester, pool exercise is well tolerated. Wear a good supportive bathing suit.

• Drink plenty of fluids before and after you exercise.

CAUTIONS

• Do not take part in a strenuous exercise program (such as a marathon) when pregnant, if you were not doing it regularly before pregnancy.

• Avoid sudden or forceful movements that will severely stress ligaments and joints that are already relaxed under hormonal influence.

• Contact sports or extreme sports should be avoided.

• Do not perform any exercises that put pressure on the lower back, curve of the spine, or cause excess compression of the uterus.

• Don't exercise outdoors in hot, humid weather.

• Don't bend too deeply or stand up abruptly.

• Stop any exercise right away if you develop signs of dizziness, bleeding, faintness, abdominal or back pain, overly rapid heart rate, or shortness of breath. If symptoms continue, call our office.

• Discuss your exercise program with your obstetric care provider to be sure that there are no factors that may cause problems. This is very important if you have any chronic medical disorder, or if the pregnancy is considered high-risk.

 NOTIFY OUR OFFICE IF

• You or a family member is pregnant and has questions or concerns about exercising.

• During pregnancy, you want to start a new exercise program or change an existing routine.

• You experience vaginal bleeding or spotting, abdominal cramping, absence of fetal movement or prolonged contractions, light-headedness or dizziness, serious headache, shortness of breath, heart palpitations, fast resting heart rate, or chest pain.

Special notes:

_____

_____

_____

More notes on the back of this page ☐

R.I.C.E. THERAPY

(Rest, Ice, Compression, Elevation)

 BASIC INFORMATION

R.I.C.E. is an acronym (a word coined from first letters) for the most important elements—rest, ice, compression and elevation—in first aid for many injuries. This acronym appears in medical information in reference to athletic injuries. Use the word R.I.C.E. to jog your memory if you have injuries, such as contusions, sprains, strains, dislocations, or uncomplicated fractures.

REST

Stop using the injured part, and rest it (for about 48 hours) as soon as you realize an injury has taken place. Continued exercise or other activity could cause further injury, delay healing, increase pain, and risk bleeding. Use crutches to avoid bearing weight on injuries of the foot, ankle, knee, or leg. Use splints for injuries of the hand, wrist, elbow or arm. After medical care, the injured part may require immobilization with splints or a cast to keep the area at rest until it heals.

ICE

Ice helps stop internal bleeding from injured blood vessels. Sudden cold causes small blood vessels to contract. This contraction of blood vessels decreases the amount of blood that can collect around the wound. The more blood that collects, the longer the healing time. Ice can be safely applied in several ways using the following instructions:

• For injury to a small area, such as a finger, toe, foot, or wrist, immerse the injured area in a bucket of ice water. Use ice cubes to keep the water cold, as ice dissolves.

• For injury to a larger area, use ice packs. Avoid placing ice directly on the skin. Before applying the ice, place a towel, cloth, or one or two layers of an elasticized compression bandage (Ace bandage) on the skin to be iced. To make the ice pack, put ice chips or ice cubes in a plastic bag, or wrap them in a thin towel. Place the ice pack over the cloth. The pack may sit directly on the injured part, or it may be wrapped in place.

• Ice the injured area for about 20 minutes at a time.

• Repeat the icing four to eight times a day, while following the instructions below for compression and elevation. After 48 to 72 hours, you may add heat as a treatment. Or you might try both. Alternate five minutes of hot water with five minutes of ice water. Continue to ice the injured area until it is healed.

COMPRESSION

Compression decreases swelling by slowing the bleeding and limiting the accumulation of blood near the injured site. Without compression, fluid from adjacent normal tissues seeps into the injury area. The more blood and fluid that accumulate around an injury, the slower the healing. The following are instructions for safely applying compression to an injury:

• Use an elasticized bandage (Ace bandage) for compression, if possible. If you do not have one available, any kind of cloth will suffice for a short time. Wrap the injured part firmly, wrapping over the ice also. Begin wrapping below the injury site, and extend above the injury site.

• Be careful not to compress the area so tightly that the blood supply is impaired. Signs of deprived blood supply include pain, numbness, cramping, and blue or dusky-colored nails. Remove the compression bandage immediately if any of these symptoms appear. Leave the bandage off until all signs of impaired circulation disappear. Then rewrap the area—less tightly this time.

ELEVATION

Elevating the injured part to, or above, the level of the heart is another way to decrease swelling and pain at the injury site. Elevate the iced, compressed area in whatever way is most convenient. Prop an injured leg on solid objects or pillows. Elevate an injured arm by lying down and placing pillows under the arm or placing them on the chest with the arm folded across. The whole upper part of the body may be elevated gently with pillows or a reclining chair or by raising the head of the bed on blocks.

 NOTIFY OUR OFFICE IF

• You have questions about R.I.C.E. therapy.

• After 24 hours of R.I.C.E., the symptoms don't improve or they become worse.

• Anytime severe pain occurs.

• There is a visible deformity of the injured area.

Special notes:

_____

_____

_____

More notes on the back of this page ☐

SCREENING TESTS & IMMUNIZATIONS, ADULT

 BASIC INFORMATION

DESCRIPTION
Certain routine screening tests are sometimes recommended for healthy persons. Those listed here are very general guidelines for healthy adults who have no symptoms of disease. They are not standards to be used in every patient. Your own screening exams may differ.

SCREENING RECOMMENDATIONS
Age 18 to 39:
- Blood pressure (every 2 years).
- Cholesterol and triglycerides (every 5 years).
- Female: clinical breast exam (every 1 to 3 years).
- Female: pelvic exam and Pap smear (every 1 to 3 years).
- Female: Chlamydia test for sexually active under 25.
- Dental exam (every 6 to 12 months).
- Eye exam (every 3 to 5 years).

Age 40 to 64 (middle years):
- Blood pressure (every 2 years).
- Cholesterol levels (every 5 years).
- Digital rectal exam (yearly, or as advised).
- Fecal occult blood test or FOBT (yearly after age 50).
- Sigmoidoscopy, colonoscopy, or barium enema (every 3 to 5 years after age 50).
- Female: clinical breast exam (yearly).
- Female: mammogram (every 1 to 2 years beginning at age 40).
- Female: pelvic exam and Pap smear (yearly).
- Female: Bone density (age 60 if weigh 154 lbs. or less).
- Male: prostate specific antigen (yearly if risk factors).
- Dental exam (every 6 to 12 months).
- Eye exam (every 2 to 4 years).

Age 65 and over (senior years):
- Blood pressure (every 2 years, or yearly if have hypertension, or have risk factors).
- Hearing exam (yearly).
- Fecal blood occult test (FOBT) (yearly).
- Sigmoidoscopy, colonoscopy, or barium enema (every 3 to 5 years).
- Cholesterol levels (every 5 years).
- Digital rectal exam (yearly).
- Female: mammogram (every 1 to 2 years until age 75, unless an abnormality detected).
- Female: clinical breast exam (yearly until age 75, unless an abnormality is detected).
- Female: Bone density test (once, and then as recommended).
- Male: prostate specific antigen (yearly if risk factors, or if advised; up to age 75).
- Dental exam (every 6 to 12 months).
- Eye exam (every 1 to 2 years).

RECOMMENDED IMMUNIZATIONS
- Tetanus-diphtheria booster—once, between ages 14 to 16, then a booster every 10 years.
- Influenza vaccine—yearly.
- Pneumococcal vaccine—once, everyone over 65; and for below age 65 for medical or other indications.
- Measles, mumps, rubella (MMR) or varicella (chickenpox)—1 to 2 doses, for persons without proof of immunity with occupational or other indications. Once, for women of childbearing age without proof of rubella immunity.
- Hepatitis A and hepatitis B vaccine—once, for persons in health care occupations or working with blood, intravenous drug users, those having multiple sexual partners or having sex with a hepatitis-infected person.
- Meningococcal (polysaccharide)—once, for persons with medical indications or other specific indications.

 NOTIFY OUR OFFICE IF

You have questions about screening tests, the results of screening tests, or immunizations.

Special notes:

_____

_____

_____

More notes on the back of this page ☐

SKIN SELF-EXAMINATION

 BASIC INFORMATION

Skin self-exam means checking your own skin regularly for any abnormal growths or unusual changes. This helps you detect and treat skin cancer (or other skin abnormalities) as early as possible. Two types of skin cancer (basal cell carcinoma and squamous cell carcinoma) are almost always cured once correctly diagnosed. With melanoma (the most serious type of skin cancer), early diagnosis is essential to start treatment before it spreads.

The National Cancer Institute (NCI) and the American Academy of Dermatology (AAD) recommend that people should perform a skin self-exam once a month. It may take about 10 to 15 minutes. Along with your self-exam, always practice sun-protection care by using a sunscreen (SPF of 15 or higher) with both UVA and UVB protection. Wear protective clothing, and limit exposure time to the sun.

Get to know your skin, so you know what is normal for you. The first time you do the self-examination, locate all moles, warts, birthmarks, scars, spots, bumps, lumps, or other skin markings. It may be difficult to remember the color, shape, and size of each, so you may want to write down the information or draw a sketch of each area and abnormality.

HOW THE TEST IS PERFORMED
• The easiest time to do the exam may be after you take a bath or shower. Women may wish to perform their skin self-exam at the same time that they perform their monthly breast self-exam.
• Ideally, the room should have a full-length mirror and bright lights so that you can see your entire body well. Use a hand-held mirror also. It is very important to be able to examine all areas of your skin, including hard-to-see areas, such as the genitals, buttocks, scalp, and back.

WHEN YOU ARE PERFORMING THE TEST, LOOK FOR:
• New skin markings (e.g., moles, blemishes, colorations, bumps).
• Moles that have changed their size, texture, color, or shape.
• Moles or lesions that won't heal or that continue to bleed.
• Moles with ragged edges, differences in colors, or lack of symmetry.
• Observe and examine your entire body, both front and back, in the mirror.
• Check under your arms and both sides of each arm.
• Examine your forearms after bending your arms at the elbows, and then look at the palms of your hands and underneath your upper arms.
• Look at the front and back of both legs.
• Look at your buttocks and between your buttocks.
• Examine your genital area.
• Observe your face, neck, back of neck, and scalp. It is best to use both a hand mirror and full-length mirror, along with a comb, to see areas of your scalp.
• Look at your feet, including the soles and the space between your toes.
• Have a partner, friend, or relative help by examining hard-to-see areas. You may want to them to take photographs of your body (or certain moles) every six months to one year. Sometimes it is difficult to tell if a mole has grown or changed, or a new one has developed, and a photo may help.

 NOTIFY OUR OFFICE IF

You find any new abnormalities on your skin, or if you see changes in size, color, or texture of old moles or skin lesions. You should also call if you have a skin lesion (sores) that won't heal.

Special notes:

_____

_____

_____

More notes on the back of this page ☐

STRESS, HOW TO COPE

 BASIC INFORMATION

CAUSES OF STRESS

• There are numerous ways to reduce stress in your life; the correct answer is finding what works for you. A certain amount of stress is not always bad. It varies from person to person how much stress one can handle easily. Sometimes, stress can push us on to greater achievement. But excessive stress or chronic stress can be self-defeating. Many health professionals believe that stress has a role in almost any disorder. Stress can complicate an illness by preventing normal recovery, prolonging pain, and adding to disability.

• Reducing stress could be as simple has adding exercise to your daily routine or making new friends. To make the most of your life, limit your stress, and for that stress that you cannot avoid, learn to manage it.

TIPS FOR COPING

Here are some tips that may help you reduce stress:

• Learn a meditation technique and practice it regularly—daily if possible. There are many methods available. Most of them include "tuning in to" and giving complete attention to a word, sound, sentence, or concept that you silently repeat to yourself. Don't try to banish other thoughts that enter your mind during your period of concentration, but don't focus on them enough to stop you from meditating. The purpose of meditation is to empty your mind of all disturbing thoughts for a given period of time to aid in mental relaxation. Mental relaxation, in turn, will help reduce stress.

• Take a short period of time away from any stressful situation you meet up with during a day. Practice a muscle-tensing and muscle-relaxing technique. Close your eyes. Take a series of deep breaths. Then start with the muscle groups in your face. Consciously tense them and hold the tension for a few seconds. Then consciously relax them. Continue through all major muscle groups in the body: neck, shoulders, hands, abdomen, back, and legs. You can use this technique to help you relax quickly any time you need to.

• Begin an exercise program. People who are physically fit are less likely to suffer the negative effects of stress, anxiety, or depression. One form of exercise is yoga. Yoga involves both stretching exercises and deep breathing techniques. However, any form of exercise is helpful in reducing the affects of stress on the body.

• Humor is another way of dealing with stress. Having the ability to find humor in a stressful situation and being able to laugh about it releases all the tension that is building inside. Even if the situation cannot be made light of, think of something else that will make you laugh.

• Healthy lifestyle changes can reduce the level of stress. A few suggestions include reducing caffeine intake, making new friends, eating healthy, and avoiding alcohol. Healthy lifestyle changes can help manage the stress as well as improve your overall well being.

• Get enough sleep. Avoid taking your problems to bed with you. At the end of the day, spend a few minutes going back over your entire day's experiences, event by event, as if you're replaying a tape. Release all negative emotions you have built up (anger, feelings of insecurity or anxiety). Relish all good energy or emotion (loving thoughts, praise, feeling good about your work or yourself). Reach a decision about undone events, and release mental or muscular tension. Now you're ready for a relaxing and emotionally healing sleep.

• Avoid self-medication or escape. Alcohol or other drugs of abuse can mask stress. They don't help deal with the problem.

• Set realistic goals for yourself. Reduce the number of events going on in your life and you may reduce the feeling of being overloaded.

• Don't overwhelm yourself by fretting about your entire workload. Handle each task as it comes, or selectively deal with matters in some priority.

• Do something for others to help get your mind off yourself.

• Avoid extreme reactions. Think about disliking something rather than hating it. Be a little nervous, not anxious. Don't be full of rage when anger will do the job. Don't be depressed when you can just be sad.

• Try to be positive. Give yourself messages as to how well you can cope rather than how horrible everything is going to be.

• Keep a stress diary. Write down stressful events, how they made you feel, what caused the event, and how you coped. On a scale of 0 (very relaxed) to 10 (extremely stressed), put down a number for your stress level.

• Research has shown that cognitive-behavioral therapy can be effective in reducing stress. Ask your health care provider about this option.

 NOTIFY OUR OFFICE IF

You or a family member wants help to cope with stress.

Special notes:

_____

_____

_____

More notes on the back of this page ☐

TESTICULAR SELF-EXAMINATION

BASIC INFORMATION

This is an exam of the testicles to look for lumps that may be testicular cancer. The testicles are the male reproductive organs, and produce sperm and the hormone testosterone. They are located in the scrotum under the penis.

The exam should be performed on a monthly basis, especially if you have a family history of this cancer, have had a previous testicular tumor, or have an undescended testicle.

NORMAL TESTICLES

Each testicle should feel firm but not rock hard. One testicle may or may not be lower or slightly larger than the other. Normal testicles contain blood vessels and other structures that can make the exam confusing. Performing the self-exam monthly allows you to become familiar with your normal anatomy. Then, if you notice any changes from the previous exam, this will alert you to contact your health care provider. Always ask you health care provider if you have any doubts or questions.

HOW THE TEST IS PERFORMED

• Perform this test during or after a shower. This way, the scrotal skin is warm and relaxed. The test is best done while standing.

   1. Gently feel your scrotal sac to locate a testicle.

   2. Firmly, but gently roll the testicle between the thumb and fingers of both hands to examine the entire surface. Feel the testicle for lumps, swellings, or other changes in consistency.

   3. Repeat the procedure with the other testicle.

• Examine the epididymis for lumps. This is a rope-like cord that is located behind each testicle. This area is fairly tender, so be cautious with your touch.

• Examine the spermatic cord for lumps. This is the sperm-carrying tube that extends from the epididymis of each testicle.

ABNORMAL FINDINGS

A lump, swelling, or other change on the testicle, epididymis, or spermatic cord may be the first sign of testicular cancer. Therefore, if you find a lump, see a health care provider right away. Keep in mind that some cases of testicular cancer do not show symptoms until they reach an advanced stage.

NOTIFY OUR OFFICE IF

• You find a small hard lump (like a pea), have an enlarged testicle, or notice any other differences from your last self-exam.

• You can't find one or both testicles. The testicles may not have descended properly in the scrotum.

• There is a soft collection of thin tubes above the testicle. It may be a collection of dilated veins (varicocele).

• There is pain or swelling in the scrotum. It may be an infection or a fluid-filled sac (hydrocele) causing blockage of blood flow to the area.

• Acute pain in the scrotum or testicle is a surgical emergency. If you experience acute pain in the scrotum or testicle, seek immediate medical help.

Special notes:

_____

_____

_____

More notes on the back of this page ☐

BASIC INFORMATION

Travel may consist of a short weekend trip or a journey of several months to foreign countries. It can bring great joy for many people, but can quickly turn into a nightmare if an unexpected illness or other health problem happens to you or a traveling companion. Chronic health problems, disabilities, or aging should not deter you from enjoying the benefits of travel. Preparation and prevention can help prevent some health problems and lessen the impact of others.

TIPS FOR PLANNING AHEAD FOR A HEALTHY TRIP

• Know the physical demands involved in making the trip. Prepare yourself as much as possible before you leave on the trip.

• Have a medical and dental check before you embark on a lengthy trip within the United States and before any foreign travel. Discuss the trip with your health care provider. Ask about possible changes in how or when you take any prescribed drugs. Have your health care provider write a letter stating why you are traveling with certain drugs or medical equipment (such as insulin and syringes). Get information about recommended and required immunizations for your destination.

• Carry a supply of your prescription drugs to last the entire trip. Don't pack the whole supply. Keep some on your person or carry them in a purse, camera bag, or briefcase. Always keep drugs in an original prescription container. This is particularly important in foreign travel. Carry a copy of the written prescription. This will help in buying drugs if needed, and sometimes, getting drug containers through customs in some countries.

• Take copies of specific medical records with you in case you need medical help. Ask your health care provider which ones would be appropriate.

• Check your medical insurance to see if it covers care outside the United States. If not, consider buying special travel insurance. Medicare will not cover medical expenses outside the United States.

• If traveling to a non-English speaking country, get the names of doctors available there who do speak English.

• Plan your schedule so that you will have time to recover from jet lag symptoms.

• Notify the airline about any special dietary needs you have.

• Follow all food and water safety guidelines for the areas you visit.

• Have a personal medical kit with you. Consider including aspirin and/or acetaminophen, antacid, antibiotic, antihistamine, decongestant, diarrhea medicine, mild laxative, motion sickness drug, antifungal and antibacterial ointments, 1% cortisone cream, sunscreen, insect repellent, antiseptic sprays or ointments, cotton balls, tweezers, bandages, elastic bandage, alcohol-based hand wipes (or waterless gels or sprays), oral rehydration solution packets, safety pins, corn plasters, sanitary pads/tampons, and an extra pair of prescription eyeglasses (plus a written copy of the prescription). Consider things such as mild sedatives, antianxiety drugs, high-altitude preventive drugs, and water purification tablets.

• If you have a special health problem or allergy, wear or carry a medical-alert type information pendant or tag.

RESOURCES FOR ADDITIONAL INFORMATION

• The federal government has a variety of publications available about travel. Contact the Federal Citizen Information Center, P.O. Box 100, Pueblo, CO 81002; (888) 878-3256; website: www.pueblo.gsa.gov.

• Your local or state health department is a good source of information. If traveling within the United States, consider contacting the health department at your destination for specific information about that location.

• For a directory of English-speaking doctors in foreign countries, contact The International Association for Medical Assistance to Travelers (IAMAT), 417 Center St., Lewiston, NY, 14092; (716) 754-4883 (not toll-free); website: www.iamat.org.

• Contact the Centers for Disease Control (CDC) hotline (877) FYI-TRIP for recorded messages about travel. Visit the website: www.cdc.gov/travel for a variety of useful travel information. Get a copy of Health Information for International Travel. It is written for health care providers, but others may find it useful.

• International SOS Assistance provides international doctor referral and other services with varying fees. Eight Neshaminy Interplex, Suite 207, Trevose, PA 19053; (800) 523-8930; website: www.internationalsos.com.

• Special travel insurance companies provide insurance as well as other medical help. Ask your travel agent for information or do a web search.

• Your credit card company may offer medical assistance for travelers. Check with them before your trip.

 ## NOTIFY OUR OFFICE IF

You or a family member wants copies of prescriptions or medical records or needs a physical before traveling.

Special notes:

_____

_____

_____

More notes on the back of this page ☐

WALKING FOR EXERCISE & FITNESS

BASIC INFORMATION

ADVANTAGES OF WALKING

· Almost everyone can do it.

· You can do it almost anywhere.

· You can do it almost anytime.

· It doesn't cost anything.

· Walking is the most popular form of exercise. When done briskly on a regular schedule, it can improve the body's ability to consume oxygen during exertion, lower the resting heart rate, reduce blood pressure, and increase the efficiency of the heart and lungs. It also helps burn excess calories. Walking burns about the same amount of calories per mile as does running.

· Since obesity and high blood pressure are among the leading risk factors for heart attack and stroke, walking offers some protection against two of our major killers.

· Walkers feel better and sleep better, and their mental outlook improves.

· Walking can exert a favorable influence on personal habits. For example, smokers who begin walking often cut down or quit. There are two reasons for this. One, it is difficult to exercise vigorously if you smoke, and two, better physical condition encourages a desire to improve other aspects of one's life.

· What makes a walk a workout? It's largely a matter of pace and distance. When you're walking for exercise, you don't saunter, stroll, or shuffle. Instead, you move out at a steady clip that is brisk enough to make your heart beat faster and cause you to breathe more deeply.

WHAT SHOES TO WEAR

· A good pair of shoes is the only "special equipment" required by the walker. Any shoes that are comfortable, provide good support, and don't cause blisters or calluses will do. Here are some suggestions:

- Good running shoes (the training models with heavy soles) are good walking shoes, as are some of the lighter trail and hiking boots, and casual shoes with heavy rubber or crepe rubber soles.

- Whatever kind of shoe you select, it should have arch supports and should elevate the heel one-half to three-quarters of an inch above the sole of the foot.

- Choose a shoe with uppers made of materials that "breathe," such as leather or nylon mesh.

WALKING STYLE

· Hold the head erect and keep the back straight and the abdomen flat. Toes should point straight ahead and arms should swing loosely at sides.

· Land on the heel of the foot and roll forward to drive off the ball of the foot. Walking on the ball of the foot, or in a flat-footed style, may cause fatigue and soreness.

· Take long, easy strides, but don't strain for distance. When walking up or down hills, or at a very rapid pace,

lean forward slightly.

· Breathe deeply (with mouth open, if that is more comfortable).

STARTING YOUR WALKING PROGRAM

· No one can tell you exactly how far or how fast to walk at the start, but you can determine the proper pace and distance by experimenting. Begin by walking for 20 minutes at least four or five times a week at a pace that feels comfortable to you. If that proves to be too tiring, or too easy, reduce or lengthen your time.

· Some people begin by walking for one or two minutes, resting a minute, and repeating this cycle until they begin to be fatigued. Where you have to start isn't important; it's where you're going that counts.

· Gradually increase your time and pace. After you have been walking for 20 minutes several days a week for one month, start walking 30 minutes per outing. Eventually, your goal should be to get to the place where you can comfortably walk three miles in 45 minutes, but there is no hurry about getting there.

· The speed at which you walk is less important than the time you devote to it, but try to walk as briskly as your condition permits. It takes about 20 minutes for your body to begin realizing the "training effects" of sustained exercise.

· A "talk test" helps you find the right pace. You should be able to carry on a conversation while walking. If you're too breathless to talk, you're going too fast.

· The more often you walk, the faster you will improve. Three workouts a week are a "maintenance level" of exercise. More frequent workouts are required for swift improvement.

CAUTION

If you develop dizziness, pain, nausea, or other unusual symptoms, slow down or stop. If the problem persists, see your health care provider before walking again.

MAKING IT WORK FOR YOU

The most important thing is simply to set aside part of each day and walk. No matter what your age or condition, it can make you healthier and happier.

NOTIFY OUR OFFICE IF

You or a family member has questions about walking for exercise and fitness.

Special notes:

_____

_____

_____

More notes on the back of this page ☐

BRONCHIAL TREE & LUNGS

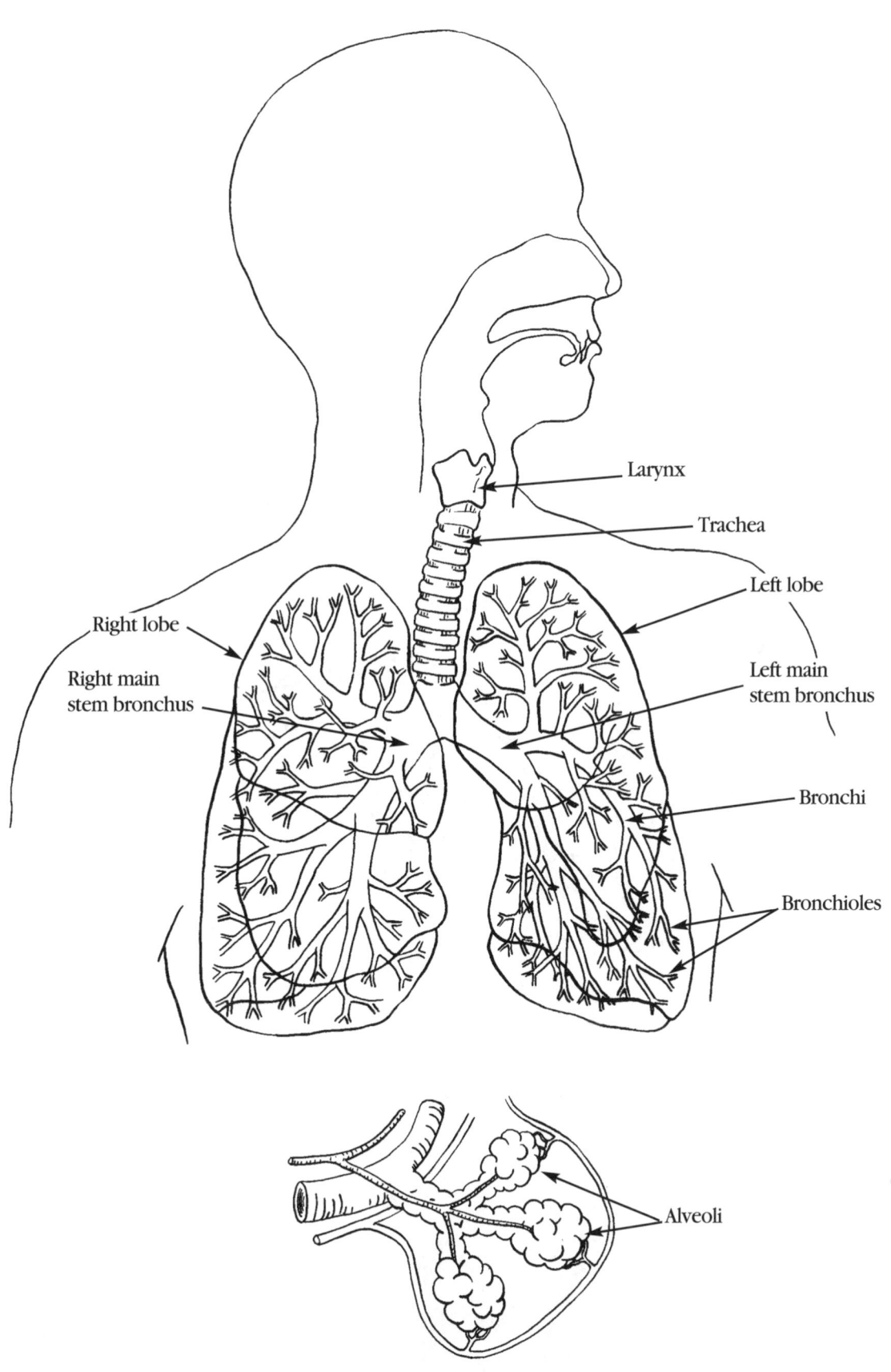

Larynx

Trachea

Right lobe

Left lobe

Right main
stem bronchus

Left main
stem bronchus

Bronchi

Bronchioles

Alveoli

613

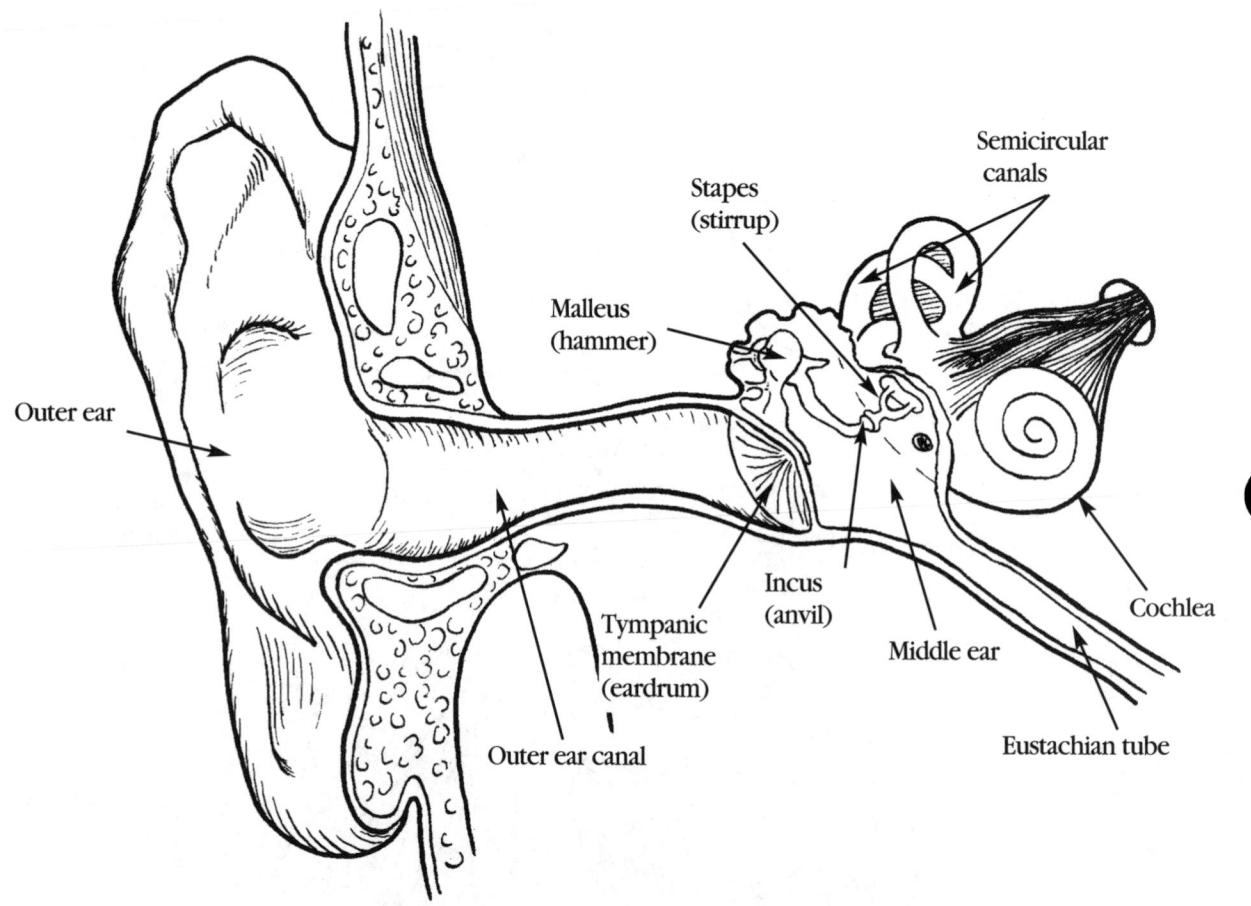

Outer ear

Stapes
(stirrup)

Semicircular
canals

Malleus
(hammer)

Tympanic
membrane
(eardrum)

Incus
(anvil)

Middle ear

Cochlea

Outer ear canal

Eustachian tube

ENDOCRINE SYSTEM, MALE & FEMALE

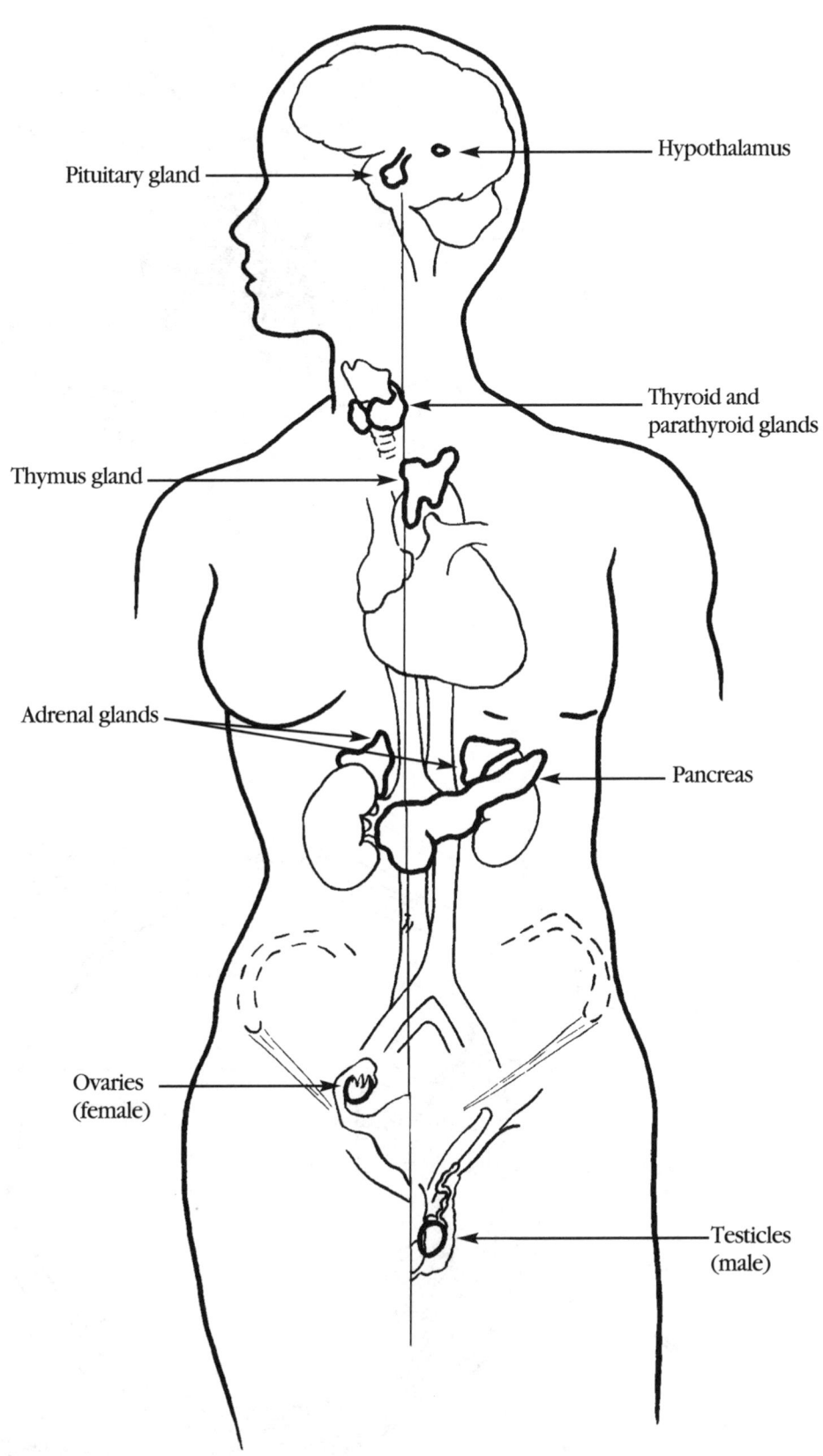

Hypothalamus

Pituitary gland

Thyroid and
parathyroid glands

Thymus gland

Adrenal glands

Pancreas

Ovaries
(female)

Testicles
(male)

615

Information From Your Health Care Provider

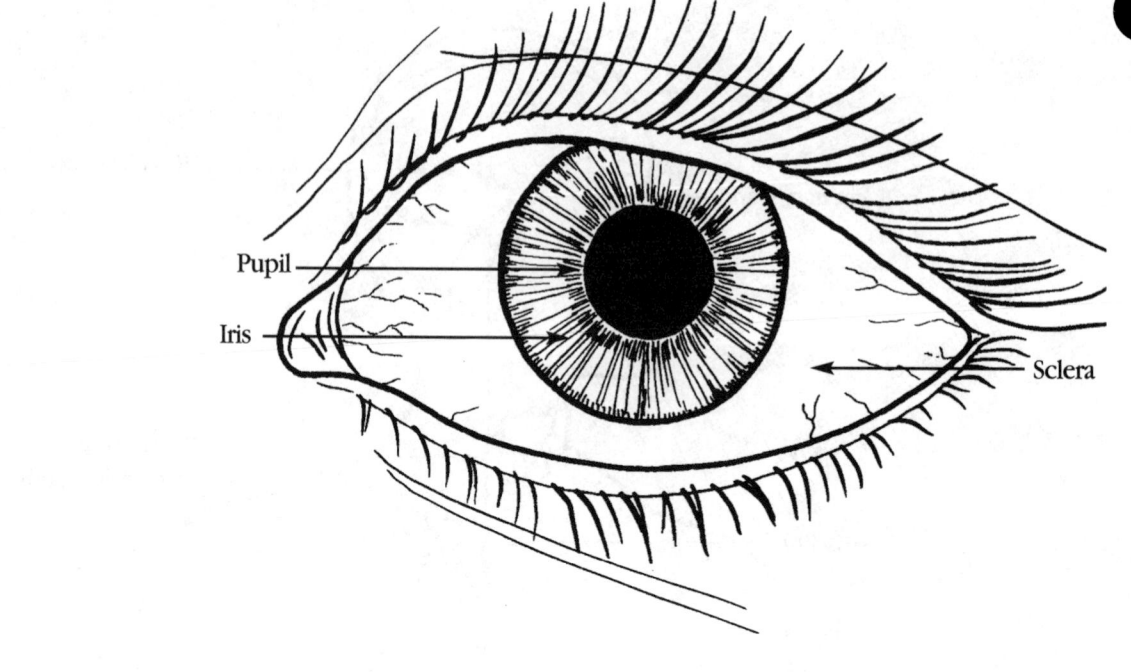

Pupil
Iris
Sclera

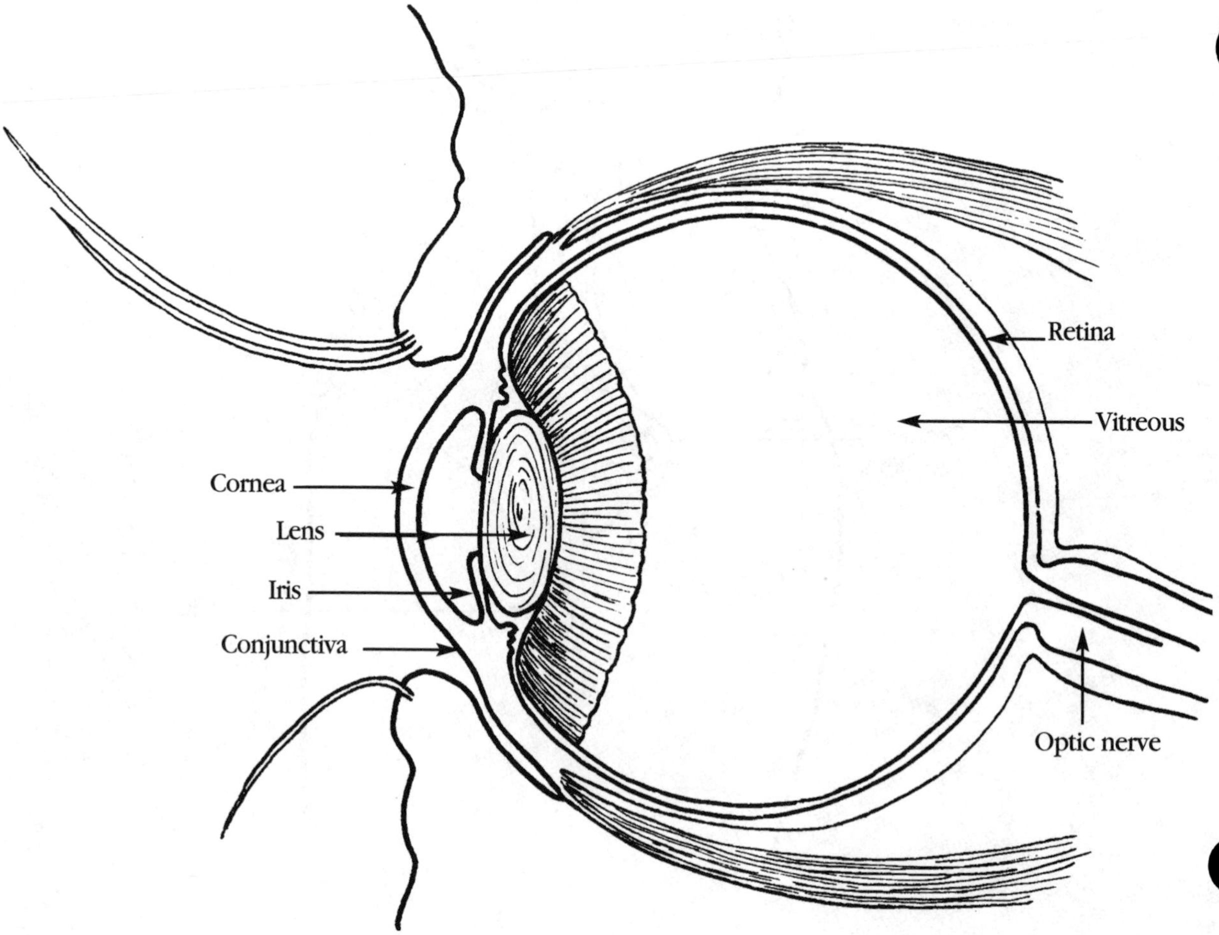

Retina
Vitreous
Cornea
Lens
Iris
Conjunctiva
Optic nerve

FEMALE GENITAL ORGANS

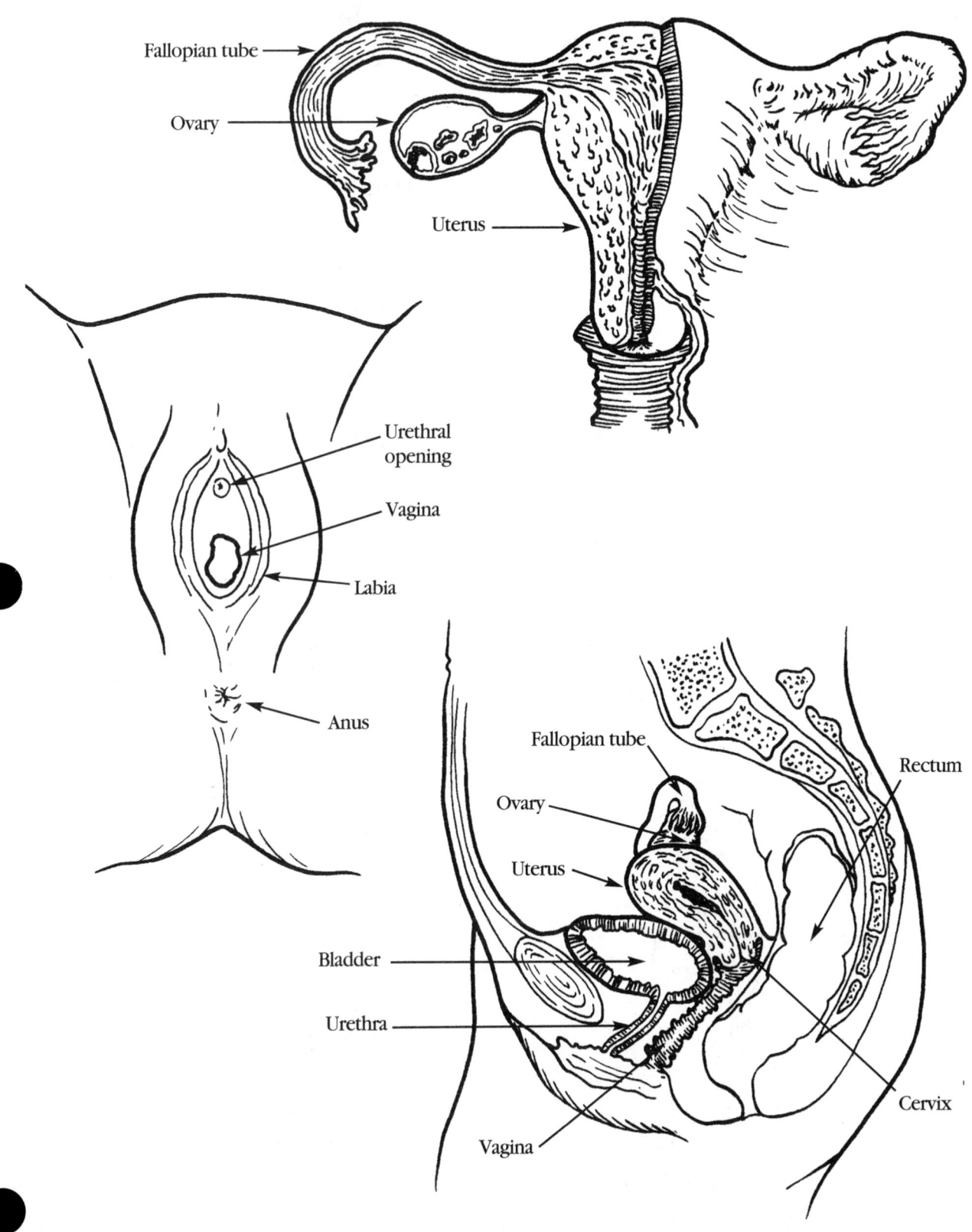

FRACTURES

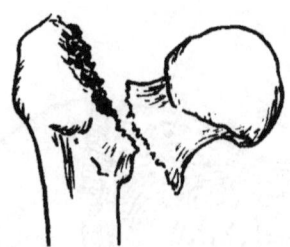

Hip Fracture Through
Trochanter of Femur

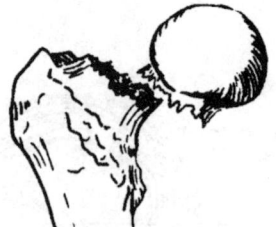

Hip Fracture Through
Neck of Femur

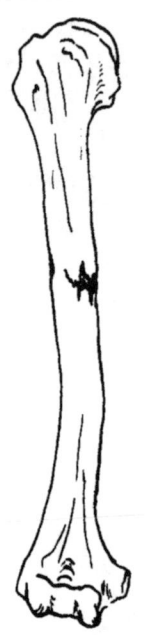

Greenstick

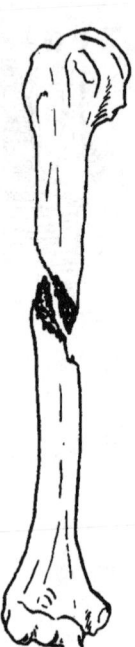

Spiral

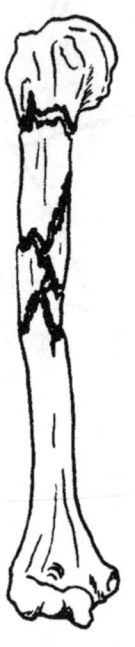

Comminuted

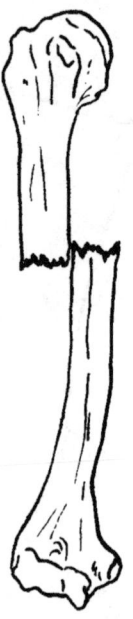

Transverse

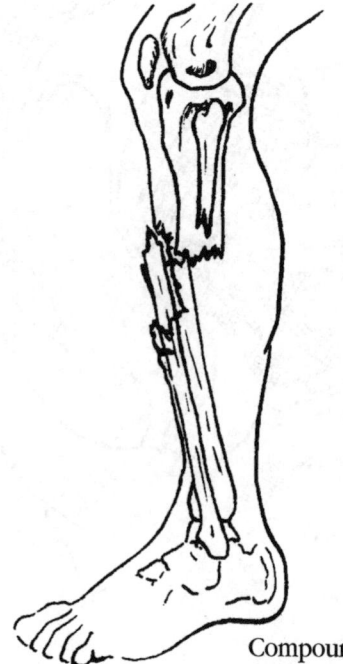

Compound

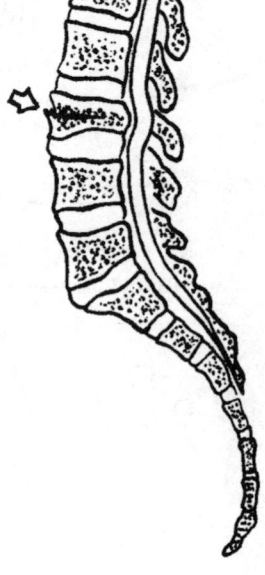

Compression

GASTROINTESTINAL TRACT

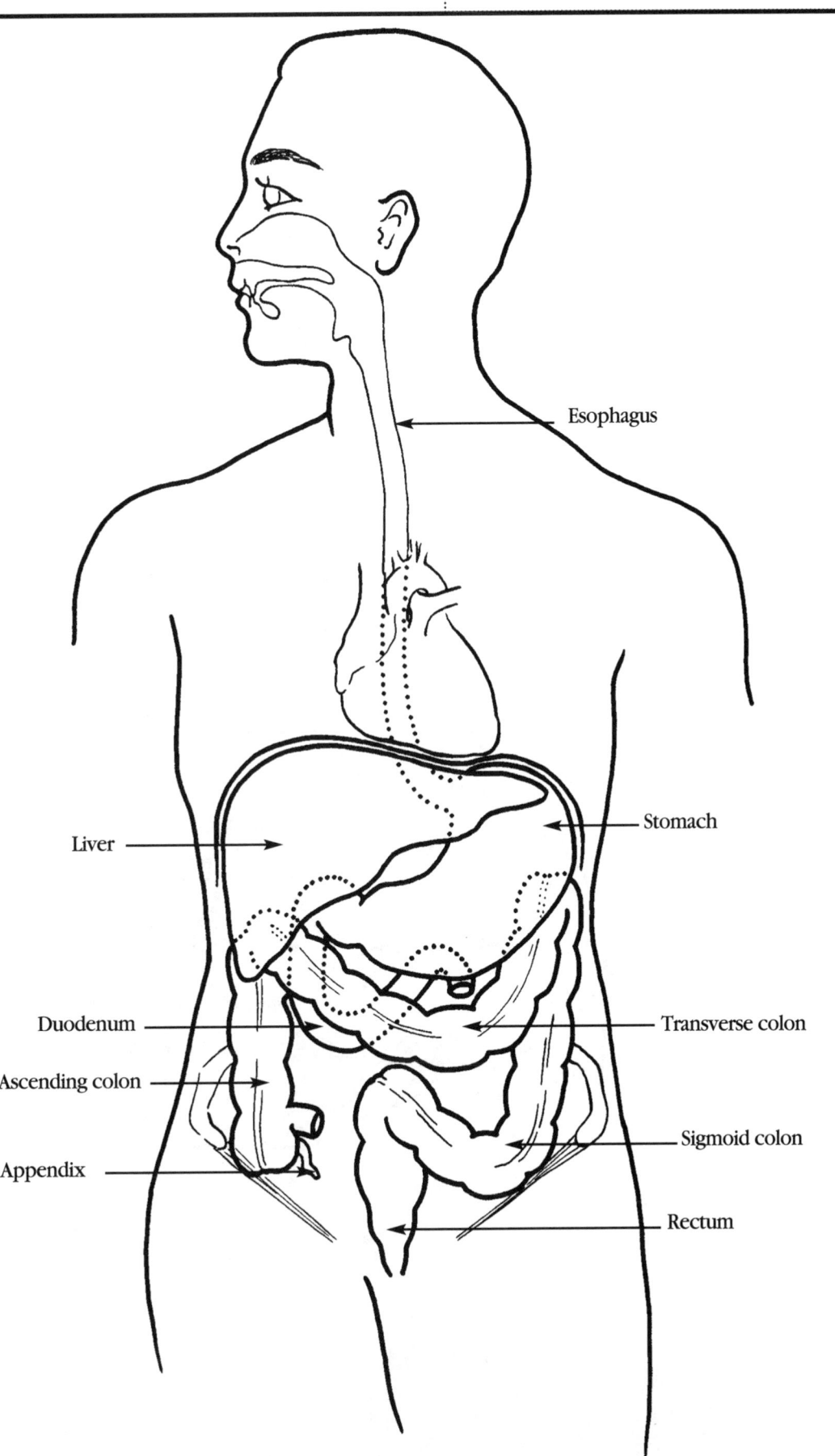

Esophagus

Liver

Stomach

Duodenum

Transverse colon

Ascending colon

Sigmoid colon

Appendix

Rectum

HEART SHOWING CORONARY ARTERIES

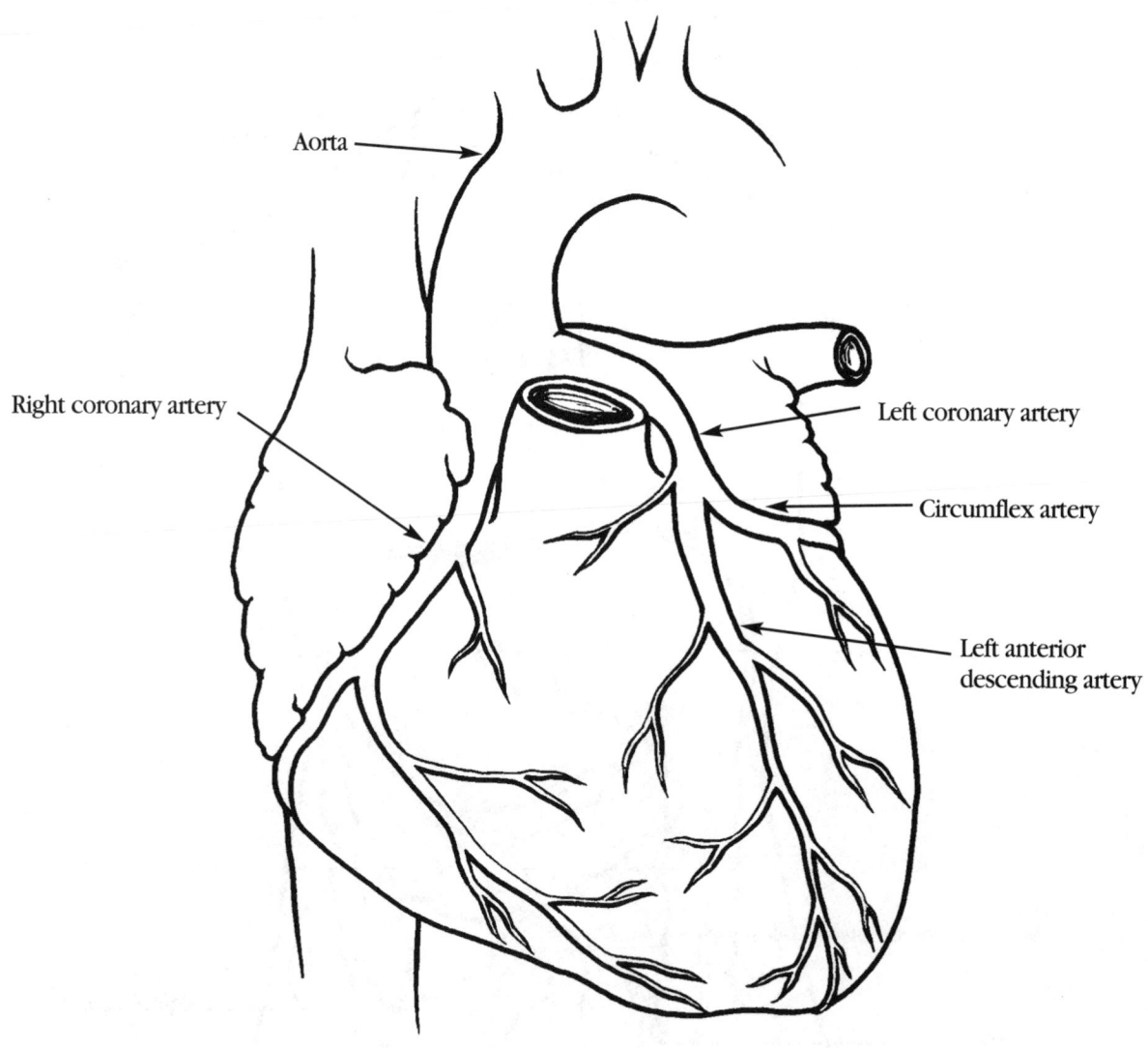

Aorta

Right coronary artery

Left coronary artery

Circumflex artery

Left anterior descending artery

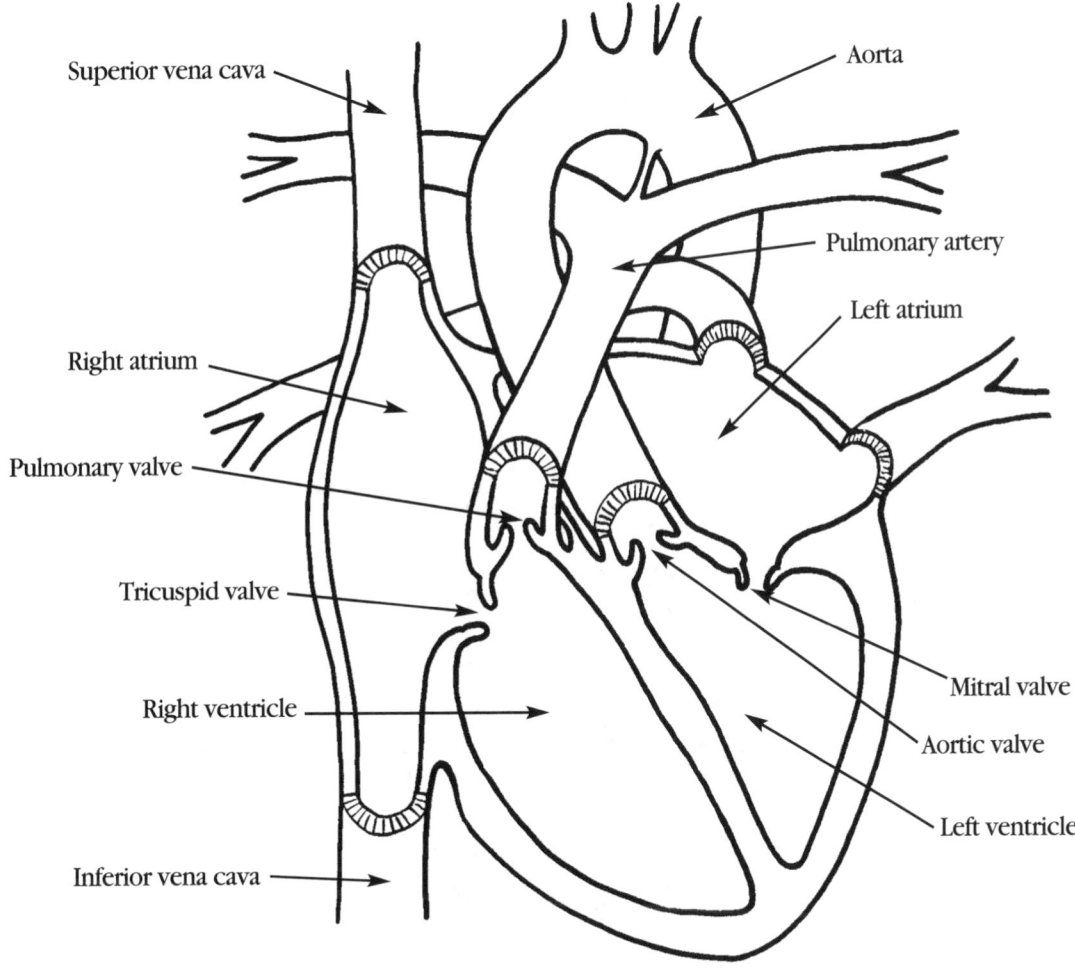

Superior vena cava

Aorta

Pulmonary artery

Left atrium

Right atrium

Pulmonary valve

Tricuspid valve

Mitral valve

Right ventricle

Aortic valve

Left ventricle

Inferior vena cava

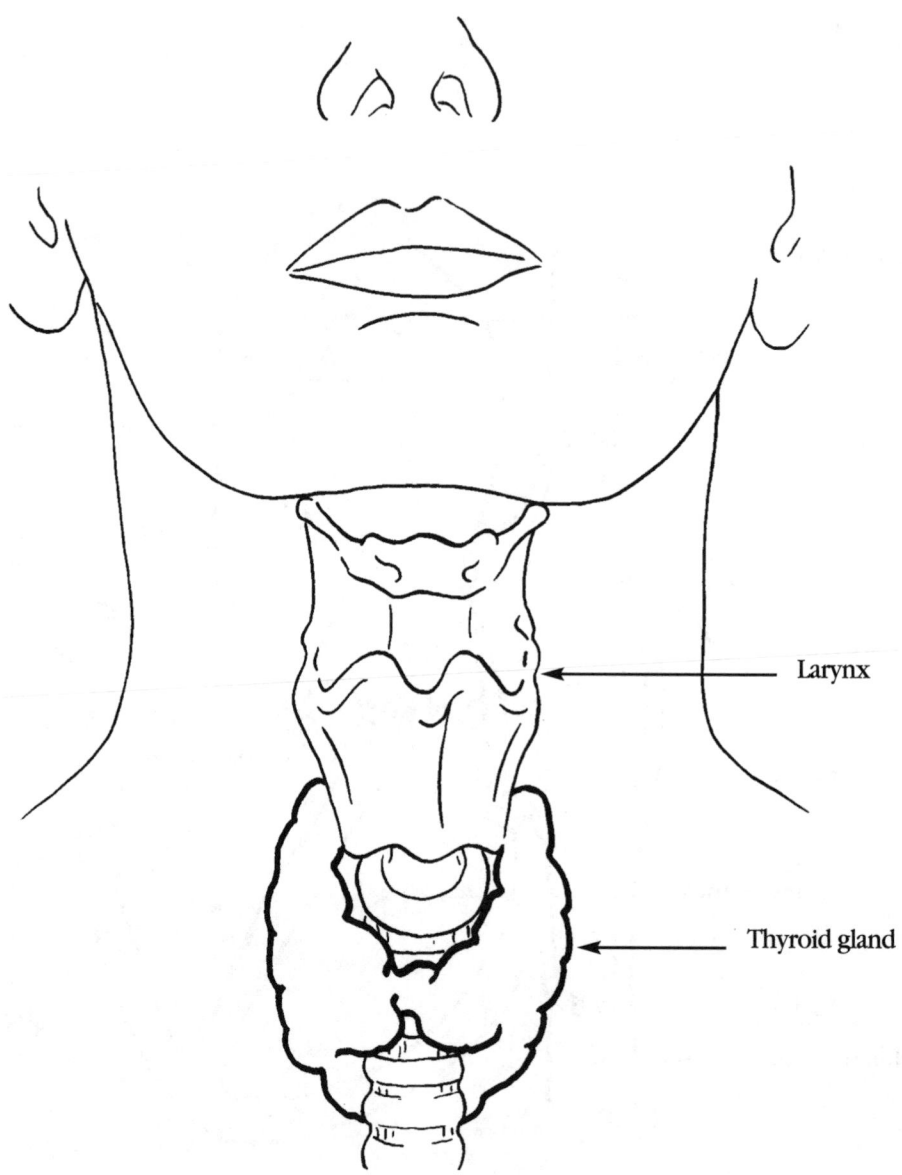

Larynx

Thyroid gland

MALE GENITAL ORGANS

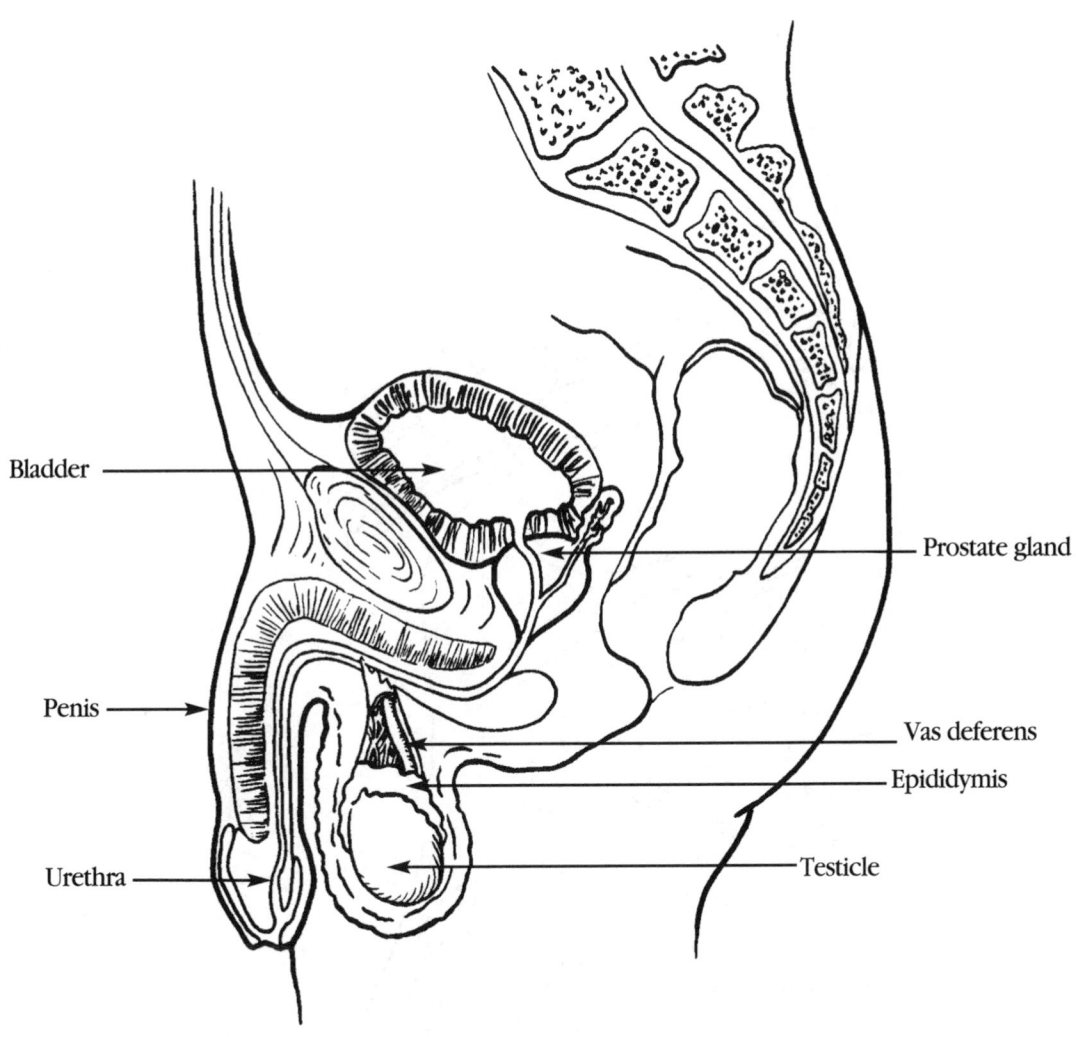

Bladder

Prostate gland

Penis

Vas deferens

Epididymis

Urethra

Testicle

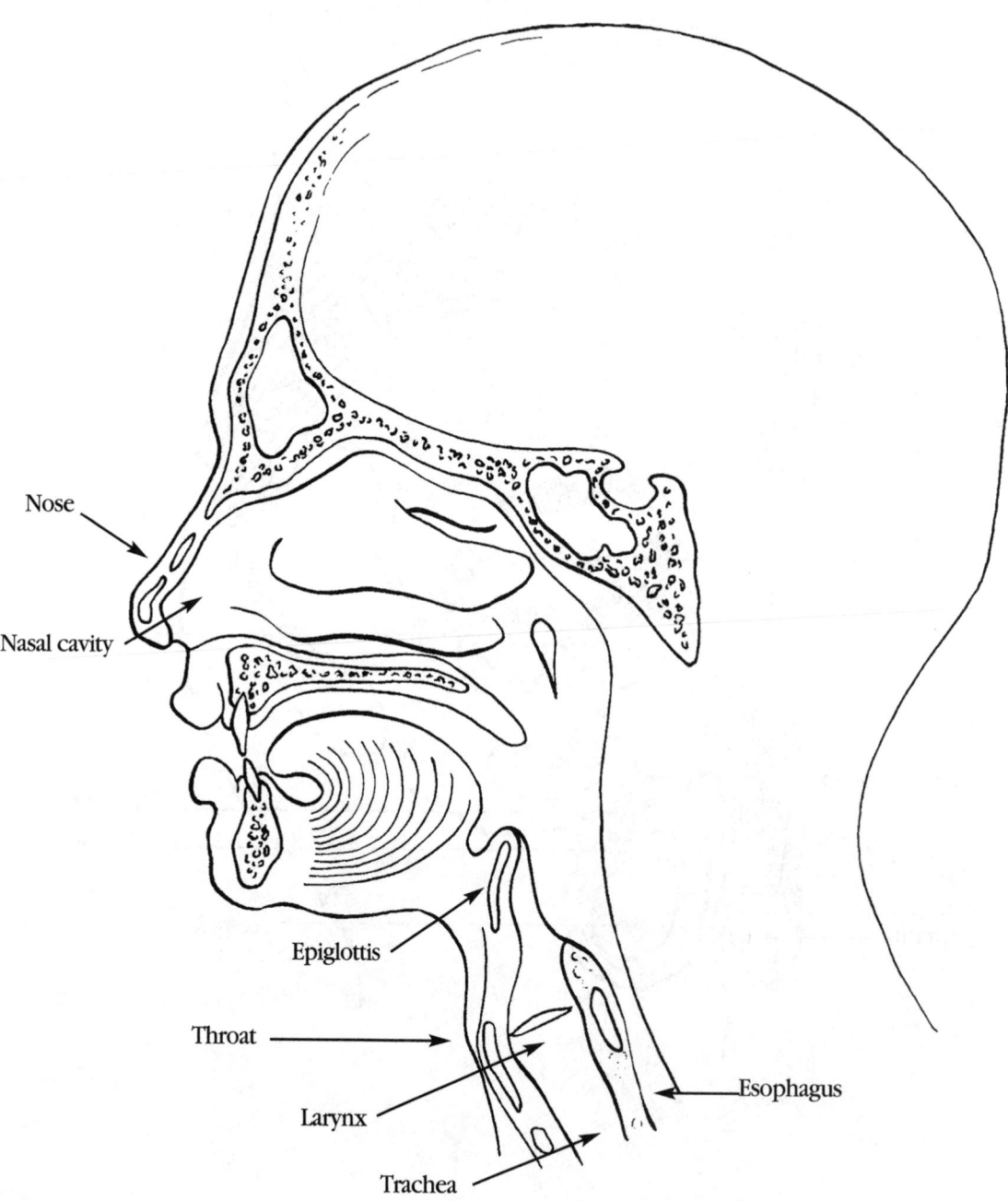

Nose

Nasal cavity

Epiglottis

Throat

Larynx

Trachea

Esophagus

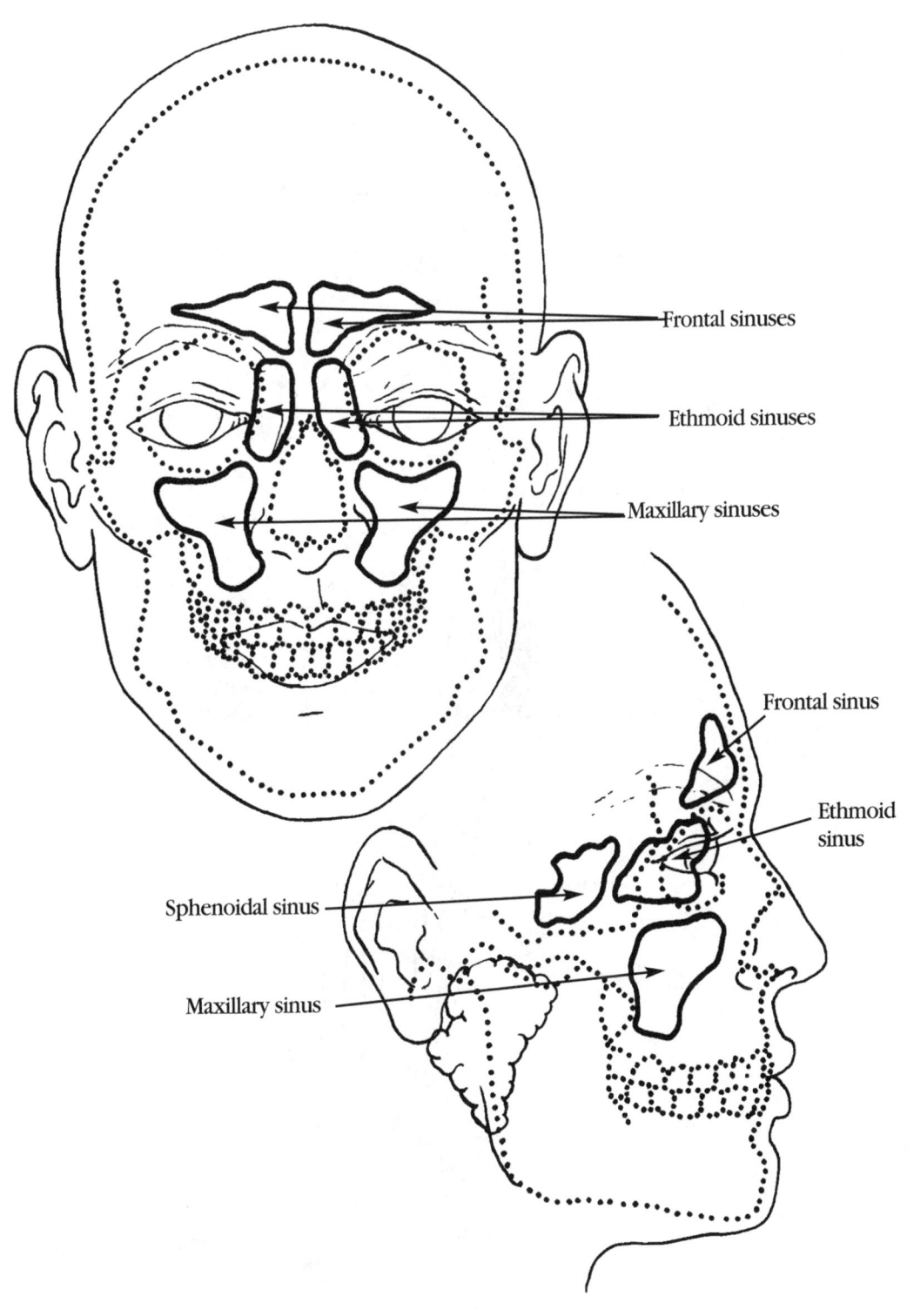

Frontal sinuses

Ethmoid sinuses

Maxillary sinuses

Frontal sinus

Ethmoid sinus

Sphenoidal sinus

Maxillary sinus

SKELETAL SYSTEM
Showing major Bones & Joints

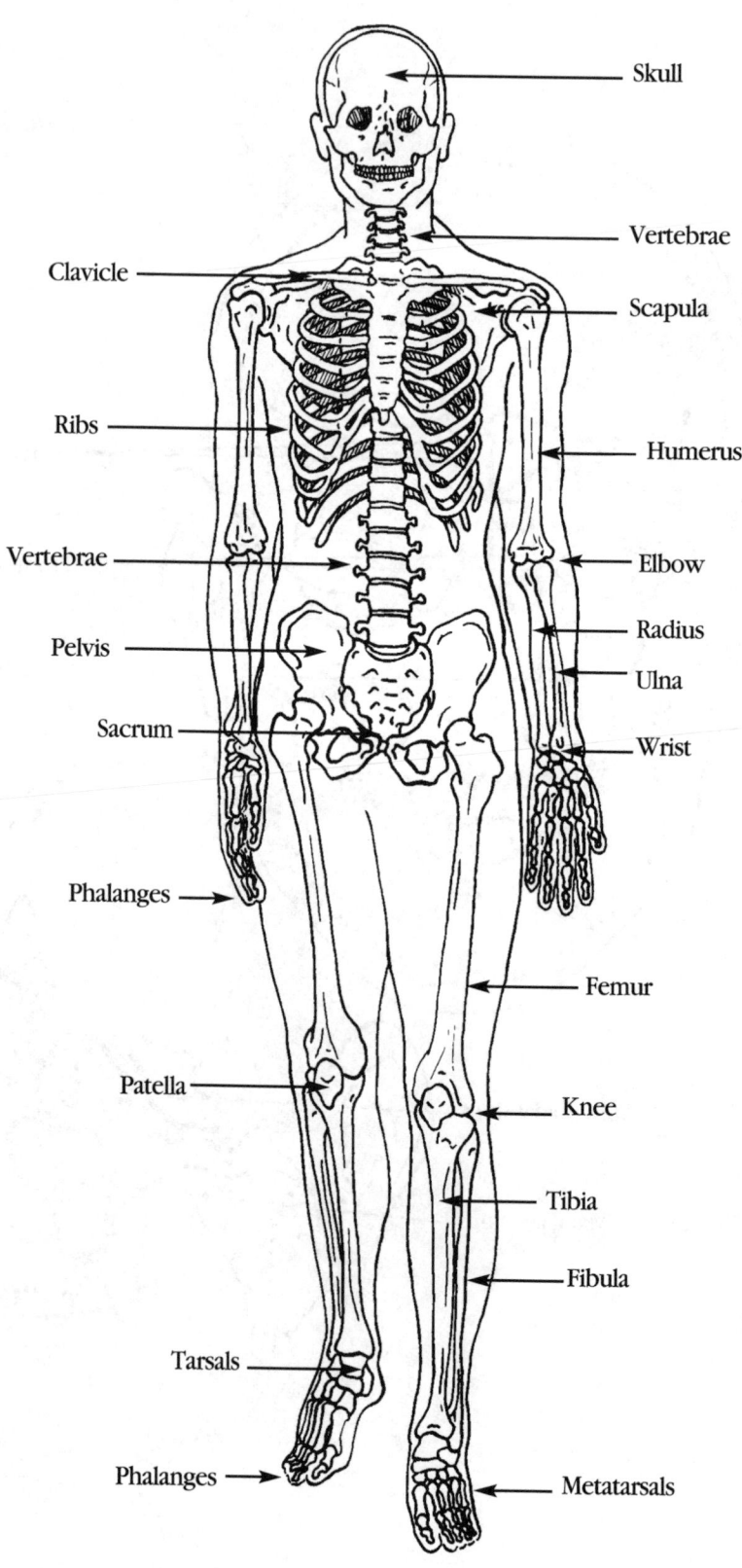

Skull

Vertebrae

Clavicle

Scapula

Ribs

Humerus

Vertebrae

Elbow

Radius

Pelvis

Ulna

Sacrum

Wrist

Phalanges

Femur

Patella

Knee

Tibia

Fibula

Tarsals

Phalanges

Metatarsals

STOMACH, LIVER, GALLBLADDER & DUODENUM

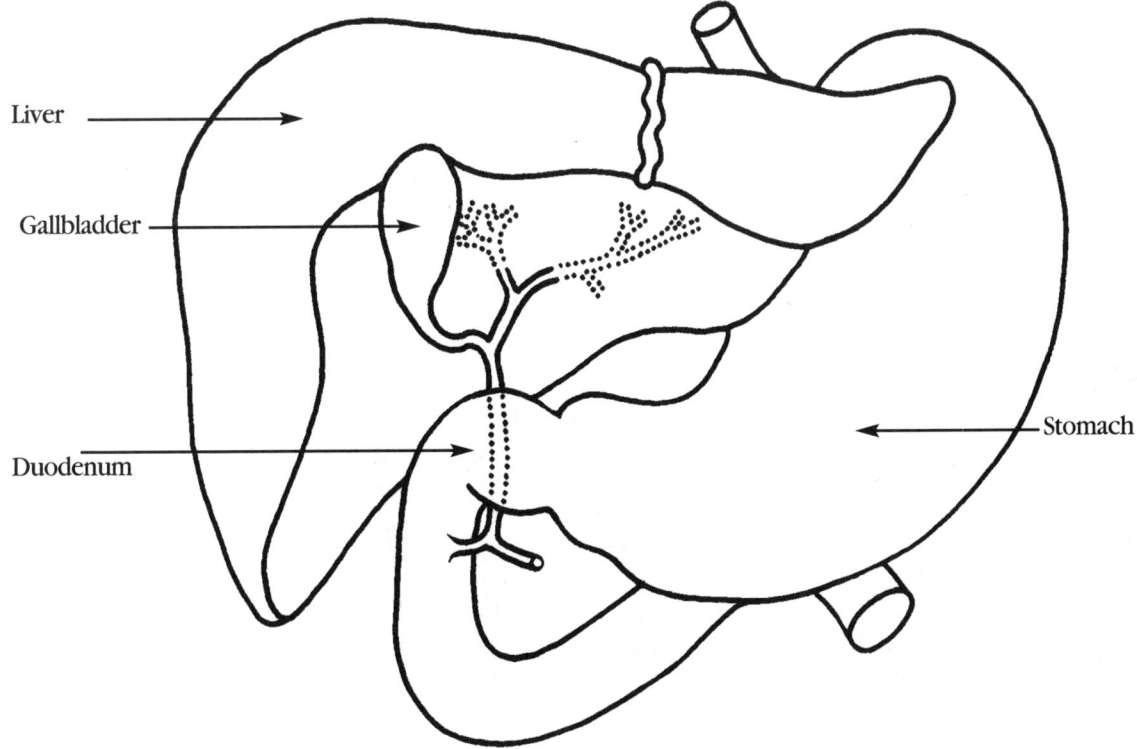

Liver

Gallbladder

Duodenum

Stomach

TRACHEA & LARYNX

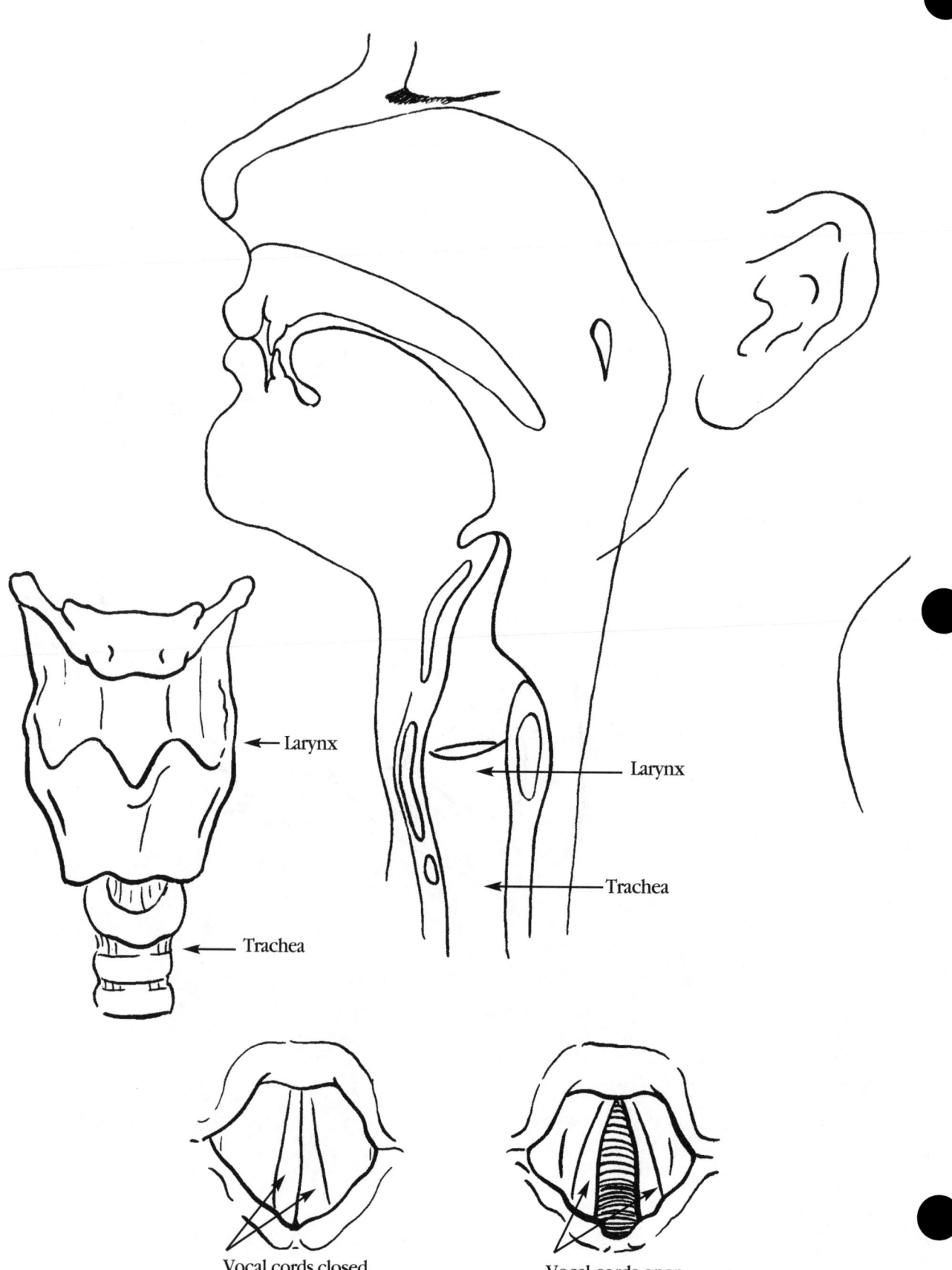

Larynx

Larynx

Trachea

Trachea

Vocal cords closed

Vocal cords open

628

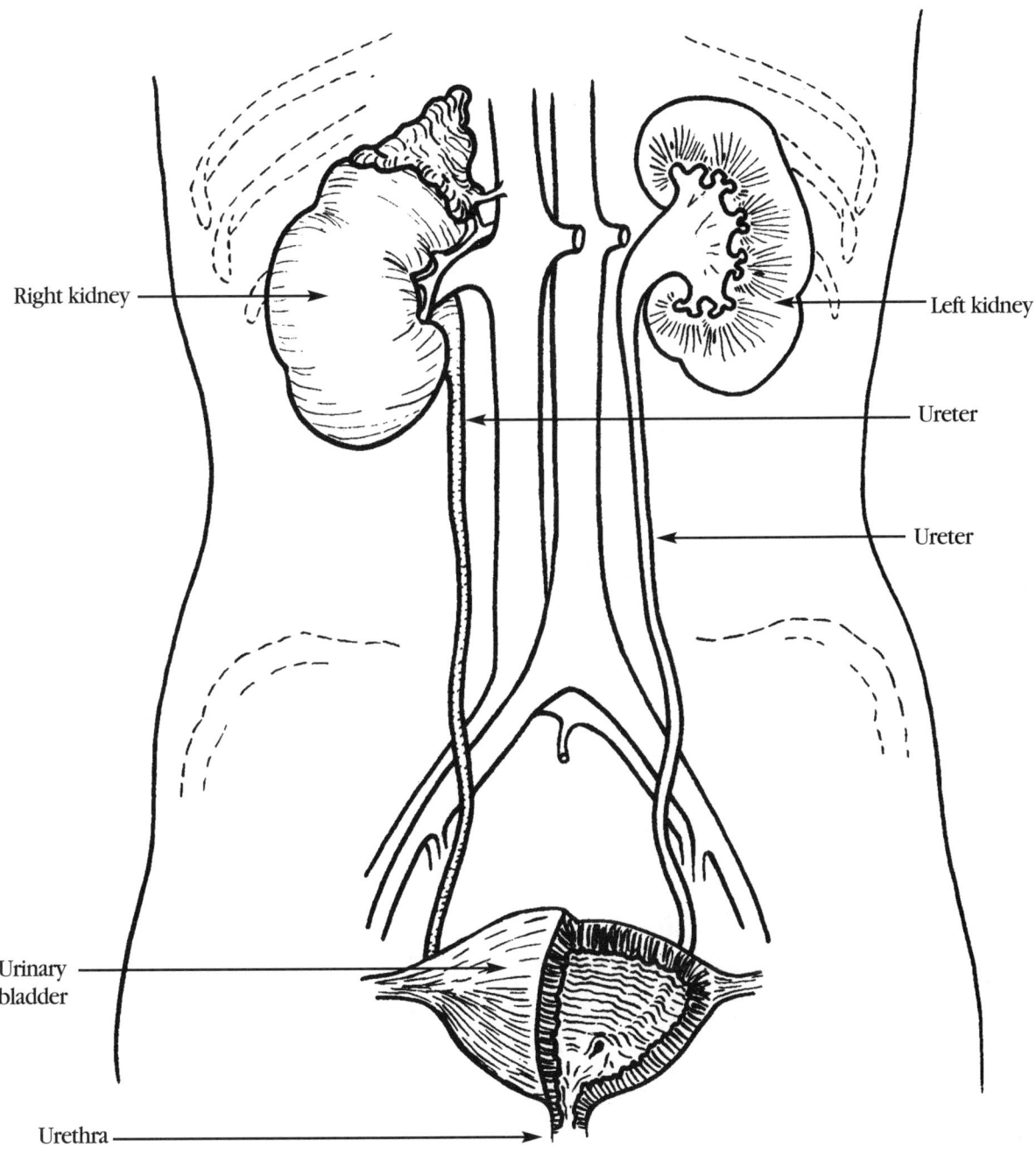

Right kidney

Left kidney

Ureter

Ureter

Urinary
bladder

Urethra

INDEX

Note: Page numbers in *italics* refer to illustrations

632